Imaging Modalities in Spinal Disorders

Morrie E. Kricun, M.D.

Associate Professor
Department of Diagnostic Radiology
Skeletal Radiology Section
Hospital of the University of Pennsylvania
Philadelphia, Pennsylvania

W.B. SAUNDERS COMPANY
Harcourt Brace Jovanovich, Inc.

1988

Philadelphia   London   Toronto   Montreal   Sydney   Tokyo

W. B. SAUNDERS COMPANY
Harcourt Brace Jovanovich, Inc.

West Washington Square
Philadelphia, PA 19105

Library of Congress Cataloging-in-Publication Data

Imaging modalities in spinal disorders.

1. Spine—Abnormalities—Diagnosis.   2. Diagnostic
imaging.   I. Kricun, Morrison E., 1938–   .
[DNLM: 1. Spine—radiography.   2. Spine—radionuclide imaging.   3. Tomography, X-Ray
Computed.   WE 725 I31]

RD768.I44   1988   617'.3750757   86–22063

ISBN 0–7216–1587–2

Editor: Dean Manke
Designer: Patti Maddaloni
Production Manager: Carolyn Naylor
Manuscript Editor: Martha Tanner
Illustration Coordinator: Walt Verbitski
Indexer: Dorothy Stade

Imaging Modalities in Spinal Disorders   ISBN 0–7216–1587–2

Last digit is the print number: 9   8   7   6   5   4   3   2   1

To my friend Seymour Saxanoff, M.D., who in his lifetime shared with me the comfort of friendship, the joy of humor, and the brilliance of his mind.

To Bernard J. Ostrum, M.D., mentor, teacher, friend. His brilliant teaching instilled a desire to learn.

To Ginny Kricun. Her vision gives direction. Her energy makes it possible.

Contributors

Michael André, Ph.D.
Assistant Adjunct Professor of Physics, University of California, San Diego, School of Medicine. Medical Physicist, Veterans Administration Medical Center and University of California Medical Center, San Diego, California.
Three-Dimensional Computed Tomography

Neil Chafetz, M.D.
Associate Professor, Department of Radiology, University of California, San Francisco, California.
Magnetic Resonance Imaging

Robert H. Cleveland, M.D.
Assistant Professor of Radiology, Harvard Medical School. Pediatric Radiologist, Massachusetts General Hospital, Boston, Massachusetts.
Digital Imaging in Scoliosis

Robert O. Cone, M.D.
Clinical Assistant Professor, Department of Radiology, The University of Texas Health Science Center at San Antonio. Attending Radiologist St. Luke's Lutheran Hospital, Southwest Texas Methodist Hospital, Nix Memorial Hospital, Medical Center Hospital, San Antonio, Texas.
Anatomy

Judy M. Destouet, M.D.
Associate Professor of Radiology, Musculoskeletal Section, Edward Mallinckrodt Institute of Radiology, Washington University School of Medicine. Radiologist, Barnes Hospital, St. Louis Children's Hospital, St. Louis, Missouri.
Arthrography and the Facet Syndrome
Percutaneous Biopsy of the Spine

Charles M. Elkin, M.D.
Assistant Professor of Radiology, Albert Einstein College of Medicine of Yeshiva University. Director of Neuroradiology, Montefiore Medical Center, Bronx, New York.
Myelography

Harry K. Genant, M.D.
Professor of Radiology, Medicine and Orthopaedic Surgery, Department of Radiology, University of California, San Francisco, California.
Magnetic Resonance Imaging

Raziel Gershater, M.B., Ch.B., F.R.C.P.(C)
Chief, Department of Diagnostic Imaging, North York General Hospital, Toronto, Canada
Lumbar Epidural Venography

Bernard Ghelman, M.D.
Associate Professor of Radiology, Cornell University Medical College. Attending Radiologist, Hospital for Special Surgery; Associate Attending Radiologist, The New York Hospital, New York, New York.
Discography

Thurman Gillespy III, M.D.
Assistant Professor, Department of Radiology, University of Florida College of Medicine, Gainesville, Florida.
Magnetic Resonance Imaging

Barry B. Goldberg, M.D.
Professor of Radiology, Jefferson Medical College of the Thomas Jefferson University, Philadelphia, Pennsylvania.
Sonography

Stephen A. Kieffer, M.D.
Professor and Chairman, Department of Radiology, Health Sciences Center, State University of New York, Upstate Medical Center at Syracuse, Syracuse, New York.
Myelography

Morrie E. Kricun, M.D.
Associate Professor, Department of Diagnostic Radiology, Skeletal Radiology Section, Hospital of the University of Pennsylvania, Philadelphia, Pennsylvania.
Anatomy
Conventional Radiography
Computed Tomography
Algorithms

Robert Kricun, M.D.
Clinical Assistant Professor, Department of Radiology, Hospital of the University of Pennsylvania, Philadelphia, Pennsylvania. Attending Radiologist, Department of Radiology, Lehigh Valley Hospital Center, Allentown, Pennsylvania.
Computed Tomography

David C. Kushner, M.D.
Assistant Professor of Radiology, Harvard Medical School. Director, Pediatric Radiology Section, Massachusetts General Hospital, Boston, Massachusetts.
Digital Imaging in Scoliosis

Norman E. Leeds, M.D.
Professor of Radiology, Mount Sinai School of Medicine of the City University of New York. Director, Radiology, Beth Israel Hospital, New York, New York.
Myelography
Algorithms

Eduardo Leon, M.D.

Instructor, Residency Training Program, Radiology Department. Radiologist, Instituto Diagnostico and Clinica El Avila, Caracas, Venezuela.
Myelography

Jesse Littleton III, M.D.

Professor of Radiology, University of South Alabama College of Medicine. Attending Radiologist, University of South Alabama Medical Center, Mobile, Alabama.
Conventional Pluridirectional Tomography

Gerald A. Mandell, M.D., F.A.A.P.

Adjunct Associate Professor of Radiology, Hospital of the University of Pennsylvania, Philadelphia, Pennsylvania. Associate Director, Medical Imaging, and Chief, Radiology, Alfred I. du Pont Institute, Wilmington, Delaware.
Radionuclide Imaging

David McLone, M.D.

Professor of Surgery (Neurosurgery), Northwestern University Medical School. Head, Division of Pediatric Neurosurgery, Children's Memorial Hospital, Chicago, Illinois.
Growth and Development

William A. Murphy, M.D.

Professor of Radiology, Washington University School of Medicine. Codirector, Musculoskeletal Section, Edward Mallinckrodt Institute of Radiology; Radiologist, Barnes Hospital, St. Louis Children's Hospital, St. Louis, Missouri.
Arthrography and the Facet Syndrome
Percutaneous Biopsy of the Spine

Thomas P. Naidich, M.D.

Professor of Radiology, Northwestern University Medical School. Director, Neuroimaging, Children's Memorial Hospital, Chicago, Illinois.
Growth and Development

Matthew E. Pasto, M.D.

Associate Professor of Radiology, Jefferson Medical College of The Thomas Jefferson University, Philadelphia, Pennsylvania.
Sonography

Deborah Pate, D.C.

Research Fellow, Radiology Service, Veterans Administration Medical Center, San Diego, California.
Three-Dimensional Computed Tomography

Rubem Pochaczevsky, M.D.

Professor of Radiology, Health Sciences Center, State University of New York at Stony Brook. Chief, Diagnostic Radiology, Long Island Jewish Medical Center, New Hyde Park, New York.
Thermography

Donald Resnick, M.D.

Professor of Radiology, University of California Medical Center, San Diego. Chief, Radiology Service, Veterans Administration Medical Center, San Diego, California.
Anatomy
The Aging Vertebral Column: Pathologic-Radiographic Correlation
Three-Dimensional Computed Tomography

David J. Sartoris, M.D.

Assistant Professor of Radiology, University of California, San Diego, School of Medicine. Staff Radiologist, Chief, Musculoskeletal Imaging, University of California Medical Center, San Diego, California.
Three-Dimensional Computed Tomography

Steven M. Schonfeld, M.D.

Clinical Assistant Professor of Radiology, University of Medicine and Dentistry of New Jersey, Robert Wood Johnson School of Medicine. Attending Radiologist, Robert Wood Johnson University Hospital, St. Peter's Medical Center, New Brunswick, New Jersey.
Myelography

Joachim F. Seeger, M.D.

Professor of Radiology, University of Arizona College of Medicine, Arizona Health Sciences Center, Arizona.
Angiography

Eugene L. St. Louis, M.D., F.R.C.P.(C)

Associate Professor, University of Toronto. Radiologist-in-Chief, The Wellesley Hospital, University of Toronto, Toronto, Canada.
Lumbar Epidural Venography

Mark Winkler, M.D.

Assistant Professor of Radiology, Clinical Director, Radiologic Imaging Laboratory, University of California, San Francisco. Attending Radiologist, University of California, San Francisco, San Francisco General Hospital Medical Center, San Francisco, California.
Magnetic Resonance Imaging

Foreword

This book, of almost 700 pages, constitutes a highly detailed exposition of disorders of the spine while incorporating all imaging modalities at the command of the radiologist. The scope of the work is best appreciated by listing the 19 subjects considered in chapter form, most of major importance. Included are chapters on growth and development, normal anatomy, the aging vertebral column, conventional radiography of the spine, conventional pluridirectional tomography, myelography with and without computed tomography, computed tomography, a special variant of computed tomography (three-dimensional [3D CT]), imaging with magnetic resonance, imaging with radionuclides, discography (including chemonucleolysis), lumbar epidural venography, angiography (particularly arterial), digital imaging in examinations for scoliosis, sonography, arthrography and the facet syndrome, thermography, percutaneous biopsy of the spine, and a final chapter on algorithms.

Of special interest are the sections on conventional radiography (Chapter 4) and computed tomography (Chapter 7). The former chapter is approximately 230 pages in length and in fact constitutes a "book within a book." This chapter deals with normal variants and virtually all important disorders that affect the spine. It is particularly gratifying to note that Dr. Kricun has not fallen into the trap of focusing completely on the newer imaging devices (e.g., CT, MR, ultrasonography). The data and information detailed in Chapter 4 of this book, even without the rest, would establish this work as an important scholarly treatise. The material dealing with disorders affecting the spine in Chapter 4 is beautifully organized and written. Conventional CT is discussed in Chapter 7 in approximately 90 pages. Herein the techniques of computed tomography and the pitfalls inherent in its use are emphasized. The advantages of CT are excellently detailed and illustrated, with considerable stress on the subjects of herniated discs and spinal stenosis. Indeed, infections, neoplasms, and spinal anomalies, defined by CT, also are considered in depth in Chapter 7 as a logical extension of Chapter 4.

The final chapter on algorithms is concise but highly informative and interesting. It constitutes a fitting conclusion to an excellent work in its discussion of which imaging modality (or modalities) to utilize for a variety of clinical problems.

It must be noted that the book is multiauthored, but the important chapter on conventional radiography (Chapter 4) is written entirely by the chief author (and editor), Morrie Kricun, and Chapter 7 on CT is written by

Dr. Morrie Kricun and his brother, Robert. All other chapters have authors other than Morrie Kricun, although in some instances he is a coauthor. Yet, this work does not suffer from problems indigenous to many multiauthored texts—namely, a lack of continuity and a change in emphasis in the writing of each chapter. Indeed, the chapters in this work flow one into the other in a highly effective manner. Obviously, achieving such continuity requires heavy involvement of the major author (and editor) in the construction of all the subject matter and a coherent and intelligent division of the material into individual chapters, as is found in this work. It must also be emphasized that Morrie Kricun has made superb selections, so that virtually every chapter with an author (or authors) other than Dr. Kricun is written by an authentic expert in the field. To name but a few would be unjust to the others, but it must be emphasized that virtually all the authors are among the best. Dr. Kricun is to be congratulated on (a) having selected them and (b) having them agree to contribute. Diagnostic radiology gains enormously as a result, because this is a major work.

The book is not only a reference work in depth but also a highly readable text, containing enough material to keep any reader busy for a long time. The emphasis on plain film radiography and, to a somewhat lesser extent, on CT serves as a focus around which the rest of the work is designed. The reader, be he or she a neuroradiologist, a radiologist not specializing in neuroradiology, a neurologist, a neurosurgeon, an orthopedic surgeon, a resident in training, or a medical student, can only gain immeasurably from reading this work and using it as a reference.

The author of this foreword considers himself most fortunate to have been asked to write it, because assenting to such an invitation obviously required the reading of the work. I have gained enormously in an area that cuts across my two major fields of interest in diagnostic radiology—skeletal radiology and neuroradiology. I thank Dr. Kricun for asking me, and I would like to express my appreciation to him further for constructing a work from which I have learned considerably.

HAROLD G. JACOBSON, M.D.

Preface

Medical imaging has become an increasingly important part of patient evaluation and treatment planning. Great advances have occurred as new imaging technologies have been developed, causing major impact in various fields of medicine. This is especially true in the imaging of spinal disorders, where many modalities have importance—some having been developed only recently. The need for appropriate preoperative and postoperative imaging as well as meticulous evaluation of the images obtained is extremely important for high-quality medical care.

The purpose of this book is twofold: to present all of the imaging modalities that are currently available for the evaluation of spinal disorders, and to discuss their indications, limitations, technical features, complications, and utilization. In-depth discussions of spinal and intraspinal disorders as well as high-quality images are presented, and the pathophysiology of radiographic signs is emphasized. Differential diagnoses and pitfalls encountered during evaluation of the images are included when appropriate.

The early chapters of the book cover the growth, development, and anatomy of the spine and the pathologic-radiographic correlation of the degenerative spinal disorders. These chapters lay the foundation upon which the imaging chapters are based. The next chapter, *Conventional Radiography*, is the longest chapter in the book. Its length is due mainly to the ease with which the plain film lends itself to a thorough discussion of local and systemic spinal disorders, thus obviating similar discussions in other chapters. This allows the authors of the other chapters to concentrate on their specific imaging modality. The chapters that follow *Conventional Radiography* are *Conventional Pluridirectional Tomography, Myelography, Computed Tomography, Three-Dimensional Computed Tomography, Magnetic Resonance Imaging, Radionuclide Imaging, Discography, Lumbar Epidural Venography, Angiography, Digital Imaging in Scoliosis, Sonography, Arthrography and the Facet Syndrome, Thermography,* and *Percutaneous Biopsy of the Spine*. The last chapter in the book discusses suggested algorithms for the imaging work-up and evaluation of various clinical conditions. A few topics were repeated in several chapters in order to provide continuity for the reader.

The availability and utilization of various imaging modalities has changed dramatically since this book was conceived. Magnetic resonance imaging (MRI) has risen to the forefront in the evaluation of disorders of the spinal canal as well as other abnormalities. However, even as this book is published, protocols for spinal imaging with MRI are changing, and protocols vary throughout the country. On the other hand, epidural venography, which was mainly an adjunctive modality for most imagers and a primary modality for some imagers in the work-up of patients with suspected herniated disc, has been virtually abandoned with the advent of high-resolution CT and MRI. Nevertheless, epidural venography is included in this book for completeness and its possible occasional use in problem cases in some imaging practices.

Choosing the contributing authors was not difficult, for they are all experts in their respective fields of imaging. These authors have produced informative, comprehensive chapters, which have been enhanced by fine-quality illustrations. Medical art, tables of differential diagnosis, and selected correlation with anatomic specimens have been utilized when appropriate. The lists of references at the end of the chapters are current and comprehensive.

It is my hope that the reader will find the book both enjoyable and informative and will appreciate the complexities that are encountered in the imaging work-up of patients with spinal disorders.

MORRIE E. KRICUN

Acknowledgments

Producing a book of this scope required the expertise of many authors, all experts in their fields. I am deeply indebted to these authors, who willingly gave of their time and knowledge to ensure manuscripts of the highest quality. Each author in turn had the help of secretaries, technologists, and photographers, whose assistance is greatly appreciated. I am particularly grateful to Patricia Cephus for her secretarial and organizational skills.

I have had the opportunity to glean knowlege from many outstanding radiologists and would like at this time to thank two of my finest teachers, Harold J. Isard, M.D., and Bernard J. Ostrum, M.D. I am indebted to Harold G. Jacobson, M.D., an internationally recognized authority in radiology of orthopedic disorders. He graciously agreed to write the foreword, for which I am deeply appreciative.

I wish to thank the individuals of W. B. Saunders Company who were instrumental in accepting this book for publication as well as those who were influential in bringing the book from the early stages to completion. Lisette Bralow was the initial medical editor who gave encouragement and assistance when the project first began. Dean Manke, her successor, made valuable contributions. I am grateful to Martha Tanner, a very competent copy editor, who performed her duties superbly. Carolyn Naylor, a diligent production manager, organized and completed the production of the book. Walter Verbitski, the illustration coordinator, and Patti Maddaloni, the book designer, made significant contributions. Indeed, I am appreciative of all the effort and work performed by those on the staff of W. B. Saunders who played a role in bringing this book to its completion.

Contents

18
William A. Murphy, M.D.
Judy M. Destouet, M.D.

19
Morrie E. Kricun, M.D.
Norman E. Leeds, M.D.

1

Thomas P. Naidich, M.D.
David McLone, M.D.

Growth and Development

The subject of embryology provides great intellectual satisfaction, for, of all subjects, it explains how we came to be what we are, in health and in disease. Our knowledge is far from complete. Mysteries remain to delight the curious. What is known, however, already provides a framework for understanding why specific abnormalities have similar patterns.

NORMAL EMBRYOGENESIS

The following discussion of normal embryogenesis is based largely upon the works of numerous authors.* In an attempt to date embryonic age accurately, different authors have used different criteria for the stages of development. The measures most commonly used include the estimated embryonic age (for example, day 7), the size of the embryo from crown to rump (for instance, 3 mm crown-rump length [CRL]), and the number of somites visible (for example, 25-somite stage). These criteria are not always interchangeable. In this discussion, therefore, it must be remembered that the precise rate of growth and development varies from individual to individual, so embryos of the same fertilization age may differ in size (that is, crown-rump length) and embryos of the same size may differ in age.

Overview of Early Development

Union of sperm and ovum forms the new zygote within the distal third of the fallopian tube on day 1.[34] The single-celled zygote passes down the tube toward the uterus and cleaves into two blastomeres about 30 hours after fertilization.[34] Successive cell divisions create a ball of 16 or more blastomeres, designated the morula, that enters the uterine cavity about 60 hours after fertilization. Within the morula, a group of centrally located cells forms the inner cell mass that develops into the embryoblast and then the embryo itself, while a group of peripherally located cells forms the outer cell mass that gives rise to the trophoblast and then part of the placenta.[34] Fluid from the uterine cavity passes into the extracellular spaces of the inner cell mass and expands these spaces into a single cavity called the blastocele.[34] As a result, the zygote now consists of an outer layer of cells (the trophoblast), a large central cavity (the blastocele), and a group of adherent cells of the inner cell mass situated at one pole of the blastocele (the embryoblast).[34] This stage is designated the blastocyst. Implantation of the blastocyst into the maternal endometrium occurs at the end of the first week of development (Fig. 1–1).[34] Implantation and subsequent growth occur in such fashion that the pole of the blastocyst containing the embryoblast comes to lie most deeply within the uterine wall, whereas the blastocele itself lies near to and partially bulges into the uterine cavity.[34] The portion of the trophoblast between the uterus and the embryoblast proliferates markedly and differentiates into two layers: the syncytiotrophoblast (situated against the maternal surface) and the cytotrophoblast (situated against the embryoblast).

At about day 7 or 8, the cells of the embryoblast begin to differentiate into two distinct cell layers.[34] Those cells situated

*Reference numbers 2, 6, 7, 15, 18, 30, 31, 33–37, 40–44, 46, 57, 65, 68.

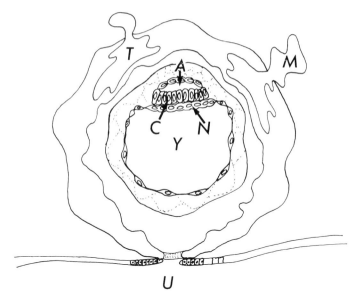

Figure 1–1. Diagrammatic representation of the blastocyst at 12 days shows the trophoblastic lacunae (**T**) and maternal sinusoids (**M**). The bilaminar germ disc is composed of ectoblast (**C**) and entoblast (**N**) separating the amniotic cavity (**A**) from the primitive yolk sac (**Y**). The uterine cavity is labeled (**U**).

immediately against the blastocele form a cell layer called the hypoblast.[18] Those cells situated immediately adjacent to the cytotrophoblast (and thus one layer more peripheral from the blastocele) form the epiblast.[18] The hypoblast and the epiblast have an overall disc shape and together are designated the bilaminar disc.[18] Shortly thereafter, small intercellular clefts and vacuoles form between the epiblast and the cytotrophoblast. These spaces coalesce into a single, large cavity lined by amnioblasts: the newly formed amniotic cavity.[34] The embryo is then a bilaminar disc with the hypoblastic layer facing the blastocele and the epiblastic layer facing the amniotic cavity.[18, 34] With subsequent growth of the trophoblast, a layer of cells delaminates from the cytotrophoblast to form a thin membrane (Heuser's membrane) that encloses the blastocele.[34] This converts the blastocele into the primary yolk sac.[34] By day 13, the hypoblastic layer has proliferated to form a layer of flat epithelial cells that lines the inside of Heuser's membrane, thereby creating a new, smaller cavity now designated the secondary yolk sac. Thus by the end of the second week of gestation, the embryo is composed of two apposed cell discs: (1) the epiblast, which forms the floor of a continuously expanding amniotic cavity, and (2) the contiguous, immediately subjacent hypoblast, which forms the roof of the secondary yolk sac (future gut).[34] The epiblast gives rise to all or nearly

all of the cells of the embryo.[18] The hypoblast becomes displaced laterally and does not contribute to embryonic cell development.[18] In the cephalic region at the future site of the mouth, the hypoblast shows a slight circular thickening known as the prochordal plate.[34] Appearance of the prochordal plate establishes the first cranial-caudal, left-right axes of the embryo.

Initial Stages of Formation of the Spine and Spinal Cord

By day 12 or 14, certainly by day 15, epiblastic cells in the caudal region of the bilaminar disc form a linear midline thickening on the amniotic side of the epiblastic disc. This thickening is designated the primitive streak (Fig. 1–2).[18, 34] It is the source of the majority of the cells that will form the middle and inner layers of the embryo.[18] A midline depression or primitive groove appears along the length of the primitive streak. Epiblastic cells enter the primitive streak, invaginate under the epiblastic layer, and then migrate rostrally and laterally between the epiblastic and the hypoblastic layers to form an intermediate mesoblastic (primary mesenchymal) layer.[18, 34] This migration converts the previous bilaminar disc into a trilaminar disc.[18, 34] Some of the cells of the mesoblastic layer invade and displace the early hypoblastic cells, so the epiblast is, in fact, the original source of the three significant layers of the trilaminar embryo: the outer embryonic ectoderm, the middle intraembryonic mesoderm, and the inner embryonic entoderm.[18] The epiblast (ectoderm) will form the central nervous system (neuroectoderm) and the epidermis (cutaneous ectoderm).[18] The mesoblast (mesoderm) will form the skeleton, striated and smooth muscles, connective tissues, blood vessels, blood cells, bone marrow, the reproductive system, and the excretory organs. The (replaced) hypoblast will form the endoderm that develops into the epithelial linings of the respiratory and digestive systems and the glandular cells of the liver and pancreas.[18]

The new mesoblastic (primary mesenchymal) layer is continuous except that no mesoderm occupies the portion of the midline between the primitive streak and the prochordal plate.[34] This space remains free of mesoderm until after the spinal cord has formed.

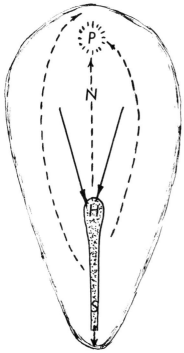

Figure 1–2. Diagrammatic representation of the germ disc shows the movement of surface cells (solid arrows) toward the primitive streak (**S**) and Hensen's node (**H**). The surface cells then migrate between the epiblast and hypoblast (broken arrows) toward the prochordal plate (**P**). **N** is the course along which the notochord will develop.

As the epiblastic cells migrate, the cephalic end of the primitive streak shows a substantial thickening and elevation designated (variably) the primitive node, primitive knot, or Hensen's node (see Fig. 1–2).[34] Hensen's node consists of a slightly elevated area surrounding a small, central, primitive pit that is situated at the cephalic end of the primitive groove. At days 16 and 17, epiblastic cells enter the primitive pit and then migrate cephalically in the midline to reach the prochordal plate.[18, 34] By day 17, these cells have formed a new midline structure, the notochordal process, which extends cephalically to Hensen's node beneath the surface epiblast and above the hypoblast. The primitive pit deepens and extends into the previously solid notochordal process, creating the notochordal canal.[18] By day 18, the notochordal process fuses with the subjacent entoderm forming a ridgelike notochordal plate in the roof of the yolk sac.[34] At the point(s) of fusion, degeneration of cells opens the notochordal canal to the yolk sac. As a result, a temporary canal is created between the amniotic cavity and the yolk sac via the primitive pit, notochordal canal, and point(s) of degeneration. This canal is designated the neurenteric canal or Kovalevsky's canal. Soon thereafter, the cranial end of the notochordal plate infolds and reunites along its longitudinal axis to form a solid cord of cells designated the true notochord or the notochord.[18] This process starts cranially and extends caudally, becoming complete by the end of the fourth week (4 mm CRL, 25 somite stage). The entoderm again detaches from the notochord and re-forms a continuous roof layer for the yolk sac.[34]

As the notochord forms, the entodermal germ layer becomes firmly attached to the ectoderm in the region immediately caudal to the primitive streak. This establishes a bilaminar cloacal membrane by day 16.[34] The cloacal membrane will give rise to the urogenital and anorectal membranes, so it is significant in the pathogenesis of diverse anomalies of the caudal spine.

After approximately day 19, the primitive streak regresses caudally.[34] However, invagination of the surface ectoderm and subsequent migration of these cells forward and laterally continue until about the end of the fourth week. Thereafter, the primitive streak and Hensen's node show regressive changes and decrease in size rapidly. The exact time and site of disappearance of the primitive pit and Hensen's node are not known.[46] Sacrococcygeal teratomas may have their origin in persistent totipotential cells of the primitive streak.[18]

Formation of the Spinal Cord

The cephalic and caudal portions of the spinal cord are formed by distinctly different mechanisms and are therefore heir to distinctly different types of malformation. The cephalic, majority portion of the spinal cord forms by an orderly sequence of (1) creation of neural folds, (2) flexion of those folds, and (3) closure of the folds into a neural tube. This process is designated neurulation.

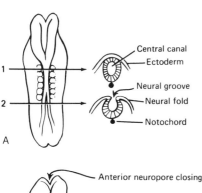

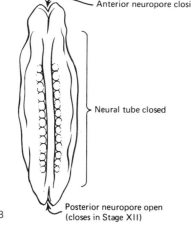

Figure 1–3. Neurulation. *A*, Dorsal view of a 22 day embryo (stage X) during initial fusion of the neural folds. Cross sections on the right represent levels 1 and 2. *B*, Dorsal view of a 24 day embryo (stage XI). Much of the neural tube has closed. The anterior neuropore, although still open in the illustration, closes during this stage. The posterior neuropore closes at about 26 days (stage XII). (From Lemire RJ, Leoser JD, Leech RW, et al: Normal and Abnormal Development of the Human Nervous System. Hagerstown, Maryland: Harper & Row Publishers, Inc, 1975.)

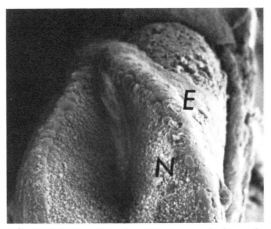

Figure 1–4. Scanning electron micrograph shows the closing of the neuroectoderm (**N**) and superficial ectoderm (**E**) at the caudal end of an embryo.

The caudal, minority portion of the cord forms by far less well-organized mechanisms of (1) agglomeration of cells, (2) canalization of the cell mass, and (3) involution of unused portions of the distal cord. This process is designated canalization and retrogressive differentiation. The two processes will be discussed separately.

Neurulation

By the start of the third week, when the embryo is approximately 1.4 mm crown-rump length (CRL), the notochord induces formation of a slipper-shaped plate of ectodermal cells in the midline just cephalic to Hensen's node.[34] This is the neural plate. The edges of the neural plate are directly continuous at all sides, with the superficial ectoderm of the ectodermal germ layer from which the plate differentiated. During the next few days, the lateral edges of the neural plate begin to elevate and become the neural folds, while the midline remains depressed and becomes the ventral neural groove (Figs. 1–3, 1–4).[34, 44] Progressive elevation and rolling over of the neural folds creates a neural tube (the future spinal cord) with a central cavity (the future central canal)[34, 44] (Fig. 1–5). Such flexion and fusion do not occur along the entire length of the neural plate simultaneously. Rather, the neural folds first meet and fuse together at the level of the third or fourth somite when the embryo is at the 6 to 7 somite stage. After this, flexion and fusion progress cephalically and cau-

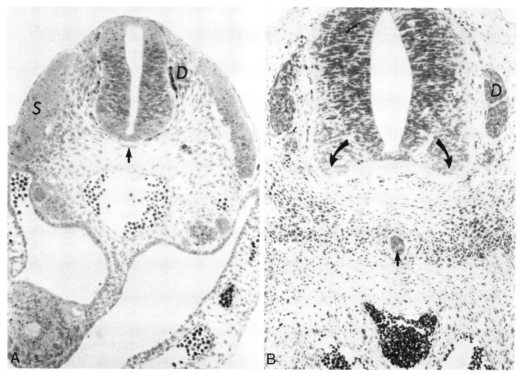

Figure 1–5. *A*, Light micrograph of a mammalian embryo shortly after closure of the neural tube shows early formation of the dorsal ganglion (**D**) from neural crest. The notochord (arrow) is not yet surrounded by mesenchyme. Mesenchyme has not yet gained access to the dorsal midline between the closure of the neural tube and the superficial ectoderm. **S** = somite. *B*, Light micrograph of a mammalian embryo recorded a few days after that of Figure 1–5*A*. The mesenchyme now surrounds the notochord (straight arrow), the initial stage in formation of the vertebrae. The dorsal ganglion (**D**) is much more advanced. The basal plates of the spinal cord are expanding ventrally (curved arrows) and will grow toward the midline to form the anterior fissure.

dally in an orderly sequence or "wave"[34] such that the level of fusion corresponds to the level of the most recently formed somite. At approximately 23 days' gestation (18 to 20 somite stage), the cephalic end of the neural tube closes at the anterior neuropore (site of the primitive lamina terminalis).[34] At approximately 26 days of gestation (3 to 5 mm CRL, 21 to 29 somite stage), the caudal end of the neural tube closes at the posterior neuropore.[34, 46] The exact site of the posterior neuropore remains unknown but is believed to lie between the eleventh thoracic and fourth lumbar segments.[37]

The mechanism by which the neural plate elevates, flexes into neural folds, and then fuses into a tube merits further discussion. The cells of the neural plate are tightly joined together by intercellular desmosomes.[44] Intracellular microfilaments of actin cross each cell from desmosome to desmosome to link the entire surface of the neural plate into a coherent structure. These micro-filaments are most concentrated in the midline and along two lateral areas of the neural plate.[44] An extracellular surface layer of complex carbohydrates covers the external (amniotic) surface of the neural plate to form the superficial cell surface coat.[44]

The neural plate begins to elevate into neural folds prior to formation of the first somite.[44] Such elevation appears to result from calcium-dependent contraction of the actin filaments and flexion of the neural plate at two major sites: (1) in the midline, deepening the ventral neural groove, and (2) along two lateral lines, creating the lateral sulci (future sulci limitans of the central canal).[44] Progressive infolding and flexion then bring the lateral edges of the neural plate into the midline, dorsal to the embryo, in preparation for fusing the folds into a neural tube. During the entire process of flexion, the superficial ectoderm has remained attached to the lateral edge of the neural ectoderm. As the neural folds approach each other in the midline, the superficial ectoderm slides slightly ventrolaterally, away from the advancing edge, to expose a greater amount of neural ectoderm. The superificial cell surface coat appears to bridge the gap between the apposing neural ectodermal cells and is believed to be the signal for cell to cell recognition and fusion.[44] Immediately following fusion of the neural folds into the tube, the superficial ectoderm of each side separates from the neural ectoderm (a process designated disjunction). The left and right portions of the disjoined superficial ectoderm then fuse together across the midline, dorsal to the already closed neural tube. This entire sequence is repeated seriatim until the posterior neuropore closes, completing neurulation. The neural tube is then sealed, and the central canal no longer communicates with the amniotic cavity. Lack of adhesion between the apposing neural folds, reopening of the closed neural folds, focal premature disjunction of superficial from neural ectoderm, and focal failure of the superficial ectoderm to separate from neural ectoderm all lead to clinically common pathologic states such as myelomeningocele, lipomyelomeningocele, and dorsal dermal sinus.

Canalization and Retrogressive Differentiation

The lowermost lumbar, sacral, and coccygeal segments form by the process of canalization and retrogressive differentiation.

Canalization. At the start of canalization, the caudal end of the neural tube and the caudal end of the notochord lie within a large aggregate of undifferentiated cells that extends into the tailfold.[33, 35, 37] These cells are designated the caudal cell mass. The distal end of the hindgut and the mesonephros also lie within the tailfold and are ventral to the notochord.[35–37]

During canalization, those caudal cells situated near the end of the neural tube begin to orient themselves around small vacuoles (days 22 to 23)[37] By 4 to 7 mm CRL, the cells have begun to resemble ependymal cells.[37] With time, other vacuoles form, vacuoles coalesce, and two to three layers of cells surrounding the vacuoles begin to resemble neural cells.[37] The coalescing vacuoles then make contact with and become continuous with the central canal formed by neurulation.[37] During this process, accessory lumina lateral to or dorsoventral to the true lumen also form and become surrounded by cells. For example, accessory lumina have been found in 35% of embryos that are between 4 and 32 mm CRL.[37] Similarly, major forking of the central canal of the conus medullaris was discovered in 10% of normal patients and minor forking in 31%.[38] Major forking of the central canal was present in 35% of normal fila terminale.[38]

Retrogressive Differentiation. In human embryos, the greater part of the cord formed by canalization later undergoes involution to the filum terminale. In very young embryos, the spinal cord reaches the extreme tip of the tail[33] and is uniform in structure throughout its length.[65] At about 8 to 11 mm CRL, while canalization still continues, the tailfolds and the distal spinal cord show the first signs of regression.[33, 37] The lumen of the neural tube caudal to the 32nd somite (future coccygeal 2) becomes distinctly narrower than the lumen of the neural tube cephalic to the 32nd somite, and the difference becomes progressively more marked with time.[33, 37] By 15.5 mm CRL, the distal neural tube is formed of only a single ependymal zone, while the proximal neural tube is made of three distinct concentric layers: an ependymal zone abutting on the canal, an intermediate mantle zone, and a marginal zone at the periphery.[65]

From approximately 5 mm to approximately 30 mm CRL (60 days), the notochord and neural tube are temporarily longer than the vertebral column and project into the tail caudal to the last vertebra.[33, 46] The distal end of the notochord is attached to the ventral surface of the neural tube and appears to kink and corrugate the ventral face of the tube. By 30 to 37 mm CRL, the embryo has entirely lost its external tail, and the spinal cord and notochord are about the same length as the vertebral column.[33]

Thereafter, the portion of the spinal cord distal to the 32nd somite begins to thin and involute. Typically, the canal of the neural tube becomes obliterated at one or several points below the 32nd somite. At the 32nd somite, the central canal widens focally to become the early ventriculus terminalis (terminal ventricle) (Fig. 1–6). This space is clearly evident by 22 mm CRL and remains

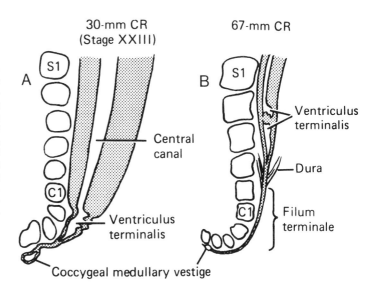

Figure 1–6. Diagrammatic representation of the human spinal cord at (**A**) the 8th week and (**B**) the 25th week demonstrates the disproportion in growth of the spinal cord and vertebral column and the regression of the spinal cord distal to the ventriculus terminalis. (From Lemire RJ, Leoser JD, Leech RW, et al: Normal and Abnormal Development of the Human Nervous System. Hagerstown, Maryland: Harper & Row Publishers, Inc, 1975. Adapted from Streeter GL: Factors involved in the formation of the filum terminale. Am J Anat 25:1–11, 1919.)

throughout life as a distal true ventricle situated within the lower conus medullaris or the upper filum terminale.[31] It communicates with the central canal of the spinal cord.[31]

The distalmost portion of the involuting neural tube frequently remains hollow for long periods of time as the coccygeal medullary vestige.[33] As a rule, this vestige lies within the connective tissue dorsal to the last two vertebrae.[33] The caudal end of the vestige merges into the caudal ligament.[33] It is not adherent to the epidermis. It is not known when the vestige disappears. A similarly formed epithelial sac frequently also develops at a more cranial site.[33]

After 30 mm CRL, the portion of cord containing the ventriculus terminalis does not dedifferentiate further.[65] That is, there is no further shortening of this portion of the cord. The glioependymal strand that is the remnant of the involuted distal cord is designated the filum terminale (see Fig. 1–6).[65, 68] The primitive filum terminale first appears at approximately 30 to 37 mm CRL, as a bundle of nerve fibers visible on the ventral side of the distal cord.[33] This extends caudally from the apex of the primitive conus medullaris at the level of the 29th–30th vertebrae. By 39, 46, and 52 mm CRL, the filum terminale is quite distinct. The transition from normal cord to filum terminale is usually very abrupt and takes place over one segment.[65]

Once the filum forms, it then elongates and thickens by interstitial growth, not by simple stretching out or further involution of the spinal cord.[65]

Further Development of the Spinal Cord

As indicated previously, the portion of the spinal cord that persists to term is formed of three concentric layers: an inner ependymal zone, a mantle zone, and an outer marginal zone.[34] The ependymal zone contains columnar ependymal cells, which border the lumen of the central canal, and a large number of intercalated, actively proliferating cells believed to be stem or germinal cells.[34] These stem cells give rise to neuroblasts and glioblasts that migrate into the mantle layer and differentiate into the neurons and supporting cells of the gray matter of the cord. The neurons within the mantle layer then send axons into the outer marginal zone, forming the white matter of the spinal cord. The marginal zone contains no cell bodies, only afferent and efferent nerve fibers. As the neuroepithelial cells proliferate and differentiate, the lateral walls of the neural tube thicken.

Each lateral wall is divided into a dorsal and a ventral half by the sulcus limitans that grooves the inner wall of the central canal (see Fig. 1–5B).[34] This probably corresponds to the lateral sulcus along which the neural tube is flexed. The portion of the lateral wall dorsal to the sulcus limitans is designated the alar plate. Together with the neural crest, this will form the dorsal horns and other structures of the sensory apparatus. The portion of the lateral wall ventral to the sulcus is designated the basal plate. This will form the ventral horn neurons and ventral roots of the motor apparatus. In the midline, the dorsal "roof" plate and the ventral "floor" plate remain thin and appear to serve only as pathways for fibers that cross side to side (see Fig. 1–5).[34]

The basal plates thicken and bulge forward on each side of the midline, leaving a deep midline longitudinal groove—the ventral median fissure (see Fig. 1–5B).[15] The alar plates grow predominantly medially and ultimately fuse in the midline to form the posterior medium septum. As a result, the dorsal portion of the lumen of the neural tube is nearly obliterated, leaving only the far smaller central canal of the spinal cord.

The marginal layer of the spinal cord becomes further thickened by the development of longitudinally coursing bundles of nerve fibers: the tracts.[15] The first tracts to form are short intersegmental tracts designated the fasciculi proprii.[15] Later, the major ascending and descending pathways arise to connect the spinal cord with the brain.[15] Myelination begins at about week 17 or 20 and continues until the infant is about 1 year old.

Spinal Ganglia

During the period that the neural tube is closing and the superficial ectoderm separates from the neural ectoderm, cells at the junction of the neural and the cutaneous ectoderm differentiate into neural crest cells.[40, 41] These migrate into the adjacent mesoderm (primary mesenchyme). Some of these neural crest cells form segmental aggregations outside the spinal cord that develop into the dorsal root ganglia (see Fig. 1–5).[15] Other cells remain as a part of the mesenchyme, now designated secondary mesenchyme.[40, 41]

In embryos of 5 to 10 mm CRL, there are usually 32 pairs of ganglia.[33] From 12 to 14 mm CRL, there may be 33 pairs, but, if so, the caudalmost pair is usually very small and has no associated nerves.[33] From 15 to 33 mm CRL, there are usually 31 pairs of spinal ganglia and, often, a 32nd pair of nerve roots without associated ganglia (the ganglia are believed to have degenerated).[33] In embryos of from 35 to 67 mm CRL and older, there are usually only 30 pairs of ganglia (occasionally 31 pairs with the last pair showing signs of degeneration).[33]

The dorsal root ganglia contain the primary sensory neurons. Processes that arise from these neurons grow centrally into the developing alar plates to form the dorsal nerve roots.[15] The point of entry of these roots is significant and is designated the dorsal root entry zone (DREZ). Other processes of the dorsal ganglion neurons grow peripherally toward the sensory receptors as sensory nerves. This situation is distinctly different from that obtaining in the basal plate, where motor neurons situated within the ventral horns give rise to processes that grow out from the spinal cord, join to form the ventral motor roots, and continue to grow peripherally into each somite.

Ascent of the Cord

In the early embryo, the spinal cord extends to the distal end of the tail. By approximately three months post partum, the tip of the conus medullaris lies at approximately the L1–L2 interspace. This ascent results from two processes: (1) retrogressive differentiation, and (2) disproportionately more rapid growth of the vertebral column. By 30 mm CRL, involution of the distal cord has formed the distal conus medullaris and ventriculus terminalis. These lie opposite the second or third coccygeal segment. Thereafter the spinal cord does not shorten further by retrogressive differentiation, so all further ascent of cord results from disproportionate longitudinal growth of the vertebral column (see Fig. 1–6). In the first 25 weeks of gestation, the ventriculus terminalis ascends from the second coccygeal level to approximately the third lumbar level—a distance of nine segments. Only two more segments are traversed before adult position is reached. The principal portion of ascent is accomplished during the first half of fetal life. In collected series totaling 801 patients, the tip of the conus medullaris at birth has been found to lie at or above the L2–L3 intervertebral disc space in 97.8% of cases.[28] It lies over the L3 vertebra in 1.8% of cases.

Formation of the Meninges

Meningeal formation follows closure of the neural tube and investment of the tube in mesenchyme. It proceeds through three stages: (1) vascularization of the neural tissue, (2) delineation of the subarachnoid space, and (3) ensheathment of neural and vascular surfaces by pia-arachnoid.[6, 7, 40–42, 44] In human embryos, endothelial channels appear on the cord surface by 8 mm CRL.[62] By 8 to 15 mm CRL, a well-defined primitive meninx is present. The dura is evident by 20 mm CRL, and the meninges assume nearly adult configuration by 65 mm CRL.[32] Based on experimental studies in mice,[6, 7, 40–42, 44] it would appear that the process proceeds as follows:

1. Period of vascularization. Increased metabolic demands by the growing cord induce the surrounding mesenchyme to form a vascular tunic consisting of lake-like spaces delimited by primitive endothelium. With time, the vascular tunic becomes continuous over the neural surface. Larger vessels form, and some penetrate into the neural tissue. No meningeal elements are visible, except for the vessels.

2. Period of delineation. Superficial (external) to the vascular tunic, the mesenchyme condenses into a distinct, compact cellular layer by reducing the size of the intervening extracellular spaces (Fig. 1–7). This cellular lamina separates the loose mesenchyme situated near the vascular tunic from the loose mesenchyme situated external to the compact lamina. The mesenchyme deep to the compact layer will form the pia, the inner layer of arachnoid, and the subarachnoid space. The compact cellular layer will form the outer arachnoid and the dura. Simultaneous with these events, (a) progressive vascularization of the brain leads to development of the choroidal epithelium and intraventricular cerebrospinal fluid, and (b) progressive vascularization of the cord supplies metabolites to the neural tissue, so these no longer have to be supplied by diffusion across the extracellular space of the mesenchyme. As a result, the nature of the ground substance within the extracellular spaces of the perineural mesenchyme changes. As watery fluid percolates into and replaces the new ground substance, the extracellular spaces of the mesenchyme are converted into a subarachnoid space situated between the vascular tunic and the compact cell layer.

3. Period of ensheathment of the neural surface and blood vessels. The vascular tunic has now divided into larger, discontinuous blood vessels. Slender arachnoid trabeculae traverse the subarachnoid space, extend to cover the neural surface, and surround the vessels within the subarachnoid space (Fig. 1–8). The pia never completely invests the neural surface. In some areas, the neural tissue is exposed directly to the subarachnoid space. The inner portion of the compact cell layer becomes more electron lucent, establishing the outer arachnoid or "hydrated cell" layer. Later this

Figure 1–7. Light micrograph of an embryo shows the compaction of the mesenchyme to delineate the limits of the subarachnoid space (arrows).

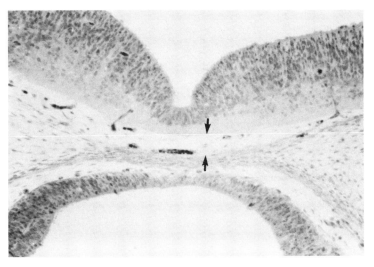

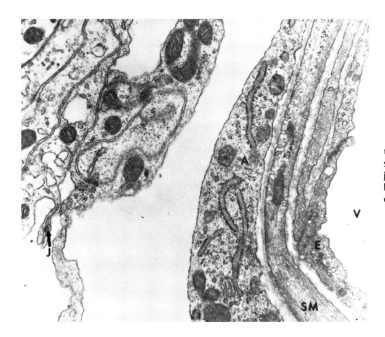

Figure 1–8. Electron micrograph of the early formation of elements in the subarachnoid space demonstrates tight junctions (**J**), a vessel (**V**) with endothelium (**E**), smooth muscle (**SM**), and an ensheathing arachnoid cell (**A**).

simple lamina develops complex interdigitations. There is no great distinction between "pia" and "arachnoid" cells. The ensheathing cells seem to be of a single cell type similar to mature pia-arachnoid. In some areas, single cells send processes to both the "pia" and the "arachnoidal" layer. However, at least some cells remain multipotential, since they supply the smooth muscle, the pericytes, and the pia-arachnoidal sheath of the blood vessels.

The outer portion of the compact cellular layer forms the dura. In most areas, it is difficult to define a distinct boundary between arachnoid and dura. Rather, there is a gradual change in morphology from arachnoid to what is obviously dura. The cells become progressively more dense and contain increasing numbers of collagen fibrils. Contrary to expectation, there is no distinct subdural space. This space is potential, not real. In some areas, a dense granular substance occupies the extracellular space at one point, which is designated the transition point. In the 67 mm CRL fetus, the dura adheres to the filum terminale at the lower end of the S4 vertebra, sealing off the lower end of the subdural space.[65] This relationship changes little by adulthood. In the 111 mm CRL fetus, the dura extends to about the same level and ends in the same manner.[65] In the adult, the dural sac ends approximately two segments higher.[65] Thus the

dural sac conforms more to its bony environment than does the spinal cord. The dural sac shows less migratory adjustment of position than does the ventriculus terminalis or conus. In the cranial region, the outermost layer of the compact cell zone forms the calvarium. In the spine, the bony vertebral column forms by a different mechanism.

Formation of the Vertebral Column

Development of the Mesoderm

Invagination of the surface cells at the primitive streak and migration of these cells between the epiblastic and the hypoblastic germ layers begins to form the mesoblast and the trilaminar germ disc by the end of the second week.[34] Initially the mesoblast (mesoderm) forms a thin, continuous sheet of tissue immediately lateral to the notochord.[34] By day 17 (1.4 mm CRL), mesodermal cells at the cephalic end of the embryo begin to proliferate and form a thick mass of tissue lateral to the notochord and subjacent to the neural plate.[34] This is the paraxial mesoderm. The paraxial mesoderm is directly continuous laterally with intermediate mesoderm and, through that, with the mesoderm of the lateral plate.[34, 36]

As the neural plate flexes and folds into the neural tube, the paraxial mesoderm thickens progressively at each side of the notochord and the closing neural folds. Because the notochord is contiguous with both the ectoderm above and the entoderm below, no mesenchyme is able to enter the space between notochord and ectoderm or the space between notochord and entoderm (see Fig. 1–5A). Similarly, because the neural plate ectoderm is directly continuous with the superficial ectoderm along the neural crest until after the neural folds fuse into the neural tube, no mesoderm is able to enter the groove of the neural folds or the cavity of the neural tube.[44]

Formation of the Spine

Development of the vertebrae proceeds through three stages: membrane development, chondrification, and ossification.[46, 60]

Membrane Development (Days 22–39).[46] During the third week, the paraxial mesoderm forms bilaterally symmetrical, longitudinal strips of solid paraxial mesoderm and begins to segment into paired blocks of somites by day 20.[15] The first somites appear in the midportion of the embryo just caudal to the cranial end of the notochord.[46] This site corresponds to the future occipital region.[46] The first 38 pairs of somites are formed between days 20 and 30.[15] Thereafter, new pairs of somites appear in the craniocaudal wave. By the end of the fifth week, 42 to 44 pairs are formed.[34] There are 4 occipital pairs, 8 cervical pairs, 12 thoracic pairs, 5 lumbar pairs, 5 sacral pairs, and 8 to 10 coccygeal pairs.[34] The first occipital pair and the last 5 to 7 coccygeal pairs later disappear.[34]

Each somite has a cavity—the myocele—that quickly disappears. The ventromedial portion of each somite, called the sclerotome, ultimately differentiates into cartilage, bones, and ligaments[34] (Fig. 1–9). The dorsolateral portion of each somite, called the dermatomyotome, ultimately forms skeletal muscle and dermis.[15] The medially situated cells of the dermatomyotome differentiate into myoblasts that will form skeletal muscle. The laterally situated cells become mesenchymatous and spread under the overly-

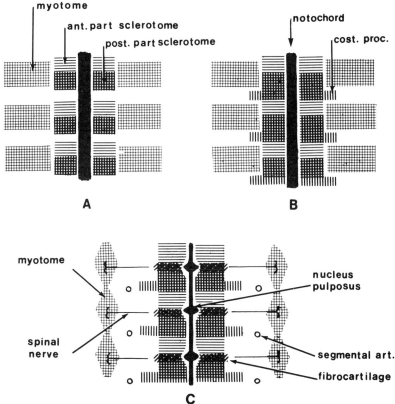

Figure 1–9. Schematic representation of the development of the vertebral column. A, Each sclerotome consists of a cranial mass of loosely packed cells (horizontal lines) and a caudal mass of densely packed cells (bold, cross-hatched lines). Notice the relationship of the myotome to the sclerotome. B, The caudal, dense cell mass of one sclerotome unites with the cranial, loose cell mass of the adjacent caudal sclerotome. C, The mesenchymal cells have formed an intersegmental structure that has received equal contributions from adjacent sclerotomes. These will become the centrum. Note the relationship of the intersegmental structure to the myotome, the spinal nerve, and the segmental artery. (From Rothman RH, Simeone FA (eds): The Spine, 2nd ed. Philadelphia: W. B. Saunders Company, 1982.)

ing ectoderm to form the dermis and subcutaneous tissue of the skin.

The intermediate mesoderm later helps to form the excretory units of the urinary system.

During the fourth week of development, the notochord separates from the ectoderm and the entoderm to form two zones: the ventral subchordal zone between the notochord and the entoderm, and the dorsal epichordal zone between the notochord and the neural tube.[44] As the notochord separates away, sclerotomic cells migrate medially into the subchordal and epichordal zones to form a dense longitudinal column of mesenchyme—the perichordal sheet (see Fig. 1–5B). This process starts in the cervical region on day 23 at 3 mm CRL and proceeds caudally.[46] The column retains traces of its segmental origin as the sclerotomic blocks are separated by less dense areas containing the segmental arteries. As the superficial ectoderm separates from the closed neural tube during the next 7 to 10 days, sclerotomic cells also migrate dorsally around the neural tube to form the membranous neural arches of the vertebra. Migration of the sclerotomic cells ventrolaterally forms the membranous costal processes and the membranous ribs. Thus, at the end of the membranous stage, cell migration from the sclerotomes forms the membranous anlagen of the vertebrae.[46]

Starting on approximately day 24, a major resegmentation occurs in the membranous vertebral bodies (see Figs. 1–9, 1–10).[6] The cells within the caudal half of each sclerotome proliferate more actively than those within the cranial half of each sclerotome. Thus the more cellular, dense, caudal "half-sclerotome" becomes easily distinguishable from the less cellular, cephalic "half-sclerotome." Sclerotomic clefts (the fissures of von Eber) arise at the midportion of each sclerotome, between the dense, caudal half-sclerotome and the less dense cephalic half-sclerotome. The sclerotomes then cleave along the sclerotomic cleft and reunite in a complex fashion such that (1) the dense caudal cells of one sclerotome unite with the less dense cells of the next most caudal sclerotome to form the new precartilaginous primitive vertebral body; (2) the intersegmental arteries are thereby trapped within the centers of the new vertebral bodies; and (3) those cells from the

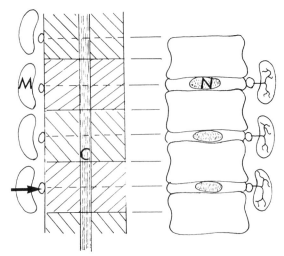

Figure 1–10. Diagrammatic representation of the formation of the vertebral column. Sclerotomes (left) and adult spinal column (right). The sclerotomes (diagonal hatching) surround the notochord (**C**). Note the relationship of the myotomes (**M**) and segmental nerves (arrow), which bridge the intervertebral disc in the adult spinal column. The notochord persists as the nucleus pulposus (**N**).

denser half-sclerotome that abut upon the sclerotomic fissure contribute the basic cells that form the annulus fibrosus of the intervertebral disc and the enchondral growth plates of the centrum.[46] This entire process proceeds bilaterally and symmetrically at each segment so that cleavage and fusion of the sclerotomes on each side form the ipsilateral halves of each vertebral body. The process probably starts in the lower cervical-upper thoracic region and spreads sequentially cranially and caudally.[46]

During this stage, the notochord also undergoes change. Initially the notochord has uniform caliber along its length.[46] During formation of the membranous vertebrae and resegmentation, notochordal cells in the region of the future centrum become compressed and degenerate, while notochordal cells in the region that will become intervertebral disc proliferate, undergo mucoid degeneration, and convert into the nucleus pulposus.[46] Additional notochordal tissue persists as the apical ligament of the dens and as occasional remnants within the skull base, sacrum, and vertebral bodies (ecchordoses).

Chondrification (Days 40–60).[37] The newly formed membranous (precartilaginous) vertebrae gradually become chondrified (Fig. 1–11). From day 39 (11 to 14 mm CRL), centers of chondrification appear in the mesenchyme of the membranous vertebral column.[37] The process of chondrification begins at the cervicothoracic level and extends upward and downward along the vertebral column. The process starts earlier in the centra and later in the neural arches. In the centrum, chondrification usually begins in two centers, one on each side of the midline. A chondrification center also appears in each half of the neural arch lateral to the neural tube and unites with its mate to form the chondral neural arch and spinous process. Two additional centers appear at the junction of the neural arch with the centrum and extend laterally into the transverse processes.[46]

"The cells dorsal to the neural tube initially have two layers. The outer layer of cells forms the arches by proliferation at the tips of the processes. This proliferation extends dorsally. The inner layer (of cells) is called the closure membrane."[46] These inner cells form the dura mater by fusing across the midline.[46] At about 50 mm CRL, the tips of the processes "are almost united across the dorsal surface of the spinal cord in the upper cervical region."[46] They are in contact in the lower cervical region and are completely fused in the thoracic and lumbar regions.[46]

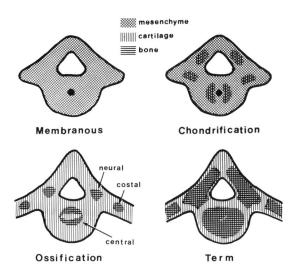

mesenchyme
cartilage
bone

Membranous   Chondrification

neural
costal

central

Ossification   Term

Figure 1–11. Schematic illustration showing the various phases and distribution of tissues in the development of a typical vertebra, vertebral arch, and transverse processes. (From Rothman RH, Simeone FA (eds): The Spine, 2nd ed. Philadelphia: W. B. Saunders Company, 1982.)

"During the seventh and eighth weeks, the anterior and posterior longitudinal ligaments form from the mesenchymal cells that surround the cartilaginous vertebrae."[46] As in the adult, "the anterior longitudinal ligament is strongly adherent to the anterior surface of the centrum, while the posterior longitudinal ligament is attached only to the edge of the disc."[46]

"Between the cartilaginous centra, a ring of cells establishes the annulus fibrosus around the portion of the notochord that will become the nucleus pulposus."[46] Further chondrification in the centra is associated with destruction of the notochord in this area, although the notochord remains within the intervertebral disc area. Despite later ossification, small remnants of notochord also remain in the centrum as the mucoid streak.[46]

Ossification (From Second Month into Postnatal Life). "The stage of ossification overlaps that of chondrification"[46] (Fig. 1–11). The vertebral arches have two ossification centers for each side (total: four). Ossification of the arches starts in the cervical and thoracic regions and extends caudally.[46] However, union of the laminae into a bony arch first occurs in the lumbar region and progresses cranially.

Ossification of the vertebral bodies starts in the low thoracic and upper lumbar regions at 34 mm CRL and then extends both cranially and caudally.[46] The vertebral bodies initially have two ossification centers for each centrum, one anterior to and the second posterior to the vestigial mucoid streak. These coalesce into a single ossification center that enlarges progressively, from the 20th to the 24th week. The residual unossified cartilage cephalic and caudal to the ossification center then forms two cartilaginous plates that face the adjacent intervertebral discs. A C-shaped cartilaginous ring develops at the ventral and lateral aspects of the centrum-disc interface, forming the ring apophysis that will ossify postnatally during the second decade. The ring anchors the annulus to the body firmly, and, once ossified, receives the Sharpey fibers of the annulus.[46] Secondary ossification centers develop in the tips of the transverse processes and spinous processes and in the ring apophyses during the 15th to 17th years.

Throughout the vertebrae, the eventual fusion of the vertebral arches and the centrum occurs well anterior to the pedicles at the site of the neurocentral synchondroses.[46] Thus the definitive vertebral body includes more than just the bone derived from the ossific center of the centrum. The terms vertebral body and centrum are not interchangeable.[46]

Formation of Vertebrae at the Caudal End of the Skeleton

At the caudal end of the embryo, the vertebrae are formed by a different, apparently less well-organized process. The caudal cell mass formed by notochord, mesoderm, and neural tissue simply segments into somites to form the sacral, coccygeal, and tail vertebrae. Retrogressive differentiation leads to reduction and fusion of most of these segments with loss of the tail. The notochord commonly loops and coils in the distalmost regressing vertebrae. The extent of this coil appears to reflect the extent of fusion of the residual primitive vertebrae.[33]

DISORDERED EMBRYOGENESIS

Nearly all the discussion that follows is educated conjecture and, therefore, highly controversial. Its merit is in focusing attention on how potential derangements of embryogenesis may serve to explain the diverse anatomic deformities observed clinically.

Failures of Neurulation

Myelocele and Myelomeningocele

The term myelocele signifies a midline, oval plaque of moist, soft, reddish neural tissue that lies exposed at and flush with the skin surface.[50] The surrounding skin is deficient. A thick, variably epithelialized fibrous tissue joins the edge of the plaque with the nearby skin margins. The term myelomeningocele signifies a myelocele that has been elevated away from the skin surface by expansion of the subarachnoid space ventral to the neural plaque.

Evidence from animal experiments[44] suggests that most myeloceles and myelome-

ningoceles represent focal failures of neurulation. The neural plate flexes into neural folds, but the folds fail to fuse in the midline. As a result, the nervous tissue has the embryonic form of a flat disc. The surface exposed to view represents the amniotic surface that would have become the interior of the cord. A midline groove on the myelocele corresponds to the ventral neural sulcus and is directly continuous above, and occasionally below, with the central canal of the portion of cord that formed normally cephalic and caudal to the myelo(meningo)cele.

Clinically, myelo(meningo)celes most commonly appear as focal defects in the lumbosacral region and are nearly always associated with the Chiari II hindbrain deformity.[49] In a study of 92 human embryos and 4 human fetuses, however, it has been shown[52, 53] that in utero, myeloschisis is often diffuse (holocord) (13%), frequently involves the cervical region (29%), and is commonly associated with holoprosencephaly (20%). These more severe forms appear incompatible with life and are likely aborted spontaneously. Thus the greater incidence of focal lumbosacral myelo(meningo)cele does not reflect its greater frequency, but its lesser severity, permitting survival to term and clinical discovery. The Chiari II malformation is not present in the embryonic period but develops later during fetal life. It is not known why some infants have a larger meningocele component of the lesion than do others.

A second possible explanation for myelocele and myelomeningocele suggests that fetal hydrocephalus causes gross distention of the central canal of the spinal cord. The closed spinal cord then ruptures open to form the myelo(meningo)cele.[20] This theory has recently received some support from experimental work in mice. Vitamin A was administered to pregnant mice during the period in which the neural tube was closing.[44] Approximately half the number of mice born exhibited myeloceles or encephaloceles. A few demonstrated, instead, gross distention of the central canal of the spinal cord and rupture of the cord in the midline ventrally, where it is never open normally.[44] Embryonic hydrocephalus and consequent rupture of the closed neural tube, therefore, might be another mechanism by which myeloceles form in humans.

Lipomyelomeningoceles and Spinal Lipomas

Spinal lipomas are distinct collections of fat and connective tissue that appear at least partially encapsulated and that have a definite connection with the leptomeninges or spinal cord.[14] The lipomyelomeningoceles are a group of lipomas intimately attached to a spinal cord that herniates through a widely bifid spinal canal to form a dorsal subcutaneous mass composed of fat, fibrous tissue, neural tissue, and meningocele.[50]

Recent work suggests that spinal lipomas and lipomyelomeningoceles may also result from deranged neurulation.[43, 44, 50, 51] The major anatomic features of lipomyelomeningoceles may be explained by postulating that spinal lipomas arise by focal premature disjunction of the neuroectoderm from the superficial (cutaneous) ectoderm at the stage immediately preceding closure of the neural tube.[43, 44, 50, 51] Such premature disjunction would allow paraxial mesenchyme to gain access to the dorsal surface of the yet-unclosed neural ectoderm. From this position, it could extend cephalically within the central canal of the closed cord above. Such mesenchyme, in contact with the dorsal neural surface, might impede or prevent closure of the neural tube in the midline dorsally, accounting for the association of lipoma with partial dorsal myeloschisis.

It is further postulated that the dorsal surface of the neural ectoderm (which would have formed the interior of the neural tube) can only induce the adjacent mesenchyme to form fat. Thus the lipoma forms dorsal to the cord between the splayed dorsal columns and often extends into the central canal of the spinal cord cephalic to the myeloschisis. The notochord and the ventral surface of the neural ectoderm (which would have formed the exterior of the neural tube) would still induce the surrounding mesenchyme to form normal pia-arachnoid and dura. Thus the dura, pia-arachnoid, and subarachnoid space would lie ventral to the neural plate. The neural crest that lies at the junction of the dorsal and ventral surfaces of the neural plate is, necessarily, the junction of the fat-inducing and meninges-inducing surfaces of the cord and, therefore, is also the junction of the lipoma, neural tissue, and meninges. The lipoma would be bounded laterally by the neural crest and meninges. No lipoma would be found within the subarachnoid space, since lipoma and arachnoid form separately in relation to different surfaces of the neural plate. Because the cord is cleft dorsally, the outer, meninges-inducing surface of cord is deficient dorsally. Consequently, no dura forms in the midline dorsally, leaving a focal dorsal dural defect. The portion of lipoma attached to cord could then pass into the extradural soft tissue of the back.

Other theories of the formation of spinal lipoma include overgrowth of fat cells normally present in the pia-arachnoid,[67] fatty differentiation of perivascular mesenchyme that normally invades the cord during embryonal vascularization, and overgrowth of embryonic rests of ectodermal origin.[50]

Dorsal Dermal Sinus

The term dorsal dermal sinus signifies an epithelial-lined tube that extends inwardly from the dorsal skin surface for varying distances.[45, 48] One half to two thirds of these extend intraspinally. Approximately 50% terminate in deep dermoid or epidermoid cysts. Embryologically, dorsal dermal sinuses most likely represent segmental adhesions of cutaneous and neural ectoderm that result from incomplete disjunction as the neural tube closes. This segmental adhesion is then drawn inwardly and cephalically as the neural ectoderm becomes buried beneath paraxial mesenchyme and as the spinal cord ascends. The sinus tract thus characteristically ascends as it passes deeply.

Failures of Canalization and Retrogressive Differentiation

Lipomas of the filum terminale, tight filum terminale syndrome, sacrococcygeal teratomas, rare residual tails, and, perhaps, terminal myelocystoceles may result from disordered canalization and retrogressive differentiation.

Tight filum terminale syndrome signifies tethering of the spinal cord in an abnormally low position by a filum terminale that is too short and too thick (greater than 2 mm in diameter).[23, 24, 48, 50] The term specifically excludes cases in which the cord is also tethered by concurrent bone spur, lipoma, and so forth. In one series, all such patients had spina bifida occulta of L4, L5, or S1.[24] Fourteen percent had kyphoscoliosis, and 25% had (nontethering) lipomatous tissue within the thickened filum. These cases appear to represent incomplete retrogressive differentiation of the distal spinal cord.

Disorders of Notochordal Formation

Split Notochord Syndrome[1, 3, 9, 17, 58, 61]

The term split notochord syndrome signifies the spectrum of anomalies believed to represent sequelae of splitting or deviation of the notochord with persistent connection between the gut and the dorsal skin.[9] The archetype of this anomaly is the dorsal enteric fistula, which is the most severe form of split notochord syndrome. The dorsal enteric fistula is a persistence of the entire patent communication between the intestinal cavity and the skin surface in the midline dorsally. Any portion(s) of the dorsal enteric fistula may become obliterated, or persist, leaving apparently isolated diverticula, duplications, cysts, fibrous cords, and sinuses at any point along the segmental tract of the anomaly. Such anomalies may arise as follows.

As the notochord grows cephalically toward the prochordal plate, it must separate the dorsal ectoderm (future skin) from the ventral entoderm (future gut). If the ectoderm fails to separate focally, leaving a strand or adhesion, the notochord must either split around the adhesion or deviate to the left or right of it. The mesoderm that normally envelops the notochord to form the segmental vertebrae is directed by the anomaly to form a split or deviated spinal column, with a persisting connection between the dorsal surface of the gut and the external surface of the body in the dorsal midline. With growth and variable degrees of migration, the adhesion may become quite long and connect segmentally related but topographically distant sites.[1] Because the notochord may split or deviate, the connection of the "cysts" to vertebrae may be midline or paramedian. As a variation of this concept, it has been postulated that the focal duplication or deviation of the notochord is

the primary defect, following which the yolk sac entoderm herniates dorsally, through the defect, to become adherent to the neuroectoderm.[4] Cleft notochords with so-called ring embryos have been observed in mammals.[4]

Other theories as to the embryogenesis of "split notochord" syndrome include intercalation of entoderm between notochord and ectoderm with later (a) detachment of the cells from the entodermal tube as it is drawn away during the descent of the foregut; (b) detachment of totipotential cells of Hensen's node during its migration, giving rise to enteric cysts without associated closure defect; and (c) failure of separation of notochord from entoderm, drawing out an enteric diverticulum.[4, 8, 11, 16, 69]

Disorders with Unknown Embryogenesis

Diastematomyelia and Diplomyelia

Diastematomyelia is a form of occult dysraphism characterized by sagittal clefting of one or more portion(s) of the spinal cord, conus medullaris, or filum terminale, resulting in two, frequently asymmetric "hemicords," each of which contains a central canal, one dorsal horn that receives the ipsilateral dorsal nerve root, and one ventral horn that gives rise to the ipsilateral ventral nerve root.[10, 25, 26, 39, 45, 47, 50] In 50% to 60% of cases, the two hemicords are contained in a single subarachnoid space enveloped in a single arachnoid and single coaxial dural tube. In 40% to 50% of cases, the meninges are also cleft focally, so each hemicord lies within its own pial-arachnoidal-dural tube. Bone spurs occur only in this second type of diastematomyelia.[28, 50]

Diplomyelia is a more or less perfect duplication of the spinal cord, producing two true cords. Each cord contains a central canal, two dorsal horns, two dorsal roots, two ventral horns, and two ventral roots.

The pathogenesis of diastematomyelia is unknown. The primary derangement could be in the extraneural tissues, with consequent clefting of the neural plate, or the primary derangement could be in the neural tissues, with later induction of changes in the surrounding bone and soft tissue. It has been suggested that persistence of the neurenteric canal may create a connection between the gut and dorsal skin that prevents normal midline fusion of prevertebral tissue, vertebral column, spinal cord, subcutaneous tissue, and skin.[8] Such a connection might explain the multiple segmentation anomalies, hemivertebrae, butterfly vertebrae, spina bifida, skin lesions, cleft dura, cleft cord, and midline cysts associated with diastematomyelia. Since the site of the neurenteric canal is believed to come to lie, finally, at the tip of the coccyx, other authors[22] have suggested that there may be accessory neurenteric canals that create the same defects.

Alternatively, others have suggested that as the lateral edges of the neural folds begin to approximate in the midline, they may curl too far ventrally, touch the ventral portion of the plate, and form two, not necessarily symmetric neural tubes, one to each side of the midline.[25] Persistence of the midventral tissue between the curls would yield a partial dorsal myeloschisis. Disappearance of the midventral portion would yield two neural tubes that could remain close together or migrate laterally. The mesenchyme would then grow in to surround the two tubes. If the distance between tubes were small, the mesenchyme between the hemicords might be induced to form only pia, creating a narrow diastematomyelia in which both hemicords lie within a single arachnoid and dural tube. If the distance between the hemicords were greater, the intervening mesenchyme might be induced to form arachnoid, dura, and bone, creating a wide diastematomyelia with cleft meninges and interposed bone spur. The other vertebral changes would then arise by disordered induction. Diastematomyelia could also arise as an abortive form of twinning.

Syndrome of Caudal Regression

The term syndrome of caudal regression defines a spectrum of anomalies that includes sirenomelia (fusion of the lower extremities), lumbosacral agenesis (absence of the caudalmost spine), anal atresia, malformed external genitalia, bilateral renal aplasia (or severe dysplasia), and pulmonary hypoplasia with Potter facies.[5, 13, 29, 57] Syndrome of caudal regression appears to result from disturbances in the caudal mesodermal axis prior to the fourth week of gestation. In chickens, complete rumplessness may be induced by exposing developing eggs to high temperature[12] or by injecting insulin or other sulfur-containing molecules into the yolk sac of incubated eggs.[54] In these animals, the degree of tail suppression depends upon the precise period of gestation at which the insult occurs.

In humans, lack of caudal vertebrae may be secondary to nondevelopment of the lower portions of the spinal cord and notochord. It has been shown that in vertebrates, extirpation of part of the neural tube (leaving the notochord intact) causes development of the vertebral bodies but absence of the vertebral arches.[27] If the notochord is removed but the neural tube is preserved, vertebral arches develop without distinct bodies.

Sixteen percent of infants with caudal regression syndrome have diabetic mothers.[55, 56] Sacral agenesis is expected in 1% of offspring of diabetic mothers.[59] Paternal diabetes may also play a role.[54]

Partial Failures of Formation or Segmentation of the Spinal Column

Incomplete Fusions of the Neural Arches

Radiologically demonstrable "incomplete fusions" of the neural arches may represent true failures to form complete membranous or chondral neural arches or failure to ossify completely a neural arch that is present in membranous or chondral form. The reported incidence of lumbosacral spina bifida is 0.2% to 34%.[19, 21, 66] The osseous defects may be midline or paramedian.

Transitional Vertebrae

In 6.4% of patients, the last lumbar vertebra develops winglike transverse processes that may (a) remain separate from the homologous segments of the first sacral vertebra—incomplete sacralization (2.9%) or (b) lie next to or articulate with the first sacral vertebra—complete sacralization (3.5%).[64] Lumbarization of S1, unilaterally or bilaterally, is present in 2% of patients.

Ribs

In 2% of patients, T12 lacks ribs.[64] L1 carries ribs in 6% to 11.3% of cases, usually bilaterally.

References

1. Abell MR: Mediastinal cysts. Arch Pathol 61:360–379, 1956.
2. Barson AJ: The vertebral level of termination of the spinal cord during normal and abnormal development. J Anat 106:489–497, 1970.
3. Beardmore HE, Wiglesworth FW: Vertebral anomalies and alimentary duplications: Clinical and embryological aspects. Pediatr Clin North Am 5:457–473, 1958.
4. Bentley JFR, Smith JR: Developmental posterior enteric remnants and spinal malformations: The split notochord syndrome. Arch Dis Child 35:76–86, 1960.
5. Berdon WE, Hochberg B, Baker DH, et al: The association of lumbosacral spine and genitourinary anomalies with imperforate anus. AJR 98:181–191, 1966.
6. Bondareff W, McLone DG: Glial limiting membrane in the *Macaca*: ultrastructures of the glial epithelium. Am J Anat 136:277–296, 1973.
7. Bondareff W, McLone DG, Decker S: Ultrastructure of glioepithelia in brains of mice and men. Anat Rec 175:487, 1973.
8. Bremer JL: Dorsal intestinal fistula, accessory neurenteric canal, diastematomyelia. Arch Pathol 54:132–138, 1952.
9. Burrows FGO, Sutcliffe J: The split notochord syndrome. Br J Radiol 41:844–847, 1968.
10. Cohen J, Sledge CB: Diastematomyelia: An embryological interpretation with report of a case. Am J Dis Child 100:257–263, 1960.
11. D'Almeida AC, Stewart DH Jr: Neurenteric cyst: Case report and literature review. Neurosurgery 8:596–599, 1981.
12. Danforth CH: Artificial and hereditary suppression of sacral vertebrae in the fowl. Proc Soc Exp Biol Med 30:143–145, 1932.
13. Duhamel B: From the mermaid to anal imperforation: The syndrome of caudal regression. Arch Dis Child 36:152–155, 1961.
14. Emery JL, Lendon RG: Lipomas of the cauda equina and other fatty tumours related to neurospinal dysraphism. Dev Med Child Neurol 11 (Suppl 20): 62–70, 1969.
15. England MA: Color Atlas of Life before Birth. Normal Fetal Development. Chicago: Year Book Medical Publishers, Inc, 1983.
16. Fallon A, Gordon ARG, Lendrum CC: Mediastinal cysts of foregut origin associated with vertebral abnormalities. Br J Surg 41:520–533, 1954.
17. Feller A, Sternberg H: Zur Kenntnis der Fehlbildungen der Wirbelsäule. I Die Wirbelkörperspalte und ihre formale Genese. Virchows Arch (Pathol Anat Physiol) 272:613–640, 1929.
18. French BN: The embryology of spinal dysraphism (in) Proceedings of the Congress of Neurological Surgeons in Toronto, Ontario, Canada 1982. Clinical Neurosurgery. Baltimore: Williams & Wilkins, 1983, pp 295–340.
19. Friedman MM, Fischer FJ, VanDemark RE: Lumbosacral roentgenograms of one hundred soldiers: A control study. AJR 55:292–298, 1946.
20. Gardner WJ: The Dysraphic States from Syringomyelia to Anencephaly. Amsterdam: Excerpta Medica, 1973.
21. Hadley HG: Frequency of spina bifida. Virginia Med Monthly 68:43–46, 1941.
22. Hamilton WJ, Boyd JD, Mossman HW: Human Embryology. Prenatal Development of Form and Function, 2nd ed. Baltimore: Williams & Wilkins, 1952.
23. Hendrick EB, Hoffman HJ, Humphreys RP: Tethered cord syndrome. In McLaurin RL (ed): Myelomeningocele. New York: Grune & Stratton, 1977, pp 369–376.
24. Hendrick EB, Hoffman HJ, Humphreys RP: The tethered spinal cord (in) Proceedings of the Congress of Neurological Surgeons in Toronto, Ontario, Canada 1982. Clinical Neurosurgery. Baltimore: Williams & Wilkins, 1983, pp 457–463.
25. Herren RY, Edwards JE: Diplomyelia (duplication of the spinal cord). Arch Pathol 30:1203–1214, 1940.
26. Humphreys RP, Hendrich EB, Hoffman JH: Diastematomyelia (in) Proceedings of the Congress of Neurological Surgeons in Toronto, Ontario, Canada 1982. Clinical Neurosurgery. Baltimore: Williams & Wilkins, 1983, pp 436–456.
27. Ignelzi RJ, Lehman RAW: Lumbosacral agenesis: Management and embryological implications. J Neurol Neurosurg Psychiatry 37:1273–1276, 1974.
28. James CCM, Lassman LP: Spinal Dysraphism; Spina Bifida Occulta. New York: Appleton-Century-Crofts (London: Butterworth & Co), 1972.
29. Kallen B, Winberg J: Caudal mesoderm pattern of anomalies: From renal agenesis to sirenomelia. Teratology 9:99–112, 1974.
30. Keim H: The Adolescent Spine. New York: Grune & Stratton, 1976.
31. Kernohan JW: The ventriculus terminalis: Its growth and development. J Comp Neurol 38:107–125, 1924.
32. Klicka E: L'ultrastructure des meninges en onlogenese de l'homme. Z Mikrosk Anat Forsch 79:209–222, 1968.
33. Kunitomo K: The development and reduction of the tail and of the caudal end of the spinal cord. Contrib Embryol 8:161–198, 1918.
34. Langman J: Medical Embryology. Baltimore: Williams & Wilkins, 1963.
35. Lemire RJ, Beckwith JB: Pathogenesis of congenital tumors and malformations of the sacrococcygeal region. Teratology 25:201–213, 1982.
36. Lemire RJ, Graham CB, Beckwith JB: Skin-covered sacrococcygeal masses in infants and children. J Pediatr 79:948–954, 1971.
37. Lemire RJ, Leoser JD, Leech RW, et al: Normal and Abnormal Development of the Human Nervous System. Hagerstown, Maryland: Harper & Row Publishers, Inc, 1975.
38. Lendon RG, Emergy JL: Forking of the central canal in the equinal cord of children. J Anat 106:499–505, 1970.
39. Lichtenstein BW: Spinal dysraphism: Spina bifida and myelodysplasia. Arch Neurol Psychiatry 44:792–810, 1940.
40. McLone DG: Development of the limiting glial membrane of the brain. Childs Brain 6:150–162, 1980.
41. McLone DG: The subarachnoid space. A review. Childs Brain 6:113–130, 1980.
42. McLone DG, Bondareff W: Developmental morphology of the subarachnoid space and contiguous structures in the mouse. Am J Anat 142:273–294, 1975.
43. McLone DG, Mutluer S, Naidich TP: Lipomeningoceles of the conus medullaris (in) Concepts in

Pediatric Neurosurgery. Vol 3. Basel: S Karger, 1982, pp 170–177.

44. McLone DG, Suwa J, Collins JA, et al: Neurulation: Biochemical and morphological studies on primary and secondary neural tube defects (in) Concepts in Pediatric Neurosurgery, Vol 4. Basel: S Karger, 1983, pp 15–29.

45. Matson DD, Jerva MJ: Recurrent meningitis associated with congenital lumbo-sacral dermal sinus tract. J Neurosurg 25:288–297, 1966.

46. Moe JH, Winter RB, Bradford DS, et al: Scoliosis and Other Spinal Deformities. Philadelphia: WB Saunders Company, 1978.

47. Naidich TP, Harwood-Nash DC: Diastematomyelia. Part I. Hemicords and meningeal sheaths, single and double arachnoid and dural tubes. AJNR 4:633–636, 1983.

48. Naidich TP, Harwood-Nash DC, McLone DG: Radiology of spinal dysraphism. Clin Neurosurg 30:341–365, 1983.

49. Naidich TP, McLone DG, Fulling KH: The Chiari malformations: Part IV. The hindbrain deformity. Neuroradiology 25:179–197, 1983.

50. Naidich TP, McLone DG, Harwood-Nash DC: Spinal dysraphism. (in) Newton TH, Potts DG (eds): Modern Neuroradiology. Vol I. Computed Tomography of the Spine and Spinal Cord. San Anselmo, California: Clavadel Press, 1983, pp 299–353.

51. Naidich TP, McLone DG, Mutleur S: A new understanding of dorsal dysraphism with lipoma (lipomyeloschisis): Radiological evaluation and surgical correction. AJNR 4:103–116, 1983.

52. Osaka K, Matsumoto S, Tanimura T: Myeloschisis in early human embryos. Childs Brain 4:347–359, 1978.

53. Osaka K, Tanimura T, Hirayama A, et al: Myelomeningocele before birth. J Neurosurg 49:711–724, 1978.

54. Pang D, Hoffman JH: Sacral agenesis with progressive neurological deficit. Neurosurgery 7:118–126, 1980.

55. Passarge E: Congenital malformations and maternal diabetes. Lancet 1:324–325, 1965.

56. Passarge E, Lenz W: Syndrome of caudal regression in infants of diabetic mothers: Observations of further cases. Pediatrics 37:672–675, 1966.

57. Potter EL, Craig JM: Pathology of the Fetus and the Infant, 3rd ed. Chicago: Year Book Medical Publishers, Inc, 1975.

58. Rhaney K, Barclay GPT: Enterogenous cysts and congenital diverticula of the alimentary canal with abnormalities of the vertebral column and spinal cord. J Pathol Bacteriol 77:457–471, 1959.

59. Sarnat HB, Case ME, Graviss R: Sacral agenesis: Neurologic and neuropathologic features. Neurology 26:1124–1129, 1976.

60. Sarwar M, Kier EL, Virapongse C: Development of the spine and spinal cord. (in) Newton TH, Potts DG (eds): Modern Neuroradiology. Vol I. Computed Tomography of the Spine and Spinal Cord. San Anselmo, California: Clavadel Press, 1983, pp 15–30.

61. Saunders RL deCH: Combined anterior and posterior spina bifida in a living neonatal human female. Anat Rec 87:255–278, 1943.

62. Sensenig EC: The early development of the meninges of the spinal cord in human embryos. Contrib Embryo 34:147–157, 1951.

63. Sherk HH, Parke WW: Developmental anatomy. In The Cervical Spine. Philadelphia: JB Lippincott Company, 1983, p 108.

64. Southworth JD, Bersack SR: Anomalies of the lumbosacral vertebrae in five hundred and fifty individuals without symptoms referable to the low back. AJR 64:624–634, 1950.

65. Streeter GL: Factors involved in the formation of the filum terminale. Am J Anat 25:1–11, 1919.

66. Sutow WW, Pryde AW: Incidence of spina bifida occulta in relation to age. AMA J Dis Child 91:211–217, 1956.

67. Swanson HS, Barnett JC Jr: Intradural lipomas in children. Pediatrics 29:911–926, 1962.

68. Tarlov IM: Structure of the filum terminale. Arch Neurol Psychiatry 40:1–17, 1938.

69. Veeneklaas GMH: Pathogenesis of intrathoracic gastrogenic cysts. Am J Dis Child 83:500–507, 1952.

2

Robert O. Cone, M.D.
Morrie E. Kricun, M.D.
Donald Resnick, M.D.

Anatomy

OSSEOUS ANATOMY

General Considerations

The human spine consists of a complex arrangement of osseous and soft-tissue elements that function to provide support and mobility for the axial portion of the human body as well as to create a protective shell for neural structures. On the basis of anatomic and functional aspects, the 33 bony vertebrae are subdivided into five segments: cervical, thoracic, lumbar, sacral, and coccygeal.[44] In order to gain a useful understanding of the anatomy of the spine, it is necessary to consider functional characteristics as well as the anatomic similarities and differences of the spine as a whole and of its individual elements.

Early in fetal development the spine assumes a single smooth curvature with dorsal convexity (kyphosis). In the adult, these kyphotic curvatures persist in the thoracic and sacrococcygeal segments and thus are termed the primary curvatures of the spine. Compensatory (secondary) curvatures develop in the cervical and lumbar segments in order to facilitate the erect posture, resulting in the typical sigmoid shape of the adult vertebral column.

Although each individual vertebra shares certain anatomic characteristics with all other vertebrae, functional requirements dictate that the vertebral elements of different segments of the spine vary in their anatomic make-up. An understanding of the similarities as well as the differences between the individual bony elements of the spine is

essential in order to comprehend and recognize pathologic derangements.

The typical vertebra consists of a body, an arch, and a variable number of bony appendages. It is separated from adjacent vertebrae by means of a fibrocartilaginous intervertebral disc and paired synovial apophyseal articulations. The vertebral body is a cylindrical structure with slightly concave cranial and caudal end-plates. The surfaces of these end-plates are slightly roughened for attachment of the fibers of the intervertebral disc. The periphery of the vertebral body consists of a relatively thin shell of cortical bone, and the large central space is composed of cancellous bone, marrow elements, and fat. The cortical surface of the vertebral body is pierced anterolaterally by a variable number of small foramina and dorsomedially by a single large foramen, which provide points of entrance and egress for neurovascular elements. The vertebral arch arises from the superior dorsolateral margins of the vertebral body and forms the dorsal and lateral margins of the spinal canal. The pedicles are short ovoid bony bars that attach to the vertebral body at the neurocentral synchondroses. Dorsally, the vertebral arch consists of a broad flattened plate of bone that fuses with the pedicle ventrally and with its contralateral mate dorsally in the midline. The division of the vertebral arch into pedicles and laminae is based on anatomic rather than embryologic criteria, because both pedicles and laminae arise from the same ossification center. The point of transition between the pedicle and lamina is the site of origin of the superior and inferior articular

20

ANATOMY • 21

facets (apophyseal joints) and of the transverse process. Gross pathologic evaluation of the spine reveals that the superior articular facet and transverse process arise from the ventral (pedicular) side of this point and the inferior articular facet arises from the dorsal (laminar) side. The pars interarticularis is that portion of the neural arch that lies between the superior and inferior articular facets; it is a common site of osseous defects, especially in the lower lumbar spine. The spinous process is a dorsally oriented bony process that arises from the posterior site of fusion of the laminae.

Cervical Spine

The cervical spine consists of seven vertebrae and functions primarily to provide mobility to the head. On an anatomic basis the cervical spine can be divided into two main segments; the craniocervical junction (C1 and C2) and the lower cervical spine (C3–C7).[18, 21]

Craniocervical Junction

The craniocervical junction consists of the base of the skull, the atlas (C1), and the axis (C2). The atlas, a ring-shaped vertebra, is unique in that it lacks a vertebral body and has an anterior arch (Fig. 2–1). The anterior arch of the atlas represents the only site of persistence of the fetal hypochordal bow, which bridges the fetal vertebral body ventrally to connect the neural arches. A small conical protuberance (anterior tubercle) is present at the ventral midline of the anterior arch of the atlas and provides a site for ligamentous attachment. The lateral masses of the atlas represent enlargements of the ventral (pedicular) portions of the vertebral arch. The superior articular facet of the atlas is concave, ovoid, and angulated medially to provide a stable base for the occipital condyles. The inferior articular facets are flattened and angulated medially to allow rotation of the atlas on the lateral articular facets of the axis. Short cervical bony tubercles on the medial border of the lateral

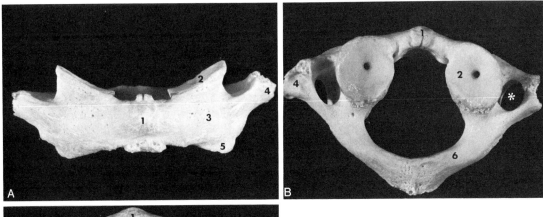

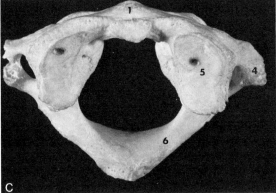

Figure 2–1. Atlas (C1). Anatomic specimen. A, Frontal view. B, View from above. C, View from below. *Key:* **1** = anterior arch and anterior tubercle of C1; **2** = superior articular facet; **3** = lateral mass; **4** = transverse process; **5** = inferior articular facet; **6** = lamina; **asterisk** = foramen transversarium.

masses of the atlas represent the insertion points of the transverse band of the cruciate ligament. Short, broad transverse processes arise from the lateral masses of the atlas and are perforated by the foramina transversaria, through which pass the vertebral arteries. The vertebral arches of the atlas are thin and rounded, with notches in their anterosuperior borders over which the vertebral arteries pass to enter the foramen magnum.

The axis is characterized by the presence of a fingerlike superior process (odontoid process, dens), which arises from the superior aspect of the vertebral body and represents the embryologic equivalent of the body of the atlas (Fig. 2–2). In young children, a synchrondrosis may be identified between the odontoid process and the body of the atlas (subdental synchondrosis). The odontoid process articulates with the posterior aspect of the anterior arch of the atlas and serves as the axis for rotatory motion of the craniocervical junction and as a stabilizing bar (Fig. 2–3). The distance between the anterior surface of the odontoid process and the posterior surface of the anterior arch of the atlas is an important radiographic observation and should not exceed 3 mm in the adult or 5 mm in the child, regardless of the degree of flexion of the head. In young children, a diamond-shaped ossification center may be identified at the superior pole of the odontoid process (ossiculum terminale); it occasionally persists into adulthood. A shallow horizontal cartilage-filled groove on the posterior surface of the odontoid process marks the site of articulation with the transverse band of the cruciate ligament. The anterior aspect of the body of the axis is characterized by a triangular bony promi-

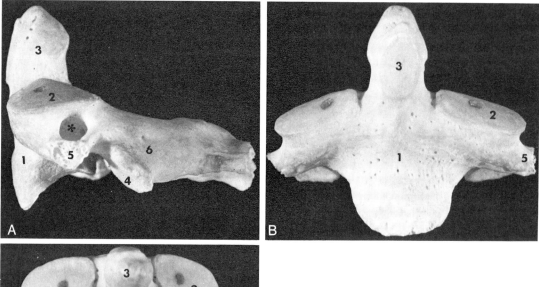

Figure 2–2. Axis (C2). Anatomic specimen. *A,* Lateral view. *B,* Frontal view. *C,* View from above. *Key:* **1** = body; **2** = superior articular facet; **3** = odontoid process; **4** = inferior articular facet; **5** = transverse process; **6** = lamina; **7** = spinous process; **asterisk** = foramen transversarium.

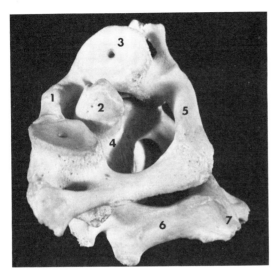

Figure 2–3. Atlas and Axis. Anatomic specimen demonstrating the relationship of the bony structures. *Key:* **1** = anterior arch of C1; **2** = odontoid process; **3** = superior articular facet of C1; **4** = body of C2; **5** = lamina of C1; **6** = lamina of C2; **7** = spinous process of C2.

nence upon which the tendon of the longus colli muscle inserts. It extends inferiorly as a bony lip to articulate with the anterosuperior aspect of the third cervical vertebral body. The facets of the axis possess large flattened articular surfaces that are oriented superolaterally to articulate with the lateral masses of the atlas. Short transverse processes are perforated by the foramen transversarium. The inferior articular facets of the axis are oriented obliquely in the anterior direction. The vertebral arch is completed posteriorly by thick ovoid laminae and a small, usually bifid, spinous process.

Lower Cervical Spine

The vertebral bodies of the lower cervical spine are characterized by a thin vertical ridge of bone arising from the periphery of the posterior and lateral aspects of the superior vertebral margin (uncinate processes, uncus) (Fig. 2–4). The uncinate processes are larger laterally than posteriorly and articulate with the rounded inferior aspect of the adjacent cranial vertebral body. The pedicles of the cervical vertebra arise from the posterolateral aspect of the cranial half of the vertebral body, forming an angle of ap-

proximately 45 degrees with the body. The superior articular facets are directed posteriorly and cranially, but the inferior articular facets are directed anteriorly and caudally. The neural foramina are oriented posterolaterally and best visualized in the 45 degree oblique radiographic projection of the cervical spine. The laminae are flattened and platelike, with small, frequently bifid spinous processes that become progressively larger in the lower cervical spine. The transverse processes of the lower cervical vertebrae have a grooved cranial surface with cranially directed anterior (carotid) and posterior tubercles. The carotid tubercle tends to be largest at the C5 and C6 levels and may be projected anteriorly to the vertebral body on lateral radiographs, simulating a fracture fragment. The medial margins of the transverse processes are pierced by the foramina transversaria.

Thoracic Spine

The bony thoracic spine consists of 12 vertebrae aligned in a long, gradual kyphotic curvature.[44] The thoracic vertebral bodies (Fig. 2–5) increase in size in the craniocaudal direction, forming a gradual transition between the smaller cervical and larger lumbar vertebral bodies. The anterior and lateral margins of the thoracic vertebral bodies form a smooth ovoid shape, with the posterior vertebral margin being slightly concave. Demifacets are present at the posterolateral margins of the vertebral body both superiorly and inferiorly for articulation with the articular facets of the heads of the ribs. The superior demifacet is directed cephalad, and the inferior demifacet is directed caudad. The first thoracic vertebra is atypical, in that the superior demifacet is enlarged and directed inferiorly because the first rib articulates only with this vertebra and not with the seventh cervical vertebra. The demifacets of the lower thoracic vertebra (T10–T12) are variable in appearance and frequently consist of single large demifacets at the level of the pedicles. The pedicles of the thoracic vertebrae are directed posterosuperiorly, and the articular facets lie in the coronal plane with slight obliquity in a superoventral to inferodorsal direction. The margins of the neural foramina consist of the inferior sur-

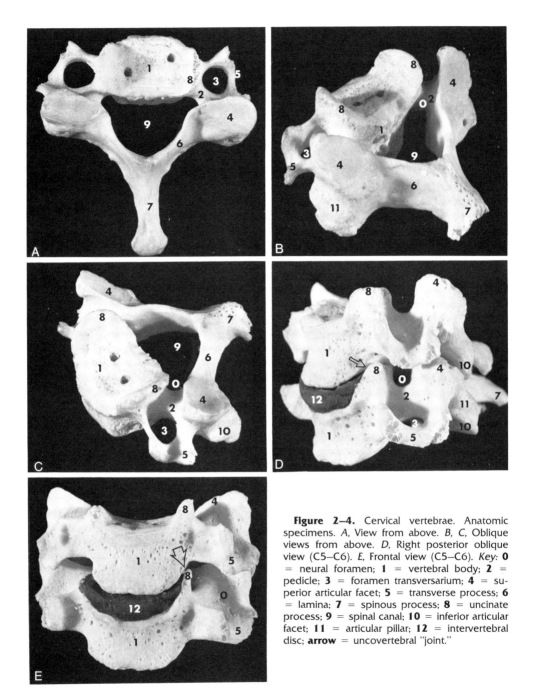

Figure 2–4. Cervical vertebrae. Anatomic specimens. *A,* View from above. *B, C,* Oblique views from above. *D,* Right posterior oblique view (C5–C6). *E,* Frontal view (C5–C6). *Key:* **0** = neural foramen; **1** = vertebral body; **2** = pedicle; **3** = foramen transversarium; **4** = superior articular facet; **5** = transverse process; **6** = lamina; **7** = spinous process; **8** = uncinate process; **9** = spinal canal; **10** = inferior articular facet; **11** = articular pillar; **12** = intervertebral disc; **arrow** = uncovertebral "joint."

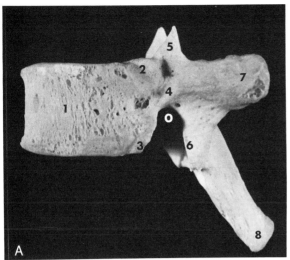 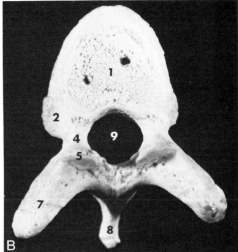

Figure 2–5. Thoracic vertebra (T8). Anatomic specimen. *A,* Lateral view. *B,* View from above. *Key:* **0** = neural foramen; **1** = body; **2** = superior demifacet for head of rib; **3** = inferior demifacet for head of rib; **4** = pedicle; **5** = superior articular facet; **6** = inferior articular facet; **7** = transverse process; **8** = spinous process; **9** = central spinal canal.

face of the cranial pedicle superiorly, the posteroinferior aspect of the cranial vertebra anteriorly, the superior aspect of the caudal pedicle inferiorly, and the superior articular facet of the caudal vertebra posteriorly. The alignment is such that the foramina are oriented in the coronal plane and best visualized in the lateral radiographic projection. The transverse processes of the thoracic vertebrae are oriented posterosuperiorly, with articular facets on their ventral aspects for articulation with the ribs. The laminae of the thoracic vertebrae are broad flattened plates that completely enclose the posterior aspect of the spinal canal. The spinous processes at this level are directed posteroinferiorly.

Lumbar Spine

The lumbar spine consists of five vertebrae aligned with a smooth lordotic curvature.[44] The lumbar vertebral bodies resemble the thoracic vertebral bodies, except for increased mass and the lack of demifacets (Fig. 2–6). The lumbar pedicles are short, broad bony bars oriented posteriorly in the parasagittal plane, as are the lumbar articular facets, although there may be a great deal of variability in facet orientation at the lumbar levels, with the articular planes varying between the sagittal and coronal planes. The transverse processes of the lumbar vertebrae

progressively enlarge in the lower lumbar spine and are oriented laterally. The lumbar laminae are broad and flat but, in contrast to the thoracic spine, have U-shaped defects inferiorly between the inferior articular facets, resulting in an incomplete bony posterior wall of the lumbar spinal canal. Lumbar spinous processes are large, rounded, and oriented posteriorly.

Sacrum and Coccyx

The sacrum is a triangular bone composed of the fused bony elements of the five embryologic sacral vertebrae (Fig. 2–7). It lies interposed between the paired iliac bones of the pelvis and provides a stable articulation between the spine and the pelvis. There is bony fusion between the sacral vertebral bodies and laterally directed pedicles (alae), such that the neural foramina of the sacrum are oriented in the parasagittal plane and best visualized in the anteroposterior radiographic projection. The ventral surface of the sacrum is concave and oriented in a posterior position at an average of 40 degrees relative to the coronal plane. At upper sacral levels, vestigial remnants of intervertebral disc substance may persist in the midline. The sacral laminae are short, broad, and fused with those of adjacent sacral levels. Short spinous processes are present at the upper sacral levels, whereas at the lower

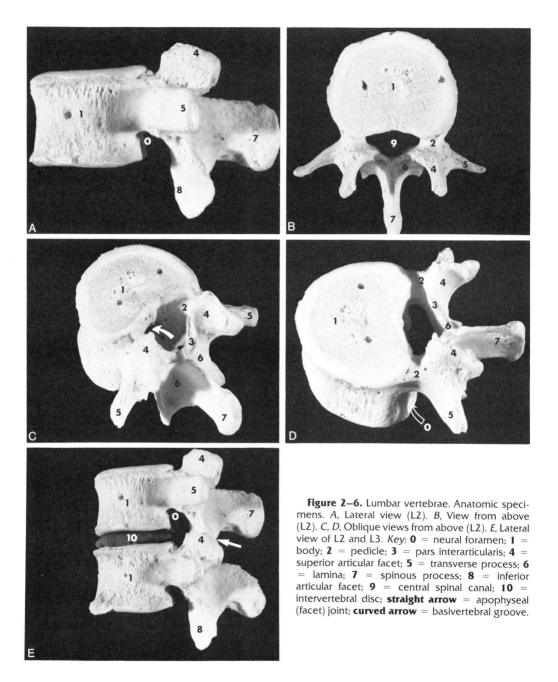

Figure 2–6. Lumbar vertebrae. Anatomic specimens. *A,* Lateral view (L2). *B,* View from above (L2). *C, D,* Oblique views from above (L2). *E,* Lateral view of L2 and L3. *Key:* **0** = neural foramen; **1** = body; **2** = pedicle; **3** = pars interarticularis; **4** = superior articular facet; **5** = transverse process; **6** = lamina; **7** = spinous process; **8** = inferior articular facet; **9** = central spinal canal; **10** = intervertebral disc; **straight arrow** = apophyseal (facet) joint; **curved arrow** = basivertebral groove.

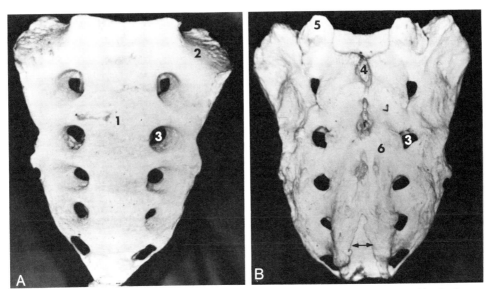

Figure 2–7. Sacrum. Anatomic specimen. *A,* Anterior view. *B,* Posterior view. *Key:* **1** = sacral body; **2** = sacral ala; **3** = sacral foramen; **4** = spinous process; **5** = articular process; **6** = lamina; **arrows** = sacral hiatus.

sacral levels, the laminae do not meet in the midline, but form the margins of inferior sacral hiatus.

The coccyx consists of three to five small ovoid vertebrae, each possessing a small rudimentary vertebral body, articular facets, and transverse processes. Each lacks pedicles, laminae, and a spinous process.

Central Spinal (Vertebral) Canal

The spinal canal is a tunnel containing the thecal sac and epidural space and their contents. It is bordered anteriorly by the posterior aspect of the vertebral bodies and intervertebral discs, posteriorly by the ligamentum flavum and bony vertebral arch, and laterally by the pedicles and facet joints.[35]

The size and shape of the spinal canal vary with age and location. In the adult cervical spine, the spinal canal is rounded in the upper spine and triangular in the lower cervical region, and its greatest dimension is the transverse diameter[35] (see Fig. 2–4A). The sagittal diameter varies widely and is greatest at the level of the atlas.[4] It decreases caudally until C5–C7, where it becomes relatively uniform in size. In the infant, the canal is relatively large compared with the vertebral bodies. It is oval, and its largest dimension is the transverse diameter.[23] By late childhood and teenage years,

the cervical spinal canal assumes a more triangular configuration.

The thoracic spinal canal in the infant is oval but becomes slightly triangular by the teenage years.[23] In the adult, the thoracic spinal canal is round at most levels (see Fig. 2–5B).

The lumbar spinal canal of the infant is oval in the transverse dimension and becomes more triangular by the teenage years.[23] In the adult, the upper lumbar spinal canal is round or oval. A trefoil configuration due to thickening of the midlaminae may be found at L5 and less commonly at L4.[17] Deltoid and triangular shapes may be encountered and are also more common at L5 than at other lumbar levels (see Fig. 2–6B). The trefoil configuration is not in itself a cause of spinal stenosis.[17] In the adult, the sagittal diameter of the lumbar spinal canal is relatively uniform from L1 to L5, but the interpedicular diameter increases from L1 to L5.[42] The sacral spinal canal is triangular.[17]

Intervertebral (Neural) Foramen

The intervertebral foramen is the "window" through which nerve roots and veins emerge and arteries enter the spinal canal (Figs. 2–8, 2–9, 2–10). It is bounded above and below by the pedicles. The floor of the

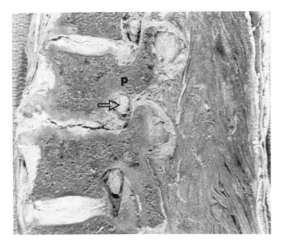

Figure 2–8. Neural foramen. Gross specimen of paraspinal section of the lumbar spine demonstrating the relationship of nerve roots and neural foramina. Notice the abundant fat within the neural foramina. *Key:* **arrow** = nerve root; **P** = pedicle.

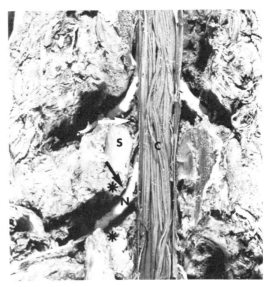

Figure 2–10. Thecal sac with cauda equina and emerging nerve roots. Gross specimen. Notice the relationship of the nerve root to the "lateral recess" and neural foramen. *Key:* **C** = cauda equina; **N** = nerve root; **S** = superior articular facet; **arrows** = lateral recess (approximately); **asterisk** = neural foramen.

foramen is formed from above downward by the posteroinferior margin of the superior vertebral body, the intervertebral disc, and the posteriosuperior margin of the inferior vertebral body.[12] The roof of the intervertebral foramen is formed by the ligamentum flavum above and the superior articular process below.[35]

The height of the intervertebral foramen

is determined by the height of the intervertebral disc.[12] In the upper portion of the intervertebral foramen are found the dorsal nerve root ganglion, ventral nerve root, sinuvertebral nerve, veins, and the spinal branch of the segmental artery.[35] The inferior aspect of the intervertebral foramen contains suprapedicular veins. Fat surrounds all structures in the intervertebral foramen.[12]

Nerve Root Canal ("Lateral Recess")

The nerve root canal is a tubular canal of variable length[12] through which the nerve root travels on its way from the thecal sac to the neural foramen (see Fig. 2–10). The concept of nerve root canal is most applicable for the L3–S1 nerve roots, because the cervical, thoracic, and upper lumbar nerve roots have a more horizontal course as they emerge from the thecal sac and do not enter a nerve root canal.[12]

The borders of the nerve root canal depend on the length of the nerve root.[12] The medial border of the S1 nerve root is the thecal sac. The lateral borders from above downward are: the fifth lumbar nerve root, the L5 neural foramen, and the pedicle of S1. The anterior borders from above downward are: the pos-

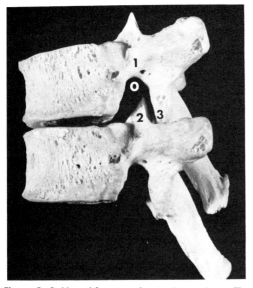

Figure 2–9. Neural foramen. Anatomic specimen. Thoracic vertebrae (T7–T8) demonstrating the neural foramen and its relationship to surrounding bony structures. *Key:* **0** = neural foramen; **1** = pedicle; **2** = superior articular process; **3** = inferior articular process.

terior aspect of L5, the L5–S1 intervertebral disc, and the posterior aspect of the S1 vertebral body. The posterior borders from above down are: the lamina of L5, ligamentum flavum, and the anteromedial aspect of the superior articular process of S1.[12] The nerve roots are surrounded by epidural fat throughout their course in the nerve root canal.

The concept of "lateral recess" has also been used to describe the course of the nerve root as it leaves the thecal sac.[9, 30] It refers to that portion of the nerve root that is bounded by the superior articular process posteriorly, the pedicle laterally, and the vertebral body anteriorly.[9, 30]

The depth of the subarticular portion of the nerve root canal ("lateral recess") diminishes from the upper lumbar level to the S1 level. A measurement of 5 mm is considered normal, but a measurement of less than 3 mm is considered stenotic.[30]

ARTICULATIONS OF THE SPINE

Craniocervical Junction

The craniocervical junction consists of a complex set of synovial articulations that allow a high degree of rotatory motion as well as flexion and extension of the head while still maintaining stability.[18, 21, 37, 44] Five distinct synovial articulations are present at this level. Although the atlanto-occipital joints allow a small amount of flexion and extension, the primary function of the atlas is as an extension of the occiput to provide a means of rotation of the head upon the axis.[28] In most instances the synovial space of the atlanto-occipital and anterior and posterior median atlantoaxial joints are continuous.[9] The median atlantoaxial joints are located between the odontoid process of the axis and the anterior arch of the atlas (anterior median atlantoaxial joint) and between the odontoid process and the transverse band of the cruciate atlantoaxial ligament (posterior median atlantoaxial joint) (Figs. 2–11, 2–12). These joints allow rotation of the atlas relative to the odontoid process. The lateral atlantoaxial joints are obliquely oriented, with both of the articular surfaces being slightly convex (Fig. 2–13). This allows a great deal of free rotation, so that approximately 50% of the rotation of the

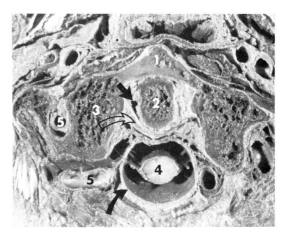

Figure 2–11. Atlantoaxial articulation. Gross specimen. Axial section. *Key:* **1** = anterior arch of C1; **2** = odontoid process; **3** = lateral mass of C1; **4** = spinal cord; **5** = vertebral artery; **curved open arrow** = transverse ligament; **straight arrow** = posterior median atlantoaxial joint space; **curved black arrow** = thecal sac. (From Kricun R, Kricun M: Computed Tomography of the Spine: Diagnostic Exercises. Rockville, Maryland: Aspen Publishers, Inc, 1987. Reprinted with permission of Aspen Publishers, Inc.)

cervical spine occurs at this level. A small amount of gliding motion also occurs at these joints, in both the sagittal and coronal planes. There is also slight vertical mobility at the atlantoaxial level owing to the con-

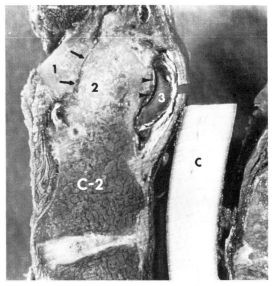

Figure 2–12. Atlantoaxial articulation. Gross specimen. Sagittal section. *Key:* **1** = anterior arch of atlas (C1); **2** = odontoid process; **3** = transverse ligament; **C** = spinal cord; **arrows** = anterior median atlantoaxial joint; **arrowheads** = posterior median atlantoaxial joint.

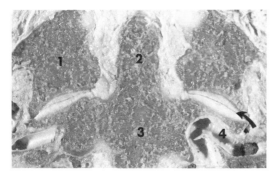

Figure 2–13. Atlantoaxial articulation. Gross specimen. Coronal section. *Key:* **1** = lateral mass of C1; **2** = odontoid process; **3** = body of C2; **4** = vertebral artery; **arrow** = lateral articulation of C1–C2.

vexity of the apposing articular surfaces. The atlantoaxial level is also unique in that it is the only mobile intervertebral articulation that lacks an intervertebral disc.

Intervertebral Discs

Intervertebral discs are present between each pair of cervical, thoracic, and lumbar vertebrae, with the exception of the atlantoaxial level. Each intervertebral disc comprises two component layers: annulus fibrosus and nucleus pulposus (Fig. 2–14). The cartilaginous end-plate may be considered the third component layer.[10] The outer circumferential layer (annulus fibrosus) is composed of fibrous tissue bands and fibrocartilage elements arranged in a cruciate pattern. The annulus fibrosus is firmly anchored to the circumference of the adjacent vertebral end-plates and less firmly to the cartilaginous surface of the midportion of the end-plate.[37, 44] The outermost fibers of the annulus fibrosus are continuous with the fibers of the anterior and posterior longitudinal ligaments. The internal structure of each intervertebral disc (nucleus pulposus) consists of a yellowish pulpy material that is maintained in a state of turgor by the dense surrounding fibers of the annulus fibrosus. The nucleus pulposus is derived from the primitive notocord and functions as a shock absorber between adjacent vertebral bodies.[10, 40] The thin cartilaginous plate serves as a barrier between the pressure of the nucleus pulposus and the adjacent vertebral body. Enchondral growth of the vertebral body occurs in an ossification layer at the edge of the cartilaginous plate, adjacent to the cancellous bone of the vertebra.[11]

Uncovertebral Joints ("Joints" of Luschka)

The uncovertebral joints are the articulations between the uncinate processes of the superolateral margins of the third through seventh cervical vertebral bodies and the beveled inferolateral margins of the adjacent vertebral bodies above[27] (see Fig. 2–4D, E). It may also be seen in the first thoracic vertebra.[27] The nature of these articulations has been a source of great controversy since their initial description as true synovial joints by von Luschka in 1858.[32] However, it has been demonstrated that no synovium exists in the "joints" of Luschka, so they are not considered true joints.[27, 32, 33] Some authors have believed that the uncovertebral cleft or fissure forms as a result of degeneration in the lateral extension of the intervertebral disc.[20, 33, 39] Recently, other authors have shown that in the fetus, intervertebral disc tissue is related to the vertebral bodies and does not extend laterally to involve the vertebral arch.[27] The area between the vertebral arches contains loose fibrous tissue that during the second decade of life resorbs and leaves a cleft that appears similar to an

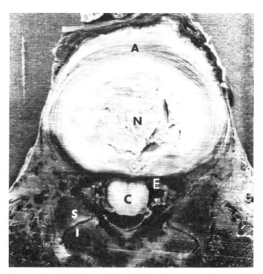

Figure 2–14. Intervertebral disc. Gross specimen. Axial section. *Key:* **A** = annulus fibrosus; **E** = epidural space; **I** = inferior articular process; **N** = nucleus pulposus; **S** = superior articular process.

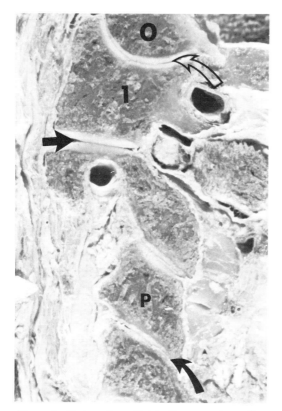

Figure 2–15. Apophyseal joints. Gross specimen. Parasagittal section of cervical apophyseal joints and cranial cervical junction. *Key:* **0** = occipital condyle; **1** = lateral mass of atlas (C1); **P** = articular pillar; **curved black arrow** = apophyseal joint; **straight arrow** = lateral atlantoaxial articulation; **open arrow** = atlanto-occipital articulation.

articulation. This cleft is the "joint" of Luschka.

Apophyseal (Zygapophyseal) Joints

Apophyseal joints are encountered at each vertebral level between the third cervical and first sacral vertebrae. All are true synovial joints consisting of the hyaline cartilage articular surfaces of the inferior articular facet of the craniad vertebra and the superior articular facet of the caudad vertebra[7] (Figs. 2–14, 2–15). At all levels, the apophyseal joints are continuous with the dorsal border of the neural foramina, and thus degenerative changes of these articulations may be associated with foraminal encroachment and radiculopathies. In terms of motion of the spine, the intervertebral disc functions as a passive element, and the ori-

entation of the apophyseal articular surfaces determine the preferred motion of each spinal segment. The cervical apophyseal joints are oriented in an oblique axial plane, which facilitates rotatory motion while allowing a great deal of flexion-extension with lesser degrees of lateral flexion. In the thoracic spine, the oblique coronal orientation of the apophyseal joints facilitates flexion-extension and lateral flexion to a much greater degree than rotation. In the lumbar spine, the facet joints at L3–L4 are oriented sagittally, and those at L5–S1 are oriented more toward the frontal plane.[43] Sagittal inclination of these articulations allows very active flexion-extension while severely limiting rotation. It should be emphasized that other factors may exert a limit on spinal motion. For example, the large cervical spinous processes limit the amount of achievable extension of the cervical spine. The ribs and paravertebral ligaments also exert important limits on spinal motion.

Costovertebral and Costotransverse Articulations

The thoracic vertebrae possess true synovial articulations between the ribs and the vertebral bodies (costovertebral joints) (Fig. 2–16) and between the ribs and the transverse processes (costotransverse joints).[37, 44]

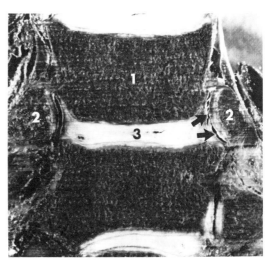

Figure 2–16. Costovertebral articulation. Gross specimen. Coronal section. *Key:* **1** = vertebral body; **2** = rib head; **3** = intervertebral disc; **arrows** = costovertebral articulation.

These articulations allow a rocking type of motion that facilitates chest wall expansion and contraction.

Sacroiliac Joints

The sacroiliac joints (Fig. 2–17) are complex multiplanar articulations that provide a stable point of attachment between the pelvis and the spinal column.[37, 44] In general, the joints are angulated approximately 10 to 30 degrees posteriorly, relative to the coronal plane, and 10 to 20 degrees medially, relative to the sagittal plane. The apposing articular surfaces demonstrate a convoluted, interlocking anatomy, which increases the stability of the joint. The sacroiliac joints are composed of two anatomic types of articulations.[37, 44] A syndesmotic articulation, in which the sacral and iliac surfaces are attached by means of a dense fibrous interosseous ligament, constitutes the cranial 25 to 50% of the joint.[37] In the lower half of the joint, the syndesmosis lies posterior to the synovial portion and gradually decreases in size inferiorly. The synovial portion of the articulation, consisting of bony surfaces lined by thick hyaline cartilage (sacrum) or thinner fibrocartilage (ilium), occupies the caudal 50 to 75% of the articulation.[38] The sacroiliac joints allow virtually no motion in the normal individual but, rather, function to absorb and transmit force between the lower extremities and the spine. In pregnancy, ligamentous laxity produces slightly increased mobility of the sacroiliac joints, which aids in allowing the fetus to pass through the bony pelvic ring.

LIGAMENTS

The ligamentous structures of the spine provide stability while allowing mobility of the bony spinal column. For the most part, the ligamentous structures at different spinal levels are similar and thus may be considered to be a single unit. However, specialized soft-tissue structures at the craniocervical junction[18, 21] and at the sacroiliac level[37, 44] deserve individual mention.

Craniocervical Junction

The atlas is circumferentially attached to the occipital bone by the anterior and posterior atlanto-occipital membranes (Fig. 2–18). The anterior atlanto-occipital membrane passes from the anterior border of the foramen magnum to the cranial aspect of the anterior arch of the atlas.[44] Ventrally it forms a distinct thickened band that attaches to the tubercle of the anterior arch of the atlas and is continuous with the anterior longitudinal ligament. Laterally, the anterior atlanto-occipital membrane is continuous with the capsular fibers of the atlanto-occipital joints. The posterior atlanto-occipital ligament passes from the posterior margin of the foramen magnum to the posterior arch of the atlas. Its anterior fibers are continuous with the capsule of the atlanto-occipital joint, and it is pierced by the vertebral artery at the level of the vertebral artery groove on the cranial border of the posterior arch of the atlas. The lateral atlanto-occipital ligaments are fibrous bands that pass from the jugular process of the occipital bone to the base of the transverse process of the atlas. The alar (check) ligaments are rounded fibrous cords passing from the lateral margins of the tip of the odontoid process to the medial aspect of the occipital condyles. A smaller ligament, the apical dental ligament, passes from the apex of the odontoid process superiorly to blend with the fibers of the anterior atlanto-occipital membrane. The cruciate ligament consists of a vertical band

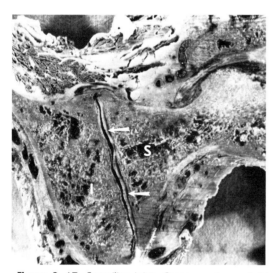

Figure 2–17. Sacroiliac joint. Gross specimen. Axial section of the sacroiliac joint. *Key:* **I** = ilium; **S** = sacrum; **arrows** = sacral articular cartilage.

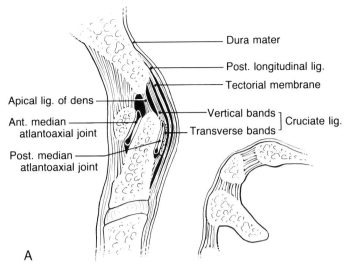

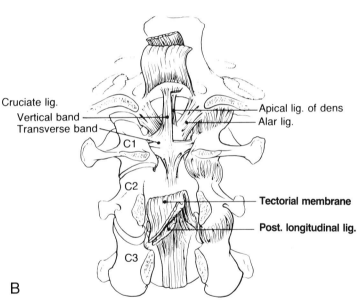

Figure 2–18. Soft tissue anatomy of the craniocervical junction demonstrating the ligaments and surrounding structures. *A,* Sagittal plane. *B,* Coronal plane. Posterior view of vertebrae. The laminae have been removed.

and a horizontal band (transverse ligament) that blend together posterior to the odontoid process and form the posterior wall of the posterior median atlantoaxial joint. The horizontal band of the cruciate ligament, better known as the transverse atlantoaxial ligament, passes between the medial aspects of the lateral masses of the atlas; it checks posterior motion of the odontoid process during flexion of the head. The vertical component attaches to the posterior surface of the body of the axis caudally and blends into the tectorial membrane cranially. The tectorial membrane is a broad, flat fibrous band that passes over the anterior margin of

the foramen magnum posterior to the cruciate ligament and becomes continuous with the posterior longitudinal ligament at the level of the body of the axis. Cranially, the tectorial membrane is continuous with the dura mater overlying the clivus.

Cervicothoracolumbar Spine

The anterior longitudinal ligament is a strong broad ligamentous band that passes along the anterior surfaces of the vertebral bodies from the level of the axis to the sacrum[44] (Figs. 2–19, 2–20). It is only loosely

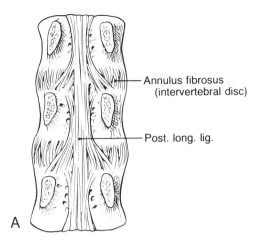

A

Annulus fibrosus
(intervertebral disc)

Post. long. lig.

Figure 2–19. Soft tissue anatomy of the thoracic spine demonstrating the ligaments and adjacent structures. *A,* Coronal plane. Posterior view of vertebrae. The laminae have been removed. *B,* Sagittal plane.

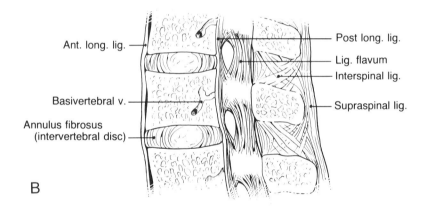

Ant. long. lig.

Basivertebral v.

Annulus fibrosus
(intervertebral disc)

Post long. lig.

Lig. flavum

Interspinal lig.

Supraspinal lig.

B

Figure 2–20. Soft tissue anatomy of the thoracic spine. Gross specimen. Sagittal section. *Key:* **A** = annulus; **B** = vertebral body; **C** = spinal cord; **L** = interspinal ligaments; **N** = nucleus pulposus; **S** = spinous process; **black arrow** = anterior longitudinal ligament; **white arrow** = posterior longitudinal ligament.

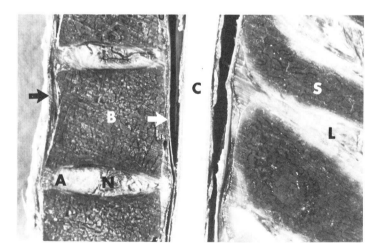

adherent to the midportions of the vertebral bodies but is densely adherent to the thickened bony ridges at the cranial and caudal margins of the vertebra and the outermost fibers of the annulus fibrosus of the intervertebral discs. The posterior longitudinal ligament extends as a continuation of the tectorial membrane from the level of the axis to the sacrum (see Figs. 2–18, 2–20). It is situated within the vertebral canal and extends over the dorsal surfaces of the vertebral bodies. Like the anterior longitudinal ligament, it adheres most densely to the cranial and caudal margins of the vertebral

bodies as well as to the fibers of the annulus fibrosus. At the level of the midportion of the vertebral body, the basivertebral vein is interposed between the posterior longitudinal ligament and the dorsal surface of the vertebral body. The articular capsules of the vertebral apophyseal joints consist of relatively thin fibrous tissues that connect the superior and inferior articular facets of adjacent vertebral levels. The articular capsules are looser at cervical levels than at thoracolumbar levels, potentiating the greater mobility of the cervical segment. The ligamenta flava are yellowish fibroelastic lig-

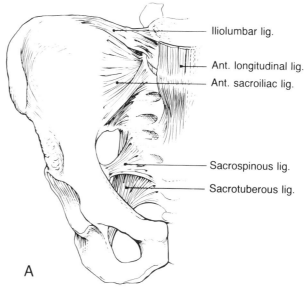

Figure 2–21. Sacral ligaments. *A,* Anterior. *B,* Posterior.

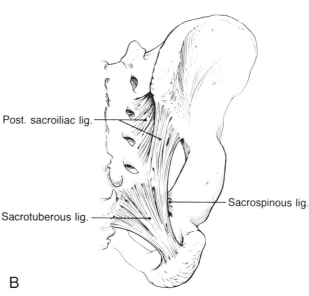

aments that connect the lamina of adjacent vertebral levels and pass from the ventral surface of the cranial laminae to the dorsal surface of caudal laminae[45] (see Fig. 2–19B). The ligamenta flava are thinnest in the cervical spine and become progressively more substantial in the thoracic and lumbar levels. The supraspinous ligament is a dense fibrous cord that connects the apices of the spinous processes from the level of the seventh cervical vertebra to the sacrum (see Fig. 2–19B). Above C7, the ligamentum nuchae is a continuation of the supraspinous ligament and passes as a dense cord from the apex of the spinous process of the seventh cervical vertebra to the external occipital protuberance of the occiput. The spinous processes of the first through seventh cervical vertebrae are connected to the ligamentum nuchae by means of a fibrous lamina that forms a midline septum between the posterior paraspinal musculatures. The intraspinal ligaments are thin fibrous membranes that pass between the caudal and cranial surfaces of adjacent spinous processes. The intertransverse ligaments are short, vertically oriented bands that pass between the transverse processes of adjacent vertebrae.

Sacral Ligaments

The ventral sacroiliac ligament is a broad, flat band that overlies the ventral aspect of the sacroiliac joint and is continuous with the joint capsule.[37, 44] The dorsal sacroiliac ligament consists of a number of dense fibrous fascicles that traverse the dorsal aspect of the sacroiliac joint. The syndesmotic portion of the articulation is bridged by a short, strong sacroiliac interosseous ligament. The iliolumbar ligament passes from the transverse process of the fifth lumbar vertebra to insert as two bands on the anterior aspect of the sacrum and on the iliac crest (Fig. 2–21). The sacrotuberous ligament is a broad flat ligamentous band passing from the posterior inferior iliac spine and posterior aspect of the sacrum and coccyx to insert on the posterior margin of the ischial tuberosity (Fig. 2–21). The sacrospinous ligament is a small triangular ligamentous band that arises from the lateral margin of the sacrum and coccyx and inserts on the apex of the ischial spine.

NEUROLOGIC ELEMENTS

Meninges

The spinal cord is enclosed by a protective covering consisting of three layers of membranous structures (Fig. 2–22). The spinal dura mater, a continuation of cranial dura, is the outermost meningeal layer and is composed of dense fibrous connective tissue arranged in interwoven bundles.[44] The arachnoid is a highly vascular areolar membrane that is loosely connected to the dura

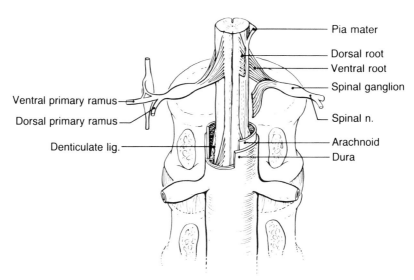

Figure 2–22. Meninges and nerve roots.

and that together with the dura forms a tubelike structure, the thecal sac. The pia mater is a thin, highly vascular membrane closely applied to the surface of the spinal cord. Triangular bands of pial tissue, the denticulate (dentate) ligaments, extend laterally and attach to the arachnoid and dura, thereby helping to secure the spinal cord to the dura.[6] The pia mater continues caudad below the level of the conus medullaris as the filum terminale, a thin strand of tissue that blends with the dura at the level of the second sacral vertebra to form the coccygeal ligament.[6]

Meninges-Related Spaces

Three spaces related to the spinal meningeal coverings are important in understanding spinal anatomy. The epidural (extradural) space lies between the dura mater and the intraspinal ligaments and periosteum[44] (Fig. 2–14). It extends laterally to surround the spinal nerve roots within the neural foramina. It is filled with loose fibrofatty areolar tissue containing numerous small vascular elements, particularly veins and venules of the rich intraspinal venous plexus. The fatty tissue of the epidural space is predominantly responsible for inherent contrast in computed tomography and magnetic resonance imaging. Fat tissue is more abundant in the epidural space at the lumbar level than at the cervical and thoracic levels. The subdural space, a potential space between the dura mater and arachnoid, contains a thin film of cerebrospinal fluid (CSF).[44] The subarachnoid space exists between the arachnoid and the pia mater and is filled with CSF, which is in direct communication with the fourth ventricle of the brain via the foramen of Magendie and the foramina of Luschka.[6] The subarachnoid space is widest in the proximal cervical and lower lumbar levels.

Spinal Cord

The spinal cord is an elongated tubular structure continuous with the caudal end of the medulla oblongata at the brain stem. It begins at the foramen magnum and extends caudally to end as the cone-shaped conus medullaris (Figs. 2–23, 2–24). The tip of the conus medullaris lies at the L3 level at birth.[1] By the age of 2 months postnatally, the conus usually resides at the "adult" level—that is, between the L1 and L2 vertebral bodies.[1] The conus is considered low lying if it is still below L2 at the age of 5 years.[19]

Within the spinal cord is the central canal lined by ependymal cells. It can be well defined in the newborn but not in the adult. It represents the vestigial lumen of the embryonic neural tube.[6]

The diameter of the spinal cord varies. It is widest in the upper cervical region and at the cervical and lumbosacral expansions, where the largest nerve roots emerge to supply the extremities. The cervical expansion

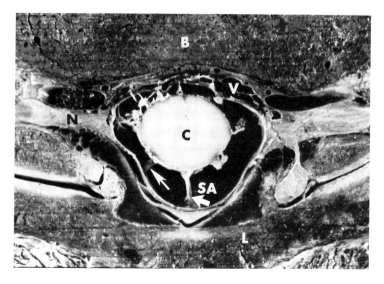

Figure 2–23. Thoracic spinal cord. Gross specimen. Axial section of spinal cord proximal to the conus medullaris. *Key:* **B** = vertebral body; **C** = spinal cord; **L** = lamina; **N** = thoracic nerve root; **SA** = subarachnoid space; **V** = anterior internal vertebral veins; **long arrow** = denticulate ligament; **short arrow** = longitudinal subarachnoid septum.

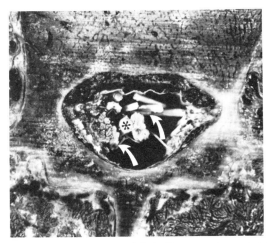

Figure 2–24. Conus medullaris. Gross specimen. Axial section caudad to the section shown in Figure 2–23 through the conus medullaris and cauda equina. *Key:* **asterisk** = conus medullaris; **arrows** = cauda equina.

consists of the lowest four cervical segments and the first thoracic segment and gives rise to the brachial plexus.[6] The lumbar expansion consists of the L1–L4 nerve roots that form the lumbar plexus and the L4–S2 nerve roots that form the sacral plexus.[6] At the level of these expansions, the spinal cord occupies a much greater proportion of the volume of the spinal canal, and the epidural fat is considerably diminished. As a result, processes such as trauma, neoplasm, and degenerative diseases that encroach on the spinal cord are much more likely to result in spinal cord compression earlier at these sites. The spinal cord is widest at the C5 vertebral level, measuring up to 15 mm.[31] The sagittal diameter of the spinal cord is relatively large at birth and increases rapidly during the first 10 years.[31] By the age of 9 years, it is close to adult size (9.6 mm at C5). The cervical cord is oval during childhood and elliptic in adult life.[23, 31]

The thoracic spinal cord is fairly uniform in size and is round from T2 to T10.[31] This is the narrowest segment of the entire spinal cord, not only in adults but in neonates and children as well.[31, 36]

The lumbar enlargement extends from T10 to L1.[6] Caudal to the lumbar enlargement, the spinal cord ends as the tapered conus medullaris at the level of L1 (occasionally L2) vertebral body in the adult (Fig. 2–24). The conus contains nerve roots of the distal three sacral segments and the single coccy-

geal segment.[6] Normally, the conus is square on cross-section in the child, but has an oval (less frequently, round) configuration in the adult.[22] Additionally, the conus demonstrates an anterior indentation or sulcus and a mild posterior prominence.[22]

Extending caudally from the tip of the conus medullaris is the filum terminale, a condensation of connective tissue and pia mater[6, 41] (Figs. 2–24, 2–25). Surrounding the conus medullaris are lumbosacral nerve roots that have emerged from the spinal cord above. These nerve roots surround the filum terminale and represent the cauda equina.

Spinal Nerves

Thirty-one pairs of spinal nerves arise from the spinal cord and exit the spinal canal via the neural foramen.[6, 44] There are eight cervical, twelve thoracic, five lumbar, five sacral, and one coccygeal spinal nerves. Multiple fine dorsal and ventral nerve rootlets emerge from the cord and form corresponding nerve roots.[44] As the nerve roots emerge from the thecal sac, they are covered by all three meningeal layers.[6] The nerve roots travel variable distances in the spinal canal until they reach their neural foramina. Here, the dorsal root swells to form the dorsal (spinal) ganglion containing the cells of origin of the afferent fibers (Figs. 2–22, 2–

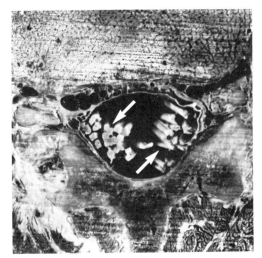

Figure 2–25. Cauda equina. Gross specimen. Axial section of gross specimen caudad to the section shown in Figure 2–24 through the cauda equina. *Key:* **arrows** = nerve roots (cauda equina).

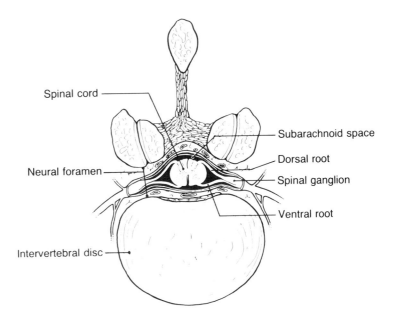

Figure 2–26. Spinal nerve roots. Diagrammatic composite representation of the spinal cord, nerve roots, and spinal ganglia.

Spinal cord

Subarachnoid space

Dorsal root

Neural foramen

Spinal ganglion

Ventral root

Intervertebral disc

26). The dorsal ganglion also contains cells and afferent fibers of the autonomic nerves.[6] Just beyond the ganglion, yet still within the neural foramen, the dorsal and ventral nerve roots unite to form the peripheral spinal nerve (common nerve trunk, mixed spinal nerve).

As each dorsal and ventral root emerges from the spinal cord, it is covered by connective tissue as it passes through the pia.[6] Additional connective tissue is applied to each nerve root as it passes through the arachnoid and dura. These layers form a connective tissue sleeve covering the nerve roots. The dura surrounding the dorsal ganglion is continuous with the epineurium of the peripheral nerve.

The first cervical nerve, made up of only the ventral nerve, emerges between the occiput and atlas.[6] The spinal nerves of C2–C8 emerge from the neural foramina with the same numbers as the vertebrae above (i.e., C8 spinal nerve emerges from the neural foramen between C7 and T1). The nerve roots caudal to T1 emerge from the neural foramina beneath the vertebral bodies of the same numbers.

The upper cervical nerve roots travel a short distance and pass along a relatively horizontal course within the spinal canal. At distal spinal levels, the intraspinal course of the nerve roots becomes progressively more vertical. The cauda equina has a long vertical intraspinal course (see Fig. 2–26).

Peripheral Nerves

The peripheral nerve divides into four branches (rami) just beyond the point of union of the dorsal and ventral nerve roots[6] (Fig. 2–22). These branches inlcude: the dorsal ramus, which supplies the muscles and skin of the back; the larger ventral ramus, which supplies all the extremities and the ventrolateral portion of the body wall; the ramus communicans, which joins the sympathetic ganglion to the common spinal nerve; and the sinuvertebral (meningeal) nerve.[6]

Sinuvertebral Nerve

The sinuvertebral nerve is formed in the neural foramen by the union of a branch of the ventral nerve root and a branch from an autonomic nerve (Fig. 2–27). It ascends in the spinal canal and is distributed to the ventral aspect of the dural sac, blood vessels, posterior longitudinal ligament, and annuli fibrosi (above and below).[3] Branches of the sinuvertebral nerve accompany the basivertebral vein into the vertebral bodies. Nerve fibers have also been discovered deep in the annulus fibrosus.[3, 46] The sinuvertebral nerve is not visible by current imaging modalities. Nevertheless, it is important to realize that disorders may affect the sinuvertebral nerve, causing low back pain without affecting nerve roots or spinal cord.[3]

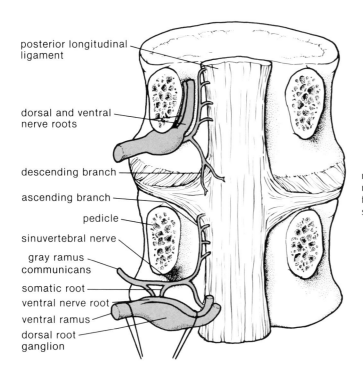

posterior longitudinal ligament

dorsal and ventral nerve roots

descending branch

ascending branch

pedicle

sinuvertebral nerve

gray ramus communicans

somatic root

ventral nerve root

ventral ramus

dorsal root ganglion

Figure 2–27. Sinuvertebral nerve. Diagrammatic representation of the sinuvertebral nerve and some of its branches. (Adapted from Bogduk N: The innervation of the lumbar spine. Spine 8:286–293, 1983.)

ARTERIES AND VEINS

Epidural Veins

A complex, freely communicating system of intraspinal veins exists throughout all spinal levels[2] (Fig. 2–28). Venous drainage of the vertebral body begins in the region of the cartilage end-plate and continues vertically either into a subchondral vein or into the centrally located Y-shaped basivertebral vein.[15] The subchondral vein may drain posteriorly into the anterior internal vertebral vein or anteriorly to join the external vertebral venous plexus.[13] The single or paired basivertebral veins drain anteriorly through fenestrations into the external vertebral venous plexus, or posteriorly, merging into the retrovertebral plexus of veins (RPV),[26] a part of the internal vertebral venous plexus. Each RPV is joined to retrovertebral plexuses above and below by the longitudinally oriented anterior internal vertebral veins (AIVV). These intraspinal veins reside in the epidural space. Radicular (interpedicular, transvertebral) veins arise from the AIVV and run along the superior and inferior aspects of the pedicles in the intervertebral canal. They emerge from the neural foramen and join vertebral, intercostal, ascending lumbar, and lateral sacral veins in the cervical, thoracic, lumbar, and sacral regions, respectively.[35] These latter veins are a component of the external vertebral venous plexus. The veins in the posterior aspect of the spinal canal and posterior external vertebral veins also communicate freely.

Arteries

The arterial supply to the spinal column is derived from the vertebral, deep cervical, intercostal, lumbar, iliolumbar, and lateral sacral arteries.[5] These arteries send branches to supply the anterior and lateral portions of their corresponding vertebral bodies.[14, 35] Other branches supply the posterior spinal elements, and still other radicular branches enter the spinal canal through the neural foramen to supply the spinal cord, other intraspinal structures, and the vertebral column.[5, 14] Once these radicular arteries enter the spinal canal, they send ascending and descending branches to the intraspinal structures, the anterior and posterior walls of the spinal canal, and the vertebral body. Arteries run proximally along the nerve roots to the spinal cord.[14]

The vertebral body is supplied by the basi-

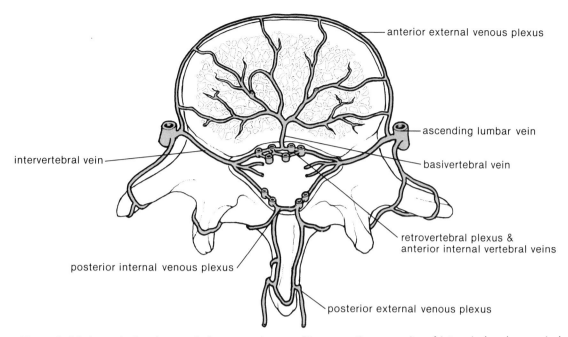

anterior external venous plexus

ascending lumbar vein

intervertebral vein

basivertebral vein

retrovertebral plexus &
anterior internal vertebral veins

posterior internal venous plexus

posterior external venous plexus

Figure 2–28. Intraspinal and paraspinal venous plexuses. Diagrammatic composite of intraspinal and paraspinal venous drainage in the axial plane.

vertebral branch, which enters the vascular groove beneath the posterior longitudinal ligament.[14, 35] Thus, an arterial grid is formed in the center of the vertebral body from branches of the perforating arteries that enter anterolaterally and branches of the basivertebral artery that arise posteriorly.[5, 14] Ascending and descending branches of the basivertebral artery supply the central third of the vertebral body and its end-plates.[14] The anterior and posterior aspects of the cartilage plates are supplied by anterolateral and dorsal arterial branches, respectively.[5, 14]

MARROW DISTRIBUTION

At birth, all marrow in the skeleton is red marrow.[29] Conversion of red (hematopoietic) to yellow (fat) marrow begins in the extremities just before birth and is a continuous process until the age of 25 years, when the adult pattern of red marrow distribution is achieved.[24, 29, 34] At this stage, red marrow exists in the skull, spine, ribs, pelvis, sternum, and proximal humeri and femora.[24, 29, 34] In the adult, the vertebral body is rich in red marrow. However, the pedicles and vertebral arch contain little red marrow.[29] The spine retains red marrow throughout life, although there is a progressive mild conversion of some vertebral red marrow to fat marrow.[16] When the marrow system is stressed, fat marrow becomes hyperplastic or is converted back to hematopoietic marrow.[24, 29] The spine responds more rapidly to marrow stress disorders than other skeletal sites.[16]

References

1. Barson AJ: The vertebral level of termination of the spinal cord during normal and abnormal development. J Anat 106:489–497, 1970.
2. Batson OV: The vertebral vein system. AJR 78:195–212, 1957.
3. Bogduk N: The innervation of the lumbar spine. Spine 8:286–293, 1983.
4. Brandner ME: Normal values of the vertebral body and intervertebral disc index in adults. AJR 114:411–414, 1972.
5. Brookes M: The Blood Supply of Bone. London: Butterworths, 1971.
6. Carpenter MB, Sutin J: Human Neuroanatomy. Baltimore: Williams & Wilkins, 1983.
7. Carrera GF, Williams AL: Current concepts in evaluation of the lumbar facet joints. CRC Crit Rev Diag Imag 21:85–104, 1984.
8. Cave AJE: Anatomical notes: On the occipito-atlanto-axial articulation. J Anat 68:416–423, 1934.
9. Ciric I, Mikhael MA, Tarkington JA, et al: The lateral recess syndrome. J Neurosurg 53:433–443, 1980.

10. Coventry MB, Ghormley RK, Kernohan JW: The intervertebral disc: Its microscopic anatomy and pathology. Part I. Anatomy, development, and physiology. J Bone Joint Surg 27:105–112, 1945.
11. Coventry MB, Ghormley RK, Kernohan JW: The intervertebral disc: Its microscopic anatomy and pathology. Part II. Changes in the intervertebral disc concomitant with age. J Bone Joint Surg 27:233–247, 1945.
12. Crock HV: Normal and pathological anatomy of the lumbar spinal nerve root canals. J Bone Joint Surg 63B:487–490, 1981.
13. Crock HV, Goldwasser M: Anatomic studies of the circulation in the region of the vertebral end-plate in adult Greyhound dogs. Spine 9:702–706, 1984.
14. Crock HV, Yoshizawa H: The blood supply of the lumbar vertebral column. Clin Orthop 115:6–21, 1976.
15. Crock HV, Yoshizawa H, Kame SK: Observations on the venous drainage of the human vertebral body. J Bone Joint Surg 55B:528–533, 1973.
16. Custer RP, Ahlfeldt FE: Studies on the structure and function of bone marrow. J Lab Clin Med 17:960–962, 1932.
17. Eisenstein S: The trefoil configuration of the lumbar vertebral canal. A study of South African skeletal material. J Bone Joint Surg 62B:73–77, 1980.
18. Epstein BS: The Spine. 4th ed. Philadelphia: Lea & Febiger, 1976.
19. Fitz CR, Harwood-Nash DC: The tethered conus. AJR 125:515–523, 1975.
20. Frykholm R: Lower cervical vertebrae and intervertebral discs. Surgical anatomy and pathology. Acta Chir Scand 101:345–359, 1951.
21. Gehweiler JA, Osborne RL, Becker RF: The Radiology of Vertebral Trauma. Philadelphia: W. B. Saunders Company, 1980.
22. Grogan JP, Daniels DL, Williams AL, et al: The normal conus medullaris: CT criteria for recognition. Radiology 151:661–664, 1984.
23. Harwood-Nash DC: Computed tomography of the pediatric spine: A protocol for the 1980's. Radiol Clin North Am 19:479–494, 1981.
24. Hashimoto M: The distribution of active marrow in the bones of normal adult. Kyushu J Med Sci 11:103–111, 1960.
25. Hasue M, Kikuchi S, Sakuyama Y, Ito T: Anatomic study of the interrelation between lumbosacral nerve roots and their surrounding tissues. Spine 8:50–58, 1983.
26. Haughton VM, Syvertsen A, Williams AL: Soft-tissue anatomy within the spinal canal as seen on computed tomography. Radiology 134:649–655, 1980.
27. Hayashi K, Yabuki T: Origin of the uncus and of Luschka's joint in the cervical spine. J Bone Joint Surg 67A:788–791, 1985.
28. Jirout J: The dynamic dependence of the lower cervical vertebrae on the atlanto-occipital joints. Neuroradiology 7:249–252, 1974.
29. Kricun ME: Red-yellow marrow conversion: Its effect on the location of some solitary bone lesions. Skel Radiol 14:10–19, 1985.
30. Mikhael MA, Ciric I, Tarkington JA, et al: Neurological evaluation of lateral recess syndrome. Radiology 140:97–107, 1981.
31. ·Nordqvist L: The sagittal diameter of the spinal cord and subarachnoid space in different age groups. A roentgenographic post-mortem study. Acta Radiol [Suppl] 227:1–96, 1964.
32. Orofino C, Sherman MS, Schechter D: Luschka's joint—a degenerative phenomenon. J Bone Joint Surg 42A:853–858, 1960.
33. Payne EE, Spillane JD: The cervical spine. An anatomico-pathological study of 70 specimens (using a special technique) with particular reference to the problem of cervical spondylosis. Brain 80:571–596, 1957.
34. Piney A: The anatomy of the bone marrow. Brit Med J 2:792–795, 1922.
35. Rauschning W: Correlative multiplanar computed tomographic anatomy of the normal spine. In Post MJ (ed): Computed Tomography of the Spine. Baltimore: Williams & Wilkins, 1984.
36. Resjo IM, Harwood-Nash DC, Fitz CR, et al: Normal cord in infants and children examined with computed tomographic metrizamide myelography. Radiology 130:691–696, 1979.
37. Resnick D, Niwayama G: Diagnosis of Bone and Joint Disorders. Philadelphia: W. B. Saunders Company, 1981.
38. Resnick D, Niwayama G, Georgen TG: Degenerative disease of the sacro-iliac joint. Invest Radiol 10:608–621, 1975.
39. Sartoris DJ, Resnick D, Guerra J Jr: Vertebral venous channels: CT appearance and differential considerations. Radiology 155:745–749, 1985.
40. Schmorl G, Junghanns H: The Human Spine in Health and Disease. 2nd ed. New York: Grune & Stratton, 1971.
41. Streeter GL: Factors involved in the formation of the filum terminale. Am J Anat 25:1–11, 1919.
42. Ullrich CG, Binet EF, Sanecki MG, et al: Quantitative assessment of the lumbar spinal canal by computed tomography. Radiology 134:137–143, 1980.
43. Van Schaik JPJ, Verbiest H, Van Schaik FDJ: The orientation of laminae and facet joints in the lower lumbar spine. Spine 10:59–63, 1985.
44. Williams PL, Warwick R: Gray's Anatomy. 35th ed. Philadelphia: W. B. Saunders Company, 1980.
45. Yong-Hing K, Reilly J, Kirkaldy-Willis WH: The ligamentum flavum. Spine 1:226–234, 1976.
46. Yoshizawa H, O'Brien JP, Smith WT, et al: The neuropathology of intervertebral discs removed for low-back pain. J Pathol 132:95–104, 1980.

3

Donald Resnick, M.D.

The Aging Vertebral Column: Pathologic-Radiographic Correlation

As a response to advancing age, the human vertebral column undergoes tissue degeneration, resulting in a variety of processes that possess characteristic pathologic abnormalities, each with a radiographic counterpart. Although involutional changes occur in bones as well as soft tissue structures, the articulations of the spine are a primary site of involvement. A discussion of the degenerative processes that affect the spinal articulations is best organized according to the type of joint that is affected.

CARTILAGINOUS ARTICULATIONS

Of the cartilaginous joints of the vertebral column, the intervertebral disc is the most important site of tissue degeneration. Abnormalities occur in the nucleus pulposus, the annulus fibrosus, the cartilaginous end-plate, or any combination of these.

Intervertebral Osteochondrosis

With advancing age, dehydration and desiccation occur in the intervertebral disc, principally in the nucleus pulposus.[2] The process that appears is termed intervertebral chondrosis when limited to cartilage, and intervertebral osteochondrosis when affecting both bone and cartilage. On gross pathologic examination, the nucleus is friable

and reveals a yellow or yellow-brown discoloration. Its onion-skin configuration begins to unravel, and linear clefts or cracks occur in its substance. Gas, predominantly nitrogen, from surrounding tissue collects within the clefts, producing one fundamental and early radiographic feature of the disease, a radiolucent shadow termed a "vacuum" phenomenon (Fig. 3–1). This phenomenon is first evident as a small lucent collection within the nucleus pulposus of the intervertebral disc, but it soon enlarges, extending into the adjacent annulus fibrosus. It should be differentiated from a second type of "vacuum" phenomenon that, in rare circumstances, is evident in the vertebral body itself. This latter finding generally indicates ischemic necrosis of bone, and it is usually observed in patients who are receiving corticosteroid medication and in whom fracture and fragmentation of vertebral bone create intraosseous spaces that subsequently become sites of gas accumulation (Fig. 3–2).

As the process of intervertebral osteochondrosis progresses, the intervertebral disc diminishes in height—a finding that is readily apparent on both pathologic and radiologic investigations. The cartilaginous end-plate reveals concomitant degeneration; it becomes destroyed by the processes of calcification of deeper cartilage, resorption of the calcified cartilage by vessels from the bone marrow, and microfractures through the thin

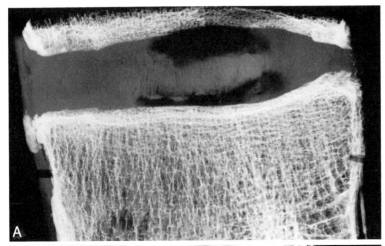

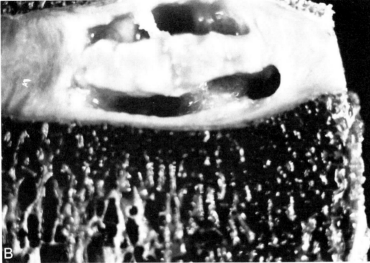

Figure 3–1. Intervertebral osteochondrosis: "Vacuum" phenomenon. A radiograph (*A*) and a photograph (*B*) of a sagittal section of the spine document clefts or cracks within the nucleus pulposus producing radiolucent collections, termed "vacuum" phenomena.

cartilage.[7] The adjacent trabeculae become thickened and contain irregularly arranged cartilaginous proliferative zones.

In addition to "vacuum" phenomena and loss of height of the intervertebral disc, the radiographic abnormalities of intervertebral osteochondrosis at this stage include sclerotic abnormalities of the subchondral bone of the vertebral body (Fig. 3–3). Bone sclerosis or eburnation is typically well defined, triangular in shape, and borders on the intervertebral disc. Although the radiodense areas may be homogenous, they may also contain small radiolucent foci, representing areas of intravertebral herniation of disc material, termed cartilaginous or Schmorl's nodes.

In summary, the process of intervertebral osteochondrosis is related to degeneration principally in the nucleus pulposus of the intervertebral disc. Its typical radiographic features are "vacuum" phenomena, loss of intervertebral disc height, sclerosis in the vertebral body, and cartilaginous nodes. This degenerative disorder is first encountered in the third or fourth decade of life, and it increases in frequency and extent with progressing age. It is most prominent in the lower lumbar and cervical regions, although the disorder can be widespread in distribution. Men are affected more frequently than women, and the clinical manifestations include pain and stiffness.

Spondylosis Deformans

A second common degenerative process of the intervertebral disc is termed spondylosis deformans. Its major radiographic sign is spinal osteophytosis.[1] Considerable debate exists as to the precise etiology and pathogenesis of spondylosis deformans, although most investigators regard it as a disease whose origin is related to tissue degeneration in the outer fibers of the annulus fibrosus, specifically in Sharpey's fibers, which normally anchor the intervertebral disc to the vertebral cortex.[12] Deterioration of these fibers is associated with loss of attachment of disc to bone and a characteristic sequence of radiographic and pathologic events.

The major morphologic characteristic of spondylosis deformans is discal displacement related to the loss of anchorage of the intervertebral disc to the vertebral body (Fig.

3–4). This displacement is accentuated when the nucleus pulposus is relatively normal and saturated with fluid, retaining most of its turgor, and when spinal motion is abnormally accentuated. Discal displacement is most prominent in an anterior and anterolateral direction, and it eventually leads to stretching of the overlying anterior longitudinal ligament. Stress is created where this ligament is attached to the vertebral body—a site that is located several millimeters from the discovertebral junction. Bone excrescences, termed osteophytes, develop at the site of stress; therefore, the osteophytes appear at a short distance from the discovertebral junction and grow ini-

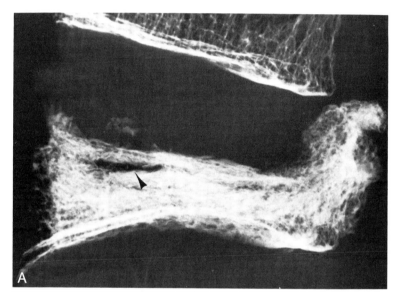
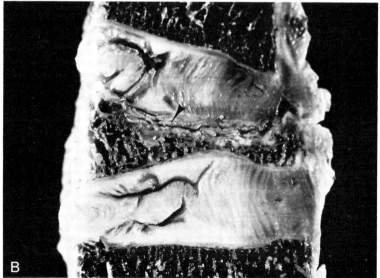

Figure 3–2. Ischemic necrosis of the vertebral body: "Vacuum" phenomenon. A radiograph (A) and photograph (B) of a sagittal section of the spine in a rheumatoid cadaver demonstrate vertebral collapse due to ischemic necrosis with fracture and a "vacuum" phenomenon (arrowheads).

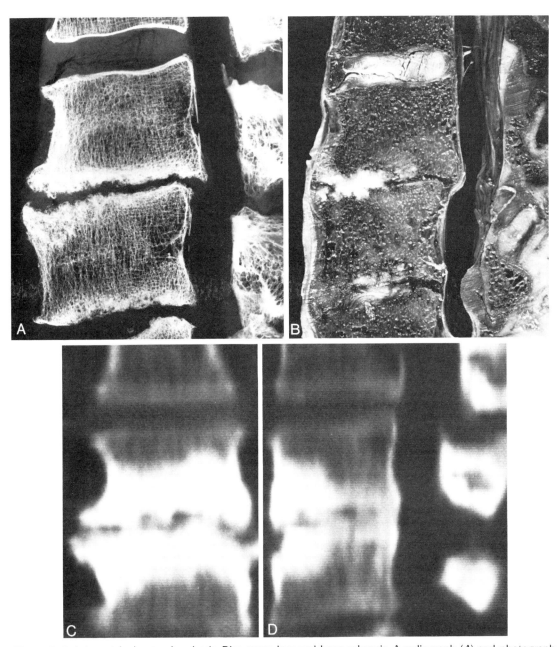

Figure 3–3. Intervertebral osteochondrosis: Disc space loss and bone sclerosis. A radiograph (A) and photograph (B) of a sagittal section of the lumbar spine reveal, at multiple levels, loss of height of disc space, irregularity of the vertebral margin, bone sclerosis, and minor degrees of vertebral subluxation. In a patient, reconstructed computed tomographic images in the coronal (C) and sagittal (D) planes demonstrate the degree of bone sclerosis that can accompany intervertebral osteochondrosis. (Courtesy of Dr. S. Rothman, Long Beach, California.)

Figure 3–4. Spondylosis deformans: Radiographic-pathologic correlation. A radiograph (A) and a photograph (B) of a sagittal section of the spine indicate mild anterior discal displacement with the development of a small osteophyte (arrowheads). Observe that the outgrowth begins several millimeters from the discovertebral junction and extends first in a horizontal direction and then in a vertical one. C, In a similar section in a different cadaver, the osteophytes are much larger and are almost bridging the intervertebral disc. D, A radiograph of a section similar to that depicted in C reveals prominent osteophytes and a "vacuum" phenomenon (arrow) in the annulus fibrosus. (D, From Resnick D, Niwayama G (eds): Diagnosis of Bone and Joint Disorders, Vol 2. Philadelphia: W. B. Saunders Company, 1981.)

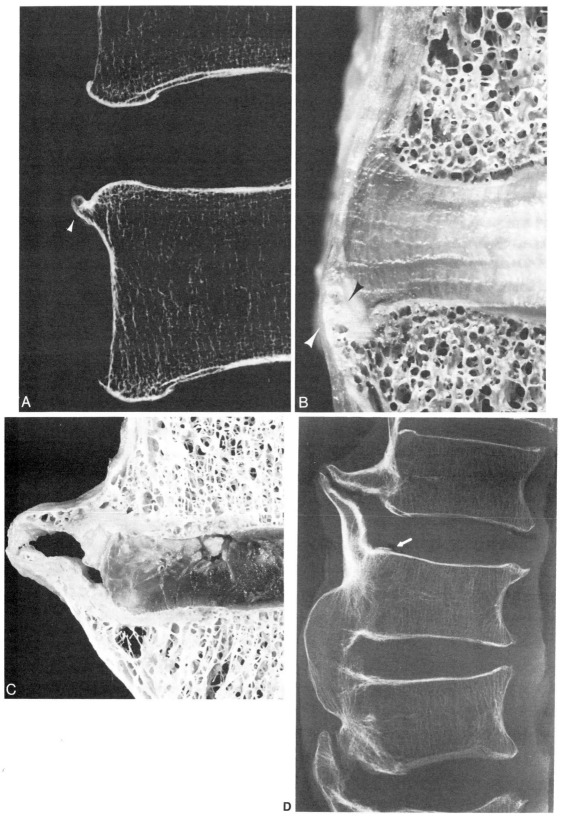

Figure 3–4 *See legend on opposite page*

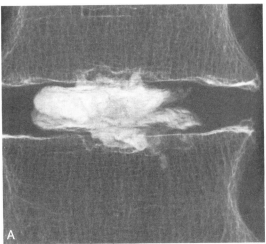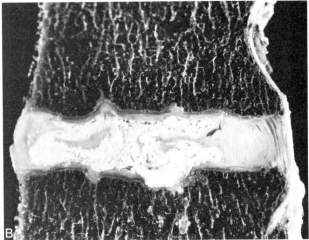

Figure 3–5. Discal calcification. A radiograph (A) and photograph (B) of a coronal section of the spine reveal hydroxyapatite crystal deposition, principally within the nucleus pulposus, associated with small cartilaginous nodes.

tially in a horizontal direction and subsequently in a vertical one. This configuration differs from that of a syndesmophyte, which is a bone excrescence that accompanies ankylosing spondylitis. The syndesmophyte represents ossification in the annulus fibrosus itself and is characterized by a vertical course extending from the margin of one vertebral body to the adjacent vertebral body.

The radiographic findings of spondylosis deformans differ from those of intervertebral osteochondrosis (see Fig. 3–4). In the former disease, osteophytes occur in the absence of narrowing of the intervertebral disc space, "vacuum" phenomena, and subchondral eburnation, whereas in intervertebral osteochondrosis, the latter findings are typical. It should be remembered, however, that both conditions are commonly encountered in the aging spine and, therefore, can coexist. Furthermore, it is difficult to separate the clinical manifestations of one from those of the other. Both may lead to pain and stiffness, although restricted back motion and dysphagia are abnormalities that would be expected to occur more frequently in spondylosis deformans than in intervertebral osteochondrosis.

Discal Calcification

Dystrophic calcification of the nucleus pulposus, annulus fibrosus, or cartilaginous

end-plate is a frequent finding in the aged skeleton when examined by either routine radiographic technique or postmortem inspection (Fig. 3–5). The crystalline deposit is generally calcium hydroxyapatite, although other calcium salts, especially pyrophosphate dihydrate, can produce similar discal deposits.[10] The routine identification of calcification of the intervertebral disc at one or several spinal levels by roentgenographic or pathologic techniques emphasizes the fact that such calcification is usually an incidental finding, unrelated to significant clinical symptoms or signs. Displacement or herniation of calcified intervertebral discs has been recorded and may be associated with back pain.[14]

Conversely, the identification of discal calcification isolated to one or several levels in the cervical region in children, particularly those between 6 and 10 years of age, has greater significance. In this age group, calcification predominantly within the nucleus pulposus of the intervertebral disc is associated in the majority of instances with pain, stiffness, limitation of motion, and even torticollis.[13] Single or multiple, oval or flat radiodense areas are evident on radiographic examination. Rupture of the calcific collections into the adjacent vertebral bodies or soft tissues is occasionally observed.[6] The temporary or transient nature of the clinical and radiologic findings in this condition should be recognized, as the prognosis for complete recovery is excellent. In most cases, pain resolves within a few days to weeks, and the calcification disappears within a few weeks to months.

Widespread or diffuse discal calcification in the adult is a manifestation of a variety of diseases, including alkaptonuria, hyperparathyroidism, and idiopathic calcium pyrophosphate dihydrate crystal deposition disease.[15]

SYNOVIAL ARTICULATIONS

Any of the synovium-lined joints of the vertebral column, including the apophyseal, sacroiliac, and costovertebral articulations, may undergo degeneration resulting in osteoarthritis. With regard to the apophyseal joints, virtually everyone after the age of 50 or 60 years will demonstrate, at the very least, pathologic evidence of degeneration. Changes predominate in the middle and lower cervical spine, upper thoracic and midthoracic spine, and the lower lumbar spine.[4] The accompanying radiologic and histologic characteristics of osteoarthritis of the apophyseal articulations are similar to those seen in other joints. Fibrillation and erosion of articular cartilage, and chondral irregularity and denudation are the observed alterations and are associated with roentgenographically apparent loss of joint space, bone sclerosis or eburnation, and osteophytes (Fig. 3–6). Intra-articular osteocartilaginous bodies, capsular laxity, and bony ankylosis of the joint may be evident. Clin-ical manifestations include pain, tenderness, and restricted motion.

Osteoarthritis is the most common affliction of the sacroiliac joint and can occur in a unilateral or bilateral distribution. Radiographically and pathologically, abnormalities predominate in the ilial side of the articulation. As in the apophyseal region, such abnormalities are evident both in the cartilage and in the bone, and they consist of cartilage erosion, bone eburnation, and osteophyte formation (Fig. 3–7). Of these features, it is the last, osteophytosis, that requires emphasis. Bone excrescences develop in the anterosuperior and anteroinferior aspects of the synovium-lined portion of the sacroiliac joint. These excrescences extend partially or completely around the front of the joint and, in the latter situation, result in para-articular bone ankylosis. On frontal radiographs, such ankylosis is easily misinterpreted as intra-articular osseous fusion, and the diagnosis of ankylosing spondylitis may be incorrectly applied. Conventional or computed tomography allows accurate analysis, delineating the juxta-articular nature, rather than the intra-articular nature, of bone ankylosis.

The costovertebral articulations, which exist between the heads of the ribs and the vertebral bodies and between the necks and tubercles of the ribs and the transverse processes of the vertebrae, are subject to degenerative joint disease. Degenerative abnormalities predominate in the articulations of the 11th

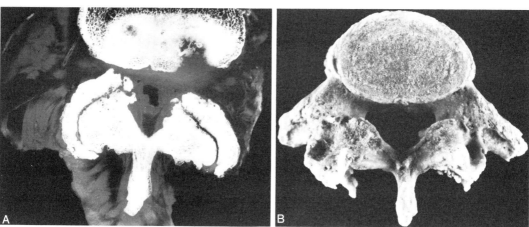

Figure 3–6. Osteoarthritis: Apophyseal joint. *A*, A radiograph of a transverse section through the apophyseal joints of a lumbar vertebra shows severe osteoarthritis with a "vacuum" phenomenon, joint space narrowing, and osseous fragmentation. *B*, In this photograph of a macerated vertebra, bone hypertrophy about the degenerating apophyseal joints has led to narrowing of the neural foramen.

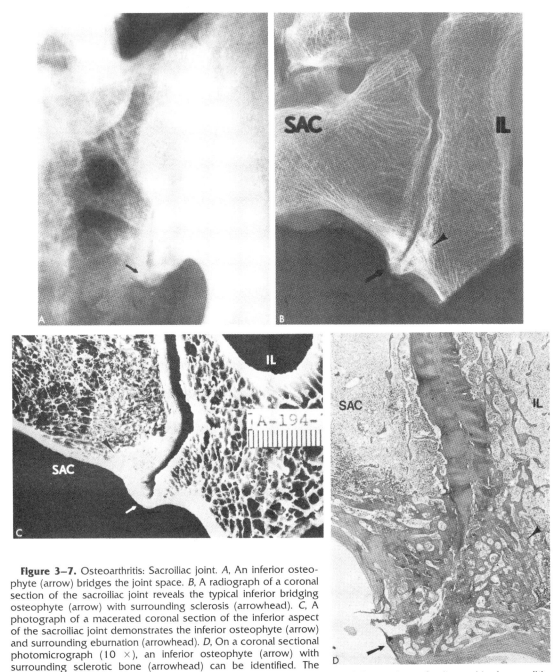

Figure 3–7. Osteoarthritis: Sacroiliac joint. *A,* An inferior osteophyte (arrow) bridges the joint space. *B,* A radiograph of a coronal section of the sacroiliac joint reveals the typical inferior bridging osteophyte (arrow) with surrounding sclerosis (arrowhead). *C,* A photograph of a macerated coronal section of the inferior aspect of the sacroiliac joint demonstrates the inferior osteophyte (arrow) and surrounding eburnation (arrowhead). *D,* On a coronal sectional photomicrograph (10 ×), an inferior osteophyte (arrow) with surrounding sclerotic bone (arrowhead) can be identified. The articular space has narrowed with cartilaginous fusion. (From Resnick D, et al: Comparison of radiographic abnormalities of the sacroiliac joint in degenerative disease and ankylosing spondylitis. AJR 128:189, 1977. Copyright 1977 by the American Roentgen Ray Society.)

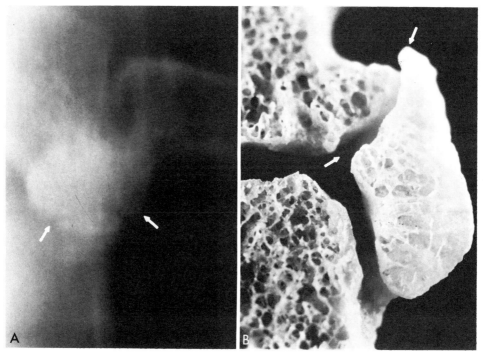

Figure 3–8. Osteoarthritis: Costovertebral joint. *A*, At the articulation between a lower thoracic rib and the transverse process of the vertebra, a large osteophyte can be seen (arrows). *B*, A photograph of a macerated coronal section of two thoracic vertebral bodies indicates degenerative abnormalities at the articulation of the vertebrae with the head of the rib (arrows). (From Resnick D, Niwayama G (eds): Diagnosis of Bone and Joint Disorders, Vol 2. Philadelphia: W. B. Saunders Company, 1981.)

and 12th ribs and consist of joint space narrowing, bone eburnation, and osteophytosis (Fig. 3–8). Ligamentous ossification in the costovertebral articulation has also been noted. Despite the presence of significant pathologic aberrations, radiographic demonstration of changes is made difficult by the existence of adjacent osseous densities, such as the vertebral bodies and the ribs.

UNCOVERTEBRAL (NEUROCENTRAL) ARTICULATIONS

The five lowest cervical vertebral bodies contain bone ridges, the uncinate or lunate processes, on each side. Between the processes of adjacent vertebral bodies exists an articulation, termed the uncovertebral joint or joint of Luschka. Although they have been described in great detail, the precise classification of the joints of Luschka is not clear. Some regard them as a synovial articulation, whereas others believe they are unique in histologic configuration, sometimes possess-

ing synovium-like characteristics. They are not present at birth and, when formed, consist of intervertebral disc tissue between the uncinate ridge and its opposing vertebral margin. With increasing degeneration of intervertebral disc tissue and progressive collapse of the disc space, disc tissue between the uncinate process and opposing vertebral margin also degenerates. The bony protuberances about the uncovertebral joints approach each other and, eventually, are firmly pressed together.[5] The ridges become prominent (osteophytes) and appear as rounded or pointed outgrowths that project from the posterior edge of the vertebral body into the disc space and into the intervertebral foramina (Fig. 3–9). Compromise of adjacent nerve roots or vascular structures such as the vertebral artery may ensue.

FIBROUS ARTICULATIONS AND ENTHESES

The fibrous structures of the vertebral column also undergo tissue degeneration. De-

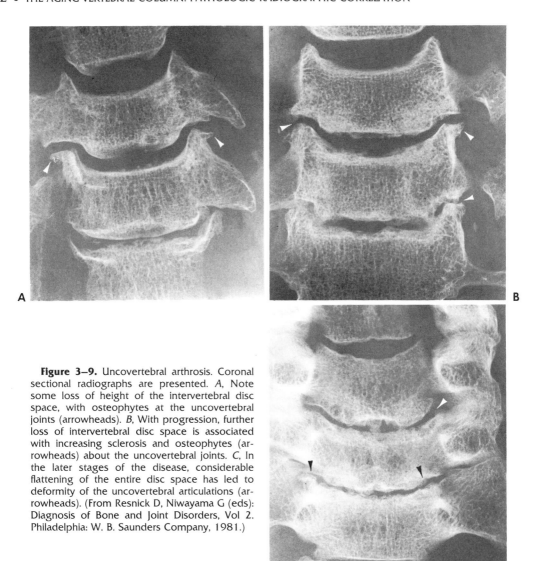

Figure 3–9. Uncovertebral arthrosis. Coronal sectional radiographs are presented. *A*, Note some loss of height of the intervertebral disc space, with osteophytes at the uncovertebral joints (arrowheads). *B*, With progression, further loss of intervertebral disc space is associated with increasing sclerosis and osteophytes (arrowheads) about the uncovertebral joints. *C*, In the later stages of the disease, considerable flattening of the entire disc space has led to deformity of the uncovertebral articulations (arrowheads). (From Resnick D, Niwayama G (eds): Diagnosis of Bone and Joint Disorders, Vol 2. Philadelphia: W. B. Saunders Company, 1981.)

terioration of ligaments, calcification, and even ossification may become evident.

Ligamentous Degeneration

Virtually every type of ligament in the vertebral column undergoes degeneration. Changes are observed in the anterior longitudinal ligament, posterior longitudinal ligament, ligamenta flava, interspinous, supraspinous, and intertransverse ligaments, ligamentum nuchae, and iliolumbar and interosseous sacroiliac ligaments. As many of these ligaments provide spinal stability, ligamentous laxity is expected in the presence of abnormalities in the intervertebral disc and apophyseal articulations. Histologically, loss of elastic tissue is seen.

Ligamentous Calcification and Ossification

Calcification and ossification of the anterior longitudinal ligament are part of the ossifying diathesis known as diffuse idiopathic skeletal hyperostosis (DISH) (see subsequent discussion). Similar changes are seen in other ligamentous structures, especially the posterior longitudinal ligament and ligamenta flava.

The process of calcification and ossification of the posterior longitudinal ligament (OPLL) deserves special emphasis (Fig. 3–10). These changes have been well described in Japanese individuals, although they occur throughout the world as well.[11] OPLL occurs more frequently in men than in women, and the diagnosis is usually established in the fifth to seventh decades of life. Although individuals with OPLL may be entirely asymptomatic, neurologic manifestations are well known and are influenced by the location and the degree of ossification. Alterations predominate in the cervical spine. Subtle findings are easily overlooked on routine radiographs unless scrutiny of the lateral roentgenogram is undertaken. An ossified plaque is apparent, especially in the mid-cervical region (C3–C5), although any cervical level or, more rarely, a thoracic or lumbar level may be affected. The ossified ligament may be confined to a single verte-bral body or extend for several vertebrae. It is commonly separated from the vertebral body by a thin radiolucent zone, although elsewhere the ossification may merge with the posterior portion of the vertebral body or vertebral bodies. In the thoracic spine, OPLL is most common in the fourth to seventh vertebral levels.[3]

The extent of OPLL and the degree of spinal canal compromise are best delineated utilizing computed tomography and myelography. The axial image format of the former diagnostic modality is ideal in the identification of the disorder, whereas the latter modality accurately demonstrates the degree of involvement of the spinal cord.

Diffuse Idiopathic Skeletal Hyperostosis (DISH)

DISH is a name recently applied to a peculiar and frequent disorder of unknown

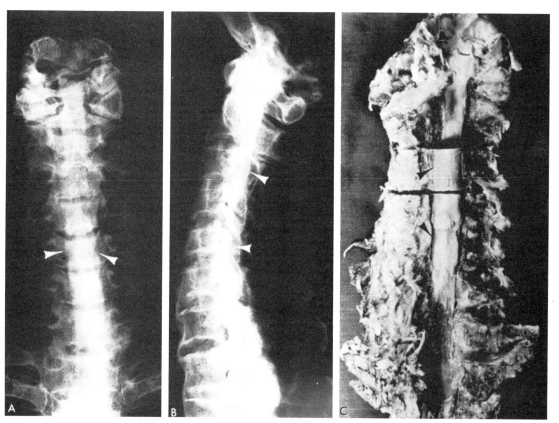

Figure 3–10. Ossification of the posterior longitudinal ligament (OPLL). *A, B,* Frontal and lateral radiographs of the removed cervical spine reveal the extent of ossification (arrowheads). Note the central location of the ossific deposits and presence of anterior vertebral osteophytes. *C,* A photograph of the anterior aspect of the spinal canal viewed from behind following extensive laminectomy demonstrates OPLL extending from the second through the sixth cervical vertebrae (arrowheads).

Illustration continued on following page

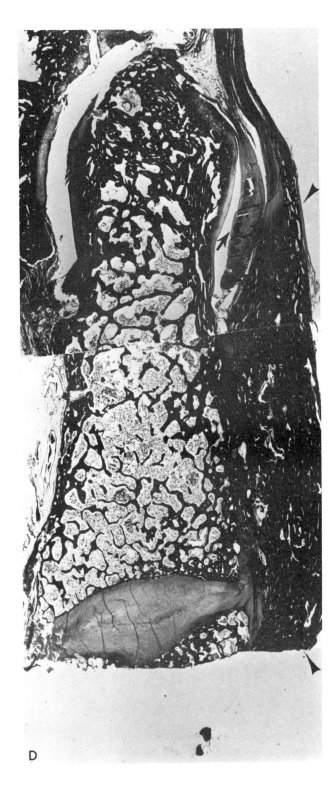

D

Figure 3–10 *Continued D,* A composite photomicrograph (6 ×) of a sagittal section of the axis and anterior arch of the atlas demonstrates the extent of OPLL (arrowheads). Note that the ossified ligament is separated from the posterior aspect of the odontoid process by the transverse ligament (arrow), although it is firmly attached to the posterior aspect of the second cervical vertebral body. Hyperostosis of the posterior margin of the axis is evident. (From Resnick D, Niwayama G (eds): Diagnosis of Bone and Joint Disorders, Vol 2. Philadelphia: W. B. Saunders Company, 1981.)

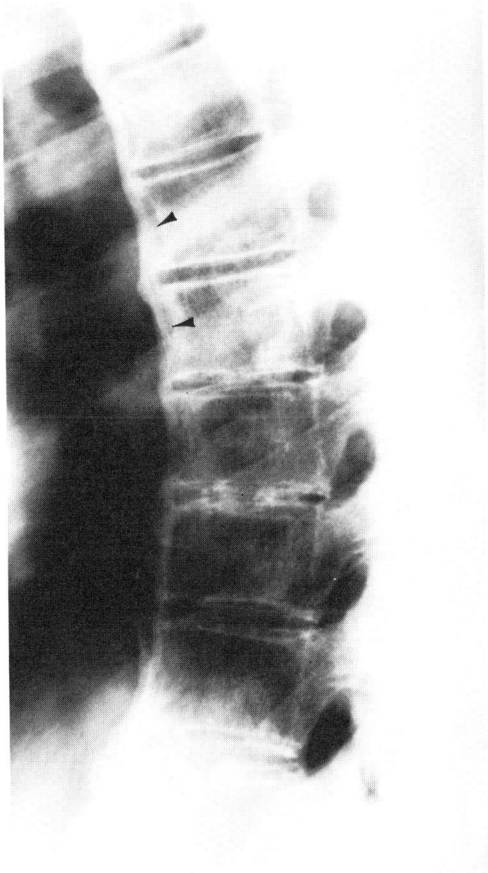

Figure 3–11. Diffuse idiopathic skeletal hyperostosis (DISH): Radiographic abnormalities. This lateral radiograph of the thoracic spine demonstrates the flowing ossification along the anterior aspect of the vertebral column that is a requirement for the diagnosis of DISH. Observe the lucency beneath the deposited bone (arrowheads).

etiology that affects the aging skeleton.[8, 9] The condition, which is also called Forestier's disease and ankylosing hyperostosis of the spine, appears to represent an ossifying diathesis leading to osseous proliferation at sites of tendon and ligament attachment to bone (entheses), ligamentous calcification and ossification, and para-articular osteophytes. Although the spine is the principal site of involvement, other portions of the axial skeleton (pelvis) and areas of the appendicular skeleton (elbow, knee, heel) are affected in a large percentage of cases.

A requirement for the diagnosis of DISH is the presence of flowing ossification along the anterior aspect of at least four contiguous vertebral bodies (Fig. 3–11). This criterion, although arbitrary in nature, allows separation of DISH from typical spondylosis deformans. Other criteria, including the absence of intra-articular bone ankylosis of apophyseal and sacroiliac joints and of disc space narrowing, effectively eliminate ankylosing spondylitis and intervertebral osteochondrosis.

In almost all cases, it is the spinal alterations that predominate. The bone production occurs primarily in the anterior surfaces of the vertebral bodies and sweeps across the intervertebral discs; it is better seen on lateral radiographs than on frontal radiographs of the spine. Sites of involvement, in order of decreasing frequency, are the thoracic spine, the lumbar spine, and the cervical spine. The resulting vertebral contour is bumpy and irregular, differing from the smooth contour that characterizes ankylosing spondylitis. A radiolucent line is commonly noted between the ossified anterior longitudinal ligament and the subjacent vertebral bodies. Radiolucent extensions are apparent at the level of the intervertebral disc. In a significant number of cases, OPLL is also apparent.

The extraspinal manifestations of DISH are most evident in the pelvis, calcaneus,

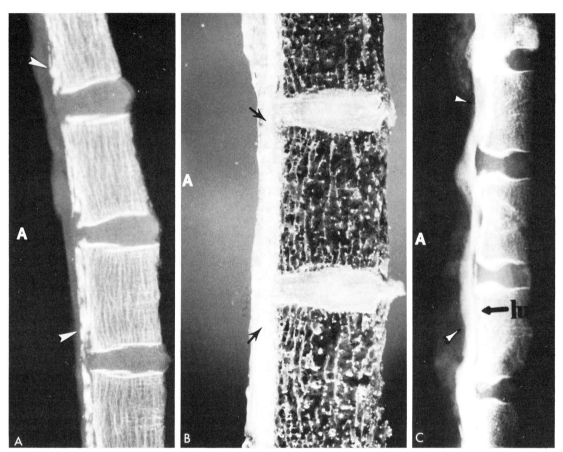

Figure 3–12. Diffuse idiopathic skeletal hyperostosis (DISH): Pathologic abnormalities. *A, B,* On a corresponding radiograph and photograph of a sagittal section of the thoracic spine, note ribbon-like calcification (arrowheads) along the anterior (A) surface of the vertebral bodies. This represents calcific deposits within the anterior longitudinal ligament (arrows). (*A, B,* From Resnick D, Niwayama G: Radiographic and pathologic features of spinal involvement in diffuse idiopathic skeletal hyperostosis (DISH). Radiology 119:559, 1976.) *C,* Progressive anterior longitudinal ligament calcification and ossification (arrowheads) are observed on the anterior (A) surface of the vertebrae with subjacent radiolucent areas (lu). (*C,* From Resnick D, Niwayama G (eds): Diagnosis of Bone and Joint Disorders, Vol 2. Philadelphia: W. B. Saunders Company, 1981.)

and olecranon process of the ulna. Well-defined bone excrescences, called whiskering, are seen in the iliac crest, ischial tuberosities, and femoral trochanters on frontal radiographs of the pelvis. Para-articular osteophytes occur near the acetabulum and sacroiliac articulation. Iliolumbar and sacrotuberous ligament ossifications are characteristic. Bone outgrowths appear at sites of tendon and ligament attachment to the calcaneus, ulnar olecranon, and patella.

The precise nature of DISH and its relationship to spondylosis deformans are not known. On pathologic examination, changes of spondylosis deformans are evident but, in addition, calcification and ossification of the anterior longitudinal ligament and bone pro-liferation where the ligament attaches to the vertebral body are distinctive (Figs. 3–12, 3–13). With this in mind, it is best to regard DISH as a common ossifying diathesis of the elderly, leading to enthesopathic alterations in both spinal and extraspinal sites.

Other Disorders

An enthesopathy affecting the osseous attachments of the interosseous sacroiliac ligament is a frequent finding in middle-aged and elderly patients. Irregular but well-defined bone excrescences occur in the ilial and sacral portions of the ligamentous space above the true synovium-lined portion of

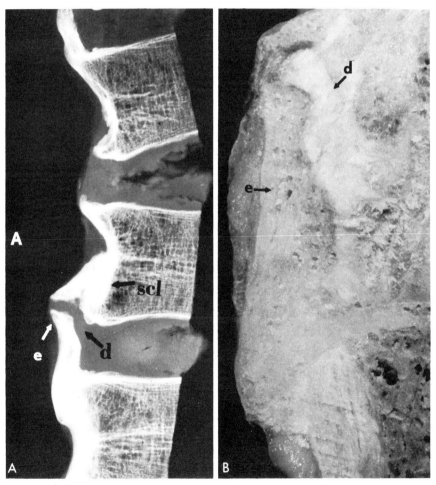

Figure 3–13. Diffuse idiopathic skeletal hyperostosis (DISH): Pathologic abnormalities. *A,* Sagittal sectional radiograph (A, anterior surface) outlines radiolucent disc extensions (d), pointed excrescences (e), and vertebral sclerosis (scl). *B,* On a photograph of the specimen, observe disc extension (d), osteophytes, and excrescences (e). (From Resnick D, Shapiro RF, Wiesner KB, et al: Diffuse idiopathic skeletal hyperostosis (DISH) [ankylosing hyperostosis of Forestier and Rotes-Querol]. Semin Arthritis Rheum 7:153, 1978.)

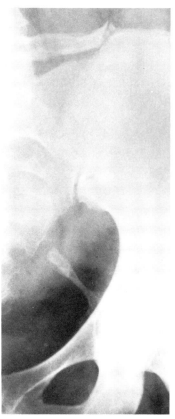

Figure 3–14. Ossification of the iliolumbar and sacro-tuberous ligaments. Note bone formation within both of these ligaments.

the sacroiliac joint. Complete bone bridging of the space is occasionally encountered.

Excessive lumbar lordosis in an elderly individual may lead to approximation and contact of the spinous processes and to degeneration of intervening ligaments. The "kissing spines" develop reactive eburnation (Baastrup's disease) and may be associated with considerable pain and discomfort.[16] The condition is appropriately regarded as an "insertion tendonopathy."

Isolated ossification of the ligamentum nuchae or iliolumbar and sacro-tuberous ligaments is occasionally encountered (Fig. 3–14). The changes appear to be degenerative in nature, although the possibility of DISH or fluorosis must be considered.

References

1. Bick EM: Vertebral osteophytosis. Pathologic basis of its roentgenology. AJR 73:979, 1955.
2. Coventry MB, Ghormley RK, Kernohan JW: The intervertebral disc: Its microscopic anatomy and pathology. II. Changes in the intervertebral disc concomitant with age. J Bone Joint Surg 27:233, 1945.
3. Hiramatsu Y, Nobechi T: Calcification of the posterior longitudinal ligament of the spine among Japanese. Radiology 100:307, 1971.
4. Kirkaldy-Willis WH, Wedge JH, Yong-Hing K, et al: Pathology and pathogenesis of lumbar spondylosis and stenosis. Spine 3:319, 1978.
5. Macnab I: Cervical spondylosis. Clin Orthop 109: 69, 1975.
6. Mainzer F: Herniation of the nucleus pulposus. A rare complication of intervertebral-disc calcification in children. Radiology 107:167, 1973.
7. Pritzker KPH: Aging and degeneration in the lumbar intervertebral disc. Orthop Clin North Am 8:65, 1977.
8. Resnick D, Shaul SR, Robins JM: Diffuse idiopathic skeletal hyperostosis (DISH): Forestier's disease with extraspinal manifestations. Radiology 115: 513, 1975.
9. Resnick D, Niwayama G: Radiographic and pathologic features of spinal involvement in diffuse idiopathic skeletal hyperostosis (DISH). Radiology 119:559, 1976.
10. Resnick D, Pineda C: Vertebral involvement in calcium pyrophosphate dihydrate crystal deposition disease. Radiographic-pathologic correlation. Radiology 153:55, 1984.
11. Resnick D, Guerra J Jr, Robinson CA, et al: Association of diffuse idiopathic skeletal hyperostosis (DISH) and calcification and ossification of the posterior longitudinal ligament. AJR 131:1049, 1978.
12. Schmorl G, Junghanns H: The Human Spine in Health and Disease, 2nd ed. Translated by EF Besemann. New York: Grune & Stratton, 1971, p 138.
13. Silverman FN: Calcification of intervertebral disks in childhood. Radiology 62:801, 1954.
14. Smith DM: Acute back pain associated with a calcified Schmorl's node. A case report. Clin Orthop 117:193, 1976.
15. Weinberger A, Myers AR: Intervertebral disc calcification in adults: A review. Semin Arthritis Rheum 8:69, 1978.
16. Yamada K, Nishiwaki I, Yasukawa H: Supplemental study upon the pathogenesis of low back pain in Baastrup's disease. Arch Jap Chir 23:384, 1954.

4

Morrie E. Kricun, M.D.

Conventional Radiography

The conventional radiograph of the spine plays an integral part in the work-up and follow-up of patients with spinal disorders and, in most clinical settings, is the first imaging modality performed. It is the simplest, least expensive method of examining the spine. The conventional radiograph is often the mirror to systemic disease and, on occasion, may give the only clue to an underlying disorder. Not infrequently, a diagnosis may be established by examining the spine on a routine chest radiograph. The purpose of this chapter is to discuss the plain radiographic signs of the normal spine and of the diseased spine as well as the pathophysiology and differential diagnosis of these signs. In addition, the radiographic features of the spine in various disorders will be discussed.

INDICATIONS

The conventional radiograph of the spine is often the initial imaging study performed in the evaluation of patients with neck and back pain syndromes, suspected spinal dysraphism or other congenital abnormalities, spinal trauma, infection, tumor, spondylitides, and a number of other disorders. The conventional radiograph is also an adjunct to other imaging modalities, particularly radionuclide scanning. Conventional radiography is the modality often chosen in the follow-up of patients with certain spinal disorders.

LIMITATIONS

The main limitation of the conventional radiograph is a lack of visibility of extraspinal and intraspinal soft tissues, including spinal cord, nerve roots, nucleus pulposus and annulus fibrosus, ligaments, blood vessels, thecal membranes, and subarachnoid and epidural spaces. Another limitation is a lack of visibility of early bone destruction. Both spinal and intraspinal lesions usually must be extensive before causing radiographically visible signs.

COMPLICATIONS

There are no known complications from the routine radiographic examination of the spine.

RADIATION BURDEN

Compared with other conventional radiographic procedures, the radiographic examination of the lumbosacral spine delivers one of the highest doses of radiation to the skin, bone marrow, and gonads.* The mean value of radiation to the gonads from a lumbosacral examination is exceeded only by urography and colon examinations.[125, 956] Table 4–1 lists the calculated doses in millirads (mrad) for different organ systems during varius spinal examinations.[1295] Notice that

---

*Reference numbers 125, 333, 511, 1295, 1312.

Table 4–1. ORGAN DOSE (ADULT) FROM DIAGNOSTIC X-RAY EXAMINATIONS*

	Number of Films	Total Body	Thyroid	Active Bone Marrow M	F	Lung M	F	Gonads M	F	Uterus-Embryo
Cervical Spine	3.7	23	404	11	11	14	14	+	+	+
Thoracic Spine	2.1	116	81	43	43	263	263	+	0.6	0.6
Lumbar Spine	2.9	272	0.3	126	126	133	133	7	405	408
Lumbosacral spine	3.4	386	+	224	224	35	35	43	640	639
Entire Spine	1.0	81	271	35	35	149	117	10	100	128

*Based on data from 1970. Doses are in mrad.
Key: + = Less than 0.1 mrad.
Reprinted with permission from Waggener RG, Kereiakes JG, Shalek RJ: CRC Handbook of Medical Physics, vol 2. Boca Raton: CRC Press, Inc, 1984. Copyright CRC Press, Inc., Boca Raton, Florida.

for women the radiation dose to the gonads is higher than that for men during the lumbosacral examination. The current dose can be 1.5 to 4 times lower if newer film-screen combinations are used. Table 4–2 lists the gonadal doses received from different radiographic projections at various ages.[1312] It is probably accurate to state that gonadal doses are higher when there is poor centering or poor coning or poor calibration of x-ray equipment or when repeated films are taken. Radiographs frequently ordered to evaluate acute low back pain ("strain") in young adults unfortunately deliver a high direct gonadal dose of radiation in this self-limiting disorder.[510] Because of the high radiation dose of the lumbosacral examination, various authors have stressed the need for eliminating unnecessary radiographic examinations and limiting the number of views per radiographic study.* Among these suggestions are the following: a single, well-centered lateral spine radiograph to replace the combination of lateral and cone lateral views;[333] obtaining only AP and lateral views in adults[874, 1110] and in children;[1059] and eliminating oblique views in adults.[874, 1045] On the other hand, some authors feel that oblique radiographs should be part of the routine examination in young patients.[735]

In patients with scoliosis who receive repeated follow-up examinations, there is also increased radiation to the gonads,[316, 917] thyroid gland,[316] and breast (in girls).[281, 900] However, proper selection of screen-film-grid combinations, collimation of x-ray beam, proper technical factors, and proper shielding reduce the radiation burden.* Utilizing posteroanterior exposure reduces the radiation to the breasts[28, 900] but increases the absorbed dose to bone marrow.[281]

Eliminating unnecessary examinations, limiting the number of repeated films, and practicing accurate centering and coning of the x-ray beam will obviously drastically

*Reference numbers 125, 333, 510, 511, 822, 874, 1045, 1054, 1059, 1109, 1110, 1277.

*Reference numbers 33, 165, 281, 316, 900, 1090.

Table 4–2. GONADAL DOSE DURING SPINAL EXAMINATIONS*

	Adults M	F	10 Years Old M	F	3 Years Old M	F
Cervical, anteroposterior	0.025	0.012	—	—	—	—
Cervical, lateral	0.003	0.006	—	—	—	—
Thoracic, anteroposterior	0.4	0.2	0.14	0.14	0.1	0.13
Thoracic, lateral	0.5	1.0	0.06	0.14	0.06	0.15
Lumbar, anteroposterior	12.0	150.0	150.0	65.0	80.0	50.0
Lumbar, lateral	40.0	240.0	145.0	180.0	190.0	111.0
Lumbosacral (spot)	6.0	50.0	—	—	—	—

*Doses are in mrad.
From Webster EW, Merrill OE: Radiation hazards. II. Measurements of gonadal dose in radiographic examinations. N Engl J Med 257:811–819, 1957. Reprinted by permission of the New England Journal of Medicine.

reduce the radiographic burden to the general population.[42, 1312]

UTILIZATION

An estimated 4 million cervical spine and 7 million lumbar spine examinations are performed yearly in the United States.[1278] A great number of these examinations are performed on patients with disorders that are often self-limiting or in which the radiographic observations do not alter patient treatment.[125] The overutilization of radiographic examinations leads to unnecessary radiation and adds to the economic burden of the cost of medical care in this country. Unnecessary examinations may be performed because of medical-legal conditions, inadequate history provided to the radiologist, and for inappropriate and controversial indications.[510]

Neck and Back Pain

The clinical problem of neck and low back pain is a challenge to the examining physician. Approximately 80% of the population will experience back pain to some extent during their lifetime.[893] Men and women are affected equally, as are blue collar and white collar workers. Yet the information obtained from the radiographic examination to determine the cause of neck and low back pain is for the most part irrelevant.* The most common causes of acute low back pain are muscle strain and ligamentous strain, and they are usually self-limiting.[510] The radiograph in this clinical situation as well as in the less common acute herniated disc is unrewarding. In patients 20 to 50 years of age with chronic low back pain, only 1/2500 (0.04%) of lumbar spine radiographic examinations yield significant positive findings that were not suspected clinically.[893]

A number of observations may be discovered on the radiographic examination that occur with equal frequency in patients with and in patients without acute or chronic low back pain. These include spina bifida occulta, transitional vertebra, Schmorl's nodes, vacuum disc, narrow disc, osteophytes, ac-

cessory ossicles, spondylolisthesis, and mild to moderate scoliosis.* However, some authors found spondylolisthesis[893, 1271] and disc narrowing[580, 893, 1271] more common in the symptomatic group. Observations of degenerative change in the cervical spine with or without encroachment of neural foramina rarely influence initial conservative treatment of neck pain.[510]

The previously described inconsistencies in assessment may be due to conflict in data obtained from the radiographic examination as well as interobserver and intraobserver differences in the interpretation of the radiographs.[434] Radiographic examination for neck and low back pain should be reserved for those with chronic or atypical symptomatology and for those with suspected fracture.

Disability

Back pain is the most common single complaint of applicants for compensation for disability alleged to be related to occupation.[335] In the Veterans Administration (VA) system, and probably other disability compensation programs throughout the country, compensation awards can be based solely on radiographic findings of degenerative disease of normal aging,[334] even in the absence of an objective physical abnormality.[335] "According to most state statutes, an ordinary disease of life resulting from the general risks and hazards common to every individual regardless of the type of employment is not an occupational disease and therefore is not compensable."[334] Establishment of criteria of normal aging would help reduce the number of instances in which patients are awarded compensation unjustifiably and would aid those who deserve compensation. This could result in an enormous monetary savings.

There are risk factors for the development of severe low back pain based on health care, occupation, exposure to vehicular vibration, and sports activities.[435, 664] The incidence of low back pain in cigarette smokers is higher than that in nonsmokers. This may be due in part to excessive coughing or reduction in blood flow to the vertebral body

*Reference numbers 427, 434, 510, 893, 1361.

*Reference numbers 427, 434, 437, 893, 1204, 1211, 1266, 1361.

and intervertebral disc, rendering the disc more susceptible to mechanical stresses.

Although cervical and lumbar disc degeneration is more common in those who perform arduous labor such as mining, the incidence of disc narrowing does not seem to be related to such occupations. There is an increase, however, in severity and prevalence of osteophytes in coal miners.[172] No specific radiographic changes develop following prolonged exposure to occupational or vehicular vibratory stresses.[434]

Pre-employment

According to some authors, the spine radiograph is of little value in predicting those who are at risk for low back pain or disability in an industrial setting.[434, 985] In a series of pre-employment radiographs of relatively young men, the incidence of spondylolysis was 2.8% and that of spondylolisthesis was 4%. These observations were considered normal variations for this age group.[876]

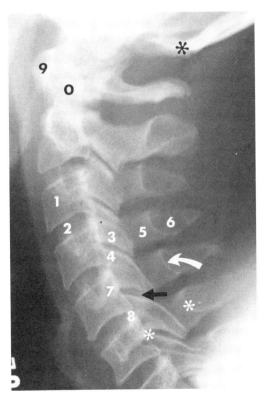

Figure 4–2. Lateral radiograph—cervical spine. *Key:* **1** = vertebral body; **2** = intervertebral disc; **3** = inferior articular process; **4** = superior articular process; **5** = lamina; **6** = spinous process; **7** = transverse process; **8** = uncovertebral articulation; **9** = anterior arch of C1; **0** = odontoid process; **black asterisk** = posterior margin of foramen magnum; **white asterisks** = sagittal diameter of spinal canal; **white arrow** = spinolaminar line; **black arrow** = facet joint.

RADIOGRAPHIC EXAMINATION

There is no *routine* examination when it comes to evaluating patients with suspected spinal disorders. The radiographic examination should ideally be tailored so that the highest diagnostic accuracy is achieved while the level of radiation exposure and cost of medical care are diminished. The choice of radiographic projections should be dictated by the clinical setting, the information desired, the age of the patient, and the anatomic site involved. A number of radiographic views are available in the arsenal of diagnostic conventional radiographic imaging, yet only a few are needed to solve most clinical problems. The other views may be obtained if additional information is sought, or if on the routine examination areas of suspicion arise that demand

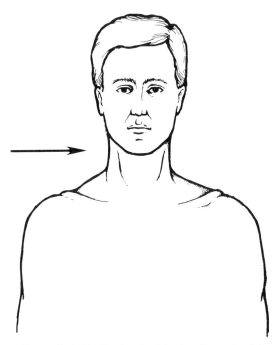

Figure 4–1. Positioning for lateral radiograph of the cervical spine. Arrow indicates direction of the x-ray beam. This artist's drawing of radiographic positioning, as well as those that follow, is based on photographs of patient positioning from Merrill V: Atlas of Roentgenographic Positions and Standard Radiographic Procedures, vol I. St. Louis: C. V. Mosby Company, 1975.

clarification. A selection of many radiographic projections is presented below.

Cervical Spine[851]

Lateral. The patient is seated or standing and is lateral to the x-ray cassette. The cassette is centered over the 4th cervical segment (Figs. 4–1 and 4–2).

Cross-Table Lateral. For initial evaluation of neck trauma. The patient is not moved but remains supine. X-ray beam is directed perpendicular to the neck and cassette at the level of the 4th cervical vertebra (Fig. 4–3). Adaptations for prefusion localization in the operation room[1259] and for patients in a halo device[53] have been reported.

Lateral With Flexion and Extension. Patient is in similar position as for lateral, but head is flexed or extended. This examination should not be performed routinely on patients who have sustained severe neck trauma.

Anteroposterior (AP). The patient is either supine or erect and the x-ray tube is angled 15 to 20 degrees cephalad (Figs. 4–4 and 4–5). Motion of the mandible during film exposure allows better visualization of the upper cervical vertebrae.[613] Modification with angling the tube can better demonstrate the anterior arch of C1.[356]

Oblique. The patient is usually sitting or standing, and the entire body is rotated 45 degrees toward the cassette for each oblique view. The x-ray beam is perpendicular to the cassette and centered over the midline (Figs. 4–6 and 4–7). The examination may

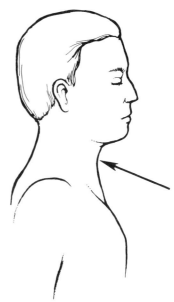

Figure 4–4. Positioning for anteroposterior cervical radiograph.

be performed either posteroanterior (PA) or anteroposterior (AP). The x-ray beam may also be angled 15 to 20 degrees caudad, with the patient in a semiprone position of 45 degrees (Fig. 4–8). In seriously injured or ill patients, supine AP oblique radiographs may be accomplished by angling the tube toward the patient, who is supine.

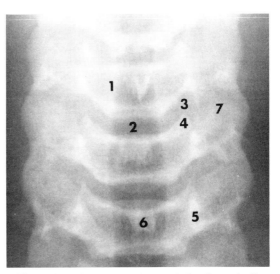

Figure 4–5. Anteroposterior cervical radiograph. *Key:* **1** = vertebral body; **2** = intervertebral disc; **3** = uncovertebral "joint"; **4** = uncinate process; **5** = pedicle; **6** = spinous process; **7** = cervical pillar.

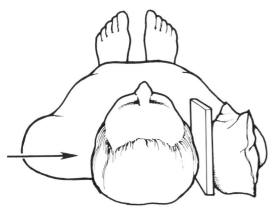

Figure 4–3. Positioning for cross-table lateral cervical radiograph.

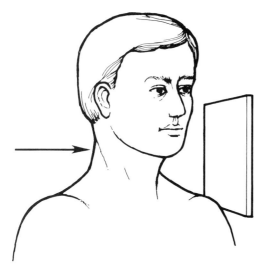

Figure 4–6. Positioning for oblique cervical radiograph. Erect position.

Angled Oblique. Special angle views of the oblique cervical spine at 45 degrees and 60 degrees can be performed in the supine position to evaluate better the articular processes, pedicles, and neural foramina.[2]

Open-Mouth Atlas and Axis (A & A). The patient is supine, and the mouth is open. The x-ray beam is perpendicular to the cassette and centered vertically over the open mouth (Figs. 4–9 and 4–10).

Vertebral Arch (Pillar). The patient is supine or prone. If the patient is supine, the neck is in extension and the x-ray beam is angled 20 to 30 degrees caudad (Fig. 4–11). There are modifications to this view in the AP projection that include 10 degree rotation of the head to either side so that the mandible does not overlie the spine.[1184] This allows

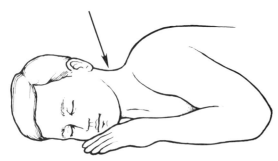

Figure 4–7. Positioning for oblique cervical radiograph. Semiprone position.

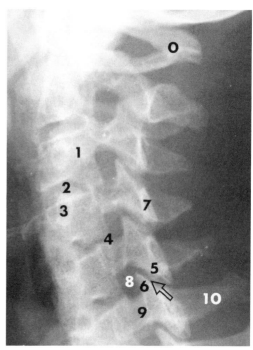

Figure 4–8. Oblique cervical radiograph. Right posterior oblique view. *Key:* **0** = posterior arch of C1; **1** = vertebral body; **2** = intervertebral disc; **3** = pedicle (right); **4** = uncovertebral articulation; **5** = inferior articular process; **6** = superior articular process; **7** = lamina; **8** = neural foramen; **9** = pedicle (left); **10** = spinous process; **arrow** = facet joint (left).

better visualization of upper cervical laminae and articular processes (Fig. 4–12). An adaptation to the AP projection with the mouth open aids in visualization of the laminae and articular processes of the upper cervical spine.[1184] Exaggerated supine oblique views with 60 degree angulation of the x-ray beam enable adequate visualization of the articular processes and neural foramina.[2] The patient may also be placed supine with the head turned 45 to 50 degrees and the chin extended (Fig. 4–13). The x-ray beam is angled 35 to 45 degrees cephalad for direct PA projection.[851] For an oblique PA projection, the head is adjusted so that its median sagittal plane is at 45 degrees and the x-ray beam is 30 to 40 degrees toward the head (Fig. 4–14).

Cervicothoracic Area (Swimmer's View). The patient is in the lateral recumbent position, with the head slightly elevated. The dependent arm is extended so that the humeral head is behind or in front of the vertebrae. The upper arm is placed in the

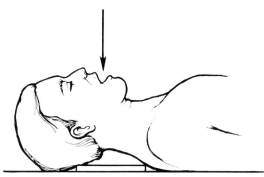

Figure 4–9. Positioning for anteroposterior projection of the atlas and axis (open-mouth view).

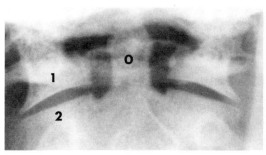

Figure 4–10. Anteroposterior radiograph of the atlantoaxial articulation (open-mouth view). *Key:* **0** = odontoid process; **1** = lateral mass of C1; **2** = articular surface of C2. Note the normal alignment between the lateral margins of the lateral mass of C1 and the opposing articular surface of C2.

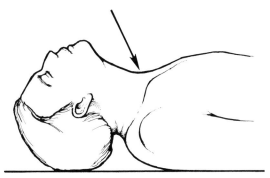

Figure 4–11. Positioning for vertebral arch radiograph (pillar view). Anteroposterior projection.

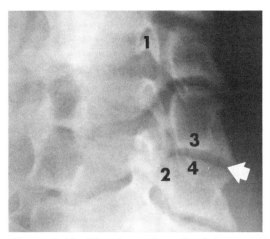

Figure 4–12. Pillar view radiograph of the cervical spine. *Key:* **1** = spinous process; **2** = lamina; **3** = inferior articular process; **4** = superior articular process; **arrow** = facet joint.

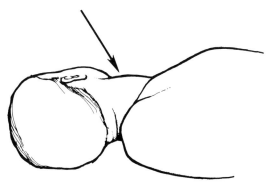

Figure 4–13. Positioning for vertebral arch radiograph. Oblique anteroposterior projection.

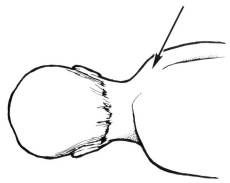

Figure 4–14. Positioning for vertebral arch radiograph. Oblique posteroanterior projection.

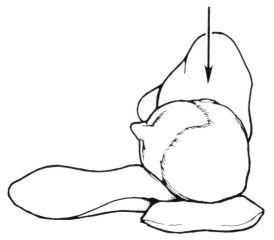

Figure 4–15. Positioning for cervicothoracic region radiograph (swimmer's view). Lateral projection.

opposite direction. The x-ray beam is directed 3 to 5 degrees caudad and centered over the 2nd or 3rd thoracic vertebra. The radiograph may also be taken with the patient in the upright position (Figs. 4–15 through 4–17).

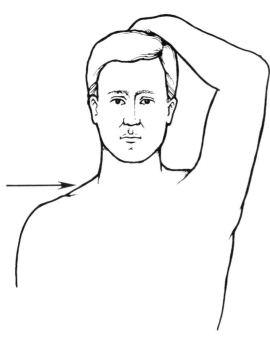

Figure 4–16. Positioning for cervicothoracic region radiograph (swimmer's view). Lateral projection upright position.

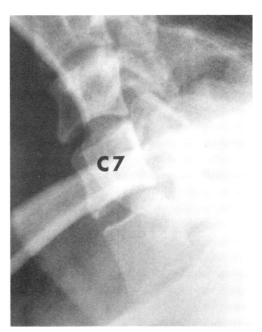

Figure 4–17. Radiograph of the cervicothoracic region (swimmer's view).

Thoracic Spine[851]

Lateral. The patient is in the lateral position, either erect or recumbent. When the patient is recumbent, the knees and hips are flexed. The x-ray beam is perpendicular to the cassette.

Anteroposterior. The patient is erect or supine. If the patient is supine, the knees and hips are flexed. The x-ray beam is perpendicular to the cassette (Fig. 4–18).

Oblique View. The patient is recumbent or standing. The body is rotated slightly so that the coronal plane forms an angle of 70 degrees with the plane of the cassette. The x-ray beam is directed 3 to 5 degrees caudad and centered over the 2nd or 3rd thoracic vertebrae. The x-ray beam is directed perpendicular to the cassette.

Lumbar Spine[851]

Anteroposterior. The frontal projection of the lumbosacral spine is usually examined from the AP direction. The patient may be recumbent or erect. If the patient is supine, the knees and hips are flexed. The x-ray

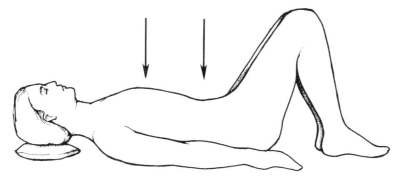

Figure 4–18. Positioning for anteroposterior radiograph of the thoracic spine (left arrow) and lumbar spine (right arrow).

beam is centered over the iliac crests and is perpendicular to the cassette (Figs. 4–18 and 4–19).

Lateral. The patient is erect or recumbent and turned onto the side. The x-ray beam is centered at the iliac crest. If the patient is recumbent, the knees and hips are flexed to diminish the degree of lordosis. The x-ray beam is perpendicular to the cassette (Figs. 4–20 and 4–21).

Coned Lateral. The patient is recumbent and turned onto the side, with the hips extended. The x-ray beam is centered at the level of the transverse plane that passes midway between the iliac crest and anterior superior iliac spines. The x-ray beam is directed perpendicular (Fig. 4–22).

Modified Lateral. This is similar to the lateral view previously described, but the x-ray beam is centered 1 cm above the iliac crest.[333] The advantage of this view is that L5–S1 is visualized as well as it is with the coned lateral in 93% of cases. Therefore, it could be performed instead of routine lateral plus coned lateral, thus reducing the gonadal radiation dose.

Oblique. The patient is either erect or recumbent, and the body is rotated 45 degrees to the cassette (semiprone position is favored as it allows more immobilization). The x-ray beam is perpendicular to the cassette. The L5–S1 facet joints are better visualized with the body rotated 30 degrees, but this additional radiograph is not usually necessary routinely (Figs. 4–23 through 4–25).

Angled Anteroposterior. The position of the patient is similar to that of the AP projection previously described. The x-ray beam is angled 30 degrees craniad and centered at the superior border of the pubic symphysis.[734] It may also be angled 45 degrees caudad and centered to the lower sternum so that the exiting beam is at the tip of the spinous process of L3,[5] or the beam can be centered over the area of primary clinical concern.[6]

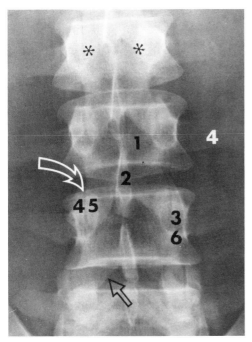

Figure 4–19. Anteroposterior radiograph of the lumbar spine (L1 omitted). *Key:* **1** = vertebral body; **2** = spinous process; **3** = pedicle; **4** = superior articular process; **5** = inferior articular process; **6** = pars interarticularis; **straight arrow** = lamina; **curved arrow** = facet joint; **asterisks** = interpedicular distance.

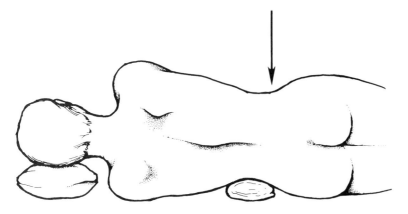

Figure 4–20. Positioning for lateral lumbosacral radiograph.

Figure 4–21. Lateral radiograph of the thoracolumbar junction. *Key*: **1** = vertebral body; **2** = intervertebral disc; **3** = pedicle; **4** = neural foramen; **5** = pars interarticularis; **6** = lamina; **7** = superior articular process; **8** = transverse process; **arrows** = lateral recess.

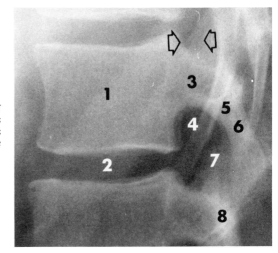

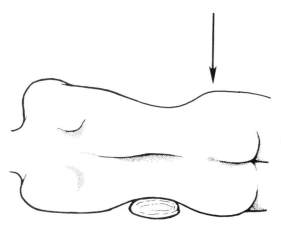

Figure 4–22. Positioning for coned lateral radiograph of the lumbosacral junction.

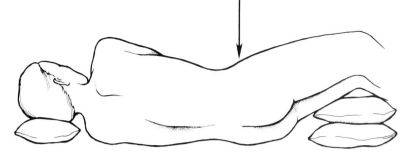

Figure 4–23. Positioning for oblique radiograph of the lumbar spine. Left posterior oblique projection for visualization of the left posterior elements.

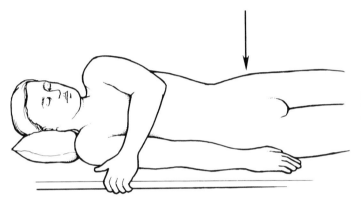

Figure 4–24. Positioning for oblique radiograph of the lumbar spine. Right posterior oblique projection for evaluation of the posterior elements on the right.

Figure 4–25. Oblique view of the lumbar spine. Right posterior oblique projection. Notice the outline of the "Scotty dog." *Key:* **1** = vertebral body; **2** = pedicle; **3** = superior articular process; **4** = inferior articular process; **5** = pars interarticularis; **6** = lamina; **7** = spinous process; **arrow** = facet joint.

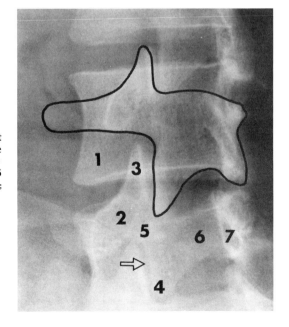

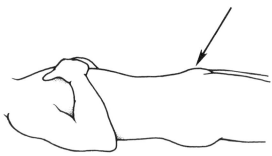

Figure 4–26. Positioning for a radiograph of the sacrum.

Sacrum

The sacrum is examined in the AP and lateral projections. In the frontal projection, if the patient is supine, the x-ray beam is directed 15 degrees cephalad and centered between the symphysis pubis and the level of the anterior superior iliac spines[851] (Fig. 4–26). If the patient is prone, the beam is directed 15 degrees toward the feet and centered to the sacral curve. For the lateral sacrum, the patient is recumbent and lateral, and the hips and knees are flexed. The x-ray beam is directed perpendicular to the cassette.

Sacroiliac Joints

The sacroiliac joints may be demonstrated on the angled view of the sacrum or on oblique views. The sacroiliac joints may be viewed twice owing to their oblique course (Fig. 4–27). For the oblique views, the patient is semiprone, with the upper side of the body 25 degrees from the table.[851] The x-ray beam is centered at the level of the anterior superior iliac spine of the side closest to the table and is directed perpendicular to the cassette. A craniocaudal axial view has been described.[306] By this method, each sacroiliac joint is examined separately. The patient sits on the x-ray table, with the trunk flexed and knees dangling. The x-ray tube is angled 10 to.20 degrees caudad using fluoroscopic control. The gonadal radiation dose in males is 2 to 5 mrad.

Coccyx

Examination of the coccyx can be performed in the AP and lateral projections. With the patient supine, the x-ray beam is angled 10 degrees caudad and centered 2 inches proximal to the pubic symphysis[851] (Fig. 4–28). If the patient is prone, the x-ray beam is angled 10 degrees craniad. For the lateral view, the x-ray beam is perpendicular to the cassette.

RADIOGRAPHIC SIGNS OF THE NORMAL AND DISEASED SPINE

Soft Tissues

The examination of radiographs of the spine consists of a meticulous evaluation of the soft tissues, vertebral alignment, bony

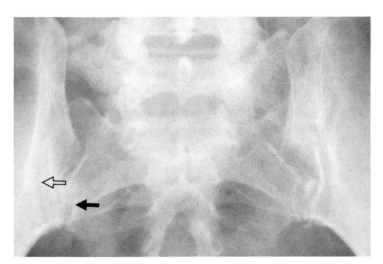

Figure 4–27. Radiograph of the sacrum and sacroiliac joints in the anteroposterior projection. The joint is uniform in size, and the articular margins are smooth and regular. *Key:* **open arrow** = anterior portion of the joint; **closed arrow** = posterior portion of the joint.

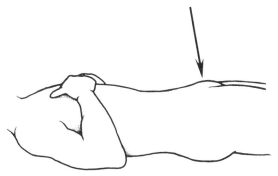

Figure 4–28. Positioning for a radiograph of the coccyx.

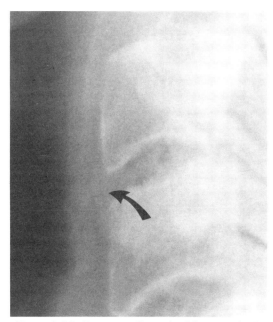

Figure 4–30. Close-up radiograph of the cervical spine in the lateral projection demonstrating a normal prevertebral fat stripe (arrow).

parts, spinal canal, neural foramina, and abnormalities of the ligaments. All vertebrae in the anatomic area should be visualized. The prevertebral soft tissues of the cervical spine are best evaluated on the lateral radiograph. In children, the retropharyngeal space between the posterior pharyngeal wall and the anteroinferior margin of C2 should be no more than 7 mm, with an average around 3.5 mm.[1337] In adults, it measures no more

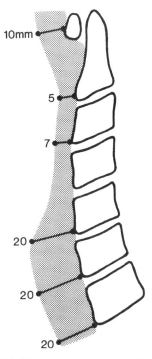

Figure 4–29. Diagrammatic representation of the cervical spine demonstrating normal measurements (in millimeters) for the prevertebral soft tissues of the neck in an adult. (Adapted from Penning L: Prevertebral hematoma in cervical spine injury: Incidence and etiologic significance. AJR 136:553–561, 1981. Copyright 1981 by the American Roentgen Ray Society.)

than 10 mm at C1, 5 to 7 mm at C2, and 7 mm at C3 and C4.[959, 1337] The soft tissue space between the posterior tracheal wall and the anteroinferior aspect of C6 should be less than 14 mm in children, with an average of 7.9 mm, and 20 to 22 mm in adults (Fig. 4–29).[959, 1337] Increase in this space may occur with hemorrhage, edema, infection, infiltration, tumor, or morbid obesity. Endotracheal and nasogastric tubes preclude accurate measurement of the prevertebral soft tissue space.

Alterations in the prevertebral fat stripe offer a more subtle clue to underlying soft tissue abnormalities and may be the only clue to an underlying local disorder. The prevertebral fat stripe is a thin radiolucent line that is adjacent to the anterior surface of the vertebrae, lying parallel to the anterior longitudinal ligament[1331] (Fig. 4–30). It is seen in most lateral cervical radiographs and is observed most frequently in adults. Displacement or blurring of the fat stripe may occur in hemorrhage, edema, infection, or tumor, sometimes without increase in the prevertebral space. It is difficult to evaluate prevertebral soft tissues in the thoracic and lumbar portions of the spine. Paravertebral soft tissue swelling, or mass, can be visualized on the AP thoracic spine radiograph owing to its contrast with air in the lungs. The medial pleural reflection is normally visualized as a paraspinal line.[342] Displacement of the pleural reflection may indicate paravertebral mass due to abscess, hematoma, or tumor[342, 862] (Fig. 4–31).

Alignment

Alignment of the normal spine is maintained by the integrity of the ligaments, joints, vertebral complex (vertebral bodies and intervening disc), and surrounding musculature. Alterations in these structures either alone or in combination may lead to abnormality in alignment. The degree of lordosis, kyphosis, and anterior or posterior subluxation is best evaluated on the lateral radiograph, whereas the degree of scoliosis, torticollis, and lateral subluxation is best evaluated on the AP radiograph.

Bony structures should align with those above and below. The posterior vertebral line is an imaginary line connecting the posteroinferior margin of the vertebral body above with the posterosuperior margin of the vertebral body below (Fig. 4–32). The spinal laminar line joins the base of adjacent laminae and follows a smooth arc extending upward to the posterior aspect of the foramen magnum. Voluntary flexion of the head

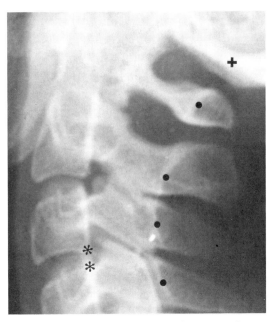

Figure 4–32. Normal alignment of the cervical spine. Lateral view. The posterior margins of the vertebral bodies (asterisks) are aligned, and the arc-shaped spinolaminar line (dots) is continuous up to the posterior margin of the foramen magnum (plus sign).

on the neck ("military position") or muscle spasm may cause loss of the normal lordotic curve (Fig. 4–33).

Atlantoaxial Subluxation

The atlantoaxial relationship can be evaluated on the lateral radiograph and is the space between the posterior margin of the anterior arch of C1 and the anterior margin of the odontoid process (Fig. 4–34). It should measure no more than 3 mm in the adult[568] and 5 mm in children.[754] Increase in this distance indicates atlantoaxial subluxation and is most likely caused by laxity or disruption of the transverse ligament from rheumatoid arthritis.[464, 794] Other causes include psoriatic arthritis,[668] other rheumatoid variants, Behçet's syndrome,[688] trauma, Down's syndrome,* chondrodysplasia punctata,[9] Morquio's syndrome,[961] achondroplasia,[494] neurofibromatosis,[236] spondyloepiphyseal dysplasia,[961] congenital atlantoaxial anomalies such as os odontoideum,[268] and a number of other disorders. Atlantoaxial sublux-

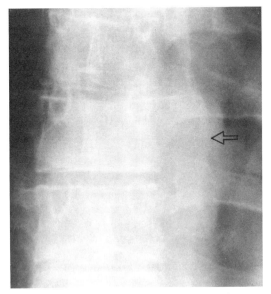

Figure 4–31. Enlargement of paravertebral soft tissues (arrow) caused by lymphoma. Notice the indentation on the pleural reflection in the mediastinum.

---

*Reference numbers 147, 268, 397, 598, 676, 801, 988, 1150, 1167.

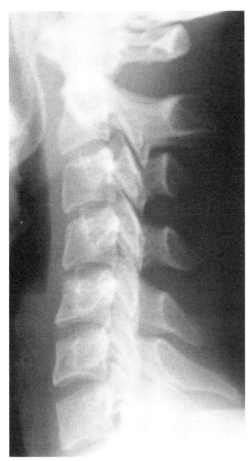

Figure 4–33. Reversal of the lordotic curve of the cervical spine. This may be due to muscle spasm or, as in this case, due to positioning. Notice the proximity of the mandible to the cervical spine.

ation may develop following metastasis to C1.[535] It has been reported in patients following upper respiratory infection, since there is a direct connection of pharyngeal drainage

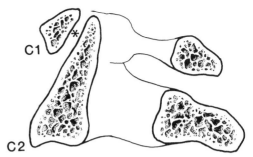

Figure 4–34. Diagrammatic representation of the anterior atlantoaxial articulation (asterisk).

to the upper cervical spine via the retropharyngeal nodes.[78, 1240] Joint effusion leads to laxity of the joint capsule and surrounding ligaments.

Pseudospread of the Atlas

Normally on the AP open mouth view, the lateral masses of C1 are aligned with the opposing articular surfaces of C2 (see Fig. 4–10). Bilateral displacement (offset) of the lateral mass of C1 with C2 may be seen following the Jefferson fracture (a burst fracture of the atlas).[630] However, in children around 5 to 7 years of age[140] and occasionally in adults,[984] a similar displacement may be noted and is a normal variant—the pseudo-offset (pseudospread) of C1 (Fig. 4–35). The offset is usually not greater than 2 mm.[984] It is due to an unequal rate of growth of the lateral masses of C1 and should not be mistaken for fracture.[140] Additionally, pseudospread of the atlas may be due to congenital

Figure 4–35. Pseudospread of the atlas. The lateral mass of C1 (**1**) is not in alignment with the articular surface of C2 (**2**).

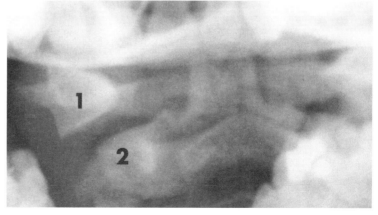

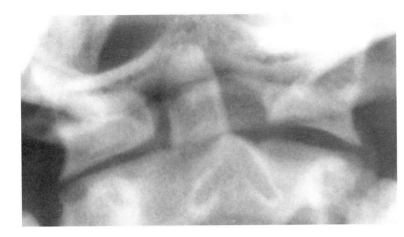

Figure 4–36. Pseudodisplacement of the odontoid process. There is a discrepancy in distance between the odontoid process and the right and left lateral masses of C1. In this patient, it was caused by tilting of the head to the right.

clefts in the anterior and posterior arches of C1[140] or to primary or metastatic tumor of the atlas, causing abnormalities in the atlantoaxial relationship.[984] Unilateral offset of the atlas on the axis up to 4 mm[581] may occur normally with lateral bending and rotation of the head.[582, 947]

Pseudodisplacement of the Odontoid Process

Normally, with the spine in neutral position, the odontoid process is equidistant from the lateral masses of C1 on the AP open mouth view (see Fig. 4–10). However, lateral flexion of the head without rotation may normally cause an asymmetry in the distance between the odontoid process and the lateral masses of C1[947] (Fig. 4–36).

If the head is turned forcibly, tilted to the side, or if muscle spasm is present, the odontoid process appears asymmetrically positioned between the lateral masses of the atlas, and the offset may be 2 to 4 mm.[582] This is within normal limits and should not be mistaken for a Jefferson fracture.

Pseudosubluxation of the Axis

The posterior border of cervical vertebral bodies is aligned in the neutral position. During infancy and childhood up to the age of 10 years, flexion and extension are centered on the 2nd and 3rd vertebrae.[616] With flexion, the fulcrum of motion is at the C2–C3 level and there is a gliding motion in the anteroposterior direction facilitated by the

horizontal plane of the facet joints and the laxity of intervertebral ligaments.[616, 1249] The amount of anterior displacement of C2 and C3 may be 0 mm to 5 mm in a normal child.[48, 185, 616] This is called pseudosubluxation of the axis[185, 525, 616, 1249] and should not be mistaken for a serious injury (Fig. 4–37). It occurs in 19% of children from 1 to 7 years of age.[185] Posterior displacement of C2 on C3 caused by hyperextension is less common in the normal child.[616] By the age of 10 years, the fulcrum of flexion and extension

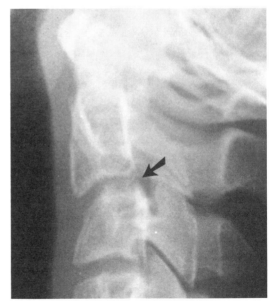

Figure 4–37. Pseudosubluxation of C2. The C2 vertebral body is displaced slightly anterior to C3 (arrow), and there is slight kyphosis of this articulation. However, the spinolaminar line is continuous and smooth. This is a normal variant in children and in some adults.

is shifted to the C4–C5 or C5–C6 level.[525, 616] Nevertheless, similar anterior displacement of C2 on C3 by 2 to 3 mm may be noted during flexion in patients in the 14 to 21 year age range.[525]

A line can be drawn that is helpful in differentiating physiologic subluxation of C2 on C3 from true dislocation or fracture dislocation.[1249] In the extended or neutral positions, the posterior arch of C2 lies behind the posterior arches of C1 and C3. However, in the flexed position, the entire C2 complex moves forward, so that its posterior arch lies in a straight line with the posterior arches of C1 and C3. This line is drawn from the anterior cortex of the posterior arch of C1 to C3, and it is designated the *posterior cervical line*.[1249] In relation to the posterior arch of C2, the posterior cervical line may normally pass through or just behind, touch, or pass within 1 mm of the anterior margin of the posterior arch of C2 (Fig. 4–38). The anterior margin of the posterior arch of C2 lies behind the spinolaminar line of C1 and C3 in 34% of children and 2 to 3 mm behind the line in up to 10% of children.[651] Physiologic subluxation exists if the above criteria are met. Pathologic subluxation is considered if the posterior cervical line misses the posterior arch of C2 by 2 mm or more, and it should be suspected if it misses by 1.5 mm.[1249] There are several pitfalls in this measurement. The posterior arch of C1 may be hypoplastic; the cortex may be poorly defined; the patient may not be in a true lateral position; or anterior angulation of the cervical spine may exist because of muscle spasm, not displacement.

Vertebrae

Size and Shape

The size and shape of vertebrae vary with age (Fig. 4–39). In the neonate, vertebral body ossification centers (centra) are ovoid on the lateral radiograph, with slightly rounded anterior margins,[473, 517] and centrum height is equal to intervertebral disc height (Fig. 4–40). There is gradual increase in growth of the primary ossification center.[223] Anterior and posterior central indentations represent vascular channels.[785, 1297] At about the age of 2 to 3 years, the vertebral body assumes a rectangular shape, which continues throughout life, with the anteroposterior dimension greater than the vertebral height.[473] Intervertebral disc height is less than vertebral height. The ossified vertebral body and pedicles begin to fuse between 3 and 6 years of age.[1084] The neurocentral synchondroses should not be mistaken for fracture (see Fig. 4–40B).

Between the ages of 6 and 8 years, superior and inferior steplike recesses on the vertebral margin are produced by the outer annular rim of cartilage[88] (Figs. 4–41 and 4–42). They are more noticeable anteriorly on the lateral radiograph.[473] The cartilage rim develops outside the cartilage plate[88] and begins to calcify at 6 to 7 years (somewhat later in males)[88, 473] (Fig. 4–43) Calcification has been noted as early as 2 years in girls.[573] Between the ages of 17 and 22 years, the calcifications coalesce, ossify by puberty,[176] and then fuse with the vertebral body.[86–88, 223] As the calcified rim becomes visible anteriorly, the superior and inferior vertebral indentations disappear radiographi-

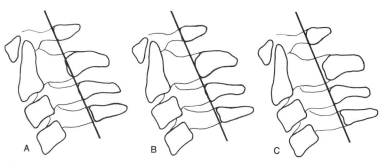

Figure 4–38. Posterior cervical line, normal limits. The posterior cervical line is drawn through the base of spinous processes of C1, C2, and C3. Normally, the line may (A) pass through or just behind the anterior cortex of C2, (B) touch the anterior aspect of the cortex of the base of the spinous process of C2, or (C) pass anterior to the anterior cortex of C2 by 1 mm or less. Pathologic dislocation of C2 or C3 may be considered if the line passes more than 3 mm in front of the posterior arch of C2. (From Swischuck LE: Anterior displacement of C2 in children: Physiologic or pathologic? A helpful differentiating line. Radiology 122:759–763, 1977.)

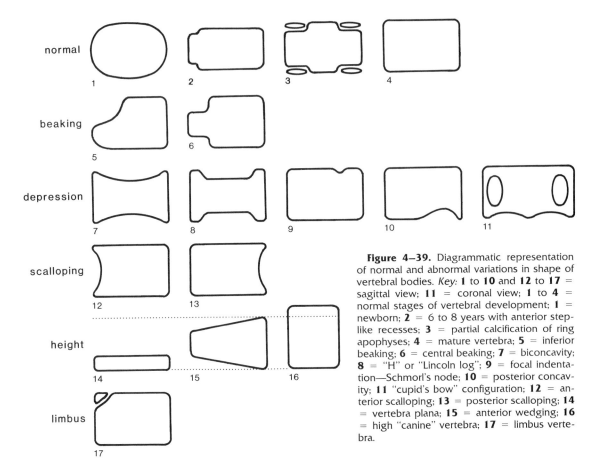

Figure 4–39. Diagrammatic representation of normal and abnormal variations in shape of vertebral bodies. *Key:* **1** to **10** and **12** to **17** = sagittal view; **11** = coronal view; **1** to **4** = normal stages of vertebral development; **1** = newborn; **2** = 6 to 8 years with anterior step-like recesses; **3** = partial calcification of ring apophyses; **4** = mature vertebra; **5** = inferior beaking; **6** = central beaking; **7** = biconcavity; **8** = "H" or "Lincoln log"; **9** = focal indentation—Schmorl's node; **10** = posterior concavity; **11** "cupid's bow" configuration; **12** = anterior scalloping; **13** = posterior scalloping; **14** = vertebra plana; **15** = anterior wedging; **16** = high "canine" vertebra; **17** = limbus vertebra.

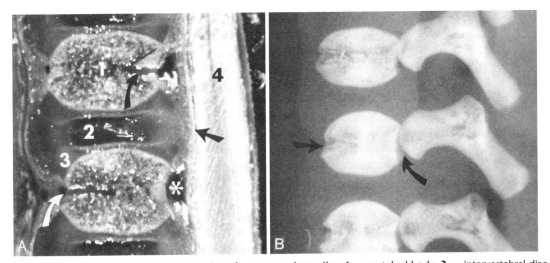

Figure 4–40. *A,* Sagittal section thoracic spine of a term newborn. *Key:* **1** = vertebral body; **2** = intervertebral disc; **3** = unossified cartilage; **4** = spinal cord; **asterisk** = retrovertebral plexus; **straight arrow** = posterior longitudinal ligament; **curved white arrow** = anterior vascular groove; **curved black arrow** = posterior vascular (basivertebral) groove. *B,* Lateral radiograph of the thoracic spine of a term stillborn. *Key:* **Straight arrow** = anterior vascular groove; **curved arrow** = neurocentral synchondrosis joining the vertebral body with the posterior elements.

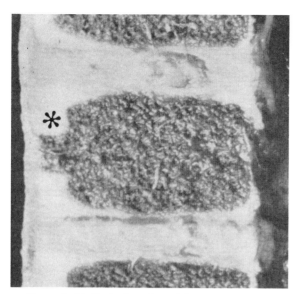

Figure 4–41. Sagittal section of the spine in a 7 year old boy. Cartilaginous rims (asterisk) appear as steplike recesses on the anterior and, to a lesser extent, on the posterior aspects of the vertebral body. This mild form of beaking is normal for patients this age. (From Schmorl G, Junghanns H: The Human Spine in Health and Disease. New York: Grune & Stratton, 1971. Copyright 1971 by Georg Thieme Verlag.)

cally. The bony rim is the attachment site for fibers of the longitudinal ligaments.[86]

Vertebrae enlarge in the vertical dimension by growth from layers of the hyaline cartilage "plate" adjacent to the superior and

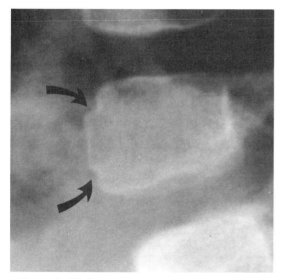

Figure 4–42. Lateral radiograph of the lumbosacral spine in a 5 year old girl. Steplike recesses (arrows) are a normal appearance at this age.

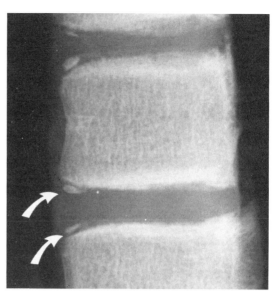

Figure 4–43. Lateral radiograph of thoracic vertebrae demonstrating ossification of ring apophyses (arrows).

inferior osseous margins.[86, 87, 500, 1129a] The growth of vertebral bodies is analogous to the longitudinal growth in long bones.[86, 87] The superior and inferior aspects of the vertebral body grow at the same rate.[473, 681] The cartilage rim does not participate in longitudinal vertebral growth, and acting histologically like an apophysis, it should not be considered an epiphysis.[87, 88, 1129a] An increase in vertebral body height in males takes place during the age range of 20 to 45 years.[17, 120] The size of normal vertebrae increases gradually from the cervical vertebrae to the L5 vertebra in response to the additional progressive load of weight-bearing at lower levels.[223] Abnormalities in vertebral size and shape may give a clue to the underlying disorder (see Fig. 4–39).

High Vertebra. Pressure or stress occurring parallel to the axis of growth inhibits the rate of long bone growth, whereas decrease in pressure or stress allows bone growth to proceed.[39] This phenomenon also applies to the spine.[176] Children who, for a number of reasons, do not stand erect during the growing years, do not stress their vertebrae in a normal manner along the vertebral axis of growth. This leads to overgrowth of the vertebral body in the cephalad-caudad direction, causing a high-appearing vertebra, the so-called canine vertebrae[473] (Fig. 4–44). Radiographically, the cephalad-caudal di-

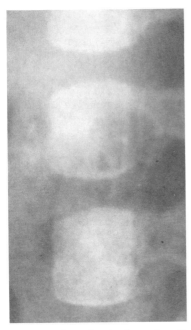

Figure 4–44. High, or "canine," vertebra. Notice the increase in vertebral height compared with the anteroposterior diameter. This patient has trisomy 21 syndrome (Down's syndrome).

mension of the vertebral body is greater than the anteroposterior dimension. The greatest alterations occur in the lumbar vertebrae, since they normally bear the greatest weight in the erect posture and have the greatest ability to respond to the lack of stress by increasing in height.

Increase in vertebral height may develop in a number of disorders, including Trisomy 21 (Down's syndrome)[990] and polio,[576] and in children with other primary nervous system disorders, such as Trisomy 18, amyotonia congenita, myelomeningocele, cerebral palsy, and hydrocephalus, and in any children who might not have walked for a significant time during the period of vertebral growth.[473] It may also develop in fibrodysplasia ossificans progressiva.[1262] High vertebrae may be detected as early as infancy.[990] Partial increase in height of vertebrae may develop in growing patients who have kyphosis or scoliosos[473] and has been shown in cervical and lumbar vertebrae of a patient who had previous tuberculosis of a thoracic vertebra.[1129a] Increase in vertebral height is reversible during the years of spinal growth. Return of normal pressures and stress on the spine before skeletal maturation causes inhibition of vertical growth and al-

lows affected vertebrae to obtain normal proportions.[450]

Flat Vertebrae (Vertebra Plana). Flat-appearing vertebral bodies in children (vertebra plana) occur most frequently from histiocytosis, metastasis (particularly neuroblastoma), leukemia, Gaucher's disease, and infection* (Fig. 4–45). Diffuse multiple vertebra plana occurs in Morquio's disease, spondyloepiphyseal dysplasia, and other disorders.[713, 1212]

The earlier in life vertebra plana caused by histiocytosis occurs, the more likely the involved vertebral body will achieve normal or close to normal height, since there are more years available for bone growth.[608] If the vertebral body collapses after or near the end of the vertebral growth period, it will not recover its normal height.

In adults, flattened vertebral bodies occur in the presence of metastasis, myeloma, infection, Paget's disease, renal osteopathy, and other disorders,[996] but the degree of collapse is usually not as severe as that in children.

Beaked (Notched) Vertebrae. Vertebrae may demonstrate an anterior beak (notch) configuration, which may be located inferiorly or centrally (Table 4–3).

---

*Reference numbers 253, 286, 430, 996, 1164, 1330, 1359.

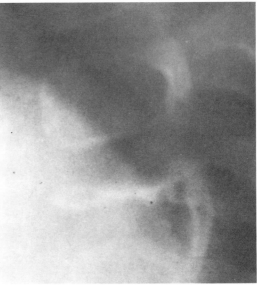

Figure 4–45. Vertebra plana. There is marked loss of vertebral height in this patient with histiocytosis.

Table 4–3. VERTEBRAL BEAKING

Inferior	Central
Hurler's syndrome	Morquio's syndrome
Cretinism	Achondroplasia
Morquio's syndrome	Spondyloepiphyseal
Achondroplasia	dysplasia
Diastrophic dwarfism	Normal (6–8 years, mild)
Trisomy 21	
Phenylketonuria	
Muscle hypotonia	
Trauma	
Normal children—early	
sitting	

Inferior Beaking. Anteroinferior beaking or notching of vertebral bodies usually occurs in children with neuromuscular disorders and muscle hypotonia and results from anterior herniation of the nucleus pulposus rather than primary hypoplasia (dysplasia) of the vertebral body[1248] (Figs. 4–46 and 4–47). Muscle hypotonia allows the child to be hyperflexed with exaggerated thoracolumbar kyphosis. This causes stress on the anterior disc with subsequent anterior disc herniation, thus preventing normal ossification in the herniated disc site.[70, 1248] This

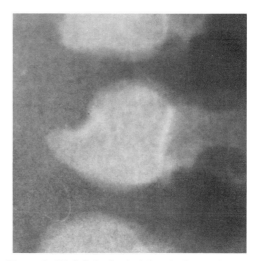

Figure 4–47. Inferior beak deformity in a patient with Hurler's syndrome. Lateral radiograph of the thoracolumbar junction.

leads eventually to a beaking deformity of the vertebra and a decrease in adjacent intervertebral disc space height. Beaking is more marked in the thoracolumbar region, particularly at the L1 level.[357a, 1248] Another possible cause of vertebral beaking found in the mucopolysaccharidoses might be the abnormal connective tissue that allows anterior disc protrusion in these disorders. Actual anterior disc herniation has been shown in a case of Hurler's syndrome[70, 1129a] (see Fig. 4–46).

Inferior beaking occurs in Hurler's syndrome,[70] cretinism,[357a, 370] Morquio's disease,[713, 1248] diastrophic dwarfism,[1085] achondroplasia, and in nondysplastic disorders such as Trisomy 21 and phenylketonuria, and in mentally retarded hypotonic children.[1248] It has been described in battered children[1129a, 1247] and following acute hyperflexion compression spinal injuries.[1247] Anterior vertebral beaking can develop in normal children, probably in those who are placed in or attain a sitting position before their paravertebral muscles are able to support them.[1248] This leads to exaggerated kyphosis of the thoracolumbar spine, with eventual inferior beaking.

While it is possible that bone dysplasia is responsible for the anteroinferior beaking deformity in some disorders, the occurrence of beaking in nondysplastic conditions speaks against this as a sole cause.

Central Beaking. In normal children around the age of 6 to 8 years, the annular

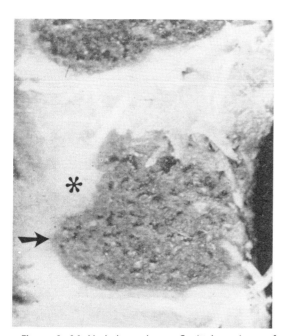

Figure 4–46. Hurler's syndrome. Sagittal specimen of a lumbar vertebral body demonstrating inferior beak deformity (arrow). Disc tissue has herniated anteriorly and inferiorly (asterisk). (From Strauss L: The pathology of gargoylism. Report of a case and review of the literature. Am J Pathol 24:855–887, 1948.)

cartilage rim produces an indentation on the upper and lower anterior vertebral margins on the lateral spine radiograph that causes a mild flat anterior depression superiorly and inferiorly[88, 160] (see Figs. 4–41 and 4–42). This gives the central portion of the vertebral body a "beaked" shape. This is present in many vertebrae and not more pronounced in the thoracolumbar junction. More pronounced abnormal anterior central beaking occurs in patients with Morquio's disease and achondroplasia (Fig. 4–48). Other radiographic signs can differentiate these disorders from normal patients with mild central beaking.

Concave Vertebrae. Diffuse weakening of vertebrae may lead to vertebral collapse. The appearance of the collapse depends upon the underlying process, integrity of the intervertebral disc, and the location in the vertebral column.

Concave-appearing vertebrae (Figs. 4–49 and 4–50) are found in disorders associated with diffuse weakening of bone, such as osteoporosis, osteomalacia, Paget's disease, uremic osteopathy (osteitis fibrosa cystica), diffuse metastatic disease, and multiple

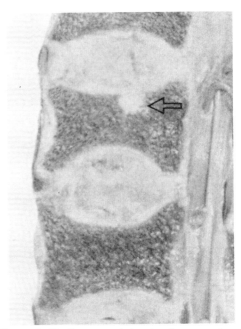

Figure 4–49. Biconcave deformity. Gross specimen of the spine. There is depression of superior and inferior vertebral margins in a patient with osteoporosis. Notice that the intervertebral discs have expanded. Intraosseous herniation of disc tissue (Schmorl's node) is present (arrow). (From Schmorl G, Junghanns H: The Human Spine in Health and Disease. New York: Grune & Stratton, 1971. Copyright 1971 by Georg Thieme Verlag.)

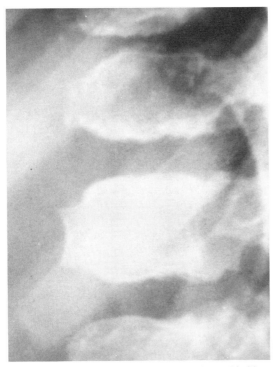

Figure 4–48. Central beaking in a patient with Morquio's syndrome. Lateral radiograph of the thoracolumbar junction demonstrating flattening of vertebral bodies and anterior central beak deformity.

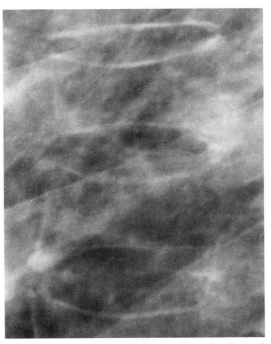

Figure 4–50. Biconcave deformity. Lateral radiograph of the spine demonstrates marked diminution in bone density (osteopenia). Biconcave deformity is noted, and vertebral margins are sharply defined.

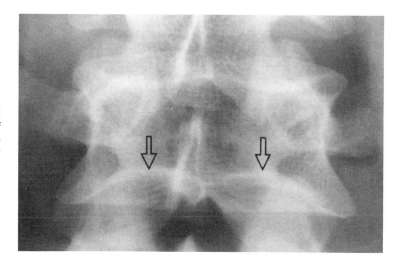

Figure 4–51. Cupid's bow configuration. Normal inferior parasagittal indentations on the inferior aspect of the vertebra (arrows), which when observed sideways, resemble the frame of an archer's (Cupid's) bow.

myeloma. The concave depressions are the result of the expansion of an intervertebral disc with normal turgor against the adjacent soft vertebral body.[1129a] This results in a smooth depression extending from vertebral end to vertebral end, with the central portion deepest. Both the upper and lower vertebral surfaces are involved. Concavity is most notable in the lower thoracic–upper lumbar spine.[1035] In the upper- and midthoracic spine, similar bone weakening processes cause anterior collapse (wedging), since the center of gravity, because of normal kyphosis, is located more toward the anterior aspect of the vertebrae in the erect posture. The term *fish vertebrae* is sometimes used to describe biconcavity of vertebrae, since the vertebrae of fish, which are cartilaginous, have a similar appearance radiographically.[1035] Concavity of the vertebral margin that appears with a sharply angled depression rather than with the smooth depression previously described has been observed in vertebrae invaded by tumor, even in the absence of visible bone destruction.[1099] However, caution should be used, since trauma may produce a similar result.

Cupid's Bow Configuration. In almost two thirds of normal individuals, parasagittal depressions develop in the posterior aspect of the inferior surface of at least one of the lower three lumbar vertebrae, forming the so-called Cupid's bow configuration on the AP radiograph and posteriorly on the lateral radiograph[401, 993] (Fig 4–51). The L4 level is most commonly affected. The deformity is usually symmetric, and there is no signifi-

cant difference in incidence from the late second decade to 60 years of age.[290] Although the etiology is unclear, Cupid's bow configuration may be caused by the turgor of the nucleus pulposus.

Posterior Concavities. Sometimes concavities occur on the upper and lower posterior margins of adult vertebrae and result from localized expansion of disc tissue.[1129a] These changes occur in the thoracic and lumbar portions of the spine and are best visualized on the lateral radiograph (Fig. 4–52). In the

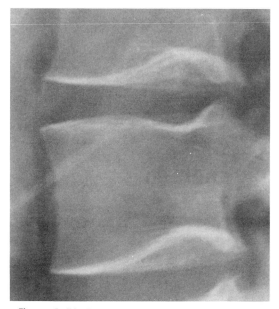

Figure 4–52. Posterior indentations of lumbar vertebrae caused by focal expansion of disc tissue. This is a normal variant.

thoracic spine, the focal concavities are smaller and more posterior, whereas on the lumbar spine, they are larger and extend to the anterior half of the vertebral body. Biconcavity may appear on the AP radiograph.[290] These depressions are easily differentiated from the cupid's bow depressions, which are parasagittal on the AP radiograph and only occur in the L3–L5 levels.

Focal Depressions (Schmorl's Nodes). Focal, asymptomatic depressions may develop in vertebrae and are due to intraosseous herniation of disc tissue (Schmorl's or cartilaginous nodes)[1026, 1129a] (Fig. 4–53). Any disorder that is associated with weakening of the cartilage end-plate or the subchondral zone of bone beneath the cartilage plate may allow disc tissue to herniate superiorly or inferiorly into the vertebral body.[1026, 1129a] Schmorl's nodes are detected in 38% of postmortem examinations and in 13.5% of radiographic examinations.[1129a] They occur most commonly in the lower thoracic and upper lumbar portions of the spine, and the lower cartilage plate is involved more commonly.[1026]

The cartilaginous plate may be weakened focally, causing decreased resistance to the pressure of the adjacent nucleus pulposus. These weak areas may lead to fissuring and subsequent intraosseous disc herniation.[1129a] Schmorl's nodes may also occur following degeneration of cartilage plates from aging.

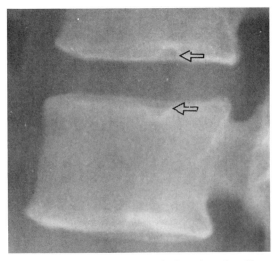

Figure 4–53. Schmorl's (cartilaginous) nodes. There are small radiolucencies surrounded by sclerotic margins in the subchondral region (arrows). These represent intraosseous herniation of disc tissue (Schmorl's nodes).

Disorders that cause weakening of subchondral bone destroy support of the cartilage plates, leading to collapse of the cartilage plate into the vertebra. Intervertebral disc follows the collapsed plate and protrudes into the vertebral body. Subchondral bone may be weakened by osteomalacia, Paget's disease, hyperparathyroidism and renal osteopathy, infection, tumor, or trauma.[1026] Schmorl's nodes may develop in about 8% of patients with osteoporosis; however, there is no association between the two.[114]

Radiographically, Schmorl's nodes appear as focal indentations or tiny radiolucencies in subchondral bone. The margins are usually sclerotic, and the degree of sclerosis is variable. Occasionally, the margins may be indistinct and may mimic a focal area of infection.

Limbus Vertebra. Intervertebral disc tissue may be displaced obliquely into the vertebral body between the cartilaginous end plate and the border of the adjacent vertebral rim[1129a] (Fig. 4–54). This is called the limbus vertebra and should not be mistaken for a fracture or destructive lesion,[458] particularly in younger patients whose ring apophyses have not fully developed.[383] It occurs most frequently in the anterosuperior corner of midlumbar vertebrae, but the inferior, posterior, and lateral vertebral margins may be affected less frequently.[1129a] Limbus vertebra is asymptomatic.[1377] Radiographically, limbus vertebra appears as a triangular or oval bone density adjacent to the vertebra, with sclerotic margins on either side of the separation. Tiny densities representing callus formation may be present in the region.

Central Depression ("H" Vertebra). In this type of vertebral depression, the superior and inferior ends of vertebral bodies are depressed centrally, manifesting sharp, flat margins (Fig. 4–55) (Table 4–4). The central nature of the depression forms an "H" shape, or "Lincoln log" configuration. This type of vertebral depression is characteristic of sickle cell hemoglobinopathy[1041] but has also been reported in renal osteopathy,[1384] Gaucher's disease,[1138] homocystinuria,[1329] in two individuals without hemoglobinopathy (one with hereditary spherocytosis and the other with osteopenia),[1072] and in one case of thalassemia major.[181]

To understand the pathophysiology for the development of the H-shaped vertebra in

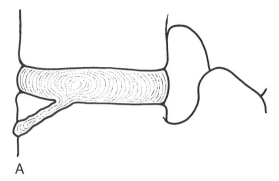

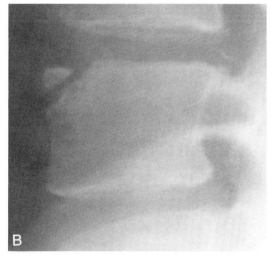

Figure 4–54. Limbus vertebra. *A,* Diagrammatic representation of the lateral aspect of the discovertebral junction demonstrating anteroinferior herniation of disc tissue separating a bone fragment. *B,* Lateral radiograph of the thoracic spine demonstrating a limbus vertebra with the bony separation at the anterosuperior vertebral margin.

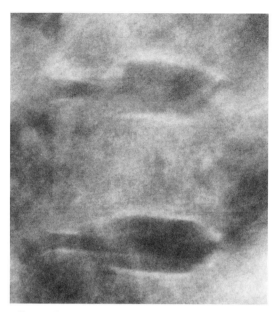

Figure 4–55. Central vertebral depression. There is depression of the central portion of the superior and inferior aspects of the vertebral body. The floor of the depression is flat and smooth, and the margins are sclerotic and distinct. This configuration resembles the letter "H" and has been called the "H" or "Lincoln log" vertebra. This patient has sickle cell anemia.

sickle cell hemoglobinopathy better, it is important to review the changes that take place in the intraosseous arterial blood supply of the subchondral zone of the vertebral body.

In both children and adults, the bone beneath the cartilage end plate may be divided into zones of arterial supply composed of nutrient arteries centrally and branches of metaphyseal, periosteal, and peripheral arteries peripherally[1000, 1001] (Fig. 4–56). The metaphyseal branches arise from the metaphyseal anastomoses that incompletely surround the vertebral body, and the peripheral arteries arise from secondary periosteal arteries[998] that run along the vertebral surface (Fig. 4–57).

In infants and small children, all of the intraosseous arteries are joined by widespread anastomoses[999–1001] (Fig. 4–58). By the age of 7 years, the anstomoses are less abundant, and by the age of 15 years, they have progressively involuted. When adult age has been reached, the intraosseous anastomoses have involuted completely.[1000, 1001] Thus, in the adult as well as the adolescent,[1001] branches from the nutrient, segmental, metaphyseal, and peripheral arteries are end-arteries.[133, 1000, 1341]

In sickle cell hemoglobinopathy, intra-arterial sickling has the potential to produce bone ischemia and cause interference with vertebral growth. However, the vertebrae of young children are unaffected owing to abundant intraosseous anastomoses. With involution of anastomoses, vertebrae are

Table 4–4. CENTRAL VERTEBRAL DEPRESSION ("H" VERTEBRA)

Sickle cell anemia
Uremic osteopathy (renal osteodystrophy)
Gaucher's disease
Homocystinuria
Hereditary spherocytosis (rare)
Thalassemia (rare)
Normal (mild)

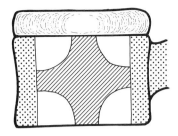

A

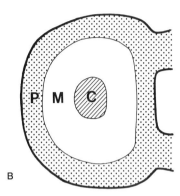

B

Figure 4–56. Zones of intraosseous arterial supply of an adult lumbar vertebral body. *A,* Sagittal view. *B,* Axial view of the subchondral region. The hatched area in *A* represents the central core and equatorial zone supplied by nutrient arteries and anterolateral equatorial arteries, respectively. The hatched area in *B* represents the central core supplied by nutrient arteries. The clear area represents the midzone supplied by the metaphyseal anastomoses. The dotted area represents the peripheral zone supplied by peripheral anastomoses. (Adapted from Ratcliffe JF: The arterial anatomy of the adult human lumbar vertebral body: A microarteriographic study. J Anat 131:57–79, 1980.)

CORONAL SECTION

METAPHYSEAL SECTION

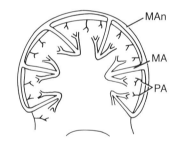

Figure 4–57. Diagrammatic representation of intraosseous arteries of an adult lumbar vertebral body. *Key:* **ALEA** = anterolateral equatorial artery; **LA** = lumbar artery; **MA** = metaphyseal artery; **MAn** = metaphyseal anastomosis; **NA** = nutrient artery; **PA** = peripheral artery; **PPA** = primary periosteal artery; **SPA** = secondary periosteal artery. (Adapted from Ratcliffe JF: The arterial anatomy of the adult human lumbar vertebral body: A microarteriographic study. J Anat 131:57–79, 1980.)

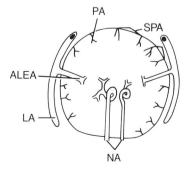

SAGITTAL SECTION

EQUATORIAL SECTION

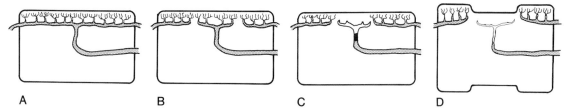

Figure 4–58. Diagrammatic representation of changing intraosseous arterial supply to the subchondral (metaphyseal equivalent) zone in a patient with sickle cell hemaglobinopathy to demonstrate the formation of central vertebral depression ("H" vertebra). *A,* Arterial supply in a child demonstrating anastomoses among the peripheral, midzone, and central core arteries. Anastomoses prevent ischemia by vascular occlusion. *B,* Partial involution of anastomoses. This begins by about the age of 7 years. *C,* Involution of anastomoses continues, so that the central portion of the subchondral region becomes vulnerable to intraosseous occlusion of the nutrient arteries in the central core. *D,* Formation of the "H" vertebra. During the growth spurt, growth is inhibited in the central section owing to ischemia, whereas growth continues unabated in the peripheral and midzones.

more susceptible to the effect of the sickling process and the production of ischemia. Enchondral bone growth may be inhibited in the central portion of subchondral bone and cartilaginous growthplate, which are supplied by end-arterial branches of the nutrient arteries. In the peripheral portions of the subchondral zone, where the vessels are more numerous and are in direct communication with paravertebral anastomoses, bone ischemia does not occur, and bone growth proceeds unhindered. It is not until the spine undergoes rapid growth, usually after the age of 10, that the central depression deformities become apparent,[1041] and this corresponds to progressive involution of collateral circulation.[1000, 1001] Thus, the central depression alterations develop before adult life.

There is another theory as to the etiology of "H" vertebrae. Ischemia of subchondral bone causes weakening and partial collapse of subchondral bone, with subsequent indentation by normal intervertebral disc tissue (Fig. 4–59).[60, 292, 554] Peripheral subchondral bone is not involved, owing to collateral circulation. However, the symmetry of depressions on numerous vertebrae in sickle cell hemoglobinopathy may militate against the theory of stress of weight-bearing and disc protrusion on ischemic weakened bone as the sole cause of "H' vertebrae.

There are differences between the radiographic appearance of the "H" vertebra in sickle cell disease and biconcave vertebrae (see Fig. 4–39). In sickle cell hemoglobinopathy, the depression is flat and the degree of central depression is equal in both superior and inferior aspects of each vertebral body as

well as throughout most of the spine.[1041] This is not so in bone softening disorders such as osteoporosis and osteomalacia, where the degree of depression is smooth and extends from one edge of the vertebra to the other.

In other disorders that demonstrate the "H" vertebrae, such as homocystinuria and Gaucher's disease, underlying vascular compromise also causes ischemia, although the etiology and mechanism may be different. The

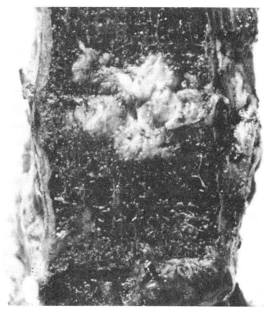

Figure 4–59. Gross section of lumbar vertebrae from a patient with sickle cell anemia. There is marked hyperplasia of the marrow. Note the central depression and intraosseous disc tissue protruding in both directions into the depressions. (From Diggs LW: Bone and joint lesions in sickle-cell disease. Clin Orthop 52:119–143, 1967.)

degree of depression is not as pronounced as that found in sickle cell hemoglobinopathy. In homocystinuria, ischemia is the result of vaso-occlusive disease caused by narrowing of the lumen from intimal and medial fibrosis in addition to occlusion by thrombosis.[1329] In Gaucher's disease,[516, 1138] glucocerebroside-laden cells (Gaucher's cells) infiltrate and pack red marrow, compressing intraosseous vessels. This leads to ischemia and deficient endochondral ossification beginning early in life.[516] Pressure atrophy of bone also occurs. Serial examinations of patients with Gaucher's disease demonstrate initial collapse of the entire vertebral body, possibly caused by infarction with subsequent weakening of bone under normal weight-bearing stress. This is followed by a differential rate of recovery—normal at the periphery of the body where collateral peripheral vessels exist, and minimal at the central depressed site.[1138] Continued recovery leads to the "H" vertebral body.

In patients with uremic osteopathy (renal osteodystrophy), the cause of central depression is unknown. There is resorption of subchondral bone, with associated weakening and collapse, allowing intervertebral discs to expand against or herniate into the vertebral body.[1024] The peripehral annular portion of the vertebral body does not participate in this depression, probably since it is stronger cortical bone that does not undergo resorption to any significant degree. On the other hand, it is difficult to imagine that the central depression, which is so symmetric at multiple levels, is caused solely by disc protrusion. Subchondral bone may be weakened by ischemia, since patients on prolonged hemodialysis develop accelerated atherosclerosis.[1384] The administration of steroids to patients during treatment may cause ischemia either by fat embolism or by hypercoagulability of blood.

Radiographically, in uremic osteopathy the degree of depression of the end-plate is mild, and the subchondral margin of bone may be poorly defined, thus differentiating this disorder from sickle cell disease. The central depression alterations need not be associated with the characteristic "rugger jersey" appearance of renal osteopathy, although its presence easily establishes the correct diagnosis. Subchondral bone resorption occurs in adults (after spinal growth has ceased), so it seems that in this disorder,

central vertebral depression is not related to inhibition of bone growth.

Central vertebral depression has also been reported in normal patients without hemoglobinopathy.[1072] Radiologic changes of depression were extremely mild in a case of congenital hereditary spherocytosis and in a patient with osteopenia.

Vertebral Scalloping. Scalloping is a descriptive term that refers to an exaggeration in the normal concavity of a vertebral body surface. It occurs most frequently in the posterior aspect of the vertebral body, however, anterior and lateral forms also occur.

Posterior Scalloping. The pathophysiologic causes of posterior scalloping (Table 4–5) vary and may be divided into broad categories: physiologic, increased intraspinal pressure, dural ectasia, small spinal canal, and bone disorders[868] (Figure 4–60).

Physiologic. Fifty-six percent of normal individuals have mild to moderate posterior scalloping[868] that occasionally may resemble pathologic scalloping. However, it only occurs in the lower lumbar spine and is not associated with other alterations, such as pedicle erosion and wide interpedicular distance.

Increased Intraspinal Pressure. It should be recalled that during development the spinal canal adapts to the presence of the growing spinal cord. Normal intraspinal pressure on a small canal or abnormal pressure on a normal canal can cause posterior scalloping, particularly if present during the growing years. Posterior scalloping may oc-

Table 4–5. POSTERIOR VERTEBRAL SCALLOPING

Physiologic
Increased Intraspinal Pressure
  Tumor
  Syringohydromyelia
  Uncontrolled communicating hydrocephalus
Dural Ectasia
  Neurofibromatosis
  Marfan's syndrome
  Ehlers-Danlos syndrome
  Morquio's syndrome
Narrow Spinal Canal
  Achondroplasia
Bone Disorders
  Neurofibromatosis
  Hurler's syndrome
  Morquio's syndrome
  Acromegaly

Adapted from Mitchell GE, Lourie H, Berne AS: The various causes of scalloped vertebrae with notes on their pathogenesis. Radiology 89:67–74, 1967.

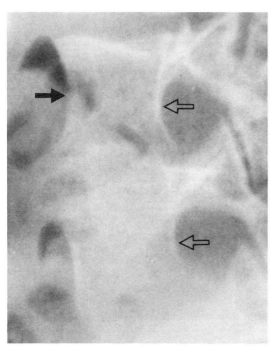

Figure 4–60. Vertebral scalloping. Posterior (open arrows) and anterior vertebral scalloping (closed arrow) of thoracic vertebrae in a patient with neurofibromatosis.

cur from intraspinal tumors, such as ependymomas, astrocytomas, congenital lipomas (since they were present early in life during growth of the canal), as well as syringohydromyelia and uncontrolled communicating hydrocephalus.[868, 1160]

Dural Ectasia. In patients with connective tissue disorders, the dura may not be structurally strong. Thus, normal pulsations of cerebrospinal fluid (CSF) cause bulging of a weakened dura and consequently allow for pulsations and increased pressure on the posterior aspect of the vertebral body, leading to posterior scalloping. Disorders of connective tissue that cause posterior scalloping include neurofibromatosis[182, 548, 1096] (see Fig. 4–60), Marfan's syndrome,[404, 904] Ehlers-Danlos syndrome,[868] hypertrophic neuropathy,[74] and possibly Hurler's syndrome and Morquio's disorder. Neurofibromatosis is probably the most common cause of posterior scalloping in patients whose scalloping is not physiologic. In neurofibromatosis, the scalloping is more likely to result from dural ectasia from a primary mesodermal dysplasia of meninges[1096] or primary bone dysplasia[548] or both[182, 1096] than from pressure erosion by a neurofibroma.[182]

Narrow Spinal Canal. In achondroplasia there is congenital narrowing of the spinal canal (canal stenosis) due to the presence of short pedicles and a decrease in the interpedicular distance.[712] The dura is normal, but the pulsations of the growing thecal sac on the confined spinal canal cause posterior scalloping.

Bone Disorders. In neurofibromatosis, posterior scalloping could be due to a primary bone dysplasia, resulting in a softened, weakened vertebra that is slowly eroded by normal pulsations of CSF pressure transmitted by the dura. It may develop in the mucopolysaccharidoses of Hurler's syndrome and Morquio's disease[868] from either structurally weakened vertebrae or bone dysplasia in addition to connective tissue abnormalities.

In acromegaly, moderate posterior scalloping occurs in two thirds of the cases, and some degree of scalloping is present in all cases.[1236] There is overgrowth of bone and soft tissues,[1221] so that the dura becomes thickened and along with CSF pulsations may erode the vertebra posteriorly. Also, as the vertebra enlarges, there is no resistance to growth anteriorly and laterally, but there is resistance posteriorly. Thus the vertebra is confronted by the pulsating thecal sac, which not only prevents its posterior growth but at the same time erodes the posterior vertebral margin. However, it has been reported that there is a lack of periosteum on the posterior vertebral surface, so that periosteal new bone growth occurs anteriorly and laterally but not posteriorly.[681]

Anterior Scalloping. Anterior erosions of vertebral bodies may be caused by pulsations of a thoracic aneurysm (thoracic and upper lumbar spine),[730, 1083] pulsations of tortuous iliac arteries, paravertebral tumor (metastasis, lymphoma, neurofibroma, and sarcoma), abscess, or bony dysplasia of neurofibromatosis[182] (see Fig. 4–60). A pseudoscalloping appearance may occur on the lateral radiograph in patients with osteopenia and anterolateral osteophyte formation[1296] or in those with overlying densities.

Lateral Scalloping. Erosion of the lateral margin of the vertebral body is usually caused by tumor (metastasis, lymphoma, neurofibroma, sarcoma), abscess, or bony dysplasia of neurofibromatosis. Tortuosity of vertebral arteries in the cervical region and dilated lumbar venous collaterals with or

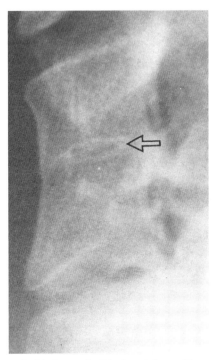

Figure 4–61. Congenital block vertebrae of the cervical spine. The vertebral bodies are fused except for a central disc remnant (arrow). Posterior elements (not visualized) were fused as well. The height of the two fused vertebral bodies and their disc remnant, as well as the disc below, is roughly equal to the height of two normal vertebral bodies, their intervertebral disc, and one adjacent disc.

without vena cava obstruction may also cause lateral vertebral scalloping.[644, 1179, 1383]

Congenital Block Vertebra. Block vertebra is a developmental disturbance in segmentation in which there is congenital fusion of two vertebral bodies in the middle of which is a thin disc remnant[655, 1129a] (Fig. 4–61). Radiographically, the height of a block vertebra with the normal disc below usually equals the height of two other nonfused vertebrae with their two discs.[655, 1129a] Trabeculae run through the fused segments, and the remnant disc space may or may not be visible. Block vertebrae occur more commonly in the cervical and thoracic regions of the spine, with C2–C3 and C5–C6 being the most common cervical sites of fusion.[135, 721] Block vertebrae do not alter the length of the spine unless there are numerous block vertebrae—a rare occurrence.[1129a] Block vertebrae usually occur in an otherwise normal individual but may be seen in patients with other skeletal abnormalities, such as dysraphism or Klippel-Feil syndrome.[838, 1155]

Hemivertebra. The vertebral column is composed of a right half and a left half embryologically. Persistence of one half of a vertebra at the cartilaginous stage results in unilateral ossification of the vertebral body (hemivertebra)[1129a] (Fig. 4–62). The ossification center, originally cuboid in shape, becomes wedge-shaped with the apex medially. Hemivertebra is more common in the thoracolumbar spine. Scoliosis develops following weight-bearing. Unbalanced multiple hemivertebrae have a poor prognosis for treatment. Multiple hemivertebrae may be balanced and not develop a progressive curvature. Less frequently, hemivertebra develops with ossification of the posterior half, the anterior half remaining fibrocartilaginous. This leads to kyphosis following the pressures of weight-bearing. In this form the posterior half of the vertebral body may be displaced into the spinal canal. Hemivertebra may be isolated or combined with other, often extensive, vertebral anomalies as well as congenital disorders, including congenital heart disease.

Butterfly Vertebra. This developmental abnormality represents sagittal cleavage of the vertebral body, resulting from sagittal division of the notochord, which contains disc tissue.[1129a] The vertebral surfaces become depressed, leading to the "butterfly"

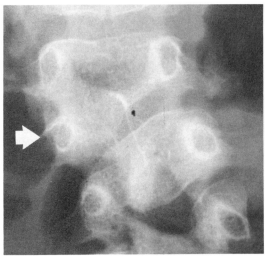

Figure 4–62. Hemivertebra. The right half of a vertebral body and its pedicle (arrow) are fused with the vertebra above. The left half is absent. Note the spinal curvature.

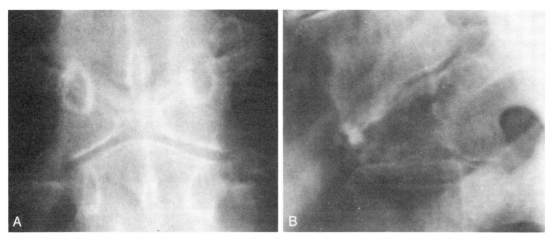

Figure 4–63. Butterfly vertebra. *A*, Anteroposterior view demonstrating wedge-shaped butterfly vertebra. The central zone consists of disc tissue. *B*, Lateral radiograph demonstrating anterior wedging and kyphotic deformity.

configuration when viewed on the AP radiograph (Fig. 4–63). The stress of walking eventually causes bilateral lateral displacement of the two halves. Butterfly vertebra is frequently associated with abnormalities of the gastrointestinal and central nervous systems.

Vascular Channels. There are focal defects (notches) in the anterior and posterior aspects of vertebral bodies that represent vascular channels for both arteries and veins[785, 1298] (see Fig. 4–40). The posterior notch is relatively larger in infants than in adults and remains visible radiographically throughout life.[1298] The notches are equidistant from the upper and lower vertebral surfaces.[681] The anterior notch is normally sharply visible up to the age of 3 to 6 years, although it may be faintly visible in older children as slitlike with sclerotic margins[1052] (Fig. 4–64). Persistence or widening of the anterior vascular notches occurs in sickle cell anemia and is due to venous engorgement from sludging of blood flow. Forty-six percent of patients with sickle cell disease in the 3 to 6 year age range demonstrated prominent anterior vascular grooves compared with 8% in a control group.[1052] Similar widening or persistence of the anterior vascular groove has been reported in other marrow hyperplastic or replacement disorders, such as thalassemia (Fig. 4–65), metastatic neuroblastoma, and Gaucher's disease, and is probably also due to venous congestion or increase in arterial requirement or both.[785] In these disorders, the margins of the anterior notch are often poorly defined, whereas in sickle cell disease they appear more sharply defined. A prominent anterior notch has also been seen in osteopetrosis and pycnodysostosis and is probably due to venous stasis caused by encroachment of the marrow space by abnormal osteoid.[319, 351, 354, 785, 849] A posterior vascular groove may be observed throughout life.

Abnormalities in Density

The density of vertebral bodies is best appreciated on the lateral radiograph, and changes in density, either increased (osteoblastic, osteosclerotic) or decreased (osteo-

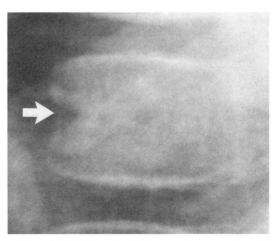

Figure 4–64. Normal anterior vascular groove (arrow). The margins are sharp and sclerotic. Compare with the gross specimen shown in Figure 4–40A.

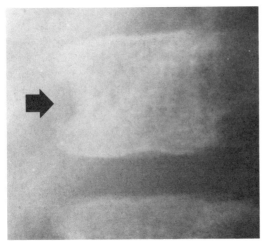

Figure 4–65. Wide persistent anterior vascular groove (arrow) in an 8 year old boy with thalassemia. The vascular groove is poorly marginated. (from Mandell GA, Kricun ME: Exaggerated anterior vertebral notching. Radiology 131:367–369, 1979.)

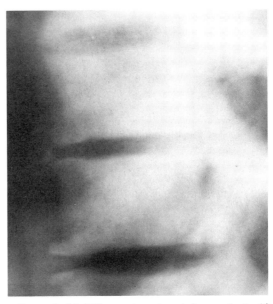

Figure 4–66. Diffuse osteosclerosis in a patient with diffuse metastatic disease from carcinoma of the prostate gland.

penic), may be diffuse or patchy or may involve one vertebral level or part of a vertebral complex.

Diffuse Increase in Density. Diffuse osteosclerotic change at multiple spinal levels is caused by metastasis from carcinoma of the prostate in elderly males (Fig. 4–66), carcinoma of the breast, or, less commonly, leukemia[755] and other metastatic tumors. Other causes include uremic osteopathy (renal osteodystrophy), myelosclerosis, sickle cell disease in adults, Paget's disease, and a number of less common disorders, such as osteopetrosis, pycnodysostosis, mastocytosis, and fluorosis.

In patients with osteosclerotic metastasis, underlying tumor incites surrounding normal bone to produce additional new bone (reactive bone).[439, 859]

Patchy Increase in Density. Patchy areas of osteosclerotic activity more likely indicate metastasis from carcinoma of the prostate, carcinoma of the breast,[859] lymphoma (usually in a young adult), treated metastatic lesions (particularly from carcinoma of the breast), Paget's disease, and, rarely, tuberous sclerosis,[41, 1260] mastocytosis, myelosclerosis,[954] sarcoidosis,[106, 129, 1238] myeloma,* and melorheostosis.[442] Uremic osteopathy may sometimes demonstrate patchy osteosclerotic changes more frequent in secondary

hyperparathyroidism than in primary hyperparathyroidism.[701]

Ivory Vertebra. Occasionally, osteosclerotic reaction may be so extensive and uniform that the entire vertebral body is involved—the so-called ivory vertebra (Fig. 4–67 and Table 4–6). One or more vertebrae may demonstrate this abnormality, and the underlying process may include the posterior elements as well. The ivory vertebra is caused by a number of disorders but is most commonly seen in metastasis most often from carcinoma of the prostate gland or

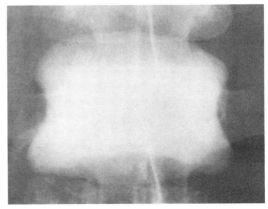

Figure 4–67. "Ivory vertebra." The L2 vertebra is diffusely sclerotic, obliterating definition of pedicles. This was caused by metastasis from carcinoma of the colon.

---

*Reference numbers 96, 137, 204, 315, 325, 355.

Table 4–6. IVORY VERTEBRA

Metastasis
Lymphoma
Paget's disease
Osteosarcoma
Chronic osteomyelitis
Melorheostosis
Chordoma (rare)
Myeloma (rare)
Osteoid osteoma (rare)

carcinoma of the breast,[1016] other metastatic tumors,[180, 372, 403] lymphoma,[479] Paget's disease,[519, 922] osteosarcoma, and, rarely, chordoma,[1140] myeloma,[1016, 1060] chronic osteomyelitis,[348, 922] melorheostosis,[442] and osteoid osteoma.[348]

Bandlike Increase in Density. Bandlike zones of osteosclerotic density in the superior and inferior subchondral regions of the vertebral body represent the so-called rugger jersey spine and are seen in patients with

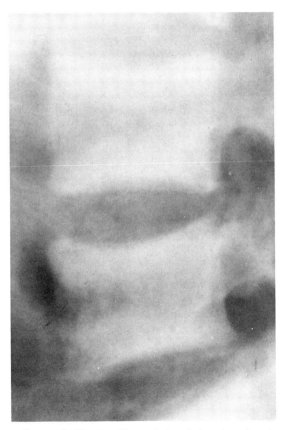

Figure 4–68. Bandlike subchondral osteosclerosis ("rugger jersey spine") in a patient with uremic osteopathy. The inner margin of the sclerotic zone is poorly defined.

uremic osteopathy (renal osteodystrophy) and secondary hyperparathyroidism,[1015] although they rarely may develop in primary hyperparathyroidism[701] (Fig. 4–68). The exact etiology is unknown. It has been shown that parathormone in small doses stimulates osteoblastic activity.[1149] Osteosclerosis may be related to the inhibiting effect on the resorption of bone by thyrocalcitonin,[701] the resistance of osteoid to the action of parathormone,[1157] or the high calcium-phosphate product with deposition of mineral into the metaphyseal equivalent subchondral region.

Another manifestation of bandlike sclerosis occurs in patients on long-term steroid therapy or in patients who have Cushing's disease. Microfractures due to associated osteoporosis undergo healing in the subchondral region, leading to osteosclerosis.[1035] However, the remainder of the vertebral body is osteopenic and often demonstrates biconcave depressions. Subchondral bandlike osteosclerosis may occur in mild forms of osteopetrosis and pycnodysostosis and in Paget's disease.

Focal Osteosclerosis. Osteosclerotic metastasis may appear as a focal round or oval area of increased density and again most commonly results from carcinoma of the prostate, carcinoma of the breast, or lymphoma. The margins are often irregular.

Benign focal areas of osteosclerosis, such as enostoses, or bone islands, occur within the vertebral body (Fig. 4–69). These occur in the spine in 1%[931] to 14%[1023] of individu-

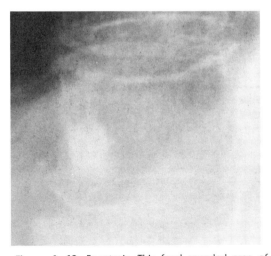

Figure 4–69. Enostosis. This focal rounded area of vertebral sclerosis represents a benign bone island (enostosis).

als and are of no clinical significance. Only about 30% can be visualized on the radiograph. They vary in size from 2 × 2 mm to 6 × 10 mm and usually appear as a single round or oval area of sclerosis, with spiculated margins often close to the vertebral margin. They may increase or decrease in size and even disappear.[95, 128, 1174]

Osteosclerosis occurs with underlying intervertebral osteochondrosis (degenerative disease of the disc) (Fig. 4–70). The intervertebral disc is narrow, and the discovertebral margin is sharply defined.[95, 1016] Intraosseous herniation of disc tissue (Schmorl's node) may produce focal areas of sclerosis.[1016] Occult discovertebral trauma may stimulate osteosclerotic reaction, forming large areas of sclerosis adjacent to the anteroinferior vertebral margin.[799, 1107] The configuration may be dome-shaped ("hemispherical" sclerosis)[295] and is often present in opposing vertebrae. The intervertebral disc is diminished in height in around 90% of cases. A central lucency is frequently present.[1107] Other similarly large areas of sclerosis may be observed without disc narrowing.[819] In osteomyelitis, osteosclerosis and disc narrowing are prominent features; however, the discovertebral margin is poorly defined.

Bone Within Bone. A "bone within a bone" configuration refers to either a scle-

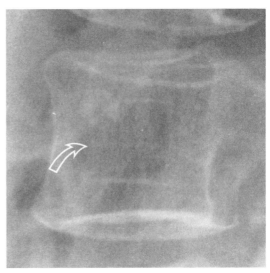

Figure 4–71. "Bone within bone." There is a faint sclerotic outline in the shape of the smaller vertebra within an adult-sized vertebral body (arrow). This patient had tuberculosis of the hip around the age of 5 years, and the inner outline of the vertebral body approximates the size of the vertebral body when the tuberculous insult took place.

rotic smaller-shaped vertebral body image ("ghost" vertebra [see Fig. 4–231]) or the sclerotic outline of a smaller vertebra within the vertebral body itself (Fig. 4–71 and Table 4–7). The linear form of the "bone within bone" appearance can be seen in 50% of normal infants under 2 months of age.[127] It could also indicate a previous severe systemic illness or chronic intermittent disease.[414] It occurs after radiation therapy[127] and in various conditions, including osteopetrosis, generalized infection, heavy metal intoxication,[414] such as from bismuth or lead,[155] and numerous other disorders.[414] These latter disorders may cause cessation of bone growth (growth arrest) followed by recovery when the problem is resolved. With recovery, chondroblastic and osteoblastic activity resumes, leading to the sclerotic lines.

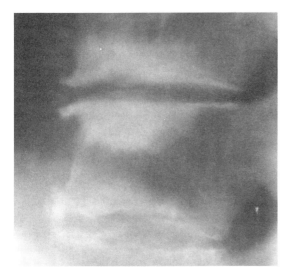

Figure 4–70. Intervertebral osteochondrosis. In addition to intervertebral disc narrowing, there is intense sclerosis in the anterior two thirds of opposing subchondral regions of adjacent vertebrae.

Table 4–7. BONE WITHIN BONE

Normal
Severe systemic illness
Osteopetrosis
Heavy metal intoxication
Generalized infection
Following radiation therapy
Thorotrast
Other disorders

The size of the "bone in bone" configuration is similar to the size of the vertebra at the time of insult. The "bone within bone" appearance in long bones has also been attributed to nutritional disturbances,[938] but this has not been so in the spine. "Bone within bone" may persist into adult life.[414]

A sclerotic "ghost" vertebra within a vertebral body has been described in patients who have received previous Thorotrast (thorium dioxide in dextran) contrast during childhood.[1176, 1261] In these patients, thorium (an alpha emitter) is taken up by the reticuloendothelial system and remains there throughout life because of its long radiation half-life. Only a small amount, however, is found in bones, and that amount is located almost entirely within cancellous bone. Radiographically, the "ghost" vertebra is similar in size and appearance to the vertebra seen at the time the Thorotrast was administered. The "ghost" vertebra is thought to be caused by chronic radiation osteitis from continuous local radiation.[1261] Similar "ghost" vertebral changes can be seen in osteopetrosis.

Diffuse Decrease in Bone Density. The vertebral bodies consist of cancellous (trabecular) bone surrounded by relatively thin cortical (compact) bone. Vertical and horizontal trabeculae are present within cancellous bone and are surrounded by marrow. Significant trabecular bone destruction or resorption must take place before changes are visible radiographically.[38] Technical factors in obtaining the radiograph may cause normal vertebrae to "appear" osteopenic or cause osteopenic vertebrae to "appear" normal in density.

Decrease in the number of trabeculae is a reflection of decrease in bone mass (osteopenia) and is difficult to assess radiographically in its early stages, although it may be appreciated in more advanced disease. Osteopenic changes occur as a result of normal aging, multiple myeloma, metastatic disease, excessive endogenous or exogeous steroids, marrow replacement, disuse, and other disorders.

Focal Osteopenia. Localized areas of decreased bone density may occur from bone destruction, either from tumor or tumorlike conditions, infection, or histiocytosis. Focal radiolucency in subchondral bone may represent Schmorl's node and should not be mistaken for metastasis or infection[1026] (see

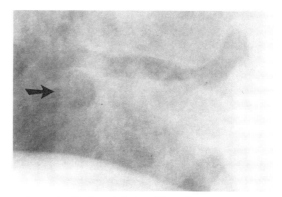

Figure 4–72. Pseudolesion. There is an apparent osteolytic lesion in the vertebral body (arrow). This is a pseudolesion composed of outlining pulmonary vessels and aerated lung tissue.

Fig. 4–53). Occasionally the combination of osteopenia and overlying osteophytes[1296] or pulmonary vessels may cause a "pseudolesion" appearance (Fig. 4–72) on the lateral radiograph.

Intraosseous Vacuum Phenomenon. Gas density may be observed within the vertebral body associated with vertebral collapse[134, 782] (Fig. 4–73). This represents a vacuum phenomenon and may be caused by local bone ischemia associated with vertebral fracture, collapse, and nonhealing.[782] Osteopenia, trauma, exogenous steroids, and disorders with vasculitis are associated underlying factors.[871] Occasionally gas density may be associated with underlying primary or metastatic tumor,[694, 1033] and, rarely, it may be produced by gas-forming organisms.[89, 963]

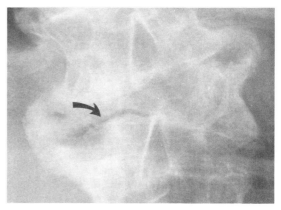

Figure 4–73. Intraosseous vacuum phenomenon. There is a cleft containing air density (arrow) within a collapsed vertebral body.

Pedicles

During the period of chondrification, each vertebral segment develops from six chondrification centers (three pairs): two for the vertebral body, two for the costal elements, and one for each side of the vertebral arch.[504, 670] In each neural arch, outgrowths form the pedicle, superior and inferior articular processes, and transverse process.

Ossification of the neural arch begins in the single center during the tenth fetal week and eventually extends anteriorly to form the pedicles.[1129a] The pedicles are not ossified until a few months after birth[923] and are separated from the centrum by a zone of cartilage (neurocentral synchondroses), which should not be mistaken for a fracture. Fusion of pedicle with the vertebral body occurs between the third and sixth years.[1129a] The pedicles contain red marrow in childhood but little red marrow in adult life.[692] Arterial and venous blood supply to and around the pedicle region is abundant.[387, 692]

Views

Thoracic and lumbar pedicles are best visualized on the AP radiograph.[352] Additionally, in the lumbar spine, they are well defined on the oblique radiograph as the "eye of the Scotty dog," which is made up by the bony cortex of the pedicle viewed on end.[136] Cervical pedicles are not as well defined on the anteroposterior radiograph as thoracic and lumbar pedicles, so it may be necessary to obtain 45 degree oblique views in order to evaluate anomalies of cervical pedicles.[48, 670]

Normal

The upper three cervical pedicles are rarely visualized, and the fourth through sixth cervical pedicles are difficult to examine.[352, 1175] Pedicles are more or less round in the lower cervical, upper thoracic, and lumbar spines, although lumbar pedicles may also appear triangular[352] (see Figs. 4–19 and 4–25). Lumbar pedicles are larger than cervical and thoracic pedicles, since they sustain greater stress from weight-bearing. The margin of pedicles is sclerotic, is well defined, and measures 1 to 2 mm in thickness. The medial border is

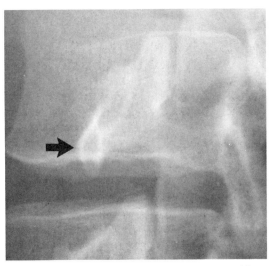

Figure 4–74. "Two-eyed Scotty dog." In this oblique radiograph of the lumbar spine, the "Scotty dog" has a double eye appearance (arrow). This represents a prominent mamillary process.

usually convex but may normally be flat[1175] from C4 to C7.[352] In the thoracolumbar region, thinning of pedicles is normal,[76, 194] and the medial border may occasionally be mildly concave.[352, 1175] The medial border of the pedicles above the level of T7, however, is never concave, and the observation of such concavity probably indicates underlying intraspinal mass.[352] Occasionally on the oblique lumbar radiograph, the pedicle has an unusual configuration, such as the "two-eyed Scotty dog," which represents a prominent mamillary process[1038] (Fig. 4–74).

Abnormalities in Size and Shape

Congenital abnormalities of pedicles are rare. None were discovered in the lumbosacral spine of 4200 skeletons.[1065] In a series of 12 cases of solitary kidneys, 16.6% had pedicle abnormalities.[1379a] Since development of the pedicle is closely related to that of other surrounding neural arch structures, it is not surprising to find pedicle abnormalities associated with those of the laminae, articular processes, and transverse processes.[670, 1220] Various abnormalities in pedicle size and shape may give a clue to the underlying disorder (Table 4–8).

Hypoplasia and Aplasia. These abnormalities may develop in otherwise normal in-

Table 4–8. PEDICLE ABNORMALITIES

Absent
  Tumor
  Congenital
  Histiocytosis
  Infection (rare)
Hypoplasia
  Neurofibromatosis
  Congenital
  Renal abnormalities
  Following radiation therapy
Narrow
  Normal (T Spine)
  Intraspinal tumor
  Dural ectasia
  Dysraphism
  Scoliosis
  Spondylolisthesis
Large
  Contralateal abnormalities of vertebral arch
  Neurofibromatosis
  Paget's disease
  Expansile tumors and tumorlike conditions
  Infection
  Histiocytosis
  Normal

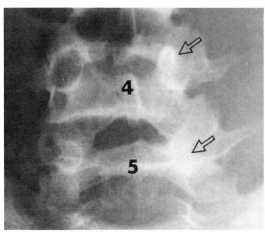

Figure 4–75. Hypoplasia of pedicles. The pedicles of L4 and L5 are hypoplastic (arrows). Corresponding transverse processes are hypoplastic as well. This patient has neurofibromatosis. (From Mandell GA: The pedicle in neurofibromatosis. AJR 130:675–678, 1978. Copyright 1978 by the American Roentgen Ray Society.)

dividuals or may be associated with disorders such as neurofibromatosis,[784] renal abnormalities,[1379a] and other conditions. Hypoplasia (Fig. 4–75) and aplasia (Fig. 4–76) may occur alone but are almost always associated with a deficiency in the ipsilateral neural arch,* particularly the superior articular process.[781] Deficiency in the dorsal transverse process[259, 504, 923, 1220] and ipsilateral inferior articular process above may be noted.[1332] These alterations lead to increased stress on the opposite neural arch, causing compensatory hypertrophy of the contralateral arch and contralateral pedicle with or without sclerosis.[56, 781, 1342] The spinous process is frequently tilted toward the unhypertrophied side,[781] and the ipsilateral transverse process may be small.[718] In addition, there may be widening of the neural foramen in the anteroposterior dimension as the superior articular process is displaced dorsally.[259] Sometimes narrowing of the foramen may be present, and it is caused by depression of the poorly supported neural arch.[504] Infants and children rarely develop hypertrophy or sclerosis of the contralateral pedicle.[1379a]

Radiographically, the hypoplastic pedicle is small in all dimensions (Fig. 4–75) and,

if extremely small, may not be visible on the AP radiograph, simulating an absent pedicle.[1332] However, a hypoplastic pedicle may be identified on the lateral radiograph as an "hourglass" constriction, an observation not present with pedicle aplasia.[56] Oblique views and, if necessary, conventional or computed tomography can often outline a hypoplastic pedicle in the setting of an apparently absent pedicle.[229, 716, 783, 1371]

Aplasia of the pedicle is rare, and its presence is more common in the cervical

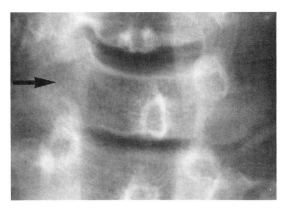

Figure 4–76. Congenital absence of the pedicle. The right pedicle of C7 is absent (arrow). The margin of the pedicle below is thicker than normal, probably formed as a response to additional stress on that side. Congenital absence of pedicles is usually associated with other congenital anomalies on the ipsilateral side and reactive response by bone on the contralateral side.

---

*Reference numbers 56, 504, 670, 781, 923, 1220, 1269, 1348.

spine,* particularly the lower part[259] (see Fig. 4–76), than in the lumbar† and thoracic portions of the spine.[718, 783, 1269] Because of the absence of the pedicle, the neural foramen may appear enlarged on the oblique radiograph.[923] The posterior displacement of the articular process or other associated congenital anomalies should rule out tumor as the etiology of the widened neural foramen.[923] Many reported cases of pedicle aplasia are probably manifestations of severe pedicle hypoplasia. Cervical spondylolysis associated with absent pedicle may rarely be observed.[1139]

Congenital aplasia of the pedicle must be differentiated from the absent pedicle due to pedicle destruction. Metastasis, myeloma, other malignant or benign tumors, infection, or histiocytosis and other tumorlike conditions can all destroy the pedicle.[72, 618] The pedicle is destroyed early in patients with metastatic disease owing to a rich peripedicular blood supply.[692] Myeloma does not destroy the pedicle early, owing to the paucity of red marrow in pedicle,[618] but will destroy the pedicles late in disease, as fat marrow in the pedicle reconverts to red marrow.[692] Infection is a rare cause of an absent pedicle, although about 2% of patients with spinal tuberculosis may demonstrate this finding.[72] In the destructive disorders, there are no associated congenital abnormalities of the ipsilateral side, nor is there hypertrophy of the contralateral pedicle, thus helping to differentiate a destroyed pedicle from congenital aplasia.[1269]

Narrow Pedicle. Narrow pedicles occur normally in the thoracolumbar junction.[194] A pedicle may appear narrow owing to destruction or erosion by an intraspinal tumor or by dural ectasia of dysraphism and other disorders (Fig. 4–77). A narrow pedicle by itself may not necessarily be indicative of pathology unless associated with other signs of canal widening, such as a wide interpedicular distance.[352] Narrow pedicles may be observed in scoliosis (more pronounced on the concave side of the curve[54] and with spondylolisthesis as the vertebra slips anteroinferiorly). Asymmetric pedicle erosion is suggestive of an intraspinal mass.[1175] Rarely, a cervical pedicle may be eroded by a tor-

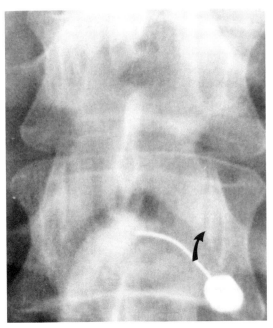

Figure 4–77. Narrow pedicles. In this patient, there is bilateral thinning of pedicles at a single vertebral level (arrow). This has been caused by an intraspinal ependymoma. Compare with pedicles above this vertebral level.

tuous vertebral artery.[30] This is caused by a loop of the vertebral artery protruding into the neural foramen and causing pedicle erosion as well as compression of the nerve root.[30, 1182] Pedicles in the lower cervical spine may be narrowed by subperiosteal resorption in hyperparathyroidism.[468]

Large Pedicle. Large pedicles may develop secondarily to a contralateral pars defect or contralateral hypoplasia or aplasia of a segment of the vertebral arch.[526, 781] Eighty-six percent of patients with unilateral arch hypertrophy have an associated contralateral pars defect.[781] Rarely a large pedicle(s) may develop congenitally in an otherwise normal patient without any other skeletal abnormalities and with a normal-appearing contralateral pedicle and neural arch.[526] Other causes of unilateral pedicle enlargement include Paget's disease, slow-growing expansile metastasis and myeloma, primary tumors and tumorlike conditions (aneurysmal bone cyst, osteoblastoma, fibrous dysplasia), infection or histiocytosis,[526] and neurofibromatosis.[784]

Sclerotic Pedicle. Sclerosis of the pedicle may be unilateral or bilateral (Fig. 4–78). Metastasis, particularly from carcinoma of the prostate and of the breast (particularly treated tumors), lymphoma, and Paget's disease are

---

*Reference numbers 229, 259, 504, 716, 832, 923, 1139, 1220, 1348.
†Reference numbers 273, 781, 878, 915, 1371, 1379a.

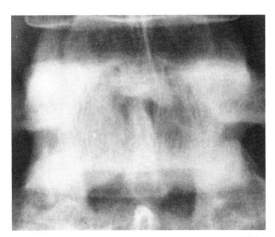

Figure 4–78. Osteosclerosis of the pedicles. In addition to bilateral osteosclerosis of the pedicles, note the presence of osteosclerosis of the vertebral body, thickened trabeculae, and thickened cortex, which are diagnostic of Paget's disease.

the most frequent causes of unilateral or bilateral sclerosis. In metastasis, the pedicle appears amorphous, and the cortical rim and trabeculae may not be visible. In Paget's disease, the cortex is usually thickened. Tuberous sclerosis, sarcoidosis, and myeloma are less common causes. Unilateral pedicle sclerosis is also caused by osteoid osteoma, osteoblastoma, and reactive change due to stress from a contralateral pars defect or, less frequently, hypoplasia or aplasia of the contralateral pedicle or vertebral arch.[1166, 1342] Diffuse bone sclerosing disorders such as myelosclerosis and osteopetrosis may have osteosclerotic pedicles, but vertebral bodies and vertebral arches are also diffusely sclerotic radiographically.

Height and Length. The vertical height of thoracic and lumbar pedicles should be evaluated and compared with the opposite pedicle on the anteroposterior radiograph. Cervical pedicles are difficult to evaluate in this manner. A pedicle with a short vertical measurement and without a sclerotic margin could indicate erosion by a mass in the neural foramen[54] (Fig. 4–79). Pedicle length can be roughly examined on the lateral radiograph of the thoracic and lumbar regions of the spine. Short pedicles are encountered in achondroplasia and contribute to spinal stenosis. Congenital elongation of the pedicle may be associated with a grade I spondylolisthesis without a defect in the pars interarticularis.[186]

Interpedicular Distance. The interpedicular distance (IPD) is measured on the AP radiograph from the medial border of one pedicle to the medial border of the opposite pedicle. This can be accomplished accurately in the thoracic and lumbar spine (see Fig. 4–19). However, the IPD in the cervical spine is difficult to evaluate[352] because pedicles become progressively oblique in position from C7 to C2.[303] Even so, what appears to be the medial border of the pedicle in the cervical spine is in fact the margin of the most ventral parts of the laminae.[103]

The interpedicular distance from C7 to L5 has been determined in children from birth to 12 years[1139a, 1175] and in individuals older than 12 years of age (Figs. 4–80 and 4–81).[352, 1139a] The lumbar IPD from birth to 6 years has also been recorded.[787] Lower limits of normal measurement have been evaluated in children[787, 1175] but not in adults.[352] In one method,[787] an IPD in the lumbar spine of children of +2 SD is strongly predictive of an intraspinal mass.[788] The IPD changes with age and varies with location, being wider in the cervical and lumbar regions (see Fig. 4–97, p. 110).[352, 567, 1175] It increases from vertebra to vertebra from C2 to C5 and becomes progressively smaller from C5 to T2 and again from T2 to T5. The canal remains the same size from T5 to T9 and then becomes progressively wider down to L5[352] and S1.[787] The increases in size of the cervical and lower thoracic canals are due to the presence of the cervical and lumbar plexuses, respectively.[352] The increase in size of the lumbar canal, even with less neural tissue, may be

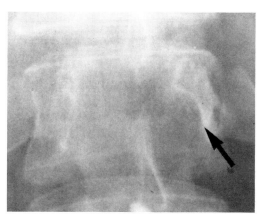

Figure 4–79. Short pedicle. There is apparent shortening of the T12 pedicle on the left (arrow). This has been caused by erosion from an intraspinal neurofibroma.

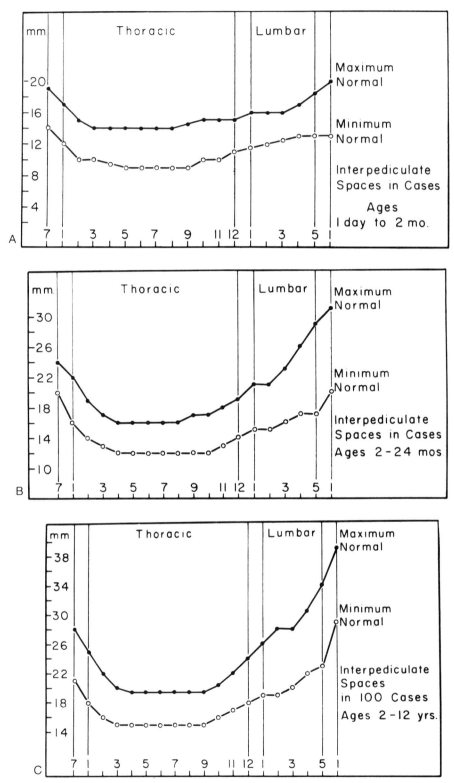

Figure 4–80. Diagrammatic representation of normal maximum and minimum interpedicular distance in children of different ages. *A*, 1 day to 2 months of age. *B*, 2 months to 2 years of age. *C*, 2 years to 12 years of age. (From Simril WA, Thurston O: The normal interpediculate space in the spines of infants and children. Radiology 64:340–347, 1955.)

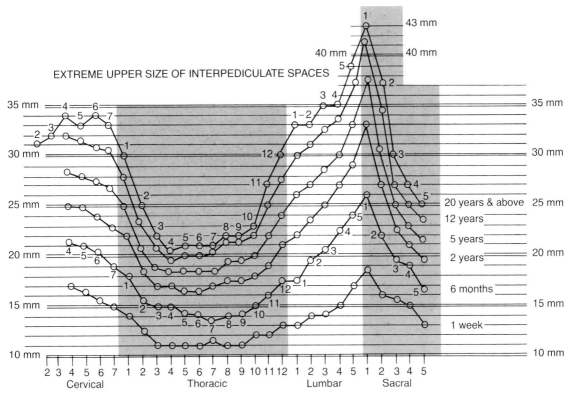

Figure 4-81. Composite graph designating the composite maximum measurement for the interpedicular distance at various levels throughout the spine and sacrum and for various age groups. (Redrawn from Schwarz GS: The width of the spinal canal in the growing vertebra with special reference to the sacrum: Maximum interpediculate distances in adults and children. AJR 76:476–481, 1956. Copyright 1956 by the American Roentgen Ray Society.)

due to the upright posture of humans and the accumulation (caused by gravity) of CSF in the lower spine region. It is not unusual for the IPD of several contiguous vertebrae to remain the same. Although the IPD at each vertebral level increases slightly with age,[567, 790, 1175] the relative width patterns are similar. Growth of the spinal canal ceases at all vertebral levels at the same time, between 18 and 25 years of age.[1139a] A sudden increase in the IP distance of 2 to 4 mm at a spinal level where the IP measurement should be the same or smaller from vertebra to vertebra (i.e., in the midthoracic spine and upper lumbar regions) is particularly significant[352, 1175] and may indicate an expanding intraspinal mass (Table 4–9; see Fig. 4–77). It is important that the IPD be measured, for a 2 to 4 mm enlargement of the canal often cannot be appreciated by visual examination.[352] Underlying intraspinal tumor may be present in patients with an abnormal IPD and only mild signs and symptoms, yet it may not be detected clinically for years.[1175]

A 1 mm increase in width of an IP space is considered within the margin of possible error and of no significance.[352, 567] On the other hand, abnormal widening of one or more IP spaces is strongly suggestive of an intraspinal mass even though the absolute measurements are within the normal limits.[1175]

In the lower lumbar spine, tumors have more room to grow before causing changes in the width of the canal, and the cauda equina may be easily displaced early in disease. In the thoracic spine, the spinal

Table 4–9. ABNORMAL INTERPEDICULAR DISTANCE

Wide
  Intraspinal tumor
  Dural ectasia
  Dysraphism
Narrow
  Achondroplasia
  Diastrophic dwarfism
  Thanatophoric dwarfism

canal is smaller and the spinal cord becomes compressed, so that patients with intraspinal tumor in this region present clinically earlier, before widening of the canal occurs. This stresses the importance of careful pedicle evaluation. Intradural-extramedullary tumors (mainly neurofibromas) widen the IPD in about 30% of cases, and most occur below the level of T10.[352]

In the presence of a defect in the neural arch (spina bifida), the IPD may be wide owing to underdevelopment of the pedicles or to an obtuse angle that the pedicles form with the vertebral body[54] (Fig. 4–82). This should not be mistaken for an underlying intraspinal lesion. On the other hand, spina bifida associated with some forms of dysraphism may demonstrate wide IPD due to dural ectasia, diastematomyelia, or congenital intraspinal lesions.[629, 1343]

The IPD may narrow progressively in the lumbar spine in the caudal direction in achondroplasia[83] (Fig. 4–83) and sometimes in diastrophic[1253, 1302] and thanatophoric dwarfism.[722]

Neural Foramina

The neural foramen is bounded by the vertebral bodies and the posterolateral surface of the disc anteriorly, by pedicles above

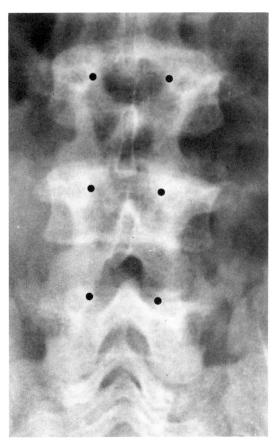

Figure 4–83. Narrow interpedicular distance. The interpedicular distance in this patient with achondroplasia becomes narrower caudally (dots). Normally, this distance becomes wider caudally.

and below, and by superior and inferior articular processes and ligamentum flavum posteriorly.[502] In the cervical spine, the nerve occupies one fifth to one fourth of the diameter of the neural foramen.[503]

Views

The neural foramina of the cervical spine are best evaluated on the oblique radiograph (see Fig. 4–8). Those of the thoracic and lumbar regions of the spine are best seen on the lateral radiograph.

Narrow Neural Foramina

In the normal cervical spine, extremes of extension, lateral flexion, or rotation may normally diminish the size of the neural

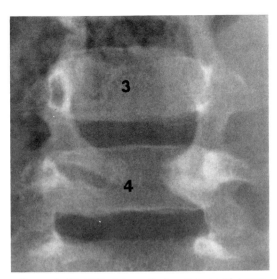

Figure 4–82. Wide interpedicular distance. The interpedicular distance is focally wider at L3 and L4 in this patient with wide spina bifida and previously treated myelomeningocele. Other congenital anomalies such as hypoplastic pedicles and fused laminae are also present.

foramen by as much as one third on the side toward the involvement.[502, 503] In the lumbar spine, similar findings occur with extension or lateral bending, while flexion widens the foramina.[502]

Narrowing of neural foramina may occur congenitally in patients with congenital block vertebrae, particularly in the Klippel-Feil syndrome, and in achondroplasia owing to the short pedicles associated with this disorder. Aplasia of the pedicle, while theoretically causing enlargement of the adjacent neural foramen, may produce narrowing of the foramen due to anterior depression of the poorly supported neural arch.[504] In addition, the neural foramen may be narrowed in the rostral-caudal direction and also in the AP direction as the superior articular process is displaced dorsally.[259] More commonly, neural foramina become narrow because of acquired alterations in surrounding tissue and adjacent bony structures. In the cervical spine, neural foraminal stenosis is caused by hypertrophy or osteophyte formation of articular processes or osteophyte formation of the uncovertebral "joints" and margins of the vertebral bodies.[502] Alterations in the uncovertebral articulation follow degeneration of disc tissue, with subsequent disc narrowing. This allows the vertebral bodies and pedicles to approximate and the superior articular process to move cephalad, thus encroaching on the neural foramen. On the oblique radiograph of the cervical spine, enlarged osteophytes of the uncovertebral "joints" encroach on the anteroinferior aspect of the neural foramen,[503] usually in the lower half of the cervical spine. Enlarged prominent articular processes may encroach on the posterosuperior aspect of the neural foramen,[503] usually in the upper cervical spine (Fig. 4–84). Osteophytes projecting laterally add to the degree of encroachment. As vertebral bodies approximate, the ligamentum flavum buckles and thickens and may become calcified[502] (Fig. 4–85). Bony spurs are larger than they appear on the radiograph. In the lumbar spine, osteophytes arising from the posterior vertebral margin or hypertrophy and osteophyte formation of articular processes in the presence of narrowing of the intervertebral disc cause encroachment on the neural foramen (Fig. 4–86). Narrowing of disc height also causes displacement of nerve roots caudally in the neural foramina,

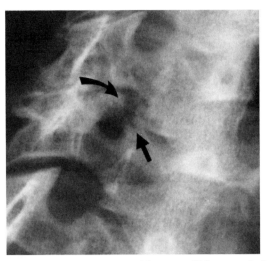

Figure 4–84. Narrow neural foramen. Oblique cervical radiograph demonstrates encroachment of the neural foramen by osteophyte formation about the uncovertebral articulation (straight arrow) as well as encroachment posteriorly by enlargement of the articular process (curved arrow).

allowing them to be subjected to pressure caused by the bony margin of the foramen.[1258]

Technical factors, such as incorrect positioning of the patient in the oblique position, may cause a false appearance of narrowing of the neural foramen. The presence and degree of narrowing or encroachment of the neural foramina may not be correlated clinically.[427, 506, 510] Patients with advanced narrowing of the neural foramen may be entirely asymptomatic, and patients with a normal-

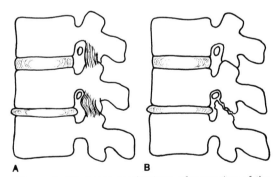

A   **B**

Figure 4–85. Some mechanisms of narrowing of the neural foramen. *A,* Degeneration of intervertebral disc allows approximation of adjacent vertebrae and infolding of the ligamentum flavum, which may encroach on the nerve. *B,* Degeneration of the intervertebral disc and degenerative osteoarthritis of the apophyseal joint may allow osteophytes of the articular process to encroach on the nerve.

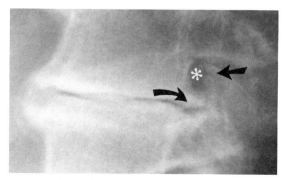

Figure 4–86. Narrow neural foramen. In this patient with intervertebral osteochondrosis, disc narrowing and sclerosis are apparent. The extensive disc narrowing has allowed the superior articular process (straight arrow) to move cephalad, encroaching on the neural foramen (asterisk). Osteophyte development posteriorly (curved arrow) may also encroach on the foramen.

appearing spine may have radiculopathy. If necessary, computed tomography can better evaluate the degree of neural foraminal stenosis.

Neural foraminal stenosis can result from retrolisthesis and sometimes from spondylolisthesis.[362, 502] In retrolisthesis, the superior articular process from below is subluxated anteriorly and cephalad into the foramen.[502] This is best appreciated on the lateral radiograph in the lumbosacral region. Inflammatory disorders usually spare the neural foramina if intervertebral discs are maintained. Fracture fragments of the vertebral arch or vertebral body may encroach on the neural foramen following trauma.

Wide Neural Foramina

An abnormally large neural foramen, either single or multiple, is often a sign of neurofibromatosis[183, 303, 784] (Fig. 4–87). The neural foramen may be enlarged by tumor (neurofibroma, schwannoma), dural ectasia, or bone dysplasia. The neural foramen may also become enlarged in patients without neurofibromatosis. A neurofibroma or schwannoma developing in the neural foramen widens the foramen. Intraspinal tumors such as meningioma and ependymoma may extend through the neural foramen into the extraspinal compartment, or extraspinal tumors such as metastasis, lymphoma, and neural tumor may extend through the neural foramen into the spinal canal. The neural

foramen may be widened by lateral thoracic meningoceles, which occur frequently in patients with neurofibromatosis;[183, 723] arachnoid diverticula; tortuosity of the vertebral artery[30, 258, 423, 745, 1182, 1339] or widening and tortuosity of the vertebral artery produced by increased blood flow;[258] aplasia[259] or severe hypoplasia of the pedicle; hyperparathyroidism (resorption of pedicles);[468] and hypertrophic interstitial polyneuritis (Dejerine-Sottas syndrome), which cuses thickening of nerves due to hyperplasia of the sheath of Schwann[943] and may cause widening of the neural foramen if the nerve root within the foramen is involved.

Intervertebral Discs

The intervertebral disc contains a central, gelatinous nucleus pulposus, which is surrounded by a fibrocartilaginous annulus fibrosus.[223, 226, 1129a] The height of the intervertebral disc changes with age. At birth, it is the same height as the ossification center and, therefore, is relatively higher than in adult life, when the intervertebral disc is one third to one quarter the height of the adjacent vertebral body.[1129a] As a general rule, the height of the intervertebral disc in each anatomic area (cervical, thoracic, lumbar) does not normally

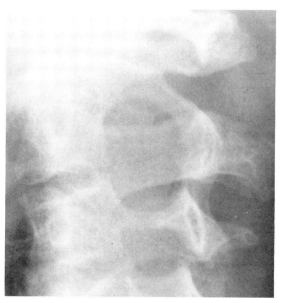

Figure 4–87. There is widening of the neural foramen in this oblique view of the cervical spine. This patient has neurofibromatosis.

diminish from cephalad to caudad, except at the L5–S1 level, where it is normally less than that at the L4–L5 level. Intervertebral disc height is greatest in the lumbar spine and least in the thoracic spine. Exact measurement of disc height can be accomplished but with difficulty.[976] Disc height is greatest anteriorly in the cervical and lumbar regions and greatest posteriorly in the thoracic spine, which accounts for the natural cervical and lumbar lordosis and thoracic kyphosis.[1191]

Decrease in Disc Height

The most frequent cause of loss of intervertebral disc height is intervertebral (osteo)chondrosis during which the disc loses water content and hyaluronidase[1129a] (see Fig. 4–70). The adjacent vertebral margins remain sharp and sclerotic. This may develop during normal aging or occur secondarily to trauma, ochronosis, calcium pyrophosphate dihydrate crystal deposition disease (CPPD-CDD), and other disorders. Decrease in disc height may occur following protrusion of disc tissue in any direction. Posterolateral herniation of nucleus pulposus is not recognizable on the plain radiograph unless the herniated disc or disc fragment is calcified. Disc narrowing may occur in association with Schmorl's nodes as disc tissue protrudes into subchondral bone.[1026, 1129a] Infection, either direct extension from osteomyelitis in the adjacent vertebral body or direct hematogenous invasion to the disc itself (discitis),[1142] leads to disc destruction, with subsequent loss of disc height. Vertebral margins are poorly defined when there is associated osteomyelitis. Intervertebral disc is not, as a rule, destroyed by tumor, since the annulus fibrosus, nucleus pulposus, and cartilage end-plate are relatively avascular (except the peripheral portion of the annulus) and therefore are resistant to tumor invasion.[227, 1027] However, loss of disc height may be associated with metastatic tumor.[593, 1027] Several mechanisms may account for this. Tumor can lead to decrease in disc height by invading or weakening subchondral bone and allowing disc tissue to protrude into the weakened vertebral body (Schmorl's node). Tumor in subchondral bone may occlude blood supply to the disc, interfering with disc nutrition and leading to disc degeneration and loss of disc height (intervertebral chondrosis).[1027] Tumor may invade a disc either by direct extension from adjacent tumor or by hematogenous spread; however, disc metastasis without contiguous vertebral tumor has not been observed.

Increase in Disc Height

The most common cause of increase in height of the intervertebral disc occurs when a disc with normal turgor expands against a cartilage end-plate or bone or both, forming focal indentations. These occur in normal individuals, usually teenagers or young adults, and are more common in the lower lumbar spine.[1275] They take the form of Cupid's bow configuration on the AP view and appear as posterior indentations on the lateral view. Disc height may also increase as healthy disc expands against bone that lacks normal resistance. This occurs in any bone softening disorder, such as osteoporosis, osteomalacia, Paget's disease, and other disorders.[1129a] The expansion of disc forms a smooth central depression and focal increase in disc height. Focal increase in disc height also may occur anteriorly following a hyperextension injury and posteriorly following a hyperflexion injury. In acromegaly, there may be increase in disc height at multiple levels due to cartilage overgrowth from excessive growth hormone.[98, 1221] Additionally, patients may be positioned so that the angle of the x-ray beam projects a false positive appearance of increase in disc height.

Calcification

Disc calcification occurs in 6% of the adult population[154, 429] and may be focal or diffuse within the disc (Fig. 4–88). It is usually the result of intervertebral chondrosis, may be isolated or occur at multiple levels, and usually develops in the midthoracic and upper lumbar regions of the spine. Calcification within the disc is much more common in the annulus fibrosus than in the nucleus pulposus, although either or both may be involved.[223, 1134] Calcification is usually permanent and asymptomatic, although herniation of calcified disc tissue may occur.[224, 777] Six to sixty percent of ruptured

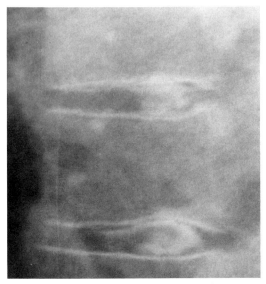

Figure 4–88. Calcification of nucleus pulposus.

thoracic discs with cord compression demonstrate calcification of the protruded nucleus.[953]

In children, disc calcification has a different significance and is a distinct clinical entity.[953, 1314] It is usually in the nucleus pulposus, usually single, occurs most frequently in the cervical spine, is temporary, and is usually symptomatic (particularly that in the cervical spine)[777, 846, 1200] (Fig. 4–89). Disc calcification may be asymptomatic for a considerable period of time prior to clinical presentation.[1314] It usually presents between the ages of 6 and 10 years, although it may develop at any age.[777] It is an incidental observation in 13% of cases, with over half discovered in early

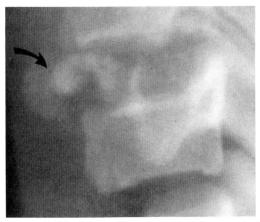

Figure 4–89. Calcification of a cervical intervertebral disc with extrusion of calcified disc fragment (arrow).

infancy.[846] Multiple levels have been involved in about one third of the cases. Calcified discs in children resolve spontaneously and completely, usually within weeks or months,[846, 1314] and one case demonstrated resolution in 9 days.[846] It is interesting that, once symptoms develop, the calcification begins to resolve.[1314] This may be due to the richer blood supply of discs in children.[1134] The etiology of disc calcification is uncertain, although infection, trauma, aseptic necrosis, and generalized metabolic disorders have been postulated.[555, 1200, 1314]

Herniation of calcified disc tissue may occur in both children[777, 1200] and adults and may produce symptoms of cord compression, particularly in the thoracic spine.[953, 1282] Dysphagia may develop from anterior disc herniation in the cervical region.[224, 1200]

Calcification of intervertebral discs may be diffuse and involve multiple levels in a number of systemic disorders, such as ochronosis,[224, 705, 953, 1315] calcium pyrophosphate dihydrate crystal deposition disease (CPPD-CDD), hyperparathyroidism, hemochromatosis,[154, 1315] and acromegaly.[1315] Hydroxyapatite crystals are found in the discs of patients with ochronosis, whereas calcium pyrophosphate dihydrate crystals are found in the other above-mentioned systemic disorders.[154] Patients with poliomyelitis[233] or other causes of paraplegia may develop disc calcification in one or multiple levels. It may develop in systemic disorders associated with spinal ankylosis, such as ankylosing spondylitis,[320] juvenile rheumatoid arthritis,[797] and fibrositis ossificans progressiva, and may be due to a lack of normal stress between fused vertebrae.[320] Calcification of one or more discs may occur in focal areas of fusion such as postoperative spine fusion,[1315] congenital block vertebrae, and Klippel-Feil syndrome.[320]

Air (Vacuum Phenomenon)

The most frequent cause of air within the intervertebral disc (vacuum phenomenon) is degeneration of disc tissue[456, 1033] (Fig. 4–90). It is found in 2% of all spines examined[791] and in 20% of elderly patients.[456] It is most common in the lower lumbar and lumbosacral regions of the spine. The gas, which is mainly nitrogen (90 to 92%),[409] is visible in the nucleus pulposus and may extend

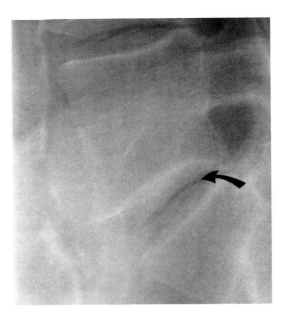

Figure 4–90. Vacuum disc phenomenon. There is a cleft containing air within the intervertebral disc at the lumbosacral junction (arrow). Disc height is maintained, but this vacuum phenomenon indicates early intervertebral disc degeneration.

into the annulus fibrosus.[456] The vacuum phenomenon usually represents the earliest radiographic sign of disc degeneration. As disc degenerates and fissures form, a partial vacuum occurs, and gas from surrounding tissues fills the fissures.[1033] Radiographically, the vacuum phenomenon appears linear, jagged, or round and may be small or extensive.[1039] Single or multiple levels may be involved,[456] and multiple levels of involvement may be associated with calcium pyrophosphate dihydrate crystal deposition disease.[798] The appearance of disc air is accentuated with extension of the spine. Associated disc narrowing and spondylosis are visible in around 94% of those with vacuum phenomenon.[791]

Gas may develop within a cervical disc (annulus) following a hyperextension injury.[101, 1039] It is formed as the disc is partially avulsed from the cartilaginous end-plate. In this clinical setting, the gas appears linear, smooth, and adjacent to the cartilaginous end-plate. Its appearance is also accentuated with extension of the cervical spine and may disappear with flexion. Gas may appear within hours of acute trauma and persist unchanged from 2 months to 5 years.[1039] It indicates a less severe injury, since a complete tear of the disc

or rupture of the anterior longitudinal ligament would be associated with hemorrhage, which would immediately fill any air space.

It should be noted that a cervical annulus vacuum sign may be observed in the absence of trauma, particularly in patients with degenerative disease of the annulus.[101] It occurs at the site of attachment of the annulus and is noted on lateral radiographs with the neck in extension.

Frequently, a linear lucency is noted in the superior margin of the intervertebral disc in 65% of adults and 50% of children.[240] This represents a normal variant—the pseudovacuum phenomenon—the Mach band. It occurs more frequently with flexion and therefore should not be mistaken for the vacuum phenomenon adjacent to the cartilage end-plate that occurs following a hyperextension injury. Also, in patients who sustain trauma, there are almost always other associated signs of trauma, such as widening or displacement of the prevertebral soft tissue and fat stripes, and widening or narrowing of the intervertebral disc space.[1039]

The presence of gas within the intervertebral disc should rule out infection, since pus would replace any air space. Thus, a vacuum phenomenon that disappears in the presence of progressive disc narrowing may indicate underlying infection within the disc.[1033] Rarely, in some forms of infection, gas may be produced by organisms within the disc, causing a vacuum phenomenon.[70a, 89, 942] The vacuum phenomenon has also been observed in almost 30% of patients with metastatic disease to the spine from carcinoma of the breast, and, in over half of these patients, the vacuum phenomenon was adjacent to vertebrae involved with metastasis and free of any significant degenerative alterations.[1113]

Ligaments and Capsules

Ligaments are not visualized on the conventional radiograph because they are soft tissue density. Disorders affecting ligaments may be suspected when malalignment or malposition of bony structures is apparent even when ligaments are not visible. Ligaments may be radiographically visible when calcified or ossified, and the type of calcification may help establish the underlying diagnosis.

Posterior Longitudinal Ligament

Calcification or ossification of the posterior longitudinal ligament (OPLL) occurs more commonly in Japanese and Eastern Asiatic people[577, 1276] and in patients with diffuse idiopathic skeletal hyperostosis (DISH)[1022] (Fig. 4–91). It is found in 2% of the Japanese population and in 0.16% of Caucasians, and the incidence may reach 20% of older Japanese people.[1276] It occurs in almost 25%[1276] to 50%[1022] of patients with DISH. Rarely, OPLL occurs in fluorosis.[1177] The etiology of OPLL is unknown. It may develop at any level, although it is more common in the cervical spine, particularly in the upper region[1022] and in the C4–C6 levels.[1276] However, all cervical levels may be involved.[515] Almost 10% develop OPLL in the thoracic or lumbar spine.[1276] OPLL is often difficult to visualize radiographically owing to overlying bone. On the lateral radiograph, it appears as a focal or continuous linear ossification parallel to the posterior aspect of the vertebral body and disc

margins.[1017, 1276] Two types of OPLL have been described. A focal type of ossification is more common in the lower cervical spine, whereas the continuous form occurs in the upper cervical region.[1276] The dorsal surface of the ossification may have an undulating configuration.[1022, 1276] Sagittal thickness of the ossification varies from 1 to 8 mm.[198] OPLL may appear adjacent to or separated from the vertebral body and disc, and it may enlarge on serial radiographs.[1276] Associated ossification of the ligamentum flavum occurs in almost 7% of cases, but the true incidence is probably higher since it is often difficult to visualize ossification of the ligamentum flavum. A thick ossified or calcified posterior longitudinal ligament may narrow the spinal canal and cause cord compression.[198, 1276] Symptoms are usually noted when ossification occupies more than 60% of the sagittal diameter of the spinal canal.[932] Asymptomatic patients with OPLL may be compromised by acute disc herniation.[936] Approximately 25% have considerable difficulty in ambulation.[1276] Patients treated with 13-cis-retinoic acid, a synthetic retinoid, may develop OPLL.[957] The posterior longitudinal ligament may become calcified or ossified in ankylosing spondylitis and less commonly in other inflammatory spondylitides, such as psoriatic spondylitis.

Anterior Longitudinal Ligament

Diffuse calcification of the anterior longitudinal ligament occurs most frequently in ankylosing spondylitis and is best visualized on the lateral radiograph. The calcified ligament in this disorder always appears thin compared with the thick paravertebral ossification found in DISH. Care should be taken not to mistake these focal calcifications for fractures. Calcification of the anterior longitudinal ligament may occur in psoriatic spondylitis, acromegaly,[357a] and fluorosis[1177] and may occur focally, associated with underlying vertebral lymphoma.[317] Focal calcification and ossification of the anterior longitudinal ligament or annulus appear frequently in the cervical spine of older patients and are probably manifestations of aging or early mild changes of DISH. Bands of ossification in soft tissues are observed in fibrodysplasia ossificans progressiva[1262] (Fig. 4–92).

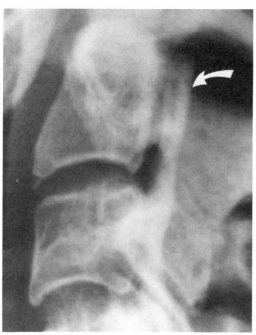

Figure 4–91. Ossification of the posterior longitudinal ligament (arrow) is noted in the cervical spine. This 60 year old patient demonstrated radiographic signs of DISH elsewhere in the spine.

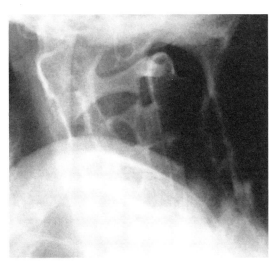

Figure 4–92. Ossification of soft tissues and ligaments in the cervical spine in a patient with fibrositis (myositis) ossificans progressiva. Facet joint fusion is noted as well.

Interspinous Ligaments

Midline calcification or ossification of the interspinous ligaments in the lumbosacral region is usually a sign of ankylosing spondylitis. Occasionally, it may occur in normal individuals. Ossification may develop within the supraspinous and interspinous ligaments as a degenerative response in patients with Baastrup's disease[1103] as the spinous processes of the cervical or lower lumbar spine approximate and may appear enlarged and focally sclerotic.[46, 652]

Ligamentum Flavum

The ligamentum flavum may calcify or ossify (LFO) physiologically in normal individuals and as part of the aging process,[502] but this is usually not visualized on the radiograph. Ossification may develop in fluorosis[1177] or be associated with CPPD with[154] or without underlying hemochromatosis.[350] Almost 8% of cases of OPLL may have associated LFO.[1276] LFO has been observed on the lateral chest radiograph in about 5% of women and men and is more commonly noted from T9 through L1.[698] Although LFO could cause neurologic symptoms, no cases were reported in one large series.[698] They are usually first visualized from 20 to 40 years of age. LFO occurs at the attachment of the ligamentum flavum to the inferior facet, superior facet, or both.

Radiographically, the ossification most commonly takes the form of a hook-shaped radiodensity that protrudes inferiorly from the articular facet into the intervertebral foramen. Other forms of ossification include beak-shaped, linear, or nodular forms.[611, 698]

Normally during extension, the ligamenta flava fold into the cervical spinal canal,[1232] so that in the presence of an anterior mass (disc, osteophyte) the cord may be compressed between the anterior mass and the infolded ligamenta flava posteriorly whenever the neck is extended.

Capsules

The capsules of facet joints may calcify or ossify in ankylosing spondylitis and appear as bilateral bands of increased density oriented in the cephalad-caudad direction (Fig. 4–93).

Ligamentum Nuchae

The ligamentum nuchae is a midline structure extending from the occiput to the spinous process of the 7th cervical vertebra.[732] Focal calcification or, more commonly, ossification in the ligamentum nuchae is identical histologically to sesamoid bones, with the ligament inserting into the bony mass by means of an adjacent fibrocar-

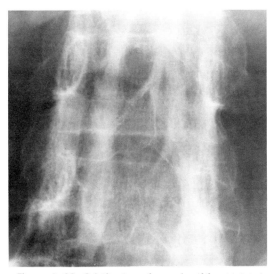

Figure 4–93. Calcification of capsules if facet joints in this patient with ankylosing spondylitis. The facet joints are fused as well.

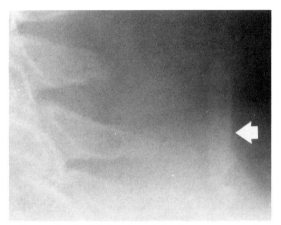

Figure 4–94. Calcification of the ligamentum nuchae in the posterior lower cervical spine (arrow).

tilaginous layer (Fig. 4–94). Therefore, it may actually be a normal sesamoid, or it may have developed as a result of previous trauma. The ossified density may be oval or triangular in shape and should not be mistaken for an acute fracture.

Stylohyoid Ligament

Calcification of the stylohyoid ligament often occurs in patients without associated spinal disorders. However, it has a higher incidence in patients with DISH (Fig. 4–95),

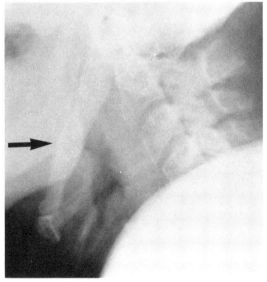

Figure 4–95. Calcification of the stylohyoid ligament (arrow), which is quite prominent in this patient with DISH.

and large calcified stylohyoid ligaments have been noted in patients with Hurler's syndrome.[922a]

Sacral Ligaments

Calcification or ossification of sacral ligaments may develop in 15% of patients with fluorosis.[881] The sacrospinous and sacrotuberous ligaments calcify initially in the inferior portion of the ligament. Calcification may be asymptomatic.

Central Spinal Canal

The central spinal canal should be evaluated for size, shape, and the presence of intraspinal calcifications. Abnormalities in width have been discussed earlier in this chapter (see *Interpedicular Distance*, pp. 97–100), so the evaluation of the spinal canal in the sagittal plane only is considered here.

The size of the spinal canal varies with age, anatomic site, and race. Normally, the spinal canal and lateral recess are large enough to accommodate neural tissue and allow some degree of gliding movement, molding, and traction of neural tissue during motion, without causing symptoms.[1323] The lack of space within the canal, caused by bony or soft tissue encroachment of the canal or both, or abnormalities that cause restriction of motion of neural tissue (fibrosis) may lead to symptoms. The limitations of the conventional radiograph in the evaluation of the size of the spinal canal are the difficulty in accurate measurement of the canal due to overlying bony densities, the lack of visualization of soft tissue parts, and the frequent lack of correlation of radiographic observations with symptomatology, as in spondylosis.

Measurement of the Sagittal Diameter

Cervical Spine. The sagittal diameter of the cervical spine is measured at each vertebral level from the middle of the posterior surface of the vertebral body to the nearest point of the anterior margin at the junction of the spinous processes with the laminae[103, 571] (Fig. 4–96). In the region of the atlas, a line is drawn from the posterior surface of

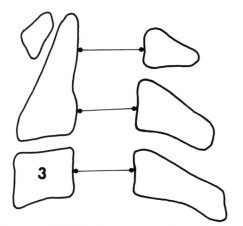

Figure 4–96. Method of measuring the sagittal diameter of the central spinal canal of the upper cervical spine. The method of measurement for the lower cervical spine is similar.

the odontoid process at the lower level of the atlantoaxial articulation to the anterior margin of the point of fusion of the posterior arches of C1.[103, 149, 571] A sagittal diameter below 13 mm is significant, whereas a measurement above 15 mm is normal.[359] A sagittal diameter of 10 mm or less is likely to be associated with cord compression if due to posterior osteophyte formation.[1363]

Generally speaking, in children and teenagers[571, 790] and in adults,[103, 1363] there is a progressive decline in sagittal diameter from C1 to C3 followed by a mild decline or no change in size from C3 to C5[571] or C7.[103, 149, 1363] Thus, the canal assumes a funnel shape. However, in 30% of children less than 11 years of age, and in 1.6% of patients between the ages of 11 and 25 years, there is nonpathologic relative widening of the sagittal diameter of the cervical canal below the level of C3 or C4 (Fig. 4–98).[1380] The mean and range of sagittal diameters observed in adults and children are listed in Tables 4–10 and 4–11. The sagittal diameters are a few millimeters less in women[103] and 2.5 millimeters less in the Japanese population.[886]

Lumbosacral Spine. There are several methods used for measuring the sagittal diameter of the lumbosacral canal on the lateral radiograph in adults,[336, 337, 362, 569] and this may lead to discrepancies in measurement results (Fig. 4–99).

A line may be drawn from the midpoint of the posterior vertebral margin perpendicular to the anterior margin of the vertebral

arch.[569] In adults, the lumbar canal ranges from 16 mm to 27 mm in the sagittal diameter. However, it is often difficult to identify the anterior margin of the vertebral arch accurately, owing to the overlying articular facets and transverse processes,[337, 639] so that the sagittal measurement of the lumbar spinal canal is often a rough guide to its size.[639]

Another method is to draw an interfacet line from the apex of the superior articular facet to the apex of the inferior articular facet of the same vertebral body and then join it with another line from the midposterior vertebral border, from L1 to L4.[336, 337] For the sagittal diameter measurement at the L5 level a line is placed 1 to 2 mm anterior to the well-demarcated anterior limit of the radiolucent spinous process.[337] By this method, the lower limits of normal are 15 mm. However, it may be difficult to identify the apices of the articular facets.[930]

In the third method, a line is drawn from the uppermost level of the neural foramen (dorsal point) to the nearest posterior margin of the vertebral body (ventral point).[362] Measurements vary between 15 mm and 23 mm, and those below 13 mm are considered abnormal.[362] This measurement can be easily obtained from L1 to L3, but it is more difficult to measure at L4 and L5.[360] This measurement is not an estimate of the sagittal plane of the central canal,[360] since it really corresponds anatomically to the measurement of the lateral recess below the pedicle.[362] Although patients with central canal stenosis frequently have stenosis of the lateral recess in the lumbar region, this measurement does not give an accurate assessment of the midsagittal diameter.[569, 930]

When these measurement methods are compared, they all demonstrate some false positive and some false negative examples of spinal stenosis,[930] so that no method is ideally suited for evaluation of the sagittal diameter of the spinal canal. Probably, evaluation of both the midsagittal plane and the height of the neural foramen should be performed to give a more accurate assessment.[569] The sagittal diameter of the lumbosacral spinal canal at different ages as measured on the lateral radiograph is shown in Fig. 4–100. The measurement is largest at L1, but below L1 the diameter varies by only 1 to 2 mm.[569] The canal is narrowest at the L2–L4 levels.[336, 569]

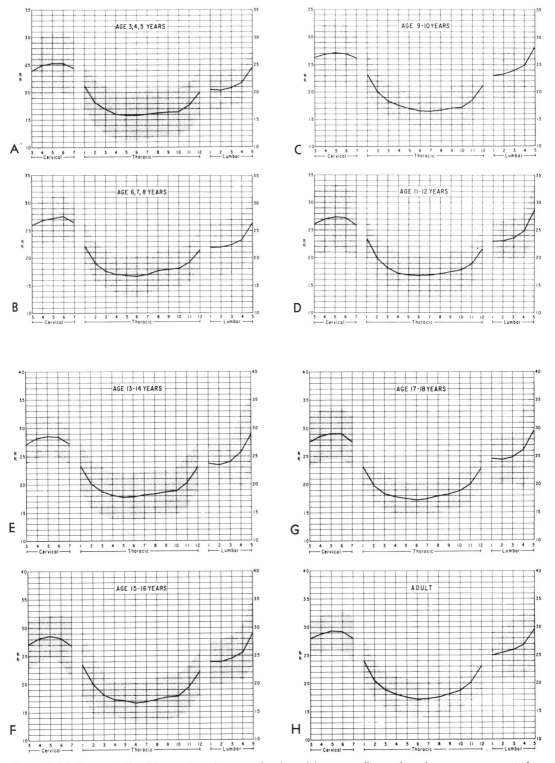

Figure 4–97. Interpedicular distance at varying ages showing minimum, median, and maximum measurements from C3 to L5. *A*, 3 to 5 years. *B*, 6 to 8 years. *C*, 9 to 10 years. *D*, 11 to 12 years. *E*, 13 to 14 years. *F*, 15 to 16 years. *G*, 17 to 18 years. *H*, Adult. See page 97 for discussion of interpedicular distance. (From Hinck VC, Clark WM Jr, Hopkins CE: Normal interpediculate distances (minimum and maximum) in children and adults. AJR 97:141–153, 1966. Copyright 1966 by the American Roentgen Ray Society.)

and those of 10 mm or less are indicative of absolute stenosis.[1286]

Wide Sagittal Diameter

The lower cervical spinal canal may widen normally in the sagittal plane in about 30% of children under 10 years of age.[1380] In the absence of symptoms, this should be of no clinical concern. Pathologic widening of any segment of the canal results from intraspinal tumors and tumorlike conditions and sometimes from syringomyelia.

In the cervical spine, the sagittal diameter is a more important measurement for canal widening than the IPD because the IPD is normally larger than the sagittal diameter, and a lesion enlarging diffusely is more likely to demonstrate changes in the sagittal diameter before demonstrating changes in the pedicles.[303] In the thoracic and lumbar spines, in which the IPD and sagittal diameter are fairly similar in size, both measurements may increase equally with intraspinal masses. As intraspinal lesions enlarge, the earliest bony alteration is at the base of the spinous processes (roof of the canal) as the cortical margin becomes flattened.[303] With further erosion, the posterior vertebral margin may become concave, and there is decrease in sagittal measurement of the vertebral body, as the expanding mass may enlarge anteriorly, causing posterior vertebral scalloping.

Narrow Sagittal Diameter

Spinal stenosis indicates narrowing of the central spinal canal, the lateral nerve root

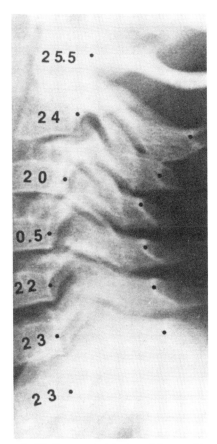

Figure 4–98. Reversed widening of the caudal cervical spinal canal in a normal individual. (From Yousefzadeh DK, El-Khoury GY, Smith WL: Normal sagittal diameter and variation in the pediatric cervical spine. Radiology 144:319–325, 1982.)

In summary, the lumbar canal in adults ranges from 15 mm to 23 mm[362] or 16 mm to 27 mm[569] in the sagittal diameter, with the lower limits of normal at 13 mm,[362] 15 mm,[337] or 16 mm.[569] Measurements below 10 to 12 mm are indicative of relative stenosis,

Table 4–10. SAGITTAL MEASUREMENTS CERVICAL SPINAL CANAL—ADULTS

	Mean* (mm)	Range* (mm)	Mean† (mm)	Range† (mm)
C1	22	16–31	25	19–32
C2	20	14–27	22	16–27
C3	17	12.5–23	19.5	15–25
C4	17	12–22	18.5	14–24
C5	17	12–22	18	14–23
C6	17	12–22	18	14–23
C7‡	17	12–22	18	14–23

*Data from Wolf BS, Khilnani M, Malis L: The sagittal diameter of the bony cervical spinal canal and its significance in cervical spondylosis. J Mt Sinai Hosp 23:283–292, 1956.
†Data from Boijsen E: The cervical spinal canal in intraspinal expansive processes. Acta Radiol 42:101–115, 1954.
‡Measurements at T1 are the same as those listed for C7.[103, 1363]

Table 4–11. SAGITTAL MEASUREMENTS CERVICAL SPINAL CANAL—3 TO 18 YEARS

		3 Years		8 Years		13 Years		18 Years	
		Mean	Range (mm)	Mean	Range (mm)	Mean	Range (mm)	Mean	Range (mm)
C1	B	20	15–24	20	16–24	21	16–25	21	17–26
	G	17	13–21	18	14–22	19	15–23	20	16–24
C2	BG	17	14–20	18	15–21	19	15–22	19	16–23
C3	BG	15	12–18	16	13–19	17	14–20	17	14–20
C4	BG	15	12–18	16	13–19	16	13–19	17	14–20
C5	BG	15	12–18	16	13–18	16	13–19	17	14–19

Key: B = boys; G = girls; BG = boys and girls. Numbers are rounded off.

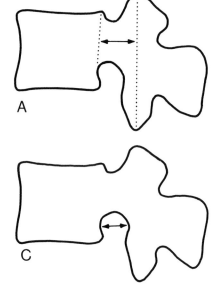

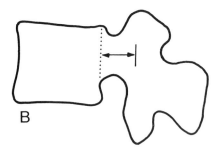

Figure 4–99. Diagram demonstrating methods of measuring the sagittal diameter of the lumbar spinal canal. A, Method of Eisenstein.[336, 337] B, Method of Hinck.[569] C, Method of Epstein,[362] which really measures the lower portion of the lateral recess. (Adapted from Omojola MF, Vas W, Banna M: Plain film assessment of spinal canal stenosis. J Can Assoc Radiol 32:95–96, 1981.)

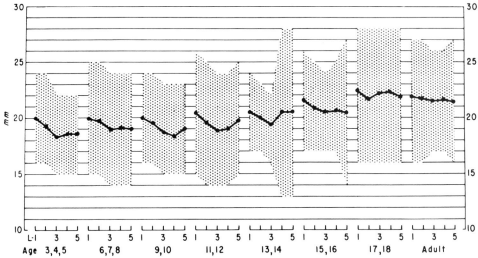

Figure 4–100. Measurements of the sagittal diameter of the lumbar spinal canal at different ages and at different levels. (From Hinck VC, Hopkins CE, Savara BS: Sagittal diameter of the lumbar spinal canal in children and adults. Radiology 85:929–937, 1965.)

canal ("lateral recess"), or the intervertebral canal (neural foramen). It includes bony and soft tissue abnormalities that act alone or in combination to reduce the volume and alter the shape of the spinal canal.

Spinal stenosis is divided into two basic categories. The first, developmental, or congenital, is subdivided into idiopathic and achondroplastic types. Acquired, the second category, is subdivided into the following types: degenerative, spondylolisthetic, iatrogenic (posterior laminectomy, posterior fusion, postchemonucleolysis), posttraumatic, osseous (Paget's disease, fluorosis, expansile bony lesions).[40, 478] Combined developmental and acquired forms occur. Disc herniation and bulging annulus are included in the classification only when they coexist with other forms of stenosis. Only central spinal stenosis with attention to the central diameter of the canal is presented at this time.

Central Spinal Stenosis. *Developmental (Congenital).* Developmental (congenital) spinal stenosis is due to abnormal development early in life[672] or achondroplasia. The degree of canal narrowing is uniform throughout most of the canal. Both the anteroposterior and midsagittal measurements are lower than normal. Achondroplasia is a classic example of this type of stenosis.[360, 362, 672] The pedicles are short and the laminae are thick, both contributing to the overall narrowing of the central spinal canal. Patients with Klippel-Feil syndrome may also have spinal stenosis.[353, 364] Congenital stenosis may develop in the cervical spine at the craniovertebral junction secondary to abnormalities in the region of the foramen magnum, atlas, and axis.[359] These anomalies include the occiptal vertebra, assimilation of the atlas, atlantoaxial fusions, and other abnormalities. Patients tend to be asymptomatic until a complicating process develops, such as spondylosis, subluxation, hyperextension injury,[572] and disc protrusion. These disorders, when combined, cause cord compression.

In the lumbar spine, congenital bony ridges may develop in the posterior vertebral surface and may cause symptomatology.[91] The canal may also be focally or diffusely narrowed, in both the sagittal and IP diameters.[264]

Degenerative (Acquired). Degenerative (acquired) stenosis develops during life and is segmental; that is, there are areas of normal canal existing between areas of stenotic canal. These stenotic changes usually occur opposite intervertebral disc and articular processes.[362] Degenerative changes of osteophyte formation (spondylosis); thicker, wider laminae; hypertrophied articular processes; midline bony bar; and large spinous processes that may protrude into the spinal canal can occur either alone or in combination.* In addition, soft tissue alterations of the degenerative process may occur and may not be visible radiographically. These changes include thickening or infolding of the ligamenta flava, herniated intervertebral disc, bulging annulus, and ossification of the posterior longitudinal ligament.[149, 359, 427, 428, 1286]

Degenerative cervical spinal stenosis is usually due to spondylosis and to osteophytes encroaching on the floor of the canal (Fig. 4–101). It occurs most often at several vertebral levels, usually developing between C4 and C6,[359] but it may also occur isolated at one level. Associated disc disease and hypertrophy or infolding of the ligamenta flava during extension, and ossification of the posterior longitudinal ligament may further compromise the already narrow canal. Although the incidence of cervical spondylosis is high, particularly in the older population, the association with neurologic symptoms is around 0.003% in the general population.[1258]

---

*Reference numbers 91, 149, 359, 360, 426–428, 1258, 1286.

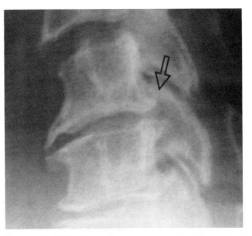

Figure 4–101. Central canal stenosis. Osteophytes (arrow) are projecting posteriorly into the cervical spinal canal. Note the osteophytes anteriorly. Intervertebral osteochondrosis is present.

Radiographically in the cervical spine, spondylosis is easily recognized, but the apparent inward extension of osteophytes may be deceptive,[359] as the osteophytes may in fact be extending laterally.[1363] In addition, a midline bony defect protruding into the canal may be obscured by overlying bony structures. Also, it is not possible to determine from the conventional radiograph alone which levels of spondylosis are related to the symptomatology.[359, 427]

In the cervical spine, myelopathy is more likely to occur if the midsagittal diameter is 10 mm or less,[1363] but the measurement is classified as premyelopathic when it is 13 mm to 17 mm.[328] Measurements above 17 mm are less prone to symptomatic disease. Sometimes the narrowest sagittal diameter in the cervical canal is between an osteophyte and the posteroinferior margin and the base of the spinous process. This distance may diminish by 2 mm in full extension compared with flexion.[1363] In addition, the posterior longitudinal ligament and ligamenta flava relax in extension with thickening (infolding)[958] of the ligamenta flava. This narrows the canal by about 2 or 3 mm.

In the lumbar spine, spinal stenosis is more frequent in the lower region, particularly at L4,[360] but may involve the L3 to L5 levels. The laminae become hypertrophied and are best viewed on the anteroposterior radiograph. Bony ridges may develop anteriorly in the canal. The pedicles appear short, probably owing to thickness of the overlying converging laminae. The spinous processes also become thick and sometimes approximate. Patients with midsagittal diameter measurements of the lumbar spine of less than 15 mm radiographically are prone to clinical spinal stenosis, whereas those with measurements of 20 mm or more are usually free of similar symptoms.[328]

There are other causes of bony spinal stenosis. These include Paget's disease, any mass expanding into the canal, postsurgical fusion, with either excessive bone formation or epidural scarring, and spondylolisthesis. Trauma may complicate a stenotic canal.[1287] Patients with acromegaly[363a] and pituitary giantism may develop spinal stenosis owing to overgrowth of bony and soft tissue parts caused by the production of excessive growth hormone. Ligamentous and dural calcifications are other intraspinal causes of spinal stenosis.

Combined. Bony spinal stenosis may be classified as combined, that is, exhibiting features of both developmental and degenerative stenosis, with or without herniation of intervertebral disc.[672] It may also be familial.[980]

Lateral Recess

The lateral recess is clinically more important in the lumbosacral spine than in the cervical or thoracic spine because lumbar nerve roots have a longer intraspinal course and run along the lateral recess in the lower lumbar spine, whereas cervical, thoracic, and upper lumbar nerve roots have a shorter, more horizontal course and do not have a relationship with the lateral recess.[230]

The lateral recess is is bordered by the superior articular facet posteriorly, the pedicle laterally, and the posterolateral surface of the vertebral body anteriorly.[858] It is difficult to evaluate on the conventional radiograph but may be identified and measured in the region of the lumbosacral spine (see Fig. 4–21). The lateral recess is the distance between the posterior vertebral margin and the anterior margin of the superior articular process as seen on the lateral radiograph. It is easier and more accurate to evaluate the lateral recess with computed tomography than with conventional radiography.[203, 804, 858] Measurements of the lateral recesses of gross specimens at the superior margin of the pedicle in the anteroposterior dimension average about 7.4 mm at L1, 3.7 mm at L5, and 4 mm at S1. Measurements in the same dimension at the inferior aspect of the pedicle change little from L1 (7.7 mm) to L5 (7 mm). Thus, measurements less than 3 mm indicate lateral recess stenosis, whereas measurements greater than 5 mm indicate the absence of stenosis.[858] Hypertrophy or osteophyte formation of the superior articular processes or both usually account for narrowing of the lateral recess.

Sacroiliac Joints

The lower one half to two thirds of the sacroiliac joint is lined by hyaline cartilage on the sacral portion and fibrocartilage on the iliac surface[209, 747]; it is surrounded by a joint capsule. The articular cartilage layer of the sacrum is thicker than that of the ilium,[1031] which accounts for earlier visualization of inflammatory changes on the iliac surface. The upper one half to one third of the sacroiliac articulation is bound by strong ligaments.

Views

The sacroiliac joints are best viewed on the anteroposterior caudal angle view (20 to 25 degrees) and on the nonangled posteroanterior view.[747] They may also be observed well on oblique views, but these are not necessary if the sacroiliac joints are satisfactorily visualized on the initial radiographs.

Normal Radiographic Appearance

The sacroiliac joints take an oblique course, so they are viewed twice on the AP radiograph.[693] The posterior aspect of the joint is medial and shorter in height than the anterior portion of the joint. The articular surfaces are smooth, with sharp, sclerotic, continuous margins. The interosseous joint space is 2 mm to 5 mm in young adults and indicates the combined thickness of the two cartilage surfaces[1031] as well as the true joint space. In the normal adolescent, the sacroiliac joints may appear irregular and slightly wider, and care should be taken so as not to misdiagnose sacroiliitis.[693]

Narrowed Joints

Narrowing of the lower one half to two thirds of the sacroiliac joints indicates loss of joint cartilage, which may occur from inflammatory, infectious, or degenerative disorders. The distribution pattern of joint narrowing may help in the differential diagnosis (Table 4–12).[1037] Bilateral ankylosis of the sacroiliac joints is most commonly due to ankylosing spondylitis. Infection should always be considered when there are radiographic features of unilateral sacroiliitis. The sacroiliac joint may appear spuriously narrow owing to patient positioning, angle of the x-ray beam, and overlying feces in the bowel.

Wide Joints

Apparent widening of the sacroiliac joints may occur normally in adolescents.[693] It may occur as an early radiographic observation in the inflammatory disorders, particularly ankylosing spondylitis, and is due to widespread osteopenia and erosions.[747] The sacroiliac joints appear wide in hyperparathyroidism secondary to subchondral bone resorption[1024] or following trauma with subluxation or dislocation of the joint. Sacroiliac joints widen normally following delivery. The sacroiliac joint may appear spuriously wide, mimicking subluxation, if the x-ray beam is not centered properly.[260]

Calcification

Calcification may occur in articular cartilage (chondrocalcinosis) but is often difficult to detect radiographically owing to the thin nature of the cartilage and the obliquity of the joint.

Table 4–12. DISTRIBUTION OF RADIOGRAPHIC FINDINGS OF SACROILIAC JOINTS

	Bilateral Symmetric	Bilateral Asymmetric	Unilateral
Ankylosing spondylitis	+	−	−
CPPD crystal deposition disease	+	+	+
Degenerative alterations	+	+	+
Familial Mediterranean fever	+	+	+
Gout	+	+	+
Hyperparathyroidism	+	−	−
Infection	−	−	+
Inflammatory bowel disease	+	−	−
Juvenile rheumatoid arthritis	+	+	+
Lupus	+	+	−
Osteitis condensans ilii	+	−	−
Psoriatic arthritis	+	+	+
Reiter's syndrome	+	+	+
Rheumatoid arthritis	−	+	+

Key: + = present; − = not present.
Adapted from Resnik CS, Resnick D: Radiology of disorders of the sacroiliac joints. JAMA 253:2863–2866, 1985.

Air

A vacuum phenomenon is commonly identified within the joint space in older patients and is nonspecific. It may be a manifestation of cartilage degeneration[798] or increased joint motion. It is more frequent in patients with calcium pyrophosphate dihydrate crystal deposition disease (CPPD-CDD).[798]

Sclerosis

Osteitis condensans ilii (OCI) is a benign form of sclerosis of the iliac side of the sacroiliac joint. It is usually bilateral and mainly symmetric, although asymmetric and unilateral appearances occur. It is unassociated with joint narrowing. OCI almost always occurs in women, with 92% having experienced pregnancy and 83% having borne children.[919] OCI occurs in over 1% of the general population. Improvement in appearance usually becomes apparent in several years, and 6% of patients demonstrate resolution of the sclerosis over a period of time.[919]

Sclerosis of subchondral bone also develops in any form of sacroiliitis as a response to healing.

THE CONVENTIONAL RADIOGRAPH IN SPINAL DISORDERS

Degenerative Disorders

The mechanical integrity of the vertebral column depends on the integrity of its components. The apophyseal joints, intervertebral discs, and ligaments that make up a structural complex are closely related mechanically, and degeneration of one component will usually cause additional stress and eventually degeneration of the other components.[378, 382, 523, 673]

The conventional radiograph can demonstrate many of the bony alterations of aging; however, their effect on the soft tissue components such as nerve roots, spinal cord, or cauda equina cannot be visualized. It is also important to realize that the radiographic signs of aging may not necessarily be the cause of the patient's symptomatology, since both symptomatic and asymptomatic groups may demonstrate similar spinal alterations due to aging.[427]

Disc Degeneration (Intervertebral Chondrosis)

With aging, degeneration of the spine may begin in any of the supporting structures but usually begins in the intervertebral disc (intervertebral chondrosis [IVC]).[1129a] Initially, there is a loss of water content and proteoglycans in the nucleus pulposus that leads to the formation of clefts that extend from the nucleus pulposus into the annulus fibrosus. With further progression, there is loss of disc height.[225–227, 1129, 1129a] With age, the discs become progressively fibrotic.[673] Chronic torsion stress seems to play an important role in initiating degeneration of the intervertebral disc.[378, 380]

The very early changes of IVC may not be visible on the radiograph.[1129a] However, the earliest radiographic finding encountered is the vacuum phenomenon[456] that forms in the clefts within the nucleus pulposus and annulus fibrosus (see Fig. 4–90). With progression of IVC, there is decrease in intervertebral disc height that can be readily detected on the radiograph. IVC is found most commonly in the L4–S1 and C5–C7 levels. There is less correlation between disc degeneration and alterations in apophyseal joints in the cervical spine than in the lumbosacral spine.[427] As the intervertebral disc degenerates, the pedicles become closer in the sagittal plane, and buckling of the ligamentum flavum may develop.[502]

Intervertebral Osteochondrosis (IVOC)

As disc degeneration progresses and IVC becomes more severe, associated degeneration of the vertebral end-plate occurs. This allows for the intraosseous herniation of disc material (Schmorl's nodes) and the formation of reactive bone (sclerosis) in the subchondral zone—intervertebral osteochondrosis (IVOC).[1129a] The sclerosis is readily visible on the radiograph (see Figs. 4–70 and 4–101). Schmorl's nodes of variable size may be noted.[1018]

Spinal Osteophytosis (Spondylosis Deformans)

In spinal osteophytosis (spondylosis deformans) osteophytes develop as bony prom-

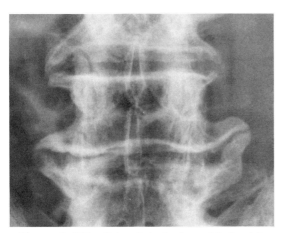

Figure 4–102. Osteophytosis (spondylosis deformans). Large osteophytes at different stages of development. At first they project horizontally, and then they may project vertically and fuse. Notice that the intervertebral disc spaces are maintained.

inences that arise from the anterior and lateral aspects of the vertebral body (Fig. 4–102). They form in response to strain that occurs at the areas of insertion of ligaments to vertebrae[85] and seem to develop in areas where stress is greater.[903] There are small tears in Sharpey's fibers, which are the outer fibers of the annulus fibrosus that attach to the rims of the vertebral bodies.[1129a] This leads to separation of fibers at their site of attachment and allows disc tissue of fairly normal turgor to be displaced anterolaterally. Protruding disc then stretches the anterior longitudinal ligament and causes stress and eventually new bone production (osteophytes) at the site of attachment of the ligament to the anterior vertebral body—a few millimeters from the vertebral edge. Osteophytes usually extend horizontally and then may extend vertically, sometimes forming a bony bridge with the adjacent osteophyte.[85, 1018] They are more common anteriorly than laterally or posteriorly.[85, 903] It takes about 1 to 3 years for osteophytes to become radiographically visible in spinal osteophytosis, although they may develop in 1 to 3 months following trauma.[1028] In osteophytosis, disc height remains normal.[85, 1018, 1129a] Spinal osteophytes are more frequent in the elderly and may develop anywhere in the axial skeleton. In the thoracic spine, pulsations of the aorta prevent significant osteophyte formation on the left side. Large osteophytes in the anterior cervical spine may cause dysphagia.[143, 1133]

Osteophytes arising from the posterior aspect of the cervical spine, particularly at the C5–C6 level, are seen frequently and may cause narrowing of the cervical spinal canal with cord compression[426] (see Fig. 4–101). This occurs particularly during extension of the neck, as the spinal cord is caught between the osteophytes and the normally infolded ligamenta flava.[1232] These osteophytes are largest in the midline and are associated with radiographic changes of disc degeneration.[426] They are not as readily detected posteriorly as they are anteriorly.[132] It is interesting, however, that osteophytes arising from the posterior surface of lumbar vertebral bodies are infrequent and usually small. This is because the posterior longitudinal ligament attaches mainly to the intervertebral disc, with only a few fibers attaching to the vertebral body.[1129a] The ligament lies separated from the midvertebral body by interposing epidural veins. Osteophytes do not form unless the ligament is overstretched. The cause of small posterior lumbar osteophytes is probably related to disc degeneration with overstretching of annulus fibers. In advanced IVOC, posterior osteophytes arise secondary to irritation by adjacent vertebrae, particularly L5–S1.

Osteophytes may develop following trauma, infection, scoliosis, or kyphosis. A form of osteophyte called the traction spur, which is horizontally directed and about 2 mm from the disc border, is felt to be a sign of spinal instability,[770] but this has not been confirmed experimentally.

Osteoarthritis of the Apophyseal Joints

The apophyseal joints are lined by synovium and frequently undergo degenerative osteoarthritis with osteophyte formation, particularly of the superior articular process.[177, 502, 507] Although any joints may be affected, osteoarthritis occurs most commonly at the C2–C3[426] or C4–C5[427] levels in the cervical spine and in the lumbosacral region. In the L4–L5 and L5–S1 levels, the apophyseal joints are aligned obliquely,[1130, 1284] placing these joints at greater risk from repeated rotational strain.[378, 380] This may eventually lead to torsional stresses and degeneration of the intervertebral disc. On the other hand, intervertebral disc narrowing may lead to additional stress on facet joints.

Asymmetry of lumbar facet joints is common, occurring in 17% to 31%[312, 382] and may lead to altered spinal mechanics and possibly premature degenerative osteoarthritis[749] or degeneration of the intervertebral disc.[382] Interestingly, in the cervical spine, the C5–C6 level has a higher incidence of IVOC, spondylosis, and disc protrusion.[426] This is possibly related to increased motion at this level, with continued stress on supporting structures. A prominent superior articular process encroaches on the posterior superior aspect of the neural foramen, whereas prominent uncovertebral articulations encroach on the anteroinferior aspect of the neural foramen. Narrowing of cervical neural foramina can be suspected on the lateral radiograph if the superior articular process is noted superimposed or anterior to the posterior vertebral margin.[542]

Radiographically, osteoarthritis of apophyseal joints is manifested by joint space narrowing, sclerosis, and osteophyte formation[1018] (Fig. 4–103). Occasionally, vacuum phenomena can be identified within the lumbosacral facet joints (Fig. 4–104), which may be related to laxity of the joint

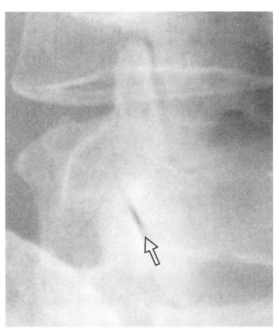

Figure 4–104. Vacuum facet. Oblique radiograph of the lower lumbar spine. There is air density within the apophyseal joint (arrow). The opposing articular surfaces demonstrate sclerosis indicative of degenerative osteoarthritis.

capsule or distraction of a normal joint due to position.[694]

Uncovertebral Arthrosis ("Joint" of Luschka)

The uncovertebral articulations exist from C3 to C7 and consist of the uncinate process (uncus) of the vertebra below and its opposing vertebral surface.[111, 543, 949] It is felt by some to represent a degenerative process.[506, 935, 949] One author felt that disc tissue extended laterally,[433] so that as intervertebral disc degenerated with age, the disc tissue between the uncovertebral articulations also degenerated.[765, 771] Others have shown that the intervertebral disc remains within the confines of the vertebral body and does not demonstrate lateral extension.[543] Other authors have noticed fibrous tissue in the uncovertebral region in fetuses and newborns[506, 543] that is resorbed during the second decade and sometimes in childhood, leaving a fissure—the "joint" of Luschka.[543, 935, 949] Thus, some feel that the uncovertebral articulation is a normal structure formed by the position of the two adjoining vertebrae.[935]

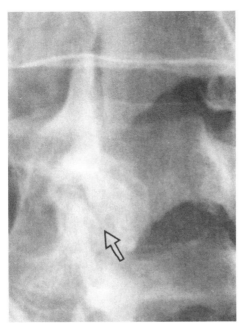

Figure 4–103. Degenerative osteoarthritis, facet joint. Oblique radiograph of the lower lumbar spine demonstrates a narrow facet joint (arrow) due to degenerative osteoarthritis with osteophyte formation and sclerosis of articular processes. Compare with the normal facet joint above.

Although this articulation has in the past been felt by Luschka and others to be lined by synovium,[111] current opinion is that they are not true joints, as no synovium has been identified normally.[506, 543, 935, 949] Adventitious "synovium" in the uncovertebral joint has been noticed in patients with rheumatoid arthritis.[1028] As intervertebral disc degenerates and the opposing uncovertebral surfaces come into apposition, reactive new bone is produced in the form of osteophytes.[506, 771, 935]

There seems to be a correlation between decrease in intervertebral disc height and the severity of the uncovertebral deformities.[949] The osteophytes arise from the posterolateral and lateral vertebral margins and may encroach upon the neural foramen and the existing nerve root[506, 771] or encroach on the adjacent vertebral artery in the foramen transversarium.[506, 771, 949, 1161]

The degenerative alterations of uncovertebral arthrosis are easily identified on the oblique, AP, and lateral radiographs (Fig. 4–105). Bony prominences extend laterally or posterolaterally and may encroach on the neural foramen, particularly in the lower cervical region. On the lateral radiograph, large bony prominences may cause a radiographic appearance resembling a fracture.[465, 506] It should be emphasized that the presence of uncovertebral alterations may not necessarily be associated with symptomatology[427] and that both asymptomatic and symptomatic patients may demonstrate similar abnormalities.

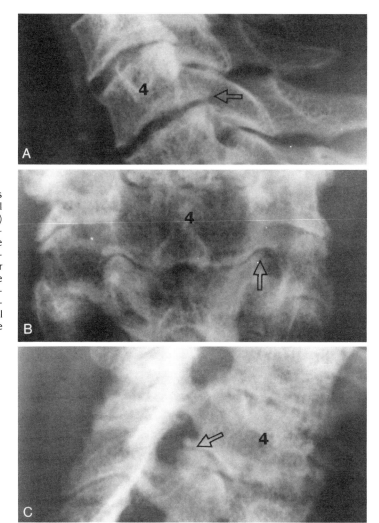

Figure 4–105. Uncovertebral arthrosis of the cervical spine (C4–C5). *A*, Lateral radiograph. Bony prominences (arrow) of the uncovertebral articulation are apparently projecting posteriorly into the spinal canal. Intervertebral osteochondrosis is present. *B*, Anteroposterior radiograph. Bony prominences of the uncovertebral articulation are noted (arrow). *C*, Oblique radiograph demonstrates prominence of the uncovertebral articulation (arrow) projecting into the neural foramen.

Diffuse Idiopathic Skeletal Hyperostosis (DISH)

Diffuse idiopathic skeletal hyperostosis (DISH),[1018] Forestier's disease,[410] is a degenerative disorder of unknown etiology that is frequent in the elderly, occurring in about 12 to 20%[1018, 1274] and being more common in the sixth and seventh decades.[1274] DISH affects both whites and blacks.[641] Male preponderance, noted in whites,[1025] is not present in blacks.[641] In this disorder, there is excessive ligamentous calcification and ossification (enthesopathy)[1029] in the spine and extraspinal locations. Any level of the spine may be involved either alone or in combination, although the thoracic spine is involved more commonly.[411, 1274] Alterations of DISH occur earlier and are more advanced in men.[411] Strict criteria for radiographic diagnosis have been established.[1025] These include (1) flowing calcifications and ossifications along the anterolateral aspect of at least four contiguous vertebral bodies with or without small osteophytes, (2) preservation of disc height in the involved areas and an absence of excessive "degenerative" disc disease, (3) absence of bony ankylosis of facet joints and absence of sacroiliac erosion, sclerosis, or bony fusion, although narrowing and sclerosis of facet joints are acceptable. Although these criteria are admittedly strict,[1025] this author feels that DISH can be

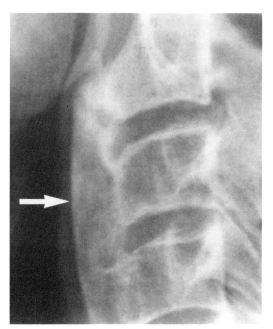

Figure 4–107. DISH. Cervical spine. Thick bony mass that appears fused with the vertebral bodies and is characteristic of more advanced DISH (arrow).

diagnosed even without contiguous vertebral involvement, provided other characteristic features are evident.

Radiographically, there are calcifications or ossifications along the anterolateral aspects of the vertebrae that bridge the intervertebral discs (Fig. 4–106). They are particularly prominent anteriorly at the disc level. They may reach the size of 1.2 cm in the cervical spine and 2 cm in the thoracic and lumbar spines. In advanced cases, the ossifications are large and irregular with a bumpy configuration[411] and may join one vertebra with the next. A characteristic linear lucency may be identified on the lateral radiograph between the anterior vertebral margin and the calcified or ossified density.[1025] (Fig. 4–106). It occurs most commonly in the thoracic spine and may be present in 87% of cases. It represents portions of the anterior longitudinal ligament that have not as yet ossified. In DISH the intervertebral disc remains normal in height.

In the cervical spine, bony prominence may become so extensive that a thick bony plate is formed anteriorly and may cause dysphagia (Fig. 4–107). Sometimes a large bony ossicle is noted anterior to the intervertebral disc.

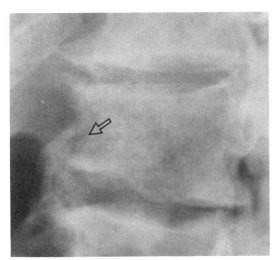

Figure 4–106. DISH. Upper lumbar spine. Thick calcification-ossification in the prevertebral region. Note the clear space between the calcific density and the vertebral body (arrow).

Alterations may develop on the posterior aspect of vertebral bodies, usually in the cervical spine in about 75% of cases.[1022] These radiographic features include osteosclerosis of the posterior vertebral margin (41%), posterior vertebral osteophytosis (34%), and calcification or ossification of the posterior longitudinal ligament (OPLL) (50%). Cervical cord compression has been caused by large posterior osteophytes[14] and by OPLL.[198, 932, 1095, 1276] DISH may occur alone or in patients with intervertebral osteochondrosis, spinal osteophytosis, or rheumatoid arthritis.[1019] Fracture of the odontoid process has been reported in DISH.[376]

Occasionally, the syndesmophytes of psoriatic arthritis and Reiter's syndrome may resemble the bony prominences of DISH. However, the alterations of DISH are predominantly anterior, whereas those of psoriatic arthritis and Reiter's syndrome are lateral. Also, the sacroiliac joints are uninvolved in patients with DISH.

Disc Herniation

Disc herniation cannot be visualized on the plain radiograph unless the disc is cal-cified, and even then the relationship of the herniated nucleus pulposus and annulus fibrosus to the adjacent neural structures cannot be determined. Loss of the normal spine curvature may be seen on the lateral radiograph and may indicate muscle spasm, but this is a nonspecific finding.

Degenerative Alterations of the Sacroiliac Joint

Osteophytes, sclerosis, and joint space loss are the hallmarks of degenerative osteoarthritis and are frequently observed in the sacroiliac joints in patients over the age of 40.[1227] These alterations are most common in males, particularly black males, and may be unilateral or bilateral in distribution. Osteophytes form as a result of stress on the sacroiliac joints. The incidence and distribution differ in males compared with females. In males, the site of stress from weight-bearing is the superior part of the joint.[1227] In women, sacroiliac joints retain more mobility for child-bearing owing to a hormonal effect causing ligament relaxation.[126, 209] Thus, women develop osteophytes in the anteroinferior part of the joint,

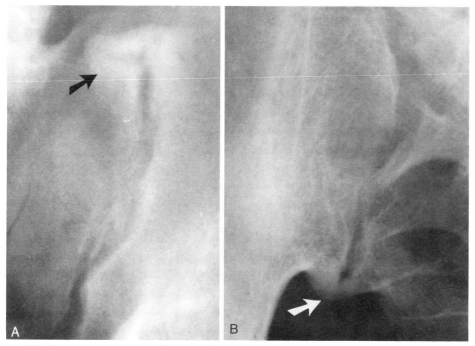

Figure 4–108. Degenerative osteoarthritis, sacroiliac joint. A, Degenerative osteophyte formation (arrow) of the upper portion of the sacroiliac joint simulating a sclerotic bone lesion. B, Para-articular osteophytes are fused in the lower aspect of the joint (arrow). The true joint space is normal in width.

the site that reflects the stress caused by the mobility of the sacroiliac joints.[1227]

Radiographically, osteophytes occur at any level but are more common in the anterosuperior margin of the joint, where they may appear as large bony densities on the AP radiograph (sometimes mimicking an osteosclerotic bone lesion) (Fig. 4–108A), or in the anteroinferior margin, where they appear triangular in shape and associated with subchondral sclerosis and joint narrowing[1030, 1031] (Fig. 4–108B). Para-articular osteophytes may bridge the joint and fuse, but intra-articular fusion does not occur.[1030] Anterior osteophytes superimposed over the sacroiliac joint may simulate intra-articular fusion. Sclerosis appears in the subchondral region in response to stress, most commonly in superoinferior aspects of the articulation, particularly on the iliac side, and may appear focal or linear alongside the articular surface.[1031] Subchondral cystlike defects and erosions are not commonly visualized.[209, 1031] The joint space usually narrows focally and asymmetrically, particularly inferiorly, although more diffuse joint narrowing may occur.[1031] The joint margins may be smooth or irregular.

In patients with DISH, the incidence of superior and inferior capsular ossification is 87.5% in males, and the incidence does not increase over the age of 50.[126] The bridging may be incomplete or complete. Intra-articular fusion does not occur.

Spondylolysis and Spondylolisthesis

Spondylolysis

Spondylolysis refers to a defect in the pars interarticularis. It occurs in 3.5%[338] to 6.4%[1063, 1065] of the population and is equal in incidence in whites and blacks in one series[338] and more common in whites in others.[1063, 1065] The most frequent occurrence is in Eskimo skeletons.[1065] Spondylolysis is most common in the L5 vertebra[338, 1063] but may occur at other lumbar levels. It rarely occurs in the cervical spine.[45, 536] It is unilateral in over one sixth to one third of cases[338, 1065] and, when unilateral, may be associated with hypoplasia of the vertebral body and neural arch[979] or congenital absence of the pedicle.[1139] Spondylolysis may occur at multiple lumbar levels in about 0.2% to 5.6% of

the population.[1003] The defects may occur in sequence or be separated by one or more normal vertebrae.

Spondylolysis is probably caused by repeated trauma (stress fractures)[508, 1352] to a pars interarticularis that has been inherently weakened by a hereditary defect or dysplasia[1350] rather than by a single acute traumatic event. Some families have a higher incidence of spondylolysis.[1352] Although the neural arch is a relatively strong structure, it has been demonstrated experimentally that a defect can be produced in the pars interarticularis by fatigue loading.[604] Thus, in vivo, fatigue fractures may occur over a long period of time if bone repair cannot keep pace with the microscopic injury caused by repeated loading of the pars interarticularis by an unaccustomed activity.[604] Torsional stresses are most disruptive to the neural arch.[381] Such fatigue fractures could theoretically occur in a pars interarticularis unaffected by any hereditary defect or dysplasia. There are others that feel that a defect could possibly develop following an acute traumatic event[677, 1062, 1352] and that bilateral defects represent nonunion of fractures of the pars interarticularis caused by excessive mobility.[338]

Spondylolysis is not present at birth[1350] and usually occurs in childhood by the age of 6 years or by early adult life. Spondylolysis has been reported in young children[1327] even as early as 4 months of age.[113] The discovery of spondylolysis in infants suggests that it is of congenital origin, although this has not been documented.[1350] The incidence increases up to adulthood in most cases, after which the incidence remains the same.[338, 1063] However, the incidence rises up to the age of 40 years in Eskimos.[1350] Spondylolysis has been noted to occur following spinal fusion, usually occurring in the uppermost vertebra included in the fusion.[69, 524] Metastasis may attack the pars interarticularis, causing bone destruction and a pathologic fracture. Spina bifida occulta associated with defects in the pars interarticularis in the lower lumbar region is 13 times as common as it is in normal spines.[1350]

Radiographically, lumbar spondylolysis is best viewed on the oblique radiograph but may be identified on the lateral and, to a lesser extent, the anteroposterior views (Fig. 4–109). It appears as a radiolucent band across the neck of the "Scotty dog," resem-

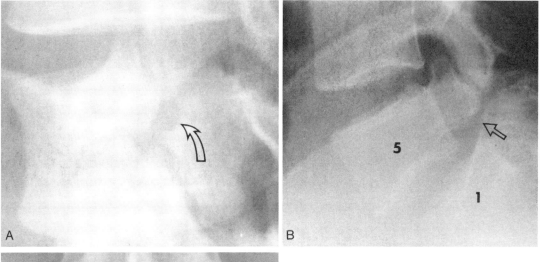

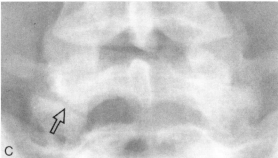

Figure 4–109. Spondylolysis. Lumbar spine. *A,* Oblique view. There is a linear radiolucency (fracture) in the region of the pars interarticularis resembling a collar on the neck of the "Scotty dog" (arrow). Lateral *(B)* and anteroposterior *(C)* views demonstrate the pars defect (arrows) in other patients. Note the anterior slip of L5 on S1 in *B.*

bling the dog's "collar." The margins of the defect are sclerotic, and occasionally calcific densities representing calcified callus formation are noted about the defect.[22] Rarely, a mass of new bone formation about a healed defect may cause spinal stenosis.[338] A similar radiolucent band can be identified on the lateral projection just caudad to the pedicle at the involved level. The defect is less obvious on the anteroposterior radiograph. When there is a unilateral pars defect, sclerosis, cortical thickening, and/or enlargement of the contralateral lamina and/or pedicle may be identified as a response to stress on those elements.[781, 1166, 1342] Enlarged superior articular facets and elliptic inferior articular facets of the involved arch have been observed in specimens.[338] Healing of the pars defect can occur but usually remains as a pseudarthrosis.[1352] Spondylolisthesis may or may not be present with spondylolysis.

Occasionally, on a true lateral lumbar radiograph, an apparent radiolucent defect with sclerotic margins is noted overlying the region of the pars interarticularis. It may not be visible on oblique radiographs and represents superimposed transverse processes—the so-called pseudospondylolysis.[347]

Spondylolysis of the cervical spine is rare.[45, 536] The etiology is unknown but may be congenital.[45] It is most common at the C6 level but has also been noted from C2 to C7.[45, 536] Radiographically, the margins of a defect are sharply defined and rounded in appearance.[536] In the axis, there is a small, peglike, bony prominence of the midanterior border of the defect.[536]

Spondylolisthesis

Spondylolisthesis is defined as subluxation of one vertebral body on another[1350, 1353] and occurs most commonly in the lower lumbar and lumbosacral regions. Displacement may be classified as anterior slippage (spondylolisthesis) or posterior slippage (retrolisthesis) of the vertebral body above on the vertebral body below. Spondylolisthesis may be classified as isthmic, degenerative,

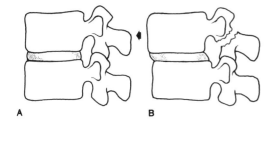

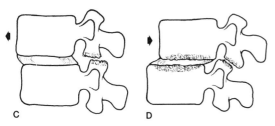

Figure 4–110. Diagrammatic representation of spondylolisthesis. Arrows denote direction of slippage. *A*, Vertebral bodies are aligned, and the pars interarticularis and facet joints appear normal. *B*, Isthmic spondylolisthesis with anterior slippage of a vertebral body due to a defect in the pars interarticularis. *C*, Degenerative spondylolisthesis with anterior slippage of a vertebral body secondary to degenerative osteoarthritis of facet joints. *D*, Retrolisthesis with posterior displacement of a vertebral body secondary to intervertebral osteochondrosis and degenerative osteoarthritis of apophyseal joints.

dysplastic, traumatic, and pathologic[1351] (Fig. 4–110).

In isthmic spondylolisthesis, the lesion is in the pars interarticularis. There may be a bilateral pars defect (fatigue fracture)[35, 1350, 1351] that occurs most often at L5,[1063] an elongated but intact pars,[1351] or an acute fracture of the pars.[677, 1352] In patients with bilateral pars defect, the vertebral slippage is greater than in those without a defect.[16] In the adolescent or child with a listhesis of 50% or more there is greater chance for progression of slippage.[1206] Familial occurrence has been noted in about 33% of cases asociated with pars defects.[1376] Scoliosis occurs in 42% of patients with symptomatic spondylolisthesis.[836]

There are other lesions of the pars interarticularis. The pars interarticularis may be intact but elongated either congenitally or secondary to repeated fatigue microfractures that heal with elongation as the L5 vertebral body slips forward.[1351] A pars defect may also occur from acute severe trauma.[677, 1351, 1352]

In degenerative spondylolisthesis, there are alterations in the biomechanics of the lumbosacral region that develop with age.[16] There is progressive stress and degeneration of intervertebral discs, facet joints, and posterior spinous ligaments. The degenerative process causes the axis of rotation to move posteriorly from the nucleus pulposus to the facet joints, and increased movement in the anteroposterior direction occurs, aggravated by the erect posture. These stresses and movement are produced by degenerative alterations and deformity of the facet joints, which, when angled more sagittally,[1350] allow more mobility,[16] less ligamentous support,[1028] and therefore listhesis. Facet joints become thickened and irregular.[16] Another reason that listhesis might occur with degenerative change is that small microfractures may occur in the inferior articular process.[1351] This causes the articular process to change direction and become more horizontal in position. Degenerative spondylolisthesis is most evident at the L4–L5 level.[16, 379] In this disorder, the entire vertebral body and posterior elements slip forward.[1350] The degree of listhesis is not always related to the degree of disc degeneration and rarely is greater than 1 cm.[16] It is usually accompanied by rotational displacement of about 6 degrees.[379] Forward listhesis may cause impingement of the existing nerve roots by the prominent displaced superior and inferior articular processes.

In retrolisthesis, degenerative spondylolisthesis associated with intervertebral osteochondrosis occurs. In this disorder, degeneration of intervertebral disc leads to closer placement of vertebral bodies and increased motion of articular processes, leading to posterior displacement of the vertebra on the one below.[1028] Retrolisthesis is most frequent in the cervical and upper lumbar regions of the spine—anatomic areas that demonstrate increased motion.

In the dysplastic type of spondylolisthesis, there is congenital dysplasia of the upper sacrum or neural arch of L5.[1351] A wide spina bifida is often present. The stresses of weight-bearing cause the vertebral body to slip forward on the one below, leaving the pars interarticularis intact. Bilateral congenital absence of pedicles of C6 has been observed with cervical spondylolisthesis.[73]

In traumatic spondylolisthesis, severe trauma causes an acute fracture of the articular processes and not the pars interarticularis.[1351]

In the pathologic type of spondylolisthesis, disease of the pars, pedicle, or articular processes causes alterations in these structures.[1351] This can be seen in metastasis (pathologic fracture), Paget's disease (unilateral elongation of the pedicle or pathologic fracture), and in some forms of arthrogryposis.

Radiographically, the posterior margin of vertebrae should line up with those above and below (see Fig. 4–109B). In spondylolisthesis, there is anterior slippage of one vertebral body on the one below. In cases where the diagnosis of listhesis is uncertain, alignment of facet joints[35] and widening of the facet joints on the oblique radiograph are additional clues to the correct diagnosis. Another sign is that of isolated lateral deviation of the spinous process viewed on the anteroposterior radiograph. This has been noted in most cases of spondylolisthesis with abnormality of the pars interarticularis.[1002] The pars abnormality may be a defect or an unequally elongated pars without a defect. In spondylolisthesis associated with defects in the pars interarticularis, there is forward displacement of the vertebral body, pedicles, transverse processes, and superior articular processes. The inferior articular processes and neural arch remain behind. In degenerative spondylolisthesis, there is anterior displacement of the vertebra and posterior elements, with associated degenerative osteoarthritis of facet joints (sclerosis, osteophyte formation, and joint-space narrowing). The degree of spondylolisthesis or retrolisthesis can be determined either by noting the percentage of slippage (0% to 100%)[1353] or by dividing the surface into four equal sections (grades 1 through 4) (Fig. 4–111). The angle of the slip (kyphosis) can be measured.[1206] Severe fourth degree spondylolisthesis of L5–S1 can be diagnosed on the AP radiograph as the "upside-down Napoleon hat" sign (Fig. 4–112). This is due to superimposition of the L5 vertebral body on S1. Hypoplasia of a lumbar vertebral body may simulate spondylolisthesis.[417]

The radiographic appearance of retrolisthesis includes posterior displacement of the vertebra above along with radiographic features of intervertebral osteochondrosis (loss of disc height, vacuum phenomenon, subchondral sclerosis) and subluxation of facet joints. In the lumbosacral region, the depth of the L5 vertebral body is greater than that of S1 in one third of normal patients. This may create an illusion of retrolisthesis;[1347] however, the anterior vertebral margin of L5 will be aligned with S1 in this situation.

Spondylolisthesis of the cervical spine is rare.[57, 193, 390, 448, 912, 1162] Most cases demonstrate spina bifida,[448] while defects of the pars interarticularis and pedicles are unusual.[193, 377, 1162] Patients rarely present with neurologic deficit.[390] Cervical spondylolisthesis has been reported to be associated with the basal cell nevus syndrome.[57]

Osseous Tumors and Tumorlike Conditions

The conventional radiograph is not helpful in the early detection of bone tumors and

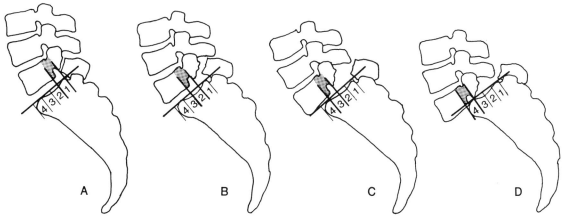

Figure 4–111. Grading of degree of spondylolisthesis by dividing the sacral surface into four equal parts. *A*, First degree. *B*, Second degree. *C*, Third degree. *D*, Fourth degree. (From Meyerding HW: Spondylolisthesis. Surg Gyn Obstet 54:371–377, 1932. By permission of Surgery, Gynecology & Obstetrics.)

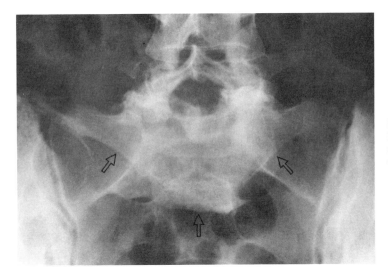

Figure 4–112. Inverted "Napoleon hat" sign (arrows) of severe spondylolisthesis. This image is caused by the superimposed anteriorly and inferiorly displaced L5 vertebra on the sacrum.

tumorlike conditions, as significant bone destruction must take place before they are radiographically visible. In addition, the plain radiograph is not helpful in demonstrating the intraspinal extent of tumor.

Malignant Tumors

Metastasis. Metastasis is the most frequent tumor of bone[775] and the most frequent tumor of the spine in both children and adults. The high incidence of metastasis to bone is interesting when one realizes that bone receives a relatively small proportion (5% to 10%) of cardiac output.[80, 634] Metastasis may occur as a solitary lesion in 29% of solitary tumors of the spine.[210] Seventy to ninety percent of all metastases are multiple.[755] Carcinomas of the breast, prostate, and lung are the most frequent primary carcinomas that invade the spine in the adult;[634] neuroblastoma and leukemia are the most common malignancies that involve the spine in the infant and child, respectively. Skeletal metastases eventually develop in around 50% to 70% of patients with prostatic carcinoma, in 25% to 45% of those with lung carcinoma, and in 50% of patients with breast carcinoma. However, it should be recalled that carcinoma of the lung is the most common primary carcinoma in men and its incidence in women is rising rapidly.

The spine is the most common skeletal site involved by metastasis,[863] with the thoracic spine affected most often.[104] Metastasis

invades the spine by hematogenous route or by direct extension.[80, 104] Hematogenous spread is almost always by the arterial route, although spinal metastasis may develop via venous spread, particularly from tumors in the pelvic region[62, 80, 216] or carcinoma of the breast.[80]

Metastasis may involve any bone and any portion of the bone; however, in the spine, the vertebral body is attacked earliest and most frequently owing to its rich vascular and red marrow supply.[531, 692] The subchondral regions and anterior margin are involved early owing to the vascular supply. The pedicles may also be involved early because of the rich vascular supply in the pedicle–transverse process junction[387, 692] (Figs. 4–113 through 4–115). The sacrum is

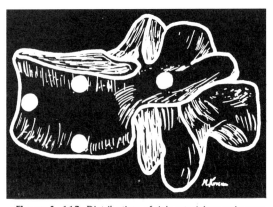

Figure 4–113. Distribution of rich arterial vascular supply and sites of early metastasis to the vertebral segment (solid white circles). These are the subchondral, anterior vertebral, and pedicle–transverse process regions.

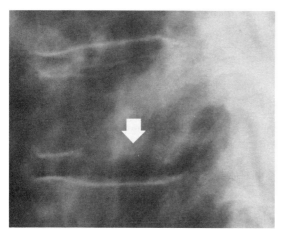

Figure 4–114. Early visible metastasis to the thoracic spine. Notice the absence of the vertebral margin (arrow).

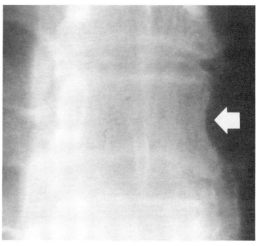

Figure 4–115. Metastasis. The left pedicle is absent (arrow). No other visible destruction is noted in this vertebral segment.

also a common site for metastasis, and many lesions are often not diagnosed.[26] Normally, the upper margins of the sacral foramina are sharply defined, arc shaped, symmetric bony densities. They should be carefully examined, as asymmetry or absence of a foraminal margin usually indicates bone destruction, most likely from metastasis[26] (either from hematogenous spread of tumor elsewhere or from direct extension from carcinoma of the rectum) (Fig. 4–116), or invasion by a primary sacral tumor. Feces in overlying bowel can occasionally obscure visualization of the sacral foramen, causing a false appearance of bone destruction.

Radiographically, it is difficult to detect metastasis on the conventional radiograph. Approximately 50% to 75% of cancellous bone thickness must be destroyed before a lesion can be detected on the lateral radiograph, and even greater destruction must occur before a lesion becomes visible on the AP radiograph[326] or in osteopenic patients. Cortical lesions 1 cm in size may not be detected.[1299] Thus, metastasis to bone may be widespread and not radiographically visible, since most bony metastases occur in cancellous bone and range in size from 1 cm to 3 cm[755] (Fig. 4–117). Lesions in the sacrum

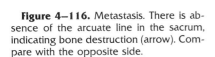

Figure 4–116. Metastasis. There is absence of the arcuate line in the sacrum, indicating bone destruction (arrow). Compare with the opposite side.

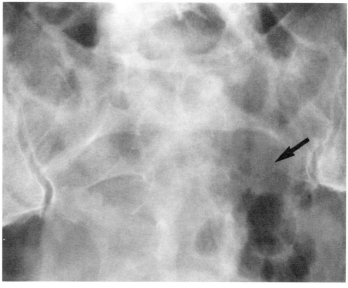

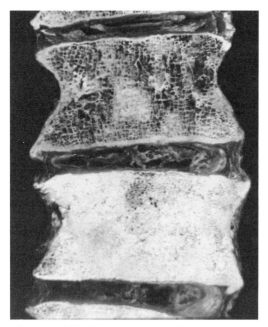

Figure 4–117. Gross specimen of metastasis to the spine from carcinoma of the prostate. Coronal section. There has been marked replacement of marrow with tumor in the lower vertebra. Focal areas of metastasis are noted in the upper vertebra, and lesions of this size may not be visualized on the radiograph.

may be difficult to detect, owing to the curved nature of this bone and the presence of overlying bowel gas and feces. Metastasis is usually osteolytic in appearance, and the margins of a metastatic lesion are often poorly defined, owing to its aggressive behavior. Early changes may be noted in the upper, lower, and anterior vertebral margins (see Fig. 4–114). Metastasis to bone usually reflects the level of aggressiveness of the primary tumor from which it originated, and marked destruction may be noted. It may also appear slow-growing, with sclerotic margins, and may "expand" bone, particularly with slow-growing primary tumors such as carcinoma of the kidney or thyroid gland. Tumor involvement of C1 or C2 may lead to atlantoaxial subluxation.[535] Intervertebral discs usually remain normal in height, although collapse of disc into bone weakened by tumor may occur.[593, 1027] A radiolucency in the posterior aspect of the vertebral body of C2 in the off-lateral projection is the costotransverse foramen and should not be mistaken for a pathologic lesion.[911] Similarly, a tortuous vertebral artery may cause erosion of the cervical vertebral arch, mimicking a lesion.[1339]

"Osteoblastic" metastasis is a misnomer, as it represents reactive normal bone stimulated by the presence of underlying tumor and does not represent the tumor itself.[34, 597, 859, 974, 1362] It may appear patchy, involve the entire vertebral body ("ivory vertebra")[372, 403, 1016] (see Fig. 4–67), or appear diffuse throughout the axial skeleton[180] (see Fig. 4–66). While any primary metastatic tumor may incite osteoblastic response, carcinoma of the prostate is by far the most common cause of osteosclerotic metastasis. About 90% of patients with metastatic prostatic tumor have purely osteosclerotic lesions.[615] There seems to be an osteoblastic factor that is found in prostatic tissue, both in hyperplastic and in tumor tissue.[615] Carcinoma of the breast is the second most common cause of osteosclerotic metastasis,[615] either untreated (9% of metastatic breast carcinoma to bone)[615, 733] or treated[59] cases. Lymphoma and rare lesions such as metastatic medulloblastoma, metastatic carcinoid, and mucin-secreting tumors of the gastrointestinal tract may appear osteosclerotic.[906] An unusual but characteristic pattern of spinal metastasis from carcinoma of the cervix may occur with bone destruction or osteosclerosis.[403] There is unilateral involvement of one or several contiguous vertebrae, usually on the left side, possibly from tumor extension directly from adjacent lymph nodes. This can be explained by the closer proximity of left para-aortic nodes to the lumbar spine, compared with those on the right.

Osteosclerotic alterations may develop in response to treatment, particularly metastasis to bone from carcinoma of the breast.[59] Treatment of metastatic carcinoma of the breast by either surgical or "medical" adrenalectomy, hormonal therapy or chemotherapy, or local radiotherapy may produce osteoblastic response in previous osteolytic lesions and indicates remission.[59, 615] The response may develop within a period of 6 weeks following onset of treatment.[59] Response of lytic metastases to chemotherapy can be appreciated, as the lytic lesions initially form a sclerotic rim and then progressively become uniformly sclerotic. The lesions then begin to fade in appearance uniformly. Increase in size of lytic lesions or destruction within a previously osteosclerotic lesion indicates progression of metastasis.[59, 615]

The radiographic changes that occur during treatment of patients with bony metastasis from carcinoma of the prostate vary. Increasing osteosclerotic or osteolytic lesions usually accompany progressive disease, although osteoblastic response occasionally may be seen during clinical remission.[974] The radiographs of patients who respond favorably to treatment usually remain unchanged in about one half of the cases. Resolution of sclerosis or recalcification of osteolytic lesions may develop as well.

Myeloma. Myeloma is the second most frequent malignant tumor of bone, second only to metastasis. It usually occurs in individuals over the age of 40 years and is most common in the spine, particularly in the vertebral body, which has a rich red marrow supply.[531, 692] Myeloma does not involve pedicles early in the course of disease, since there is little red marrow in pedicles,[618] but it does involve pedicles in advanced disease, as fat marrow is reconverted to red marrow.[692] Pedicle involvement may explain radicular pain in some patients.[756]

Like metastasis, myeloma is not visualized radiographically early in the course of disease, and it usually presents radiographically with single or multiple osteolytic lesions with sharply defined margins. The myeloma cell produces an osteoclast activating factor that facilitates bone resorption.[884] In more advanced disease, there may be marked bone destruction resembling metastasis (Fig. 4–118). Myeloma may form an "expansile" multiloculated lesion, and sometimes a soft tissue mass may be present. Occasionally, myeloma may be so widespread that the spine appears diffusely osteopenic without any focal areas of visible destruction (Fig. 4–119). Although these difficulties in detecting myeloma are well recognized, the conventional radiograph is still more sensitive overall in detecting myeloma lesions than is radionuclide scanning.[762, 1370] Rarely, myeloma may invade the intervertebral disc when there is extensive tumor in contiguous vertebrae.[853] Disc narrowing associated with myeloma could also be due to vertebral end-plate collapse from the underlying tumor, with subsequent interosseous disc herniation and narrowing. There is a close correlation between the skeletal changes of myeloma and the serum immunoglobulin levels and postabsorptive urinary hydroxyproline levels.[1144a]

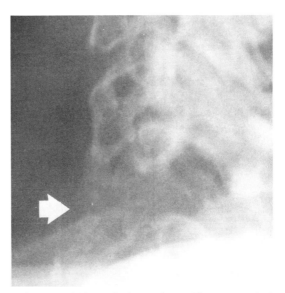

Figure 4–118. Multiple myeloma. There is marked destruction of a lower cervical vertebral body (arrow). Multiple osteolytic lesions are noted in the vertebrae above. Metastasis may have a similar appearance.

Rarely, a "solitary" bone lesion of myeloma may be the only identifiable evidence of this disorder.* Solitary myeloma is defined as a single osteolytic bone lesion without evidence of myeloma cells on the bone marrow examination.[1368] Although "solitary lesions" (plasmacytoma) have been reported, some are probably solitary manifes-

*Reference numbers 179, 211, 235, 475, 731, 948, 1270, 1281, 1346.

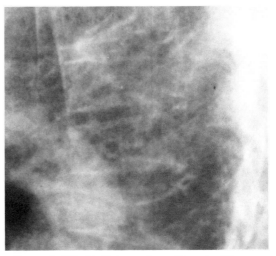

Figure 4–119. Multiple myeloma. There is diffuse osteopenia without visible bone destruction. Collapse of a thoracic vertebra is noted.

tations of more widespread and as yet un-detected myeloma.[1368] Solitary myelomas are most frequent in the spine and pelvis.[475, 756, 853, 948] They appear either as multicystic os-teolytic lesions with thick trabeculae or as an osteolytic lesion similar in appearance to metastasis.[853] Patients with true solitary plas-macytoma of the spine without epidural ex-tension have the potential for long-term re-mission,[201, 211, 756] even up to 21 years.[211] Some forms of so-called benign solitary mye-loma may actually be focal hyperplasia of histiocytes induced from an inflammatory process.[635] Rarely, untreated myeloma may appear osteosclerotic.* The radiographs may demonstrate multiple patchy sclerotic le-sions or diffuse uniform bone sclerosis. Sol-itary uniform vertebral sclerosis ("ivory ver-tebra") may develop in myeloma.[1060] Osteosclerotic-appearing myeloma is fre-quently associated with a clinical syndrome of polyneuropathy, organomegaly, endocri-nopathy, M protein, and skin changes—the so-called POEMS syndrome.[1021] Osteoscle-rosis may also develop in osteolytic lesions following treatment.[269, 756]

Chondrosarcoma. Chondrosarcomas ac-count for 1.2% of all primary bone tumors of the spine and sacrum other than mye-loma.[242] Only 8% to 12% of chondrosarco-mas occur in the spine and sacrum.[242, 245, 461, 553] Chondrosarcoma arises de novo or from malignant degeneration in Paget's disease[97, 1239] from an osteochondroma or following irradiation to bone.[36] Patients with spinal chondrosarcoma usually present with pain, pathologic fracture, or symptoms of spinal cord or cauda equina compression.[578] Chon-drosarcomas may occur at any level but are more frequent in the thoracic spine and sacrum.[210] They usually occur during the fourth through sixth decades, but those that develop secondarily to osteochondroma present at an earlier age.

Chondrosarcoma may grow to a large size prior to clinical presentation. Radiographi-cally, there is bone destruction with frequent extensive punctate or ringlike calcification in the matrix[97, 166, 691] (Fig. 4–120). Occasion-ally, calcifications may appear amorphous in more aggressive tumors.[755] The tumor margin may or may not be sclerotic. Verte-bral body compression is not uncommon. The underlying osteochondroma may not be

---

*Reference numbers 96, 137, 204, 315, 325, 355, 371.

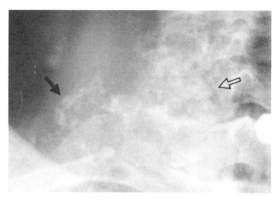

Figure 4–120. Chondrosarcoma. There is bone de-struction (open arrow) in the lower cervical spine. Punc-tate and ringlike calcifications (closed arrow) are noted in the paravertebral soft tissues. Calcifications of this nature represent cartilage matrix. (Courtesy of Dr. J. George Teplick, Philadelphia, Pennsylvania.)

visible radiographically. Very rarely, a highly malignant form of mesenchymal chondrosarcoma may develop extradurally outside of bone and cause a spinal cord compression.[191]

Chordoma. Chordomas are the most fre-quent primary tumor in the axial skeleton other than myeloma.[210] They usually de-velop during the sixth and seven decades. Chordomas arise from notochord rests and are found most commonly in the sacrococ-cygeal region (50% to 65%), clivus (25% to 35%), and vertebral column (15%) (cervical, lumbar, and thoracic, in that order).[242, 365, 564, 1242] The axis may be a common site for cervical chordomas,[100, 266, 1028] although a chordoma has been reported in the atlas.[1374] The relative frequency in the axis has not been demonstrated in all series of cervical chordomas.[885] In the sacrum, chordomas usually occur in the S4 and S5 segments.[564] They are slow-growing, destructive tumors that may achieve considerable size.

Radiographically, chordoma is an osteo-lytic or osteoblastic lesion or both, arising from the midline portion of the vertebral body or sacrum (Figs. 4–121 and 4–122). The margin about the tumor is sclerotic in around 45% of cases.[400] Calcifications occur in 14% to 50%[365, 400, 560, 854, 1239, 1280] and occur more frequently in tumors of the sacrum than in those of the spine.[695] Tumor may also displace and engulf fragments of bone as it grows.[1280] This may appear on the radio-graph as matrix calcification. Chordomas

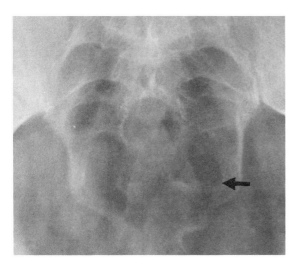

Figure 4–121. Chordoma. There is an osteolytic lesion in the central portion of the distal sacrum (arrow). This represents chordoma. Metastasis could have a similar appearance.

usually grow anteriorly, forming a large soft tissue mass.[1242] Pathologic fracture may occur.[1280] Rarely, chordoma may present with extensive sclerosis, appearing as an "ivory" vertebra[1140] and, in the sacrum, may cause scalloping with expansion in about one half of the cases.[1280] Occasionally, chordomas invade intervertebral discs and extend to the adjacent vertebra—an unusual feature of tumors in general.[400, 966]

Around 10% to 40% of chordomas metas-

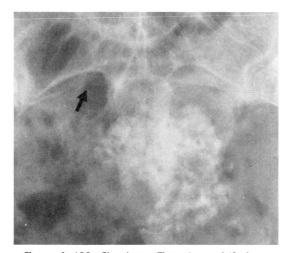

Figure 4–122. Chordoma. There is a calcified mass superimposed over the sacrum. Calcification of this type could be mistaken for uterine fibroids in a female patient; however, there is partial destruction of one of the arcuate lines of the sacrum (arrow), which indicates bone destruction and, in this case, chordoma.

tasize, and this usually occurs late in the course of disease.[189, 196, 400, 1047, 1242, 1293] In the cervical spine, chordoma may rarely present with a prevertebral mass[885] or as a pharyngeal mass.[1153] This may be due to the fact that the developing notochord passes through mesenchymal tissue and may be directly in contact with pharyngeal epithelium.[885] Chordoma rarely presents as a posterior mediastinal mass, without vertebral destruction,[220] or causes widening of the cervical neural foramen, mimicking neurofibroma.[1153, 1303]

Ewing's Sarcoma. Ewing's sarcoma of the axial skeleton is rare,* accounting for 5.6% of all primary bone tumors of the axial skeleton other than myeloma.[242] Four percent to 7.4% of Ewing's sarcoma cases involve the spine and sacrum.[242, 244, 717, 1305] In several large series of Ewing's sarcoma, ranging from 50 to 156 cases, no tumors were discovered in the axial skeleton.[84, 213, 1292] In another series of 244 cases, two occurred in the sacrum, and none developed in the spine.[981] In one series of 41 cases, 32% were present in the spine and sacrum.[1283] Most Ewing's sarcomas develop within the first 3 decades. In the axial skeleton they are twice as frequent in the sacrum as in the vertebrae,[242] with around 60% occurring in the sacrum.[1335] The lumbar, thoracic, and cervical vertebrae are affected, in that order.[1335]

Radiographically, Ewing's sarcoma is a highly aggressive osteolytic or osteosclerotic lesion. In the spine, tumor involves the vertebral body but occurs in the vertebral arch as well[690] (Fig. 4–123). Partial collapse of the body and associated paravertebral mass is frequent, even when bone destruction is not visible.[1335] There may be loss of intervertebral disc height. Calcifications within tumor matrix are rare[1317] and probably represent calcification of necrotic tissue or islands of bone placed by tumor. Tumor rarely extends to an adjacent vertebra.[772] Metastasis of Ewing's sarcoma to the spine from an extraskeletal site is more common than primary Ewing's sarcoma of the spine[1239, 1335] and may occur in around 30% of cases.[1335] The skull and spine are the most common sites of bone metastasis.[981] Intradural metastasis has been reported, and central nervous system metastasis without bone or dural involvement oc-

*Reference numbers 327, 607, 684, 690, 717, 772, 1091, 1181, 1283, 1317, 1335.

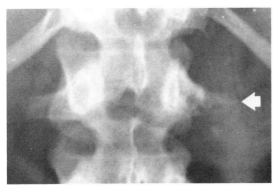

Figure 4–123. Ewing's sarcoma. There is destruction of the left transverse process of L1 (arrow). This is an unusual location for Ewing's sarcoma. Metastasis and histiocytosis could have a similar appearance.

curs in around 2% of cases.[1301] Rarely, Ewing's tumor may mimic a herniated disc clinically.[398] Overall, neurologic complications of Ewing's tumor in general occur in around 30% of cases some time during the course of disease.[1335]

Ewing's sarcomas of the sacrum have the same radiographic alterations as those in the vertebral column. However, tumor frequently extends into the pelvis and may form masses of enormous size.[1283]

Fibrous Histiocytoma. Fibrous histiocytoma is a highly malignant tumor that rarely affects the axial skeleton. It may occur as a primary[274a, 284a, 385a, 1005a] or metastatic spinal lesion[385a] or may develop secondary to irradiation.[1283a] The vertebral body or posterior elements may be involved, and the lesion may appear destructive or expansile.

Giant Cell Tumor. Giant cell tumor (GCT) (osteoclastoma) is a tumor derived either from osteoclasts[934] or from certain stromal cells that make up the bulk of the tumor.[1116] Viruslike intranuclear inclusions similar to those of Paget's disease have been observed in this tumor in 15% of cases.[1124] GCT is a rare primary spinal or sacral bone tumor,* accounting for 8.7% of all primary bone tumors in this axial skeleton other than myeloma.[242] About 12% of GCT occurs in the axial skeleton.[824] Giant cell tumors occur most frequently during the third and fourth decades, and about 60% to 70% occur in patients 20 to 40 years of age.[603, 1116] Only

10% develop in patients under the age of 20.[561] However, in one series, 29% of spinal GCT occurred in the first 2 decades, suggesting that the tumor may be basically different from giant cell tumors elsewhere.[241] GCT is 3 to 4 times as frequent in the sacrum as it is in the remainder of the vertebral column,[242, 467] and it is the second most common tumor of the sacrum[1190] (Fig. 4–124). In the spine, the cervical and thoracic regions are involved more frequently.[242, 298]

GCT is an osteolytic lesion that may demonstrate "expansion."[298, 561] Seventy percent of giant cell tumors of the spine involve the vertebral body.[241, 1141] Of these, about 40% involve the pedicle and vertebal arch.[241] Giant cell tumor may involve contiguous vertebrae[298, 1141] and may extend across the sacroiliac joint to involve the adjoining ilium.[1190] Isolated tumor in the vertebral arch may also occur.[298] Patients may present with neurologic compromise[1141] as tumor extends into the spinal canal.

Giant cell tumor may rarely develop in Paget's disease of bone;[952, 1088, 1122] however, these tumors are not as aggressive as giant cell tumors in normal bone.[1122] GCT should not be graded histopathologically[622] or radiographically as benign or malignant, as appearances are often misleading. There is around a 34% to 50% recurrence rate for giant cell tumor,[603, 824] and recurrent tumors behave more aggressively.

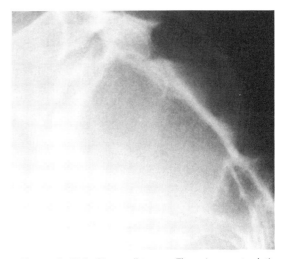

Figure 4–124. Giant cell tumor. There is an osteolytic lesion that is causing expansion in the proximal sacrum of this 28 year old patient. Aneurysmal bone cyst could have a similar appearance.

---

*Reference numbers 200, 241, 298, 412, 472, 514, 561, 666, 714a, 824, 1009, 1141, 1168, 1285.

CONVENTIONAL RADIOGRAPHY • 133

Leukemia. Leukemia is the most common malignancy of childhood.[914] The axial skeleton, which is rich in red marrow, is a frequent site for leukemia. The incidence and appearance of radiographic features of leukemia are variable, depending somewhat on the form of leukemia and the age of the patient.

The radiographic features of leukemia in the axial skeleton vary somewhat with the various types of leukemia but include generalized osteopenia, focal osteolytic lesions, thin horizontal radiolucent bands in the subchondral region, vertebral collapse, and osteosclerosis (either single, patchy, or diffuse).[271, 276, 357, 596, 647, 1067, 1114] Three percent of patients demonstrate vertebral collapse at the time of clinical presentation.[1067] Generalized osteopenia occurs from trabecular destruction by tumor, resorption by marrow hyperplasia,[1114] or steroid medication. Anterior wedging[357] and biconcavity of vertebrae may be observed. Focal osteolytic lesions are more difficult to detect in cancellous bone. They may be due to focal bone destruction by tumor or infarction secondary to vascular occlusion.[1114] Erosion of the anterior and lateral vertebral margin caused by paravertebral tumor may rarely be observed.[950] The thin horizontal radiolucent bands in the subchondral (metaphyseal equivalent) zone may be noted in the vertebrae of children with leukemia[357] (Fig. 4–125). The bands are in both the superior and inferior vertebral ends and run parallel to the vertebral margins.[914] They are comparable to the submetaphyseal lucent bands that are observed in the long bones of children with this disorder.[357] The bands represent growth arrest due to the underlying illness.

Osteosclerosis is an uncommon finding and may be single, patchy, or diffuse.[124, 271, 276, 647, 1114] If vertebrae become weakened, vertebral collapse may ensue. Severe collapse, vertebra plana, is not a common feature of leukemia. Periosteal reaction, which is observed commonly in long bones and ribs, is not observed in the spine.

Lymphoma. *Hodgkin's Disease.* Hodgkin's disease may involve bone by erosions from direct extension of tumor in adjacent paravertebral lymph nodes or, similar to other forms of metastasis, by hematogenous (arterial or venous) route.[62, 104] About 10% to 30% of patients with Hodgkin's disease demonstrate osseous involvement radiographically,[65, 121, 479, 491] even though nearly all demonstrate osseous tumor at autopsy.[479] The axial skeleton is the most frequent site for skeletal involvement of Hodgkin's disease,[121] and the thoracic and upper lumbar spines are involved most commonly.[588] About two thirds of the lesions are multiple.[950]

The radiographic appearance is variable. Lesions may appear osteolytic, osteosclerotic, or mixed[950] (Fig. 4–126). There may be bone destruction that may lead to vertebral collapse. Erosion (scalloping) caused by direct extension of tumor from paravertebral

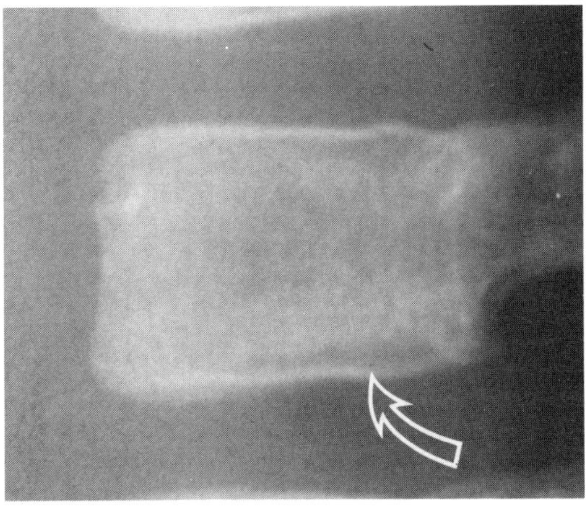

Figure 4–125. Leukemia. There are radiolucent bands in the metaphyseal equivalent zones similar to those found in the long bones of patients with leukemia (arrow). (Courtesy of Dr. Spencer Borden, IV, Philadelphia, Pennsylvania.)

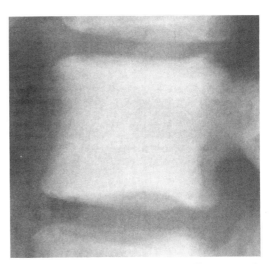

Figure 4–126. Lymphoma. There is diffuse osteosclerosis representing the "ivory" vertebra. This is one of several radiographic manifestations of lymphoma.

lymph nodes may develop on the anterior or lateral vertebral margins.[479, 950] Paravertebral mass occurs in almost 30% of spinal lesions in the thoracolumbar spine.[479] Hodgkin's disease may appear with osteosclerosis, either patchy, diffuse, or as a so-called ivory vertebra.[408, 479, 950] About one half of the sclerotic lesions occur at L1, and similar lesions are least observed in the cervical spine.[479] Osteosclerosis is most likely due to reaction of bone to the presence of tumor or to response induced by the tumor itself. Purely osteosclerotic lesions are rare in children with Hodgkin's disease.[491] Fluffy periosteal reaction has been noted along the anterior or lateral vertebral margins and occurs as a response to the adjacent paravertebral tumor.[479] Calcification of the anterior longitudinal ligament may occur associated with underlying vertebral tumor[317] or following radiation therapy.[950]

There is a correlation between the histologic type of Hodgkin's disease and the incidence of bone destruction. Patients with a tumor demonstrating nodular sclerosis histopathologically and whose prognosis is more favorable clinically develop bone destruction in 11% of cases. Those whose tumors demonstrate mixed cellularity histopathologically and who have a more aggressive tumor clinically develop bone destruction in 64% of cases.[121] In addition, the radiographic pattern of bone destruction is more aggressive in appearance in those tumors that appear more aggressive histopathologically.

Non-Hodgkin's Lymphoma. Non-Hodgkin's lymphoma (NHL) involves the axial skeleton by hematogenous spread and direct extension. Hematogenous spread by arterial or venous route is more common than with Hodgkin's disease.[950] Venous extension of tumor via intraspinal and paraspinal plexuses may account for spinal involvement in patients with deep pelvic tumor.[124] Patients with poorly differentiated tumors are more likely to develop osseous metastasis than those with well-differentiated tumors.[124] Bone involvement, which occurs in 1% to 5%[1205] or 7% to 25%[124] of patients with NHL, indicates disseminated stage IV disease. Nine percent of patients actually present initially with bone involvement.[124]

Like that of Hodgkin's disease, the radiographic pattern of NHL may be osteolytic, osteosclerotic, or mixed.[124] The osteolytic lesions are usually aggressive in appearance radiographically, thus correlating with the aggressive behavior of the tumor histopathologically and clinically. Well-differentiated tumors histologically are less likely to demonstrate bone destruction. Osteosclerotic lesions are not as frequent and, when present, are not as sclerotic as those of Hodgkin's disease.[950] About 4% of NHL cases arise within bone.[950]

Histiocytic Lymphoma (Reticulum Cell Sarcoma). Histiocytic lymphoma affects the axial skeleton more commonly by hematogenous metastasis and rarely develops as a primary lesion within the spine. A primary lesion has occurred in the spine in 0 of 46,[865] 2 of 37,[214] 3 of 33,[1349] and 0 of 17[940] cases of primary histiocytic lymphoma of bone.

Osteosarcoma. Although osteosarcoma is the most frequent primary malignant bone tumor other than myeloma, accounting for 25% of all primary bone tumors, it rarely occurs in the spine.* It accounts for 7% of all tumors in the axial skeleton other than myeloma.[242] Only 1% to 2% of osteosarcomas involve the spine and sacrum.[61, 243] Osteosarcomas usually occur during the first 3 decades but can develop in later years. They occur most frequently in the lumbar and thoracic spines.[61] They develop either de novo or, more commonly, in the axial skeleton as malignant degeneration from previous radiation,† Paget's disease,[61, 944] osteoblastoma,[242, 852, 1147a] or other bone lesions, or years later after injection with Thorotrast (thorium dioxide in dextran).[21, 1176, 1261] Osteosarcoma has been reported developing in giant cell tumor, Gaucher's disease, osteopetrosis, and myositis ossificans involving other skeletal sites.[1078a] The incidence of osteosarcomatous degeneration of Paget's disease of the spine is relatively lower than in long bones.[61] This is surprising, especially in light of the frequent occurrence of Paget's disease in the spine.[944]

Radiographically, osteosarcomas display aggressive bone destruction, usually accompanied by production of tumor bone that appears cloudlike, fluffy, and amorphous[691] (Fig. 4–127). Purely osteosclerotic forms occur and may produce the "ivory vertebra."

---

*Reference numbers 61, 311, 793, 870, 926, 944, 1170.
†Reference numbers 61, 161, 210, 311, 1170, 1187, 1243.

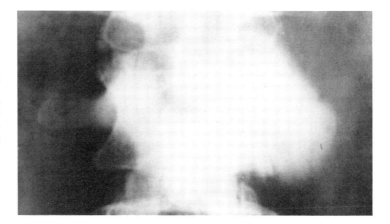

Figure 4–127. Osteosarcoma. There is a large, irregular, amorphous, osteosclerotic vertebral mass obliterating vertebral margins and extending into the paravertebral tissues. This paravertebral mass is due to tumor bone formation.

Tumor usually begins initially in the vertebral body, with tumor in one half of the vertebral body extending to the posterior elements.[61] Isolated involvement of posterior elements may occur.[1170] Purely osteolytic lesions may occur less frequently. Perpendicular or sunburst periosteal reaction, frequent with osteosarcomas in long bones,[691] is not as readily visible in the spine or sacrum. Neurologic deficit is common in patients with vertebral osteosarcoma (70% at clinical presentation,[1170] and patients do poorly clinically.[61] In the sacrum, tumor commonly extends anteriorly into the pelvis, forming a huge mass.

The development of multiple osteogenic sarcomas arising simultaneously in multiple skeletal sites is rare. It is more likely that the lesions develop from multicentric foci rather than representing osseous metastasis from an osteosarcoma at another site.[1178] The spine may be involved in this disorder, and the radiographic features are similar to those of solitary osteosarcoma.

Benign Tumors and Tumorlike Conditions

Aneurysmal Bone Cyst. Aneurysmal bone cyst is a relatively uncommon benign tumorlike condition. Sixty-five percent of aneurysmal bone cysts are primary to bone, and 35% are secondary, developing in another lesion.[107] Approximately 20% to 25% of aneurysmal bone cysts involve the axial skeleton,[174, 737, 1264] although aneurysmal bone cysts in the coccyx have not been reported.[541] Eighty percent occur in patients under the age of 20 years.[1264] There is a slight predilection for the thoracic and lumbar regions.[541] Sixty percent involve the posterior elements, particularly the spinous process. Both the vertebral body and posterior elements may be involved in up to 43% to 87% of cases when first discovered.[541, 1264]

Aneurysmal bone cyst is an osteolytic lesion that is usually eccentrically placed.[107] Classically, there may be "expansion" of cortex,[90, 541, 690, 773, 1304] particularly in thin

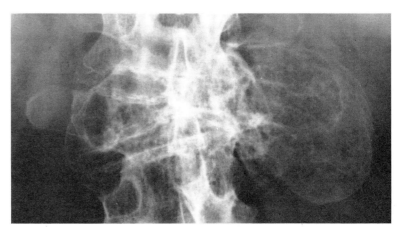

Figure 4–128. Aneurysmal bone cyst. There is a marked expansile lesion arising from the transverse process and causing vertebral collapse of L3. Slow-growing metastasis and multiple myeloma could cause a similar appearance.

elements of the spine (that is, spinous process, transverse process) (Fig. 4–128). The lacy trabeculated pattern ofen visible in aneurysmal bone cyst of tubular bones is usually not observed.[1264] Only 25% of aneurysmal bone cysts demonstrate septations along the margins.[107] The rim of aneurysmal bone cyst may be so thin that it may not be visible on the conventional radiograph. When vertebrae are involved, there is osteolytic destruction and sometimes partial collapse. Extensive vertebral destruction may lead to vertebra plana.[541] Paravertebral and intraspinal extension occur but may not be visible radiographically.

Patients usually present with vague pain, often radicular in nature,[649] and may present with other neurologic signs and symptoms.[432, 743, 1151, 1228, 1264] Aneurysmal bone cyst may involve several contiguous vertebrae,[170, 541, 773, 1228, 1285] and in one case involvement of four adjacent vertebrae was reported.[541] Kyphosis may develop if there is pronounced destruction of the anterior aspect of the vertebral body.[1228] Aneurysmal bone cysts recur in about 30% of cases.[1086a] In young adults, aneurysmal bone cysts of the sacrum may appear highly expansile, resembling giant cell tumor.

Chondroblastoma. Chondroblastoma is a benign primary tumor that rarely involves the spine. It has been reported in 0 of 69,[1118] 1 of 126,[246] and 1 of 70[1213] cases of chondroblastoma based on large series of this tumor. It accounts for 0.25% of tumors of the spine and sacrum other than myeloma.[242] Radiographically, it is an osteolytic lesion that involves the vertebral body and posterior elements.[145] About 60% of chondroblastomas demonstrate sclerotic margins. Chondroblastoma may "expand" bone and form a calcified rim, and it may extend into the spinal canal and cause cord compression.[145] Twenty-five percent of chondroblastomas demonstrate matrix calcification on the conventional radiograph.[830]

Chondromyxoid Fibroma. Chondromyxoid fibroma rarely involves the spine.* It accounts for 0.25% of tumors of the axial skeleton other than myeloma.[242] Five-tenths percent to 3% of chondromyxoid fibromas involve the spine.[384, 1119]

---

*Reference numbers 75, 384, 808, 920, 991, 992, 1119, 1214.

Radiographically, chondromyxoid fibroma appears as an osteolytic lesion that more commonly involves the posterior elements but may involve the vertebral body as well.[808, 920, 1214] The spinous process is a common site for chondromyxoid fibroma.[808, 920] The tumor may extend into the spinal canal and cause cord compression.[75, 920, 992, 1214] Malignant degeneration is exceedingly rare.[242] Only 2% of chondromyxoid fibromas demonstrate matrix calcification.[384]

Enchondroma. Enchondroma (chondroma) is a rare spinal tumor, accounting for 1.5% of all primary axial tumors other than myeloma.[242] Only 3.7% of enchondromas occur in the axial skeleton. Enchondroma is an osteolytic lesion that frequently calcifies. It may develop anywhere in the spinal column and, if large enough, may extend into the spinal canal and cause cord compression.[557, 1183] Cartilage tissue occurs in the growth plate, intervertebral disc, and notochord tissue, so theoretically enchondroma could develop from cartilage rests anywhere in the spine.[557] Rarely, an enchondroma of the rib may also extend into the spinal canal and cause cord compression.[1267]

Eosinophilic Granuloma. Eosinophilic granuloma is an uncommon tumorlike condition of children and young adults that involves the reticuloendothelial system.[1123] It is more common in the appendicular skeleton than it is in the spine, and it occurs most frequently in the first 3 decades, with a peak incidence in individuals between 5 and 10 years of age.[1101] Although 71% of cases are solitary when first discovered,[566] the spine is an uncommon site of solitary involvement. Yet, 14% of multiple lesions affect the spine.[197] Eosinophilic granuloma may involve any portion of the spinal column. The spinal lesion is often discovered on a routine chest radiograph in asymptomatic patients.[1147]

Radiographically, eosinophilic granuloma of the spine is an aggressive-appearing osteolytic lesion most frequently affecting the vertebral body. The most common features are bone destruction in the cervical spine and vertebral collapse in the thoracic spine.[1098] Vertebral collapse is common in younger children. Since a considerable portion of the vertebral body is often involved, collapse may be so extensive that the vertebral body appears extremely thin (waferlike), with a characteristic appearance of vertebra

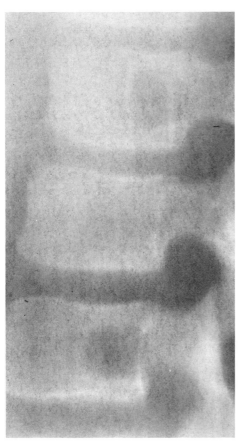

Figure 4–129. Eosinophilic granuloma. There are well-defined osteolytic lesions with sclerotic margins in two vertebral bodies. There is no evidence of vertebral collapse. This is not as characteristic of eosinophilic granuloma as is vertebra plana (see Fig. 4–45).

plana* (see Fig. 4–45). Rarely, as many as five vertebral levels may be affected.[286] In older children, there is relatively less destruction, so that complete collapse is less likely.[1147] Vertebral bodies may be involved without evidence of collapse[657] (Fig. 4–129). Sometimes following collapse, the width of the vertebral body is greater than normal, and the degree of flatting may be asymmetric. Eosinophilic granuloma may occur in any portion of the vertebral arch. Pedicle destruction occurs[1164] but is not common.[389, 1330] Rarely, bone "expansion" is present.[187] Fusiform paravertebral soft tissue mass is an uncommon finding[187] but may occur.[389, 1164] It usually extends one vertebral level above and below the lesion.[164] Intervertebral disc spaces are spared,[164, 187] but the intervertebral

*Reference numbers 164, 187, 286, 389, 430, 1164, 1330.

disc may collapse into an involved vertebral body, causing decrease in disc height.

Eosinophilic granuloma of the spine may be associated with neurologic signs if spinal cord block is present.[484, 1098, 1164] Eosinophilic granuloma tends to resolve spontaneously, regardless of whether therapy is instituted[599] and regardless of the type of therapy instituted.[164, 1101, 1147] The degree of restoration of vertical vertebral height is variable. The rate of healing is also variable and depends on patient age, size and location of the lesion, and the amount of bone removed during biopsy or curettage.[1101] Interestingly, the earlier in life the vertebra plana occurs, the more likely it is that the vertebra will reconstitute its full or near full height following healing.[608] This is due to the fact that there is more time for continued vertebral growth. The mean resolution time for reconstitution is 11 to 14 months.[1101] In older children whose vertebral growth is complete, reconstitution of vertebral collapse is less likely, and healing may occur without height being regained.[1147]

Fibrous Dysplasia. Fibrous dysplasia may be monostotic or polyostotic. The spine is infrequently involved with fibrous dysplasia. Monostotic lesions of the vertebral body occur in 7% of patients with this disorder.[441] The matrix is usually radiolucent[1077] but may develop a faint increase in density, representing mineralized osteoid (Fig. 4–130). The margins are sclerotic and may be partially scalloped. Osteosclerotic and mixed sclerotic and radiolucent lesions occur.

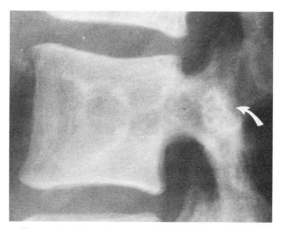

Figure 4–130. Fibrous dysplasia. There is a well-defined, scalloped osteolytic lesion in the vertebral body. A sclerotic margin surrounds the lesion. A smaller scalloped lesion is noted in the posterior elements (arrow).

Varying degrees of vertebral collapse may be present, often producing neurologic signs, and paraplegia has been reported.[441] Intervertebral discs may narrow both above and below the lesion, and bone softening may allow the formation of Schmorl's nodes.

Hemangioma. Hemangioma is the most common "benign" tumor of the vertebral column and occurs in 10% of the population, usually developing in the thoracic and lumbar spines.[1129a] It is usually discovered as an incidental observation on the conventional radiograph or through computed tomography or magnetic resonance imaging. Hemangioma is not a true tumor but consists of dilated venous channels (venules) and capillaries reflecting venous stasis.[738] Fat tissue has been observed within the lesion.[694, 889a] Hemangioma develops in the vertebral body and may extend into the posterior elements. Occasionally it may be isolated to the vertebral arch.[1129a] Hemangioma occurs occasionally in children, the youngest reported being 10 years of age.[873]

Radiographically, the appearance is characteristic. There are thickened vertical trabeculae that appear as a "honeycomb" pattern and form in response to mechanical stress caused by the loss of adjacent trabeculae, which are resorbed by the dilated venous channels[695] (Fig. 4–131). The vertebrae may appear radiolucent if the lesion is extensive. Spinal cord, cauda equina, or nerve root compression may rarely develop secondary to encroachment by hemorrhage or the expanding lesion, particularly when the lesion involves the posterior elements.[786, 873, 1129a, 1133a] Paravertebral masses are noted in one half of cases with symptomatology and

are possibly due to associated compression fractures.[873]

There are true hemangiomas (angiomas), hemangiopericytomas (angiosarcomas), and hemangioendotheliomas of bone, which are rare and more aggressive in their behavior.[1279] They may appear similar to benign hemangiomas,[64, 210] but they are often osteolytic and expansile and may be associated with vertebral collapse.* They are more likely to cause neurologic signs and symptoms than is benign "hemangioma." Benign "hemangioma" is of no clinical significance and requires no further imaging investigation unless there are symptoms of spinal cord block or the radiographic appearance is more aggressive, suggesting a true hemangioma or angiosarcoma.

Osteochondroma. Osteochondroma accounts for 4.3% of all primary tumors of the axial skeleton other than myeloma.[242] Only 3.2% of osteochondromas (exostoses) develop in the axial skeleton. It may develop as a solitary lesion or as part of hereditary multiple exostoses.[175, 774, 1073] Seven percent of patients with hereditary multiple exostoses have spinal involvement.[367] Osteochondroma almost always involves the vertebral arch[918] and spinous processes,[367] although one case involved the lateral mass of the atlas.[1372] It occurs more commonly in the cervical and thoracic regions of the spine,[748] although the lesions in patients with hereditary multiple exostoses are more common in the thoracic and lumbar regions.[1291]

Radiographically, the mass may demonstrate coarse trabeculation as it arises from bone[748, 918, 1372] (Fig. 4–132). Underlying bone may be intact.[918] Exostoses may enlarge to extend the length of over two or more vertebral levels.[1291] Spinal cord compression may develop, particularly if the lesion arises from the vertebral arch.[748, 774, 1291] Exotoses arising from the costovertebral junction may also cause spinal cord compression.[175, 272, 466, 648] Sometimes the radiograph appears normal in the presence of spinal cord compression and may be due to compression on the cord by the radiolucent cartilaginous cap of the osteochondroma.[1073] Clinically, patients with spinal osteochondromas may present with pain, neurologic symptoms, or a non-

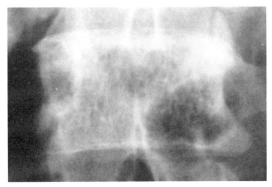

Figure 4–131. Hemangioma. There is thickening of trabeculae causing a "honeycomb" appearance. This is characteristic of hemangioma.

---

*Reference numbers 64, 547, 645, 724, 1128, 1279, 1381.

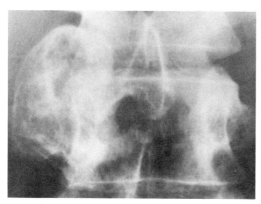

Figure 4–132. Osteochondroma. There is a large mass that is partially calcified and centered over the transverse process–vertebral body junction. (Courtesy of Dr. Roger Kerr, Los Angeles, California.)

tender mass in the neck that may reach a large size. Osteochondroma of the spinous process may enlarge sufficiently to involve the spinous process of the adjacent vertebra, causing fusion.[394]

Osteoblastoma. Osteoblastoma is a rare primary bone tumor of the spine.* It comprises about 5% of primary bone tumors of the axial skeleton other than myeloma.[242] Seventy-five percent of osteoblastomas occur during the first 2 decades,[831] and 97% occur in individuals under 30 years of age.[627] Around 36% to 54% of osteoblastomas occur in the axial skeleton.[612, 792, 971] They are most common in the lumbar, thoracic, and cervical spines and sacrum, in that order.[627, 831]

Osteoblastoma involves the vertebral arch alone in 62% of cases.[831] The laminae and pedicles are most commonly affected,[792] representing 50% of vertebral arch osteoblastomas.[627] Both the vertebral arch and vertebral body may be involved (11% to 24%),[627, 831] but osteoblastoma of the vertebral body alone is uncommon.[285, 363, 463, 627] About one quarter to one half of cases demonstrate neurologic symptoms[627, 831] and about one half have epidural extension of tumor.[627] They may increase rapidly in size even within several months.[620] Scoliosis occurs in one third of cases,[627] and osteoblastoma is one of the causes of painful scoliosis.[12, 744, 844, 995] The lesion occurs on the concave side of the scoliotic curve.[844]

---

*Reference numbers 12, 285, 363, 463, 486, 610, 709, 744, 995, 1309.

Radiographically, osteoblastoma is an osteolytic lesion that is greater than 1 cm[627] to 2 cm[620] in diameter. Almost 60% are 2.5 cm or larger.[627] The margin is frequently well defined.[831] Around one third to one half of the cases demonstrate increased density (ossification) within the matrix,[627, 831] which usually appears punctate, globular, or amorphous. Osteoblastomas are frequently expansile (78%)[831] but may appear entirely osteosclerotic (Fig. 4–133). Paraspinal mass with a calcified rim can be identified in around 10% of cases.[627] Approximately one quarter of cases have an aggressive appearance that may resemble malignancy.[831]

Osteoblastoma is similar histologically to osteoid osteoma,[247, 285, 620, 739] and because of this, the two lesions have sometimes been grouped together as the osteoid osteoma–osteoblastoma complex.[64] However, in some lesions, the histologic picture varies[620, 739] in that there seem to be a greater number of osteoblasts present with osteoblastoma.[620] Osteoblastomas are usually greater than 2 cm in diameter when initially discovered, whereas osteoid osteomas are rarely over 1 cm in size.[620, 627] Osteoid osteoma is almost always confined to the vertebral arch, does not expand bone, and has extensive sclerosis as well as a small radiolucent nidus.

On extremely rare occasions, osteoblastoma has undergone malignant degeneration into osteosarcoma.[252, 809, 852, 869, 1147a] Whether these tumors actually became malignant or whether they were low-grade osteosarcomas that appeared histologically similar to osteoblastoma is uncertain.[252, 852] Osteoblastoma may be difficult or even impossible to dif-

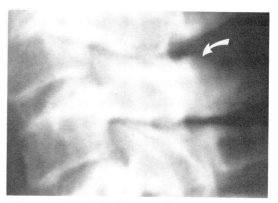

Figure 4–133. Osteoblastoma. There is osteosclerosis in the spinous process and lamina of C4 (arrow). (Courtesy of Dr. Robert Kricun, Allentown, Pennsylvania.)

ferentiate histopathologically from osteosarcoma. Cases of aggressive or "malignant" osteoblastoma have been described.[869, 1121] These tumors resembled osteoblastomas histologically; however, they displayed a more aggressive histologic pattern and behaved more aggressively locally. It was felt that these tumors were the malignant counterparts of osteoblastoma. No cases resembled osteosarcoma histologically, and none developed metastasis.

Computed tomography is more accurate than conventional radiography in assessing the full extent of osteoblastoma.[363, 627, 674, 929]

Osteoid Osteoma. Osteoid osteoma accounts for 2.3% of all primary bone tumors of the axial skeleton other than myeloma.[242] About 4% to 10% occur in the spine and sacrum,[421, 612] and 80% to approximately 90% develop in individuals under the age of 25 years.[242, 421]

The diagnosis of osteoid osteoma can be established on the conventional radiograph in 75% of the cases.[1246] Osteoid osteoma is more common in the lumbar and thoracic spines and almost always involves the vertebral arch,[64, 421] with about 50% developing in the laminae or pedicles and 20% occurring in the articular processes.[627] The nidus of osteoid osteoma is always 1 cm or smaller,[242, 620, 627] is almost always radiolucent, and may not be visible on the spine radiograph, owing to its small size and overlying bony structures.[64, 1246] Occasionally, the center of the nidus calcifies, but this is not as well visualized with conventional radiography as it is with computed tomography.* Osteoid osteoma often incites extensive new bone formation,[612] which may be the only visible radiographic feature; however, even focal sclerosis may not be visible on the plain radiograph. Thus, osteoid osteoma may appear as a radiolucent lesion (nidus) with or without central calcification and with or without surrounding sclerosis,[769] or it may appear as a purely osteosclerotic lesion (Fig. 4–134). Osteoid osteoma does not progress in size, "expand," or destroy bone, although bone elements may enlarge slightly, owing to periosteal response.[64, 627] As a matter of fact, osteoid osteoma is self-

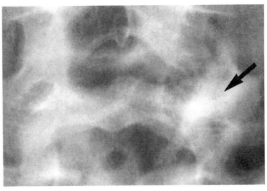

Figure 4–134. Osteoid osteoma. There is an osteosclerotic lesion in the region of the pars interarticularis and lamina of L5 (arrow). There is no visible bone destruction. (Courtesy of Dr. Jay Mall, San Francisco, California.)

limiting,[627] and spontaneous remission in 2 to 8 years has occurred,[162, 612] possibly through infarction of the nidus.[612] However, it is difficult to document such reports without pathologic proof.[1173, 1246] Rarely, osteoid osteoma in one vertebral body is associated with sclerosis in an adjacent vertebral body.[552, 763] Scoliosis is a frequent finding, with the lesion occuring on the concave side of the scoliotic curve.[663, 844, 995] Neurologic abnormalities occur in over 20% of cases.[627] The characteristic intense nature of the pain induced by osteoid osteoma is related both to the vascular nature of the lesion, causing increased local edema, and to the presence of nerve fibers within the nidus.[1135]

Since osteoblastomas and osteoid osteomas represent a common basic process histologically, it may be that location of the lesion determines the nature of the reaction by surrounding bone.[285, 1120] Osteoid osteomas tend to occur in or near cortical bone, whereas osteoblastomas tend to develop in cancellous bone.[612, 1120] Lesions in or near cortical bone tend to elicit more intense osteosclerosis than those that develop in cancellous bone.[612] This may be due to the fact that cortical bone has an intimate relationship with the periosteum and endosteum, which respond with new bone formation. Cancellous bone does not demonstrate the same intense response to the presence of the lesion.[1120] Early, lesions in the vertebral body elicit little or no osteosclerotic response.[324] Later, an occasional thin sclerotic margin may be evident.[1120] The

---

*Reference numbers 52, 64, 440, 627, 674, 905, 928, 1313.

size of the lesion may be determined by the location and bony response. Lesions in the cortex are probably confined by the reactive response of the surrounding bone and possibly by the compactness of cortical bone, whereas lesions developing in more porous spongy bone are less restricted by the natural lack of bony response and possibly by the relative ease of growth and expansion in the less compact cancellous bone.

Other Benign Lesions. Any tumor or tumorlike condition may develop in the axial skeleton, although they are rare. Unicameral bone cyst of the spinous process,[1373] neurilemoma of the vertebral body,[288] primary amyloidoma,[725] and lymphangiomatosis[329, 1010] have been reported.

Osteomyelitis

Infection of the spine usually occurs from hematogenous spread of organisms and may develop following lumbar puncture, spinal surgery, penetrating trauma, paravertebral abscess, urinary tract infection with instrumentation, incomplete abortion, colorectal surgery, superficial sepsis, or respiratory infection.[291, 420, 469, 487, 1105, 1219] Drug addicts, debilitated patients, those whose immune system is suppressed, and various immigrating populations are more likely to acquire spinal osteomyelitis.[399, 469, 685, 1208, 1219] The spine is the most common site of bone and joint infection in patients on renal dialysis,[1208] even though the incidence is low. Pyogenic spinal infection has been reported following dental extraction,[964] acupuncture,[501] and compression fractures of the spine.[861]

Although 70% to 80% of all osteomyelitis occurs in children,[1219] spinal osteomyelitis in this age group is unusual.[304, 1001, 1272] Vertebral osteomyelitis is more common in late adolescence (10 to 15 years)[1219] and in adults (20 to 60 years.)[1001, 1272, 1308] About 2% to 4% of osteomyelitis occurs in the spine.[469] Infection of the spine almost invariably involves the vertebral bodies[487, 1219] and may extend to involve posterior elements; however, isolated involvement of posterior elements is rare.[72, 487] Anteroposterior and lateral views usually suffice for the conventional radiographic evaluation of spinal infection.

The location of osteomyelitis at any age is dependent on marrow distribution and marrow vascular supply.[692] In children, all marrow is red marrow, and the axial skeleton possesses a certain portion of the total marrow system. After marrow conversion is completed by the age of 20 to 25 years, the axial skeleton has a greater proportion of the body's red marrow. Since marrow blood supply is related to red marrow distribution,[692] it is not surprising that infection of the spine is relatively more frequent in adults than in children.

The lumbar, thoracic, and cervical spines are affected by osteomyelitis in descending order of frequency.[1219, 1308] In the vertebrae, it is the subchondral zone, the metaphyseal equivalent region,[913] that is involved early and most often by infection.

Hematogenous spread of infection to the spine is usually by the arterial route,[1001, 1341] although venous spread via the paraspinal and communicating intraspinal venous plexuses has been implicated.[62, 1341] Intraosseous arterial supply to the subchondral (metaphyseal equivalent)[1341] zone is vastly anastomotic in infants and young children,[1000, 1001] and by adult life anastomoses have involuted completely, leaving arterial branches as end-arteries[133, 1000, 1341] (see Fig. 4–57).

It is postulated that a septic microembolus traveling in the arterial system of an adult may lodge in the metaphyseal arteries of the vertebral body[1001] within the subchondral zone (Fig. 4–135). The overlying cartilage plate and intervertebral disc are readily invaded early in disease, either from direct extension of infection from the vertebral body or from hematogenous spread to tiny capillaries that enter the disc directly.

The septic microembolus that had lodged in the metaphyseal arteries forms a wedge-shaped septic infarct within bone.[1001] It extends retrograde to the metaphyseal anastomoses so that other regions of the subchondral zone may then be affected. In addition, the vast collateral circulation along the outer aspect of the vertebra favors the extension of infection (Figs. 4–136 and 4–137). Transdiscal arteries,[1001, 1341] which join opposing metaphyseal anastomoses across the disc, may also aid in the spread of infection to the disc. Newly observed small arteries (intermetaphyseal communicating arteries) running anteriorly along the vertebrae and discs in the longitudinal direction connect the various metaphyseal anastomoses (Fig.

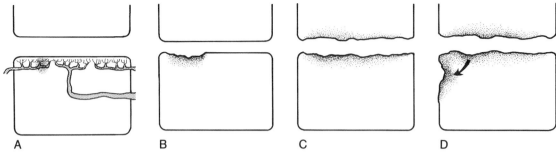

A   B   C   D

Figure 4–135. Diagrammatic representation of the formation and spread of infection in the vertebral body, adjacent disc, and prevertebral region in the adult. *A*, Infection (shaded area) begins in the subchondral region. Disc height is normal. *B*, Further subchondral destruction and extension into the intervertebral disc, causing diminution of disc height. *C*, Extension of infection to involve the opposing vertebral margin. *D*, Infection extends anteriorly into the prevertebral subligamentous region, forming an abscess.

4–137).[1001] These arteries help explain the occurrence of infection in skip vertebrae, away from the site of origin.

However, in infants and children, vast intraosseous anastomoses in the subchondral zone prevent the formation of infarction found in older patients, and it is felt that infarction must form if osteomyelitis is to

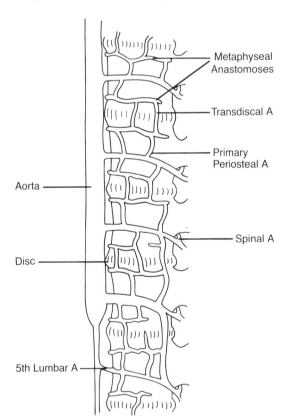

Figure 4–136. Diagram of the lateral surface of the lumbar spine demonstrating anterolateral longitudinal anastomoses. Notice that the transdiscal arteries that lie in the adventitia of the disc join metaphyseal anastomoses of adjacent vertebrae. The primary periosteal arteries join the lumbar arteries to the metaphyseal anastomoses. (Adapted from Ratcliffe JF: Anatomic basis for the pathogenesis and radiologic features of vertebral osteomyelitis and its differentiation from childhood discitis: A microarteriographic investigation. Acta Radiol [Diagn] 26:137–143, 1985.)

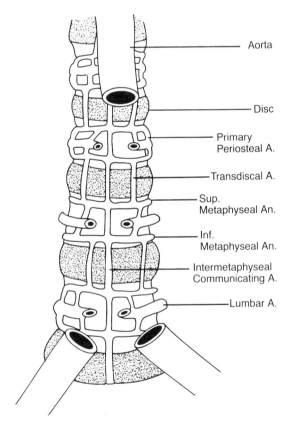

Figure 4–137. Diagram of the anterior surface of the lumbar spine. The aorta has been removed, exposing the intermetaphyseal communicating artery. Notice the intervertebral anastomoses. (Adapted from Ratcliffe JR: Anatomic basis for the pathogenesis and radiologic features of vertebral osteomyelitis and its differentiation from childhood discitis: A microarteriographic investigation. Acta Radiol [Diagn] 26:137–143, 1985.)

develop.[1001] Thus, in infants and children, the clinical and radiographic changes are usually mild compared with those found in adults. The rate and degree of progression of infection in the spine depend on the virulence of the organism and the response of the host.

Pyogenic Infection

The most common offending organism in children and adults is *Staphylococcus aureus*.[469] Gram-positive organisms, such as pneumococcus and streptococcus, and gram-negative organisms, such as *Escherichia coli, Pseudomonas*, salmonella, and *Klebsiella*, are less common. Beta-hemolytic streptococcus usually develops in patients from a few weeks to 2 months of age;[823] however, *Staphylococcus aureus* is still the most common offending organism in this age group.[340] Pyogenic osteomyelitis tends to behave aggressively as a rule, although some infectious organisms and those partially treated will behave less so.

The conventional radiograph may appear normal initially, as infection begins in the subchondral zone. The earliest radiographic finding of spinal infection is narrowing of the intervertebral disc[291] caused by the proteolytic effect of enzymes, which rapidly destroy the disc.[1308] This may occur within days or weeks of the onset of infection. The margins of the end-plate become indistinct, and destruction of subchondral bone may become evident within 1 to 2 weeks following the insult[1028] (Fig. 4–138). Osseous changes are more prominent in the anterior two thirds of the vertebral body.[469] Another early site of involvement is the anterior vertebral margin, which becomes indistinct early in disease. As infection progresses, disc height continues to diminish, and there may be involvement and indistinctness of the opposing vertebral end-plate (Fig. 4–139). Disc narrowing and opposing end-plate indistinctness or destruction are the hallmarks of infection.

Continued vertebral destruction may lead to vertebral collapse and, when severe, may cause gibbous deformity, which is usually mild. Reparative sclerosis with new bone formation becomes evident in 8 to 12 weeks.[469] Spontaneous fusion may develop in about 40% of cases.[487] Rarely, the infectious process may extend to the posterior

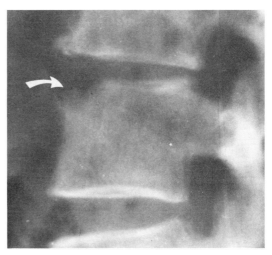

Figure 4–138. Pyogenic spinal osteomyelitis. Lumbar spine. There is destruction of the anterosuperior vertebral margin (arrow) associated with diminution in intervertebral disc height.

elements,[469, 933] and isolated involvement of these elements is rare (Fig. 4–140). In infants, there may be marked destruction of vertebral bodies with normal or nearly normal-appearing adjacent vertebral end-plates.[340] Rapid spontaneous fusion may develop. Years later, kyphosis resembling the congenital form may occur. Rarely, infants develop paraparesis.

Paravertebral abscess occurs in 18% to 23% of cases of pyogenic spinal osteomylitis;[469] however, the incidence of abscess formation is not as great as occurs with tuberculosis.[1308] Paravertebral infection in the

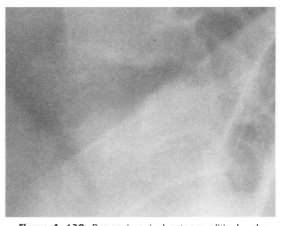

Figure 4–139. Pyogenic spinal osteomyelitis. Lumbar spine. Further progression of infection in this patient compared with the patient in Figure 4–138. There is also destruction of opposing vertebral margins as well as diminution in intervertebral disc height.

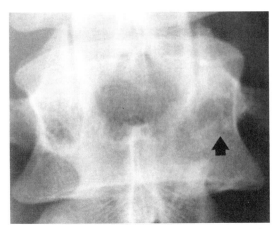

Figure 4–140. Pyogenic osteomyelitis involving the pedicle (arrow). There is no other radiographic evidence of bone destruction.

cervical spine causes soft tissue fullness and obliteration and displacement of prevertebral fat planes. In the thoracic spine, infection forms a paravertebral mass that may erode into the vertebra, causing a "gouge" defect. In the lumbosacral spine, paravertebral abscesses usually do not form, as the pus escapes into the psoas sheath. However, the psoas margin may become indistinct and bulge.[1308] Calcification may develop within abscesses[1265] that are long-standing.

Complications may develop following spinal infection. Paraplegia may occur in 0.2% to 0.9% of cases[469] and is most common in the cervical spine.[341] Factors that predispose to paraplegia include diabetes, rheumatoid arthritis, increased age of the patient, and a more cephalad level of infection. Paraplegia may develop if the abscess extends into the epidural space.[1265] Atlantoaxial subluxation has been reported with infection involving the 2nd and 3rd cervical vertebrae.[487]

Pyogenic Sacroiliitis. Pyogenic infection of the sacroiliac joints is more common in children than in adults and is almost always unilateral in distribution. However, it occurs in only 1.5%[1111] to 4.3%[913] of all joint infections in children and presents most frequently in late childhood.[1111] Adult drug abusers and those whose immune systems are suppressed are more likely to develop infection. Although it is possible that infection may originate within the sacroiliac joint, it is more likely that infection originates as osteomyelitis in the adjacent metaphyseal equivalent bone of the ilium, which

is more vascular than the synovium of the joint.[914] Infection may then spread readily to the joint space.

The conventional radiograph may appear normal in about two thirds of patients on the initial examination. Radiographic abnormalities begin to appear about 2 to 6 weeks following the onset of symptoms in 95% of cases.[1111] Initially, there may be focal juxta-articular osteopenia. The margins of the sacroiliac joint may appear indistinct (Fig. 4–141). As infection advances, there are erosions of the articular surface, sometimes causing apparent widening of the sacroiliac joint. Bone destruction progresses in adjacent bone, and reactive sclerosis occurs in response to healing. The articular cartilage becomes destroyed, and the joint space narrows. Bony ankylosis may develop even after treatment.[1037]

Brucellosis. Brucellosis infection of the spine is rare.[741] However, the spine is involved in 30% of cases of brucellosis, and

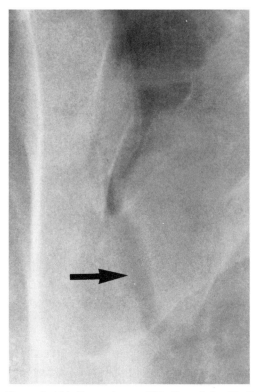

Figure 4–141. Pyogenic sacroiliitis. There is focal indistinctness of the joint margin (arrow), and sacroiliac joint width is normal. This is an "early" plain film sign of infection. The patient had pain for 3 weeks prior to this radiograph.

50% of these have radiographically detectable spinal lesions that are similar in appearance to other causes of spinal infection.[1097] The lumbar, thoracic, and cervical spines and sacroiliac joints are involved with decreasing frequency.[741] Early, the findings are nonspecific, appearing months after the onset of symptoms. Radiographic features include indistinctness and erosion of vertebral end-plates, disc narrowing, paravertebral abscesses that are smaller than those of tuberculosis, and occasionally erosions of the anterior vertebral margin.[741] With progression, further vertebral destruction and disc narrowing occur. Reparative sclerosis is very pronounced, and large osteophytes and vertebral fusion may develop. Up to four vertebral levels may be involved. Infection in the posterior elements is rare.

Tuberculosis

Tuberculosis infection of the spine is almost always caused by *Mycobacterium tuberculosis*.[469] It reaches the spine by hematogenous spread from either pulmonary infection (17% to 29%) or gastrointestinal tract (8%) or from an abscess without spinal involvement (7%).[307] The site of origin may not be evident. Lymphatics have been implicated in the spread of tuberculosis, as the thoracic duct is in contact with the anterior longitudinal ligament.[307]

Tuberculosis may develop in patients who have received chemotherapy and in those whose immune system is suppressed. Younger patients are affected more severely and more rapidly than older patients.[1311] The average duration from onset of symptoms to evaluation is 20 months. Tuberculosis may occur at any age but is more common in patients under 5 years of age and in the third decade.[1219] It occurs most commonly in the thoracic spine of children and in the thoracolumbar spine of adults. Involvement of the cervical spine is unusual at any age.[469] Tuberculous infection is more indolent and less aggressive than pyogenic infection. Results of tuberculin skin testing may be negative in 14% of adult patients with spinal tuberculosis.[742]

Radiographically, the earliest sign of tuberculous infection resembles pyogenic infection in that there is diminution of disc height,[255, 307, 469, 1219] which may occur without physical signs of vertebral involvement.[307] Indistinctness of margin of the upper and lower vertebral end-plates[1219] and abscess formation are other early radiographic signs.[1311] With progression, further erosion of vertebral end-plates and vertebral destruction and collapse occur, often sparing the posterior articulations.[307, 1219, 1311] Vertebral destruction may allow intervertebral disc and vertebral body above to collapse into the lower vertebral body.[1311] Bony fusion sometimes occurs and is usually located in the lumbar spine[487] (Figs. 4–142 and 4–143).

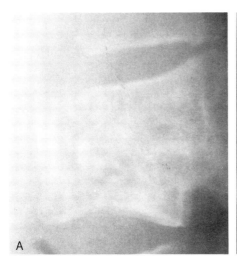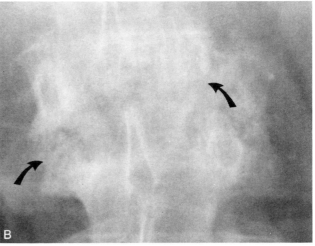

Figure 4–142. Tuberculous osteomyelitis. *A* and *B*, There is vertebral destruction as well as collapse of one vertebra into the one below, with interbody fusion. Note pedicle destruction in *B* (arrows).

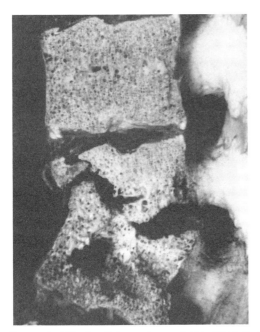

Figure 4–143. Sagittal specimen of the spine in a patient with tuberculous osteomyelitis. Note vertebral destruction, collapse, and partial interbody fusion. (Courtesy of the Mütter Museum, The College of Physicians of Philadelphia.)

Destructive lesions may develop centrally within the vertebral body rather than in subchondral bone.[978] This type of destruction may occur in children under the age of 12 years[307] or in adults,[978] and it occurs most commonly in the thoracic and lumbar spines.[307, 978] The lesions are osteolytic and well defined, with little or no marginal sclerosis.[1219] They may be single or multiple or, rarely, involve multiple vertebrae.[978] A sequestrum may be present. Central lesions usually demonstrate vertebral collapse without visible disc involvement[307, 897] and may resemble metastasis.[897] Disc narrowing, erosion of vertebral end-plates,[307] and abnormalities in adjacent vertebral bodies[255] may develop later.[307] Vertebral collapse in patients with spinal tuberculosis is more commonly associated with centrally located vertebral lesions.[307] Infection may destroy the pedicle in 2% of cases of spinal tuberculosis.[72] Rarely, tuberculosis may present with diffuse osteosclerosis ("ivory vertebrae") (Fig. 4–143).

Erosion of the anterior vertebral margin due to infection ("gouge defect") beneath the anterior longitudinal ligament is uncommon[1219] but may occur as disease progresses[307] (Fig. 4–144). Periosteal reaction

is not common.[469] Ossification of the anterior longitudinal ligament and ossification paralleling the vertebral body have been noted.[978]

Contiguous vertebral involvement is common in some series, occurring in two adjacent vertebral bodies in half of the cases and in 3 adjacent vertebrae in 25% of the cases.[1311] Infection beneath the anterior longitudinal ligament spreads to adjacent vertebrae. However, others have felt that multiple skip areas are not common, occurring in 4% to 10% of cases.[307] The degree of destruction of intervertebral disc is also variable. Some degree of loss of disc height is usually noted, and in one series the disc was completely obliterated in 83% and demonstrated definite narrowing in 17% of cases;[307] however, occasionally intervertebral disc height is maintained, particularly when the central type of bone destruction is encountered.[897]

Abscess formation is common, occurring in almost 60%[1311] to 84%[307] of cases. It is sometimes the first radiographic sign of spinal tuberculosis.[307] The abscesses are large, often out of proportion to the associated bone destruction.[469, 1311] Almost 20% of soft tissue changes occur without bone de-

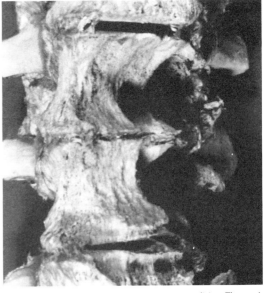

Figure 4–144. Tuberculous osteomyelitis. There is marked anterior vertebral destruction and scalloping of two adjacent vertebral bodies caused by tuberculous abscess formation in this specimen. Intervertebral disc is diminished in height. (Courtesy of the Mütter Museum, The College of Physicians of Philadelphia.)

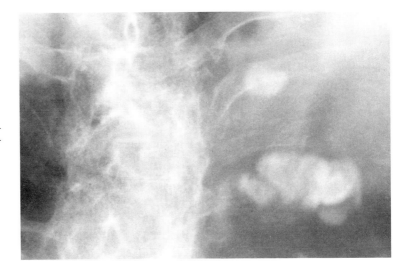

Figure 4–145. Calcified paravertebral abscess secondary to tuberculosis.

struction. Calcification is frequent in chronic abscess[469] (Fig. 4–145). Subligamentous extension of the abscess may occur without disc or vertebral destruction.[469]

There are differences in the extent and severity of spinal tuberculosis in children and adults. In children, the disease is more extensive and diffuse, abscesses are larger, and severe kyphosis is less common.[592] In adults, the disease is more localized, abscesses are small, and there is a higher incidence of severe kyphosis.

Thirteen percent to 43% of patients with spinal tuberculosis may develop cord compression,[469, 592] and 43% of children may present initially with paraplegia,[49] even without radiographically evident bone destruction.[742] Kyphosis may be as great as 90 degrees[1219] (Fig. 4–146). Spinal cord or cauda equina compression may be caused by kyphosis, caseous material, bone fragmentation, or sequestered disc tissue.[469] Tuberculosis of the neural arch and intraspinal extradural tuberculosis without bone involvement are atypical infections that may cause neurologic symptoms.[47, 897] Approximately 10% of patients with neurologic deficit have involvement of the neural arch. Less common complications include hoarseness, caused by direct extension of the tuberculosis abscess that affects the recurrent laryngeal nerve,[1195] and atlantoaxial subluxation or upward translocation of the odontoid process in patients with upper cervical disease.[310, 375, 1219] There may be widening of the retropharyngeal space, destruction of either the atlas or the axis, and atlantoaxial

subluxation of 12 mm to 4 cm.[375] Dysphagia and, rarely, asphyxia have been reported.[375] Retrolisthesis of the involved vertebral body may occur.[1311]

Tuberculous Sacroiliitis. Tuberculous sacroiliitis is less common than pyogenic infection of the sacroiliac joints[913] and usu-

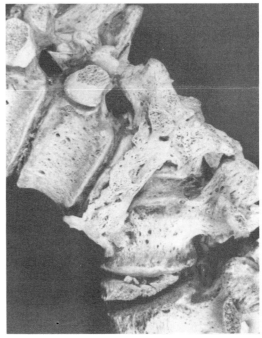

Figure 4–146. Tuberculous osteomyelitis and kyphosis. Note the marked vertebral destruction, collapse, and kyphotic angulation in this specimen. (Courtesy of the Mütter Museum, The College of Physicians of Philadelphia.)

ally occurs in young adults. About 80% of cases develop in patients between 20 and 40 years of age.[1199] Infection is usually unilateral in distribution. Tuberculosis occurring in other skeletal sites is common in patients with tuberculous sacroiliitis, and 36% to 84% have infection elsewhere.[1199] Multiple sites of infection often develop. The spine (29%), especially the lower lumbar spine, and hips (13%) are the most frequent associated sites of tuberculous infection. It may be that the psoas muscle serves as the avenue of spread among these three anatomic sites. Abscesses may form about the sacroiliac joint.

The radiographic features of tuberculous sacroiliitis are often similar to pyogenic infection. However, the clinical course of tuberculosis is more protracted.[1037] The earliest detectable radiographic findings are indistinctness of the articular surface[1199] followed by irregularity of joint margins and widening of the joint space due to erosions.[978] Focal areas of bone destruction varying in size develop in any site along the sacroiliac joint and may extend to involve the entire joint[978] (Fig. 4–147). Reactive sclerosis develops and may be extensive. As joint cartilage is further

Table 4–13. PYOGENIC SPONDYLITIS VERSUS TUBERCULOUS SPONDYLITIS

	Pyogenic	TB
Behavior (aggressiveness)	+ + +*	+
Bone destruction	+ + +	+ + +
Anterior erosion	+	+ + +
Sclerosis	+ + + (more rapid)	+
Osteophytes	+ + +	+
Vertebral collapse	+ +	+ + +
Osteopenia	+ + +	+
Disc narrowing	+ + +	+ + +
Vertebral fusion	+ + +	+ + (lumbar)
Abscess incidence	+ +	+ + +
Abscess size	+ +	+ + +
Abscess calcification	+	+ + +
Multiple vertebral segments	+	+ + +
Skip lesions	+	+ +
Posterior elements	Rare	Rare
Kyphosis	+	+ + +

*Occasionally the behavior is not aggressive.
Key: + + + = frequent; + + = moderately frequent; + = occasional.

destroyed, the sacroiliac joint narrows and proceeds to ankylosis.

Atypical Mycobacterium Tuberculosis Infection. Atypical *Mycobacterium tuberculosis* infection is rare in bone and usually involves the soft tissues and joints. Patients who have lupus erythematosus or who are receiving exogenous steroids are most susceptible to this infection.[1387]

Comparison of Pyogenic and Tuberculous Spinal Infection

The radiographic differentiation between pyogenic and tuberculous infection of the spine in an individual case may be difficult or even impossible to establish.[19, 255, 469] However, there are several features that are more commonly observed in each of the disorders (Table 4–13).

Fungal Diseases

The radiographic appearance of spinal infection caused by fungal disorders may be indistinguishable from that of pyogenic or tuberculous infection.

Actinomycosis. Spinal involvement by actinomycosis is rare[761, 1252] and usually devel-

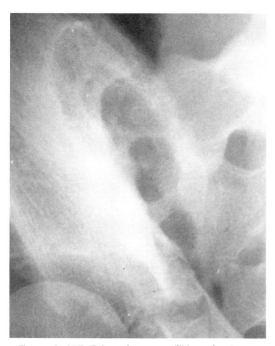

Figure 4–147. Tuberculous sacroiliitis and osteomyelitis. There is marked destruction of the sacroiliac joint and adjacent bone. Wide sclerotic margins surround the lesion.

ops from contiguous spread of adjacent infection in the soft tissues[1044] either from the mandible to the cervical spine or from pulmonary parenchymal disease to the thoracic spine.[469] Abdominal infection may spread to the spine via the psoas sheath.[63] Radiographically, there may be osteolytic destruction with sharp margination.[1252] A "honey comb"[469] or "soap bubble"[63] pattern may be present. Periosteal reaction may appear early, followed by erosion, and the anterior vertebral margin may demonstrate a "sawtooth" appearance.[761] Vertebral bodies are involved more commonly than are the posterior elements.[1252] and several vertebrae may be infected during the course of disease.[469] Vertebral destruction usually occurs without collapse or kyphosis.[1044] Bone destruction may extend to involve all posterior elements as well as adjacent ribs;[761] however, intervertebral disc height is usually preserved.[761, 1044] Paravertebral abscess is a constant finding[1252] and large osteophytes may develop in the region of abscess,[1044] probably as part of the healing process.

There is an organism, *Arachnia propionica*, that is a gram-positive rod and resembles *Actinomyces israelii*. It has an almost identical morphology and similar biochemical properties.[218] It is difficult to differentiate these two organisms by conventional laboratory techniques. Therefore, many cases of spinal actinomycosis osteomyelitis may actually be caused by *Arachnia propionica*. Radiographically, cases caused by *Arachnia propionica* resemble pyogenic osteomyelitis more than they do true actinomycosis of the spine.

Aspergillosis. Aspergillosis osteomyelitis is rare in the spine. Predisposing conditions include surgery, neoplasm, radiotherapy, suppression of the immune system, chronic debilitating disease, or adjacent pulmonary infection.[388, 807, 828] In one report, all patients were given exogenous steroids prior to onset of infection.[807] Radiographically, there may be evidence of bone destruction, but disc height is usually preserved. Paraplegia following spinal infection has been reported[388, 828] and is possibly related to epidural abscess.

Blastomycosis. Blastomycosis frequently involves the spine, with the thoracic region affected first, the lumbar region second, and the cervical region third.[469] Radiographically, blastomycosis may resemble tuberculosis in the spine.[1044] The lesions are osteo-

lytic, and destruction may extend to involve all posterior elements and even the proximal ribs, although involvement of the proximal ribs is unusual for tuberculosis. Prominent erosions of the anterior vertebrae may occur.[63] Intervertebral discs are invariably destroyed.[63] Multiple sites of spinal involvement occur in 20% to 50% of patients with disseminated disease,[469] and "skip" lesions may occur.[63] The sacrum may also be involved.[443]

Candidiasis. Candidiasis rarely involves the spine. It may occur from direct implant (injury, surgery), from contiguous spread, or by hematogenous route.[545, 579] The vertebral bodies are affected most often in adults, and long bones are involved most commonly in children.[545]

Coccidioidomycosis. Osseous lesions occur in 0.9% to 50% of patients with disseminated coccidioidomycosis.[253, 469, 826, 1044] Ten percent to 60% involve the spine.[469] Lesions are often at multiple levels.[826, 1359] Radiographically, there is vertebral destruction with cyst-like lesions that demonstrate sclerotic margins.[253, 826] The posterior elements may be involved as well. Vertebral collapse may be so extensive that it may occasionally resemble vertebra plana.[253, 1359] Paravertebral mass is often present; however, intervertebral disc height is usually spared.[253, 826, 1044] Vertebral sclerosis may be noted and reflects healing.[826] The sacrum may also be involved.[253]

Cryptococcosis (Torulosis). Skeletal involvement by *Cryptococcus neoformans* is not common but is frequently associated with either disseminated cryptococcosis or underlying predisposing disorders such as tuberculosis, sarcoidosis (20%), diabetes, and other disorders.[24, 199] Bone lesions from cryptococcosis are unusual and occur by hematogenous route or by direct extension.[469] Isolated spinal infection is rare.[24, 477] Radiographically, there are radiolucent lesions in the vertebrae and posterior elements, and paraspinal mass may develop.[469] Pedicles and laminae may be involved, but disc height is usually preserved. Periosteal reaction and sclerosis are not evident. Paraplegia has been reported.[805]

Histoplasmosis. Histoplasmosis rarely affects bone.[1044] In the spine, all bony elements may be involved.[255] Multiple lesions and paraspinal mass are frequent, and vertebral collapse may occur late in the course of disease.

Sarcoidosis

Sarcoidosis is a granulomatous disorder that involves the skeletal system in 1% to 13% of cases[1102] and in 11% to 29% of adolescents with this disorder.[1238] About 80% to 90% of patients with osseous sarcoidosis demonstrate pulmonary disease radiographically, and almost all patients with osseous sarcoidosis demonstrate skin lesions.[1102] Sarcoidosis infrequently involves the spine radiographically, even though the characteristic noncaseating granulomas have been discovered in vertebral marrow.

The radiographic pattern is variable and does not resemble the tiny characteristic radiolucencies and "lace-like" trabecular pattern discovered in the small bones of the hands and feet. There may be bone destruction surrounded by a sclerotic margin in one or several vertebrae.[77, 129, 144] Intervertebral disc height is usually maintained.[144] The posterior elements may be involved,[144] but rarely alone. Any region of the axial skeleton may be affected, but the thoracic and lumbar spines demonstrate changes most often.[129] A soft tissue mass may accompany the destructive lesion.[129, 1238] Sarcoidosis may also present as a focal, patchy, or diffuse osteosclerotic lesion,[106, 129, 1378] with or without evident bone destruction (Fig. 4–148). Radiculopathy may occur.[43]

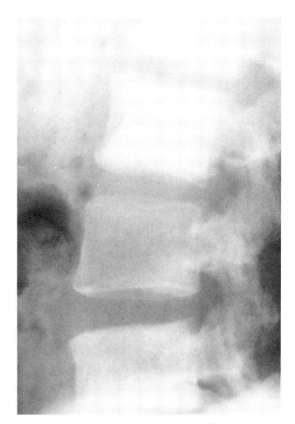

Figure 4–148. Sarcoidosis. There is diffuse osteosclerosis in multiple vertebrae. There is no visible vertebral destruction.

Discitis

Symptomatic narrowing of the intervertebral disc in children is a syndrome of uncertain etiology.[1209, 1326] It has been termed discitis,[15, 847] intervertebral disc inflammation,[1193, 1209] spondyloarthritis,[15, 872] disc infection,[665] and vertebral osteomyelitis with disc infection.[1326]

Discitis is difficult to diagnose in its very early stages, as the clinical picture often directs the physician to different areas.[872, 1209] Patients may complain of refusal to walk, vague pain in the buttock, thigh or knee pain, backache, and a variety of clinical syndromes.[847, 1209]

The mean age of onset is 4 to 6.5 years, and the age range is 11 months to almost 15 years.[1193, 1209] The clinical course is fairly constant in children. Although discitis is considered a disorder of children, similar radiographic features have been described in late teens and adults.[665] The clinical course in these older patients is more severe, probably owing to radiographic delay in diagnosis and a chronicity that is not observed in children.

The etiology of discitis is unclear and controversial, although a number of authors feel that it is presumably an infectious process.[847, 1209] Infection with variable organisms has been proved by disc biopsy and culture[1193, 1209] in 8% of cases.[15]

Infection may reach the intervertebral disc via subchondral vascular channels that perforate the vertebral end-plate and extend into the disc.[225, 387, 533, 1191] These vascular channels have been noted in children up to the age of 8 years and have persisted up to the age of 30 years.[225] Other investigators feel that capillaries located in the region of the annulus fibrosus are terminal ramifications of vessels that enter the intervertebral disc from the side.[1209] These vascular channels are arranged radially and are independent of the vascular supply to the end-plate and vertebral body. Others have noted anastomotic vascular channels in opposing metaphyseal equivalent zones, which are joined by about 20 transdiscal arteries that reside in the adventitia of the disc.[1001, 1341] It is possible that these arteries might send tiny perforating branches into the disc, although this has not yet been demonstrated. Thus, infection may find a direct route to the intervertebral disc in children and young adults (discitis), or it may extend directly to the disc through the cartilaginous plate from the metaphyseal equivalent subchondral bone (osteomyelitis with secondary discal infection).

Early, the radiograph may appear normal.[847] The initial radiographic sign is decreasing disc height that occurs during the second to fourth weeks after the onset of symptoms.[665, 847, 872, 1193, 1209] There is progression of disc narrowing in about 50% to 60% of cases[665, 872] over a 4 to 8 week period.[1193] The process may remain confined to the intervertebral disc in about one half of the cases, or it may involve adjacent vertebrae.[665] The earliest vertebral alterations consist of osteopenia in the vertebral end-plates.[872] This is followed by erosions of vertebral endplates, which become evident over a variable period of time,[665] usually during the second to sixth weeks after onset.[665, 872, 1193, 1326] The end-plates may be affected equally, or one vertebra may be affected more than the other.[665] A radiolucent defect (bone destruction) occurs in the vertebral end-plate[872] in about 77% of cases.[1193] The intervertebral disc may expand into the vertebral body.[665, 1193]

As healing takes place, there is restoration of end-plates as early as 1 to 2 months after onset[1193, 1209] and reconstitution of bone destruction occurs with or without sclerosis in 3 to 4 months after onset.[1193] In about one half of the cases, the alterations do not progress beyond the point of end-plate erosions and reactive sclerosis.[665] Intervertebral disc height may become reconstituted, remain the same,[872] or in some cases narrow progressively. Other evidence of progression of disease includes partial or almost complete vertebral fusion, which occurs in 12% to 25% of cases.[1193, 1209]

During the course of disease, there is no evidence of paravertebral abscess, anterior vertebral collapse, or extensive sclerosis.[1193] The radiolucent defect in the vertebral body may persist. There is no, or at most a mild, scoliosis in up to 42% of patients with long-term follow-up.[872, 1193, 1209] During healing, there may be overgrowth of the vertebral body in the anteroposterior direction, possibly in response to injury of the cartilage end-plates.[1193]

Discitis involves the L4–L5 region most often,[15, 1193, 1209] occurring there about 40% of the time.[1209] The thoracolumbar junction is also a common site of involvement.[1193] Discitis rarely occurs above the T8 level.[1209]

Although some authors consider the clinical syndrome of discitis as disc infection secondary to vertebral osteomyelitis,[1326] there are distinct differences in the two clinical syndromes.[665] Discitis runs a much milder clinical course; there is partial restoration of disc height; and interbody fusion is not as common as occurs with osteomyelitis with disc infection[15, 665, 1193] (Table 4–14).

Intraspinal Tumors and Tumorlike Conditions

Intraspinal tumors and tumorlike conditions may be detected on the plain radiograph by alterations that occur in the surrounding bony elements or if the lesion

Table 4–14. DISCITIS VERSUS OSTEOMYELITIS WITH DISC INFECTION

	Discitis	Osteomyelitis with Disc Infection
Age (Mean)	4.7 years	8.3 years
Location	L4–L5; thoracolumbar spine	Midlumbar; thoracolumbar spine
Clinical course	Mild, fairly constant	More severe, prolonged
Positive culture	8%	33% (0–7 years old)
Bone destruction	+	+ + +
Early bone destruction	−	+ +
Spontaneous fusion	+	+ +
Sclerosis	+	+ + +
Restoration disc height	+	−

Key: + + + = frequent; + + = moderately frequent; + = occasional; − = does not occur.

calcifies. Plain film detection usually depends on the size of the lesion and its location within the spine. It must be emphasized that a conventional radiograph may appear normal in 50% of cases of intraspinal lesion.[357a] This is particularly true in the upper cervical and lower lumbar regions, where the subarachnoid space is wider and can accommodate more tumor growth before tumor is manifested clinically. Also, a tumor growing in a relatively narrow spinal canal, such as the lower throacic spine, has little room to grow and may, therefore, present earlier, with a tumor of smaller size and no bone erosion.

The radiographic examination of patients with suspected intraspinal lesion could begin with a plain radiograph in the AP and lateral projections. Careful attention should be paid to the size and shape of the canal on both projections as well as the presence of vertebral and posterior element abnormalities. This includes widening of the intrapedicular distance, erosion of pedicles, thinning of laminae, increase in sagittal diameter of the canal, and widening of neural foramina (Figs. 4–149 and 4–150; see also Fig. 4–77). Careful evaluation is important, for it has been shown that earlier radiographs of patients with intraspinal tumors

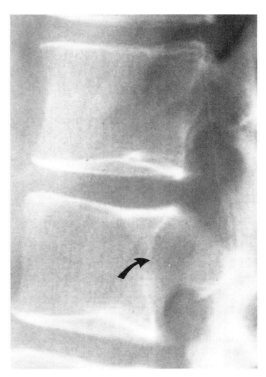

Figure 4–150. Ependymoma. There is posterior scalloping (arrow) in the lumbar spine caused by an ependymoma. Compare with the vertebral body above. This is the same patient as the one shown in Figure 4–77.

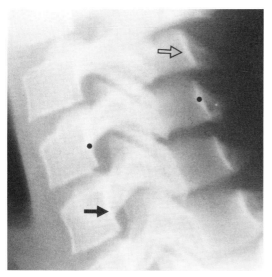

Figure 4–149. Intramedullary tumor. Astrocytoma. Eleven year old patient with widening of the sagittal diameter of the spinal canal (dots). Note the flattening of the lamina (open arrow) and the posterior scalloping (closed arrow) compatible with an intraspinal mass.

often demonstrate radiographic changes of wide, sagittal diameter that went undetected.[571] Intraspinal lesions are classified as intramedullary, intradural-extramedullary, and extradural.

Intramedullary

The most frequent intramedullary (IM) lesions are ependymomas, astrocytomas, and syringohydromyelia. Ependymomas are the most frequent IM tumor, accounting for about 50% of all IM tumors[997] (see Figs. 4–77 and 4–150). They usually occur in the region of the conus medullaris and filum terminale, where ependymal cells are more abundant. Astrocytomas are the second most common IM tumor. They develop anywhere within the spinal cord but are common in the cervical region (see Fig. 4–149). Syringohydromyelia is most frequent in the mid- and lower cervical cord but may extend distally to involve the entire cord.[695] When IM lesions enlarge, they do so uniformly. When large enough, they expand against the bony spinal canal, widening it in all directions.[54, 303] Radiographic signs of IM lesions may be focal or extend over several vertebral levels. On the lateral radiograph, there may be increase in the sagittal diameter of the canal with associated thinning of the laminae and scalloping of the posterior surface of the vertebral body.[54, 103, 303] On the AP radiograph, there may be widening of the interpedicular distance, thinning of the medial pedicle margin, and erosion of its adjacent vertebral margin.[54, 352, 567, 1175] About 40% of cases with intramedullary tumors demonstrate widening of the IPD,[352] and 54% demonstrate skeletal changes.[103] In children, disproportional widening may occur posteriorly, presumably owing to the development of tumor prior to fusion of laminae[1363] or prior to ossification of growth centers.[103] As a rule, intramedullary lesions do not calcify. In syringohydromyelia, the cord is more often normal in size or collapsed,[695] so the plain radiograph often will not demonstrate bony alterations.

Intradural-Extramedullary

The most frequent intradural extramedullary lesions are neurofibromas and meningiomas, which account for 54% of all intraspinal lesions in adults.[997] Neurofibromas and meningiomas are rare in children.[54]

Plain radiographic changes of meningioma and solitary neurofibroma are usually unrewarding. Meningiomas, which occur most frequently in the thoracic spine (80%) of women, present clinically with smaller tumors long before bone changes become evident. Meningiomas may calcify radiographically in 3.3%[141] and occasionally may incite adjacent bony (vertebral) sclerosis, although not as frequently as intracranial meningiomas.[357a] They cause bone erosion, and widening of the IPD occurs in less than 10% of cases.[141, 352]

Neurofibromas may occur anywhere within the spinal canal and may be solitary or multiple. Solitary neurofibromas may become large enough to cause bone erosion and other radiographic findings, depending on tumor location. If the tumor involves the dorsal root ganglion, then pedicle erosion or widening of the neural foramen or both occur (see Fig. 4–79). Neurofibromas widen the IPD in 56% of cases.[352] Neurofibromas

may become large and erode the canal asymmetrically. In some cases, widening of the IPD may be the only plain radiographic clue. Neurofibromas do not calcify and do not incite reactive change found in meningiomas. Neurofibromas may be multiple and are often associated with neurofibromatosis.[760, 1089]

Extradural

Extradural tumors and tumorlike conditions almost always include epidural metastasis and herniated disc tissue. The plain radiographic detection of epidural lesions is unrewarding unless the lesion calcifies, as occurs occasionally with disc herniation. Epidural metastases are usually associated with adjacent vertebral destruction, which may or may not be evident radiographically. Epidural tumor should be suspected in patients with a known primary malignancy who develop clinical signs of spinal cord block. Isolated epidural metastases are not detected on the plain radiograph.

Congenital Anomalies

The conventional radiograph is helpful in demonstrating the location and extent of skeletal abnormalities that may occur as isolated events in otherwise normal individuals or that may develop in association with dysraphism or congenital malformation syndromes. In some forms of dysraphism, the conventional radiograph not only can identify skeletal abnormalities but often can give clues to the location of underlying associated intraspinal anomalies.[695] The spine can be evaluated adequately on the AP and lateral radiographs, although additional views may occasionally be necessary. The entire spine should be examined in cases of suspected dysraphism and congenital malformation syndromes, since skeletal abnormalities may occur at multiple levels. In some disorders, additional examinations should include the skull, occipitoatlantal articulations, and the atlantoaxial relationships.

Craniocervical Junction

Congenital abnormalities of the craniocervical region are not uncommon.[838] They may be unassociated with neurologic signs or symptoms, sometimes being discovered incidentally on the radiograph, or they may be associated with severe neurologic disability. Often, malformations of the craniovertebral junction exist in combination[297] and may cause neurologic symptoms that may mimic other neurologic disorders.[505] This is true of basilar invagination, assimilation of the atlas, abnormalities of the odontoid process, atlantoaxial dislocation, Klippel-Feil syndrome, and other anomalies.

Obtaining a true lateral view of the upper cervical spine or skull is extremely important for the evaluation of a number of these disorders. The posterior lip of the foramen magnum (opisthion) is an anatomic landmark that is observed when evaluating several abnormalities or measuring for basilar invagination. It is identified on 84% of lateral cervical spine radiographs as a teardrop-shaped density.[898] The spinolaminar line is an unreliable indicator of the position of the opisthion, since it often passes anterior to it.

Basilar Invagination. Basilar invagination (basilar impression) is a deformity of bony structures at the base of the skull in the region of the foramen magnum in which the margins of the foramen magnum are turned upwards, reducing the volume of the posterior cranial fossa.[570, 838] This allows the odontoid process and cervical spine to assume a more cephalad location. The odontoid process may protrude into the foramen magnum and encroach upon and compromise the brain stem[827] and possibly the vertebral arteries. Basilar invagination is a rare disorder that may be congenital or developmental. Congenital basilar invagination is the most common type[977] and is often associated with other congenital anomalies,[297] such as Klippel-Feil syndrome, atlantoaxial fusion, hypoplasia of the atlas, odontoid abnormalities, block vertebra, and other deformities.[827, 1294]

Basilar invagination may be developmental, as it is associated with disorders that cause softening of the bony structures at the base of the skull. The most common cause of developmental basilar invagination is Paget's disease,[301] occurring in 30% of cases of Paget's disease in one series.[977] Basilar invagination has been reported to cause sudden death in a patient with Paget's disease.[358] Other bone softening disorders that

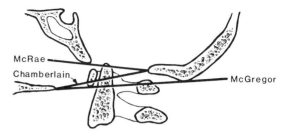

Figure 4–151. Diagrammatic representation for measurement of basilar invagination.

have been associated with basilar invagination include osteoporosis, osteomalacia (rickets), cretinism, renal osteopathy, and osteogenesis imperfecta.[301, 827] It may develop in achondroplasia,[764] cleidocranial dysostosis (as a result of delayed ossification), Morquio's syndrome (as a result of defective ossification,[827] or osteogenesis imperfecta.[983] It has been reported in hydrocephalus and following either sudden trauma[301] or chronic trauma, such as is caused by carrying heavy loads on the head.[827] Primary or secondary tumor as well as infection (in the years prior to antibiotics) has been implicated as causing basilar invagination.[301] Basilar invagination is difficult to evaluate radiographically and several methods have been utilized (Figs. 4–151 and 4–152).

Chamberlain's Line. Chamberlain's line extends from the "dorsal lip of the foramen magnum to the dorsal margin of the hard palate"[190] as determined on the lateral skull radiograph (see Fig. 4–151). Although it was originally felt that extension of the odontoid process or of C1 above this line represented basilar invagination,[190] it has subsequently been shown that in normal individuals, the mean position of the tip of the odontoid process is 1 mm below[1106] to 0.6 mm above[977] Chamberlain's line, with a standard devia-

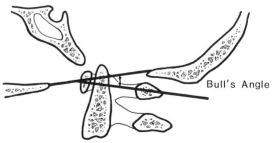

Figure 4–152. Bull's angle.

tion of 3.5 mm[1106] or 3.3 mm.[977] Some of the limitations of using this line in the measurement of basilar invagination are that the posterior margin of the foramen magnum may not be visualized on the radiograph and that the posterior margins of the foramen magnum may also themselves be invaginated.[1210] Chamberlain's line is considered relatively unreliable.[570]

McGregor's Line. McGregor's line is "the line drawn from the upper surface of the posterior edge of the hard palate to the most caudal point of the occipital curve in the true lateral x-ray"[827] (see Fig. 4–151). The advantage of McGregor's line is that the occiput is easy to visualize and is a fixed point of reference. The mean position of the odontoid process is 1.3 mm above the line, with a standard deviation of 2.62 mm (examining African Bantu skulls). A measurement of the tip of the odontoid process of 4.5 mm or greater above the line is considered abnormal.[827] Others have found significantly different values. In one series, the mean value for position of the odontoid process in males was 0.33 mm above the line, with a standard deviation of 3.81 mm and in females the mean value was 3.67 mm above the line, with a standard deviation of 2.62 mm.[570] In another study, the normal value is 9 mm or less.[1007] The differences between these results and those of McGregor may be due to the difference in racial population studied and in the positioning of the patients.[570] In 90% of normal children of either sex from age 3 to 18 years, the odontoid process is 2 mm above McGregor's line, with a range of 0 to 5 mm. However, wide variations exist among children and within the same patient.

One of the arguments against using Chamberlain's and McGregor's lines for determining basilar invagination is that they are drawn from the hard palate, which is not related to the base of the skull.[1210] The position and plane of the hard palate are variable, altered by development of the facial bones.[570] For instance, a low palate may give a false impression of basilar invagination, whereas a high palate may cause the correct diagnosis to be missed.[1210] Also, an odontoid process may appear high in position without basilar invagination. This may occur in patients with a congenitally abnormal, long odontoid process or in those with occipitalization of the atlas.

Bull's Angle. This angle occurs when lines are drawn in the plane of the hard palate and in the central plane of the anterior and posterior portions of the atlas[142] (see Fig. 4–152). An angle of more than 13 degrees is considered indicative of basilar invagination. However, a limitation to this evaluation is that the angle varies with flexion and extension of the head.[570]

Digastric Line. This line is drawn between the two digastric grooves, which lie in the lateral part of the base of the skull[402] (Fig. 4–153). The line is the rostral limit for the position of the tip of the odontoid process.[301] The distance from this line to a line drawn from the middle of the atlanto-occipital joints is normally 10 mm and diminishes with basilar invagination.[570]

McRae's Line. McRae's line is drawn from the anterior lip of the foramen magnum (basion) to the posterior lip of the foramen magnum (opisthion) on the lateral view (see Fig. 4–151). This line measures the anteroposterior dimension of the foramen magnum. Normally on the true lateral view, "the

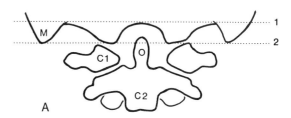

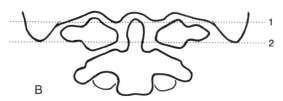

Figure 4–153. Digastric line. Diagrammatic representation of the atlanto-occipital articulation and a measurement for basilar invagination. Key: **1** = digastric line joining the digastric grooves; **2** = mastoid line joining the tips of the mastoid processes; **M** = mastoid process; **O** = odontoid process. A, Normal appearance. The digastric line (**1**) is well above the odontoid process, and the mastoid line (**2**) passes through the tip of the odontoid process. B, Basilar invagination. Both lines **1** and **2** pass through the odontoid process.

occipital squama on each side of the foramen magnum is seen as a thin dense plate of bone convex downward" and lies below the line.[839] Basilar invagination is present "if the line of the occipital squama is convex upward or if it lies above the line of the foramen magnum or if the occipital condyles lie on or above the line of the foramen magnum."[839]

In addition, the dorsal displacement of the odontoid process relative to the foramen magnum can also be evaluated.[839] In one series in which patients with both symptomatic basilar invagination and an odontoid process 5 to 25 mm above Chamberlain's line were evaluated, no cases demonstrated an odontoid process above McRae's line.[837] Thus, it can be assumed that an odontoid process above the level of the foramen magnum (McRae's line) could be associated with symptomatic basilar invagination. Also, in the same series, none of the cases demonstrated an anteroposterior diameter of the spinal canal behind the atlas or axis of less than 20 mm.

Platybasia. Platybasia ("flattening of the skull")[827] is a term often incorrectly used synonymously with basilar invagination. It is an anthropologist's term referring to the degree of obtuseness of the basal angle of the skull.[1210] The angle is created by the intersection of the plane of the sphenoid with the plane of the clivus, as seen on the lateral view of the skull. This is accomplished by drawing a line from the nasion (naso-frontal suture) to the tuberculum sellae or the center of the pituitary fossa or the posterior clinoids. A line drawn from the tuberculum sellae, center of the pituitary fossa, or posterior clinoids to the anterior tip of the foramen magnum delineates the plane of the clivus.

The normal basal angle varies between 103.5 degrees and 131.5 degrees[1210] Platybasia may be diagnosed when the basal angle equals or exceeds 145 degrees.[839] The majority of patients with basilar invagination do not demonstrate platybasia,[1210] although the two conditions may coexist.[837, 977]

Occipitalization of the Atlas. Occipitalization of the atlas represents partial or complete fusion of the atlas with the occiput and is the most common abnormality of the craniovertebral junction[837, 1294] (Fig. 4–154). Fusion may occur anteriorly or posteriorly or both anteriorly and posteriorly. In one

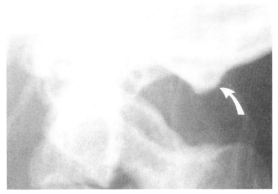

Figure 4–154. Occipitalization of the atlas. Lateral radiograph of the occipitocervical junction demonstrates fusion of the posterior arch of the atlas with the occiput (arrow).

series, all cases demonstrated fusion of the anterior arch of C1 with the anterior lip of the foramen magnum.[839] Evidence of a posterior arch is usually present, often as a bony ridge at the posterior edge of the foramen magnum. The lateral masses of C1 may fuse with the occiput either unilaterally or bilaterally and often asymmetrically.[839, 1210] Assimilation (or complete occipitalization) of the atlas refers to complete fusion of all components of the atlas with the base of the skull.[1210] The transverse process of C1 is usually abnormal, being either fused or partially absent.[839] Occipitalization is frequently associated with other abnormalities of the craniovertebral junction,[297, 1210] with fusion of cervical vertebrae, basilar invagination, and atlanto-axial dislocation being the most common.[1210, 1294] Fusion of C2–C3 occurs in 68% of cases of occipitalization.[839] Posterior fusion usually can be detected on the lateral radiograph; however, focal fusion with the edge of the foramen magnum may be difficult to visualize.

Occipitalization in children may be difficult to evaluate radiographically. At birth, the anterior arch of the atlas is not ossified in about 80% of cases,[1268] and there is a normal unossified portion of the posterior arch of C1.[1294]

Basilar invagination may be present. The space between the posterior margin of the odontoid process and the nearest bony part posteriorly (either the posterior arch, bony ridge, or foramen magnum) should be measured. Patients who are symptomatic and whose spinal canal posterior to the odontoid

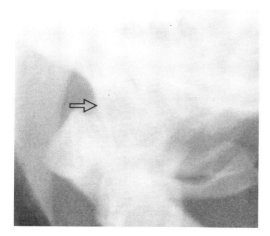

Figure 4–155. Third condyle. There is bone formation that appears fused with the anterior aspect of the foramen magnum (arrow). This represents the "third condyle," the most common manifestation of the occipital vertebra.

process measures 19 mm or less probably have signs caused by the bony abnormality,[839] although a similar measurement may occur without neurologic signs.[1210]

Occipital Vertebra. The occipital vertebra, or proatlas, is the most caudal of the primitive vertebrae. It normally fuses with other primitive vertebrae and aids in forming the basilar process of the occipital bone.[757, 1234] Failure of such fusion of the occipital vertebra leads to abnormal bone formation on the outer surface of the skull in the region of the foramen magnum.

The occipital vertebra is a rare congenital abnormality, occurring in 0.47% of the general population.[757] It may exist alone or in combination with other local congenital abnormalities.[757, 1234] The most frequent manifestation of the occipital vertebra is the so-called third condyle[757] (Fig. 4–155). It is a median formation of bone of exocranial development. It is adjacent to but detached

from the anterior margin of the foramen magnum. It may be either an articular depression or a single tuberosity with an anterior facet.[505] It is usually small but may appear 14 mm or larger[757] and is best observed on the lateral radiograph. Other forms of the occipital vertebra include a hypochordal arch, a neural arch, and transverse processes that may fuse with the margin of the base of the skull.[503, 505]

Odontoid Process (Dens Axis). Embryologically, the body of the odontoid process is continuous with the centrum of C1, from which it separates during development, moves caudally, and fuses with C2.[393] The odontoid process of the axis is not visualized in the neonate because it is cartilaginous. It is not until later infancy and early childhood that it begins to calcify.[357a] At the age of 2 to 3 years, the odontoid process is visualized on the radiograph with a vertical V-shaped cleft at the proximal tip. A lucent cartilaginous line, present in all children under 4 years of age,[393] separates the odontoid process and the body of the axis.[357a] Fusion of the odontoid process with the body of C2 occurs around the age of 10 to 12 years.[357a, 393] A separate ossification center (os terminale) may develop within the "V" cleft around the age of 3 years and is present in about 25% of children between 5 and 11 years of age (Fig. 4–156). It usually fuses with the odontoid process by the age of 12 years.[393] The lucent line at the odontoid base, the "V" cleft, and the os terminale should not be mistaken for fractures.[357a] Rarely, the odontoid process may remain as the body of C1.[1250] A normal odontoid process may occasionally be tilted posteriorly, owing to variation in growth.[1251]

Occasionally in adults, an optical phenomenon, the Mach band, may appear as a lucent line at the base of the odontoid proc-

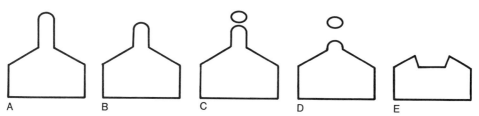

Figure 4–156. Diagrammatic representation of abnormalities of the odontoid process. *A*, Normal. *B*, Hypoplasia. *C*, Os terminale. *D*, Os odontoideum. *E*, Aplasia. (From von Torklus D, Gehle W: The Upper Cervical Spine. New York: Grune & Stratton, 1972. Copyright 1972 by Georg Thieme Verlag.)

ess on the anteroposterior open-mouth radiograph and simulate a fracture.[237, 238] A repeat radiograph in the atlantoaxial or lateral projection confirms that no fracture exists.

Os Odontoideum. Os odontoideum is a small round or oval ossicle separated from and cranial to a hypoplastic odontoid process (Fig. 4–157). The ossicle may be in a normal position adjacent to the tip of the odontoid process, or it may exist more cephalad near the basion—either separate from or fused to the basion.[393] There are conflicting opinions as to the origin of os odontoideum, although most authors feel that it is congenital.[449, 867, 1294, 1364] It may develop in otherwise normal individuals or in those with congenital syndromes, such as trisomy 21 (Down's syndrome),[393, 598] Klippel-Feil anomaly,[393, 1163] chondrodystrophia calcificans congenita,[81] or other syndromes. It may be associated with other cogenital anomalies of the occipitocervical region.[497] Cases have been reported following trauma to patients with a previously normal-appearing odontoid process[392, 393, 422, 540] and following infection.[499] It is felt by some that an unrecognized fracture of the base of the odontoid process in infancy is followed by nonunion, compromise of the vascular supply above the fracture, and partial or complete failure of development of the fractured segment.[392, 540] Os odontoideum has also been reported after acute ligamentous disruption followed by atlantoaxial instability.[1046] Complete separation of the odontoid process from the axis has been reported in a patient with rheumatoid arthritis[464] and should not be mistaken for os odontoideum.

Subluxation is frequent with os odontoideum.[867] Flexion and extension radiographs can help determine the degree of motion and of canal compromise, and whether the transverse ligament is intact. Although narrowing of the spinal canal at C1–C2 may occur from excessive motion in patients with os odontoideum, there is no constant correlation between symptomatology and the degree of atlantoaxial instability.[449]

Hypoplasia. The mean height of the odontoid process is 18 mm in males and 16.8 mm in females, and height measurement less than 11.9 mm indicates hypoplasia.[833] Hypoplasia of the odontoid process may be congenital or acquired. It may be associated with os odontoideum, as has just been discussed (see Fig. 4–157). Hypoplasia without os odontoideum may be seen in a number of disorders and may be associated with abnormal mobility of the atlantoaxial relationship. These include Morquio's disease, pseudoachondroplasia, metatrophic dwarfism, Down's syndrome, spondyloepiphyseal dysplasia, and other disorders.[357a, 713, 1150]

A small or tapered or a small and tapered odontoid process is frequently the result of inflammatory erosions in adult or juvenile rheumatoid arthritis or any of the rheumatoid variants, such as psoriatic arthritis, Reiter's syndrome, and ankylosing spondylitis.

Absence. Absence of the odontoid process may occur following severe erosion in rheumatoid arthritis or any of the rheumatoid variants. Metastasis, trauma,[422] and infection[499] are less common causes. Congenital absence is extremely rare, and those reported cases probably were examples of os odontoideum that was not well visualized on plain radiographs.[449]

Fusion of Atlas and Axis. Rarely, the anterior arches of the atlas and axis may be fused congenitally, either alone[496, 927] or in association with fusion of the occiput.[497] Atlantoaxial fusion of the lateral articulating surfaces may develop following inflammatory disease, such as rheumatoid arthritis or psoriatic arthritis.[321]

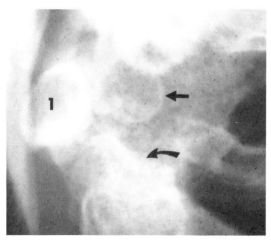

Figure 4–157. Os odontoideum. There is a somewhat rounded bone density (straight arrow) posterior to the anterior ring of C1, which is larger than normal and demonstrates a thickened cortex. The odontoid process is hypoplastic (curved arrow). *Key:* **1** = anterior arch of atlas. (Courtesy of Dr. Robert Kricun, Allentown, Pennsylvania.)

Klippel-Feil Deformity

This disorder comprises a broad spectrum of skeletal deformities that vary in severity and characteristically involve the cervical spine.

Clinically the neck is short. There are extensive segmentation anomalies, the most common of which is the fusion of two or more cervical vertebrae (block vertebra)[302] (Fig. 4–158). This may occur without fusion of thoracic or lumbar vertebrae.[994] In the classic description, all the cervicothoracic vertebrae carried ribs, giving the appearance of complete absence of the cervical column.[679] The fusions were so extensive that the vertebral column extending from the occiput to the sacrum was formed by 12 differentiated vertebrae and an osseous mass of fused vertebrae.

Other cervical anomalies may be present. These include spina bifida, hemivertebra, vertebral body clefts, large neural foramen,

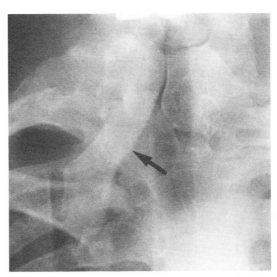

Figure 4–159. Omovertebral bone. There is bone bridging the spine with the scapula (arrow).

atlanto-occipital assimilation, deformed odontoid process, and basilar invagination.[302] Fusion of posterior elements may be present, causing narrowing of neural foramina. Although the central spinal canal is usually normal or large, cases of central spinal stenosis do occur.[987] Other more common skeletal abnormalities include scoliosis,[1358] the presence of an omovertebral bone[302] (Fig. 4–159), and Sprengel's deformity.[925] Associated congenital anomalies of the genitourinary,[994] cardiovascular, neurologic, and dermatologic systems may be present.[302, 994] Hypermobility of unfused cervical segments adjacent to fused segments may occur and may lead to spinal cord or nerve root compression[353, 364, 1201] even with minor injury,[353] and the omovertebral bone may possibly contribute to cervical subluxation and cord compression.[1202]

Lumbosacral Transitional Vertebra (LSTV)

In the normal spine, the 24th vertebra is the last presacral vertebra, and the 25th is the first sacral vertebral body.[1129a] The term sacralization refers to a unilateral or bilateral enlargement of the transverse process or to partial or complete fusion of a transverse process or vertebral body of the presacral vertebra with the sacrum. Lumbarization indicates elevation of S1 above the sacrum,

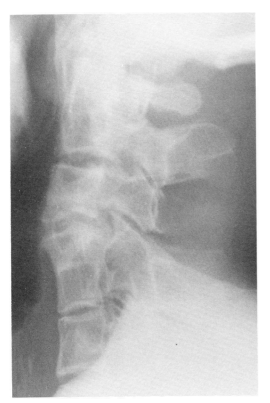

Figure 4–158. Klippel-Feil deformity. There is evidence of congenital block vertebra and fusion of posterior elements in this patient who also had Sprengel's deformity.

with unilateral or bilateral lack of formation of its lateral masses and the vertebral body either being assimilated or becoming the last presacral vertebra.[1129a] It is much less common than sacralization. These patients demonstrate 12 thoracic vertebrae and 6 lumbar vertebrae without changes in the transverse process of the presacral vertebra. Since it is often difficult to determine whether the transitional vertebra observed is the 24th or 25th without additional spinal radiographs, the term lumbosacral transitional vertebra (LSTV) is helpful.

One of the clues that may help in determining which vertebra is L5 is that, generally speaking, the transverse process of L3 is the largest of the transverse processes, is directed horizontally or downward, and has a vertical border. The transverse process of L4 is shorter and thinner than those of L1 and L3 and is directed upward, and its end demonstrates a pointed shape.[1129a, 1204] In 3% of cases, the transverse process of L4 is larger than that of L3.[1204] LSTV occurs in about 5% of the general population.[1266] There are various forms of LSTV, ranging from hyperplasia of the transverse processes to large transverse processes that articulate with the sacrum to fusion of the transverse process and vertebral body with the sacrum (Figs. 4–160 and 4–161). These abnormalities may be partial or complete and unilateral or bilateral.

The type I form of LSTV is characterized by a unilateral or bilateral enlarged (dysplastic) transverse process that measures at least 19 mm in width.[1266] The bilateral form is more common than the unilateral form.[184] This anomaly is considered a "forme fruste,"[184] or an attempt at sacralization,[1204] and is the most common form.[1266] There is an increased incidence of type I in families with true LSTV.[1266]

Type II is the second most common form of LSTV and is the most frequent form of true sacralization.[184] In this form of incomplete sacralization/lumbarization, there may be unilateral or bilateral, large, wing-shaped transverse processes that follow the margin of the sacral ala and form an articulation with the sacrum (see Fig. 4–161). The articulation is a diarthrodial joint with a hyaline cartilage articular surface, and it is surrounded by a joint capsule.[1129a] Therefore, it is not surprising that these joints may undergo degenerative changes of osteoar-

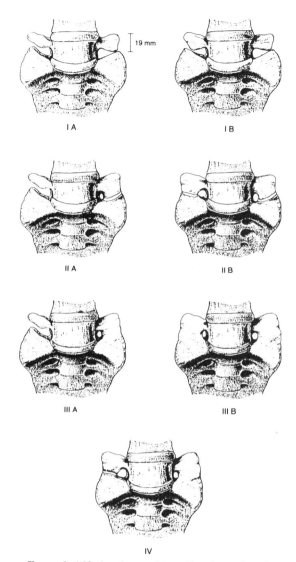

Figure 4–160. Lumbosacral transitional vertebra classification. (From Castellvi AE, Goldstein LA, Chan DPK: Lumbosacral transitional vertebrae and their relationship with lumbar extradural defects. Spine 9:493–495, 1984.)

thritis, with osteophyte formation and sclerosis.[1129a]

In the type III form of LSTV there is unilateral or bilateral complete sacralization or lumbarization (or both) that demonstrates complete bony fusion of the large, wing-shaped transverse processes with the sacrum.[184]

Type IV LSTV is a mixed form, in that it comprises type II on one side and type III on the other.[184]

The overall incidence in the general population of types II through IV is 6.7%.[1266]

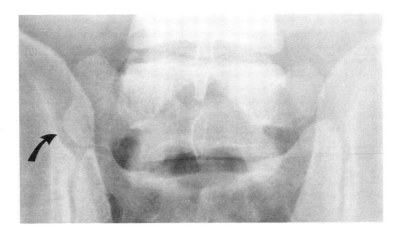

Figure 4–161. Type IIA lumbosacral transitional vertebra with articulation on the right (arrow). The transverse process of L5 on the left is broad (type IA).

Although the incidence of low back pain is not greater in patients with LSTV compared with the normal population,[1266] there is increased incidence of disc herniation just above the transitional vertebra in about 17% to 83% of type II LSTV.[184] This increased incidence is probably due to abnormal torque movements, with disc degeneration at that level. However, in types I, III, and IV LSTV, the incidence and location of disc herniation are similar to incidence and location of disc herniation in the general population, except there is no disc herniation at the levels of type III and IV LSTV. In patients with herniated nucleus pulposus in the lumbosacral region, about 30% demonstrate lumbosacral abnormalities, and about one half of these demonstrate true transitional appearances.[184]

Sacrum

Clinically significant sacral anomalies, such as sacral agenesis and hemisacrum, are rare, occurring in around 0.004% of hospital admissions,[683, 1087] but developing in 16% of all children born to diabetic or prediabetic mothers or to mothers who will eventually develop diabetes.[1215] However, only about 4% to 5% of patients with severe sacral anomalies had mothers who had diabetes during pregnancy.[1087, 1215] The exposure to fat solvents, particularly acetone, during early pregnancy and the experimental administration of insulin during pregnancy have also been implicated.[1215] Sacral anomalies have also been reported as an inherited defect.[1011]

There is an association between these sacral anomalies and other congenital abnormalities, including hemivertebra, scoliosis, tracheoesophageal fistula, imperforate anus, and renal or musculoskeletal anomalies.[263, 683, 686, 1011, 1215] Neurogenic bladder is common.[1011] Absence of the pituitary gland has been reported in a patient with sacral agenesis.[31]

In patients with sacral agenesis (Fig. 4–162), there is relative neurologic sparing and a relatively low incidence of visceral congenital abnormalities.[1215] There may be as-

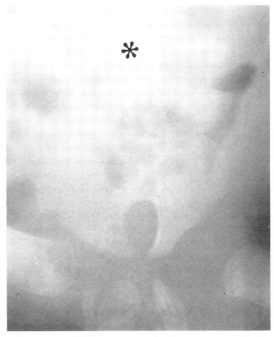

Figure 4–162. Sacral agenesis. There is complete absence of the sacrum, and the iliac bones are fused centrally. The lumbar vertebrae are also congenitally absent (asterisk).

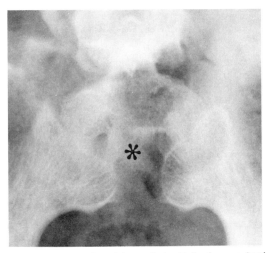

Figure 4–163. Sacral hypoplasia. Only the proximal portion of a small sacrum is present (asterisk). The distal aspect of the sacrum and the coccyx are absent.

sociated partial or complete lower vertebral agenesis, so that the iliac bones articulate with the lowest vertebra, and the medial iliac borders may approximate. The degree of agenesis of the sacrum is variable. It may be partial, sparing S1 (the most common form), or complete (associated with partial or complete agenesis of caudal lumbar vertebrae).[1011] In this latter form, the iliac bones articulate with the lowest lumbar vertebra, and if severe, the iliac bones approximate medially.[1011]

Hemisacrum is not as common as sacral agenesis. In this disorder, there is partial or total unilateral sacral agenesis (Fig. 4–163). There is a high incidence of visceral anomalies; however, there is little neurologic deficit other than denervation of the bladder.[1215]

Dysraphism

Spinal dysraphism represents an inadequate or improper fusion of embryonal tissues (ectodermal, mesodermal, and neural) in the dorsal median plane of the developing embryo that leads to anomalies of the skin, bones, dura, spinal cord, and nerves.[736] Spinal dysraphism includes a number of abnormalities that vary in severity and may occur alone or in combination. They may be clinically overt, such as myelomeningoceles, lipomyelomeningoceles, and most meningoceles, or clinically occult, such as diaste-

matomyelia, tethered cord, some meningoceles, and intraspinal and extraspinal masses such as lipomas and cysts. The conventional radiograph is usually the initial imaging modality obtained whenever dysraphic disorders are suspected[424] and imaging is desired. Spina bifida, wide sagittal diameter of the spinal canal, wide interpedicular distance, abnormal vertebral segmentation (butterfly vertebra and hemivertebra), bony spur (in diastematomyelia), fused laminae, and other anomalies may give clues to the possible location of an underlying associated dysraphic abnormality.[694]

The entire spine should be evaluated, since dysraphic disorders may exist at multiple levels.[916] Evaluation is performed in the AP and lateral projections. The conventional radiograph is abnormal in 95% of patients with occult dysraphism, although bony defects may be difficult to appreciate in infants.[424] The conventional radiograph is always abnormal in patients with overt spinal dysraphism.

Spina Bifida. Spina bifida refers to a fusion defect in the posterior elements, or, rarely, a defect in the vertebral body (Figs. 4–164 and 4–165). The severity of the defect varies from a narrow cleft in the lamina to splaying or absence of laminae at multiple levels. Mild, narrow posterior spina bifida at L5 or S1 is a common anomaly in otherwise normal, asymptomatic patients and is called spina bifida occulta[1204] (Fig. 4–164). It occurs in 22% of the general population and is of no clinical significance.[110]

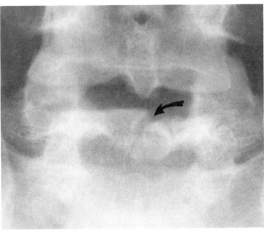

Figure 4–164. Spina bifida. There is a defect in the posterior neural arch (arrow). This represents spina bifida occulta in an otherwise normal individual.

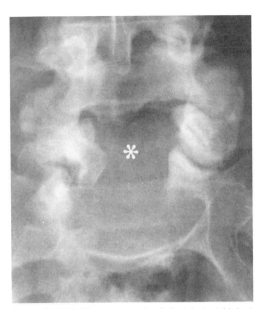

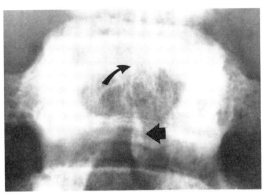

Figure 4–166. Diastematomyelia. There is an ossified septum (spur) in the midline (straight arrow) that is diagnostic of diastematomyelia and is differentiated from the spinous process above (curved arrow). The spur indicates the site of cord splitting. (Courtesy of Dr. Gerald Mandell, Wilmington, Delaware.)

Figure 4–165. There is a wide defect (asterisk) (spina bifida) in the posterior elements of the lumbosacral spine. In addition, there are deformities of the pedicles and possible fusion deformities on the right. A defect this size is compatible with an underlying dysraphic abnormality. This 30 year old patient had a myelomeningocele that was repaired shortly after birth.

Diastematomyelia. Diastematomyelia is an uncommon form of occult spinal dysraphism in which the spinal cord or filum terminale or both are divided sagittally or parasagittally into two nearly equal parts, often separated by a fibrous band or by a cartilaginous or an osseous spur.[565, 896] Although usually detected in children, diastematomyelia may escape detection until adult life.[1104]

The plain radiograph may play an important role in the diagnosis of diastematomyelia and in the attempt to locate the site of cord splitting. Vertebral abnormalities occur in all cases.[586]

The ossified spur, a diagnostic sign of diastematomyelia and the actual site of the split spinal cord, is visualized in around 20% of cases[565] (Fig. 4–166). The septum is probably calcified from an ossification center separate from the vertebra and does not arise from the vertebral body. The spur is larger at its dorsal end. The length of the fibrous or osteocartilaginous septum varies from 1 mm to the length of four vertebrae. The septum may be composed of mesodermal tissues other than bone.[1108]

Abnormalities of the posterior elements are common in diastematomyelia, occurring in 91% of cases.[565] Intersegmental vertical fusion of laminae associated with spina bifida occurs in around 60% of cases and is a strong predictor of the site of cord splitting (Fig. 4–167). Widening of the interpedicular distance with or without flattening of pedicles occurs in the region of diastematomyelia in 88% of cases. However, the widest interpedicular distance is at the same level as the septum in only one half of the cases.

Abnormalities of vertebral bodies occur in

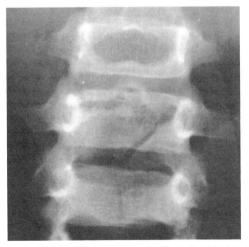

Figure 4–167. Diastematomyelia. There is widening of the interpedicular distance, as well as vertical fusion of laminae. Spina bifida and a cleft in the lamina are noted. An ossified spur is not visible. Nevertheless, the site of diastematomyelia can be suggested at the level of vertical laminar fusion. (Courtesy of Dr. Spencer Borden, IV, Philadelphia, Pennsylvania.)

85% of patients with diastematomyelia and include narrowing of the vertebral bodies in the AP diameter (at the level of the spur), partial or complete splitting of vertebrae in the sagittal plane, hemivertebra, narrowing of the intervertebral disc, and fusion of multiple vertebrae.[565]

Thus, a calcified or ossified septum with a combination of vertically fused laminae and spina bifida at or near the level of lamina fusion is strongly suggestive of diastematomyelia and correlates frequently with the level of the spur.

Diastematomyelia occurs in 5% of cases of congenital scoliosis and should be ruled out in this clinical setting.[460] Scoliosis, on the other hand, occurs in 60%[586] to 80%[67] of patients with diastematomyelia and is more frequent in patients with a more rostral septum.[565] Diastematomyelia may rarely occur at more than one level.[821]

Meningocele and Myelomeningocele.
Meningoceles and myelomeningoceles occur more commonly in the lower lumbar and lumbosacral regions,[424] whereas cervical and thoracic locations are less common. Myelomeningoceles also occur frequently in the thoracolumbar region. Spina bifida is always present, but the degree of severity varies. In meningoceles, the posterior spina bifida is localized and varies from a narrow cleft to absence of several vertebral arches[916] (see Fig. 4–165). The spinal canal may or may not be widened focally at the level of the lamina defect. The radiograph may indicate the presence of other dysraphic abnormali-

ties.[424] Radiographs of the skull do not reveal alterations of increased intraspinal pressure, since hydrocephalus is not frequently associated with meningocele.

In patients with myelomeningocele, the spinal alterations are more pronounced and devastating than with simple meningocele. There is a markedly wide spina bifida, and the pedicles and lamina are widely separated and everted.[424] If spina bifida involves T12–L1, the entire lumbar and sacral regions are also bifid; however, if T12 and L1 have normal-appearing posterior elements, the spina bifida is localized to the lumbar, sacral, or thoracic spine.[424] Vertebral anomalies include wedge vertebra, hemivertebra, vertebral body aplasia, and unilateral or bilateral fused vertebrae. Kyphosis and scoliosis may develop and are observed more frequently, as children are surviving longer.

Congenital Malformation Syndromes

Congenital malformation syndrome (CMS) is a broad term that includes a number of disorders that demonstrate skeletal malformations. The general categories of disorders include those with chromosomal abnormalities, dysplasias, dystrophies, and metabolic disorders with biochemical deficiencies. The spine is commonly involved in a number of the congenital malformation syndromes and may offer a characteristic appearance that enables the diagnosis to be made radiographically.

Table 4–15. SOME CONGENITAL MALFORMATION SYNDROMES: SPINAL ABNORMALITIES

	Achondroplasia	Conradi	Diastrophic Dwarfism	Hurler	Morquio	Spondyloepiphyseal Dysplasia Congenita	Tarda
Scoliosis	−	+	+	−	+	+	+
Kyphosis (C)	−	−	+	−	−	−	−
Kyphosis (TL)	+	−	+	+	+	+	+
AA instability	−	+	−	+	+	+	−
↓ IP distance	+	−	+	−	−	+/−	−
Inferior beak	+ (occ)	−	−	+	+/−	−	−
Central beak	+	−	+	−	+	+	+
Spina bifida	−	−	+	−	−	−	−
Disc	N	N	N	N	↑	↓	N, ↑
Vertebral shape	Biconcave		Flat		Flat	Pear, flat	Posterior hump; flat
Posterior scalloping	+	−	+	+	+	+	−

Key: AA = atlantoaxial; C = cervical; IP = interpedicular; N = normal; TL = thoracolumbar; + = present; − = not present; +/− = may or may not be present; ↑ = increased; ↓ = decreased.

Adapted in part from Bethem D, Winter RB, Lutter L, et al: Spinal disorders of dwarfism: review of the literature and report of eighty cases. J Bone Joint Surg 63A:1412–1425, 1981.

Congenital malformation syndromes are rare, yet their exact incidence in the general population is difficult to estimate. Identification of the incidence at birth does not take into consideration those syndromes that become manifest in childhood or adult life and does not take into consideration the possibility of early death.[1375] A number of congenital malformation syndromes are easily diagnosed clinically; however, radiographic evaluation can establish the diagnosis in some cases. In other cases, the radiographic examination demonstrates the full extent of skeletal anomalies (Table 4–15). Examination should include all segments of the spine, as abnormalities occur at multiple levels. AP and lateral radiographs are usually sufficient for spinal evaluation.

Achondroplasia

Achondroplasia is the most common form of short limb dwarfism.[50, 712] It is a hereditary disorder with an autosomal dominant mode of transmission. The basic error is in the zone of proliferating cartilage in the cartilage growth plate.[1085] This leads to a failure of enchondral bone formation in all bones, although it is more pronounced in long bones, particularly at the sites of more active growth. Thus, all ossification centers in the spine are small, and the intervertebral discs are larger than vertebral bodies.[159] Normally in the postnatal period, vertebrae grow in all directions to a greater degree in the lumbar spine than in the thoracic spine. They increase gradually in size from L1 to L5. In achondroplasia, the cartilage defect is accentuated in the sites of greater growth, so that alterations of failure of enchondral bone formation are more pronounced in the lumbar spine (particularly L5) than in the thoracic spine. Thus, the spine tapers from L1 to L5 (Fig. 4–168). With the smaller vertebral size, the interpedicular distance (IPD) is narrower.[83, 1085] In addition, the pedicles also experience inadequate longitudinal growth, so they become shortened to about one half their normal length.[159] Also, there may be premature fusion between the pedicles and the ossification centers of the vertebral body, also causing short pedicle growth.[357a] These features, along with the narrower IP distance, lead to failure of normal development of the spinal canal (spinal stenosis), particularly in the lumbosacral region.

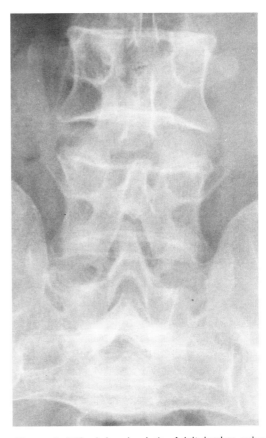

Figure 4–168. Achondroplasia. Adult lumbar spine. There is progressive narrowing of the interpedicular distance in the caudal direction characteristic of achondroplasia. This observation may also be made in some cases of diastrophic and thanatophoric dwarfism.

Some abnormalities are radiographically visible at all ages, although the degrees of severity may alter with age. Other anomalies appear radiographically as the patient becomes older.

At birth the IPD of L5 is narrower than that of L1 in most cases, but occasionally the IPD is similar throughout the lumbar spine.[712] However, in the second 6 months of life, actual relative narrowing of the IPD can be demonstrated, and this becomes progressively more pronounced by adult life. The pedicles are short at birth, and the progressive relative degree of shortening becomes more pronounced by adult years as well.

Wedge-shaped or hypoplastic vertebral bodies may be observed in early infancy and in early childhood, usually in the thoracolumbar and upper lumbar regions of the spine[712] (Fig. 4–169). In the older child, mild concavity of the posterior vertebral body

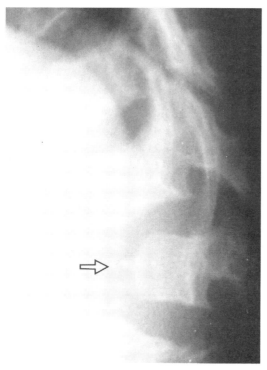

Figure 4–169. Achondroplasia. In this 27 month old child there is beaking deformity anteriorly of L1 (arrow) along with kyphotic deformity. Posterior scalloping is evident.

The degree of stenosis of the spinal canal is related to the diminished IP distance and the shortenend pedicles and is most evident in the lumbosacral region by adult life. The normal developing thecal sac, spinal cord, and cauda equina are confined by the narrow canal. Yet, the average age of onset of neurologic symptoms in achondroplastic dwarfs is 38 years, and such symptoms are not common before the age of 15 years.[83] It therefore seems that a narrow canal alone may not be sufficient to cause neurologic complications in the adult, but bulging of the annulus fibrosus, disc protrusion, osteophyte formation, progressive lumbar lordosis, and thoracolumbar kyphosis are contributory factors in the development of neurologic symptoms, as they compromise an already narrowed spinal canal.[83, 712, 877] Almost one half of achondroplasts develop spinal complications.[877] Intervertebral discs in achondroplastic dwarfs are congenitally hyperplastic and bulge laterally and posteriorly. Multiple protruding discs are common.

may be observed, and this becomes more pronounced by adult years. Posterior vertebral scalloping is caused by the pulsations of a normal thecal sac on the small spinal canal. Vertebral bodies appear smaller and cuboid-shaped in the lateral projection, and irregularity of the anterior vertebral margin of T12–L1 vertebrae can be observed.[1085]

Mild kyphosis may develop at the thoracolumbar junction before the infant begins to stand. This is not associated with any vertebral abnormality[712] and is thought to be due to muscle hypotonia, which resolves once the child begins to walk and muscle strength develops[83] (Fig. 4–170). The development of kyphosis in the older child is associated with a hypoplastic vertebra.[712] Kyphosis may present in about one third to one half of the cases,[83, 642] and in about one third of these, it may become severe.[83]

Angulation at the L5 junction is increased compared with that of the normal neonate.[712] Once the child begins to walk, the degree of lumbar lordosis increases.[83] Exaggerated lumbar lordosis occurs in about 70% of patients.[50]

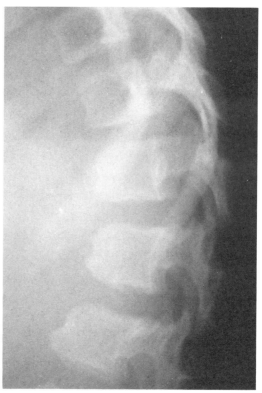

Figure 4–170. Achondroplasia. Eighteen month old patient with kyphosis. There is no deformity of vertebral bodies at the site of kyphosis.

There are parameters that may be helpful in predicting which achondroplasts are at risk for developing severe neurologic symptoms when adult life is reached. These parameters include thoracolumbar kyphosis, an IP distances less than 20 mm at L1 and less than 16 mm at L5, and a prominent lumbar lordosis.[642]

The foramen magnum may be small, and occipitalization of C1 may be present and lead to cervical myelopathy.[83, 877] Basilar invagination[83] and atlantoaxial dislocation[494] have been reported to cause quadriplegia.

Chondrodystrophia Calcificans Congenita (Conradi's Disease)

Chondrodystrophia calcificans congenita (CCC), otherwise known as chondrodysplasia punctata (Conradi's disease), is a rare congenital disorder in which there is a disturbance in enchondral ossification, particularly in epiphyses of long bones.[1085] The administration of warfarin to pregnant women may result in CCC. There are two forms: a lethal form in which the infant usually dies before the age of 1 year, and a more benign form with which individuals may live into adult life.[617] The disorder is characterized by multiple stippled calcifications in epiphyses, which are more pronounced in long bones. In the spine, stippled calcifications may be seen along the lateral margins of the vertebral bodies in coronal clefts[357a, 1085] and in primary ossification centers[1085] (Fig. 4–171). Stippling may disappear if the child survives, or it may persist into adolescence.[357a, 1085] Similar calcifications are common in the sacrum, particularly the sacral ala and distal sacral segment.[1085] Calcifications may be noted in the intervertebral discs,[150] which, along with vertebral bodies, are usually normal in size.[1085] Double ossification centers have been described.[212]

In those who survive, calcifications disappear, and irregularity of the superior and inferior vertebral margins may occur. Anterior vertebral wedging and scoliosis may develop.[1085] These vertebral alterations, although milder, are comparable to those changes that occur in epiphyses of long bones in those children that survive.

Atlantoaxial dislocation, cervical kyphoscoliosis, reduction in vertebral height, fusion of vertebral arches with the occiput,

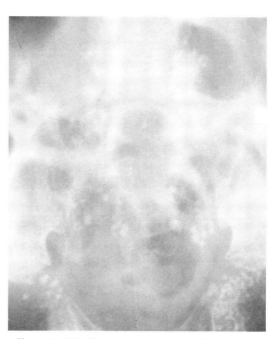

Figure 4–171. Chondrodystrophia calcificans congenita. In this 3 month old patient there are multiple stippled calcifications in coronal clefts alongside vertebral bodies, in the sacrum, and in the epiphyses of the proximal femora.

and butterfly vertebrae have been reported.[9, 803]

Diastrophic Dwarfism

Diastrophic dwarfism is a rare autosomal recessive hereditary disorder associated with short stature, micromelia, bilateral clubfoot, and a characteristic abducted, hypermobile, proximally placed thumb ("hitch-hiker thumb").[82]

Scoliosis is present in most patients and develops by the age of 8 years,[83, 558] although it has been reported in children as young as 6 months of age.[558] It is unassociated with underlying vertebral abnormalities[1233] but may lead to vertebral deformity.[1085] Progression of scoliosis may be slow or rapid and may become severe. Kyphosis develops in the cervical spine and may become so severe[27, 82, 711, 1302] that the odontoid process becomes aligned parallel to the foramen magnum[711] (Fig. 4–172). No abnormalities of the odontoid process have been noted, although cervical subluxation has been observed.[27] Lumbar lordosis is also a common observation in diastrophic dwarfs, and it

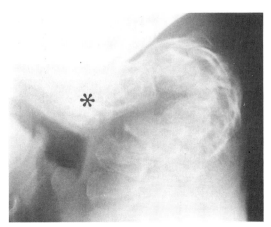

Figure 4–172. Diastrophic dwarfism. There is marked kyphosis of the cervical spine in this 11 year old patient. The odontoid process (asterisk) is parallel to the foramen magnum. (Courtesy of Dr. Gerald Mandell, Wilmington, Delaware.)

becomes prominent in childhood.[82, 558, 1253] Spina bifida occulta is a common observation in the cervical spine in some series[82, 558] but not in others.[1302] The defect varies from a small cleft in the spinous process to large defects in the vertebral arch.[82] The lower cervical spine is affected most commonly, but up to all seven cervical vertebrae may be involved. There is no correlation between spina bifida and cervical kyphosis.[1085]

Vertebral bodies are usually normal in width and height, although some flattening may be evident in cervical vertebrae,[27] and increased height may be noted in lumbar vertebrae.[990] The pedicles are short, although this is apparently limited to the lower lumbar spine.[711] Narrowing of the IP distance is probably variable. It is reported in some patients[1253, 1302] and not in others.[1302] In infancy, the IP distance is usually normal.[711, 1085]

Ehlers-Danlos Syndrome

Ehlers-Danlos syndrome is a familial disorder of connective tissue that is transmitted by an autosomal dominant mode of inheritance.[71] Hyperextensible skin and hypermobile joints are characteristic of this disorder.[1100] Kyphoscoliosis (18%), vertebral wedging, and straightening of the thoracic spine have been observed in the thoracolumbar and cervical regions of the spine.[71, 222, 1100] Degenerative changes become more

common with age, and spondylolisthesis may occur.[71] Dural ectasia may occur in this connective tissue disorder, causing posterior scalloping.[714]

Fibrodysplasia Ossificans Progressiva

Fibrodysplasia ossificans progressiva (myositis ossificans progressiva) is a rare, inherited connective tissue disorder in which progressive ossification of soft tissues and associated skeletal abnormalities occur.[1262] Ossification of soft tissues usually begins in the neck in the paravertebral region. The steady progression of ossification may at times be rapid, particularly following biopsy. Bony bars may eventually form (see Fig. 4–92), and bands of ossification may extend from the spine to an extremity. Vertebral abnormalities include fusion of facet joints (see Fig. 4–92), high vertebrae, narrow anteroposterior vertebral diameter, scoliosis, decreased sagittal diameter of the lumbar spine, and increased sagittal diameter of the cervical canal.[1262]

Hurler's Syndrome

Hurler's syndrome (mucopolysaccharidosis I, gargoylism) is one of the mucopolysaccharidoses in which there is an error of the "structural polysaccharide" (mucopolysaccharide) of connective tissue, with mucopolysaccharide deposited into soft tissues and infiltrated into adjacent bone.[1085] Heparan sulfate and dermatan sulfate are excreted in the urine (Table 4–16).

The vertebral bodies may demonstrate osteopenia at birth.[157] Later in infancy a characteristic inferior "beak" deformity of the anteroinferior vertebral margin may be present[157, 1085, 1248] (see Figs. 4–46 and 4–47). It is usually located in the lower thoracic or upper lumbar vertebrae and is probably caused by anteroinferior herniation of disc tissue, which prevents a normal ossification of the vertebral margin.[1235] This may be explained by the fact that the T12–L1 location is a point of major stress when the crawling child changes to an upright position of sitting or standing,[1085] or by the fact that there may have been hyperflexion in these children, whose muscles may be hypotonic, accounting for anteroinferior disc hernia-

Table 4–16. CLASSIFICATION OF MUCOPOLYSACCHARIDOSES

Syndrome	Type	Genetics	Predominant Mucopolysaccharide in Urine	Impaired Mentation	Spine Abnormalities
Hurler	I	AR	Heparan sulfate; dermatan sulfate	+ + +	+ + +
Hunter	II	XR	Heparan sulfate; dermatan sulfate	+ + +	+ + +
Sanfilippo	III	AR	Heparan sulfate	+ +	+
Morquio	IV	AR	Keratan sulfate	−	+ + +
Scheie	V	AR	Heparan sulfate	+/−	+
Maroteaux-Lamy	VI	AR	Dermatan sulfate	−	+ + +

Key: AR = autosomal recessive; XR = x-linked recessive; + + + = frequent; + + = moderately frequent; + = occasional; − = does not occur; +/− = may or may not be present.

Adapted from Greenfield GB: Radiology of Bone Diseases, 4th ed., Philadelphia: J. B. Lippincott Company, 1986.

tion.[1248] The inferior beak configuration leads to thoracolumbar kyphosis,[1085] which is less prominent in children.[357a] Although thoracolumbar kyphosis is an early sign of Hurler's syndrome and has been noted as early as 2 months of age, it usually develops later than the first year of life.[157] The interpedicular distance and spinal canal are normal.

In childhood, vertebral bodies may be small and somewhat rounded.[357a] They may also appear high, with narrowing in the AP diameter due to delay in walking.[473] Posterior scalloping may occur and may be due to dural ectasia related to the connective tissue abnormalities, bone "dysplasia," or both.[868] The dura may become thickened.[357a] Calcification of the stylohyoid ligament occurs in almost 90% of children with Hurler's syndrome (compared with 25% in normal children). The stylohyoid ligament in children with Hurler's syndrome appears thicker than in normal children.[922a]

Marfan's Syndrome

Scoliosis is a frequent feature of Marfan's syndrome. In addition, there may be widening of the spinal canal[904] in all diameters, with posterior scalloping, and thinning of pedicles and laminae due to dural ectasia from the underlying diffuse connective tissue (collagen) defect.[404, 714] Widening of the sacral canal and sacral foramina may occur.[404] Vertebrae are elongated and slender,[357a] and congenital fusion, spina bifida, and hypoplasia of the spinous process may be noted.[904] Severe spondylolisthesis of L5–S1 has been observed.[1355]

Morquio's Disease (Mucopolysaccharidosis IV)

Morquio's disease (mucopolysaccharidosis IV) is one of the mucopolysaccharides with an autosomal recessive mode of transmission.[713] Although patients with Morquio's disease do have platyspondyly and proximal femoral epiphyseal alterations, the disorder should be considered one of the mucopolysaccharidoses and not placed in the category of spondyloepiphyseal dysplasia. Patients with Morquio's disease have clouding of the cornea and demonstrate keratosulfate in the urine (see Table 4–16)—observations not found in other patients with platyspondyly and epiphyseal irregularities. They are not mentally retarded. In a series of patients with universal platyspondyly, 43% had changes similar to those seen in Morquio's disease. Nevertheless, it should be stressed that platyspondyly by itself is not an adequate criterion upon which to establish a diagnosis of Morquio's disease.[713]

The alterations in the spine in patients with Morquio's disease vary with age. In early childhood, vertebrae demonstrate mild flattening and an oval configuration.[713]

There is a defect in ossification of the anterosuperior aspect of the thoracolumbar and lumbar vertebrae resembling inferior beaking. In the older child, the thoracic bodies demonstrate slow growth in height. A central "tongue" (central beak) (see Fig. 4–48) protrudes anteriorly from oval-shaped thoracic and lumbar vertebrae, except at the thoracolumbar junction, where inferior beaking persists. Intervertebral discs are wide. Kyphoscoliosis may be present. Occasionally, retrolisthesis of one of the thoracolumbar or lumbar vertebrae may be noted.

In the adult, the vertebrae remain flattened and rectangular in configuration. Vertebral height is unaltered from late childhood. The inferior beak defect persists in the region of the thoracolumbar junction. Osteopenia may be noted, and the intervertebral discs remain wide.

The odontoid process is mildly hypoplastic in early childhood and hypoplastic or "absent" in the older child[713] (Fig. 4–173). There is excessive motion of C1 on C2, and the posterior arch of C1 may approximate the posterior aspect of the foramen magnum, giving the appearance of basilar impression even though there are no abnormalities of the occipital bone itself (Fig. 4–173). The alterations of the odontoid process and its relationship to the foramen magnum remain virtually unchanged into the adult years, except for decrease in atlantoaxial motion. Death has been attributed to the underlying atlantoaxial deformity in a patient who sustained a minor accident and suffered neuroaxis compression.[632] Other disorders in the classification of mucopolysaccharidoses are listed in Table 4–16.

Neurofibromatosis

Neurofibromatosis (NF) is a congenital abnormality classified as one of the phakomatoses.[183] It is a disorder caused by maldevelopment of neuroectodermal and mesodermal tissues. The spine is frequently involved in NF. Most of the radiographic features of NF are due to mesodermal dysplasia or tumor. Occasionally, spinal alterations may be the only clue to this disorder.

The most frequent manifestations of NF are due to mesodermal dysplasia[183] and include abnormalities in the dura (dural ectasia) and possibly bone (dysplasia). Kyphoscoliosis is the most frequent skeletal abnormality, occurring in about 10% to 40% of patients with NF.[585, 723] Posterior scalloping of vertebral bodies usually results from dural ectasia and occasionally results from tumor erosion.[182, 548, 723, 1096] (see Fig. 4–60). Anterior and lateral vertebral scalloping is a less common finding and probably is due to bone dysplasia[182] (see Fig. 4–60). Adjacent paravertebral tumor may also erode bone, causing a similar appearance.

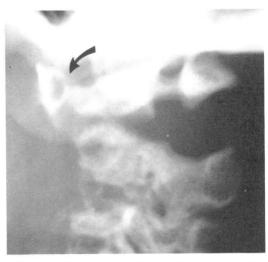

Figure 4–173. Morquio's disease. Platyspondyly, atlantoaxial subluxation (arrow), and hypoplasia of posterior arch of C1 are noted. The odontoid process appears hypoplastic. (Courtesy of Dr. Spencer Borden, IV, Philadelphia, Pennsylvania.)

Hypoplasia or aplasia of the pedicle and hypoplasia of the transverse process may occur[183, 784] (see Fig. 4–75). Lateral thoracic meningocele is usually associated with NF and is felt to be the most common cause of paraspinal mass in patients with this disorder. Up to 70% of patients with lateral thoracic meningocele have NF.[760] It may due to dural ectasia, bone dysplasia, or other factors. Widening of the neural foramen is a common finding. Paraspinal tumor may also have a similar appearance and may cause rib erosion.

Tumors of the nerve sheath (schwannomas) are the most frequent solitary intraspinal tumor in NF but may occur without this disorder.[760] Tumors of nerve roots and terminal nerve twigs (neurofibromas) are usually multiple and rarely occur without NF. Both types of tumor may develop within the spinal canal, the neural foramen, or paraspinally. Bone erosion by adjacent tumor may be detected on the conventional radiograph. There may be widening of the neural foramen or erosion of the pedicle by a "dumbbell" tumor, most frequently in the cervical and thoracic regions of the spine.[183, 694, 723] However, the wide neural foramen is usully caused by dural ectasia or bony dysplasia (see Fig. 4–87). When intraspinal tumors are large enough, they may widen the spinal canal, causing further erosion of pedicles, increase of the interpedicular distance, and thinning of laminae. Neural tumors may undergo malignant degeneration. About 50% to almost 100% of malignant degeneration of schwannomas and neurofibromas, respectively, occur in NF.[760]

There are less commonly associated congenital abnormalities that are probably coincidental when discovered with neurofibromatosis. These include atlanto-occipital fusion, spina bifida, hemivertebra, sacralization, and spondylolisthesis.[183]

Osteopetrosis

Osteopetrosis is a rare familial disorder in which the osteoclasts fail to resorb bone[789, 1146, 1156] (primarily spongiosa),[1085] and retarded or arrested osteocytic chondrolysis and osteocytic osteolysis occur.[697] Although resorption of enchondral cartilage and bone is diminished, formation of cartilage and bone continues at a normal rate, leading to accumulation of a large amount of calcification of cartilage and bone.[1156] There is evidence of an extraskeletal (hematopoietic) origin of the osteoclasts, possibly a monocyte

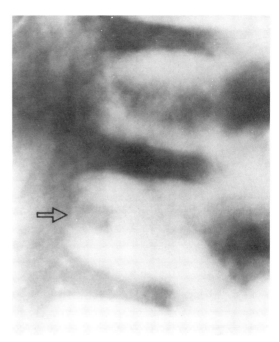

Figure 4–175. Osteopetrosis. There are bands of osteosclerosis. Widening and persistence of the anterior vascular groove are noted (arrow) in this 11 year old child. (Courtesy of Dr. Spencer Borden, IV, Philadelphia, Pennsylvania.)

or macrophage, as the responsible precursor.[1146] Radiographically, vertebrae and posterior elements exhibit varying degrees of osteosclerosis. In advanced cases, the bone marrow spaces are obliterated by unresorbed calcified cartilage and bone,[860] and this can be evident radiographically[1256] (Fig. 4–174). In milder forms, bands of osteosclerosis of varying height are present, in the superior and inferior subchondral zones[529, 759] (Fig. 4–175) and contain foci of calcified cartilage histologically.[860] A diffuse, osteosclerotic "bone within a bone" appearance may be seen within the vertebral body. Vertebral height and shape are normal,[357a] although there may be persistent widening of the anterior vascular groove of the vertebral body due to venous stasis caused by encroachment of the marrow space by abnormal osteoid[785] (Fig. 4–175). Intervertebral disc height appears normal. In the sacrum, osteosclerosis is more pronounced adjacent to the sacroiliac joints. Interestingly, bone that develops in osteophytes in older patients with osteopetrosis appears normal histologically.[860]

Two forms of osteopetrosis have been described. The more common of the two, the

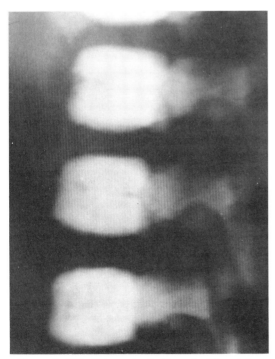

Figure 4–174. Osteopetrosis. There is diffuse intense sclerosis of all vertebrae and posterior elements. (Courtesy of Dr. Spencer Borden, IV, Philadelphia, Pennsylvania.)

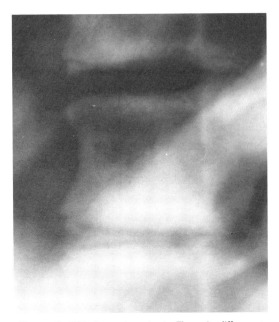

Figure 4–176. Pycnodysostosis. There is diffuse vertebral osteosclerosis with increased sclerosis in the subchondral zones similar in appearance to osteopetrosis. (Courtesy of Dr. Spencer Borden, IV, Philadelphia, Pennsylvania.)

clinically "benign" (tarda) form, is associated with normal longevity and does not demonstrate any hematologic abnormalities. It has an autosomal dominant mode of inheritance.[1256] The other form is the clinically "malignant" (congenita) form, which is rare and universally fatal, with death occurring within the first decade. It is inherited as an autosomal recessive trait.

Pycnodysostosis

Pycnodysostosis is an autosomal recessive disorder that is a variant of osteopetrosis.[849, 1255] The exact nature of the basic defect in pycnodysostosis is unknown.[849] In one patient studied by electron microscopy, no element of normal bone repair or remodeling was absent. All elements of fracture healing were present. Osteoclasts were infrequent but otherwise normal. The defect in mature bone in patients with pycnodysostosis may be due to disorganization of bone structure at the level of lamellar bone formation and of the osteon.

Changes in the spine are similar to osteopetrosis and include varying degrees of osteoclerosis, from diffuse osteosclerosis of all

components to bandlike densities in the subchondral region[319, 351, 891] (Fig. 4–176). Notching of the anterior vertebral margins may be seen.[319, 354, 351, 849] Thoracolumbar compression fractures[354] and spondylolisthesis[351] have been reported. Clinically, anemia, a common finding in osteopetrosis, is not observed in patients with pycnodysostosis.[351, 849] Patients with pycnodysostosis are short statured, a feature not present in patients with osteopetrosis.

Sclerosing Disorders

Osteopoikilosis, osteopathia striata, and melorheostosis are benign sclerosing disorders that are discovered incidentally and affect the spine less frequently and to a lesser degree than they do the long bones.

Osteopoikilosis. Osteopoikilosis is a rare, nonsymptomatic sclerosing disorder that presents with a variable number of focal osteosclerotic densities in cancellous bone, varying in size from a few millimeters to several centimeters.[482] They occur in epiphyses and metaphyses[704] and their equivalents. They are observed most frequently at the ends of long bones as well as in membranous bones and small bones of the hands and feet. The spine and sacrum are rarely involved; however, the spinous processes, transverse processes, and lateral masses of the sacrum usually demonstrate the abnormality (Figs. 4–177 and 4–178). Histopath-

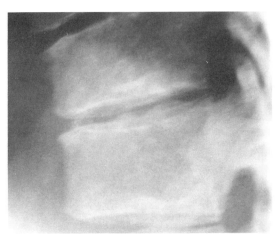

Figure 4–177. Osteopoikilosis. Multiple tiny punctate sclerotic densities are noted in the vertebral bodies and, to a lesser extent, in the pedicles.

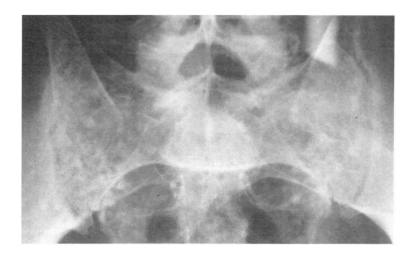

Figure 4–178. Osteopoikilosis. Multiple punctate sclerotic densities are noted in the sacrum.

ologically, the sclerotic densities represent numerous bone trabeculae, of varying thicknesses and arranged in a regular manner,[482] that correspond to old and inactive remodeling of trabeculae of cancellous bone.[704] Osteopoikilosis demonstrates a dominantly inherited mode of transmission.[845] The characteristic location of the numerous focal areas of sclerosis in epiphyses and metaphyses should obviate a mistaken diagnosis of osteoblastic metastasis.

Melorheostosis. Melorheostosis is one of the rare sclerosing disorders in which osteosclerosis appears to occur as irregular linear streaks along a sclerotome distribution in long bones.[890] Characteristically, osteosclerosis resembles melting wax flowing down the side of a candle.[167, 880] Endosteal and periosteal thickening may occur. Patients may be symptomatic,[890] particularly if periosteal thickening is present.

Melorheostosis may occasionally involve vertebral bodies or the sacrum.[7, 167, 418, 482, 880] Similar to long bones, irregular sclerosis has been noted along one side of the vertebra.[1129a] Sclerotic densities in the carpals or tarsals may be small, resembling osteopoikilosis, and changes of melorheostosis, osteopoikilosis, and osteopathia striata may coexist.[7]

Osteopathia Striata. This rare sclerosing disorder appears as linear streaks in long bones and flat bones. Its occurrence in the spine is extremely unusual.

Spondyloepiphyseal Dysplasia

Spondyloepiphyseal dysplasia (SED) is a hereditary bone dysplasia. There are two forms: the more severe congenita form[1212] and the more mild, later appearing tarda form.[710] Both forms involve striking changes in the spine and proximal femoral epiphyses and femoral necks. In this disorder, there is no clouding of the cornea or keratosulfaturia.[1212] Thus Morquio's disease does not fit into this category.

Congenita Form. SED congenita is manifest at birth[1212] and has an x-linked recessive mode of inheritance. Radiographically, in infancy, there is delay in ossification. Vertebral body height is diminished, and vertebrae may be incompletely fused and demonstrate two lateral ossification centers. On the lateral spine radiograph, the posterior aspect of the vertebral bodies is commonly shorter than the anterior aspect, causing a trapezoidal or pear-shaped appearance.[1212] In later infancy, vertebrae remain flattened and demonstrate an ovoid or "pear" shape. Ossification defects develop in the anterosuperior and anteroinferior vertebral margins and are more pronounced in the thoracolumbar spine. Here, marked hypoplasia of the anterior portion of the vertebra may occur. During childhood, vertebrae remain shortened (Fig. 4–179), particularly in the thoracolumbar region, whereas the lower lumbar vertebrae usually appear more normal with age.[1212] Thoracic kyphosis and lumbar lordosis develop. Scoliosis may occur in later childhood. The intervertebral discs are diminished in height.

By the adult years, there is marked shortening of the spine.[1212] The vertebrae remain flattened with irregular margins. Some appear wedged, and anterior vertebral hypoplasia is present in the thoracolumbar re-

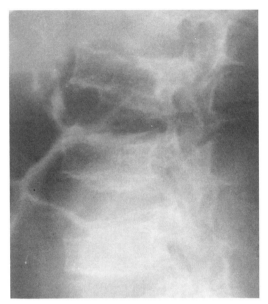

Figure 4–179. Spondyloepiphyseal dysplasia congenita. Platyspondyly is noted at multiple levels, and there is mild anterior beaking deformity as well. (Courtesy of Dr. Spencer Borden, IV, Philadelphia, Pennsylvania.)

gion. The lumbar spine is not involved as severely as are the cervical and thoracic spines. Kyphoscoliosis and pronounced lumbar lordosis are present.

The odontoid process appears unossified in childhood. By the adult years, there is a lack of bony fusion between the odontoid process and the C2 vertebra,[1212] and hypoplasia of the odontoid process is common.[83]

Tarda Form. SED tarda usually becomes evident during adolescence, although it has been discovered in childhood years.[1316] Radiographically, there is universal platyspondyly, although not as severe as in the congenita form. Universal flattening and anterior wedging are evident,[1316] and there may be increase in the AP diameter of vertebrae.[972] There is a peculiar hump shape of the posterior and central aspects of the superior and inferior vertebral margins,[643, 710] a characteristic observation allowing unequivocal diagnosis of this disorder[710, 972] (Fig. 4–180). There is variable associated anterior vertebral narrowing[643, 710] resembling the central beaking of Morquio's disease. Mild kyphosis or scoliosis may occur. It is felt that vertebrae are normal in appearance in early childhood and that the typical changes do not become evident until adolescence. Intervertebral discs are normal or high in childhood, but they narrow with progression

of disease and with age. Disc narrowing may become more pronounced posteriorly.

Patients with SED tarda develop premature osteoarthritis in major joints, particularly weight-bearing joints, and these changes are almost always present by adulthood.[643, 1316] SED tarda occurs only in males and is inherited by a recessive sex-linked mode of transmission.[643, 710]

Thanatophoric Dwarfism

This lethal dysplasia is probably a reflection of dominant mutation.[659] A fault in enchondral ossification leads to extreme lack of development of vertebral height in all vertebrae (Fig. 4–181). Radiographically, there is pronounced flattening of all vertebrae, with relative increase in disc height.

Trisomy 21 Syndrome (Down's Syndrome)

Trisomy 21 syndrome is an autosomal disorder in which there is an extra chromo-

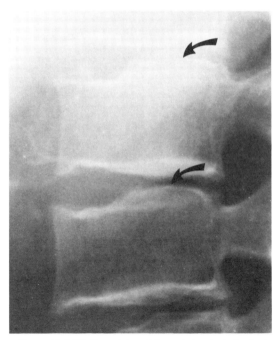

Figure 4–180. Spondyloepiphyseal dysplasia tarda. In this 26 year old male there is a hump-shaped deformity of the posterior superior vertebral margin (arrows), seen best on the lateral view, which is characteristic of this disorder. There is also an increase in the anteroposterior diameter of the vertebrae. (Courtesy of Dr. Edwin Wilson, Burlington, New Jersey.)

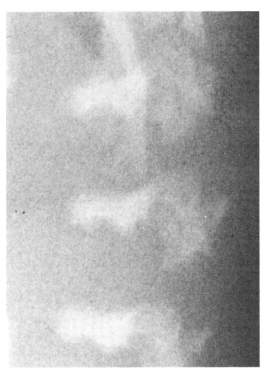

Figure 4–181. Thanatophoric dwarf. There is extreme flattening of vertebrae and extensive widening of the intervertebral disc "space." (Courtesy of Dr. Spencer Borden, IV, Philadelphia, Pennsylvania.)

some 21.[625a] Radiographically, in the axial skeleton there is increase in height of vertebral bodies probably due to poor muscle tone and delay in walking[473] (see Fig. 4–44). The anteroposterior diameter of the lumbar vertebrae may be reduced, and posterior scalloping may be evident.[990] Anterior vertebral concavity is more common and is wider and deeper than normal. The pedicles are elongated, and the spinal canal is wide.[357a] Narrowing of cervical and thoracolumbar intervertebral discs has been noted.[800]

Abnormalities of the odontoid process occur in 6% of the patients with Down's syndrome[1150] and include odontoid dysplasia or hypoplasia, os odontoideum, and os terminale. Other osseous anomalies include the third condyle, or occipital vertebra, and accessory ossicles.[147, 682] These alterations may predispose patients with Down's syndrome to atlantoaxial subluxation,[598, 800, 1150] which is a gradual progressive abnormality[147] occurring in 10% to 30% of patients with this disorder.[863a, 1167] The mean age for

the development of neurologic symptomatology is about 10.5 years, although patients may not develop neurologic symptoms until they reach their mid-40s.[988] Hemiplegia, quadriplegia, and even death have been observed.[598, 988] Nearly all patients with an odontoid–C1 interval of 4.5 to 6 mm are asymptomatic, whereas those with measurements of more than 7 mm may demonstrate neurologic symptoms.[988] In one series, the mean odontoid–C1 interval of symptomatic patients was 8.9 mm, with a standard deviation of 2.5 mm. Atlantoaxial subluxation in patients with Down's syndrome may be due to laxity,[801] malformation, or aplasia[800] of the transverse ligament, which is part of a generalized process of ligament laxity found in these patients.[1150] The presence of ligament laxity and odontoid abnormalities places a child with Down's syndrome at a high risk for atlantoaxial subluxation.[1150] Ligament laxity decreases with advancing age. Occasionally, atlantoaxial dislocation may be unreducible if it is caused by bony or soft tissue factors; the transverse ligament may slip anteriorly under the os terminale; there may be deposition of soft tissue between the odontoid process and the anterior arch of the atlas;[598] or the presence of a third condyle[801] or os odontoideum may interfere with reduction. Although atlanto-occipital instability is rare in patients with trisomy 21 syndrome, the evaluation of the atlanto-occipital articulation is important, particularly for those who wish to participate in athletic activities, especially following surgical fusion of C1–C2.[1076]

Other cervical spine alterations include a high incidence of degenerative changes at the C2–C3 and C3–C4 levels in adults, especially those over the age of 37 years; occasional subluxation at levels other than C1–C2; and congenital fusion of vertebral bodies and facet joints.[863a]

Turner's Syndrome

Turner's syndrome is a chromosomal abnormality with a karyotype pattern consisting of 45 chromosomes[357a]—an XO genotype. There is hypoplasia of C1, particularly the posterior arch.[660] Other observations include atlantoaxial fusion, square-shaped vertebrae, scoliosis, osteopenia, and occasional sclerosis along the sacroiliac joints.[357a, 396, 660]

Metabolic and Endocrine Disorders

Osteopenia

Osteopenia is a term that indicates decrease in bone mass, regardless of its quality or composition, and therefore indicates decrease in radiodensity of bone[431, 707] (Figs. 4–182 through 4–184). It occurs when bone resorption exceeds bone formation, regardless of pathogenesis.[1028] It is a collective term for a large number of disorders. Osteopenia may be diffuse, regional, or focal. Diffuse osteopenia may be observed in osteoporosis, osteomalacia, primary hyperparathyroidism, diffuse myeloma, and metastasis, may follow increased administration of exogenous or increased formation of endogenous steroids, and may occur in a number of other disorders.[1131] Senescent or postmenopausal osteoporosis is the most common cause of osteopenia.

Radiographically, bones appear less radiodense than normal, owing to diminution

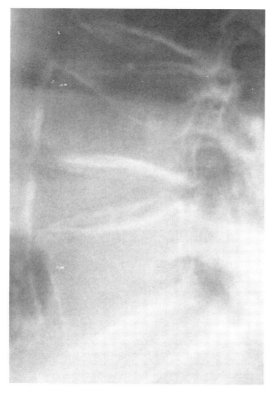

Figure 4–182. Osteopenia. There is a decrease in bone density (osteopenia) caused by thinning and diminution of trabeculae. The cortical margins are also thin in this 65 year old woman. In addition, there is depression of the superior vertebral margin. This patient had osteoporosis.

of trabeculae—particularly those running horizontally. Vertical trabeculae appear thinner and accentuated, and the vertebral end-plates demonstrate relative increase in density, even though they too are thinner. Osteopenia may not be visible early, since it is not noticed radiographically until the vertebrae have lost about 30% to 60% of calcium.[700, 840] It must be emphasized that the interpretation of the radiograph is often subjective and may be dependent upon observer differences (often leading to poor consensus),[58, 362a, 689] technical factors, patient body habitus, and patient positioning.[967] Alterations in technical factors may produce radiographs that are not representative of the true underlying bone density. Overexposure may produce a dark radiograph that simulates loss of bone density, and underexposure may produce a radiograph that simulates normal bone density, thereby possibly masking osteopenia. Alterations in the temperature or chemicals of the developing processor and film-screen combinations can also affect the radiographic density of bone. Body habitus, the amount of soft tissues, respiratory phase (during which a thoracic spine radiograph is obtained), and racial and geographic factors may alter the radiographic density image. Whites usually have less bone mass than blacks,[707] and individuals in the United States have greater bone mass than those in Europe.[967] The lateral radiograph is the preferred view when evaluating the spine for osteopenia. The conventional radiograph has an additional utilization, as it can complement dual photon absorptiometry in ruling out underlying spondylosis and aortic calcifications.[696] Although many causes of diffuse osteopenia cannot be differentiated radiographically, there are some associated signs that may suggest the proper diagnosis.

Osteoporosis and Scurvy

Osteoporosis is the most common metabolic disorder affecting the spine.[1028] It is a disorder in which there is less bone present than is normally expected for someone of comparable age, sex, race, and environment.[910, 967] There is decrease in nonmineralized bone matrix histologically, with thinning of trabeculae and cortex[910, 967] (see Fig. 4–183). Osteoporosis is found in a number of clinical settings but most commonly after

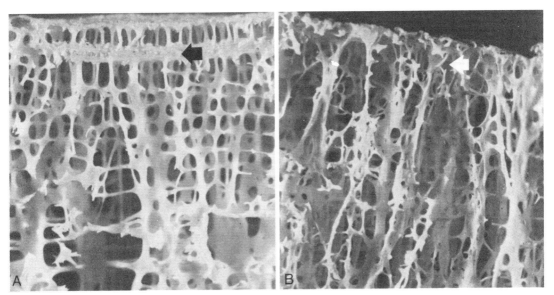

Figure 4–183. Macerated specimens. *A,* Normal vertebral body. Notice the normal thickness of vertical and horizontal trabeculae and the increased thickness of trabeculae in the subchondral zone (arrow). *B,* Osteoporosis. Notice the diminution and thinness of both horizontal and vertical trabeculae as well as diminution of trabeculae in the subchondral region (arrow). (From Schmorl G, Junghanns H: The Human Spine in Health and Disease. New York: Grune & Stratton, 1971. Copyright 1971 by Georg Thieme Verlag.)

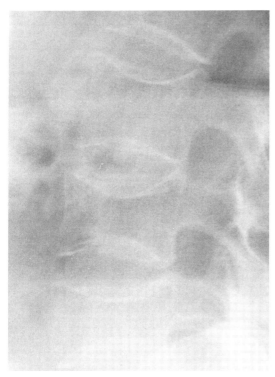

Figure 4–184. Osteomalacia. There is diffuse osteopenia (diminution of bone density) as well as symmetric biconcave deformities at all visible levels.

the menopause and during aging. The loss of cortical bone is 3 times greater in women than in men.[840] Decrease in trabecular bone begins by age 30 to 35 in both men and women, with an average decrease of 6% to 8% per decade and 10% per decade in postmenopausal women.[813] Osteoporosis may also be caused by disorders that produce increased breakdown of protein matrix (Cushing's syndrome, exogenous steroids, thyrotoxicosis, and acromegaly); failure of formation of matrix (scurvy, hypothyroidism, starvation, osteogenesis imperfecta); lack of mechanical stimulation of bone formation (immobilization, neuromuscular disorders),[476, 707, 910] and following administration of large doses of heparin.[1094] Osteoporosis is uncommon in children, although there is a rare form of osteoporosis of unknown etiology called idiopathic juvenile osteoporosis, which is self-limiting, with healing prior to puberty.[474, 589] Some cases demonstrate progression of vertebral collapse.[1192]

Radiographically, in osteoporosis, diffuse osteopenia exists, caused by thinning or loss of horizontal (secondary) trabeculae and, to a lesser extent, vertical (primary) trabeculae (see Figs. 4–50, 4–182, and 4–183*B*). Later, the surrounding cortex becomes thin[1218] but is sharply defined adjacent to osteopenic, cancellous bone. With loss of trabecular reinforcement, vertebral bodies are weakened structurally. Biconcavity deformities of vertebral bodies develop as intervertebral discs of normal turgor protrude into weakened bone (see Figs. 4–49 and 4–50). This type of vertebral depression in osteoporosis is more common in the lower thoracic and upper lumbar regions. Biconcavity is a slow remodeling process that forms as a result of multiple minor trabecular fractures that lead to weakening of subchondral bone[967] and the expansion of normal discs.[1191, 1218] In fact, degenerating discs are not associated with vertebral biconcavity.[1191] The concavity may extend from the anterior to the posterior vertebral edges. The degree of depression is characteristically asymmetric in the superior and inferior vertebral margins and does not appear uniform at different spinal levels, except in children, where biconcavity is uniform.[1074]

Anterior wedging may occur,[1131] and it is more common in the thoracic spine owing to the stress of weight-bearing being applied more anteriorly in this region of normal kyphosis. Scoliosis and kyphosis may develop related to compression fractures.[546] Almost one half of women over 64 years of age with osteoporosis develop structural scoliosis with curves of at least 10 degrees. Complete vertebral collapse may develop in patients with osteoporosis. Some authors have felt that Schmorl's nodes may be associated with osteoporosis.[114] However, others feel that there is no association between Schmorl's nodes and osteoporosis, and that Schmorl's nodes are not indicative of osteoporosis.[967] Patients with osteoporosis who are treated with sodium fluoride develop a coarse trabecular pattern and osteosclerosis in one third of the cases.[344, 1136]

Scurvy is caused by a deficiency in vitamin C. Radiographically, there are diffuse osteopenia, cortical thinning, and biconcavity of vertebrae.[633] There are diminution of horizontal trabeculae and thinning of vertical trabeculae. Compression fractures occur when adults are affected.

Cushing's Syndrome

Cushing's syndrome is caused by excessive adrenocortical steroids produced by either hyperplasia or tumor of the adrenal cortex or by the exogenous administration of corticosteroids. Radiographically, osteopenia is the most common abnormality. Subchondral sclerosis may occur in the upper and lower subchondral zones owing to exuberant callous formation in the presence of microfractures.[889, 1237] These are more readily identified in compressed or collapsed vertebrae and help differentiate Cushing's disease from other forms of osteoporosis. Anterior wedging in the thoracolumbar spine is common, and biconcave vertebrae are often identified.[889, 1237] Cushing's syndrome rarely occurs in infancy. Osteopenia and wedge fractures may or may not be present.[261]

Osteomalacia and Rickets

In osteomalacia, there is insufficient or delayed mineralization of cancellous or cortical bone.[707, 967, 1223] In rickets, there is interruption in the orderly development and mineralization of the cartilaginous growth plate.[968] Mineralization affects not only enchondral bone formation but also the formation of membranous bone and callus.[305] Osteomalacia and rickets are caused by abnormalities in vitamin D metabolism or calcium or phosphorus metabolism or both.[968] Numerous disorders produce osteomalacic or rachitic syndromes.[305, 1223] Osteomalacia may coexist with rickets, prior to fusion of the cartilaginous growth plates,[968] and with osteoporosis in adult years. Rarely, osteomalacia may develop secondary to tumor of mesenchymal origin.[221, 462] Reversal of osteomalacia occurs within 3 to 6 months after removal of the tumor.[221]

A discussion of vitamin D metabolism is beyond the scope of this chapter but is discussed comprehensively elsewhere.[970] Vitamin D is a prohormone—not a vitamin. It is hydroxylated twice before becoming physiologically active.[968, 970] The first hydroxylation to 25-hydroxyvitamin D (25-OH-D) occurs in the liver. The second hydroxylation to 1,25-dihydroxyvitamin D (1,25(OH)$_2$D), the active form of the hormone, is performed in the kidney.[970] 1,25(OH)$_2$D acts on intestine, bone, parathyroid glands, and kidneys to maintain calcium and phosphorus metabolism and to maintain mineralization of bone.[968]

The radiographic diagnosis of osteomalacia may be difficult.[188] In advanced cases, osteopenia develops in the spine but is nonspecific.[305, 968] There is a decrease in the number of secondary trabeculae, while the remaining trabeculae appear prominent.[967, 969] Trabecular margins appear indistinct owing to poor mineralization of osteoid,[969] and vertebral end-plates may also appear indistinct.[305] Intervertebral discs protrude into the vertebrae, producing biconcavity that is fairly symmetric at most levels.[968] Vertebral depression is uniform in both the superior and inferior vertebral margins (see Fig. 4–184). These vertebral alterations differ from those of osteoporosis, in which remaining primary trabeculae are often sharply defined and the degree of biconcavity varies at different levels. Kyphosis may develop in osteomalacia.[188]

Insufficiency fractures, a characteristic sign of osteomalacia in other parts of the skeleton, have not been observed in the spine in large series,[729] as they seem to occur in sites adjacent to main arteries that initially could cause pressure on the weakened bone.

Most forms of osteomalacia are diffuse in the skeleton. However, there is a rare form of osteomalacia, termed atypical axial osteomalacia, that consists of osteomalacic changes in the axial skeleton only (particularly in the cervical and lumbar spines, the pelvis, and the ribs), with a relatively normal-appearing appendicular skeleton.[415, 969]

In osteomalacia, changes in the peripheral skeleton are more characteristic than those in the axial skeleton.[188] Hand radiographs can often aid in differentiating advanced osteomalacia from osteoporosis in a patient who demonstrates nonspecific axial osteopenia.[841]

The radiographic features of rickets in the spine of children are similar to those of osteomalacia in the adult. These include generalized osteopenia and loss of secondary trabeculae.[968] Fairly uniform biconcavity associated with wide intervertebral disc spaces may be noted.[969] In very severe cases, vertebrae may be flattened and may demonstrate anterior beaking.[279] Vertebral height and density may return to normal following therapy.[357a] Scoliosis may develop with increasing age.[968] Basilar invagination caused by softening of the base of the skull has been noted.

Acromegaly

Acromegaly is a disorder caused by excessive production of growth hormone produced by pituitary tumors, such as eosinophilic adenoma and rarely chromophobe adenoma, or eosinophilic adenocarcinoma.[1221] Occasionally, hyperplasia of eosinophilic cells without tumor formation may cause acromegaly. Large amounts of growth hormone acting on the spine cause increase in periosteal apposition of bone in vertebral bodies,[1221, 1300] hyperplasia of disc tissue,[195, 1221] and hypertrophy of soft tissue structures, such as connective tissues, ligaments, perineurial and endoneurial tissues,[451] and dura. In adults, periosteal appositional bone growth is more extensive then endochondral bone formation,[1221] so that there is an increase in vertebral size in the anterior and lateral vertebral surfaces[1221, 1300] with less growth posteriorly. The lack of new bone formation posteriorly may be due to a lack of periosteum in this region[681] or due to the resistance of the pulsating thecal sac adjacent to the posterior vertebral margin as it attempts to extend posteriorly. The new bone formation anteriorly and laterally is present from the lower cervical to the lower lumbar spine but is most pronounced in the lower thoracic region.[195, 1300] Increase in vertebral height is usually not apparent.[1221] In advanced cases, the new bone formation is sometimes, clearly outlined on the radiograph.[1300]

Posterior scalloping of vertebral bodies is more common in the lumbar spine than in the cervical or thoracic spine and is more severe in patients with long-standing disease[1236] (Fig. 4–185). Moderate or marked posterior scalloping occurs in the lumbar spine in 65% of patients with acromegaly, and posterior scalloping may be noted to some degree in all patients with this disorder. Posterior scalloping may be due to pressure erosion by either enlarged soft tissues (dura) in the spinal canal or increased molding resorption caused by excessive growth hormone.[1221] It could possibly also develop as bone growing posteriorly is met by the resistance of pulsations from the thecal sac.

Osteophytes develop in patients with acromegaly and are uniformly distributed throughout the spine.[1300] They are more prominent laterally than anteriorly[98, 195] and are more irregular than those observed in

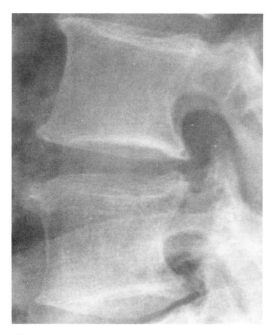

Figure 4–185. Acromegaly. Posterior vertebral scalloping is noted. The intervertebral discs are slightly increased in height.

patients with spondylosis deformans and intervertebral osteochondrosis.[451, 708] There is no associated sclerosis of vertebral endplates in patients with acromegaly and osteophytosis.[451, 708] However, some feel that the incidence of osteophytes is not greater than that which occurs in the general population.[1221] Apophyseal joints may also enlarge in acromegaly.[1221] The presence of osteopenia is variable. It is reported by some authors[195, 1236] but not observed commonly by others.[1221]

Enlargement of intervertebral disc height occurs in the lumbar and cervical spines.[98, 1221] New disc growth parallels the growth of the vertebral body.[195] Calcification of intervertebral discs has been reported in 20% of patients with acromegaly[708] and may be due to calcium pyrophosphate dihydrate crystal deposition disease (CPPD-CDD), which is associated with this disorder.

Patients with acromegaly may develop compression of the cauda equina.[451] This development may be due to hypertrophy of connective tissue and ligaments within the spinal canal as well as hypertrophy of perineurial and endoneurial tissues.[451] Osseous ridges may exist or form within the spinal canal and may cause neurologic compression. Most patients with acromegaly, however, do not develop cauda equina compression, so it may be that narrowness of a small or borderline small canal may be compounded by bony enlargement or soft tissue enlargement or both in patients with acromegaly.

Giantism results when excessive growth hormone is produced prior to closure of the cartilaginous growth plates. Vertebrae may become elongated in the rostral-caudal direction. Spinal stenosis may develop owing to bony overgrowth.[330a]

Hyperparathyroidism and Uremic Osteopathy (Renal Osteodystrophy)

Hyperparathyroidism (HPT) indicates overactivity of the parathyroid gland. Excessive production of parathyroid hormone causes osteocytic and osteoclastic bone resorption; however, in moderate amounts, parathyroid hormone may stimulate bone production.[322, 1057] Primary HPT refers to abnormalities originating in the parathyroid gland itself. Benign adenomas are the causative lesion in 91% of cases, and hyperplasia of the parathyroid gland (8%) and carcinomas are rare causes of this disorder.[1222] Secondary HPT most often occurs as a result of chronic renal failure but may develop in association with pseudohypoparathyroidism and osteomalacia.[1013] Excessive parathyroid hormones stimulate osteocytes,[322] which in turn resorb bone and mobilize calcium into the serum. Increase in parathyroid activity in the presence of chronic renal failure is caused by several factors. In chronic renal failure, progressive elevation of serum phosphate binds serum calcium and causes progressive hypocalcemia, which in turn stimulates parathyroid hormone production. In advanced chronic renal failure, there is also inhibition in the production of $1,25(OH)_2D$ (vitamin D), which diminishes the negative feedback suppression on the parathyroid glands.[1028] The resistance of bone to parathyroid hormone in chronic renal failure may be another cause of hypocalcemia.[968]

Uremic osteopathy refers to the skeletal alterations that are almost invariably present in, and develop as a result of, chronic renal failure.[265] Radiographic features of renal osteopathy commonly occur in the axial skeleton. The most common alterations in the spine include those of hyperparathyroidism (with bone resorption and, rarely, brown tumor formation), osteosclerosis, osteomalacia, and osteoporosis. They vary depending upon the duration and severity of the disease, the stress applied to bone, the anatomic site involved, and the geographic region in which the patient resides.[970]

Radiographic findings of HPT, uncommon in the spine in early chronic renal failure,[265] become evident with progression of disease and include resorption of bone and, rarely, the formation of visible brown tumors. Bone resorption develops in subchondral, subperiosteal, trabecular, intracortical, and endosteal locations[1013] and is altered by mechanical stress.[1057] Normally, the subchondral zone beneath the cartilaginous plate is reinforced by numerous trabeculae. With HPT there is resorption of trabeculae in this zone[1024] and replacement of well-mineralized lamellar bone with poorly mineralized woven bone and fibrous tissue (osteitis fibrosa).[1057] There may be focal resorption of the cartilaginous end-plate.[621] These resorptive alterations lead to weakening of subchondral bone and diminished resistance to normal stresses imposed by the intervertebral disc. The cartilage end-plate may collapse owing to the pressure of the intervertebral disc, and both disc and cartilage plate may protrude into the vertebral body as Schmorl's nodes.[1024, 1129a] Vertebrae may demonstrate mild central depression ("H"

shape), with chronic renal failure and HPT after dialysis has been instituted[1384] (Fig. 4–186). The broad central depression in the region of the end-plate may or may not be associated with poorly defined bony margins. The peripheral cortical rim is spared. Subchondral resorption in the sacroiliac joints may cause bilateral joint widening with indistinct articular margins (Fig. 4–187).

Subperiosteal resorption of bone is not as readily identified in the spine as it is in, say, the hands. It occurs in the anterior aspect of the vertebral body and has been demonstrated on histologic specimens.[1024] Rarely, the pedicles of C5 to C7 may be resorbed, as these are the sites of flexion as well as mechanical pressure in the adult.[468] Trabecular, intracortical, and endosteal resorption of bone, easily recognized on hand radiographs of patients with HPT,[842] are more difficult to identify in vertebrae. Overlying densities and the thin nature of these bony structures limit evaluation for fine detail. However, cortical bone may appear thin as a result of endosteal and intracortical resorption by osteoclastic activity.[1057] This increases the cancellous (trabecular) bone space. Trabeculae may undergo resorption, which, when pronounced, leads to the appearance of osteopenia. Cortical and trabecular margins may appear poorly defined ow-

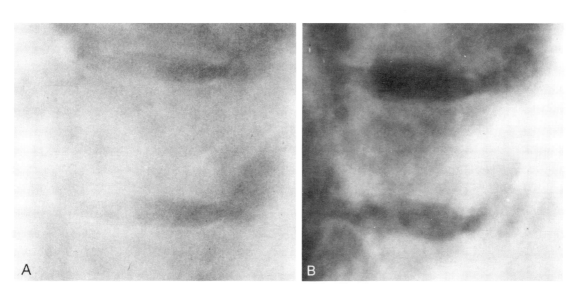

Figure 4–186. Patient with chronic renal failure. *A,* Predialysis. There is mild osteosclerosis. The vertebral margins, although not as well defined as normal, are still sharply but thinly outlined. *B,* Three years after renal dialysis was initiated. There is a central depression deformity ("H" vertebra). The margins of the floor of the central depression are poorly defined. Diffuse osteosclerosis is evident.

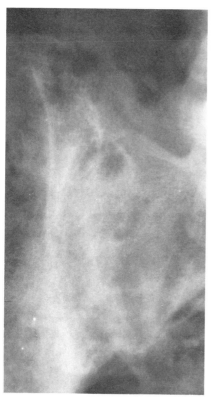

Figure 4–187. Hyperparathyroidism with widening of the sacroiliac joint(s). The margins are poorly defined owing to subchondral bone resorption.

teopathy.[1383] In uremic osteopathy, osteosclerosis may be diffuse in all bones (Fig. 4–188), appear patchy, or occur as bandlike densities of variable height in the subchondral zone, forming the so-called rugger jersey spine (see Fig. 4–68). Osteosclerosis is rare in primary HPT.[701] It has been observed in the subchondral zones of vertebrae in children[752] and adults.[11, 313, 368, 1257] Diffuse and patchy sclerosis of vertebrae, including sclerosis of posterior elements, has also been reported.[217, 453, 701, 1257] In primary HPT, osteosclerosis may regress following parathyroidectomy.[368, 701]

Osteosclerosis represents accumulation of poorly mineralized osteoid.[1028] Although each unit of osteoid is mineral deficient, the increased volume of osteoid accounts for the osteosclerosis. The etiology of osteosclerosis in primary and secondary HPT is not certain. Parathyroid hormone in small doses can stimulate osteoblastic response.[1149] Thyroid calcitonin inhibits bone resorption, which may cause bone sclerosis.[701] Another reason for osteosclerosis has been proposed. Normal increased blood supply to the subchondral region allows deposition of increased amounts of osteoid, which is more resistant to the action of parathyroid hormone than

ing to the resorptive process, although this too may be difficult to appreciate on the radiograph. Osteosclerosis may mask trabecular resorption.

Brown tumor is a rounded collection of fibrous tissue and giant cells and is more commonly a product of primary HPT, although it may be seen in patients with secondary HPT. Brown tumors are more readily apparent radiographically in the appendicular skeleton and are rarely observed in the axial skeleton. They appear as well-defined, rounded lesions that may cause bone "expansion." They may present with vertebral body and pedicle destruction and appear aggressive, simulating malignancy.[1159, 1241] Expanding brown tumors may extend into the paravertebral space and spinal canal and cause spinal cord compression.[1241] Rarely, presentation with neurologic symptoms may be the initial clinical evidence of primary HPT.[1159, 1241]

Osteosclerosis in the spine is a common feature of uremic osteopathy and secondary HPT.[701] The spine is the most common site of osteosclerosis in patients with renal os-

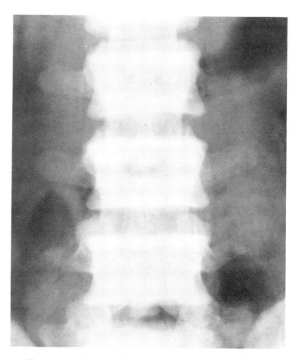

Figure 4–188. Renal osteopathy. There is diffuse osteosclerosis of the axial skeleton.

is the bone in the midvertebral body.[1157] Thus, trabeculae in the central part of the vertebra are resorbed, and osteoid in the subchondral zone is not. The bandlike radiodensities may be due to mechanical compression of trabeculae in the subchondral region or healing of the alterations caused by HPT or both.[1024] It should be noted that evidence of osteosclerosis, osteitis fibrosa cystica, and osteomalacia may be present histologically in patients with renal osteopathy, yet the radiographic examination may be normal.[270] Osteomalacia may be present histologically in 10% to 20% of patients with uremic osteopathy, yet only a small percentage demonstrate osteopenia.[322, 1157] In uremic osteopathy associated with osteomalacia, large amounts of osteoid are deposited in the subchondral areas and may be noted on the radiograph.[968] Osteosclerosis develops with thick trabecular density within cancellous bone.[1057, 1324]

Osteopenia may be seen both in primary HPT and in patients with uremic osteopathy. Generalized osteopenia can be observed in 85% of infants[331] and 17%[453] to 61% of adults[1049] with primary HPT, and the alterations are usually mild or moderate. It is often difficult to detect osteopenia in the axial skeleton because 25% to 50% of mineral loss must occur before osteopenia can be identified radiographically.[454] The recognition of osteopenia is a subjective observation, altered by technical factors. Osteopenia detected in patients over 50 years of age with primary HPT may be caused by senile or postmenopausal osteopenia. It may be due to the diminution of bone mass caused by resorption of cortex and trabeculae as well as to the presence of osteitis fibrosa cystica. In uremic osteopathy and secondary HPT, osteomalacia, although an uncommon finding, may also contribute to osteopenia. Osteomalacia in patients with chronic renal failure may be caused by the failure of the kidney to hydroxylate 25-hydroxycholecalciferol to 1,25-dehydroxycholecalciferol— the metabolite that regulates intestinal transport and absorption of calcium.[1157] Radiographically, the spine demonstrates an overall decrease in density as well as a decrease in size and number of trabeculae. Biconcavity of vertebrae may be seen in both osteomalacia and osteoporosis. Radiographic changes do not correlate with the degree of osteomalacia in patients with uremic osteopathy and HPT.[270]

In HPT, there is preferential resorption of trabeculae in the center of the vertebral body,[1057] and there is replacement with poorly mineralized fibrous bone. This puts greater stress on the vertebral trabeculae above and below, which also undergo resorption. The vertical trabeculae, which are under enormous stress, may be deflected, allowing the vertebral body to collapse, even in the presence of osteosclerosis.[1057] Vertebral collapse may also be due to the presence of accompanying senile or postmenopausal osteoporosis and is a nonspecific radiographic observation that is not diagnostic of uremic osteopathy. In fact, osteoporosis is often masked by the vertebral osteosclerosis.

The radiographic features of uremic osteopathy may be altered following renal transplantation or in patients on hemodialysis—sometimes disappearing, sometimes progressing, or sometimes remaining unchanged. In the spine, 17% of patients with subchondral osteosclerosis prior to surgery demonstrate regression of sclerosis after renal transplantation, while 83% demonstrate an increase in density.[488] Osteosclerosis often increases in patients on hemodialysis.[322] Osteopenia (25%) and compression of vertebrae may also occur following surgery and may be due to steroid-induced osteoporosis.[488] Osteopenia may develop in patients on hemodialysis.[322] The H-shaped vertebra may be identified in patients on maintenance hemodialysis. A destructive spondyloarthropathy resembling infection has been noted in patients following long-term hemodialysis.[644a] It may be secondary to hydroxyapatite and calcium pyrophosphate crystal deposition.

Calcium pyrophosphate dihydrate crystal deposition disease (CPPD-CDD) is more common in primary HPT and is rarely observed in chronic renal failure and secondary HPT.[1013] Other radiographic features seen in patients with uremic osteopathy in the appendicular skeleton are not observed in the axial skeleton. These include periosteal reaction and soft tissue and vascular calcifications.

Hypoparathyroidism

Bone density and vertebral structures are normal in 57% of patients with hypoparathyroidism and in 22% of patients with pseudohypoparathyroidism.[131, 1224] Osteopenia or focal or diffuse osteosclerosis may occur.[131, 1224, 1254] Spinal ligaments may become calcified.[1254] A "bone within bone" appearance with dense lines paralleling vertebral end-plates may be seen.[1075] The etiology of this observation in hypoparathyroidism is unclear but may be related to seizures and repeated illness, administration of vitamin D and calcium, or variations of calcium and phosphorous levels that cause bone to be laid down irregularly.

Hyperthyroidism

Radiographic features in the spine are nonspecific and include findings of osteopenia, biconcavity of vertebrae, collapse of vertebral bodies, and kyphosis.[1237] Accentuated skeletal maturation occurs.[105, 1053] The neonate with hyperthyroidism may demonstrate lucent neurocentral synchondroses that are thinner than normal as well as minimal anterior vertebral notching.[105]

Hypothyroidism

The spine is abnormal in over 90% of infants and young children with cretinism.[370] Kyphosis develops from 6 months to 2.5 years of age without vertebral abnormalities. Inferior beaking deformity of T12, L1, or L2 vertebrae occurs subsequently within 6 months or more and may diminish or resolve within 2 to 7 years following therapy[370] (Fig. 4–189).

In patients with hypothyroidism, skeletal maturation is also delayed (Fig. 4–190). The delay in maturation is more difficult to appreciate in the spine than in the more metabolically active long bones, where alterations are more pronounced. Diminished vertebral height[856] and the delay in appearance or fusion of ring apophyses may give clues to delay in skeletal maturation. In addition to delay in skeletal maturation, 13% of adult cretins may demonstrate a localized anterior vertebral deformity in the thoracolumbar region. Diffuse osteopenia, widened intervertebral disc spaces, and atlantoaxial instability may also be noted.[112]

Hemochromatosis

Patients with hemochromatosis demonstrate calcification in the intervertebral disc

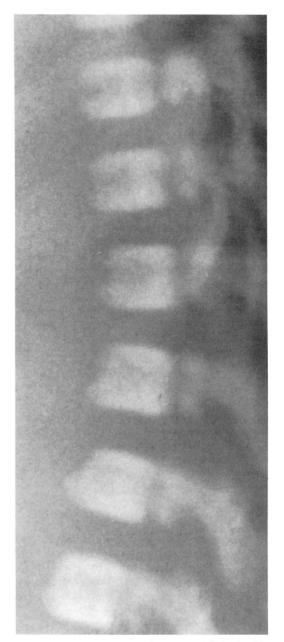

Figure 4–189. Cretinism. There is an inferior beaking deformity of the upper lumbar vertebrae.

in 15% of cases.[154] Calcification is more common in the periphery of the disc, although the nucleus pulposus occasionally calcifies as well. Calcification of the ligamentum flavum also occurs but is not easily visible on the radiograph. Discal and ligamentous calcifications in hemochromatosis are due to calcium pyrophosphate dihydrate crystal deposition disease.

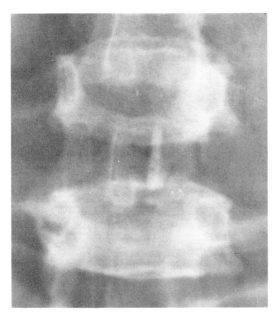

Figure 4–190. Cretinism. This adult with cretinism demonstrates underdevelopment of the vertebral body. The normal rectangular shape is not evident.

Homocystinuria

Homocystinuria is an inborn error of amino acid metabolism in which the conversion of homocystine to cystathionine is blocked owing to an absence or deficiency in the enzyme cystathionine synthase.[66, 1194] The disorder is characterized by ectopic lens (100%), mental retardation (about 75%), and skeletal abnormalities suggesting Marfan's syndrome (35%), such as kyphoscoliosis, arachnodactyly and other findings, and thrombosis of medium-sized arteries and veins.[66, 1194] However, generalized osteopenia occurs in about 40%[1194] to about 95%[879] of patients with homocystinuria with or without the features of Marfan's syndrome. Vertebral bodies demonstrate diffuse biconcavity (73%) and irregularity of vertebral endplates.[879, 766] In addition, patients with homocystinuria frequently have mental retardation (about 75%), another feature that is absent in Marfan's syndrome.[66, 1194]

Ochronosis

Alkaptonuria is a rare disorder in which homogentisic acid oxidase is absent. This leads to accumulation of homogentisic acid, which, when oxidized, forms a dark, pigmented substance (ochronosis).[1028]

Deposits of gentisic acid on intervertebral discs and ligaments lead to dystrophic calcification with hydroxyapatite crystal formation that usually begins in the third decade.[154, 705] The lumbar spine is the site of the earliest crystal deposits, although entire spinal involvement is frequent and characteristic. Calcification (hydroxyapatite crystals) is usually diffuse within discs (Fig. 4–191). Intervertebral osteochondrosis is commonly associated with ochronosis. Intervertebral disc narrowing, which may be severe, "vacuum" phenomenon, and subchondral sclerosis occur. Apophyseal joints are involved as well, with joint space narrowing, sclerosis, and even fusion.[705] Sacroiliac joints may demonstrate joint space narrowing, irregularity, subchondral cystlike defects, and sclerosis.

Spondylitis and Sacroiliitis

The plain radiograph is extremely helpful in the detection and diagnosis of inflammatory disorders of the spine and sacroiliac joints, although very early changes may not

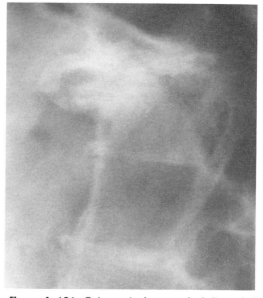

Figure 4–191. Ochronosis. Intervertebral disc calcification is noted at multiple levels. Degenerative changes of intervertebral osteochondrosis and osteophyte formation are present.

be apparent.[746, 747] The radiographic patterns and distribution of disease often aid in the differentiation of spondylitic disorders.

Ankylosing spondylitis and spondylitis associated with bowel disorders are almost always bilateral and symmetric in distribution in both the spine and sacroiliac joints. Unilateral or asymmetrically bilateral disease usually occurs in psoriatic spondylitis, Reiter's syndrome, juvenile rheumatoid arthritis, gout, and degenerative disorders. Psoriatic arthritis, Reiter's syndrome, and juvenile rheumatoid arthritis may also demonstrate bilateral symmetric involvement of the sacroiliac joints late in disease. Rarely, lupus[902] and familial Mediterranean fever[130, 727] present with bilateral sacroiliitis.

Anteroposterior and lateral spine radiographs are usually sufficient for the radiographic evaluation of spondyloarthropathies. Flexion views of C1–C2 may demonstrate subluxation not readily apparent in the neutral position. However, flexion radiographs should not be performed if neurologic signs or symptoms of cord compression are present. In evaluation of the sacroiliac joints, a cephalad-angled anteroposterior view is the best and simplest method.[249] Oblique views may help in problem cases but are not necessary for the initial evaluation.

The association between HLA-B27 antigen and spondylitic disorders is 90% to 100% in ankylosing spondylitis, around 90% in Reiter's syndrome, and 55% in psoriatic arthritis.[1137] This antigen is found in 12% of patients with DISH, in 4% to 8% of the normal white population, and in 1% to 2% of the normal black population. Sacroiliitis without spondylitis is a frequent feature of HLA-B27 arthritides.[1144] In patients with seronegative peripheral arthritis, 23% are HLA-B27 positive, compared with 7% of normal patients. Sacroiliitis is common (83%) in patients who are HLA-B27 positive and have peripheral arthritis, whereas it is less common (21%) in patients who are HLA-B27 negative.[1144]

Ankylosing Spondylitis

Ankylosing spondylitis (AS) is a chronic inflammatory disorder of unknown etiology. HLA-B27 antigen has been reported in 90% to 100% of cases;[1137] however, AS syndromes have rarely been noted in patients without HLA-B27 antigen.[625] Characteristic changes involving the spine and sacroiliac joints occur. Ankylosing spondylitis is usually considered a bilateral symmetric disease[1020] that classically begins in the sacroiliac joints[123, 294] and thoracolumbar or, less commonly, lumbosacral spine. Asymmetry, however, may occur.[1137] As AS progresses, the remainder of the thoracolumbar spine becomes involved, and disease "ascends" to involve the upper thoracic and cervical spines. This pattern is not invariable and may occur rapidly or slowly.[1020] Differences in distribution of disease and severity of syndromes exist between men and women.[123, 817, 1020] In women, the disease begins more often in the lumbar spine; onset is earlier; the clinical course is milder; extensive ankylosis rarely

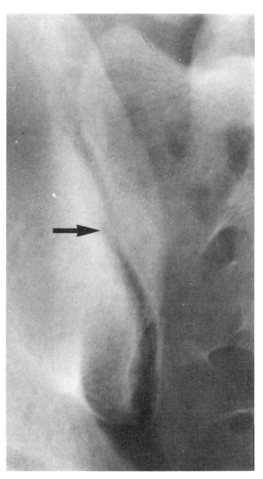

Figure 4–192. Ankylosing spondylitis. There is focal indistinctness of the sacroiliac joint (arrow) that represents early sacroiliitis.

occurs; radiographic changes are present in the peripheral joints; ligamentous calcification is less common; and there is more frequent symptomatic involvement.[817] Some authors feel that isolated cervical and sacroiliac disease, with sparing of the thoracic and lumbar spines, is found more frequently in women (about 30%);[1020] however, other authors disagree.[123] Although the radiographic features of AS are usually similar in both men and women,[1020] the radiographic changes in the sacroiliac joints may be less pronounced in women.[667]

The earliest radiographic features of AS are usually detected in the sacroiliac joints,[294] which are (almost) always involved.[728] Although very early changes of ankylosing spondylitis in sacroiliac joints may be unilateral (11.4%),[294, 1137] they are more likely to be bilateral when first discov-

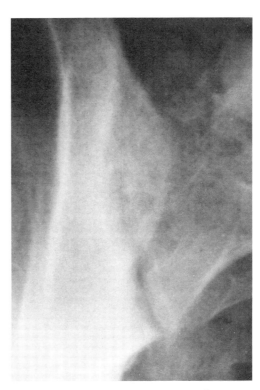

Figure 4–194. Ankylosing spondylitis. Further progression of sacroiliitis with joint space narrowing, marginal erosions, and mild sclerosis.

ered.[1014] Both the true joint and the ligamentous portion of the joint are affected.[1014] Early, there are focal areas of para-articular osteopenia that may be difficult to appreciate on the plain radiograph.[1028] The earliest detectable radiographic sign is usually indistinctness of the joint margin caused by early inflammatory erosions and focal osteopenia[747] (Fig. 4–192). Soon, joint margins become irregular owing to the continued inflammatory erosive process. This is more evident on the iliac side of the true joint, where the cartilage is thinner than on the sacral side.[1014] Progressive erosions may widen the joint, and reactive sclerosis develops in subchondral bone (Fig. 4–193). Eventually, the joint space may narrow (Fig. 4–194) or become partially or completely fused. Fusion is more characteristic of AS (Fig. 4–195). In the ligamentous portion of the joint, calcification and ossification of ligaments lead to complete ankylosis[1028] (see Fig. 4–195). Isolated sacroiliac abnormalities may occur early in disease but are uncommon in long-standing AS.[1020]

Spinal inflammation follows or occurs

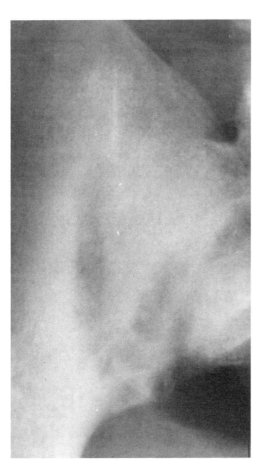

Figure 4–193. Ankylosing spondylitis. Widening of the sacroiliac joint is caused by erosions. The margins of the joint are poorly defined.

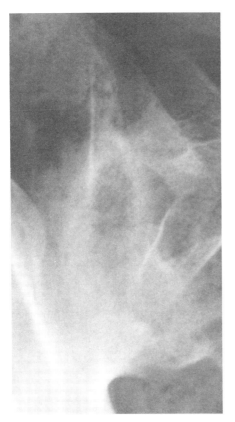

Figure 4–195. Ankylosing spondylitis. There is fusion of the sacroiliac joint, which in this patient was a bilateral process.

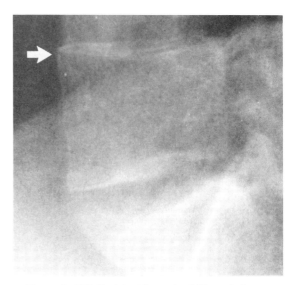

Figure 4–196. Vertebral "squaring." The anterior margin of the L5 vertebral body has a square configuration due to inflammatory change at the anterior corners of the vertebral body. This patient has ankylosing spondylitis, but similar findings can be seen in psoriatic spondylitis and Reiter's syndrome. (From Kricun ME: Radiographic approach to the arthritides. In Katz W (ed): Diagnosis and Management of Rheumatoid Disorders. Philadelphia: J. B. Lippincott Company, 1987.)

concomitantly with sacroiliac disease. The thoracolumbar and lumbosacral regions are affected initially. However, the early changes of ankylosing spondylitis are difficult to appreciate radiographically in the thoracolumbar area[746] from T10 to L2.[294] Inflammation at the anterosuperior and anteroinferior vertebral margins cause obliteration of the margins with erosions of these zones. This leads to a "square" appearance[1014] of the normally concave vertebral contour in about 40% of cases[1137] (Fig. 4–196). With healing, reactive sclerosis at these anterior vertebral margins causes the "shining corners" to appear. Inflammation in this zone also produces calcification and, later, ossification of the outer fibers of the annulus fibrosus. These are called syndesmophytes—the hallmark of inflammatory spondylitis (Figs. 4–197 and 4–198). They appear first around T10–L2.[294] In ankylosing spondylitis, they are thin, typically bilateral and symmetric, and extend vertically from

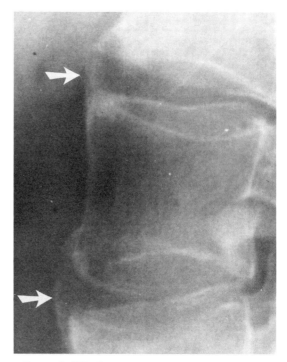

Figure 4–197. Syndesmophytes. There is calcification in the preannular tissues that represents a syndesmophyte (arrows) in this patient with ankylosing spondylitis.

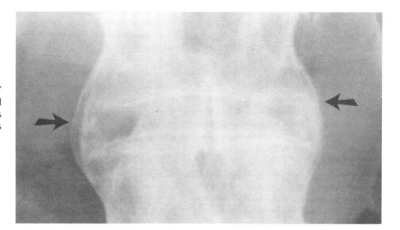

Figure 4–198. "Bamboo spine." Ankylosing spondylitis. Marginal symmetric bilateral syndesmophytes bridge the lateral vertebral margins (arrows).

near the margin of one vertebral body to the next. Eventually, when diffuse, they form the so-called bamboo spine[1014] (see Fig. 4–198). Erosions may be observed in the costovertebral articulations. Spinal involvement without sacroiliac joint disease is extremely rare and occurs in 1% of patients with AS.[946, 1020]

Early erosions of apophyseal joints from inflammation are difficult to detect[249] except in the cervical spine. With progression, there is joint space narrowing, sclerosis, and eventually ankylosis, which is easily detected and occurs in about 30% of cases[1137] (Fig. 4–199). Calcification and ossification of the apophyseal joint capsules (see Fig. 4–93) and calcification of interspinous and supraspinous ligaments are readily visible (Fig. 4–200).

Disc calcification (Fig. 4–201), spinal fractures (Fig. 4–202), pseudarthrosis (Fig. 4–203), and cranial settling are other associated, less frequent features of ankylosing spondylitis.[452, 518, 600, 794, 941, 1318] Fractures of the spine occur in 12% of patients with AS, but the injury is often insignificant.[1318] However, neurologic symptoms occur in 15% of cases, and the mortality rate from trauma is 2.8%. Fractures may be difficult to diagnose radiographically. In the cervical spine they usually occur through an ossified disc or adjacent to the cartilage end-plate and extend posteriorly through the posterior elements.[452] In the thoracolumbar spine, fractures occur most commonly at the

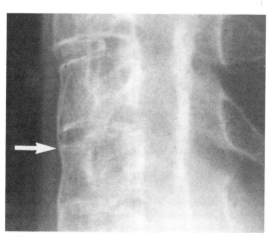

Figure 4–199. Ankylosing spondylitis. Cervical spine. There is fusion of all apophyseal joints. In addition, thin calcification of the anterior longitudinal ligament is noted (arrow).

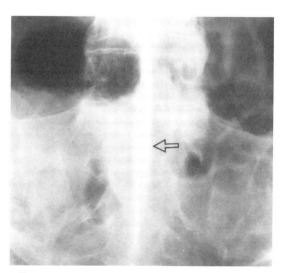

Figure 4–200. Ankylosing spondylitis. There is bilateral fusion of the sacroiliac joints and marginal syndesmophyte formation in the lumbar spine. In addition, the posterior spinous ligaments are calcified (arrow).

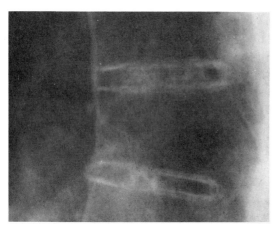

Figure 4–201. Ankylosing spondylitis. Calcification is noted within intervertebral discs. The anterior longitudinal ligament is calcified.

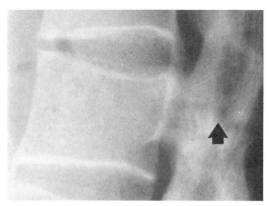

Figure 4–203. Akylosing spondylitis. A fracture with pseudoarthrosis formation is noted in the posterior elements (arrow).

thoracolumbar junction. They develop through the intervertebral disc but may occur through the vertebral body adjacent to the vertebral end-plate. Stress fractures appear to begin in the posterior elements and extend into the verteral body at a later time as pseudarthrosis develops.[452]

Alterations may develop in the atlantoaxial region, with erosions of the odontoid process and atlantoaxial subluxation.[794, 1318] These changes are not as common as in patients with rheumatoid arthritis. Odontoid erosions and sclerosis and occasionally fusion of the odontoid process to the anterior atlas or basion may be observed.[794] Cranial settling may develop.

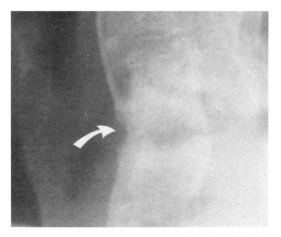

Figure 4–202. Ankylosing spondylitis. Cervical spine. There is a fracture through the intervertebral disc and calcified anterior longitudinal ligament (arrow). Focal kyphosis is noted.

More severe erosive and destructive changes at vertebral end-plates have been described in AS.[296, 941, 1143, 1318] These alterations may be due to the inflammatory process itself[296, 1338] or more probably to microfractures, particularly when the abnormalities extend through the intervertebral disc and posterior elements.[296, 452, 941, 1318] They represent changes of pseudarthrosis resulting from increased motion at the fracture site. Radiographically, there may be irregularity, bone fragmentation, and sclerosis.[452, 941] These discovertebral alterations occur in 28% of patients with AS.[294] They may be so pronounced that they may mimic infection.[941, 1338]

Dural ectasia (diverticula, cysts), with compression of the cauda equina and erosion of the posterior vertebral body and vertebral arch, can complicate AS.[151, 532, 1078] Rheumatoid arthritis coexisting with AS has been reported.[778]

Erosive Spondylopathy

It is known that patients with ankylosing spondylitis may in the course of disease develop erosions, destruction, and sclerosis of end-plates[1338] (Fig. 4–204). However, some patients may develop similar radiographic findings as an early and even initial radiographic sign of ankylosing spondylitis.[624] In one series of nine patients, seven were HLA-B27 antigen positive and in 2 to 4 years developed radiographic features of sacroiliitis, vertebral squaring, and arthritis of the apophyseal joints compatible with ankylosing spondylitis.[624] In another series of seven

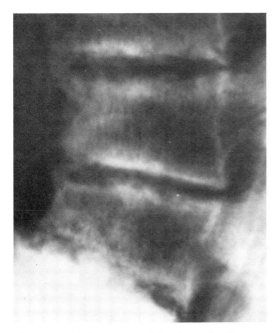

Figure 4–204. Erosive spondyloarthropathy. There are erosions of vertebral margins, with mild subchondral sclerosis.

cases, similar erosive and destructive findings were observed in the spine. Only one patient was HLA-B27 antigen positive, and two patients did not develop sacroiliitis or other radiographic features of ankylosing spondylitis even 5 and 7 years after initial symptoms occurred.[373a] Nevertheless, erosive spondylopathy in most instances is probably an early or initial manifestation of ankylosing spondylitis.[624]

Juvenile Ankylosing Spondylitis

Ankylosing spondylitis occurring in patients whose symptoms begin in the second decade (usually at about 12 years of age) may be classified as juvenile ankylosing spondylitis.[675b] Males are affected more commonly than females, and presenting symptoms are usually related to peripheral joints. The radiographic features in the axial skeleton are similar to those of ankylosing spondylitis. Sacroiliitis is unilateral[702] or bilateral and occasionally asymmetric early in disease but symmetric in advanced cases.[675b] Early, indistinct margins of the sacroiliac joints may be difficult to appreciate in this age group since sacroiliac joint margins are normally indistinct in the growing child and

adolescent owing to the lack of full development of the subchondral cortical layer.[702, 747] Also, joint widening due to erosions occurs early. This is followed by joint narrowing and eventually ankylosis. Spinal abnormalities occur in about 70% of cases.[675b] Sclerosis of anterior vertebral margins ("shining corners"), vertebral squaring, syndesmophytes, and apophyseal joint fusion may be evident. Atlantoaxial subluxation may occur and rarely may be the initial presenting manifestation of this disorder.[1263] Atlanto-occipital fusion is rare.[675b] Spinal abnormalities progress from the lumbar spine upward. Paravertebral subligamentous calcification is the last radiographic feature to develop.[702]

Psoriatic Arthritis

Approximately 25%[668] to 50%[528] of patients with psoriatic arthritis develop disease in the spine and sacroiliac joints, and 90% of these have severe generalized psoriasis and peripheral arthritis.[668] Sacroiliitis is the most common manifestation of psoriasis in the axial skeleton and is usually bilateral and symmetric in 62% of patients,[668] particularly late in disease. Bilateral asymmetric sacroiliitis occurs in about 5% to 10%.[249, 668] Sacroiliitis may occur without spondylitis, but spondylitis without sacroiliitis is unusual.[528, 668] The severity of sacroiliitis is unrelated to the severity of spondylitis.

The sacroiliac joints are involved in about 40% of cases.[728] The principles of inflammatory arthritis are manifested in the sacroiliac joints, although they are not as marked as with ankylosing spondylitis. These include erosions and initial widening of the joint space and reactive sclerosis. Destruction and narrowing of the sacroiliac joints may be followed by bony ankylosis. Both the true joint and the ligamentous portion of the joint are affected. Osseous fusion occurs in the ligamentous portion of the joint but less commonly than in ankylosing spondylitis.[1014, 1028] Asymptomatic sacroiliac alterations may be the only musculoskeletal evidence in 8% of patients with severe psoriasis.[528]

Alterations of psoriatic spondylitis, on the other hand, are almost always asymmetric in distribution. Early, there is paravertebral calcification or ossification in the form of syndesmophytes extending from one vertebra to the next[668] (Fig. 4–205). They are best visualized on the AP radiograph and may form rapidly. Syndesmophytes are most common in the lower cervical spine and in the lower thoracic, thoracolumbar, and upper lumbar spines. These ossifications arise paravertebrally and appear coarse and broad. They are unilateral or bilateral and asymmetric in appearance and may bridge adjacent vertebrae. "Squaring" of vertebrae occurs at any level but is more common in the thoracic spine in up to one third of the cases.[668] In the cervical spine, inflammatory changes may develop in the apophyseal joints (Fig. 4–206). Fusion of these joints occurs in 20% of patients and is not as common as with ankylosing spondylitis.[668] Thin or fluffy calcification of the anterior longitudinal ligament occurs occasionally (see Fig. 4–206). The atlantoaxial articulation may be involved. Atlantoaxial subluxation and sclerosis as well as erosion of the odontoid process and arch of the atlas occur in around 45% of cases. Fusion of the atlas with the axis has been reported.[321] Subaxial cervical subluxation may develop and become associated with cord compression.[374]

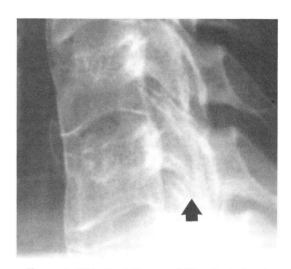

Figure 4–206. Psoriatic spondylitis. Cervical spine. There is thin calcification of the anterior longitudinal ligament and very mild indistinctness of apophyseal joints (arrow) caused by the inflammatory process.

Reiter's Syndrome

Radiographic changes in the spine and sacroiliac joints in patients with Reiter's syndrome are similar to those found in patients with psoriatic arthritis. However, changes of spondylitis are not common in Reiter's syndrome.[668, 1171] Reiter's syndrome usually affects young adult males more frequently. Sacroiliitis is common, occurring in about 36%[728] to 42% of patients.[1171] In the sacroiliac joints, unilateral or, more commonly, bilateral asymmetric disease[879, 1110] allows differentiation from ankylosing spondylitis, although bilateral symmetric changes may also occur.[796] Early, erosions and joint space widening are later followed by sclerosis and joint space narrowing. Ankylosis is less common than in ankylosing spondylitis.[1014] In the spine, asymmetric vertical unifocal or multifocal paravertebral ossifications bridge adjacent vertebrae. They are usually thick and bulky, resembling those of psoriatic spondylitis. They usually arise laterally or posterolaterally to the vertebra.[796] The anterior surface is usually spared. Lower thoracic and upper lumbar vertebrae are more commonly affected. The cervical spine is infrequently involved and may demonstrate inflammatory changes in apophyseal joints as well as atlantoaxial subluxation.[715]

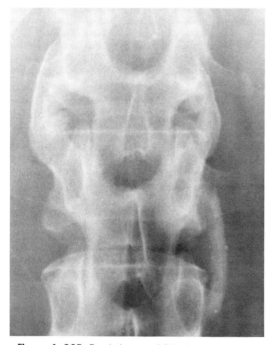

Figure 4–205. Psoriatic spondylitis. Large asymmetric paravertebral ossifications (syndesmophytes) are noted.

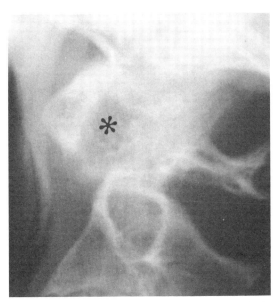

Figure 4–207. Rheumatoid arthritis. Atlantoaxial subluxation. There is widening of the space between the odontoid process and the anterior arch of the atlas (asterisk).

Rheumatoid Arthritis

Rheumatoid arthritis (RA) is a highly inflammatory disease that frequently involves the cervical spine, particularly the upper portion, and it is uncommon in the thoracic and lumbar spines and sacroiliac joints. Rheumatoid arthritis commonly involves the occipito-atlantoaxial joints.[795] It should be recalled that there are six synovial joints in the occipito-atlantoaxial region: the occipitoatlantal, atlantoaxial, the joint between the odontoid process and the anterior arch of the atlas, and the joint between the odontoid process and the transverse ligament.[795] The most common radiographic changes in the cervical spine center on the C1–C2 articulation, as approximately 45% to 85% of patients develop some form of subluxation[750] (Fig. 4–207). Anterior atlantoaxial subluxation is the most common radiographic spinal alteration in RA and may be as severe as 15 mm.[750, 795, 955] It occurs in about 35% of patients with RA and is usually due to laxity or rupture of the transverse ligament caused by the rheumatoid process. When severe, it may be associated with cervical myelopathy and compression of the vertebral artery.[638, 750] However, with erosions of the odontoid process, an apparent "subluxation" may not indicate abnormalities of the transverse ligament.[795] It is conceivable that the reduced diameter of the odontoid process resulting from erosions may cause it to fit loosely in the confines of the anterior atlas and transverse ligament, accounting for atlanto-odontoid instability.[794] However, when subluxation is severe, rupture of the ligaments can be postulated, particularly when subluxation is at least 10 mm to 12 mm.[750] Compression of the upper cervical cord may occur with atlantoaxial subluxation greater than 9 mm or when there is associated cranial settling.[1322] Lateral subluxation of C1 on C2 is associated with anterior subluxation in about 20% of cases. Posterior atlantoaxial subluxation is uncommon. For this to develop, there has to be a defect in the anterior arch of the atlas or erosion or fracture of the odontoid process or superior and posterior movement of the atlas, acting alone or in combination.[751]

Erosions about the odontoid process occur in 14% of cases but are not easily detected on the radiograph[795] (Fig. 4–208). They may be absent even when atlantoaxial subluxation exceeds 5 mm, but they are usually visible when the measurement is greater

Figure 4–208. Rheumatoid arthritis. There are erosions about the odontoid process (arrow).

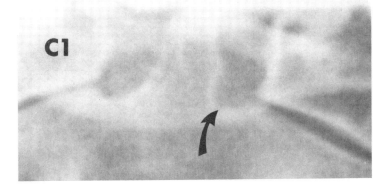

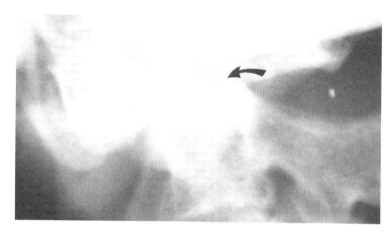

Figure 4–209. Rheumatoid arthritis. There is resorption of the odontoid process (arrow) and marked atlantoaxial subluxation. The axis has moved cephalad.

than 8 mm. Erosions usually occur anteriorly and posteriorly owing to the close relationship with surrounding synovium. The rheumatoid process may be extensive and severely erode the odontoid process, sometimes leading to complete resorption[795] (Fig. 4–209) or separation,[464] and pathologic fracture of the odontoid process has been reported.[795]

Occipitocervical abnormalities occur in about 20% of cases.[795] There may be upward movement of the odontoid process on C1, sometimes with the odontoid protruding into the foramen magnum.[346, 794, 795, 1008] The body of C2 may even reside in the ring of C1 (Fig. 4–210) owing to destruction and collapse of the occipitoatlantal and atlantoaxial articulations, particularly the lateral masses of C1. Ligamentous disruption occurs as well.[346] Less commonly, there are erosions of occipital condyles and superior processes of C2 caused by pannus from the inflamed synovium. Destruction of the occipito-atlantoaxial complex allows the skull to settle lower on the cervical spine. Consequently, the odontoid process projects above the foramen magnum. This is termed more appropriately cranial settling by some,[346] and others call it upward migration of the dens, atlantoaxial impaction,[1007] or pseudobasilar invagination.[794] Five per cent to 8% of patients with RA develop cranial settling, which, although it is life threatening, rarely causes death.[346] Severe neurologic problems may ensue, owing to the odontoid's impinging on the medulla and the vertebral arteries' becoming occluded between the odontoid process and the foramen magnum.[638] Cranial settling[346] should be differentiated from basilar invagination, which is defined as invag-

ination or upturning of the foramen magnum associated with upward movement of the spine[570, 795] and which does not occur in RA. Lateral, inferior, and, rarely, posterior subluxation of C1–C2 articulations may develop.[527, 1288] Superior migration of the odontoid process and subaxial subluxation associated with fusion of the lateral atlantoaxial articulations have been noted.[795]

It is often difficult to evaluate the degree of cranial settling, as superimposition of the mastoids and other bony structures as well as resorption of the odontoid process itself occurs. A variation of McGregor's line[827] may aid in this evaluation, obviating the need to visualize the tip of the odontoid process.[1007] This is performed by measuring the distance

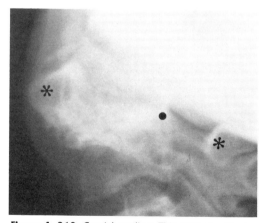

Figure 4–210. Cranial settling. This patient with rheumatoid arthritis demonstrates upward migration of the axis (dot) into the ring of the atlas (asterisks). It is difficult to evaluate the odontoid, which appears at least partly resorbed. Marked atlantoaxial subluxation is noted with the atlas displaced forward.

from the inferior end-plate of C2 to Mc-Gregor's line (Fig. 4–211). This distance is normally 34 mm or more in men and 29 mm or more in women. A value below these limits indicates cranial settling.

It should be recalled that patients with rheumatoid arthritis may have a normal C1–C2 measurement on the lateral radiograph in the neutral position and that subluxation can be elicited with the neck in flexion.[795] Even advanced subluxation may not be appreciated unless flexion views are obtained. Therefore, care must be taken when a rheumatoid patient with possible neurologic symptoms is to be positioned for the radiograph—thus avoiding additional neurologic compromise. Sclerosis of the odontoid process is an infrequent observation.[794]

Rheumatoid arthritis also involves the cervical spine below the level of C2 but less frequently. Apophyseal joints demonstrate erosions, joint narrowing, and eventually fusion[955] (Fig. 4–212). Subluxation, which occurs in about 10% of patients with RA,[795] often develops at multiple levels, sometimes forming a "step-ladder" appearance[794, 939] (Fig. 4–213). Subluxations are usually anterior and involve the C3–C5 levels most often.[939] Rarely, subaxial caudal dislocation and partial vertebral destruction of C3 can be seen in cases of severe RA.[1006] Ligamen-

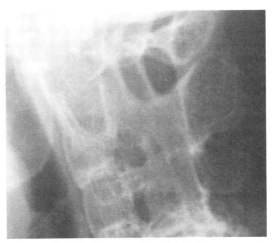

Figure 4–212. Rheumatoid arthritis. There are advanced changes of inflammatory disease in the cervical spine, with fusion of apophyseal joints. Intervertebral discs are diminished in height.

tous ossification is not a feature of rheumatoid arthritis, although inflammation of posterior spinal elements can erode the spinous processes[795, 939] (Fig. 4–214). Osteopenia is common, and patients with RA are at a greater risk for vertebral fractures.[587] Sometimes, disc narrowing associated with irregularity of subchondral margins can be observed (Fig. 4–215).

Although about 80% of patients with rheumatoid involvement of the spine demonstrate radiographic progression of disease, only about 35% demonstrate progressive neurologic abnormalities.[955]

The thoracic and lumbar spines are infrequently involved and may demonstrate apophyseal joint erosions, discovertebral changes similar to those in the cervical spine, subluxation, and vertebral collapse.[562] Involvement of costovertebral articulations may be noted, and the rheumatoid process may extend to the intervertebral disc.[562] Sacroiliac joint involvement is not an early or frequent feature of rheumatoid arthritis. Alterations are mild with unilateral or bilateral asymmetric changes. Erosions develop, but ankylosis rarely occurs.[1028] Rarely, rheumatoid cysts may cause spinal cord or cauda equina compression.[748a]

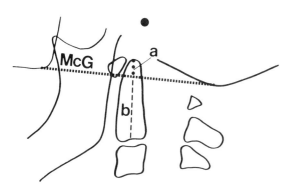

Figure 4–211. Measurement for cranial settling. The normal measurement for **b** is 34 mm in men and 29 mm in women. A measurement lower than these values is considered cranial settling. Key: **McG** = McGregor's line; **a** = distance between the apex of the odontoid process and McGregor's line; **b** = distance between the lower end plate of C2 and McGregor's line. (From Redlund-Johnell I, Pettersson H: Radiographic measurements of the cranio-vertebral region: designed for evaluation of abnormalities in rheumatoid arthritis. Acta Radiol [Diagn] 25:23–28, 1984.)

Juvenile Rheumatoid Arthritis

Like rheumatoid arthritis, juvenile rheumatoid arthritis (JRA) frequently involves

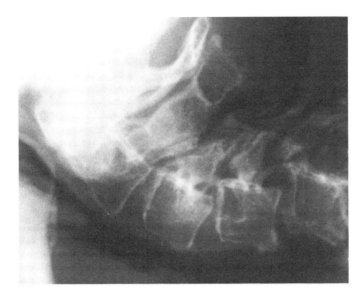

Figure 4–213. Rheumatoid arthritis with subaxial subluxations. This patient has severe kyphosis (not seen). There is subluxation of all subaxial vertebrae, forming the "step ladder" configuration.

the upper portion of the cervical spine. Symptoms of cervical spondylitis may precede symptoms in peripheral joints. Atlantoaxial subluxation, subaxial subluxation at other cervical levels (particularly C2–C4), and inflammatory changes of apophyseal joints, such as erosions, joint narrowing, and frequently fusion, are prominent features of JRA[425, 556, 797, 1165] (Figs. 4–216 and 4–217). Ankylosis of the apophyseal joints predominates in the upper half of the cervical spine, particularly at the C2–C3 level.[797] Similar changes in the lower cervical spine do not occur without ankylosis of upper cervical joints. The thoracic and lumbar spines are infrequently involved. Alterations in vertebral body growth may occur at levels where apophyseal joints have fused.[797] Both vertebral bodies and discs are reduced in height. Osteopenia and vertebral collapse may be evident because of corticosteroid therapy.[32, 797] Occasionally, lucent bands in the subchondral regions are noted; they indicate growth arrest.[797]

Ligament calcification and syndesmophytes are not features of this disorder. How-

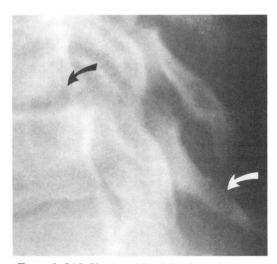

Figure 4–214. Rheumatoid arthritis. Note the resorption of the spinous processes (white arrow) and the erosion of the vertebral margin (black arrow).

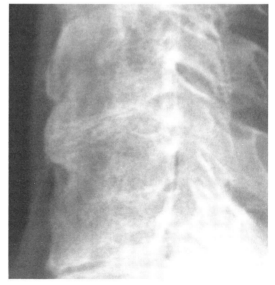

Figure 4–215. Rheumatoid arthritis with interbody fusion of the cervical spine at multiple levels.

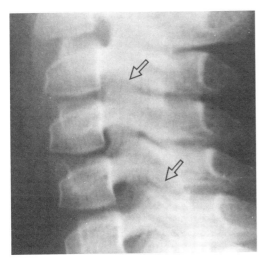

Figure 4–216. Juvenile rheumatoid arthritis. Note the indistinctness and narrowing of the apophyseal joints (arrows) of the cervical spine.

ever, focal soft tissue calcification adjacent to the anterior ring of C1 has been noted.[556] The association of JRA with disorders of laxity of ligaments, such as trisomy 21 (Down's) syndrome, may cause serious cervical instability.[1165]

Inflammatory changes of sacroiliac joints, with or without cervical spondylitis, are

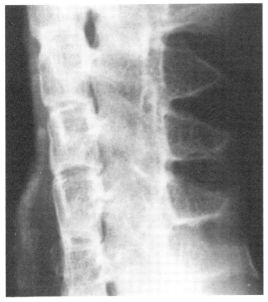

Figure 4–217. Juvenile rheumatoid arthritis. Advanced changes in the cervical spine, with fusion of apophyseal joints and diminished growth of vertebral bodies, which appear narrow in the anteroposterior diameter. Intervertebral discs are also diminished in height.

infrequent.[797] They include erosions, early joint widening, joint space narrowing, and eventually fusion. Involvement may be unilateral or bilateral and is either asymmetric or symmetric, with symmetric involvement usually occurring late in the course of disease. Care must be taken not to base the diagnoses of early juvenile rheumatoid arthritis solely on the appearance of the sacroiliac joints, since slight widening of the joints and irregularity and indistinctness of joint margins may be normal in growing children and teenagers.[32, 702, 747]

In adults with Still's disease, the cervical spine is involved, although the involvement is less extensive than it is in children.[152] Fusion of several apophyseal joints, disc narrowing, and disc calcification may be noted. The sacroiliac joints are usually spared.

Intestinal Spondylitis

Patients with ulcerative colitis and Crohn's disease develop sacroiliitis with or without spondylitis usually following or during the onset of bowel disease.[153, 206, 883] However, spondylitis may precede symptoms of colitis by a number of years.[206, 875] Spondylitis has rarely been diagnosed in Whipple's disease.[169, 875, 989] However, others feel that a number of cases previously reported to have both Whipple's disease and "spondylitis" may not have had a true spondylitis.[116] Many cases had clinical symptoms but were HLA-B27 negative and did not demonstrate radiographic abnormalities.

Four percent to 22% of patients with ulcerative colitis and around 10% of patients with Crohn's disease develop arthritic symptoms.[153, 206, 883, 1386] Although some feel that patients may demonstrate a flare-up of arthritic symptoms with a flare-up of bowel disease that may occur in 25% of patients,[825] others do not.[875] Also, there seems to be no relationship between the development of sacroiliitis and the region of bowel involvement or the occurrence of fistulae.[875]

The axial skeleton is the most frequent anatomic site of radiographically evident findings in colitic arthritis.[206] The radiographic features may resemble those of ankylosing spondylitis, demonstrating symmetric distribution in the sacroiliac joints and spine (Fig. 4–218). Bilateral symmetric ease develop spondylitis.[883] Alterations of spondylitis are most common at the thoracolumbar junction[1386] and upper lumbar spine, although the entire lumbar spine may be involved. Radiographically, there are thin vertical syndesmophytes that eventually lead to the so-called bamboo spine.[206] Apophyseal joint alterations consisting of erosions, joint narrowing, and fusion may occur. Inflammatory erosions may be noted at the costovertebral articulations (Fig. 4–219). The cervical spine is involved infrequently.[1386]

The etiology of the association of spondylitis and sacroiliitis with intestinal disorders is unclear, although it may be caused by low-grade infection from bowel or urinary tract reaching the musculoskeletal structures via venous plexuses.[946, 1225, 1386] However, the fact that spondylitis may precede bowel disease by years may detract from this theory.[883, 1386] Genetic factors have also been implicated.[875]

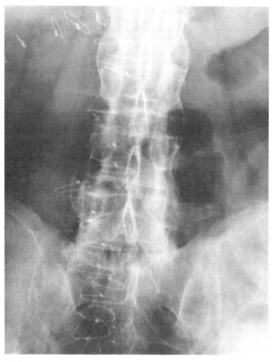

Figure 4–218. Colitic spondylitis and sacroiliitis. Symmetric marginal syndesmophytes are noted at multiple levels, and there is bilateral fusion of sacroiliac joints. This patient has Crohn's disease.

sacroiliitis is the most common osseous radiographic observation, occurring in 83% of patients with colitis. There are erosions, early joint space widening, sclerosis, joint space narrowing, and eventually ankylosis.

Spondylitis, which is usually bilateral and symmetric, occurs in about 11% of patients with colitis and clinically evident arthritis.[206] Only 3% of patients with Crohn's dis-

Gout

Gout is a crystal deposition disorder in which the affecting crystal is monosodium urate. The cervical spine is affected most often,[512] although gout rarely involves the spine. Tophi cause erosions of adjacent bone, and overhanging edges, which are characteristic of gout elsewhere, may be present. Involvement of posterior elements, erosion of vertebral margins, vertebral collapse (rare),[703] and narrowing of the intervertebral discs may occur[148, 512, 740] (Fig. 4–220). Gout rarely may involve the atlas or

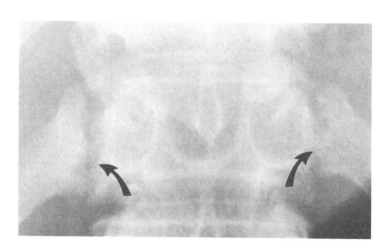

Figure 4–219. Costovertebral erosions (arrows) in a patient with ulcerative colitis.

CONVENTIONAL RADIOGRAPHY • 199

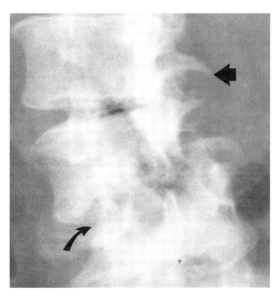

Figure 4–220. Gout. There is marked destruction of the L4–L5 intervertebral disc (curved arrow), with subluxation of L4 laterally to the right. Large bizarre-shaped bony protrusions (straight arrow) resembling overhanging edges of gout are present. Degenerative changes at the L3–L4 disc are also noted.

odontoid process, leading to atlantoaxial subluxation.[148, 1290]

The sacroiliac joints are involved in 7.3%[779] to 17% of cases with advanced disease.[13] Subchondral cystlike defects, with sclerotic margins, irregularity of articular surfaces (particularly of the lower third of the joint), and sclerosis may be present.[13, 779] Distribution is usually unilateral[13, 623] but may be bilateral and asymmetric. Fusion of the sacroiliac joint is rare in gout.[13]

Neuropathic Spinal Arthropathy

Neuropathic spinal arthropathy is associated with tertiary syphilis, syringomyelia, and diabetes.[385] Spinal injury, such as motor vehicle accidents, intraspinal tumors, and primary neuropathies, may occasionally cause neuropathic spinal arthropathy.[1180, 1198, 1360] The underlying pathologic process in patients with neuropathic spinal arthropathy is the lack of pain and proprioception. Repeated abnormal stresses to articular cartilage of the apophyseal joints may then result in a painless injury.[1360] Reactive synovitis follows. However, a patient with a sensory neuropathy may not feel the pain,

so that repeated injury leads at first to degenerative joint disease with a reduction or absence of the protective sensation in the joint synovium.[1360] Ligaments and capsules that are also insensitive to stretch stimuli may not be able to stimulate protective muscle contractions that stabilize the spine. Consequently subluxation and dislocation may result. With repeated stress, microfractures develop. They are followed by hemorrhage, inflammation, and attempts at healing, which lead to further mechanical disintegration of the spine. Repeated trauma causes additional fractures, bony fragmentation and deformity, and decreased or markedly increased mobility.[1360] Vertebral changes usually develop slowly, but they may develop rapidly, forming almost complete osteolysis within weeks.[385] Peripheral joints are affected more commonly than the axial skeleton.

Although neuropathic spinal arthropathy is typically painless, pain may develop as nerve roots are compressed by vertebral collapse, bone hypertrophy, and herniation.[385] Neuropathic axial neuropathy develops in about 5% to 15% of luetic patients with peripheral joint involvement.[385, 1180] In patients with lues, the lumbar spine is the most commonly involved, followed by the thoracic and cervical spines.[385]

Early in the course of disease, neuropathic spinal arthropathy is difficult to diagnose radiographically.[385, 1198] There are two categories of radiographic features (bone destruction and bone production), and each may occur early in the course of disease and may go unrecognized. One of the earliest changes observed radiographically is destruction of the articular facets.[1360] Reactive bone formation with sclerosis and osteophytosis may resemble degenerative disease; however, later the osteophytes caused by repeated stress and motion may become extremely prominent and out of proportion to the degree of joint disease (Fig. 4–221). The vertebral body may demonstrate irregularity at the end-plates and intense sclerosis and osteophytosis.[385, 1198] Sclerosis may mimic osteoblastic metastasis, although it usually parallels the disc and may exist in apposing vertebral surfaces. Later, frank destruction and vertebral fragmentation occur. The intervertebral disc narrows and, with associated irregularity of the vertebral end-plate, may mimic infection. Retrolisthesis, trans-

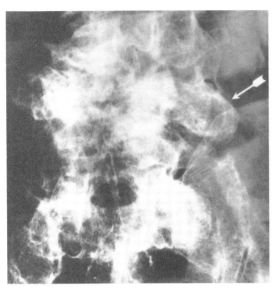

Figure 4–221. Neuropathic spondylopathy. There is disorganization, with marked disc narrowing, sclerosis, and lateral subluxation in this 53 year old patient with lues. There is extensive bone formation (arrow). (From Feldman F et al: Acute axial neuroarthropathy. Radiology 111:1–16, 1974.)

location, and pseudarthrosis may develop.[1198]

In late reparative stages, osteophytes may fuse in an attempt to stabilize the spine. However, fractures of the osteophytes and fractures of the vertebral bodies may cause multiple paravertebral bone fragments that appear similar to the bony fragments that develop in peripheral joints of patients with neuropathic disease.[385] Kyphoscoliosis may develop.

Lupus Erythematosus

About one half of the patients with lupus erythematosus develop radiographic signs of sacroiliitis. These signs include subchondral sclerosis, indistinct joint surfaces, and unevenness in joint width.[902] Bilateral ankylosis of the sacroiliac joints occurs in 16% of cases. The sacroiliitis is unrelated to the duration of disease and the age of the patient. Almost all patients with sacroiliitis have polyarthritis. There is an absence of symptomatology, and all patients are HLA-B27 negative.

Crystal Deposition Disorders

Calcium Pyrophosphate Dihydrate Crystal Deposition Disease (CPPD-CDD)

CPPD-CDD is a crystal deposition disorder in which CPPD crystals are deposited in hyaline cartilage and fibrocartilage. It may develop as a primary disorder or in association with hyperparathyroidism and hemochromatosis.[1036] Association with other disorders is probably coincidental. It usually involves the appendicular skeleton, particularly the knees, wrists, and pubic symphysis.[1032] Other joints may be involved as well. CPPD-CDD may also develop in the axial skeleton, particularly the intervertebral discs, facet joints, sacroiliac joints, posterior median atlantoaxial joint, and intraspinal and extraspinal ligaments.[1034] Approximately one third of patients with peripheral chondrocalcinosis have discal calcification.[1048] The cervical and lumbar spine are more commonly involved.[820]

Deposition of crystals begins in the outer layers of the annulus fibrosus[820] (Fig. 4–222). The nucleus pulposus is usually not calcified, although the entire disc may become calcified in those with a familial occurrence.[1315] In these patients, the posterior aspect of the disc is calcified more commonly. In patients with primary hyperparathyroidism, 55% demonstrate discal chondrocalcinosis.[1048]

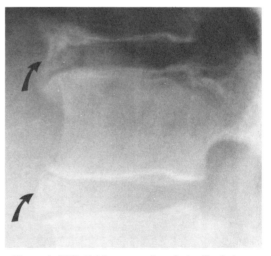

Figure 4–222. Calcium pyrophosphate dihydrate crystal deposition disease. There is calcification of the anterior portion of the annulus (arrows).

In addition, there may be signs of mild to marked degenerative change[820] consisting of disc narrowing, vacuum disc, and subchondral vertebral sclerosis.[1315] Involvement of multiple disc-vertebral levels, particularly with vacuum phenomena, may suggest this disorder.[798] Apophyseal joints may also demonstrate chondrocalcinosis of articular cartilage, although it is difficult to detect radiographically. There may be associated joint narrowing and osteophyte formation.[1034, 1036]

Spinal ligaments may be involved with CPPD-CDD. These include the posterior longitudinal ligaments, intraspinous and supraspinous ligaments, ligamenta flava, transverse ligament of the atlas, and sacroiliac ligaments.[1034] Linear and mottled calcifications are frequent in the region of the transverse ligament–odontoid process, occurring in up to 44% of patients with CPPD-CDD.[299] It is of interest that the transverse ligament contains chondroid cells and could be considered analogous to fibrocartilage.[299] Involvement of the transverse ligament may lead to atlantoaxial subluxation,[1034] and involvement of the ligamenta flava may cause spinal cord compression and myelopathy.[924] Large, tumorlike deposits of CPPD crystal within the spinal canal are rare, but when present, they may cause cord compression and erosions of surrounding bone.[345, 924]

Chondrocalcinosis may occur in the sacroiliac joints, but it is frequently not visible owing to the partial obscuring of the sacroiliac joints caused by their obliquity and by overlying feces in bowel. In addition to chondrocalcinosis, there may be subchondral cystlike defects, sclerosis, and even joint space narrowing.[798, 1034] Ankylosis of the sacroiliac joints does not occur.

Hydroxyapatite Deposition Disease (HADD)

HADD is a crystal deposition disorder that may develop as a primary disease or be secondary to various disorders, including scleroderma and hyperparathyroidism, particularly in those patients on dialysis.[109, 256] Crystal deposition is common in ligaments, tendons, and bursae. Intra-articular calcifications are less common.

Hydroxyapatite (HA) crystals have been discovered in the intervertebral discs of patients with ochronosis.[154] Calcification of the tendon of the longus colli muscle may be observed in patients with calcific tendinitis.[539, 646, 908, 909] This is represented by focal amorphous calcification adjacent to the anterior margin of C2 just below the anterior arch of C1.[79, 539] The calcification is similar in radiographic appearance to calcific tendinitis elsewhere. Prevertebral soft tissue swelling may exist from C1 to C4 or C5. Early, the calcification is well defined but becomes less defined as resorption ensues.[646] Calcification usually resorbs within 2 to 8 weeks.[79, 539] In patients with scleroderma, dystrophic calcifications may develop in the soft tissue, particularly the hands, and about large joints. Rarely, they may form in the spine both paraspinally and intraspinally[694] (Fig. 4–223).

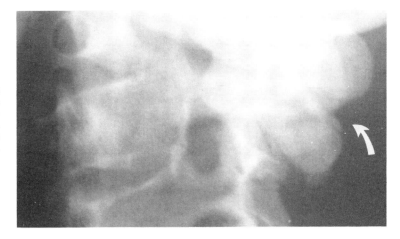

Figure 4–223. There is a large clump of calcification in the region of the apophyseal joints of the upper cervical spine (arrow). This patient has scleroderma, and the calcifications are most likely hydroxyapatite crystals.

Anemias

Anemias cause changes in the marrow that may be reflected in the radiograph of the spine. Some anemias, such as thalassemia, sickle cell disease, iron deficiency anemia, and hereditary spherocytosis, cause hyperplasia of marrow. In addition, sickle cell anemia (SSA) and the mixed hemoglobinopathies also produce focal bone marrow ischemia. Persistent widening of the anterior vertebral vascular groove, which occurs in SSA and thalassemia, and osteosclerosis, which occurs in SSA, are other spinal manifestations of anemias.

Marrow Hyperplasia

It should be recalled that just before birth, when all marrow is red (hematopoietic) marrow, conversion to fat marrow begins in the distal extremities and progresses proximally.[692] This is a steady, normally unaltered process until the age of 20 to 25 years, when red marrow normally exists in the spine, pelvis, ribs, sternum, skull, and proximal femora and humeri.[234, 530, 692, 965] Normally, red marrow is present in the vertebrae throughout life,[965] although some mild, steady, progressive conversion to fat marrow occurs, beginning about the age of 4 years[234] (Fig. 4–224). By about the age of 15 years, red marrow composes about 75% of the vertebral marrow compartment. Nevertheless, the vertebrae contain the greatest relative amount of red marrow, so that by the age of 70 years, the ratio of red marrow to fat marrow is 60% to 40%. It has been shown that in other adult mammals, the vertebrae of the tail, the sacrum, and even vertebrae of the lower lumbar contain fat marrow. This finding may be due to differences in intraosseous temperature between peripheral and more central bone marrow.[594, 595] In humans, fat marrow can be observed in the adult sacrum.

In the normal adult, the needs for hematopoiesis are met by the red (hematopoietic) marrow existing in the axial and proximal appendicular skeleton.[692] In marrow replacement or stress disorders, including chronic anemias (particularly hemolytic anemias), the body responds to the need for additional hematopoiesis by converting fat marrow back to red marrow.[234, 531, 692] This process

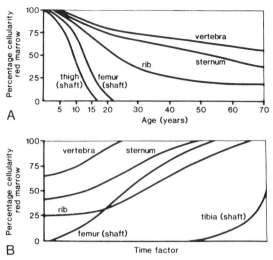

Figure 4–224. A, The relative amount of red and yellow marrow in different anatomic sites and their degree of change (conversion) over the years. B, The relative response to reconversion of red marrow by several anatomic sites following marrow stress. (From Kricun ME: Red-yellow marrow conversion: Its effects on the location of some solitary bone lesions. Skeletal Radiol 14:10–19, 1985. Adapted from Custer RP, Ahlfeldt FE: Studies on the structure and function of bone marrow: II. Variations in cellularity in various bones with advancing years of life and their relative response to stimuli. J Lab Clin Med 17:960–962, 1932.)

occurs most rapidly in the vertebrae[234] (Fig. 4–224).

In childhood, when most body marrow is red marrow, development of hemolytic anemias, which stress the marrow system, may, if severe, lead to a postponement of marrow conversion, since existing marrow becomes hyperplastic in trying to meet the body's needs for hematopoiesis.[692] This is particularly evident in thalassemia, a chronic, continuous marrow stress disorder in which severe alterations of marrow hyperplasia occur if patients are untreated. When patients with thalassemia receive transfusions, stress on the marrow system is temporarily relieved, hyperplasia diminishes, and normal conversion to fat marrow may occur. This is particularly evident in peripheral bones.[156] In patients with thalassemia it has been observed that after puberty the spine and other central portions of the skeleton (skull, pelvis) demonstrate persistence or increase in the degree of hyperplasia and that regression of marrow hyperplasia occurs in the peripheral bones. This finding has been attributed to the normal conversion process of marrow. However, this does not explain the increase in hyperplasia in the axial skeleton. This probably occurs in the spine and other central marrow sites, as they remain hyperplastic owing to the fact that they are the sites most responsive to marrow stress.[234, 692] Once the marrow in the distal bones converts to fat marrow in these patients, it takes a longer time for distal sites to respond to hyperplasia, whereas the red marrow in the spine is the first line of defense.

In sickle cell anemia, sickle cell crises are sporadic and chronic, so that the marrow system is not continually stressed as it is with untreated thalassemia. The degree of marrow hyperplasia in sickle cell disease is related to the severity of disease, the frequency of marrow crises, and the need for additional hematopoiesis. Nevertheless, the intermittency of the crises allows the marrow system to relax somewhat between crises, lessening the degree of hyperplasia.

No matter what the etiology, hyperplastic marrow encroaches on the smaller trabeculae and, by either pressure erosion or trabecular resorption,[1040] causes diminution in the size and number of the horizontal trabeculae[60, 921, 1040] (Fig. 4–225). Decrease in visible trabeculae leads to a radiographic appearance of osteopenia.[921] The remaining vertical trabeculae are stressed, react with new bone formation, and consequently ap-

pear coarsened. They are more apparent because they are contrasted with surrounding osteopenic marrow that lacks secondary smaller trabeculae.[1040] The lack of trabeculae ultimately weakens the vertebra biomechanically.[1041]

Marrow hyperplasia is most common and evident in thalassemia, although severe SSA may also demonstrate these findings. The degree of marrow hyperplasia is less common and milder in other, less severe forms of sickle cell disease, in which hemoglobin S occurs with other abnormal or normal hemoglobins, and in other chronic anemias.[882]

Ischemia and Infarction

In SSA and sickle cell–hemoglobin C disease, red blood cell sickling leads to an increase in viscosity of blood, which leads to vascular stasis.[293] Microscopically, an increase in the reticulum and an absence of fat are observed in vertebrae.[293] If the process is prolonged and severe enough, and if there is not adequate collateral blood supply, then thrombosis, ischemia, and possibly infarction may occur. This leads to the centrally depressed H-shaped vertebra that is characteristic of SSA (see Fig. 4–55). The "H" vertebra occurs in 43.6% of patients with SSA,[882] in 36.4% of those with sickle cell–thalassemia;[1042] in 32% of patients with sickle cell–hemoglobin C,[1040] and rarely in those with thalassemia.[181, 882] Massive ischemic necrosis of vertebrae may rarely develop in sickle cell anemia.[1041] Marrow infarction is not a feature of thalassemia or the mixed hemoglobinopathies unless hemoglobin S is present,[857] and the possibility of ischemia causing the rare "H" vertebra in thalassemia is uncertain.[181]

Osteosclerosis

Diffuse osteosclerosis and coarsening of trabeculae may occur in patients with SSA[293, 554] and may be due to diffuse marrow infarction with the sequential occurrence of marrow necrosis, fibrosis, granulation tissue, metaplastic woven bone, and appositional new bone formation on dead trabeculae.[293, 1028] This observation is not present in the other hemoglobinopathies. Patchy vertebral sclerosis has been observed.[332]

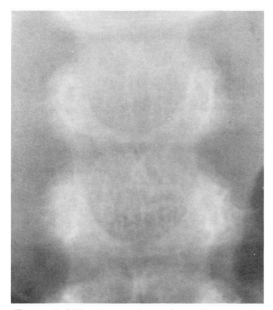

Figure 4–225. Marrow hyperplasia. Osteopenia is noted, and there is coarsening of remaining trabeculae. This patient has thalassemia.

Persistent Anterior Vascular Channels

Persistence or widening of the anterior vertebral vascular channels has been discussed earlier in this chapter (see Fig. 4–65). It occurs in SSA, thalassemia, and other disorders.[785, 1052] The anterior vertebral vascular channel is normally observed in children from 3 to 6 years of age and then may become faintly (if at all) visible in older children.[785] In normal children between 3 and 6 years of age, only 8% demonstrate this channel, whereas 46% of patients with SSA in a similar age group demonstrated this groove.

Sickle Cell Anemia

Sickle cell anemia is a chronic hemolytic anemia occurring almost exclusively in the black population. In this disorder homozygosity for an abnormal hemoglobin S occurs. More than 60% of the hemoglobin in the red blood cells is sickle hemoglobin.[921] When these red blood cells are placed in an atmosphere of low oxygen tension, they are distorted and acquire a sickle shape. This leads to clumping of red cells and thrombosis of small arteries followed by tissue ischemia. The cells are fragile and may hemorrhage easily, leading eventually to anemia.

The incidence of SSA is about 0.3% to 2% of the North American black population in the United States.[68, 921] Owing to repeated intermittent crises that cause vertebral arterial occlusion, alterations of hyperemia with osteopenia and formation of coarse, thick trabeculae occur.[178, 1041, 1052] H-shaped vertebrae[882, 1041] occur in 43.6% of patients[1042] (see Fig. 4–55). Vertebral depression is uniform both superiorly and inferiorly and demonstrates a well-defined flat margin. H-shaped vertebrae are rarely observed before the age of 10 years[882] but have been reported in patients 5[882] and 7 years of age.[1041] The H-shaped changes usually occur around the time of adolescence. There is a correlation between the level of hemoglobin S in red blood cells and vertebral changes. In a small series of patients, levels of hemoglobin S greater than 77% had characteristic vertebral changes, and those with levels less than 67% did not.[1042]

Persistence of anterior vertebral vascular grooves in children[1052] and occasionally patchy or diffuse osteosclerosis[332, 882, 1052] may develop. Alterations in SSA are more common and more severe than those that occur in the mixed hemoglobinopathies. A case of bone infarction with subsequent resolution has been observed within a lumbar vertebral body and its adjacent vertebral margin.[726] In this case, the disc space was preserved.

Sickle Cell–Hemoglobin C Disease

Sickle cell–hemoglobin C disease occurs in about 2% of the North American black population.[921] Sickle cell–hemoglobin S is combined with hemoglobin C. The radiographic features are similar to those of SSA but are less common, less severe, and occur in an older age group.[882] About 60% of the symptomatic patients demonstrate radiographic findings.[68] Thus, the radiographs may reflect the clinical course.[1040] The spine may demonstrate alterations of marrow hyperplasia, with coarse trabecular pattern in one third of the cases,[60, 68, 1040] diminution of secondary trabeculae, and osteopenia.[1040] Depressed H-shaped vertebrae occur in 17% of cases and are more common in the thoracolumbar spine.[68, 1040] Occasionally, vertebral flattening or wedging is observed.[1040]

Sickle Cell Trait

In this condition, sickle hemoglobin S is combined with normal hemoglobin A. It occurs in about 7% to 10% of the North American black population.[882, 921] Under normal physiologic conditions, the degree of hypoxia that is necessary to cause sickling of erythrocytes is not reached;[292] however, sickling of erythrocytes may occur when the patient is exposed to low oxygen tension levels. Alterations of hyperplasia are not common but occasionally occur.[882] H-shaped vertebrae do not develop in sickle cell trait.

Sickle Cell–Thalassemia Disease

In this disorder, there is inheritance of one gene for hemoglobin S and one for thalassemia.[1042] Radiographic changes are comparable to those seen with sickle cell–hemoglobin C disease.[292] Marrow hyperplasia occurs with osteopenia and coarse trabecular pattern. "H" vertebrae develop in 36.4% of cases.[1042]

Thalassemia

In this disorder, a hereditary defect in hemoglobin synthesis leads to the formation of microcytic hypochromic red cells.[882] The result is ineffective erythropoiesis followed by rapid hemolysis of newly formed red cells. In the severe homozygous form, thalassemia major (Cooley's anemia), the anemia is pronounced, and compensatory marrow hyperplasia is extensive. It is much more extensive in the central skeleton than in the peripheral bones.[156] Osteopenia and coarsened trabeculae occur,[882] with the remaining trabeculae arranged vertically. Radiographic features other than marrow hyperplasia are rare.[158] Widening or persistence of the anterior vascular groove may be observed (see Fig. 4–65).[785] The H-shaped vertebra almost never occurs; it has been reported in only one case.[181] After childhood, in severe cases, vertebrae may undergo compression deformity, and short stature associated with limb shortening may develop.[158] Extramedullary hematopoiesis may develop in severe cases and may be detected as a paravertebral mass more commonly in the thoracic spine.[1079] The masses may be unilateral or bilateral, and there is a predilection for formation below T7;[1079] however, they may occur from T2 to T11.[687] These masses of hematopoietic tissue may arise if hyperplastic marrow extrudes through the vertebral cortex.[687] In thalassemia minor, the heterozygous form, marrow hyperplasia is milder than in thalassemia major. Radiographically, osteopenia and mild coarsening of trabeculae are seen.[882]

Iron Deficiency Anemia

In this disorder, alterations of hyperplasia that occur in the spine are mild compared with those that occur in the skull.[882]

Hereditary Spherocytosis

In this hemolytic anemia, the changes of marrow hyperplasia, osteopenia, and trabec-ular coarsening are mild in the axial skeleton.[882] Central vertebral depression has been reported.[1072]

Miscellaneous Disorders

Paget's Disease

Paget's disease is a disorder characterized by various phases of bone resorption and bone formation.[614, 1217] Although the etiology is unknown, viral causes have been suggested.[416, 1124] Intranuclear viral inclusions have been found within pagetic osteoclasts, suggesting either a measles virus or a respiratory syncytial virus. Paget's disease frequently involves the axial skeleton.[287, 706] The sacrum and lumbar vertebrae are the most common sites;[498] the cervical spine is rarely affected.[626, 806, 1217] It has been suggested that when the diagnosis of Paget's disease is established radiographically, all areas of ultimate bony involvement are already affected.[416] Yet development of new areas of Paget's disease may appear from 1.5 to 3 years after treatment.[850] Vertebral bodies and posterior elements may be involved alone or in combination, although vertebral bodies are affected more commonly.[287] Paget's disease is polyostotic in 80% of cases.[605]

Early, there is excessive bone resorption, which is usually not appreciated on the spinal radiograph.[250] However, sometimes focal osteolytic changes may be observed.[323] Destruction may be so extensive that trabeculae are not visible in the vertebral body.[1217] Later, in the most commonly encountered phase,[706] the mixed phase, bone resorption by osteoclasts and bone formation by osteoblasts occur simultaneously.[416] Abnormal osteoblasts produce primitive woven bone and abnormal lamellar bone, which do not have the structural strength of normal bone.[250] As bone is produced, trabeculae become thick and coarse (Fig. 4–226), occasionally resembling hemangioma radiographically.[287] Continued trabecular thickening leads to increased bone density on the radiograph.[250, 1217] Subchondral trabeculae also thicken (see Fig. 4–226), and eventually the subchondral zone and cortex become thick, producing the so-called picture frame appearance (Fig. 4–227). Continued cortical thickening leads to enlargement of the vertebral body, which occurs in about 20% of the vertebrae in-

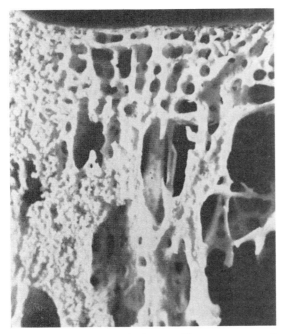

Figure 4–226. Paget's disease. There are areas of osteolysis as well as thickening of trabeculae. (From Schmorl G, Junghanns H: The Human Spine in Health and Disease. New York: Grune & Stratton, 1971. Copyright 1971 by Georg Thieme Verlag.)

volved.[706] Bone enlargement is caused by activity of multiple cellular units, with bone apposition in the endosteum and periosteum. Osteosclerosis of cancellous bone, thickening of the cortex and trabeculae, and bone enlargement represent the sclerotic inactive or healed phase of Paget's disease.[1217]

Rarely, the entire vertebral body may become osteosclerotic, causing the so-called

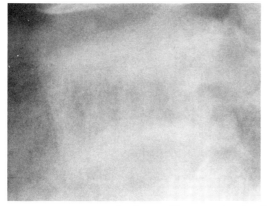

Figure 4–227. Paget's disease. There are bands of osteosclerosis surrounding the vertebral margin and forming the "picture frame" appearance. The trabeculae are thick, and the vertebral body is enlarged.

ivory vertebra.[250] Distinguishing this from other causes of "ivory" vertebra is usually not difficult, since Paget's disease demonstrates trabecular and cortical thickening, and other causes of osteosclerosis do not. Sometimes, the pedicle may appear osteosclerotic, resembling osteoblastic metastasis from carcinoma of the prostate. Again, the cortex is usually thickened in Paget's disease. Articular processes may enlarge, but facet joint spaces remain normal.[933]

Enlargement of the vertebral body posteriorly and compression fractures may cause encroachment on the thecal sac or spinal cord.[250, 323, 806] This is particularly true in the thoracic spine, where the spinal canal is relatively narrow. Cord compression occurs in 25% of patients with Paget's disease of the cervical spine.[626] Other features of Paget's disease are nonspecific and are related to the generally soft nature of pagetoid bone.[1217] Paget's bone tends to fracture when stressed by a bending force, particularly during the osteolytic phase. Pathologic fractures are most prevalent in the thoracic and lumbar spines. Other features of Paget's disease include biconcavity of vertebrae, intraosseous disc herniation (Schmorl's node), and basilar invagination.[250] Healing of pagetoid lesions has been observed following medical treatment; however, lesions remained unchanged in appearance in 64% of patients treated during the active remodeling phases and demonstrated increased sclerosis in 23% of patients.[706]

Sarcomatous degeneration rarely develops in Paget's disease,[481, 602, 605, 1117] occurring in 0.15% of the population.[1188] It is even more rare in the spine and sacrum, with 3%[1188] to 8%[1117] of the sarcomas occurring in the axial skeleton. The most common tumor that arises from malignant degeneration of Paget's bone is osteosarcoma.[481, 605] Of the osteogenic sarcomas arising in pagetoid bone, only 1.5% occur in the spine, and 3% develop in the sacrum.[605] Malignant degeneration in Paget's disease is more prevalent in the middle-aged or older patients. Fourteen percent of osteogenic sarcomas that develop in individuals over the age of 21 occur in pagetoid bone.[605] Other tumors that develop in Paget's bone include fibrosarcoma and, less commonly, chondrosarcoma, malignant fibrous histiocytoma,[481, 1117] and giant cell tumor.[602, 1117] The radiographic diagnosis of underlying sarcomatous degeneration can be suspected if the characteristic features of the specific sarcoma appear or if there is excessive bone destruction coexisting with Paget's disease.

Some authors feel that the hypervascularity of Paget's disease allows easier deposition of metastasis in pagetoid bone,[619] while others feel that the association is rare.[10, 146] Although myeloma has been reported to coexist with Paget's disease,[490, 1365] this occurrence is probably coincidental.[986]

Tuberous Sclerosis

Tuberous sclerosis is a rare disorder characterized by adenoma sebaceum of the skin, mental deficiency, and epileptiform seizures.[1260] The alterations in the axial skeleton are frequent and include multiple patchy areas of osteosclerosis, particularly in the pedicles and vertebral arches[538, 1260] (Fig. 4–228). Sclerosis of pedicles may be unilateral or bilateral.[41]

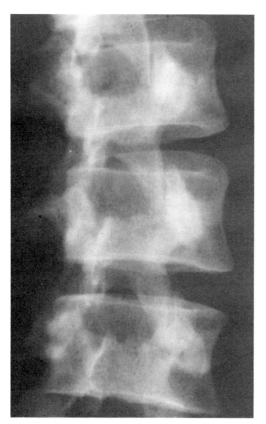

Figure 4–228. Tuberous sclerosis. There is osteosclerosis of multiple pedicles. (Courtesy of Dr. J. George Teplick, Philadelphia, Pennsylvania.)

Radiation

Radiation, either from external or internal sources, may lead to alterations in the axial skeleton. The effects of radiation depend on the dose absorbed by bone, duration of radiation, quality of radiation, area of the spine irradiated, age of the patient when irradiation was instituted, and whether irradiation occurred to abnormal bone.

Spinal complications may develop from therapeutic irradiation or occupational hazards and include alterations in vertebral architecture and growth, scoliosis, radiation necrosis or osteitis, tumor formation, and effects on fracture healing. Irradiation of tumor within bone also causes reactive changes in the underlying bone.

External irradiation from supervoltage or orthovoltage therapy for Wilms' tumor, neuroblastoma, medulloblastoma, intra-abdominal tumors, benign hemangiomas, and other disorders, particularly in growing children, can cause spinal alterations, as the vertebrae are included in the portal of treatment.[549, 1056] As a general rule, the greater the treatment dose and the younger the child at the time of therapy, the greater the radiographic alterations.[907] Children who by orthovoltage therapy receive less than 1000 rad do not develop gross, permanent spinal abnormalities (although growth retardation may occur with 800 rad); however, those who receive 1000 to 2000 rad may develop minor changes of growth arrest.[907] Those who receive over 2000 rad will probably experience growth disturbance. Patients who receive less than 2600 rad from megavoltage therapy do not develop spinal deformities, whereas those who receive more than 3070 rad do.[549] The skeletal changes observed with megavoltage therapy occur as frequently but are not as pronounced as those following orthovoltage therapy. A comparison of structural and alignment abnormalities that develop following orthovoltage or megavoltage therapy is presented in Table 4–17.

Alterations in Architecture and Growth

Irradiation to bone causes retardation of chondrogenesis and osteogenesis that leads to premature closure of epiphyses and cessation of bone growth.[549] In the growing spine, these changes are reflected in enchon-

Table 4–17. RELATIVE COMPLICATIONS OF RADIOTHERAPY

	Orthovoltage*	Megavoltage†
Growth recovery lines	28%	45%
End-plate irregularity	83%	70%
Anterior beak	20%	25%
Decreased vertebral height	83%	Data not available
Vertebral asymmetry	75%	45%
Decreased vertebral development	100%	Data not available
Scoliosis‡	70% to 81%	80% to 100%
Degree of curve	20% > 20°	100% < 20°
	61% < 25°	
	2% < 5°	69% < 5°
Kyphosis‡	26% to 30%	45% to 56%
Degree of curve (average)	21°	14°
Degree of curve (range)	7° to 57°	< 10° to 25°

*Data from Riseborough EJ, Grabias SL, Burton RI, et al: Skeletal alterations following irradiation for Wilms' tumor: with particular reference to scoliosis and kyphosis. J Bone Joint Surg 58A:526–536, 1976.

†Data from Heaston DK, Libshitz HI, Chan RC: Skeletal effects of megavoltage irradiation in survivors of Wilms' tumor. AJR 133:389–395, 1979.

‡All ages after puberty.

dral growth at the cartilaginous vertebral end-plates.[1056] Although widening of growth plates due to cessation of growth has been observed radiographically in long bones following irradiation,[283, 574] it is more difficult to appreciate such radiolucency in the spine, as the vertebral growth rate is normally slower than the growth rate of long bones. However, after irradiation is completed, bone growth begins to recover, and the radiographic findings reflect healing as well as damage to bone tissue. The earliest radiographic features are reflected in the vertebral end-plates and lead to architectural changes.

Growth Recovery Lines. Growth rate begins to recover after irradiation is completed, and thin sclerotic bands may develop adjacent to the vertebral end-plates. These represent growth recovery lines, as bone is now rapidly formed. This observation occurs in 28%[1056] to 45%[549] of patients and may form a "bone in a bone" appearance.[1056] It is felt that a dose of 1000 to 2000 rad is necessary to cause this appearance.[1092] Growth recovery lines are the mildest form of postirradiation change. These lines appear as early as 6 months after irradiation and are not confined to the field of treatment but reflect overall bone growth.

End-plates and Trabeculae. Irregularity of vertebral end-plates occurs in 70% to 83% of patients[549, 1056] and is easily recognized. Occasionally, a coarse trabecular pattern may be identified.[1056] A dose of 2000 to 3000

rad is necessary to cause these abnormalities.[1092]

Vertebral Height and Shape

Some form of failure of vertebral body development exists in all patients who receive irradiation.[1056] The most common type is an asymmetric decrease in vertebral height,[1056] although symmetric changes also occur (Fig. 4–229). Asymmetric vertebral

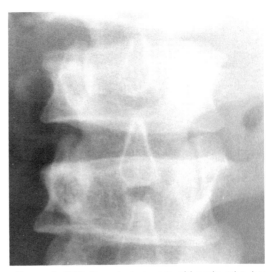

Figure 4–229. Twenty-two year old male who had radiotherapy on the right side. Notice the asymmetry in the size of the vertebral body.

height occurs in 45%[549] to 75%[1056] of patients and is more pronounced on the side of tumor receiving greatest irradiation. Lack of unilateral vertebral development leads to lateral vertebral wedging. Asymmetry in vertebral body shape is an important diagnostic observation that may help predict which side will develop a concavity of scoliosis but does not help predict the degree of severity of the scoliotic curve. Anterior vertebral narrowing and beaking deformity occur in 20%[1056] to 25%[549] of patients. A dose of 2500 rad or more is necessary to produce the beaking deformity.[1092] The configuration of the ring apophysis appears unaltered.[1056] Pedicle growth may be inhibited, and pedicles may appear asymmetric in size. In addition, bilateral irradiated pedicles may both appear symmetrically smaller than pedicles outside of the irradiated field. Intervertebral discs appear to widen on the side of vertebral body wedging. The surrounding paravertebral soft tissues are also irradiated and may develop fibrosis and contracture, which inhibit vertebral growth.

Alignment

Scoliosis. Scoliosis may develop in 70% to 100% of patients following irradiation.[549, 1056] Although scoliosis is common following megavoltage therapy, the degree of scoliotic curve is greater following orthovoltage therapy[549, 1056] (see Table 4–17). Scoliosis develops as a result of lateral vertebral wedging and paravertebral soft tissue scarring.[1056] It occurs whether or not a portion or the entire vertebra is in the field of irradiation. Scoliosis progresses rapidly during the adolescent growth spurt, and it takes about 5 years following irradiation to become manifest.[549] The degree of progression is not related to the patient's age at the onset of irradiation.[1056] The effect of the combination of chemotherapy and radiotherapy on growing bone is uncertain, although there is probably not a significant additional adverse effect.[549]

Kyphosis. Kyphosis develops in 26% to 56% of patients, and the incidence is greater in those who receive megavoltage.[549, 811, 1056] It occurs most commonly in the thoracolumbar junction.[811] The degree of kyphotic curve varies from 14 degrees with megavoltage to 21 degrees with orthovoltage. Kyphosis is usually associated with scoliosis, and when it occurs without scoliosis, it is relatively mild.[1055, 1056] When kyphosis is associated with progressive scoliosis, surgical correction with Harrington rods is made more difficult, and the incidence of pseudarthrosis increases.

Radiation Osteitis and Necrosis

Mature bone may develop atrophy when 4000 to 10,000 rad are absorbed, and radiographic changes may be demonstrated.[591] However, radiation osteitis and necrosis are not common in the spine, since the delivered dose is at levels usually lower than those that would cause these changes. When the absorbed radiation dose is high, osteoblasts, osteoclasts, and blood vessel are damaged,[119, 591, 937] although enough osteoblasts remain so that bone repair may eventually ensue. Radiographically, there is coarsening and disorganization of trabeculae as well as increased bone density of varying degree, followed by osteolysis.[591, 937] These observations are difficult to detect[119] owing to the greater amount of cancellous bone in the spine. Bone changes are usually more severe following treatment with orthovoltage than with megavoltage and are related to the higher ratio of bone to soft tissue absorption.[591] Bone weakened by irradiation and osteopenia leads to fractures that may not heal. Nonunion of fractures may lead to pseudarthrosis.[108, 591] In the presence of an already existing fracture, irradiation may inhibit callous formation.[544]

Radiographically, radiation osteitis or necrosis may at times resemble metastasis or radiation-induced tumor (Fig. 4–230). Radiation changes are diffuse and within the treatment field[591] and do not demonstrate a soft tissue mass.[119] The latent period in development of radiation osteitis is shorter than that for radiation-induced osteosarcoma.

Tumor Formation

Both benign and malignant tumors may develop secondary to external radiation (orthovoltage, megavoltage) as well as internal radiation (radionuclides, radium, and Thorotrast). Bone sarcomas may develop following single or multiple exposures to radia-

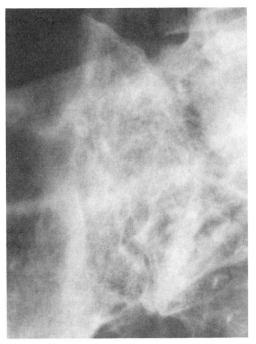

Figure 4–230. Radiation osteitis. There are focal areas of radiolucency and sclerosis about the sacroiliac joint that resemble metastatic disease. This is due to radiation osteitis.

tion.[1093] Although radiation-induced leukemia may develop within 3 to 4 years, the sarcomas and giant cell tumors have a long median latent period of 11 years following irradiation,[118] with a range of 1 to 42 years.[161, 866, 1093]

Osteochondroma (exostosis), a benign tumor, may develop following irradiation.[251, 275, 887] It usually forms in children and is more common if irradiation was initiated prior to the age of 2 years.[251] These tumors have occurred following doses of 1600 to 6425 rad.[887] No case of malignant degeneration from radiation-induced exostosis has been reported.[1092]

The incidence of radiation-induced sarcoma (RIS) is low.[118] Osteosarcoma is the most frequent radiation-induced tumor[1172, 1187, 1243] and accounts for 50% of the cases. Over 5% of all osteosarcomas occur following irradiation.[606] Fibrosarcoma, malignant fibrous histiocytoma, chondrosarcoma, giant cell tumor, spindle cell sarcoma,* and,

rarely, Ewing's tumor[1172] make up the remainder of cases. Nine percent of RISs are chondrosarcomas.[36] In one series, 16% of radiation-induced sarcomas occurred in the axial skeleton, with 11% in the spine and 5% in the sacrum.[1187] It has been reported that an increase in frequency of RIS as well as shortening of the latent period may develop with a combination of radiation therapy and multiple drug chemotherapy.[118, 1187] No RISs have developed at doses below 3000 rad delivered in a 3 week period.[118, 866] Patients who receive palliation radiotherapy for disseminated metastatic disease do not develop secondary bone sarcomas, since the dose received is usually below the minimum dose required for the induction of osteosarcoma.[118] In addition, these patients usually do not survive beyond the latent period for the development of secondary tumor.

It is well known that irradiation of benign bone tumors and tumorlike conditions may cause them to undergo malignant degeneration.[161, 1172] Aneurysmal bone cysts, osteoblastoma, fibrous dysplasia, and osteomyelitis may undergo malignant degeneration when irradiated. Giant cell tumor when irradiated may develop a more aggressive behavior or undergo a more aggressive malignant change to osteogenic sarcoma or fibrosarcoma.[1093, 1172]

RISs have variable radiographic features. Most appear purely osteolytic or purely osteosclerotic; mixed patterns are less prevalent.[1187] Some cases demonstrate peripheral sclerosis that represents radiation osteitis, although the radiographic appearance may mimic a mixed sclerotic-lytic pattern. Tumors that demonstrate dense sclerosis are usually osteosarcomas or chondrosarcomas. The tumors vary in size from 2 cm to 8 cm or larger. Soft tissue extension may be apparent but is difficult to assess fully on the conventional radiograph. Periosteal reaction is uncommon. Radiation to sites of bone metastasis inhibits tumor growth and allows the formation of reactive sclerotic bone.[108]

Radium

The ingestion of ^{226}Ra by luminous dial workers and the injection of ^{224}Ra, which was performed years ago to treat tuberculosis and ankylosing spondylitis, have caused radiation changes in bone.[118] Radiographically,

---

*Reference numbers 36, 118, 161, 513, 537, 1093, 1187, 1189.

patients who ingest [226]Ra demonstrate coarsening of trabeculae and focal areas of osteolysis and patchy osteosclerosis.[534] Avascular necrosis, pathologic fractures, and RIS may also develop. Six percent of those who received [224]Ra develop bone sarcomas after a latent period of 3.5 to 22 years.[118]

Thorotrast

Thorium dioxide in dextran (Thorotrast) is a radioactive radiographic contrast material that was abandoned in the mid-1950s.[471] It is an alpha emitter with a half-life of 400 years. Thorotrast, therefore, remains virtually unaltered throughout life.[1261] It is taken up by the reticuloendothelial system, which includes cancellous bone and, to a minor extent, cortical bone. The marrow remains preserved as Thorotrast is engulfed by macrophages that line the endosteum. Thorotrast has been associated with radiation-induced tumors not only in the skeleton but in other anatomic sites. Osteosarcomas and fibrous sarcomas have developed following a latent period of 16 to 32 years after injection of Thorotrast.[21, 1176, 1261]

Radiographically, a dense "bone within bone" configuration has been described[1176, 1261] (Fig. 4–231). The size of the dense "bone

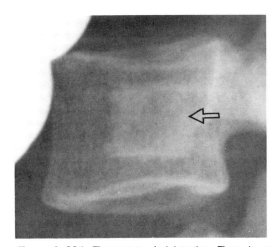

Figure 4–231. Thorotrast administration. There is an osteosclerotic "bone within a bone" appearance (arrow) in this patient who received Thorotrast at the age of 3 years. The size of the sclerotic vertebral body is the size of the vertebra at the time of Thorotrast administration. (From Teplick JG, Head GL, Kricun ME, et al: Ghost infantile vertebrae and hemipelves within adult skeleton from Thorotrast administration in childhood. Radiology 129:657–660, 1978.)

in bone" represents the size of the vertebra as it was at the time of thorotrast injection. The sclerosis represents changes caused by thickened trabeculae, and histologic alterations are characteristic of chronic radiation osteitis.[1261] The dense "bone in bone" appearance does not resemble growth recovery lines, as the entire inner vertebral configuration is sclerotic. Diffuse osteosclerosis has also been described and is possibly due to the adverse effect of Thorotrast on bone remodeling.[888]

Scoliosis and Kyphosis

Scoliosis

Scoliosis is defined as a lateral curvature of the spine. Clinically, there are two major types: structural and nonstructural.[470] Nonstructural scoliosis is nonprogressive. The curve is relatively mild and is commonly located in the thoracolumbar or lumbar spine. Spinal motion is symmetric bilaterally, and there is no evidence of rotational deformity.[815] Occasionally, this type of scoliosis may progress to the structural form.[470] In structural scoliosis, limitation and asymmetry of normal lateral bending occur, and rotational deformity is present.[815]

Scoliosis may be caused by a number of disorders (Table 4–18). The general classification of scoliosis is discussed subsequently. Spinal curvatures are designated by the apex of the curvature. The terms right and left refer to the side of convexity of the spinal curvature.

Classification

Idiopathic. Idiopathic scoliosis occurs in the absence of any significant congenital spinal abnormality or musculoskeletal disorder.[289] The etiology is unclear.[767, 894] The curvatures are usually mild and do not progress.[753] Idiopathic scoliosis may be subdivided into three categories that represent the ages at which these forms are discovered: infantile, juvenile, and adolescent.[470, 834]

Infantile idiopathic scoliosis occurs in children younger than 4 years of age and is more common in boys.[470] Left thoracic curves predominate. About 74% of patients have curves that resolve spontaneously, and the remainder have curves that progress.[834] The resolving form of infantile idiopathic

Table 4–18. CLASSIFICATION OF SCOLIOSIS

Idiopathic
1. Infantile
   a. Resolving
   b. Progressive
2. Juvenile
3. Adolescent
	Neuromuscular (e.g., poliomyelitis, syringomyelia, cerebral palsy)

Congenital Anomaly
1. Congenital scoliosis—deformity due to abnormal bone development
   a. Failure of formation
      complete unilateral (hemivertebrae)
      partial unilateral (wedge)
   b. Failure of segmentation
      partial or unilateral (bar)
      complete or bilateral (block)
   c. Mixed and miscellaneous and congenital syndromes (e.g., Klippel-Feil syndrome, Sprengel's deformity, caudal regression syndrome, diastrophic dwarfism, spondyloepiphyseal dysplasia, Morquio's syndrome)
2. Abnormalities due to abnormal bony or neural development
   a. Myelodysplasia
   b. Miscellaneous (e.g., diastematomyelia, tethered cord, lateral or anterior meningocele, neurenteric cyst)
3. Extravertebral (e.g., congenital posterior rib fusions, hypoplastic lungs, myositis ossificans progressiva)
	Skeletal Dysplasias
	
	Developmental ectodermal or mesodermal defects (e.g., neurofibromatosis, Marfan's syndrome, Ehlers-Danlos syndrome, arthrogryposis, homocystinuria)
	
	Post-traumatic
	1. Vertebral (e.g., fracture, irradiaton, surgery including intrathecal shunts)
	2. Extravertebral (e.g., thoracoplasty, burns)
	
	Inflammatory and Neoplastic (e.g., tuberculosis, osteoid osteoma, osteoblastoma)
	
	Spinal Cord Lesion and/or Canal Lesions excluding myelodysplasia (e.g., astrocytoma, arachnoid cyst, lipoma, neurofibroma)
	
	Bone Softening Disease (e.g., osteoporosis, osteomalacia, rickets, hyperparathyroidism, Cushing's disease, steroids)

Adapted from McAlister WH, Shackelford GD: Classification of spinal curvatures. Radiol Clin North Am 13:93–112, 1975.

scoliosis is relatively mild, with curves less than 30 degrees,[470] whereas the progressive form demonstrates continued progression in the spinal curvature of about 5 degrees per year, up to about 100 degrees.[815]

Juvenile idiopathic scoliosis occurs in children from 4 to 9 years of age.[470] There is a higher incidence in boys during the age range of 4 to 6 years, whereas girls are affected more commonly between the ages of 7 and 9 years.[395] A right thoracic curve is more common.

Adolescent idiopathic scoliosis is the most frequent form of scoliosis, occurring in 4.5% to 10% of the general population.[1066, 1197] It is present in about 80% of those patients who desire treatment for scoliosis.[815] Adolescent scoliosis occurs in children from the age of 10 years to skeletal maturity,[470] is 5 times as frequent in girls, and demonstrates a right thoracic curve most commonly. There is a family tendency toward this form of scoliosis in about 15% to 20% of cases[67, 228, 815] and in about 80% if radiographic evaluation is performed.[67] About one third of parents

and siblings of patients with scoliosis have curves greater than 10 degrees, whereas only 5.6% of control groups demonstrate similar spinal curves.[228, 894]

Adolescent idiopathic scoliosis is a manifestation of exaggerated disproportionate growth between the vertebral column and neural structures.[1081] Right thoracic curves predominate.[470] Around 23% of patients demonstrate progression of the curve, and the incidence is related to the severity and pattern of the curve, the age of presentation, and other features.[758] Sixty-eight percent of the curves greater than 30 degrees progress after skeletal maturity.[1319] Osteophytes may form in about 75% of patients and reflect the presence of osteoarthritis of facet joints as well as degeneration of intervertebral discs.[1051] Following fusion during the adolescent growth spurt, longitudinal growth in the posterior elements ceases, while the vertebral body continues to grow anteriorly.[551] Pulmonary function may be affected in patients with severe thoracic curves.[1320]

Congenital. This form of scoliosis is

caused by congenital abnormalities in vertebral development,[1354] such as failure of formation (hemivertebra, wedge vertebra) and failure of segmentation (bar, block vertebra), as well as by dysraphism (abnormal bone or neural development)[470, 815] (Fig. 4–232). Occult congenital intraspinal abnormalities occur in 18.3% of patients with congenital scoliosis.[834a] The most common of these abnormalities is diastematomyelia. In addition, 80% of patients with diastematomyelia develop scoliosis.[67] Syringohydromyelia may rarely present with progressive scoliosis.[51] Congenital scoliosis with vertebral anomalies has been reported in monozygotic twins.[975]

Patients who develop congenital scoliosis have a progressive type of curve, most commonly involving the thoracic spine.[1357] Thoracic and thoracolumbar curves progress more than other curves. Similar to other forms of scoliosis, congenital curves progress most rapidly during the preadolescent growth spurt, although curves may progress

in infancy even without growth. Once progression begins, it continues as long as growth is present. In general, patients with congenital scoliosis when followed to maturity demonstrate no progression of the curve in 15% of cases, moderate progression of 5 to 30 degrees in 47%, and more than 30 degrees in 35%.[1357]

Unilateral failure of segmentation leads to the formation of a unilateral unsegmented bar.[1354] It may involve two or more vertebrae and the vertebral bodies, posterior elements, or both.[1357] The bar is the most serious of the congenital anomalies. It is associated with the most progressive form of scoliosis because there is no growth potential on the side of the bar, and there is normal or excessive growth on the opposite side. Another anomaly that causes severe curvature is the presence of multiple hemivertebrae adjacent to each other on the same side.[1354] In this situation, there is severe deficiency in growth on one side, with normal growth on the opposite side. Unilateral unsegmented

Scoliosis Anomalies

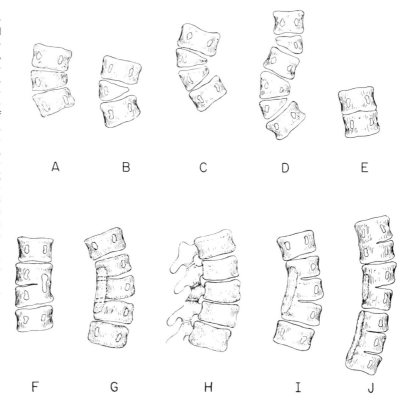

Figure 4–232. Anomalies associated with scoliosis. *A*, Partial unilateral failure of vertebral formation (wedged vertebra). *B*, Complete unilateral failure of vertebral formation (hemivertebra). *C*, Unbalanced double hemivertebra. *D*, Balanced double hemivertebra. *E*, Symmetric failure of segmentation (congenital fusion). *F*, Asymmetric failure of segmentation (unsegmented bar). *G*, Asymmetric failure of segmentation (unsegmented bar involving posterior elements only—anteroposterior view). *H*, Asymmetric failure of segmentation. Oblique view demonstrating intact disc space and lack of segmentation of posterior elements. *I*, Unsegmented bar involving both the intervertebral disc and posterior elements. *J*, Unbalanced multiple unsegmented bars. (From Winter RB, Moe JH, Eilers VE: Congenital scoliosis. A study of 234 patients treated and untreated. Part I: natural history. J Bone Joint Surg 50A:1–15, 1968.)

bar and multiple hemivertebrae on the same side of the spine are excellent predictors for severe progressive scoliosis. A single hemivertebra may cause severe or mild curves.

Additionally, progression of a scoliotic curve is more likely to occur in those curves that display a greater degree of curvature and a greater number of vertebrae within the curve.[1354] The curve of patients with congenital scoliosis progresses about 5 degrees per year on average.[815]

Eighteen percent of patients with congenital scoliosis (excluding myelomeningocele) have coexisting urologic abnormalities, the most common of which are unilateral kidney, duplication of a kidney, renal pelvis, renal ectopia, and obstructive uropathy.[768] The incidence of scoliosis in patients with congenital heart disease is between 3.3% and 19% (compared with 0.03% and 6% in the general population).[1080] Over one third of patients are over 13 years of age, and scoliosis is 3 times more common in patients with cyanotic versus noncyanotic heart disease.

Neuromuscular. Patients with syringomyelia, cerebral palsy, poliomyelitis,[576] and other neuromuscular disorders may develop scoliosis, and pronounced curvatures may occur.[815] Occasionally, these disorders may present clinically with scoliosis. In patients with poliomyelitis, unilateral paralysis of muscles, particularly the lateral abdominals and quadratus lumborum, produces the greatest degree of curvature.[576]

Congenital Malformation Syndromes. Patients with neurofibromatosis, diastrophic dwarfism, spondyloepiphyseal dysplasia congenita, chondrodystrophia calcificans congenita (Conradi's disease), and other disorders may develop severe progressive scoliosis. Just over 3% of patients with "idiopathic" scoliosis have underlying neurofibromatosis.[1043]

Tumors and Tumorlike Conditions. Spinal, intraspinal, and paraspinal lesions may cause scoliosis that is usually mild. Osteoid osteoma and osteoblastoma may actually present clinically with scoliosis, back pain, and limitation of motion.[12, 663, 744, 844, 995] Osteoid osteoma and osteoblastoma are probably the most common causes of a pain-induced scoliosis,[844] and the onset of scoliosis may be rapid.[663] The severity of scoliosis is related to the age of the patient at the time of development of symptoms and to the duration of symptoms prior to the surgical excision of the lesion.[995] Patients who present with symptoms at or around the time of skeletal maturation develop a postural scoliosis that usually resolves completely after excision of the lesion.[995] However, the initial postural scoliosis in a growing child may change to a structural form of scoliosis with vertebral rotation, particularly if the diagnosis is delayed beyond the undetermined point that might affect focal vertebral growth. Radiographically, the lesion is always on the concave side at the apex of the curvature. It may be difficult to detect small lesions in the spine, and this often leads to a delay in diagnosis. Osteoblastoma and osteoid osteoma of the rib[373, 661a] as well as other posteriorly located rib lesions may produce scoliosis.

Vertebral and paravertebral infections, particularly tuberculosis, may be associated with spinal curvatures, predominately kyphosis.

Intraspinal tumors and tumorlike conditions are more common in children,[815] and the radiographic features of an intraspinal mass may or may not be present. Severe spinal curvature may develop following surgery in patients who have continued growth potential.

Trauma. Lateral wedge compression fractures, untreated fracture dislocations, spinal cord injury, and irradiation may lead to scoliosis or kyphosis.[470, 780, 810, 1055]

Pathomechanics

Scoliosis, whether idiopathic or secondary to an underlying disorder, causes similar progressive structural alterations in the spine that progress during growth and usually cease when growth is complete.[1229] These asymmetric alterations are due to continued adaptation of the spine during the growth period. They include alterations in normal enchondral bone formation, appositional bone growth, and bone resorption. They are more pronounced during the preadolescent growth spurt.

It should be recalled that normal vertebral growth in height occurs at the growth cartilage adjacent to the vertebral body.[87, 500] It is here that cartilage matures and undergoes enchondral ossification. It should also be recalled that the stress of weight-bearing inhibits longitudinal vertebral growth, whereas lack of weight-bearing stress allows vertebral growth and height to continue.[450, 473] If weight-bearing stresses are excessive, not only is growth in height repressed but bone resorption ensues.[1229] In addition, periosteal (appositional) bone formation about the vertebra is initiated by traction on the periosteal layers.

In scoliosis, there is continued increased stress on the weight-bearing or concave side of the curve (Fig. 4–233). Eventually, in the axially loaded growing spine, chondrocyte columns are compressed, and enchondral bone formation on the concave side of the scoliotic curve is impeded.[1229] However, on the convex (tension) side of the curve, there is diminution of stress, so chondrogenesis and bone formation increase. This asymmetry of stress on the growing bone, suppressing growth on the concave side and accelerating growth on the convex side, leads eventually to lateral vertebral body wedging.

As wedging progresses, the periosteal layer is drawn away from the vertebral body on the concave side of the curve. It becomes taut and stresses the underlying Sharpey's fibers. The "space" between the periosteum and vertebral body becomes filled with vascular connective tissue and osteoblasts, and eventually bone forms, which leads to cortical thickening.[1229]

Other alterations develop as well.[1229] The periosteum and perichondrium on the convex side of the curve are stretched and often avulse. This leads to resorption of underlying cortical bone as well as hyaline cartilage on the convex side. The ring apophysis is not related to growth of the cartilaginous plate. In scoliosis, compression of the vertebral rim prior to formation of the ring apophysis prevents ossification of that portion of the apophysis. With scoliosis, the intervertebral disc is compressed on the concave side and is distracted on the convex side. Eventually, the disc moves toward the convex side of the curve. The fact that most spinal curvatures do not progress suggests that the predisposing conditions for adaptive alterations were resisted during growth and later on in years.

Imaging Evaluation

The conventional radiograph is helpful in the measurement and follow-up of patients with scoliosis, in treatment planning in the postoperative follow-up examinations, and for the evaluation of bony abnormalities that may be responsible for the curvature. The choice of radiographic views and the use of other imaging modalities vary. Reduction in radiation exposure to young patients during treatment can be achieved by utilizing high-speed screen-film combinations, the breast shield, special cassette-holders and grid, and additional filtration in the x-ray tube collimator.[281, 480] Utilizing posteroanterior radiographic projections helps reduce the amount of radiation to the thyroid and breast significantly[28, 480, 900] but delivers more radiation to bone marrow.[282] Another technique, which involves utilizing a segmented field of collimated exposure to only appropriate transitional areas of the curves, reduces the amount of radiation, particularly to the breast. This has been used in patients requiring serial radiographic examinations.[257] In addition, diminishing the number of examinations, decreasing the number of radiographs per examination, and choosing only

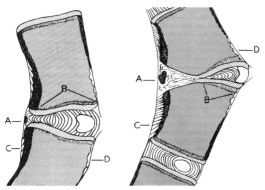

Figure 4–233. Schematic representation of bone adaption to the stresses of scoliosis. *Key:* **A** = intervertebral disc; **B** = cartilaginous plate; **C** = periosteal apposition; **D** = bone resorption. Angulation compresses the disc at the concavity and distracts it at the convexity. The nucleus of the disc moves toward the convexity. New fibrocartilage and bone may form on the left. Chondrocyte columns are compressed in the concavity and released from pressure in the convexity, thus impeding or accelerating enchondral bone formation, respectively. Vertebral wedging occurs. The periosteal apposition is drawn away from compact bone at the concavity. Bone apposition occurs about Sharpey's fibers. The vertebral body assumes an irregular quadrilateral shape from bone resorption. Underlying compact bone and cartilage are resorbed. (From Stilwell DL Jr: Structural deformities of vertebrae: Bone adaption and modeling in experimental scoliosis and kyphosis. J Bone Joint Surg 44A:611–634, 1962.)

those views that are necessary to solve the clinical problems help greatly to diminish the radiation burden further.

Opinion varies as to which views to obtain when utilizing the conventional radiograph for the initial examination. Some authors include an AP standing (without shoes), right and left lateral bending, lateral, and supine AP views.[816] The vertebrae from T1 to the iliac crest are imaged, and the sacrum is also included on the lateral view. However, AP or PA and lateral radiographs may suffice on the initial examination, and other views can be obtained if treatment is contemplated. In addition, an AP or PA radiograph alone may be acceptable if the conventional radiograph is used as a screening procedure. In older children and adults, 14 inch × 36 inch cassettes may be used to include the entire area desired. AP and lateral views in the sitting position may be used in patients with severe dysraphism or neuromuscular disorders.

The lateral bending radiograph helps differentiate structural from nonstructural scoliosis by demonstrating the degree of rigidity or mobility of the spinal curvature.[816] The type of follow-up and frequency of examinations vary. For idiopathic scoliosis, the severity of deformity and age of the patient help determine whether the interval between radiographs as part of the follow-up examination is 3 months or 6 months or longer. In patients who are in a cast, only AP radiographs are usually necessary.

Skeletal maturation should be determined in patients with idiopathic scoliosis, since progression of the curve usually ceases with skeletal maturation. Patients with idiopathic scoliosis and curves greater than 50 degrees occasionally may experience progression of a curve even after growth is complete.[816] Skeletal age of the hands and wrists and the degree of ossification of the vertebral ring apophyses and iliac apophyses are important areas to observe for skeletal maturation. Of these, the ring apophyses are the most important.[470]

Measurement of Scoliosis

Two methods for measuring the degree of scoliosis (and kyphosis) are used: the Cobb method and the Ferguson method. In the Cobb method[208a] (Fig. 4–234), a line is drawn indicating the superior surface of the end

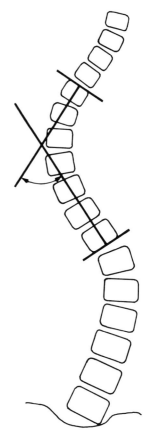

Figure 4–234. Method of Cobb for measuring the angle of scoliosis.

vertebra (the one whose superior surface demonstrates the maximal slant toward the concavity of the curve). Another line is drawn indicating the inferior surface of the lower end vertebra (the lowest vertebra whose inferior surface slants maximally toward the concavity of the curve).[208a, 1379] Lines are then drawn perpendicular to both the proximal and distal lines (superior and inferior surfaces of the top and bottom vertebrae respectively). The angle that is formed by these intersecting perpendicular lines is the angle (degree) of the curvature. All intervertbral discs within the scoliotic curve demonstrate widening on the convex side of the curve.

In the Ferguson method[385b] (Fig. 4–235), the apex of the curve is the vertebra with the greatest amount of rotation. The center of the vertebra is the intersection of lines connecting the superior corner of one side of the vertebra with the inferior corner of accurate[455] and is a more direct way of measuring the curve. It does not rely on the angle of the surface of the last vertebra of the curve.[675] However, it is more difficult to use this method with curves greater than 50 degrees.

Rotation

Rotation cannot be measured accurately. The degree of rotation may be determined by the degree of displacement of the spinous process from the midline (spinous process method [Cobb's method] [Fig. 4–236]) or by the displacement and configuration of the pedicles (pedicle method [Fig. 4–237]).[901] The pedicle method is a simplified method and consists of measuring the amount of displacement of the convex pedicle as it moves from the convex to the concave aspect of the vertebral body. This can be calculated as a percentage (0% to 100%). The pedicle measurement method is easier to perform with varying degrees of rotation, for the pedicles are less distorted in appearance than they are in the spinous process method. In addition, different methods yield different results. The values obtained by the spinous process method of measurement are usually lower than those obtained by the pedicle technique. Another method of measurement for rotation involves comparing the appearance of pedicles, transverse processes, and neural foramina with specimen radiographs

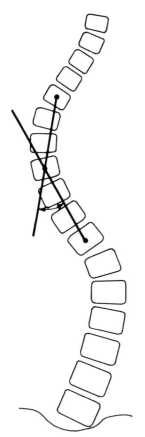

Figure 4–235. Method of Ferguson for measuring the angle of scoliosis.

the opposite side.[385b, 816] If the vertebra is wedge shaped, the wedge is altered to the shape of a rectangle and its center marked. The proximal and distal vertebrae are those that demonstrate the least amount of rotation,[675] that is, the spinous process is near or at the midline.[816] The center of these vertebrae is determined in the same way. Lines are then placed to connect the center of the end vertebrae with the center of the vertebra at the apex of the curve. The angle of the curve is the divergence of these lines from 180 degrees.[675]

The Cobb method magnifies the degree of curvature as the curve progresses, but this usually leads to earlier treatment.[815] In addition, there is a better percentage of correction with the Cobb method following surgery than with the Ferguson method.[455] On the other hand, the Cobb method cannot be used accurately with curves less than 50 degrees.[675] The Ferguson method is more

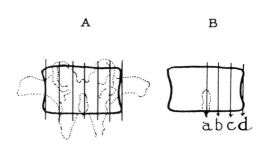

A   **B**

NORMAL VERTEBRA   ROTATION
NO ROTATION

Figure 4–236. Determining vertebral rotation by the method of Cobb (spinous process method). A, The spinous process is in the center of the vertebral body. The width of the vertebra is divided into six equal parts. B, The position of the spinous process is noted. There is no rotation if the process is at **a**; +1 rotation at **b**; +2 rotation at **c**; +3 rotation at **d**; and +4 rotation beyond **d**. (From Nash CL Jr, Moe JH: A study of vertebral rotation. J Bone Joint Surg 51A:223–229, 1969.)

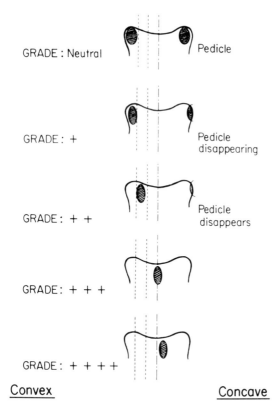

Pedicle method of determining vertebral rotation.

| | Pedicle | |
	Convex	Concave
Grade: Neutral	No asymmetry.	No asymmetry.
Grade: +	Migrates within first segment.	May start disappearing.
	Early distortion	Early distortion.
Grade: ++	Migrates to second segment.	Gradually disappears.
Grade: +++	Migrates to middle segment.	Not visible.
Grade: ++++	Migrates past mid-line to concave side of vertebral body.	Not visible.

Figure 4–237. Determining vertebral rotation by the pedicle method. (From Nash CL Jr, Moe JH: A study of vertebral rotation. J Bone Joint Surg 51A:223–229, 1969.)

through varying degrees of rotation.[843] Another method, utilizing low-dose stereoradiography and simple mathematic calculations, can be performed.[1231]

Kyphosis

Kyphosis is defined as curvature of the spine with decreased anterior angulation. A kyphotic curve of the thoracic spine measuring over 15 degrees by the Cobb method is considered abnormal.[1356] In the lumbar spine the curve is normally lordotic, so any

Table 4–19. CLASSIFICATION OF KYPHOSIS

Adolescent kyphosis (Scheuermann's disease)
Congenital kyphosis
  Failure of vertebral body formation
  Failure of vertebral body segmentation
  Mixed
Neuromuscular
Bone softening diseases
Skeletal dysplasia
Trauma
Inflammatory diseases
Arthritides
Tumors
Miscellaneous

Adapted from McAlister WH, Shackelford GD: Classification of spinal curvatures. Radiol Clin North Am 13:93–112, 1975.

loss of lordosis is relative kyphosis. There are two main types of kyphosis: congenital and acquired. Some of the disorders that result in kyphosis are listed in Table 4–19.

Classification
Congenital. Congenital kyphosis results from a congenital malformation in the vertebrae.[1273] Like scoliosis, kyphosis may be due to failure of vertebral body formation (anterior or posterior hemivertebra, aplasia), failure of vertebral body segmentation (anterior unsegmented bar), or both.[815, 1273] The degree of kyphosis is related to the amount of vertebral body or bodies that do not form.[815] All patients with anterior unsegmented bar develop progressive kyphosis at an average rate of 5 degrees yearly.[812] Scoliosis and genitourinary abnormalities are commonly associated with forms of congenital kyphosis.[815] The thoracolumbar spine and upper thoracic spine are most commonly affected. Progression of kyphosis may be rapid during the adolescent growth spurt. Paraplegia may develop with severe upper thoracic curves.

Adolescent (Juvenile). Adolescent (juvenile) kyphosis, or Scheuermann's disease, develops during the adolescent years. It results from abnormalities in the cartilage growth plate.[609] Normally the cartilaginous plate is a thick structure and is thicker in the periphery, where the annulus fibrosus inserts and the ring apophyses develop. In juvenile kyphosis, the cartilage in the vertebral plate is abnormal. This causes weakening of the vertebral plate and allows for the formation of Schmorl's nodes, which protrude into the vertebral body.[609, 1026] Vertebral growth is impaired under the areas of abnormal growth plate.[609] Ossification in ring apophyses is irregular in areas of abnormal cartilage. The kyphosis that develops is caused by anterior wedging of several vertebrae.[470, 1230] This probably results from interference with ossification, caused by the abnormal cartilage in the cartilage growth plate, and from increased stress on the anterior aspect of the vertebral body.[609]

The alterations observed in juvenile kyphosis are more frequent in the middle and lower regions of the thoracic spine, particularly the T6 to T10 levels.[815] Interestingly, juvenile kyphosis has been reported in identical twins.[92] Radiographically, the superior and inferior vertebral margins are irregular, and multiple Schmorl's nodes may be evident.[815, 1356] Disc height is diminished, and kyphosis and wedge-shaped vertebrae may be noted.[1230] Rarely, spinal cord compression may develop owing to the dorsal kyphosis associated with herniation of thoracic intervertebral disc.[675a]

Congenital Malformation Syndromes. Kyphosis develops in a number of congenital malformation syndromes and may be quite pronounced. In diastrophic dwarfism, kyphosis may be severe in the cervical spine. Kyphosis develops in 40% to 60% of patients with Marfan's syndrome,[25] 10% to 15% of patients with neurofibromatosis,[1356] and in a small number of patients with achondroplasia.

Two forms of kyphosis develop in patients with dysraphism. The congenital type, which is found in myelomeningocele, is present at birth and is usually associated with paraplegia. Kyphosis may cause significant clinical problems in those children who survive. The developmental type of kyphosis is not present at birth. It progresses slowly during the growing years[1356] and is associated with occult dysraphism.

Osseous Abnormalities. Kyphosis may develop following vertebral destruction and collapse resulting from tumor, tumorlike conditions, and infection, particularly tuberculosis. Bone destruction followed by anterior vertebral collapse leads to kyphosis. This deformity also follows both stable and unstable spinal injuries[1336] and irradiation.[1055] It has been reported in Gaucher's disease following a pathologic compression fracture.[1086]

Postoperative. Iatrogenic kyphosis may develop following Harrington's instrumentation in patients with ligament laxity syndromes, such as Ehlers-Danlos and Marfan's syndromes, and is due to ligament disruption secondary to overdistraction.[25] Kyphosis may also develop following extensive laminectomy, particularly in the cervicothoracic region.

Measurement

A modification of the Cobb method can be utilized for the measurement of kyphosis.[816] The end vertebra is defined as the one most slanted from the horizontal. Lines are drawn parallel to the end vertebral margins, and then intersecting perpendicular lines are drawn. The kyphotic angle is the angle produced by the two intersecting perpendicular lines.

POSTOPERATIVE PATIENT

The conventional radiograph may be helpful in evaluation of the postoperative patient and in the evaluation of complications following surgery. Anteroposterior and lateral radiographs usually suffice for the radiographic evaluation.

Spinal Fusion

The main objectives in performing spinal fusion are to establish normal spinal alignment, eliminate instability and excessive motion, and prevent the development of kyphosis or scoliosis or both.[406, 407] Numerous surgical procedures can be performed to achieve spinal fusion. They vary depending upon the underlying disorder, the anatomic site involved, and the personal preference of the surgeon. The advantages of surgical fusion are the rapid decompression of neural elements and the decrease in morbidity that occurs with prolonged immobilization.[407] Only a few of the numerous surgical procedures and modifications are discussed in this chapter.

Cervical Spine

Fusion of the cervical spine can be accomplished by an anterior, a posterior, or a combined approach.

Anterior Fusion. Anterior fusion of the spine is performed when it is important to remove disc tissue or osseous fragments that might be encroaching on the spinal cord or nerve root.[407] The anterior approach for spinal fusion allows the surgeon rapid direct access to the intervertebral disc and vertebral body, with relatively little need to dissect soft tissues or muscles and with little postoperative morbidity.[208, 407] This approach is usually not performed above the level of C3 owing to technical difficulties. Anterior surgical fusion should only be attempted if the spine is stable posteriorly.[407] There are three basic types of anterior fusion: the Smith-Robinson graft, the Cloward procedure, and the strut graft.[407] Following removal of a ruptured disc or bone fragment, a bone dowel or bone graft is inserted to maintain disc space height and prevent any anterior slippage of vertebrae. The strut graft is utilized when removal of a part of or removal of the entire vertebral body is desired (metastasis, trauma, infection), or when additional support is necessary.

Complications of the anterior surgical approach include pneumothorax, vocal cord paralysis, perforation of the esophagus, hematoma with tracheal compression, and possibly respiratory compromise[407] and dislodgement of the bone graft.[171]

The Smith-Robinson procedure consists of removal of the intervertebral disc and preservation of the cartilaginous end-plates with insertion of an iliac graft to maintain the intervertebral disc space.[1186] The graft is readily identified on the lateral radiograph as a wedge of bone density within the intervertebral disc space. Vertebral end-plates are preserved and sharply defined. The disc graft may extrude, but this is uncommon.[407]

The Cloward procedure is performed to decompress the intervertebral disc as well as parts of the vertebral body that protrude into the spinal canal.[208] The disc is removed, and the superior and inferior end-plates are partially removed. An autogenous (iliac bone) or heterogenous bone dowel is inserted into the end-plates and is seated between the vertebral bodies. On the anteroposterior radiograph, the bone dowel graft appears as a rounded bone density with a radiolucent center caused by the tools that remove and insert the dowel. On the lateral radiograph, the bone dowel is rectangular in shape but is not as well visualized. The superior and inferior end-plates are poorly defined in part because of their partial surgical removal. The bone dowel may not fuse and may disintegrate, causing collapse of the disc space. The bone dowel may extrude in almost one third of cases, and this may lead to kyphosis.[407]

Another method of anterior fusion is the strut graft, which is inserted to replace an entire or almost entire vertebral body or to add support. Bone graft is obtained from the ileum, rib, or tibia. The strut is inserted into vertical notches to fuse with the adjacent vertebral bodies as well as bridge the intervertebral disc space above and below. On the radiograph, the graft appears as a bony rectangular density on the anteroposterior and lateral radiographs. The strut may slip or extrude, and kyphosis may develop in about 15% of cases.[407]

Posterior Fusion. This approach is performed when there is disruption of posterior ligaments allowing anterior subluxation or dislocation.[1061] Atlantoaxial subluxation or an unstable os odontoideum may also be treated by posterior fusion of the spine. The choice of procedure is dictated by whether the laminae are intact. When posterior ligaments are disrupted, stability is achieved by the use of metallic wire and cortical onlay bone grafts.[407] Complications of posterior fusion include continued instability, hematoma, and myelopathy.

The McLaurin method of posterior fusion is performed for atlantoaxial instability.[829] In this procedure, wire secures the posterior arch of C1 and the spinous process of C2. Onlay bone graft is placed on each side of the laminae. Radiographically, the wires are easily identified. Instability is infrequent.

In the Rogers procedure, wires either penetrate or are wrapped around the base of the spinous process above and below the level of instability.[1071] The wires are also sewn through bone grafts that overlie the laminae, thus securing the posterior elements. Radiographically, the wires are easily identified. They are midline on the anteroposterior view, and they overlie the spinous processes on the lateral view. Persistent instability with possible development of kyphosis occurs in about 5% of cases.

Posterior fusion may be accomplished by placing bone graft from the iliac crest or tibia in a vertical direction on the posterior aspect of the laminae and securing the graft with loops of wire passed beneath the laminae in the epidural space.

The wires may be passed around a single lamina, forming a loop at each level, or a single wire may be placed around several consecutive laminae.[407] Bowing of the sublaminar portion of the wire into the spinal canal may cause spinal cord or nerve root injury in about 3.5% of cases. Hematoma may develop and cause cord compression.

In patients with previous multiple contiguous laminectomies, facet joints may be wired together at each level.[1061] Radiographically, the wires are noted in the region of the facet joints on the anterior, posterior, and lateral views. Complications of this procedure are uncommon.

Combined Fusion. A combined anteroposterior fusion is performed when it is necessary to remove anterior bone fragments or disc tissue or both and correct posterior instability.[407]

Nonsurgical Treatment. Cervical traction is a nonsurgical method of obtaining fusion following certain cervical fractures. It takes about 6 weeks to 2 months for fusion to occur.[407]

Radiographic Evaluation. Postoperatively, the patient is placed in one of several devices, such as a halo jacket or a cervical collar. It is important to evaluate the degree of alignment, the position of the graft or wires, and the presence and degree of fusion of the bone graft.

Bone fusion is expected to occur in 8 to 12 weeks, and plain film with conventional tomography or computed tomography can be utilized to evaluate bony fusion of the graft. It may be difficult to evaluate the cervical spine adequately on the conventional radiograph owing to the overlying device. Following removal of the neck device, evaluation of the cervical spine in flexion and extension can be performed (with the patient's physician present) to demonstrate the degree of stability. Bone grafts are usually visible on the radiograph, although it may be difficult to detect bony bridging of the graft (Fig. 4–238). Bony fusion can be diagnosed if there is continuous bone density at the junction of the graft and host vertebra. Solid fusion can be suggested if there is a lack of motion at the graft site, and this can occur with fibrous union as well as bony fusion.[115] Fibrous union is diagnosed if a radiolucent line exists at the junction of

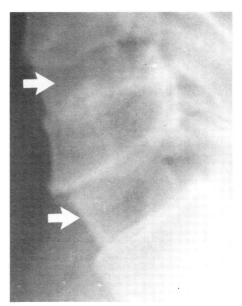

Figure 4–238. Anterior cervical fusion. Normal radiographic appearance of intervertebral bone graft (arrows) in the lower cervical spine. Intervertebral height is maintained.

the graft with the end-plates of the host vertebrae. If the graft is not incorporated into the vertebral body, resorption and collapse of the graft develop (Fig. 4–239), and fibrous tissue exists in place of the graft. Radiographically, osteopenia and decrease in size

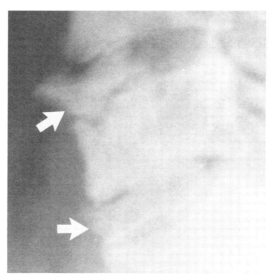

Figure 4–239. Failure of cervical bone grafts. Same patient as that shown in Figure 4–238 3 months after surgery. The height of the bone graft is diminished (arrows), and there is partial protrusion of the upper bone graft, which demonstrates nonunion.

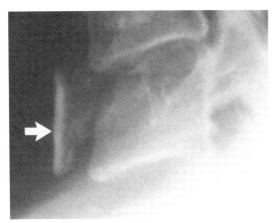

Figure 4–240. Extruded bone graft. The graft (arrow) has extruded anteriorly from the C6–C7 intervertebral space.

of the graft are seen. The graft may resorb completely.[1369] Concomitant narrowing of the intervertebral disc space develops. The radiographic features may resemble those of infection, although with infection osteopenia occurs in the adjacent vertebral body, and erosions develop at the site of graft insertion.[115] Bone graft may also extrude (Fig. 4–240). Following fusion, osteophytes and degenerative disc disease form above the level of fusion in response to altered mechanical stresses.[122] These radiographic observations may not correlate with clinical findings.

Thoracic and Lumbar Spines

Fusion of the thoracic and lumbosacral spines may be accomplished by anterior or posterior or combined methods.

Posterior Fusion. This method of fusion is performed for disruption of posterior elements that allow displacement of vertebrae above the level of dislocation[406] and for treatment of scoliosis.[1344]

Harrington distraction rods are metallic rods used in patients with scoliosis or in patients with spinal fractures who have an intact anterior longitudinal ligament, such as those with fracture dislocations of the thoracolumbar spine.[406] They aid in reducing a fracture dislocation. The rods are hooked to the laminae of the second intact vertebra below and into the facet joints of the second vertebra above the level of instability,[406] or,

in the case of scoliosis, the rods are hooked so as to include the upper and lower ends of the curves.[1344] The rods may be bent by the surgeon to conform to the kyphosis of the thoracic spine or the lordosis of the lower thoracic and lumbar spines. Two distraction rods may be used.

Complications occur in about 25% of cases, and these include an unhooked rod, overdistraction, progressive kyphosis, improper hooking of the transverse processes, and remnants of bone fragments left in the canal.[406, 814] Fractures of the Harrington rod may occur.[1085a] They develop in 12.5% of patients with Harrington distraction rods who do not have autogenous iliac bone graft and in 2.1% of patients with autogenous bone graft.[366] Distraction has been reported to cause facet dislocation and disc disruption leading to progressive kyphosis.[25] Pseudarthrosis may occur if motion of the spine is present.[814, 1344] Other complications of posterior fusion include pneumothorax and atelectasis, osteomyelitis (rare), and vascular complications.[1344] Traumatic dislocation[314] or fracture dislocation[669] in the lower cervical spine may occur following upper thoracic posterior spinal fusions with Harrington rods. The cervicothoracic junction becomes more vulnerable to trauma after fusion of the upper thoracic spine. Most of these complications can be detected radiographically. Intraoperative neurologic complications attributable to Harrington distraction rods occur in less than 1% of cases.[1340a]

Harrington compression rods are used in patients with multiple anterior compression fractures or distraction injuries caused by severe flexion injury and producing abnormal kyphosis[406] (Fig. 4–241). Fractures of Harrington compression rods occur in 3.5% of cases, mostly those without autogenous graft.[366]

Posterior fusion with autogenic or allogenic bone graft may be used to supplement Harrington instrumentation. Pseudarthrosis is a common complication of spinal fusion for scoliosis. Its incidence ranges from around 3% to 68% in patients treated without internal fixation (Fig. 4–242) and from 2% to 17% in patients treated with Harrington instrumentation.[44] There is little difference in the incidence of pseudarthrosis between those receiving autogenic grafts and those receiving allogenic grafts.

Other surgical procedures used for tho-

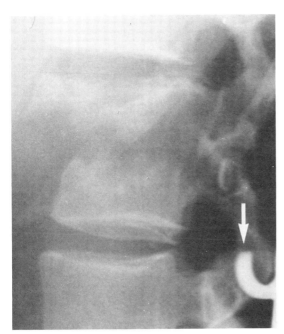

Figure 4–241. Posterior fusion with a Harrington device. The inferior hook (arrow) is in proper position in this patient with an L2 fracture.

racolumbar spine stabilization include Luque rods, which are utilized in fusion for complex neuromuscular spinal deformities,[637] scoliosis, and thoracolumbar fracture dislocations; the Weiss spring stabilization;[406] and a combination of any of the surgical procedures. Complications occur in about one third of the patients with the Luque procedure,[406] with the most common neurologic complication being sensory dysesthesia.[637] Rarely, delayed paraplegia may develop. Complications are unusual with fusions obtained by multiple devices.[406]

Anterior Fusion. Lumbar interbody fusion can be performed by an anterior approach for failed spinal surgery, certain cases of disc disease, spondylolisthesis, infection, certain vertebral fractures, and other clinical situations[231] (Fig. 4–243).

Radiographic Evaluation. Following surgery, the patient is in either a traction device or a body jacket, so an anteroposterior radiograph will suffice in the early postoperative course. Plain films and conventional tomography may be obtained 8 to 12 weeks after surgery to evaluate for bony fusion. After the body cast has been removed, flexion and extension views (with the patient's physician present) can confirm stability. The metallic devices should be intact. Bone graft is often best visualized on oblique views with the patient out of the cast and in the recumbent position.[1344] The bone graft does not appear as solid fusion until about 6 to 9 months after surgery. The diagnosis of nonunion should not be made in the early stages of healing unless there is failure of hardware or loss of correction. In the treatment of scoliosis, documentation of correction at 3 months and later is made on the anteroposterior and lateral projections with the patient in a standing position so that comparison

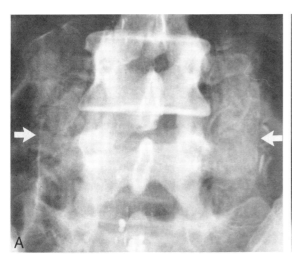
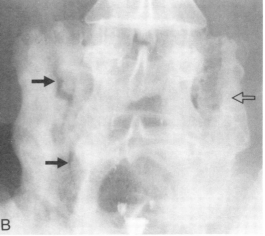

Figure 4–242. Posterior fusion of the lower lumbar spine with bone graft. *A,* Radiographic appearance of bone graft (arrows) shortly after surgery. *B,* Another patient with solid fusion of bone graft on the left (open arrow) and radiolucencies (closed arrows) on the right representing partial failure of fusion (pseudoarthrosis).

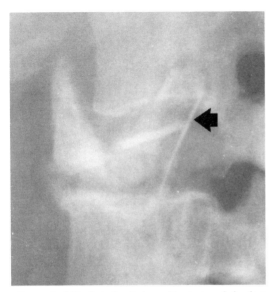

Figure 4–243. Anterior fusion with strut graft for fracture of the lumbar spine (arrow).

with preoperative radiographs can be established.

Following surgery for degenerative spondylolisthesis, 65% of patients may develop further slippage, particularly if bilateral facetectomies have been performed.[636] Twenty percent of patients with acquired spinal stenosis develop postoperative slippage.

Halo-Pelvic Traction

Patients who are placed in halo-pelvic traction for distraction and immobilization for kyphosis or scoliosis develop spontaneous posterior or interbody cervical fusion in 6% of cases[309] and may develop other cervical symptoms. Additional complications include pain, degenerative changes, avascular necrosis of the odontoid process, and atlantoaxial instability.[308] Over 50% of the patients develop cervical complications, although only 15% have significant symptoms. The incidence of complications increases if the apparatus is applied for 4 months or longer.

Disc Surgery

Osteomyelitis and intervertebral disc infection are uncommon following intervertebral disc surgery and occur in about 0.2% to

3% of operations on lumbar intervertebral discs.[1005] Patients may present with symptoms anywhere from 3 days to 8 months after surgery, with most presenting between 1 and 4 weeks postoperatively. The earliest radiographic changes occur from 1 to 8 months (average 3 months) following surgery and usually occur 4 to 6 weeks after the first symptoms appear. Radiographic features are similar to those of osteomyelitis and are described earlier in this chapter. Indistinctness and irregularity of vertebral end-plate margins and narrowing of the intervertebral disc space occur. Vertebral sclerosis often occurs. Intervertebral fusion may develop from 6 months to 2 years after surgery. Fracture of the inferior articular process of the lumbar spine may occur following laminectomy with facetectomy and may produce a radiculopathy.[1082]

TRAUMA

Conventional radiography is usually the initial imaging modality employed following trauma to the neck or back. The plain film can adequately demonstrate alignment abnormalities, vertebral body fracture fragments, and the degree of vertebral compression. In addition, it can be utilized to follow the reduction of spinal fractures. The plain film can be evaluated for underlying disorders that may complicate an injury (such as metastasis), inflammatory disorders, spondylosis, and congenital anomalies (such as os odontoideum). The limitations of the conventional radiograph include difficulty in evaluating posterior elements, intraspinal soft tissues, and position of fracture fragments within the canal.

Although most cases of spinal cord injury are due to motor vehicle and diving accidents, cervical spondylosis associated with a hyperextension injury is the commonest cause of spinal cord injury in patients over 50 years of age, and the traumatic event need not be severe.[650] Head and neck injuries are discovered in about 60% of patients who sustain a fatal accident,[99] and in 50% of these patients, cervical spinal injury is not suspected clinically.[139]

The type and location of spinal injuries depend on the severity of the traumatic event and the mechanism of injury. It is important to obtain the proper radiographs, but the choice of radiographic views is often dictated by the patient's clinical presentation. Radiographs should be evaluated in a logical manner, and there should be an understanding of the mechanism of injury. A complete discussion of the radiology of spinal trauma is beyond the scope of this chapter. However, the radiographic examination, the method of evaluating the radiograph, and the more frequently encountered lesions and their mechanism of injury are presented. For further discussion, the reader is referred to various books on the radiology of spinal trauma.[3, 449, 521]

Radiographic Examination

The decision as to whether a patient is examined radiographically depends on the history and physical examination. Spinal injuries may not be adequately assessed clinically, and other bodily injuries may detract attention from the spine,[650] particularly in the unconscious patient. In clinical situations where there is severe bodily injury, life support procedures should be instituted prior to radiographic evaluation. Only after stabilization is assured should spinal imaging be considered.

There is no routine radiographic examination for patients who sustain neck or back trauma. Ideally, the examination should be individualized for each patient.[650] The method of obtaining a satisfactory radiographic examination depends upon the severity of injury and the patient's clinical condition. The examination should be obtained with the least risk to the patient. Those who are severely injured may not be able to be positioned in the same manner as those who sustain a minor injury.

Following neck trauma, the initial radiograph should be a cross-table lateral projection with the patient supine, and it should be obtained without moving the patient. If the patient must be moved, the attending physician should be present.[1158] The radiograph is evaluated to see whether all seven cervical vertebrae are visualized. If C6 and C7 are obscured by an overlying shoulder, pulling the patient's hands downward may pull the shoulders away from the x-ray beam, thus allowing C6 and C7 to be visualized. Additional views should be considered only after the lateral radiograph is ex-

amined to ensure visualization of C7. Visualization of C7 is important because fracture dislocations at C6–C7 and C7–T1 may otherwise go unrecognized[369, 818, 1125] (Fig. 4–244).

The choice of additional views varies. Following severe neck injury, they should be obtained with the patient remaining supine and without movement. An anteroposterior (AP) view and, if necessary, oblique and AP angle views can still be performed with the patient supine and may aid in the evaluation of the C6–T1 levels.[818] If the injury is not severe, the neurologic examination normal, the patient cooperative, and the cross-table lateral radiograph unremarkable, a swimmer's view can be obtained if C6 and C7 cannot be visualized on the initial cross-table lateral radiograph. Once all cervical vertebrae are identified in this clinical situation, additional lateral, AP, AP atlantoaxial, and oblique cervical spine views can be obtained, preferably in the upright position. Angle pillar views and other angle oblique views can be performed if necessary. Flexion and extension radiographs are not performed routinely and should not be performed on patients with neurologic symptoms. If it is necessary to obtain these views, they should be performed after initial radiographs are reviewed and under the supervision of the attending physician. Flexion and extension motion should be voluntary rather than forceful.[4]

For patients who sustain severe multiple bodily injuries and who have altered cerebration, AP and cross-table lateral views of the entire spine should be obtained.[650] Radiographs taken elsewhere should be transferred with the patient and reviewed. A repeat radiographic examination should be performed to determine whether any alterations in the spine have occurred during the interval.

It should be emphasized that approximately one third of cervical fractures may not be discovered on the initial radiographic examination.[99] Fractures superimposed on normal structures or fracture lines oblique to the x-ray beam may not be visible.[654] Also, in about 50% of patients with spinal cord injury from trauma, there is no radiographic evidence of fracture or dislocation on the radiographic examination.[18] These injuries usually occur in older patients with degenerative disease who sustain a hyperexten-

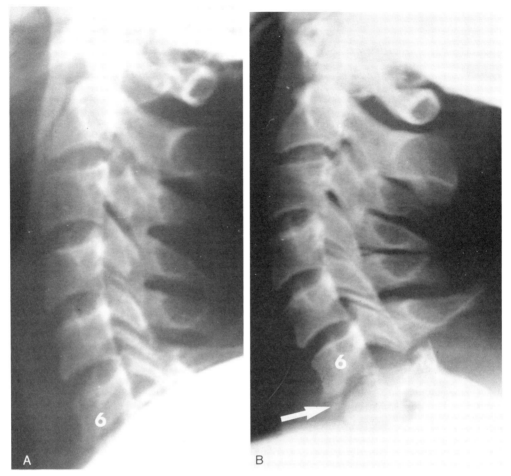

Figure 4–244. Importance of visualizing seven cervical vertebrae in a patient who has sustained neck trauma. *A,* Initial cervical radiograph following a severe vehicular accident. Only six cervical vertebrae are visualized. *B,* By pulling the shoulders downward, the fracture dislocation of C6–C7 (arrow) is exposed. This stresses the importance of visualizing all vertebral levels examined. (Courtesy of Dr. Robert Kricun, Allentown, Pennsylvania.)

sion injury. The spinal cord becomes compressed between osteophytes and the ligamenta flava, causing hematomyelia.

Following severe upper (thoracic) or lower (lumbar) back trauma or both, AP and cross-table lateral radiographs can be obtained with the patient supine and without patient movement. If the examination is unremarkable or if there are radiographic signs of vertebral arch fracture, angle oblique supine radiographs can be obtained to evaluate the vertebral arch better. If thoracic or lumbar injury is not severe and the physical and initial radiographic evaluations are unrewarding, the patient probably will not benefit from additional radiographs, although oblique views can demonstrate the posterior structures more satisfactorily.

Evaluation of the Radiograph

The conventional radiographs, even the limited initial views, offer the best overall examination of the spine.[650] The radiographs should be meticulously evaluated for abnormalities in soft tissues, alignment, vertebral bodies, and posterior elements. The following scheme is helpful.

Counting Vertebrae

All vertebral levels of the examined anatomic area should be visible on the lateral radiograph, as serious injuries may be overlooked (see Fig. 4–244). Additional views can be obtained if all levels are not identified.

Soft Tissues

The normal measurements for prevertebral soft tissue in the neck as well as alterations in the soft tissues have been discussed earlier in this chapter (see Fig. 4–29). However, it should be emphasized that it may take hours or days before the soft tissue changes appear following trauma—even in the neck. Also, alterations in soft tissues may be the *only clue* to the location of underlying traumatic lesions.[449] In the upper cervical region, a hematoma is almost always demonstrated with fractures of the odontoid process or the anterior aspect of a vertebra or following a disruptive hyperextension injury.[959] Most hematomas disappear within 2 weeks of injury. Lateral displacement of the tracheal column may be due to hemorrhage following fracture or ligamentous injury[207] but could also be due to an enlarged thyroid gland unrelated to trauma.

In the thoracic spine, evaluation of the paravertebral soft tissue planes on the anteroposterior radiograph often gives a clue to the site of fracture. The margin of the paravertebral stripe is normally sharply defined, while the width varies with the amount of underlying soft tissues. Loss of sharp definition of the paravertebral stripe or lateral displacement of the paravertebral stripe or both may occur from paravertebral hemorrhage.[445] Unilateral or bilateral widening of the paravertebral stripe is noted in 100% of patients with either stable or unstable fractures from T4 to T11.

The psoas muscle arises from the T12 to the L4 vertebrae. Normally the psoas margin (fat stripe) is well defined bilaterally, although only one side or neither side may be outlined. Radiographic technique and the patient's body habitus may determine whether the psoas margin is visible. Obscuring or widening of the psoas margin may be caused by underlying retroperitoneal hemorrhage. It is probably more significant if the psoas margin is partially obscured or widened or if a fracture is visible. It should be noted that the psoas margin may normally be bilaterally prominent distally in normal patients who engage in manual labor or extensive athletic activities. Trauma to T12 is associated with widening of the paravertebral stripe in 22% of stable and 12% of unstable fractures, and the psoas margin is obscured in 78% of stable and 88% of unstable fractures.[445] It may be difficult to evaluate the paravertebral soft tissues of T12. In the lumbar spine, the psoas margin is partially or entirely obscured in all cases of both stable and unstable fractures.

Alignment

In the cervical spine, subluxations and dislocations are easily recognized on the lateral or AP radiographs. All vertebrae should align with those above and below. The posterior vertebral margins and the spinolaminar arcs are normally smooth and continuous. The atlantoaxial relationship, atlantoaxial subluxation, pseudosubluxation, and pseudospread of the atlas have been discussed earlier in this chapter.

Loss of lordosis in the cervical and lumbar curves may be due to muscle spasm or patient positioning in otherwise normal individuals.[185, 640] In the cervical region, acute focal kyphotic angulation may be a sign of rupture of the nuchal and posterior interspinous ligaments.[207] Flexion deformity in the cervical spine greater than 11 degrees relative to adjacent vertebrae is considered abnormal and may represent instability.[650] Torticollis could also be due to muscle spasm or voluntary positioning and occurs most often in childhood and early adolescence.[520] Unstable thoracolumbar lesions may demonstrate malalignment. Vertebral displacement is observed in 56% of unstable injuries and 0% of stable fractures.[445] Scoliosis or kyphosis or both occur in 70% of stable and unstable fractures and are related to paraspinal muscle spasm.

Vertebral Bodies

The radiographic appearance of fractures of the vertebral body is variable and is influenced by the mechanism of injury. The fractures may appear linear, as cortical disruption, as decrease in vertebral body height (compression), and as triangular fragments. The conventional radiograph can accurately assess the degree of vertebral compression.[661] Fracture fragments extending posteriorly past the imaginary line that aligns vertebrae above and below may be considered within the spinal canal.

In the cervical spine, the recognition of a

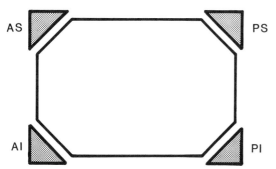

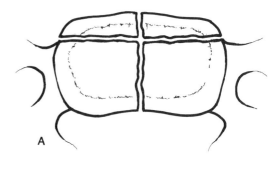

Figure 4–245. Diagram of triangular fractures that may be observed following trauma to cervical vertebrae. Posterior triangular fractures are difficult to visualize because of overlying bony structures. *Key:* **AI** = anteroinferior; **AS** = anterosuperior; **PI** = posteroinferior; **PS** = posterosuperior.

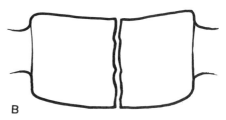

Figure 4–246. Diagrammatic representation of a sagittal fracture of a cervical vertebra. *A*, Axial view. *B*, Coronal view.

triangular-shaped fracture fragment arising from a corner of the vertebra as visualized on the lateral radiograph may give a clue to the underlying injury and stimulate a more careful search for possible associated lesions[720] (Fig. 4–245). Triangular fractures are more common anteriorly, particularly arising from the anteroinferior corner. Classically, a triangular fracture of the anteroinferior corner of the vertebral body is described as a "teardrop" fracture associated with flexion fracture dislocation injury.[1132] It is usually larger than other types of triangular fractures and may even be quadrilateral in shape, involving the anterior aspect of the vertebral body. However, the term "teardrop" has been widely used and has been applied to other triangular-shaped fractures, including those found after hyperextension[583] and other injuries.[720] In this chapter, the term "teardrop" will refer to the classic description previously noted. Posterior triangular fractures are often difficult to detect owing to overlying bone density.

Sagittal fractures are common, often unrecognized, and usually associated with quadriplegia.[719, 786a, 1050] Rarely, a patient may sustain a vertical cervical fracture without developing neurologic symptoms.[786a] Sagittal fractures may be isolated or, more commonly, a component of the flexion "teardrop" fracture dislocation. Vertical sagittal fractures are produced by a compressive force that drives the central portion of the intervertebral disc as a wedge into the vertebral body below, splitting it into two nearly equal halves[1050] (Fig. 4–246).

In the thoracic and upper lumbar spines, compression injuries often become compression flexion injuries owing to the normal kyphosis of the thoracic spine, causing anterior wedging of the vertebral body (Fig. 4–247). Usually, the superior margin is depressed, but the inferior margin may demonstrate similar findings. In the lumbar spine, where there is no kyphosis, compression force causes central collapse of the

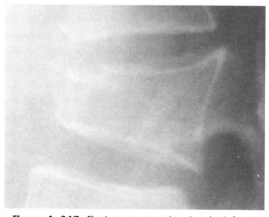

Figure 4–247. Flexion compression (wedge) fracture of L2 vertebral body. The anterior aspect of the vertebral body is collapsed, whereas the posterior aspect remains intact.

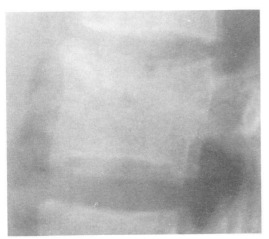

Figure 4–248. Compression fracture of L2. The superior vertebral margin is depressed and concave, while the inferior margin remains intact. In this patient with osteopenia, the forces of compression were more central along the vertebral surface compared with Figure 4–247.

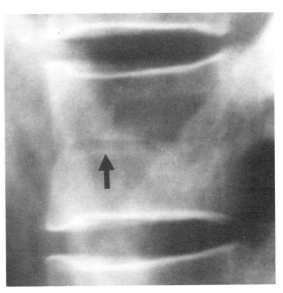

Figure 4–250. Pseudofracture (arrow), which represents a normal vascular groove.

vertebral body (Fig. 4–248). It should be emphasized that spinal fractures may be present but not radiographically visible, so that other radiographic signs (soft tissue abnormalities, alignment, and so forth) give clues to underlying trauma.

There are several normal variants and degenerative changes that should not be mistaken for vertebral body fracture. Superimposed prominent articular processes (Fig. 4–249), prominent uncovertebral articulations, vascular grooves (Fig. 4–250), air in the larynx, and skin folds may produce linear radiolucent lines simulating fracture.[239,]

[465, 653] The superimposition of the transverse process on the intervertebral disc, as seen on the lateral view of the cervical spine in children and adults, and synchondroses in children may mimic fractures.[48] The anterosuperior surface of C5 and, less commonly, C6 may normally be slightly depressed (Fig. 4–251). Partial calcification of the annulus or anterior longitudinal ligament adjacent to the vertebral margin may mimic an avulsion of an osteophyte (Fig. 4–252). However, with ligamentous calcification, no soft tissue swelling is present, and the corner of the vertebra is intact. With avulsion fractures, soft tissue swelling may be observed, and

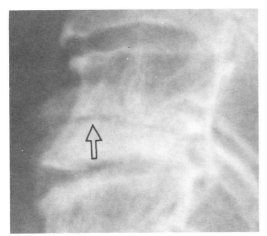

Figure 4–249. Pseudofracture (arrow) caused by prominent cervical osteophytes.

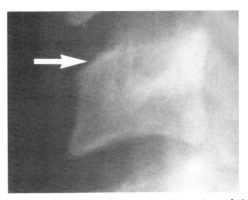

Figure 4–251. Normal-appearing depression of the anterosuperior margin (arrow) of C5 vertebra that should not be mistaken for a fracture. A similar depression may occur in C6.

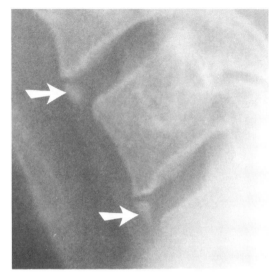

Figure 4–252. Partial calcification of the annulus or anterior longitudinal ligament (arrows) in the cervical spine, which should not be mistaken for fractures or fractures of osteophytes. Notice the adjacent sclerotic vertebral margins.

the corner of the vertebra is deficient. Calcification of ring apophyses in growing children should not be mistaken for fracture[899] (Fig. 4–253).

Pedicles

Horizontal linear fractures in the lumbar spine develop with lap belt hyperflexion injury. Focal widening of the interpedicular

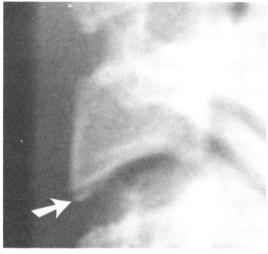

Figure 4–253. Calcification of ring apophysis (arrow) in the cervical spine.

distance and discrepancy of alignment of pedicles on the AP radiograph could indicate underlying vertebral arch disruption.[445]

Laminae

Fractures of the laminae are often not detected on the radiograph. Disruption of normal overlapping of cervical laminae on the oblique view indicates vertebral subluxation.

Spinous Process

Fractures of the spinous process may develop from direct or indirect trauma. Abnormal widening of the space between two adjacent spinous processes on the lateral radiograph suggests rupture of the posterior interspinous ligaments and is associated with hyperflexion injuries. In the cervical spine, this observation may disappear if the neck is extended, for instance, during the cross-table lateral examination. Abnormal widening of the interspinous distance on the anteroposterior radiograph suggests anterior cervical dislocation.[895] In the lumbar spine, abnormal widening of the interspinous distance could indicate a lap seat belt type of injury, and there may be associated trauma to posterior bony structures. In the cervical spine, deviation of the spinous process on the AP radiograph may indicate a vertebral arch fracture or unilateral locked facets.[207] With unilateral locked facet, the spinous process above the facet locking is tilted toward the side of locking.[117] The spinous process may also be displaced, with lamina hypertrophy,[781] disc degeneration, prolapse, facet disease,[1004] or spondylolisthesis.[1002] Spina bifida occulta should not be mistaken for fracture or displacement of the spinous process.

Apophyseal Joints, Articular Processes, Articular Pillars, and Transverse Processes

Fractures of the posterior elements are often difficult to detect on the conventional radiograph owing to overlying bony and soft tissue densities.[661] Oblique and pillar views can sometimes aid in visualizing the traumatic lesion of articular pillars of the cervical spine. Cervical articular pillar fractures occur most frequently at C6[864, 1289] and are present in around one fifth of patients with cervical vertebral arch injury.[864] Fractures of articular processes occur in about 20% of cervical spine fractures.[1366]

Widening of the apophyseal joints indicates subluxation and suggests tear or laxity of the joint capsule, usually associated with hyperflexion injuries. In thoracolumbar trauma, wide facet joints may be observed in about 30% of unstable injuries.[445] The true incidence is possibly higher, for it is difficult to evaluate these joints. Wide apophyseal joints may also be seen in patients with spondylolisthesis. Locked or perched facets can be detected on the lateral and oblique radiographs. Congenital unfused apophyses of the articular processes or transverse processes should not be mistaken for fracture (Figs. 4–254 and 4–255).

Intervertebral Disc

Widening of the intervertebral disc anteriorly may indicate a hyperextension in-

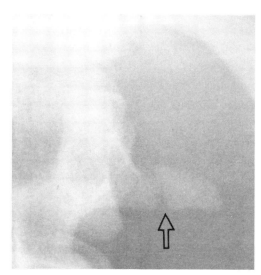

Figure 4–255. Unfused transverse process of L1 (arrow), which should not be mistaken for a fracture.

jury,[202] whereas widening of the disc posteriorly may occur following hyperflexion trauma. Diminution of disc height due to trauma may occur as disc tissue protrudes into the vertebral body following an axial compression injury. Following thoracolumbar trauma, disc narrowing occurs in 74% of stable and 69% of unstable fractures.[445] Diminution of disc height may be delayed for several weeks following trauma. Disc rupture in cervical injuries is more common in the lower cervical spine than in the upper spine.[267] Gas in the intervertebral disc of the cervical spine adjacent to the vertebral margin occurs with hyperextension injuries[1039] (Fig. 4–256). Disc narrowing from intervertebral osteochondrosis and lumbar vacuum

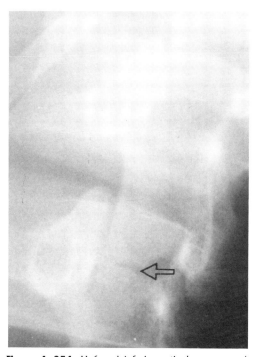

Figure 4–254. Unfused inferior articular process (arrow) of the lumbar spine, which should not be mistaken for a fracture.

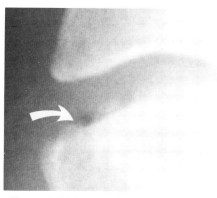

Figure 4–256. Vacuum phenomenon in the annulus (arrow) caused by a hyperextension injury.

phenomenon are frequent radiographic findings of the aging disc and should not be mistaken for a traumatic event (see Fig. 4–90).

Spinal Canal

The width of the spinal canal may be measured in the anteroposterior and lateral projections. It is difficult to evaluate the interpedicular distance in the cervical spine, and the spinolaminar line in the thoracic spine is often obscured by overlying ribs.[445] In the thoracolumbar spine, widening of the spinal canal occurs in over 44% of unstable injuries and indicates a fracture of the vertebral arch. Narrowing of the spinal canal may be caused by dislocation or fracture fragments within the canal.

Mechanisms of Injury

There are several mechanisms of spinal injury that may act alone or, more often than not, in combination. The forces of injury include compression, flexion, extension, rotation, and horizontal shear (Fig. 4–257). The spinal unit consists of two adjacent intact vertebral bodies, the interposing healthy disc with its normal turgor, the two apophyseal joints, and a group of ligaments (anterior longitudinal, posterior longitudinal, interspinous, supraspinous, and liga-

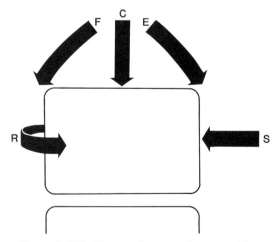

Figure 4–257. Diagram demonstrating several forces that may act upon the spine. *Key:* **C** = compression; **E** = extension; **F** = flexion; **R** = rotation; **S** = shear.

mentum flavum). Each tissue within the spinal unit will break when enough force is applied in the correct direction to a certain area over a period of time.[1058] Although spinal injuries are often thought of as force vectors that occur in one plane and can be applied to radiography, the fact remains that normal motion cannot occur in one plane. The biomechanics of injury are, therefore, more complex.[18]

Compression Forces

Compression is produced when a vertical force is applied to the spinal unit through either the head or the buttocks.[583] Pure compression causes the vertebrae to approximate, which causes a slight bulge in the annulus fibrosus. The healthy nucleus pulposus does not change in shape, since it is liquid and is not compressible.[1058] The annulus is tense and bulges only slightly against the vertebral end-plates. Blood is pressed out of the vertebral body into perivertebral sinuses, and there is an accompanying drop in pressure, thus allowing the force to be dissipated. With continued force and increase in pressure, the end-plate eventually breaks, causing a vertical fracture of the vertebral body, and this allows the nucleus pulposus to protrude into the body. Since the disc now has lost its normal turgor, the annulus is capable of significant bulging. With increased compression force, the disc is driven farther into the vertebral body, causing fragmentation—the so-called burst fracture (Fig. 4–258). The vertebral body is shattered from within outward.[583] Thus, under pure compressive forces, the vertebral body fails before the intervertebral disc fails. Pure compression fracture occurs in the cervical and lumbar spines, where the spine is mobile enough to be placed in a straight position (see Fig. 4–248). In older patients in whom the nucleus pulposus has lost its fluid content and therefore its normal turgor, compression forces cause immediate bulging of the annulus without bulging of the vertebral end-plate.[1058] Further increase in compressive force leads to disc prolapse, possible tear of the annulus, or generalized vertebral collapse with inward buckling of the sides of the vertebral body. If the force is asymmetric, a marginal depression fracture occurs.

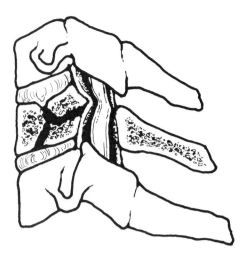

Figure 4–258. Diagrammatic representation of a compression (burst) fracture of the cervical spine. The vertebral body is shattered, and the intervertebral disc is protruding inferiorly into the body. Vertebral fragments extend posteriorly compressing the spinal cord. There is diminution of intervertebral disc height below.

Flexion Forces

With pure flexion injury, the force is transmitted to the anterior aspect of the vertebral body, causing a wedge fracture[583] (Figs. 4–259; see also Fig. 4–247), while the posterior ligament complex remains intact. Rupture of normal spinal ligaments is *not* produced by pure hyperflexion or hyperextension.[1058]

Most fractures of the thoracolumbar spine

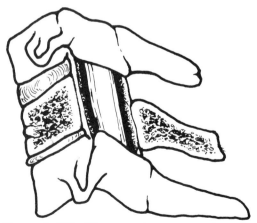

Figure 4–259. Diagrammatic representation of a compression flexion (wedge) fracture of the cervical spine. There is a slight decrease in the height of the vertebral body anteriorly, and the intervertebral disc below is narrow. There is no compression of the spinal canal.

are due to flexion trauma aided by the normal kyphosis of the thoracic spine and the relative softness and compressibility of cancellous bone of the vertebral body.[449] In the midthoracic spine, which is normally kyphotic in shape, the center of gravity is somewhat anterior. Consequently a pure compression force is transmitted into a compression flexion injury.

Extension Forces

In pure hyperextension injury, the vertebral arches fail before anterior structures fail, and rupture of the anterior longitudinal ligament does not occur.[1058]

Rotation and Shear

Intervertebral discs, apophyseal joints, and ligaments, especially in the cervical spine, are vulnerable to rotation and shear stresses, whereas they are very resistant to the stresses of compression, flexion, extension, and distraction.[1058] Rotational forces cause ligament rupture and dislocation. If the rotational force is posterior and the spine is flexed, the joint capsule ruptures. This is followed by rupture of the posterior longitudinal ligament, which is followed by dislocation. An associated fracture may be present but is dependent on the severity of the compression force. If rotation force occurs with the spine extended, the anterior longitudinal ligament ruptures.

After the nucleus pulposus has lost its turgor, rotation and horizontal shear forces may cause vertebral subluxation even without rupture of the anterior longitudinal ligament.[1058] Thus, ligaments rupture with rotation and shear forces, and vertebrae fail under compression, flexion, and extension forces. Generally speaking, compression forces cause fractures, and rotational forces cause dislocation. The classic hyperflexion and hyperextension fracture dislocations, therefore, actually are caused in part by rotational forces.

Stable Versus Unstable

A spine that can withstand stresses without progressive deformity or neurologic abnormalities or both is considered stable.[278, 386, 1336] An unstable spine, therefore, is one that leads to increased deformity or increased neurologic deficit or both. Stability of the spine depends on the integrity of the vertebral body, posterior elements, intervertebral disc, joint capsule, and ligaments (Fig. 4–260). The posterior ligamentous complex includes the supraspinous and interspinous ligaments, joint capsules, and ligamenta flava.[583] The anterior longitudinal ligament and anterior annulus fibrosus help stabilize the anterior spine, whereas the posterior longitudinal ligament and posterior annulus fibrosus help stabilize the midportion of the spinal segment.[278, 1058]

One may consider the vertebral column as divided into three "columns" in the sagittal plane[277] (Fig. 4–261). Stability of the spine may be determined by the effects of trauma on the supporting structures and the degree of involvement of these columns.

The posterior "column" is formed by alternating bony structures (posterior arch and articular processes) and the posterior ligamentous complex.[278] The middle "column" consists of the posterior longitudinal ligament, the posterior one third[386] (or posterior wall[278]) of the vertebral body, and the posterior one third of the annulus fibrosus.[386] The anterior "column" is made up of the anterior longitudinal ligament, the anterior two thirds of the annulus fibrosus, and the anterior two thirds of the vertebral body.[386]

It has been shown that rupture of the posterior ligamentous complex by itself does not produce instability.[277] If, in addition, the posterior longitudinal ligament and posterior aspect of the annulus fibrosus rupture, acute instability occurs in flexion.[277, 1058] For dislocation to occur, the intervertebral disc and anterior longitudinal ligament must be disrupted in addition.[278] Thus, the middle "column" plays an important role in the classification of fractures as stable or unstable. Minor injuries, such as fracture of the spinous processes, transverse processes, articular processes, and pars interarticularis, do not lead to acute instability.

Although the three column concept has been applied to thoracolumbar spinal injuries,[277, 278, 386] it is possible that it may be applied to cervical spine trauma with some modification in the regions of the atlantoaxial articulation and the odontoid process.

Children Versus Adults

Even though spinal injuries are uncommon in children and adolescents, there are differences between injuries sustained by young people and those sustained by adults.[835] About one half of the injuries sustained by children and adolescents involve the cervical spine, and over one third occur at multiple levels. Spinal cord injury is present in 14% of patients. Some interesting observations have been made. Reconstitution of vertebral body height may occur if the vertebral end-plates do not sustain severe injuries; the intervertebral disc is usually spared; unstable injuries may progress spontaneously; and spinal cord injury may

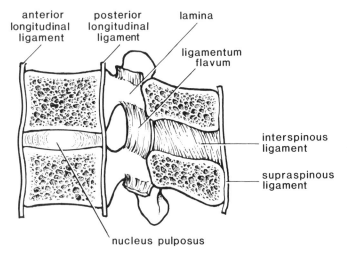

anterior longitudinal ligament   posterior longitudinal ligament   lamina

ligamentum flavum

interspinous ligament

supraspinous ligament

nucleus pulposus

Figure 4–260. Diagrammatic representation of the relationship of the vertebral bodies, intervertebral discs, and ligaments in a stable vertebral unit.

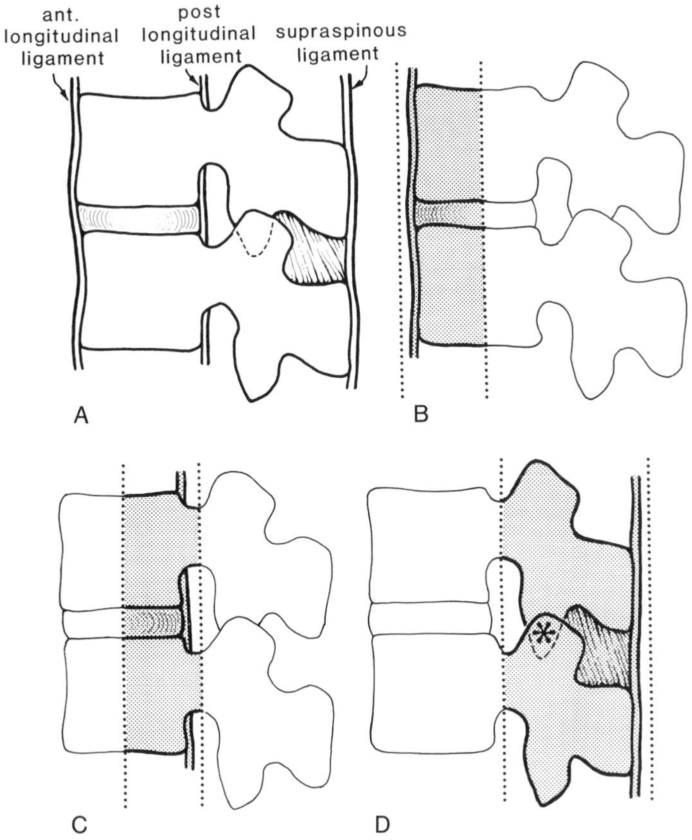

Figure 4–261. Diagrammatic representation of the three structural "columns" of the spine. The shaded areas represent the regions within the column. Dotted lines indicate the column boundaries. *A*, Normal spinal unit. *B*, Anterior column. *C*, Middle column. *D*, Posterior column. *Key:* **Asterisk** = facet joint. (Adapted from Denis F: The three-column spine and its significance in the classification of acute thoracolumbar spinal injuries. Spine 8:817–831, 1983.)

develop in the absence of radiographic findings.[835] Fracture dislocation of the cervical spine may occur following traumatic delivery and may be associated with major injury to the spinal cord.[1216] The upper cervical spine is more involved with vertex presentations and the lower cervical spine with breach presentations. Thoracic injuries are uncommon during delivery.

Multiple Spinal Injuries

Patients who sustain severe spinal trauma may simultaneously sustain noncontiguous spinal injuries at more than one level in around 4.5% of cases.[163] The primary lesion is identified as responsible for the patient's neurologic deficit. The secondary or tertiary lesions may escape early detection, leading to a mean delay in diagnosis of around 50 days. Three patterns have been described that account for over half of the cases of noncontiguous spinal injury.[163] These include a primary lesion at C5–C7 with sec-

ondary lesions at T12 or the lumbar spine; primary lesion at T2–T4 with secondary lesions in the cervical spine; and primary lesion in the thoracolumbar junction with secondary lesions at L4–L5. Additionally, a hyperextension "teardrop" injury to the upper cervical spine may be associated with an injury to the thoracic spine.[720] Since fractures of the upper and midthoracic spine are not as frequent as other vertebral levels, a primary fracture with neurologic deficit should alert the physicians to the possibility of a second spinal injury elsewhere.[163]

Upper Cervical Spine

Injuries to the cervical spine are common, for its wide range of motion renders the cervical spine susceptible to injury. The cervical spine may be functionally divided into upper and lower components. The upper cervical spine includes the occipitoatlantal and atlantoaxial articulations, and the lower cervical spine includes vertebrae C3 to C7.

The upper cervical structures are best viewed on the atlantoaxial open-mouth and lateral projections and are often not well delineated on the initial cross-table lateral radiograph. It should be emphasized that fractures may be obscured by overlying bone densities, so observation of indirect signs of cervical trauma, particularly soft tissue changes, becomes important in the radiographic evaluation. Patients who sustain upper cervical spine injury frequently have associated head injury. Seventy percent of patients with C1 and C2 injuries have neurologic signs.[300]

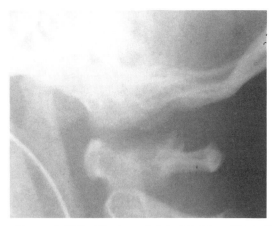

Figure 4–263. Atlanto-occipital dislocation. There is malalignment between the occiput and the spine, and distraction between the occiput and C1 is also noted.

Atlanto-occipital Dislocation

This traumatic lesion is rare, usually fatal, and most often caused by motor vehicle accidents[489, 1158] (Fig. 4–262). However, some patients survive and even present without neurologic impairment.[339, 656, 1367] Children are affected more frequently than adults.[138] Atlanto-occipital instability may also occur in rheumatoid arthritis.[794] Unilateral atlanto-occipital dislocation has been reported to be associated with a bipartite atlas.[55] Atlanto-occipital alignment can be evaluated by utilizing a ratio of the distance between the basion and the posterior arch of C1 to the distance between the anterior arch of the atlas and the opisthion[982] (Fig. 4–263). A ratio greater than 1 on the lateral radiograph indicates dislocation of the occiput on the atlas, and the ratio is unaffected by age. However, this ratio may not help detect

longitudinal atlanto-occipital dislocation[656] or the less common posterior type of atlanto-occipital dislocation.[982]

Atlantoaxial Subluxation

Atlantoaxial subluxation may be secondary to trauma with or without an odontoid fracture. However, it usually develops secondary to nontraumatic conditions, such as rheumatoid arthritis and other disorders that have been discussed earlier. Atlantoaxial subluxation is diagnosed on the lateral radiograph by displacement of the atlas from the axis by 3 mm or more in the adult and by 5 mm or more in children[568, 754] (see Fig. 4–34).

Jefferson Fracture

The Jefferson fracture is classically a bilateral fracture of both the anterior and posterior arches of the atlas and is caused by an axial compression force to the vertex of the skull with the head and neck erect[1158] (Fig. 4–264). This causes the atlas to be compressed between the occipital condyles of the skull and the superior articular surfaces of the axis. The wedge-shaped lateral masses are forced laterally owing to the obliquity of their articular surfaces,[630] and if the force is great enough bilaterally, the anterior and posterior arches of the atlas fracture and the lateral masses are displaced laterally[447, 630] (Figs. 4–264 and 4–265). Avulsion fracture

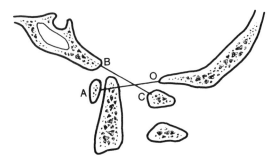

Figure 4–262. Diagrammatic representation of normal measurements that can be utlized to detect atlanto-occipital dislocation. *Key:* **A** = anterior arch of C1; **B** = basion; **C** = posterior arch of C1; **O** = opisthion. The ratio of BC to AO is normally less than 1. A ratio greater than 1 is positive for atlanto-occipital dislocation. This is valid only in the absence of associated fractures of the atlas. This ratio may not be helpful in some cases of longitudinal or posterior distraction.

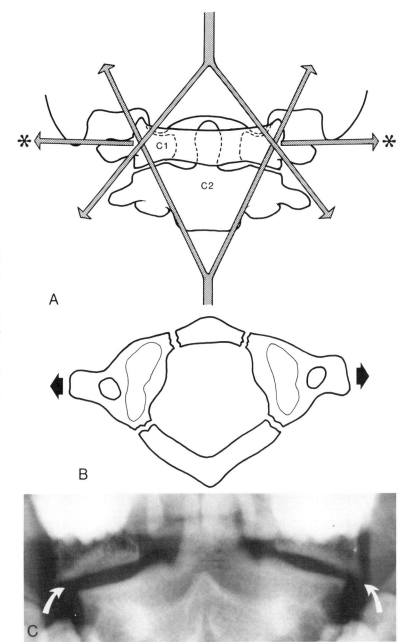

Figure 4–264. Jefferson fracture. *A,* Diagrammatic representation of the compression forces on the atlas and the formation of vector forces (asterisks) that cause the Jefferson fracture. Notice the angle of articulation between the occipital condyle and C1 as well as the articulation between C1 and C2. *B,* Diagram of C1 in the axial plane. Bilateral fractures of the anterior and posterior arches are noted. Arrows indicate vector forces. *C,* Anteroposterior radiograph of the atlantoaxial articulation showing offset (arrows) of the lateral mass of C1 on the articular surface of C2.

of the lateral masses may occur,[447, 563] but the fracture fragment may not be visible on the conventional radiograph owing to its small size and the presence of overlying bony densities. Jefferson fractures and isolated anterior or posterior arch fractures are the most common fractures of the atlas. Jefferson fracture constitutes 5% of all fractures and dislocations of the cervical spine.[447]

Normally, the lateral masses should line up with the articular surfaces of the axis (see Fig. 4–10) on the atlantoaxial open-mouth view. With the Jefferson fracture, bilateral and occasionally unilateral lateral displacement of the lateral masses occurs and is usually greater than 3 mm.[446] Displacement greater than 6.9 mm indicates probable tear of the transverse ligament.[1207] Fractures of the anterior and posterior arches of the atlas may escape detection, but in-

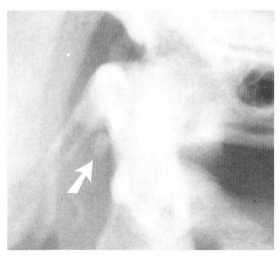

Figure 4–265. Unfused ossicle of the anterior ring of C1 (arrow) that should not be mistaken for a fracture.

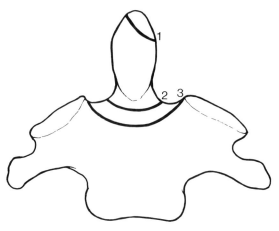

Figure 4–267. Diagram demonstrating the three types of fractures of the odontoid process.

crease in prevertebral soft tissues may provide a clue to underlying trauma. The posterior arch fractures, when visible, can be identified on the lateral radiograph.[1158] Another radiographic sign detected on the lateral radiograph is the interposition of the basion between the anterior arch of C1 and the odontoid process,[405] reflecting the closer approximation of the occiput to the axis as the lateral masses of C1 are driven outward. Isolated fractures of the anterior or posterior arch of C1 may occur.[1226]

Combined anterior and posterior spina bifida of the atlas may also lead to lateral displacement of the atlas, simulating a Jefferson fracture.[140] The anterior arch defects are midline and only a few millimeters wide, whereas the posterior arch defects are usu-

ally not midline and vary in size.[140] Focal posterior arch aplasia, unfused inferior accessory ossicles of the anterior arch of the atlas (see Fig. 4–265), and partial calcification of the arcuate ligament (Fig. 4–266) should not be mistaken for fracture of the atlas.[658]

Odontoid Process

Fractures of the odontoid process occur from sudden forward or backward head movement, with the neck rigid and erect and the facet joints locked.[959] They are the most frequent fractures of the axis,[509, 802] account for 13% of cervical spine fractures,[1112] and are usually produced by motor vehicle accidents or falls. Children may sustain an odontoid process fracture from less violent injury;[1203] however, they usually do not de-

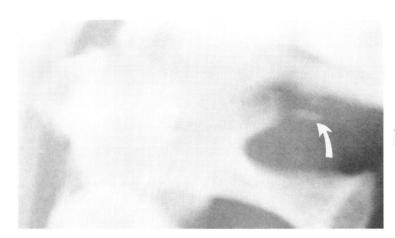

Figure 4–266. Partial calcification of the arcuate ligament (arrow) in the region of C1.

CONVENTIONAL RADIOGRAPHY • 239

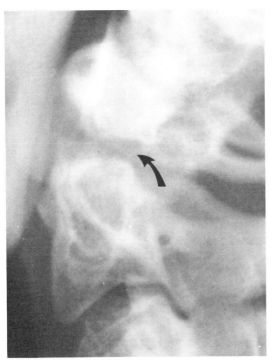

Figure 4–268. Type II fracture of the odontoid process (arrow).

velop neurologic symptomatology from this injury alone.[509]

Fractures of the odontoid process may be classified into three types[29] (Fig. 4–267). Type I is an oblique fracture of the proximal tip of the odontoid process; type II involves the junction of the odontoid process with the body of C2 (Fig. 4–268); and in type III the fracture extends into the vertebral body.[29] Most dens fractures are of type II.[29, 509] Type I fractures are uncommon. Type I and most type III fractures heal with simple immobilization. Eighty-seven percent to over 90% of type III fractures heal with conservative treatment.[29, 205] Thirty-two per-

cent to 100% of patients with type II odontoid fracture treated conservatively[29, 205, 776, 1306] and 66% of those treated with fusion develop nonunion[776] (Fig. 4–269). Fractures of the odontoid process may also be classified according to whether they develop above or below the lateral atlantoaxial joint.[864] "High" fractures that occur above the level of the lateral atlantoaxial joint are more likely to develop nonunion.[864] It should be recalled that there are two vascular arcades to the dens: one to the tip of the dens and the other to the body of the axis.[1127] This leaves an area of poor blood supply at the base of the odontoid process. In addition, the apical ligaments create a distraction effect with the fracture through the base of the odontoid process, causing a gap that prevents adequate healing.[776] Avascular necrosis of the dens may occasionally develop following fracture.

Radiographic detection of type II and type III fractures may be difficult.[520] The AP open-mouth and lateral projections aid in evaluating this region; however, it may be impossible to obtain an open-mouth view. Radiographically, there may be widening of the retropharyngeal soft tissues and obliteration of the prevertebral fat line. A fracture line or cortical disruption may be noted, and the fracture may or may not be displaced. Around 80% of odontoid fractures demonstrate displacement, and two thirds are dislocated anteriorly[864] (Fig. 4–270). If the "low" dens fracture involves the body of C2, the elongated ring density in the body of the axis normally seen on the lateral cervical radiograph is disrupted[522] (Fig. 4–271). The ring is not disrupted with "high" dens fracture.

A number of abnormalities mimic fracture of the odontoid process, including Mach

Figure 4–269. Nonunion of a fracture of the base of the odontoid process (arrow). The margin of the odontoid process is sclerotic.

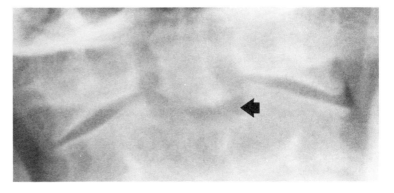

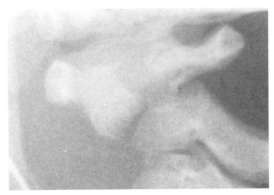

Figure 4–270. Fracture of the base of the odontoid process, with marked anterior dislocation and marked soft tissue swelling. (Courtesy of Dr. Spencer Borden, IV, Philadelphia, Pennsylvania.)

bands, overlying teeth, synchondroses in children, the ossicle terminale, congenital clefts in the anterior[973] or posterior arch of C1 or in the posterior skull, other overlapping normal structures, and a normal, posteriorly tilted odontoid process.[1251] Os odontoideum may mimic an ununited fracture of the odontoid process, since both have sclerotic margins (see Fig. 4–157). With os odontoideum, however, the shape that the os makes with the odontoid process is abnormal, whereas with ununited fracture, the overall shape of the fragment and odontoid is more normal in appearance.[449]

Hangman's Fracture

The so-called hangman's fracture is the second most common fracture of the axis[509, 802] and consists of a bilateral avulsion fracture of the posterior arch of C2 that extends into the pedicles. Occasionally, the posterior wall of the body of the axis is fractured.[330] The odontoid process and transverse ligament remain intact.[1334] The method of injury is usually an acute hyperextension of the skull on the upper cervical spine,[1148] as occurs when the chin or forehead encounters the windshield, forcing the head into hyperextension (Fig. 4–272). Patients usually do not manifest neurologic signs or symptoms,[349, 1148] probably owing to the wide spinal canal at this level,[1148] although serious injury may occur.[330] In addition, around 20% have associated cerebral concussion, and 14% have associated cervical lesions.[330] About 65% of cases are classified as stable. Rarely, the vertebral artery may become thrombosed and cause demise.[628]

Radiographically, the fractures of the pedicles and vertebral arch may be detected on the lateral radiograph (Fig. 4–273); however, oblique views may be necessary to demonstrate the pedicle fractures and to confirm the bilaterality of this traumatic lesion. The

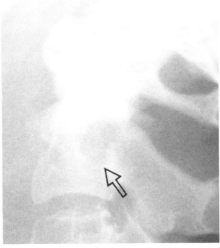

Figure 4–271. Fracture of the axis. The normal ring of C2 is interrupted (arrow), indicating a fracture. Marked soft tissue swelling is present anteriorly.

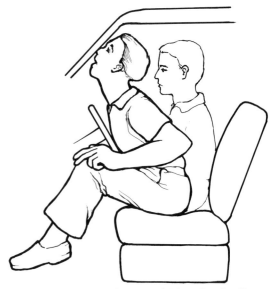

Figure 4–272. Mechanism of injury for the "hangman's" fracture. With sudden deceleration, the face impacts on the windshield and the neck is thrown into hyperextension.

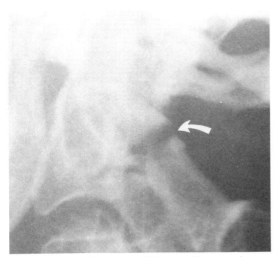

Figure 4–273. "Hangman's" fracture. There is a fracture of the lamina and pedicle of C2 (arrow). The intervertebral disc below is normal in height.

intervertebral disc of the axis and C3 may be diminished in height, and anterior subluxation of C2 on C3 may or may not be present.[330, 449] The C1–C2 relationship remains intact. A triangular fracture of the anteroinferior corner of C2 may be present occasionally.[720] Nonunion and cord compression may be late sequellae.[1334] Congenital spondylolisthesis of C2 may mimic a hangman's fracture; however, with this lesion, the margins of the bone defect are sclerotic and smooth, and the intervertebral disc is preserved.[449]

Middle and Lower Cervical Spine

Trauma to the middle and lower regions of the cervical spine (the C3–C7 vertebral levels) may produce isolated or combined fractures of the vertebral arch and vertebral bodies or even more complex fracture dislocations. Injuries to the lower cervical spine are more common than injuries to the upper cervical spine.[300]

The vertebral arch is the most frequent site of cervical spine fractures, accounting for 50% of fractures in this area. Most fractures of the vertebral arch occur in the articular pillars, particularly at C6.[864] They are often difficult to diagnose radiographically, although the pillar views are sometimes helpful. Caution should be taken in the evaluation of cervical pillars in elderly patients,

since pillars normally lose height with age.[1289]

Fractures of other elements of the vertebral arch are less common. Most fractures of the laminae occur at C5 and C6, and most fractures of the spinous process occur at C6 and C7.[864] Most pedicle fractures occur at the C2 level in the upper cervical spine. Fractures of the transverse processes are rare and difficult to identify. They usually involve C7 and, at this level, are commonly associated with brachial plexus injuries.[449]

The so-called clay shoveler's fracture is the result of indirect trauma produced by the repetitive stress of muscle pull on the dorsal spine, or it may represent an avulsion type of fracture and develop following an acute severe hyperflexion or hyperextension injury.[168, 300, 449] It appears on the dorsal tip of the spinous process of C7 but may occur from C6 to T3 (Fig. 4–274). The margins are usually sclerotic, indicating chronicity and nonunion. On the AP radiograph, the spinous process appears "double."[168] Clay shoveler's fracture is a stable injury.[520]

The vertebral body is the second most frequent anatomic site of cervical injury, and fractures of the vertebral body account for about one third of all cervical fractures.[864] Most occur in the lower three vertebrae, with over half at C6 and C7.[864]

Fracture dislocations are serious injuries that may be caused by severe hyperextension or hyperflexion trauma usually from motor vehicle accidents or falls. Fractures of the face or mandible correlate well with extension injuries.[18] Neurologic signs and symptoms of cord compression often develop but may be absent initially with some traumatic lesions.[444]

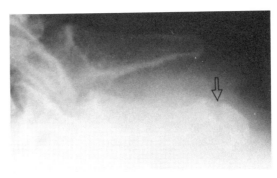

Figure 4–274. Clay shoveler's fracture. There is a fracture of the dorsal aspect of the spinous process of C7 (arrow). The margins are sclerotic, indicating that this is not an acute injury.

It should be emphasized that in patients with cervical spinal cord injury, 34% have a clinical level of injury between C6 and T1,[1125] which are areas difficult to evaluate by conventional radiography.[818, 1125]

Hyperextension Sprain

Receiving a blow to or falling on the chin or the face causes hyperextension of the cervical spine[350] (Fig. 4–275). The spinous and articular processes approximate and, acting as a fulcrum, cause the anterior longitudinal ligament[350] and the anterior aspect of the intervertebral disc[444] to rupture. Thus, the traumatic force is dissipated through soft tissues only.[202] However, a small fragment of bone may be avulsed from the anterior aspect of the vertebral body.[449] The cervical spine above the separation is displaced posteriorly, leading to compression of the spinal cord. Compression occurs because the spinal cord is trapped between the posteriorly displaced vertebral body and the lamina of the vertebra below.[202] In this injury, the dislocation is temporary and spontaneously reduces as the neck recoils in flexion.[444] Thus, the radiograph may appear entirely normal. However, more often, radiographic signs of trauma are evident and include the avulsed fragment (65%),[324a] abnormalities of soft tissue caused by edema or hemorrhage,[959] or, less frequently, a wide intervertebral disc (15%)[202] or a vacuum disc (15%)[1039] (see Fig. 4–256). Prevertebral soft tissue swelling may involve the entire cervical region, and in 30% of cases, it may be the only radiographic clue to underlying injury.[324a] Clinically, the degree of neurologic compromise is variable and may be severe.[413] Patients with spondylosis or spinal stenosis or both may sustain significant cord damage[650] without radiographic evidence of injury.

Hyperextension Fracture Dislocation

This traumatic lesion is the most frequent combined injury of the cervical spine.[444] In this injury, a blow to the forehead causes a backward and downward force on the head and neck, which are thrown into hyperextension.[413] The blow to the forehead adds compression to the force so that the head moves through a backward and downward arc, causing trauma to the posterior structures, including the articular processes, spinous processes, laminae, and pedicles. If the force is great enough and the articular processes are fractured or compressed, it may push the vertebral body anteriorly, since the articular processes, which normally prevent forward displacement, have been compro-

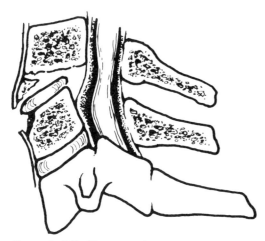

Figure 4–275. Diagrammatic representation of a hyperextension sprain injury of the cervical spine with avulsion fracture. The anterior longitudinal ligament is ruptured and there is avulsion of the anterosuperior vertebral body below. The intervertebral disc is separated from the inferior end-plate above. There is posterior displacement of the vertebral body that encroaches on the spinal cord.

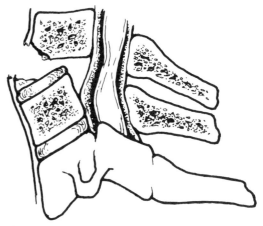

Figure 4–276. Hyperextension fracture dislocation. Diagrammatic representation of a hyperextension fracture dislocation injury. The anterior longitudinal ligament is ruptured, and there is a triangular-shaped avulsion fracture of the anteroinferior aspect of the vertebral body above. The intervertebral disc is separated from the inferior vertebral end-plate, and the vertebral body is displaced posteriorly, encroaching on the spinal cord.

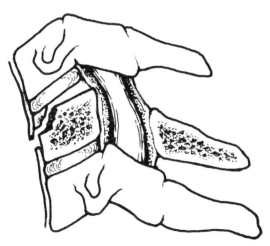

Figure 4–277. Hyperextension fracture dislocation. Diagrammatic representation. Rupture of the anterior longitudinal ligament and a triangular-shaped avulsion fracture of the anterosuperior corner of the vertebral body below occur. The intervertebral disc is separated from the superior vertebral end-plate, and there is anterior displacement of the vertebral body above.

occur.[444] Fractures of the articular pillars or spinous processes may be noted. The avulsed fragment of the anteroinferior[413] or anterosuperior[449] vertebral margin caused by rupture of the anterior longitudinal ligament may be identified. Fracture fragments may approximate, and subluxation may correct itself on flexion (Fig. 4–278). Clinically, patients are often neurologically intact, although severe cord compromise may occur.[449] Additionally, there may be a rotary component suggested by the unilaterality of the pillar fracture.[444] Hyperextension fracture dislocation is considered an unstable injury.[520]

Hyperflexion Sprain

In this injury, a force to the occiput from below causes hyperflexion of the cervical spine. The spinous processes are distracted, and the posterior interspinous ligaments and capsule of the articular facet are ruptured.[18, 449] The facets may then override, and the intervertebral disc is compressed anteriorly. Mild anterolateral displacement may occur.[483] As the force dissipates, the spine begins to recoil. When this occurs, one of three things may happen: (1) the articular facets may return to their normal position, in which case the lesion is a hyperflexion sprain; (2) the facets may lock bilaterally (locked facets); or (3) if there has been some rotation, they may lock unilaterally.[444, 1126]

mised. Additionally, the disc below may rupture.[444] The anterior longitudinal ligament may remain intact or rupture late, causing avulsion of either the anteroinferior corner of the vertebral body above the involved disc level[413, 583] (Fig. 4–276) or the anterosuperior corner of the vertebral body below the involved disc level[449] (Fig. 4–277).

Radiographically, mild to moderate anterior or posterior vertebral subluxation, fractures or compression of posterior elements,[413] and slight loss of disc height

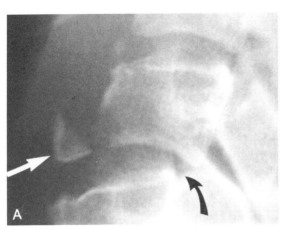
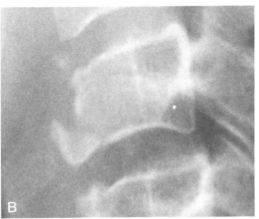

Figure 4–278. Hyperextension fracture dislocation of C3. *A,* Radiograph taken with the neck in extension. Note the triangular fracture of the anteroinferior corner of C3 (straight arrow) and the posterior displacement of C3 on C4 (curved arrow). *B,* Same patient with the neck in flexion. The subluxation is reduced, and the fracture fragment is more closely approximated to the vertebral body. The fracture could easily be seen on the view with the neck in neutral position.

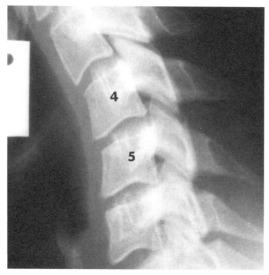

Figure 4–279. Hyperflexion sprain. Note the widening of the interspinous space and the focal hyperflexion at C4–C5.

Most hyperflexion sprains occur at the C5–C6 level in adults[864] and at the C2–C3 and C3–C4 levels in children.[449] Motor vehicle accidents account for most hyperflexion sprains. Any neurologic injury sustained is usually temporary,[444] although in 20% of cases delayed instability from impaired ligamentous healing develops.[483]

Radiographically, focal kyphotic hyper-angulation of the cervical spine caused by rupture of the posterior spinal ligaments is seen[483] (Fig. 4–279). This may not be apparent on the supine cross-table lateral projection, so obtaining the upright lateral radiograph may be necessary in order to establish this diagnosis. In addition, slight (1 to 3 mm) displacement of the subluxated vertebra, widening of the interspinous space and apophyseal joints, and anterior narrowing and posterior widening of the intervertebral disc occur.[483]

Locked Facets

The mechanism of injury that causes facets to lock is similar to that of the hyperflexion sprain.[444] A blow to the occiput from below causes hyperflexion of the cervical spine. The spinous processes are distracted, the posterior interspinous ligaments and articular capsules are ruptured, and the facets override. As the force of injury dissipates, the spine begins to recoil. However, instead of the spine moving back to its normal position, the facets lock[444] (Fig. 4–280). With locked facets, the inferior articular process is anterior to the superior articular process of the vertebra below. Locking may be bilateral or unilateral (Figs. 4–281 and 4–282).

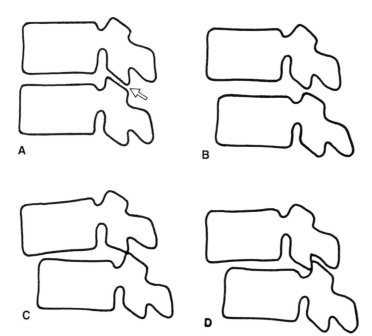

Figure 4–280. Diagrammatic representation of the normal and abnormal relationships of articular processes (arrow). *A,* Normal. *B,* Subluxation. *C,* Perched facets. *D,* Locked facets.

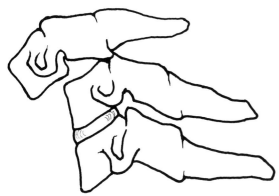

Figure 4–281. Bilateral locked facets. Diagrammatic representation of bilateral locking of articular processes. There is more than 50% anterior displacement of the vertebrae above.

An associated rotary component to the mechanism of injury leads to unilateral facet locking.[117, 1126] Neurologic deficit may or may not be present.

Most cases of facet locking occur at C5–C6 and C6–C7.[864] Sixteen percent of patients who sustain cervical cord trauma have unilateral locked facets.[1126] Six percent of patients with locked facets have an associated fracture of the cervical spine.[444] A triangular fracture of the anterosuperior corner of the vertebra with or without a fracture of the posteroinferior corner of the vertebra above may be noted with unilateral locked facet.[720] This latter combination of triangular frac-

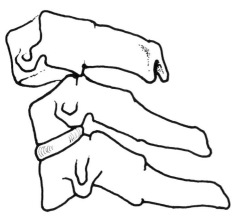

Figure 4–282. Unilateral locked facets. Diagrammatic representation of unilateral locking of articular processes. To accomplish this, an element of rotation must be present. The degree of anterior subluxation is usually 25% or less.

tures above and below the dislocation may be typical of this injury. A triangular fracture of the anterosuperior corner of the vertebra is more common in association with unilateral than bilateral locked facets.

Bilateral facet locking is more frequent than unilateral locking and is a more serious injury clinically. Anterior vertebral displacement is around 50% or greater with bilateral locked facets[18, 520] and usually is less than 25% with unilateral locked facets.[254] In addition, anterior vertebral displacement is often mild with unilateral locked facets.

The characteristic radiographic features of unilateral and bilateral facet locking are best appreciated on the oblique views, which demonstrate loss of overlapping of the laminae. On the lateral view, the locked facet is easier to detect with bilateral locking than with unilateral locking. With unilateral facet locking, the vertebrae below the displacement appear on the lateral radiograph in perfect lateral projection with a single posterior vertebral margin, and the rotated vertebrae above the dislocation demonstrate a narrow double posterior vertebral margin or other signs of rotation (Fig. 4–283). In addition, the superior articular process of the locked vertebra forms a "bow tie," or double facet, configuration with the corresponding locked inferior articular process of the vertebra above (see Fig. 4–283B). This latter radiographic sign is sometimes difficult to appreciate on the lateral radiograph but should be carefully searched for if there are vertebral displacement and double-appearing posterior vertebral margins above the level of vertebral displacement. The triangular-shaped fractures are best viewed on the lateral radiograph.

With bilateral locked facets, there is anterior subluxation of around 50% or more of the vertebral surface,[520] and the locked facets are more easily identified on the lateral view (Fig. 4–284). No "bow tie," or double-appearing, posterior vertebral walls are present, since there is no rotary component in this injury.

On the AP radiograph of patients with unilateral locked facets, the spinous process above facet locking is lateral from the midline toward the side of the locked facet[117] owing to the rotational component of this injury.[1126] This sign is present in only one third of cases[1126] and may not be present if

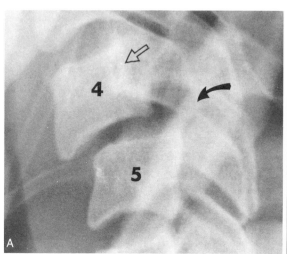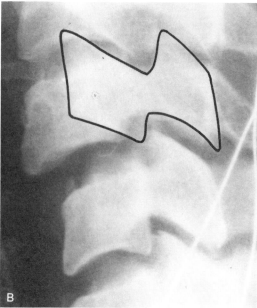

Figure 4–283. Unilateral locked facet of C4–C5. *A,* There is unilateral locking of the C4–C5 articular processes (curved arrow) as well as anterior subluxation, which is about 25% of the vertebral surface. The asymmetry of the posterior elements of C4 (straight arrow) compared with the normal-appearing posterior margin of C5 indicates an element of rotation. The so-called bow tie appearance is evident but is better demonstrated as outlined in *B.*

the spinous process is fractured.[449] With bilateral locked articular facets, there is little or no displacement of the spinous processes from the midline. Bilateral locked facet is considered an unstable injury, but unilateral locked facet is considered stable.[664]

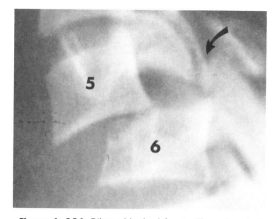

Figure 4–284. Bilateral locked facets. There is anterior displacement of C5 on C6 slightly greater than 50% of the vertebral surface. The superior articular processes of C6 are locked behind the inferior articular processes of C5 (arrow). The posterior surfaces of both vertebral bodies are uniform, and there is no evidence of rotation.

Hyperflexion Fracture Dislocation ("Teardrop")

In this injury, hyperflexion and axial compression cause the vertebra above to crush the vertebra below. There is an accompanying triangular fracture of the anteroinferior vertebral corner or, more commonly, a larger triangular or quadrilateral fracture of the anterior aspect of the vertebral body.[449, 720, 1132] (Fig. 4–285). This anterior fracture fragment has been called the "teardrop" fracture.[1132] A sagittal vertical fracture may be present in about 67% of cases, indicating a component of compression.[719, 1050] With dissipation of the force of injury, the vertebra remains displaced posteriorly, and the anterior fragment is displaced anteriorly. This injury is considered unstable.[664, 1132] The anterior aspect of the spinal cord is injured either by destruction of a portion of the cord or by compression from displaced bone or disc tissue.[1132]

Radiographically, the "teardrop" fracture and the fracture of the anterior aspect of the vertebra are easily identified on the lateral radiograph. The anterior triangular or quadrilateral fragment is displaced forward and

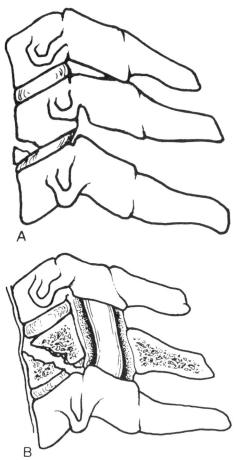

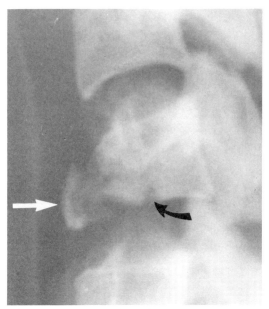

Figure 4–286. Hyperflexion fracture dislocation of C5. There is a comminuted fracture of C5 with a triangular-shaped "teardrop" fracture fragment (straight arrow). The fracture extends to the inferior vertebral surface (curved arrow). The posterior fracture fragment is displaced posteriorly, encroaching on the spinal canal.

Figure 4–285. Hyperflexion ("teardrop") fracture dislocation. Diagrammatic representation. *A*, There is a triangular-shaped fracture of the anteroinferior corner of the vertebral body. The vertebra is displaced posteriorly, and there is narrowing of the intervertebral disc below. *B*, A larger triangular-shaped fracture of the anterior aspect of the vertebral body. The major posterior fracture fragment is displaced posteriorly and encroaches on the spinal cord. The intervertebral disc below is diminished in height.

[1196] which is aided by the normal kyphosis of the thoracic spine. Pure compression acting on a kyphotic curve would result in the same type of injury. Flexion compression injury causes stress on the anterior column,

downward, and the large posterior fracture fragment is displaced posteriorly into the spinal canal and angled inferiorly (Figs. 4–286 and 4–287). The involved vertebra is compressed, and the intervertebral disc is narrow. Soft tissue changes of edema or hemorrhage or both are noted in the prevertebral area.

Thoracolumbar Spine

Compression Flexion (Wedge Fracture)

Most fractures of the thoracolumbar spine are due to compression flexion trauma,[584.]

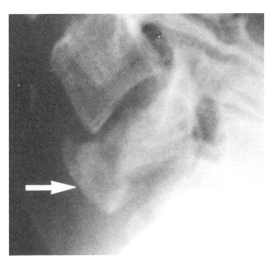

Figure 4–287. Hyperflexion fracture dislocation of C7. There is a compression fracture of C7, with the anterior aspect of C7 displaced anteriorly as a quadrilateral "teardrop" fracture fragment (arrow).

which may lead to collapse (wedge fracture),[583] while sparing the middle column.[386]
The posterior column may also be spared,
but if the compression flexion force is great
enough, there will be tension (distraction) of
the posterior column,[278, 386] with subluxation,
dislocation, or fracture dislocation of articular processes, as well as progression of
spinal deformity.[386] Usually this occurs if
the degree of anterior collapse is greater than
50% of the vertebral body height.[386] Wedge
fracture is the most frequent type of spinal
fracture. It occurs at all ages, but the incidence increases with age as the rate of osteopenia rises. Wedge fractures of the thoracolumbar spine may occur in patients who
jump from heights or fall.[1185] They usually
occur in the thoracolumbar region (T12–L1),
although the C7–T1 junction is another common site of wedge fracture.[449] In the lower
lumbar spine, a compression force acts more
toward the center of the vertebral body because of the normal lordosis. Consequently
a fracture may appear as a central vertebral
depression.

Radiographically, in the thoracic and thoracolumbar regions the anterior depression
of the vertebral body (wedge vertebra) is
usually less than 50% of the vertebral
height[386] (see Fig. 4–247). The middle and
posterior columns are intact, so the height
of the posterior vertebral body (middle column) is normal.[278] The interspinous distance
is slightly increased on the lateral projection.
There is no subluxation. This type of injury
is considered stable, since the middle and
posterior columns are spared[277] and there is
no further progression of spinal deformity.[386]
Lateral flexion compression forces may produce lateral wedging of the vertebral body.[277]

Vertical Compression (Burst Fracture)

In this injury, both the anterior and middle
columns fail under axial loading.[277, 278, 386]
The nucleus pulposus of the intervertebral
disc is driven into the vertebral body below,
which "explodes,"[583] leading to severe comminution of the vertebral body and fracture
of one (usually superior) or both vertebral
end-plates.[277] The posterior wall of the vertebral body is tilted, and the fragment is
displaced posteriorly into the spinal canal.[278]
There may be widening of the interpedicular
distance, a vertical fracture of the lamina,

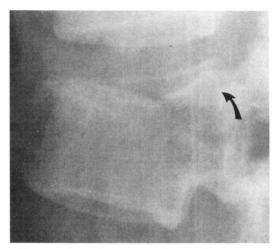

Figure 4–288. Compression "burst" fracture of L1.
There is compression of the superior aspect of L1 vertebral body with posterosuperior displacement of the
posterior fracture fragment (arrow).

and splaying of the facet joints;[277] however,
the posterior spinous ligaments remain intact.

Radiographically, loss of vertebral height
(compression) is seen, with normal or increased height of the posterior vertebral
margin[386] (Fig. 4–288; see also Fig. 4–258).
There is comminution of the superior half
of the vertebral body as well as a sagittally
oriented fracture in the inferior half.[493] The
retropulsed fragment from the posterosuperior aspect of the vertebral body may rotate
by as much as 150 degrees, with the cartilaginous end-plate facing anteriorly, and
may be displaced up to 8 mm in the cranial
or caudal direction. Almost all of the retropulsed fragments separate from the vertebral
body in its midportion posteriorly at the
level of the basivertebral groove. These observations are best appreciated through computed tomography[493] or conventional tomography.[699] The interpedicular distance may be
widened. Rarely, the fracture is from the
posteroinferior corner and rotated clockwise, suggesting that it remains attached to
the annulus fibrosus.[699]

This lesion is considered unstable[277, 386]
even though it may be present without neurologic deficit in over one half of the cases.[277]
With the weight-bearing function of the middle column already compromised, axial
loading of the spine may cause the middle
column to be forced deeper into the spinal
canal.[386] Progressive widening may be ob-

served in patients wearing a cast in the standing position. This could be an ominous sign of impending neurologic deficit during follow-up.[277]

Seat Belt Injuries

Lap Belt Injuries

In this injury, a person wearing a lap-type seat belt is subjected to sudden deceleration.* At impact, the body above the lap belt is hurled forward in hyperflexion while the body below the belt is restrained[1196] (Fig. 4–289). Since the lap belt is applied adjacent to the abdominal wall, the fulcrum of the injury is far more anterior than normal and is situated at the anterior abdominal wall rather than at the intervertebral disc. The fulcrum of injury is far anterior to the vertebral column, so the entire vertebral complex is under tension and distracted.[1068, 1196] There is failure of the posterior and middle columns under tension, initiated by flexion at the anterior column and sometimes by additional distraction[277]—a flexion distraction type of injury.[386] A similar injury may occur from injuries in which the body is thrust forward against a horizontal object, such as a fence.[1196]

Disruption of the posterior ligaments and facet joints occurs. However, if the ligaments remain intact, a transverse fracture occurs in the posterior elements and sometimes extends into the vertebral body.[1068] The dis-

*Reference numbers 274, 277, 361, 386, 495, 590, 1068, 1196.

traction begins in the posterior column and often extends into the anterior column. The anterior part of the anterior column may fail in compression, but it continues to act as a hinge[278] if the anterior longitudinal ligament remains intact. This type of lesion is unstable in flexion. It is not associated with subluxation[278] or acute neurologic compromise.[277]

However, if the distraction forces additionally tear the entire annulus fibrosus, the vertebra above may subluxate on the vertebra below. This is accompanied by stretching (without tearing) of the anterior longitudinal ligament.[277] The lesion is then unstable,[631] and neurologic compromise is proportional to the degree of subluxation. There is potential for progression of deformity and neurologic compromise in these lesions.[386] This latter type of lesion is then classified under the category of fracture dislocation.[277] The variations of the basic seat belt injuries in the lumbar region are due to various force vectors that occur at the time of rapid deceleration.[1196] These are determined by the speed and direction of the vehicle, the position of the individual, and other factors.

It should be appreciated that the force of injury may be so great that bone may be

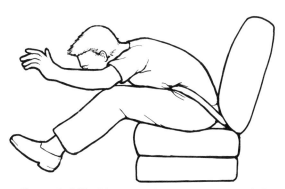

Figure 4–289. Diagrammatic representation of the mechanism of injury of the seat (lap) belt injury. Sudden deceleration causes the body above the seat belt to hurl forward. The fulcrum of injury is on the anterior abdominal wall.

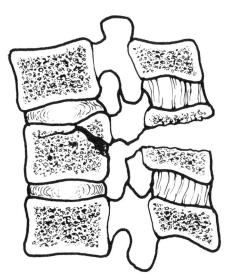

Figure 4–290. Chance fracture. There is a fracture through the spinous process extending into the postero-superior aspect of the vertebral body. The fracture fragments of the spinous process are distracted. The interspinous ligaments remain intact.

pulled apart or ripped by the distraction force.[1196] In addition, one half of the patients that sustain this type of injury have intra-abdominal injuries.[495]

Chance Fracture. The Chance fracture consists of a horizontal fracture of the neural arch, which extends anteriorly to involve the posterosuperior aspect of the vertebral body[192] (Fig. 4–290). There is widening of the interspinous distance as well as increased height in the neural foramina.

Smith Fracture. In the Smith fracture, rupture of the supraspinous and interspinous ligaments occurs (Figs. 4–291 and 4–292). The force of injury may produce varying findings. The fracture may continue anteriorly and rupture the ligamentum flavum,

joint capsule, posterior longitudinal ligament, and intervertebral disc (Fig. 4–291A); rupture the ligamentum flavum and joint capsule and avulse the posteroinferior aspect of the vertebral body (Fig. 4–291B); avulse the superior articular process (sparing the joint capsule); and rupture the posterior longitudinal ligament and intervertebral disc[1196] (Fig. 4–291C). This injury produces widening of the interspinous distance and increase in height of the neural foramina as the vertebrae are distracted.

Horizontal "Splitting" Fracture. Another form of lap belt fracture dislocation involves horizontal splitting of the vertebral arch and vertebral body[590] (Figs. 4–293 and 4–294). The posterior ligaments remain intact.

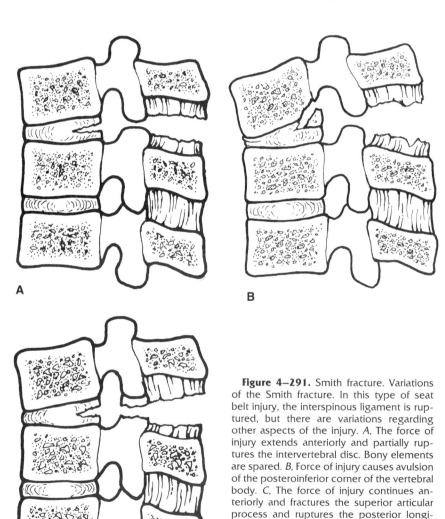

A

B

C

Figure 4–291. Smith fracture. Variations of the Smith fracture. In this type of seat belt injury, the interspinous ligament is ruptured, but there are variations regarding other aspects of the injury. A, The force of injury extends anteriorly and partially ruptures the intervertebral disc. Bony elements are spared. B, Force of injury causes avulsion of the posteroinferior corner of the vertebral body. C, The force of injury continues anteriorly and fractures the superior articular process and ruptures the posterior longitudinal ligament and intervertebral disc.

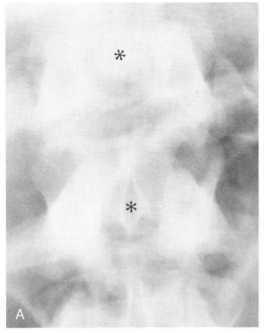

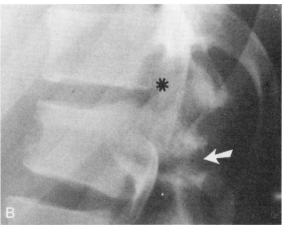

Figure 4–292. Smith fracture. *A*, Anteroposterior view demonstrating widening of the interspinous distance due to distraction injury (asterisks). The spinous processes are intact. *B*, Lateral radiograph demonstrating widening of the neural foramen (asterisk) and a horizontal fracture of the posterior elements (arrow) extending to the posterosuperior aspect of the vertebral body. There is slight anterior compression of the vertebral body. (Courtesy of Dr. Robert Kricun, Allentown, Pennsylvania.)

Lap-Sash Belt Injuries

Lap-sash belt injuries result from impact against the sash.[361] These lesions are infrequent and occasionally may cause serious injury. Lap-sash belt injuries include flexion extension fractures of the lower cervical vertebrae, fractures of the spinous and transverse processes of the lower cervical and upper thoracic vertebrae, rupture of the intervertebral disc, and avulsion of the brachial plexus.

Fracture Dislocations

Fracture dislocations are the most unstable thoracolumbar injuries in that all three columns fail under combinations of compression, tension, rotation, and shear.[277] This failure leads to subluxation or dislocation, which are both pathognomonic signs of fracture dislocation[278] (Figs. 4–295 and 4–296). Most fracture dislocations of the thoracolumbar spine result from a force applied to the dorsal aspect of the thoracic spine.[280]

With a flexion rotation type of injury, the posterior ligaments rupture, one or both articular processes fracture,[584] and the middle column fails.[277] The anterior column also fails, and vertebral wedging develops. The anterior longitudinal ligament is stripped from the vertebral body, whereas all other ligaments are usually torn by the rotational component of the injury.[277, 386] The force of rotation may go through the disc or through the vertebral body.[277]

Radiographically, subluxation or disloca-

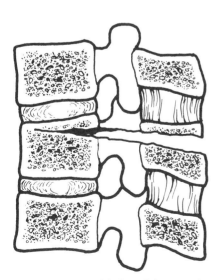

Figure 4–293. Horizontal (splitting) fracture. There is a fracture through the spinous process extending anteriorly into the vertebral body in a horizontal fashion. Separation of spinous process fracture fragments is noted.

252 • CONVENTIONAL RADIOGRAPHY

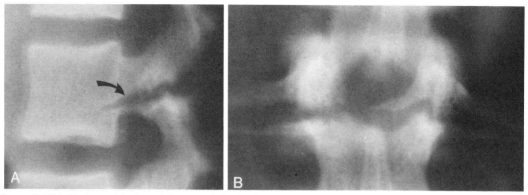

Figure 4–294. Horizontal (splitting) fracture of the lumbar spine. Conventional tomographic examination. *A,* Lateral view demonstrates a fracture (arrow) through the posterior elements extending into the vertebral body. Slight distraction of fracture fragments is noted. *B,* Anteroposterior view demonstrates a horizontal fracture through the posterior elements and transverse processes.

tion is seen, as are increase in the interspinous distance and displacement of a fracture of the superior articular process, which indicates rotation.[278] (see Fig. 4–295). A split fracture through the vertebral body may be evident if the rotation occurred there. There are often associated fractures of the ribs and transverse processes.[277]

With a shear type of fracture dislocation, all three columns are disrupted, including the anterior longitudinal ligament.[277] The subluxation or dislocation may be anterior or posterior. Vertebral bodies may even be intact without loss of height. In the posteroanterior shear injury, there is fracture of the posterior arch and spinous processes of the vertebra above and of the superior articular processes of the vertebra below. Some-

times with posterior shearing force, the lower vertebra is displaced anteriorly.[280] In the anteroposterior shear injury, all ligaments rupture, and either the bony structures remain intact or the spinous processes fracture.[277]

With fracture dislocation injuries, the spinal cord is severely compressed and often severed, causing paraplegia[699] (see Fig. 4–296). With the shear type of injury, patients usually present with paraplegia,[277] although cases of total dislocation without paraplegia or cases that demonstrate recovery have been reported.[457, 1244] In most cases of acute injury to the upper thoracic spine associated with paraplegia, a fracture dislocation is present.[1070]

Bilateral locked facets of the thoracic

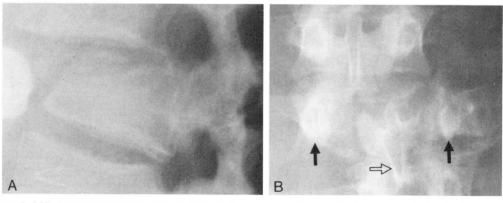

Figure 4–295. Fracture dislocation of L2. *A,* Lateral view demonstrating the fracture and posterior displacement into the spinal canal. There is also anterior displacement of the vertebra above. *B,* Anteroposterior radiograph demonstrating marked fracture dislocation. Widening of the interpedicular distance (closed arrows), indicating fracture of the posterior elements, and displacement of the spinous process (open arrow) are shown. These findings are more striking compared with the lateral radiograph in this case.

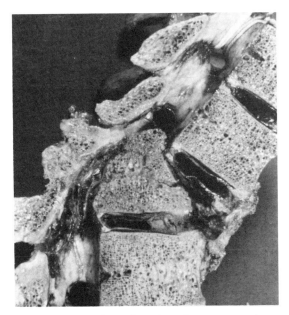

Figure 4–296. Sagittal section of a gross specimen demonstrating fracture dislocation of the spine. There is marked compression of the vertebral body, with posterior displacement into the spinal canal. There is anterior displacement of the spine above with kyphotic deformity. (Courtesy of the Mütter Museum, The College of Physicians of Philadelphia.)

sacrum may be associated with neurologic deficit[550, 1310] in 25% of cases,[1129] although clinical signs may be delayed.[173]

Fractures of the sacrum may be classified as transverse or vertical.[1310] Vertical sacral fractures almost invariably occur with severe injury to the pelvic ring, so that sacral fractures should be sought in the presence of this clinical setting. These sacral fractures are often difficult to detect radiographically, since they are often subtle and masked by overlying bowel gas and feces. Most vertical fractures are unilateral.[449] The margins of the sacral foramina normally appear as smooth arcs that are symmetric in appearance. Disruption of an arc may indicate a subtle underlying fracture. This is best detected on the AP or angled AP radiograph. The lateral margin of the sacrum and the sacral ala are also fairly symmetric, so that cortical disruption might indicate a fracture. Incomplete fusion around distal sacral or coccygeal foramina, a normal variant, should not be mistaken for fracture or bone destruction.

Transverse fractures of the sacrum are rare, occurring in 4% to 5% of all sacral fractures[173] (Fig. 4–297). They may occur in

spine are uncommon observations but should be considered in any patient who sustains a thoracic fracture dislocation injury.[1345] Lumbosacral dislocations,[1012] fracture dislocations,[262, 559] and unilateral facet dislocation[1385] are rare lesions.

Sacrum

Sacral fractures may be due to direct trauma (gunshot wound, direct blow) or indirect trauma (associated pelvic fractures).[438, 1129] Sacral fractures occur in 44% of pelvic ring fractures[449] and are associated with pelvic fractures in 90% of cases.[1129] In another series, the sacrum or sacroiliac joint was involved in 68% of pelvic fractures.[438] These fractures result as forces are transmitted through the ilium and cause disruption of the pelvic ring both anteriorly and posteriorly. The posterior disruption of the pelvic ring causes vertical sacral fractures or sacroiliac dislocation.[1310] Anterior disruption of the pelvic ring is manifested by fractures or diastasis of the pubic symphysis or fracture of the ischiopubic rami. Any fracture of the

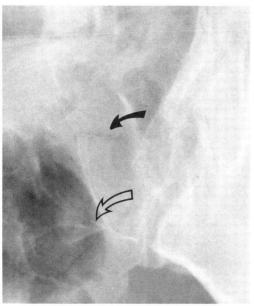

Figure 4–297. Fracture of the sacrum. There is a horizontal radiolucency (closed arrow) that represents a fracture. In addition, there is asymmetry of the arcuate (neural foraminal) line (open arrow). In a traumatic setting, disruption of the arcuate line should alert one to the possibility of an underlying fracture, even though a fracture line may not be visible.

the upper or lower aspect of the sacrum and may be isolated. Those in the upper sacrum usually occur at the S1–S2 level and are really fracture dislocations. The injury usually occurs in younger patients and results from severe traumatic flexion of the upper body on a fixed pelvis.[1310] It should be recalled that the sacral disc spaces begin to ossify from caudad to cephalad, beginning at age 15.[1310] The upper sacral interspace ossifies at 25 years of age, making it more vulnerable to trauma in younger patients.

Lower transverse sacral fractures develop from a direct blow to the coccyx. The fracture usually occurs at the angle of kyphosis of the sacrum; however, any of the lower three sacral vertebrae may be affected.[1310] Transverse fractures of the sacrum are usually detected on the lateral radiograph, and an angled AP radiograph may also demonstrate the fracture line.

Insufficiency fractures develop when the elastic resistance of bone is insufficient to withstand normal stress.[219] It may develop following irradiation or in a number of disorders, such as osteoporosis, osteomalacia, Paget's disease, and uremic osteopathy.[219, 284] These fractures invariably occur in the sacral alae, parallel to the sacroiliac joints, and are lateral to the margins of the lumbar vertebrae.[219] The weight of the body transmitted through the spine may account for the fracture in this typical location.

Radiographically, insufficiency fractures are difficult to detect. They appear as vertical, linear, sclerotic densities in the first through the third sacral segments.[219] Sacral foraminal lines may appear thickened. The sclerosis is bilateral and symmetric in 75% of cases. Occasionally, the fracture may become complete, and the fracture fragment may be displaced.[219] Sacral insufficiency fractures heal readily.[284]

INSTABILITY OF THE SPINE

Defining instability of the spine is fraught with difficulty, for opinions are varied and often conflicting.[892] Lumbar instability may be defined as "the clinical status of the patient with back problems who, with the least provocation, steps from the mildly symptomatic to the severe episode."[671] Or, spinal instability may be defined as increased abnormal spinal movement, whether it be abnormal coupling (combination of movements) or increased abnormal motion[318] under stress.[671] However, not all patients who demonstrate abnormal spinal motion are symptomatic. Abnormal motion may become important if it can be proved to be the cause of the patient's pain syndrome.[318] Some authors consider an abnormal anatomic relationship between adjacent vertebrae a sign of instability,[680] whereas other authors feel that it is abnormal spinal movement, which is determined by measuring the axis of spinal movement, that is important in defining spinal instability.[960] Thus, spinal instability may have a clinical, a "mechanical" definition or both.

Spinal instability may develop secondary to degenerative changes, trauma, spondylo-

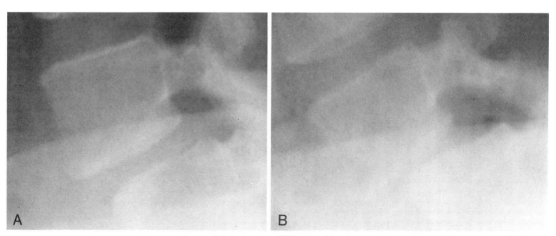

Figure 4–298. Changes in degree of spondylolisthesis of L5–S1 with changes in position of the patient. *A*, Patient is supine. Note the mild degree of anterior slippage. *B*, Patient is standing. The forward slippage of L5 has increased.

lysis, bone destruction, postoperatively, and from other causes. Degeneration of intervertebral discs and facet joints are the most common causes of spinal instability. Instability may develop postoperatively if there is excessive removal of supporting structures. For example, it may develop following removal of 30% to 50% of the facets.[436]

The conventional radiograph may be used in the evaluation for increased abnormal spinal motion in most cases in which the patient is severely symptomatic.[671] Radiographs may be obtained in the flexion, extension, and lateral bending positions. Although the various available measurements of abnormal motion are somewhat inconsistent, misleading, time consuming, and complicated to perform,[318, 671] some are easy to perform and generally reliable. However, the patient's clinical condition, difficulty in identifying anatomic landmarks on the radiographs, and technical factors can interfere with adequate radiographic evaluation.[318]

Ideally, motion should be evaluated in all planes.[892] Flexion and extension radiographs can be obtained with the patient in the lateral decubitus position, and lateral bending films can be obtained with the patient in the supine position.[318] The decubitus and

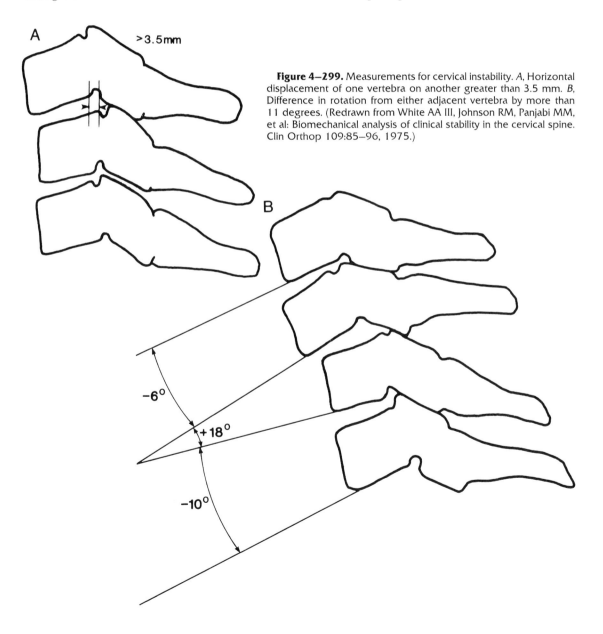

Figure 4–299. Measurements for cervical instability. *A,* Horizontal displacement of one vertebra on another greater than 3.5 mm. *B,* Difference in rotation from either adjacent vertebra by more than 11 degrees. (Redrawn from White AA III, Johnson RM, Panjabi MM, et al: Biomechanical analysis of clinical stability in the cervical spine. Clin Orthop 109:85–96, 1975.)

supine positions may help limit the degree of distortion caused by the patient's pain. Similar views can be obtained with the patient in a standing position,[436, 680] in which the stresses of weight-bearing may accentuate any deformity.[760a]

In both normal flexion and normal extension of the lumbar spine, the bony landmarks for measurement (posterior vertebral corners) remain aligned. The angles and axes of spinal movement can be determined.[960] With normal flexion, the vertebral bodies move very slightly forward in flexion and very slightly backward in extension.[459] The height of the anterior intervertebral disc is decreased, and the posterior height is increased. Increase in disc height greater than 25% to 30% of the resting disc height should be considered abnormal.[671] This increase could possibly be masked by the compression experienced in the standing position. Abnormal motion produced by flexion usually presents with anterior displacement of the vertebral body[436] (Fig. 4–298). However, posterior displacement (opposing the direction of flexion) may occur.[680]

In normal lateral bending, the lateral vertebral margins are in alignment. The normal motion of lateral bending consists of the coupling (combination) of rotation and vertebral body tilt.[671] The vertebral bodies rotate away from the site of bending, and the spinous processes move toward and fall within the opposite (concave) side of the spinal curve.[318, 671] Intervertebral disc spaces narrow on the concave side.[671] The degree of rotation is smooth, as evidenced by progressive displacement of the pedicles relative to the margin of the vertebral body. Radiographic signs of increased abnormal motion during lateral bending include lateral displacement (translation) of one vertebra on the adjacent vertebra; malalignment of spinous process and pedicles; abnormal disc narrowing on the ipsilateral side of bending; decreased bending, with loss of vertebral rotation and tilt, and widening of the disc space on the side of bending; and bending to one side to a greater degree than the other side.[671]

Another radiographic sign of instability may be the so-called horizontal ("traction") spur seen on the lateral radiograph.[770] However, this has not been correlated experimentally.

In the cervical spine, instability is immi-

nent or exists if there is more than 3.5 mm of horizontal displacement of one vertebra on the adjacent vertebra, or if there is more than 11 degrees of rotational difference to either adjacent vertebra[1333] (Fig. 4–299).

ACKNOWLEDGMENTS

I am extremely grateful to Patricia Cephas, Henry Way, and Susan Schrader for the manuscript preparation; to Steve Strommer, G. Douglas Thayer, and Juanitta James for the excellent photographic images; and to Lynn Reynolds for the superb medical illustrations.

References

1. Abdelwahab IF, Frankel VH, Klein MJ: Aggressive osteoblastoma of the third lumbar vertebra: case report 351. Skeletal Radiol 15:164–169, 1986.
2. Abel MS: The exaggerated supine oblique view of the cervical spine. Skeletal Radiol 8:213–219, 1982.
3. Abel MS: Occult Traumatic Lesions of the Cervical and Thoraco-lumbar Vertebrae. With an evaluation of the role of CT, 2nd ed. St. Louis: WH Green, Inc, 1983.
4. Abel MS: The radiology of chronic neck pain: sequelae of occult traumatic lesions. CRC Crit Rev Diagn Imaging 20:27–78, 1983.
5. Abel MS, Smith GR: Visualization of the posterolateral elements of the lumbar vertebrae in the anteroposterior projection. Radiology 122:824–825, 1977.
6. Abel MS, Smith GR, Allen TNK: Refinements of the anteroposterior angled caudad view of the lumbar spine. Skeletal Radiol 7:113–118, 1981.
7. Abrahamson MA: Disseminated asymptomatic osteosclerosis with features resembling melorheostosis, osteopoikilosis, and osteopathia striata. J Bone Joint Surg 50A:991–996, 1968.
8. Ackermann W, Schwartz GS: Non-neoplastic sclerosis in vertebral bodies. Cancer 11:703–708, 1958.
9. Afshani E, Girdany BR: Atlantoaxial dislocation in chondrodysplasia punctata. Report of the findings in two brothers. Radiology 102:399–401, 1972.
10. Agha FP, Norman A, Hirschl S, et al: Paget's disease. NJ State J Med 76:734–735, 1976.
11. Aitken RE, Kerr JL, Lloyd HM: Primary hyperparathyroidism with osteosclerosis and calcification in articular cartilage. Am J Med 37:813–820, 1964.
12. Akbarnia BA, Rooholamini SA: Scoliosis caused by benign osteoblastoma of the thoracic or lumbar spine. J Bone Joint Surg 63A:1146–1155, 1981.
13. Alarcón-Segovia D, Cetina JA, Díaz-Jouanen E: Sacroiliac joints in primary gout. Clinical and roentgenographic study of 143 patients. AJR 118:438–443, 1973.
14. Alenghat JP, Hallett M, Kido DK: Spinal cord

compression in diffuse idiopathic skeletal hyperostosis. Radiology 142:119–120, 1982.

15. Alexander CJ: The aetiology of juvenile spondylarthritis (discitis). Clin Radiol 21:178–187, 1970.
16. Alexander E Jr, Kelly DL Jr, David CH Jr, et al: Intact arch spondylolisthesis: a review of 50 cases and description of surgical treatment. J Neurosurg 63:840–844, 1985.
17. Allbrook DB: Changes in lumbar vertebral body height with age. Am J Phys Anthropol 14:35–39, 1956.
18. Allen BL Jr, Ferguson RL, Lehmann TR, et al: A mechanistic classification of closed indirect fractures and dislocations of the lower cervical spine. Spine 7:1–27, 1982.
19. Allen EH, Cosgrove D, Millard FJC: The radiological changes in infections of the spine and their diagnostic value. Clin Radiol 29:31–40, 1978.
20. Alpar EK, Karpinski M: Late stability of the cervical spine. Arch Orthop Trauma Surg 104:224–226, 1985.
21. Altner PC, Simmons DJ, Lucas HF Jr, et al: Osteogenic sarcoma in a patient injected with Thorotrast. J Bone Joint Surg 54A:670–675, 1972.
22. Amato M, Totty WG, Gilula LA: Spondylolysis of the lumbar spine: demonstration of defects and laminal fragmentation. Radiology 153:627–629, 1984.
23. Ameli NO, Abbassioun K, Saleh H, et al: Aneurysmal bone cysts of the spine: report of 17 cases. J Neurosurg 63:685–690, 1985.
24. Amenta PS, Stead J, Kricun ME: Isolated cryptococcus neoformans osteomyelitis of femur: case report 226. Skeletal Radiol 9:263–265, 1983.
25. Amis J, Herring JA: Iatrogenic kyphosis: a complication of Harrington instrumentation in Marfan's syndrome: a case report. J Bone Joint Surg 66A:460–464, 1984.
26. Amorosa JK, Weintraub S, Amorosa LF, et al: Sacral destruction: foraminal lines revisited. AJR 145:773–775, 1985.
27. Amuso SA: Diastrophic dwarfism. J Bone Joint Surg 50A:113–122, 1968.
28. Andersen PE Jr, Andersen PE, van der Kooy P: Dose reduction in radiography of the spine in scoliosis. Acta Radiol [Diagn] 23:251–253, 1982.
29. Anderson LD, D'Alonzo RT: Fractures of the odontoid process of the axis. J Bone Joint Surg 56A:1663–1674, 1974.
30. Anderson RE, Shealy CN: Cervical pedicle erosion and rootlet compression caused by a tortuous vertebral artery. Radiology 96:537–538, 1970.
31. Anderton JM, Owen R: Absence of the pituitary gland in a case of congenital sacral agenesis: J Bone Joint Surg 65B:182–183, 1983.
32. Ansell BM, Kent PA: Radiological changes in juvenile chronic polyarthritis. Skeletal Radiol 1:129–144, 1977.
33. Antoku S, Russell WJ: Dose to the active bone marrow, gonads, and skin from roentgenography and fluoroscopy. Radiology 101:669–678, 1971.
34. Aoki J, Yamamoto I, Hino M, et al: Sclerotic bone metastasis: radiologic-pathologic correlation. Radiology 159:127–132, 1986.
35. Appleby A, Stabler J: A new sign of spondylolisthesis. Clin Radiol 20:315–319, 1969.
36. Aprin H, Riseborough EJ, Hall JE: Chondrosarcoma in children and adolescents. Clin Orthop 166:226–232, 1982.
37. Arcomano JP, Karas S: Congenital absence of the lumbosacral articular processes. Skeletal Radiol 8:133–134, 1982.
38. Ardran GM: Bone destruction not demonstrable by radiography. Br J Radiol 24:107–109, 1951.
39. Arkin AM, Katz JF: The effects of pressure on epiphyseal growth: the mechanism of plasticity of growing bone. J Bone Joint Surg 38A:1056–1076, 1956.
40. Arnoldi CC, Brodsky AE, Cauchoix J, et al: Lumbar spinal stenosis and nerve root entrapment syndromes: definition and classification. Clin Orthop 115:4–5, 1976.
41. Ashby DW, Ramage D: Lesions of the vertebrae and innominate bones in tuberous sclerosis. Br J Radiol 30:274–277, 1957.
42. Aspin N: The gonadal x-ray dose to children from diagnostic radiographic techniques. Radiology 85:944–951, 1965.
43. Atkinson R, Ghelman B, Tsairis P, et al: Sarcoidosis presenting as cervical radiculopathy: a case report and literature review. Spine 7:412–416, 1982.
44. Aurori BF, Weierman RJ, Lowell HA, et al: Pseudarthrosis after spinal fusion for scoliosis. Clin Orthop 199:153–158, 1985.
45. Azouz EM, Chan JD, Wee R: Spondylolysis of the cervical vertebrae: report of three cases, with a review of the English and French literature. Radiology 111:315–318, 1974.
46. Baastrup CI: On the spinous processes of the lumbar vertebrae and the soft tissues between them, and on pathological changes in that region. Acta Radiol 14:52–55, 1933.
47. Babhulkar SS, Tayade WB, Babhulkar SK: Atypical spinal tuberculosis. J Bone Joint Surg 66B:239–242, 1984.
48. Bailey DK: The normal cervical spine in infants and children. Radiology 59:712–719, 1952.
49. Bailey HL, Gabriel M, Hodgson AR, et al: Tuberculosis of the spine in children: operative findings and results in one hundred consecutive patients treated by removal of the lesion and anterior grafting. J Bone Joint Surg 54A: 1633–1657, 1972.
50. Bailey JA II: Orthopaedic aspects of achondroplasia. J Bone Joint Surg 52A:1285–1301, 1970.
51. Baker AS, Dove J: Progressive scoliosis as the first presenting sign of syringomyelia: report of a case. J Bone Joint Surg 65B:472–473, 1983.
52. Balasubramanian E, Keim HA, Hajdu M: Osteoid osteoma of the thoracic spine with surgical decompression aided by somatosensory evoked potentials. Spine 10:396–398, 1985.
53. Bank WO, Kerlan RK Jr, Kesselring LW: Improved lateral cervical spine radiography through halo traction device. AJR 137:29–30, 1981.
54. Banna M, Gryspeerdt GL: Intraspinal tumors in children (excluding dysraphism). Clin Radiol 22:17–32, 1971.
55. Banna M, Stevenson GW, Tumiel A: Unilateral atlanto-occipital dislocation complicating an anomaly of the atlas. J Bone Joint Surg 65A:685–687, 1983.
56. Bardsley JL, Hanelin LG: The unilateral hypo-

plastic lumbar pedicle. Radiology 101:315–317, 1971.

57. Barnes DA, Borns P, Pizzutillo PD: Cervical spondylolisthesis associated with the multiple nevoid basal cell carcinoma syndrome. Clin Orthop 162:26–30, 1982.

58. Barnett E, Nordin BEC: The radiological diagnosis of osteoporosis: a new approach. Clin Radiol 11:166–174, 1960.

59. Barry WF Jr, Wells SA Jr, Cox CE, et al: Clinical and radiographic correlations in breast cancer patients with osseous metastases. Skeletal Radiol 6:27–32, 1981.

60. Barton CJ, Cockshott WP: Bone changes in hemoglobin SC disease. AJR 88:523–532, 1962.

61. Barwick KW, Huvos AG, Smith J: Primary osteogenic sarcoma of the vertebral column: a clinicopathologic correlation of ten patients. Cancer 46:595–604, 1980.

62. Batson OV: The vertebral vein system. AJR 78:195–212, 1957.

63. Baylin GL, Wear JM: Blastomycosis and actinomycosis of the spine. AJR 69:395–398, 1953.

64. Beabout JW, McLeod RA, Dahlin DC: Benign tumors. Semin Roentgenol 14:33–43, 1979.

65. Beachley MC, Lau BP, King ER: Bone involvement in Hodgkin's disease. AJR 114:559–563, 1972.

66. Beals RK: Homocystinuria: a report of two cases and review of the literature. J Bone Joint Surg 51A:1564–1572, 1969.

67. Beals RK: Nosologic and genetic aspects of scoliosis. Clin Orthop 93:23–32, 1973.

68. Becker JA: Hemoglobin S-C disease. AJR 88:503–511, 1962.

69. Beeler JW: Further evidence on the acquired nature of spondylolysis and spondylolisthesis. AJR 108:796–798, 1970.

70. Begg AC: Nuclear herniations of the intervertebral disc. Their radiological manifestations and significance. J Bone Joint Surg 36B:180–193, 1954.

70a. Beguiristain JL, de Pablos J, Llombart R, et al: Discitis due to Clostridium perfringens. Spine 11:170–172, 1986.

71. Beighton P, Thomas ML: The radiology of the Ehlers-Danlos syndrome. Clin Radiol 20:354–361, 1969.

72. Bell D, Cockshott WP: Tuberculosis of the vertebral pedicles. Radiology 99:43–48, 1971.

73. Bellamy R, Lieber A, Smith SD: Congenital spondylolisthesis of the sixth cervical vertebra: case report and description of operative findings. J Bone Joint Surg 56A:405–407, 1974.

74. Bellon EM, Kaufman B, Tucker ME: Hypertrophic neuropathy. Plain film and myelographic changes. Radiology 103:319–322, 1972.

75. Benson WR, Bass S Jr: Chondromyxoid fibroma: first report of occurrence of this tumor in vertebral column. Am J Clin Pathol 25:1290–1292, 1955.

76. Benzian SR, Mainzer F, Gooding CA: Pediculate thinning: a normal variant at the thoracolumbar junction. Br J Radiol 44:936–939, 1971.

77. Berk RN, Brower TD: Vertebral sarcoidosis. Radiology 82:660–663, 1964.

78. Berkheiser EJ, Seidler F: Nontraumatic dislocations of the atlanto-axial joint. JAMA 96:517–523, 1931.

79. Bernstein SA: Acute cervical pain associated with soft-tissue calcium deposition anterior to the interspace of the first and second cervical vertebrae. J Bone Joint Surg 57A:426–428, 1975.

80. Berrettoni BA, Carter JR: Mechanisms of cancer metastasis to bone. J Bone Joint Surg 68A:308–312, 1986.

81. Bethem D: Os odontoideum in chondrodystrophia calcificans congenita. A case report. J Bone Joint Surg 64A:1385–1386, 1982.

82. Bethem D, Winter RB, Lutter L: Disorders of the spine in diastrophic dwarfism: a discussion of nine patients and review of the literature. J Bone Joint Surg 62A:529–536, 1980.

83. Bethem D, Winter RB, Lutter L, et al: Spinal disorders of dwarfism: review of the literature and report of eighty cases. J Bone Joint Surg 63A:1412–1425, 1981.

84. Bhansali SK, Desai PB: Ewing's sarcoma. Observations on 107 cases. J Bone Joint Surg 45A:541–553, 1963.

85. Bick EM: Vertebral osteophytosis: pathologic basis of its roentgenology. AJR 73:979–983, 1955.

86. Bick EM: Vertebral growth: its relation to spinal abnormalities in children. Clin Orthop 21:43–48, 1961.

87. Bick EM, Copel JW: Longitudinal growth of the human vertebra. A contribution to human osteogeny. J Bone Joint Surg 32A:803–814, 1950.

88. Bick EM, Copel JW: The ring apophysis of the human vertebra. Contribution to human osteogeny II. J Bone Joint Surg 33A:783–787, 1951.

89. Bielecki DK, Sartoris D, Resnick D, et al: Intraosseous and intradiscal gas in association with spinal infection: report of three cases. AJR 147:83–86, 1986.

90. Billings KJ, Werner LG: Aneurysmal bone cyst of the first lumbar vertebra. Radiology 104:19–20, 1972.

91. Birkenfeld R, Kasdon DL: Congenital lumbar ridge causing spinal claudication in adolescents: report of two cases. J Neurosurg 49:441–444, 1978.

92. Bjersand AJ: Juvenile kyphosis in identical twins. AJR 134:598–599, 1980.

93. Black JR, Ghormley RK, Camp JD: Senile osteoporosis of the spinal column. JAMA 117:2144–2150, 1941.

94. Blair JD, Wells PO: Bilateral undescended scapula associated with omovertebral bone: report of a case. J Bone Joint Surg 39A:201–206, 1957.

95. Blank N, Lieber A: The significance of growing bone islands. Radiology 85:508–511, 1965.

96. Blaquière RM, Guyer PB, Buchanan RB, et al: Sclerotic bone deposits in multiple myeloma. Br J Radiol 55:591–593, 1982.

97. Blaylock RL, Kempe LG: Chondrosarcoma of the cervical spine. Case report. J Neurosurg 44:500–503, 1976.

98. Bluestone R, Bywaters EGL, Hartog M, et al: Acromegalic arthropathy. Ann Rheum Dis 30:243–258, 1971.

99. Bohlman HH: Acute fractures and dislocations of the cervical spine: an analysis of three hundred hospitalized patients and review of the literature. J Bone Joint Surg 61A:1143–1150, 1979.

100. Bohlman HH, Sachs BL, Carter JR, et al: Primary neoplasms of the cervical spine: diagnosis and treatment of twenty-three patients. J Bone Joint Surg 68A:483–494, 1986.

101. Bohrer SP: The annulus vacuum sign. Skeletal Radiol 15:233–235, 1986.
102. Bohrer SP, Klein A, Martin W III: "V" shaped predens space. Skeletal Radiol 14:111–116, 1985.
103. Boijsen E: The cervical spinal canal in intraspinal expansive processes. Acta Radiol 42:101–115, 1954.
104. Boland PJ, Lane JM, Sundaresan N: Metastatic disease of the spine. Clin Orthop 169:95–102, 1982.
105. Bonakdarpour A, Kirkpatrick JA, Renzi A, et al: Skeletal changes in neonatal thyrotoxicosis. Radiology 102:149–150, 1972.
106. Bonakdarpour A, Levy W, Aegerter EE: Osteosclerotic changes in sarcoidosis. AJR 113:646–649, 1971.
107. Bonakdarpour A, Levy WM, Aegerter E: Primary and secondary aneurysmal bone cyst: a radiological study of 75 cases. Radiology 126:75–83, 1978.
108. Bonarigo BC, Rubin P: Nonunion of pathologic fracture after radiation therapy. Radiology 88:889–898, 1967.
109. Bonavita JA, Dalinka MK, Schumacher R Jr: Hydroxyapatite deposition disease. Radiology 134:621–625, 1980.
110. Boone D, Parsons D, Lachmann SM, et al: Spina bifida occulta: lesion or anomaly? Clin Radiol 36:159–161, 1985.
111. Boreadis AG, Gershon-Cohen J: Luschka joints of the cervical spine. Radiology 66:181–187, 1956.
112. Borg SA, Fitzer PM, Young LW: Roentgenologic aspects of adult cretinism: two case reports and review of the literature. AJR 123:820–828, 1975.
113. Borkow SE, Kleiger B: Spondylolisthesis in the newborn: a case report. Clin Orthop 81:73–76, 1971.
114. Boukhris R, Becker KL: Schmorl's nodes and osteoporosis. Clin Orthop 104:275–280, 1974.
115. Bowerman JW, Hughes JL: Radiology of bone grafts. Radiol Clin North Am 13:67–77, 1975.
116. Bowman C, Dieppe P, Settas L: Remission of pseudospondylitis with treatment of Whipple's disease. Br J Rheum 22:181–182, 1983.
117. Braakman R, Vinken PJ: Unilateral facet interlocking in the lower cervical spine. J Bone Joint Surg 49B:249–257, 1967.
118. Brady LW: Radiation-induced sarcomas of bone. Skeletal Radiol 4:72–78, 1979.
119. Bragg DG, Shidnia H, Chu FCH, et al: The clinical and radiographic aspects of radiation osteitis. Radiology 97:103–111, 1970.
120. Brandner ME: Normal values of the vertebral body and intervertebral disc index in adults. AJR 114:411–414, 1972.
121. Braunstein EM: Hodgkin disease of bone: radiographic correlation with the histological classification. Radiology 137:643–646, 1980.
122. Braunstein EM, Hunter LY, Bailey RW: Long term radiographic changes following anterior cervical fusion. Clin Radiol 31:201–203, 1980.
123. Braunstein EM, Martel W, Moidel R: Ankylosing spondylitis in men and women: a clinical and radiographic comparison. Radiology 144:91–94, 1982.
124. Braunstein EM, White SJ: Non-Hodgkin lymphoma of bone. Radiology 135:59–63, 1980.
125. Brekkan A: Radiographic examination of the lumbosacral spine: an "age-stratified" study. Clin Radiol 34:321–324, 1983.
126. Brigode M, Francois RJ, Dory MA: Radiological study of the sacroiliac joints in vertebral ankylosing hyperostosis. Ann Rheum Dis 41:225–231, 1982.
127. Brill PW, Baker DH, Ewing ML: "Bone-within-bone" in the neonatal spine: stress change or normal development. Radiology 108:363–366, 1973.
128. Broderick TW, Resnick D, Goergen TG, et al: Enostosis of the spine. Spine 2:167–170, 1978.
129. Brodey PA, Pripstein S, Strange G, et al: Vertebral sarcoidosis: a case report and review of the literature. AJR 126:900–902, 1976.
130. Brodey PA, Wolff SM: Radiographic changes in the sacroiliac joints in familial Mediterranean fever. Radiology 114:331–333, 1975.
131. Bronsky D, Kushner DS, Dubin A, et al: Idiopathic hypoparathyroidism and pseudohypoparathyroidism: case reports and review of literature. Medicine 37:317–352, 1958.
132. Brooker AEW, Barter RW: Cervical spondylosis. A clinical study with comparative radiology. Brain 88:925–936, 1965.
133. Brookes M: The Blood Supply of Bone. London: Butterworth, 1971.
134. Brower AC, Downey EF Jr: Kümmell disease: report of a case with serial radiographs. Radiology 141:363–364, 1981.
135. Brown MW, Templeton AW, Hodges FJ III: The incidence of acquired and congenital fusions in the cervical spine. AJR 92:1255–1259, 1964.
136. Brown RC, Evans ET: What causes the "eye in the Scotty dog" in the oblique projection of the lumbar spine? AJR 118:435–437, 1973.
137. Brown TS, Paterson CR: Osteosclerosis in myeloma. J Bone Joint Surg 55B:621–623, 1973.
138. Bucholz RW, Burkhead WZ: The pathological anatomy of fatal atlanto-occipital dislocations. J Bone Joint Surg 61A:248–250, 1979.
139. Bucholz RW, Burkhead WZ, Graham W, et al: Occult cervical spine injuries in fatal traffic accidents. J Trauma 19:768–771, 1979.
140. Buden E, Sondheimer F: Lateral spread of the atlas without fracture. Radiology 87:1095–1098, 1966.
141. Bull JWD: Spinal meningiomas and neurofibromas. Acta Radiol 40:283–300, 1953.
142. Bull JWD, Nixon WLB, Prat RTC: The radiological criteria and familial occurrence of primary basilar impression. Brain 78:229–247, 1955.
143. Bulos S: Dysphagia caused by cervical osteophyte. Report of a case. J Bone Joint Surg 56B:148–152, 1974.
144. Bundens DA, Rechtine GR: Sarcoidosis of the spine. Spine 11:209–212, 1986.
145. Buraczewski J, Lysakowska J, Rudowski W: Chondroblastoma (Codman's tumour) of the thoracic spine. J Bone Joint Surg 39B:705–710, 1957.
146. Burgener FA, Perry PE: Solitary renal cell carcinoma metastasis in Paget's disease simulating sarcomatous degeneration. AJR 128:853–855, 1977.
147. Burke SW, French HG, Roberts JM, et al: Chronic atlanto-axial instability in Down syndrome. J Bone Joint Surg 67A:1356–1360, 1985.
148. Burnham J, Fraker K, Steinbach H: Pathologic

fracture in an unusual case of gout. AJR 129:1116–1119, 1977.

149. Burrows EH: The sagittal diameters of the spinal canal in cervical spondylosis. Clin Radiol 14:77–86, 1963.

150. Burton IF, Devine HW: Chondroangiopathia calcarea seu punctata. AJR 88:470–475, 1962.

151. Byrne E, McNeill P, Gilford E, et al: Intradural cyst with compression of the cauda equina in ankylosing spondylitis. Surg Neurol 23:162–164, 1985.

152. Bywaters EGL: Still's disease in the adult. Ann Rheum Dis 30:121–133, 1971.

153. Bywaters EGL, Ansell BM: Arthritis associated with ulcerative colitis. A clinical and pathological study. Ann Rheum Dis 17:169–183, 1958.

154. Bywaters EGL, Hamilton EBD, Williams R: The spine in idiopathic haemochromatosis. Ann Rheum Dis 30:453–465, 1971.

155. Caffey J: Changes in the growing skeleton after the administration of bismuth. Am J Dis Child 53:56–78, 1937.

156. Caffey J: Cooley's erythroblastic anemia: some skeletal findings in adolescents and young adults. AJR 65:547–560, 1951.

157. Caffey J: Gargoylism (Hunter-Hurler disease, dysstosis multiplex, lipochondrodystrophy). Prenatal and neonatal bone lesions and their early postnatal evolution. AJR 67:715–731, 1952.

158. Caffey J: Cooley's anemia: A review of the roentgenographic findings in the skeleton. AJR 78:381–391, 1957.

159. Caffey J: Achondroplasia of pelvis and lumbosacral spine: some roentgenographic features. AJR 80:449–457, 1958.

160. Caffey J: Pediatric X-ray Diagnosis, vol 2, 7th ed. Chicago: Year Book Medical Publishers, Inc, 1978.

161. Cahan WG, Woodard HQ, Higinbotham NL, et al: Sarcoma arising in irradiated bone: report of eleven cases. Cancer 1:3–29, 1948.

162. Caldicott WJH: Diagnosis of spinal osteoid osteoma. Radiology 92:1192–1195, 1969.

163. Calenoff L, Chessare JW, Rogers, LF, et al: Multiple level spinal injuries: importance of early recognition. AJR 130:665–669, 1978.

164. Calhoun JD, Thompson SB: Vertebra plana in children produced by xanthomatous disease. AJR 82:482–489, 1959.

165. Cameron JR, Wochos JF: Patient exposure from diagnostic roentgenograms. JAMA 238:28, 1977.

166. Camins MB, Duncan AW, Smith J, et al: Chondrosarcoma of the spine. Spine 3:202–209, 1978.

167. Campbell CJ, Papademetriou T, Bonfiglio M: Melorheostosis: a report of the clinical, roentgenographic and pathological findings in fourteen cases. J Bone Joint Surg 50A:1281–1303, 1968.

168. Cancelmo JJ Jr: Clay shoveler's fracture. A helpful diagnostic sign. AJR 115:540–543, 1972.

169. Canoso JJ, Saini M, Hermos JA: Whipple's disease and ankylosing spondylitis: simultaneous occurrence in HLA-B27 positive male. J Rheumatol 5:79–84, 1978.

170. Capanna R, Albisinni U, Picci P, et al: Aneurysmal bone cyst of the spine. J Bone Joint Surg 67A:527–531, 1985.

171. Capen DA, Garland DE, Waters RL: Surgical stabilization of the cervical spine: a comparative analysis of anterior and posterior spine fusions. Clin Orthop 196:229–237, 1985.

172. Caplan PS, Freedman LMJ, Connelly TP: Degenerative joint disease of the lumbar spine in coal miners—a clinical and x-ray study. Arthritis Rheum 9:693–702, 1966.

173. Carl A, Delman A, Engler G: Displaced transverse sacral fractures: a case report, review of the literature and the CT scan as an aid in management. Clin Orthop 194:195–198, 1985.

174. Carlson DH, Wilkinson RH, Bhakkaviziam A: Aneurysmal bone cysts in children. AJR 116:644–650, 1972.

175. Carmel PW, Cramer FJ: Cervical cord compression due to exostosis in a patient with hereditary multiple exostoses. J Neurosurg 28:500–503, 1968.

176. Carpenter EB: Normal and abnormal growth of the spine. Clin Orthop 21:49–55, 1961.

177. Carrera GF, Williams AL: Current concepts in evaluation of the lumbar facet joints. CRC Crit Rev Diagn Imaging 21:85–104, 1984.

178. Carroll DS: Roentgen manifestations of sickle cell disease. South Med J 50:1486–1490, 1957.

179. Carson CP, Ackerman LV, Maltby JD: Plasma cell myeloma: a clinical, pathologic and roentgenologic review of 90 cases. Am J Clin Pathol 25:849–888, 1955.

180. Carstens SA, Resnick D: Diffuse sclerotic skeletal metastases as an initial feature of gastric carcinoma. Arch Intern Med 140:1666–1668, 1980.

181. Cassady JR, Berdon WE, Baker DH: The "typical" spine changes of sickle-cell anemia in a patient with thalassemia major (Cooley's anemia). Radiology 89:1065–1068, 1967.

182. Casselman ES, Mandell GA: Vertebral scalloping in neurofibromatosis. Radiology 131:89–94, 1979.

183. Casselman ES, Miller WT, Lin SR, et al: von Recklinghausen's disease: incidence of roentgenographic findings with a clinical review of the literature. CRC Crit Rev Diag Imaging 9:387–419, 1977.

184. Castellvi AE, Goldstein LA, Chan DPK: Lumbosacral transitional vertebrae and their relationship with lumbar extradural defects. Spine 9:493–495, 1984.

185. Cattell HS, Filtzer DL: Pseudosubluxation and other normal variations in the cervical spine in children. J Bone Joint Surg 47A:1295–1309, 1965.

186. Cautilli RA, Joyce MF, Lin PM: Congenital elongation of the pedicles of the sixth cervical vertebra in identical twins. J Bone Joint Surg 54A:653–656, 1972.

187. Chacha PB, Khong BT: Eosinophilic granuloma of bone. A diagnostic problem. Clin Orthop 80:79–88, 1971.

188. Chalmers J, Conacher WDH, Gardner DL, et al: Osteomalacia—a common disease in elderly women. J Bone Joint Surg 49B:403–423, 1967.

189. Chalmers J, Heard BE: A metastasing chordoma: A further note. J Bone Joint Surg 54B:526–529, 1972.

190. Chamberlain WE: Basilar impression (platybasia): a bizarre developmental anomaly of the occipital bone and upper cervical spine with striking and misleading neurologic manifestations. Yale J Biol Med 11:487–496, 1939.

191. Chan HSL, Turner-Gomes SO, Chuang SH, et al: A rare cause of spinal cord compression in childhood from intraspinal mesenchymal chondrosarcoma. Neuroradiology 26:323–327, 1984.

192. Chance CQ: Note on a type of flexion fracture of the spine. Br J Radiol 21:452–453, 1948.
193. Charlton OP, Gehweiler JA Jr, Morgan CL, et al: Spondylolysis and spondylolisthesis of the cervical spine. Skeletal Radiol 3:79–84, 1978.
194. Charlton OP, Martinez S, Gehweiler JA Jr: Pedicle thinning at the thoracolumbar junction: a normal variant. AJR 134:825–826, 1980.
195. Chester W, Chester EM: The vertebral column in acromegaly. AJR 44:552–557, 1940.
196. Chetiyawardana AD: Chordoma: results of treatment. Clin Radiol 35:159–161, 1984.
197. Cheyne C: Histiocytosis X. J Bone Joint Surg 53B:366–382, 1971.
198. Chin WS, Oon CL: Ossification of the posterior longitudinal ligament of the spine. Br J Radiol 52:865–869, 1979.
199. Chleboun J, Nade S: Skeletal cryptococcosis. J Bone Joint Surg 59A:509–514, 1977.
200. Chow SP, Leong JCY, Yau ACMC: Osteoclastoma of the axis. J Bone Joint Surg 59A:550–551, 1977.
201. Christopherson WM, Miller AJ: A re-evaluation of solitary plasma-cell myeloma of bone. Cancer 3:240–252, 1950.
202. Cintron E, Gilula LA, Murphy WA, et al: The widened disk space: a sign of cervical hyperextension injury. Radiology 141:639–644, 1981.
203. Ciric I, Mikhael MA, Tarkington JA, et al: The lateral recess syndrome. J Neurosurg 53:433–443, 1980.
204. Clarisse PDT, Staple TW: Diffuse bone sclerosis in multiple myeloma. Radiology 99:327–328, 1971.
205. Clark CR, White AA III: Fractures of the dens: a multicentric study. J Bone Joint Surg 67A:1340–1348, 1985.
206. Clark RL, Muhletaler CA, Margulies SI: Colitic arthritis. Clinical and radiographic manifestations. Radiology 101:585–594, 1971.
207. Clark WM, Gehweiler JA Jr, Laib R: Twelve significant signs of cervical spine trauma. Skeletal Radiol 3:201–205, 1979.
208. Cloward RB: The anterior approach for removal of ruptured cervical disks. J Neurosurg 15:602–614, 1958.
208a. Cobb JR: Outline for the study of scoliosis. Am Acad Orthop Surg 5:261–275, 1948.
209. Cohen AS, McNeill JM, Calkins E, et al: The "normal" sacroiliac joint: analysis of 88 sacroiliac roentgenograms. AJR 100:559–563, 1967.
210. Cohen DM, Dahlin DC, MacCarty CS: Apparently solitary tumors of the vertebral column. Mayo Clin Proc 39:509–528, 1964.
211. Cohen DM, Svien HJ, Dahlin DC: Long-term survival of patients with myeloma of the vertebral column. JAMA 187:914–917, 1964.
212. Cohen J, Currarino G, Neuhauser EBD: A significant variant in the ossification centers of the vertebral bodies. AJR 76:469–475, 1956.
213. Coley BL, Higinbotham NL, Bowden L: Endothelioma of bone (Ewing's sarcoma). Ann Surg 128:533–560, 1948.
214. Coley BL, Higinbotham NL, Groesbeck HP: Primary reticulum-cell sarcoma of bone. Radiology 55:641–658, 1950.
215. Collins VP: Bone involvement in cryptococcosis (torulosis). AJR 63:102–112, 1950.
216. Coman DR, deLong RP: The role of the vertebral venous system in the metastasis of cancer to the spinal column: experiments with tumor cell suspensions in rats and rabbits. Cancer 4:610–618, 1951.
217. Connor TB, Freijanes J, Stoner RE, et al: Generalized osteosclerosis in primary hyperparathyroidism. Trans Am Clin Climatol Assoc 85:185–201, 1973.
218. Conrad SE, Breivis J, Fried MA: Vertebral osteomyelitis, caused by Arachnia propionica and resembling actinomycosis: report of a case. J Bone Joint Surg 60A:549–553, 1978.
219. Cooper KL, Beabout JW, Swee RG: Insufficiency fractures of the sacrum. Radiology 156:15–20, 1985.
220. Cotler HB, Cotler JM, Cohn HE, et al: Intrathoracic chordoma presenting as a posterior superior mediastinal tumor. Spine 8:781–786, 1983.
221. Cotton GE, Van Puffelen P: Hypophosphatemic osteomalacia secondary to neoplasia. J Bone Joint Surg 68A:129–133, 1986.
222. Coventry MB: Some skeletal changes in the Ehlers-Danlos syndrome: a report of two cases. J Bone Joint Surg 43A:855–860, 1961.
223. Coventry MB: Anatomy of the intervertebral disk. Clin Orthop 67:9–15, 1969.
224. Coventry MB: Calcification in a cervical disc with anterior protrusion and dysphagia: a case report. J Bone Joint Surg 52A:1463–1466, 1970.
225. Coventry MB, Ghormley RK, Kernohan JW: The intervertebral disc: its microscopic anatomy and pathology. Part I: anatomy, development and physiology. J Bone Joint Surg 27:105–112, 1945.
226. Coventry MB, Ghormley RK, Kernohan JW: The intervertebral disc: its microscopic anatomy and pathology. Part II: changes in the intervertebral disc concomitant with age. J Bone Joint Surg 27:233–247, 1945.
227. Coventry MB, Ghormley RK, Kernohan JW: The intervertebral disc: its microscopic anatomy and pathology. Part III: pathological changes in the intervertebral disc. J Bone Joint Surg 27:460–474, 1945.
228. Cowell HR, Hall JN, MacEwen GD: Genetic aspects of idiopathic scoliosis. Clin Orthop 86:121–131, 1972.
229. Cox HE, Bennett WF: Computed tomography of absent cervical pedicle: case report. J Comput Assist Tomogr 8:537–539, 1984.
230. Crock HV: Normal and pathological anatomy of the lumbar spinal nerve root canals. J Bone Joint Surg 63B:487–490, 1981.
231. Crock HV: Anterior lumbar interbody fusion: indications for its use and notes on surgical technique. Clin Orthop 165:157–163, 1982.
232. Crock HV, Yoshizawa H: The blood supply of the lumbar vertebral column. Clin Orthop 115:6–21, 1976.
233. Crosett AD Jr: Calcification of the intervertebral disc in a child. Report of a case following poliomyelitis. J Pediatr 47:481–484, 1955.
234. Custer RP, Ahlfeldt FE: Studies on the structure and function of bone marrow: II. Variations in cellularity in various bones with advancing years of life and their relative response to stimuli. J Lab Clin Med 17:960–962, 1932.
235. Cutler M, Buschke F, Cantril ST: The course of single myeloma of bone: a report of 20 cases. SGO 62:918–932, 1936.
236. D'Aprile P, Krajewska G, Perniola T, et al: Con-

genital dislocation of dens of the axis in a case of neurofibromatosis. Neuroradiology 26:405–406, 1984.

237. Daffner RH: Pseudofracture of the dens: Mach Bands. AJR 128:607–612, 1977.

238. Daffner RH: Visual illusions affecting perception of the roentgen image. CRC Crit Rev Diagn Imaging 20:79–119, 1983.

239. Daffner RH, Deeb ZL, Rothfus WE: Pseudofractures of the cervical vertebral body. Skeletal Radiol 15:295–298, 1986.

240. Daffner RH, Gehweiler JA Jr: Pseudovacuum of the cervical intervertebral disc: a normal variant. AJR 137:737–739, 1981.

241. Dahlin DC: Giant-cell tumor of vertebrae above the sacrum: a review of 31 cases. Cancer 39:1350–1356, 1977.

242. Dahlin DC: Bone Tumor, 3rd ed. Springfield, Illinois: Charles C Thomas, 1978.

243. Dahlin DC, Coventry MB: Osteogenic sarcoma: a study of six hundred cases. J Bone Joint Surg 49A:101–110, 1967.

244. Dahlin DC, Coventry MB, Scanlon PW: Ewing's sarcoma. A critical analysis of 165 cases. J Bone Joint Surg 43A:185–192, 1961.

245. Dahlin DC, Henderson ED: Chondrosarcoma: a surgical and pathological problem. Review of 212 cases. J Bone Joint Surg 38A:1025–1038, 1956.

246. Dahlin DC, Ivins JC: Benign chondroblastoma: a study of 125 cases. Cancer 30:401–413, 1972.

247. Dahlin DC, Johnson EW Jr: Giant osteoid osteoma. J Bone Joint Surg 36A:559–572, 1954.

247a. Dahlin DC, Unni KK, Matsuno T: Malignant (fibrous) histiocytoma of bone—fact or fancy? Cancer 39:1508–1516, 1977.

248. Dahlqvist SR, Nordmark LG, Bjelle A: HLA-B27 and involvement of sacroiliac joints in rheumatoid arthritis. J Rheumatol 11:27–32, 1984.

249. Dale K, Vinje O: Radiography of the spine and sacro-iliac joints in ankylosing spondylitis and psoriasis. Acta Radiol 26:145–159, 1985.

250. Dalinka MK, Aronchick JM, Haddad JG Jr: Paget's disease. Orthop Clin N Am 14:3–19, 1983.

251. Dalinka MK, Bonavita JA: Radiation changes. In Resnick D, Niwayama G (eds): Diagnosis of Bone and Joint Disorders: With Emphasis on Articular Abnormalities, vol 3. Philadelphia: WB Saunders Company, 1981, pp 2341–2362.

252. Dalinka MK, Chunn SP: Osteoblastoma—benign or malignant precursor? report of a case. J Can Assoc Radiol 23:214–216, 1972.

253. Dalinka MK, Greendyke WH: The spinal manifestations of coccidioidomycosis. J Can Assoc Radiol 22:93–99, 1971.

254. Dalinka MK, Kessler H, Weiss M: The radiographic evaluation of spinal trauma. Emerg Med Clin North Am 3:475–490, 1985.

255. Dalinka MK, Lally JF, Koniver G, et al: The radiology of osseous and articular infection. CRC Crit Rev Diagn Imaging 7:1–64, 1975.

256. Dalinka MK, Reginato AJ, Golden DA: Calcium deposition diseases. Semin Roentgenol 17:39–48, 1982.

257. Daniel WW, Barnes GT, Nasca RJ, et al: Segmented-field radiography in scoliosis. AJR 144:325–329, 1985.

258. Danziger J, Bloch S: The widened cervical intervertebral foramen. Radiology 116:671–674, 1975.

259. Danziger J, Jackson H, Bloch S: Congenital absence of a pedicle in a cervical vertebra. Clin Radiol 26:53–56, 1975.

260. Darling BC: The sacro-iliac joint: Its diagnosis as determined by the x-ray. Radiology 3:486–491, 1924.

261. Darling DB, Loridan L, Senior B: The roentgenographic manifestations of Cushing's syndrome in infancy. Radiology 96:503–508, 1970.

262. Das De S, McCreath SW: Lumbosacral fracture-dislocations: a report of four cases. J Bone Joint Surg 63B:58–60, 1981.

263. Dassel PM: Agenesis of the sacrum and coccyx. AJR 85:697–700, 1961.

264. Dauser RC, Chandler WF: Symptomatic congenital spinal stenosis in a child. Neurosurgery 11:61–63, 1982.

265. David DS: Calcium metabolism in renal failure. Am J Med 58:48–55, 1975.

266. Davidson JK, Mucci B: Chordoma of the body of C2: case report 322. Skeletal Radiol 14:76–80, 1985.

267. Davis D, Bohlman H, Walker AE, et al: The pathological findings in fatal craniospinal injuries. Neurosurgery 34:603–613, 1971.

268. Dawson EG, Smith L: Atlanto-axial subluxation in children due to vertebral anomalies. J Bone Joint Surg 61A:582–587, 1979.

269. Dawson WB: Sclerotic repair of myelomatous bony defects following chemotherapy. Clin Radiol 19:323–326, 1968.

270. Debnam JW, Bates ML, Kopelman RC, et al: Radiological/pathological correlations in uremic bone disease. Radiology 125:653–658, 1977.

271. DeBoeck M, Peeters O, Van Camp B, et al: Monocytic leukemia associated with myeloid metaplasia resembling metastatic bone disease. Skeletal Radiol 11:9–12, 1984.

272. Decker RE, Wei WC: Thoracic cord compression from multiple hereditary exostoses associated with cerebellar astrocytoma. J Neurosurg 30:310–312, 1969.

273. Degesys GE, Miller GA, Newman GE, et al: Absence of a pedicle in the spine: metastatic disease versus aplasia. Spine 11:76–77, 1986.

274. Dehner JR: Seat belt injuries of the spine and abdomen. AJR 111:833–843, 1971.

275. Delgado E, Rodriguez JI, Serrada A, et al: Radiation-induced osteochondroma-like lesion in young rat radius. Clin Orthop 201:251–258, 1985.

276. Demanes DJ, Lane N, Beckstead JH: Bone involvement in hairy-cell leukemia. Cancer 49:1697–1701, 1982.

277. Denis F: The three-column spine and its significance in the classification of acute thoracolumbar spinal injuries. Spine 8:817–831, 1983.

278. Denis F: Spinal instability as defined by the three-column spine concept in acute spinal trauma. Clin Orthop 189:65–76, 1984.

279. Dent CE, Friedman M, Watson L: Hereditary pseudo-vitamin D deficiency rickets: ("hereditare pseudo-mangelrachitis"). J Bone Joint Surg 50B:708–719, 1968.

280. DeOliveira JC: A new type of fracture-dislocation of the thoracolumbar spine. J Bone Joint Surg 60A:481–488, 1978.

281. DeSmet AA, Fritz SL, Asher MA: A method for minimizing the radiation exposure from scoliosis radiographs. J Bone Joint Surg 63A:156–158, 1981.

282. DeSmet AA, Goin JE, Asher MA, et al: A clinical study of the differences between the scoliotic angles measured on posteroanterior and anteroposterior radiographs. J Bone Joint Surg 64A: 489–493, 1982.

283. DeSmet AA, Kuhns LR, Fayos JV, et al: Effects of radiation therapy on growing long bones. AJR 127:935–939, 1976.

284. DeSmet AA, Neff JR: Pubic and sacral insufficiency fractures: a clinical course and radiologic findings. AJR 145:601–606, 1985.

284a. Destouet JM, Kyriakos M, Gilula LA: Fibrous histiocytoma (fibroxanthoma) of a cervical vertebra. A report with a review of the literature. Skeletal Radiol 5:241–246, 1980.

285. Dias L de S, Frost HM: Osteoblastoma of the spine. A review and report of eight new cases. Clin Orthop 91:141–151, 1973.

286. Dickey LE Jr, Hobbs RJW, Sherrill JD Sr: Vertebra plana and the histiocytoses: report of a case with involvement of five vertebrae. J Bone Joint Surg 37A:1261–1265, 1955.

287. Dickson DD, Camp JD, Ghormley RR: Osteitis deformans: Paget's disease of the bone. Radiology 44:449–470, 1945.

288. Dickson JH, Waltz TA, Fechner RE: Intraosseous neurilemoma of the third lumbar vertebra. J Bone Joint Surg 53A:349–355, 1971.

289. Dickson RA, Lawtown JO, Archer IA, et al: The pathogenesis of idiopathic scoliosis: biplanar spinal asymmetry. J Bone Joint Surg 66B:8–15, 1984.

290. Dietz GW, Christensen EE: Normal "cupid's bow" contour of the lower lumbar vertebrae. Radiology 121:577–579, 1976.

291. Digby JM, Kersley JB: Pyogenic non-tuberculous spinal infection: an analysis of thirty cases. J Bone Joint Surg 61B:47–55, 1979.

292. Diggs LW: Bone and joint lesions in sickle-cell disease. Clin Orthop 52:119–143, 1967.

293. Diggs LW, Pulliam HN, King JC: The bone changes in sickle cell anemia. South Med J 30:249–259, 1937.

294. Dihlmann W: Current radiodiagnostic concept of ankylosing spondylitis. Skeletal Radiol 4: 179–188, 1979.

295. Dihlmann W: Hemispherical spondylosclerosis—a polyetiologic syndrome. Skeletal Radiol 7:99–106, 1981.

296. Dihlmann W, Delling G: Disco-vertebral destructive lesions (so-called Andersson lesions) associated with ankylosing spondylitis. Skeletal Radiol 3:10–16, 1978.

297. DiLorenzo N, Fortuna A, Guidetti B: Craniovertebral junction malformations: clinicoradiological findings; long-term results and surgical indications in 63 cases. J Neurosurg 57:603–608, 1982.

298. DiLorenzo N, Spallone A, Nolletti A, et al: Giant cell tumors of the spine: a clinical study of six cases, with emphasis on the radiological features, treatment and follow-up. Neurosurgery 6:29–34, 1980.

299. Dirheimer Y, Bensimon C, Christmann D, et al: Syndesmo-odontoid joint and calcium pyrophosphate dihydrate deposition disease (CPPD). Neuroradiology 25:319–321, 1983.

300. Dolan KD: Cervical spine injuries below the axis. Radiol Clin N Am 15:247–259, 1977.

301. Dolan KD: Cervicobasilar relationships. Radiol Clin N Am 15:155–166, 1977.

302. Dolan KD: Developmental abnormalities of the cervical spine below the axis. Radiol Clin N Am 15:167–175, 1977.

303. Dolan KD: Expanding lesions of the cervical spinal canal. Radiol Clin N Am 15:203–214, 1977.

304. Donovan RM, Shah KJ: Unusual sites of acute osteomyelitis in childhood. Clin Radiol 33:222–230, 1982.

305. Doppelt SH: Vitamin D, rickets and osteomalacia. Orthop Clin N Am 15:671–686, 1984.

306. Dory MA, Francois RJ: Craniocaudal axial view of the sacroiliac joint. AJR 130:1125–1131, 1978.

307. Doub HP, Badgley CE: The roentgen signs of tuberculosis of the vertebral body. AJR 27: 827–834, 1932.

308. Dove J, Hsu LCS, Yau ACMC: The cervical spine after halo-pelvic traction: an analysis of the complications in 83 patients. J Bone Joint Surg 62B:158–161, 1980.

309. Dove J, Hsu LCS, Yau ACMC: Spontaneous cervical spinal fusion. A complication of halo-pelvic traction. Spine 6:45–48, 1981.

310. Dowd CF, Sartoris DJ, Haghighi P, et al: Tuberculous spondylitis resulting in atlanto-axial dislocation: case report 344. Skeletal Radiol 15:65–68, 1986.

311. Dowdle JA Jr, Winter RB, Dehner LP: Postradiation osteosarcoma of the cervical spine in childhood: a case report. J Bone Joint Surg 59A: 969–971, 1977.

312. Downey EF Jr, Nason SS, Majd M, et al: Asymmetrical facet joints. Another cause for the sclerotic pedicle. Spine 8:340–342, 1983.

313. Doyle FH: Some quantitative radiological observations in primary and secondary hyeprparathyroidism. Br J Radiol 39:161–167, 1966.

314. Drennan JC, King EW: Cervical dislocation following fusion of the upper thoracic spine for scoliosis: a case report. J Bone Joint Surg 60A:1003–1005, 1978.

315. Driedger H, Pruzanski W: Plasma cell neoplasia with osteosclerotic lesions: a study of five cases and a review of the literature. Arch Intern Med 139:892–896, 1979.

316. Drummond D, Ranallo F, Lonstein J, et al: Radiation hazards in scoliosis management. Spine 8:741–748, 1983.

317. Duncan AW: Calcification of the anterior longitudinal vertebral ligaments in Hodgkin's disease. Clin Radiol 24:394–396, 1973.

318. Dupuis PR, Young-Hing K, Cassidy JD, et al: Radiologic diagnosis of degenerative lumbar spinal instability. Spine 10:262–276, 1985.

319. Dusenberry JF Jr, Kane JJ: Pycnodysostosis: report of three new cases. AJR 99:717–723, 1967.

320. Dussault RG, Kaye JJ: Intervertebral disk calcification associated with spine fusion. Radiology 125:57–61, 1977.

321. Dzioba RB, Benjamin J: Spontaneous atlanto-axial fusion in psoriatic arthritis: a case report. Spine 10:102–103, 1985

322. Eastwood JB, Bordier PJ, de Wardener HE: Some biochemical, histological, radiological and clinical features of renal osteodystrophy. Kidney Int 4:128–140, 1973.

323. Edeiken J, DePalma AF, Hodes PJ: Paget's dis-

ease: osteitis deformans. Clin Orthop 46:141–153, 1966.

324. Edeiken J, DePalma AF, Hodes PJ: Osteoid osteoma (roentgenographic emphasis). Clin Orthop 49:201–206, 1966.

324a. Edeiken J, Monroe B, Wagner LK, et al: Hyperextension dislocation of the cervical spine. AJNR 7:135–140, 1986.

325. Edelman RR, Kaufman H, Kolodny GM: Multiple myeloma—blastic type: case report 350. Skeletal Radiol 15:160–163, 1986.

326. Edelstyn GA, Gillespie PJ, Grebbell FS: The radiological demonstration of osseous metastases: experimental observations. Clin Radiol 18:158–162, 1967.

327. Edland RW: Ewing's sarcoma of the spine: report of a case. Radiol Clin (Basel) 37:162–168, 1968.

328. Edwards WC, LaRocca SH: The developmental segmental sagittal diameter in combined cervical and lumbar spondylosis. Spine 10:42–49, 1985.

329. Edwards WH Jr, Thompson RC Jr, Varsa EW: Lymphangiomatosis and massive osteolysis of the cervical spine: a case report and review of the literature. Clin Orthop 177:222–229, 1983.

330. Effendi B, Roy D, Cornish B, et al: Fractures of the ring of the axis: a classification based on the analysis of 131 cases. J Bone Joint Surg 63B:319–327, 1981.

330a. Efird TA, Genant HK, Wilson CB: Pituitary giantism with cervical spinal stenosis. AJR 134:171–173, 1980.

331. Eftekhari F, Yousefzadeh DK: Primary infantile hyperparathyroidism: clinical, laboratory and radiographic features in 21 cases. Skeletal Radiol 8:201–208, 1982.

332. Ehrenpreis B, Schwinger HN: Sickle cell anemia. AJR 68:28–36, 1952.

333. Eisenberg RL, Akin JR, Hedgcock MW: Single, well-centered lateral view of lumbosacral spine: is coned view necessary? AJR 133:711–713, 1979.

334. Eisenberg RL, Hedgcock MW, Gooding GAW, et al: Compensation examination of the cervical and lumbar spines: critical disagreement in radiographic interpretation. AJR 134:519–522, 1980.

335. Eisenberg RL, Hedgcock MW, Williams EA, et al: Optimum radiographic examination for consideration of compensation awards: II. Cervical and lumbar spines. AJR 135:1071–1074, 1980.

336. Eisenstein S: Measurements of the lumbar spinal canal in two racial groups. Clin Orthop 115:42–46, 1976.

337. Eisenstein S: The morphometry and pathological anatomy of the lumbar spine in South African Negroes and Caucasoids with specific reference to spinal stenosis. J Bone Joint Surg 59B:173–180, 1977.

338. Eisenstein S: Spondylolysis: a skeletal investigation of two population groups. J Bone Joint Surg 60B:488–494, 1978.

339. Eismont FJ, Bohlman HH: Posterior atlanto-occipital dislocation with fractures of the atlas and odontoid process. Report of a case with survival. J Bone Joint Surg 60A:397–399, 1978.

340. Eismont FJ, Bohlman HH, Soni PL, et al: Vertebral osteomyelitis in infants. J Bone Joint Surg 64B:32–35, 1982.

341. Eismont FJ, Bohlman HH, Soni PL, et al: Pyogenic and fungal vertebral osteomyelitis with paralysis. J Bone Joint Surg 65A:19–29, 1983.

342. Eklöf O, Galatius-Jensen F, Damgaard-Pedersen K: Malignant versus benign paravertebral widening in children. Pediatr Radiol 11:193–201, 1981.

343. El-Khoury GY, Clark CR, Dietz FR, et al: Posterior atlantooccipital subluxation in Down syndrome. Radiology 159:507–509, 1986.

344. El-Khoury GY, Moore TE, Albright JP, et al: Sodium flouride treatment of osteoporosis: radiographic findings. AJR 139:39–43, 1982.

345. El-Khoury GY, Tozzi JE, Clark CR, et al: Massive calcium pyrophosphate crystal deposition at the craniovertebral junction. AJR 145:777–778, 1985.

346. El-Khoury GY, Wener MH, Menezes AH, et al: Cranial settling in rheumatoid arthritis. Radiology 137:637–642, 1980.

347. El-Khoury GY, Yousefzadeh DK, Kathol MH, et al: Pseudospondylolysis. Radiology 139:72, 1981.

348. Eller JL, Siebert PE: Sclerotic vertebral bodies: an unusual manifestation of disseminated coccidioidomycosis. Radiology 93:1099–1100, 1969.

349. Elliot JM Jr, Rogers LF, Wissinger JP, et al: The hangman's fracture. Fractures of the neural arch of the axis. Radiology 104:303–307, 1972.

350. Ellman MH, Vazquez T, Ferguson L: Calcium pyrophosphate deposition in ligamentum flavum. Arthritis Rheum 21:611–613, 1978.

351. Elmore SM: Pycnodysostosis: a review. J Bone Joint Surg 49A:153–162, 1967.

352. Elsberg CA, Dyke CG: The diagnosis and localization of tumors of the spinal cord by means of measurements made on the x-ray films of the vertebrae, and the correlation of clinical and x-ray findings. Bull Neurol Inst New York 3:359–394, 1934.

353. Elster AD: Quadriplegia after minor trauma in the Klippel-Feil syndrome: a case report and review of the literature. J Bone Joint Surg 66A:1473–1474, 1984.

354. Emami-Ahari Z, Zarabi M, Javid B: Pycnodysostosis. J Bone Joint Surg 51B:307–312, 1969.

355. Engels EP, Smith RC, Krantz S: Bone sclerosis in multiple myeloma. Radiology 75:242–247, 1960.

356. England AC III, Shippel AH, Ray MJ: A simple view for demonstration of fractures of the anterior arch of C1. AJR 144:763–764, 1985.

357. Epstein BS: Vertebral changes in childhood leukemia. Radiology 68:65–69, 1957.

357a. Epstein BS: The Spine. A Radiological Text and Atlas. Philadelphia: Lea and Febiger, 1976.

358. Epstein BS, Epstein JA: The association of cerebellar tonsillar herniation with basilar impression incident to Paget's disease. AJR 107:535–542, 1969.

359. Epstein BS, Epstein JA: Cervical spinal stenosis. Radiol Clin N Am 15:215–226, 1977.

360. Epstein BS, Epstein JA, Jones MD: Lumbar spinal stenosis. Radiol Clin N Am 15:227–239, 1977.

361. Epstein BS, Epstein JA, Jones MD: Lap-sash three point seat belt fractures of the cervical spine. Spine 3:189–193, 1978.

362. Epstein BS, Epstein JA, Lavine L: The effect of anatomic variations in the lumbar vertebrae and spinal canal on cauda equina and nerve root syndromes. AJR 91:1055–1063, 1964.

362a. Epstein DM, Dalinka MK, Kaplan FS, et al: Observer variation in the detection of osteopenia. Skeletal Radiol 15:347–349, 1986.

363. Epstein N, Benjamin V, Pinto R, et al: Benign

osteoblastoma of a thoracic vertebra: case report. J Neurosurg 53:710–713, 1980.

363a. Epstein N, Whelan M, Benjamin V: Acromegaly and spinal stenosis. J Neurosurg 56:145–147, 1982.

364. Epstein NE, Epstein JA, Zilkha A: Traumatic myelopathy in a seventeen year old child with cervical spinal stenosis (without fracture or dislocation) and a C2–C3 Klippel-Feil fusion: a case report. Spine 9:344–347, 1984.

365. Eriksson B, Gunterberg B, Kindblom L-G: Chordoma: a clinicopathologic and prognostic study of a Swedish national series. Acta Orthop Scand 52:49–58, 1981.

366. Erwin WD, Dickson JH, Harrington PR: Clinical review of patients with broken Harrington rods. J Bone Joint Surg 62A:1302–1307, 1980.

367. Esposito PW, Crawford AH, Vogler C: Solitary osteochondroma occurring on the transverse process of the lumbar spine: a case report. Spine 10:398–400, 1985.

368. Eugenidis N, Olah AJ, Haas HG: Osteosclerosis in hyperparathyroidism. Radiology 105:265–275, 1972.

369. Evans DK: Dislocations at the cervicothoracic junction. J Bone Joint Surg 65B:124–127, 1983.

370. Evans PR: Deformity of vertebral bodies in cretinism. J Pediatr 41:706–712, 1952.

371. Evison G, Evans KT: Bone sclerosis in multiple myeloma. Br J Radiol 40:81–89, 1967.

372. Evison G, Pizey N, Roylance J: Bone formation associated with osseous metastasis from bladder carcinoma. Clin Radiol 32:303–309, 1981.

373. Fabris D, Trainiti G, Di Comun M, et al: Scoliosis due to rib osteoblastoma: report of two cases. J Pediatr Orthop 3:370–375, 1983.

373a. Fallet GH, Courtois C, Vischer TL, et al: Erosive spondylopathy. Scand J Rheumatol 9:110–114, 1980.

374. Fam AG, Cruickshank B: Subaxial cervical subluxation and cord compression in psoriatic spondylitis. Arthritis Rheum 25:101–106, 1982.

375. Fang D, Leong JCY, Fang HSY: Tuberculosis of the upper cervical spine. J Bone Joint Surg 65B:47–50, 1983.

376. Fardon DF: Odontoid fracture complicating ankylosing hyperostosis of the spine. 3:108–112, 1978.

377. Fardon DF, Fielding JW: Defects of the pedicle and spondylolisthesis of the second cervical vertebra. J Bone Joint Surg 63B:526–528, 1981.

378. Farfan HF: Effects of torsion on the intervertebral joints. Can J Surg 12:336–341, 1969.

379. Farfan HF: The pathological anatomy of degenerative spondylolisthesis: a cadaver study. Spine 5:412–418, 1980.

380. Farfan HF, Cossette JW, Robertson GH, et al: The effects of torsion on the lumbar intervertebral joints: the role of torsion in the production of disc degeneration. J Bone Joint Surg 52A:468–497, 1970.

381. Farfan HF, Osteria V, Lamy C: The mechanical etiology of spondylosis and spondylolisthesis. Clin Orthop 117:40–55, 1976.

382. Farfan HF, Sullivan JD: The relation of facet orientation to intervertebral disc failure. Can J Surg 10:179–185, 1967.

383. Feldman F: Miscellaneous localized conditions: a whirlwind review of the "oh my aching back" syndrome. Semin Roentgenol 14:58–75, 1979.

384. Feldman F, Hecht HL, Johnston AD: Chondromyxoid fibroma of bone. Radiology 94:249–260, 1970.

385. Feldman F, Johnson AM, Walter JF: Acute axial neuroarthropathy. Radiology 111:1–16, 1974.

385a. Feldman F, Lattes R: Primary malignant fibrous histiocytoma (fibrous xanthoma) of bone. Skeletal Radiol 1:145–160, 1977.

385b. Ferguson AB: Roentgen Diagnosis of the Extremities and Spine. New York: Hoeber Publishers, 1945, pp 360–365.

386. Ferguson RL, Allen BL Jr: A mechanistic classification of thoracolumbar spine fractures. Clin Orthop 189:77–88, 1984.

387. Ferguson WR: Some observations on the circulation in foetal and infant spines. J Bone Joint Surg 32A:640–648, 1950.

388. Ferris B, Jones C: Paraplegia due to aspergillosis: successful conservative treatment of two cases. J Bone Joint Surg 67B:800–803, 1985.

389. Ferris RA, Pettrone FA, McKelvie AM, et al: Eosinophilic granuloma of the spine: an unusual radiographic presentation. Clin Orthop 99:57–63, 1974.

390. Ferriter PJ, O'Leary P, Block J, et al: Cervical spondylolisthesis: a case report. Spine 9:830–832, 1984.

391. Fielding JW, Cochran GVB, Lawsing JF III, et al: Tears of the transverse ligament of the atlas: a clinical and biomechanical study. J Bone Joint Surg 56A:1683–1691, 1974.

392. Fielding JW, Griffin PP: Os odontoideum: an acquired lesion. J Bone Joint Surg 56A:187–190, 1974.

393. Fielding JW, Hensinger RN, Hawkins RJ: Os odontoideum. J Bone Joint Surg 62A:376–383, 1980.

394. Fielding JW, Ratzan S: Osteochondroma of the cervical spine. J Bone Joint Surg 55A:640–641, 1973.

395. Figueiredo UM, James JIP: Juvenile idiopathic scoliosis. J Bone Joint Surg 63B:61–66, 1981.

396. Finby N, Archibald RM: Skeletal abnormalities associated with gonadal dysgenesis. AJR 89:1222–1235, 1963.

397. Finerman GAM, Sakai D, Weingarten S: Atlanto-axial dislocation with spinal cord compression in a mongoloid child: a case report. J Bone Joint Surg 58A:408–409, 1976.

398. Fink LH, Meriwether MW: Primary epidural Ewing's sarcoma presenting as a lumbar disc protrusion: case report. J Neurosurg 51:120–123, 1979.

399. Firooznia H, Golimbu C, Rafii M, et al: Radiology of musculoskeletal complications of drug addiction. Semin Roentgenol 18:198–206, 1983.

400. Firooznia H, Pinto RS, Lin JP, et al: Chordoma: radiologic evaluation of 20 cases. AJR 127:797–805, 1976.

401. Firooznia H, Tyler I, Golimbu C, et al: Computerized tomography of the cupid's bow contour of the lumbar spine. Comput Radiol 7:347–350, 1983.

402. Fischgold H, David M, Brégeat P: La tomographie de la base du crâne en neuro-chirurgie et neuro-ophtalmologie. Paris: Masson & Cie, 1952. Cited by Hinck VC, Hopkins CE, Savara BS: Diagnostic criteria of basilar impression. Radiology 76:572–585, 1961.

403. Fisher MS: Lumbar spine metastasis in cervical carcinoma: a characteristic pattern. Radiology 134:631–634, 1980.

404. Fishman EK, Zinreich SJ, Kumar AJ, et al: Sacral abnormalities in Marfan syndrome. J Comput Assist Tomogr 7:851–856, 1983.

405. Flournoy JG, Cone RO, Saldana JA, et al: Jefferson fracture: presentation of a new diagnostic sign. Radiology 134:88, 1980.

406. Foley MJ, Calenoff L, Hendrix RW, et al: Thoracic and lumbar spine fusion: postoperative radiologic evaluation. AJR 141:373–380, 1983

407. Foley MJ, Lee C, Calenoff L, et al: Radiologic evaluation of surgical cervical spine fusion. AJR 138:79–89, 1982.

408. Foley WD, Baum JK, Wheeler RH: Diffuse osteosclerosis with lymphocytic lymphoma: a case report. Radiology 117:553–554, 1975.

409. Ford LT, Gilula LA, Murphy WA, et al: Analysis of gas in vacuum lumbar disc. AJR 128:1056–1057, 1977.

410. Forestier J, Rotes-Querol J: Senile ankylosing hyperostosis of the spine. Ann Rheum Dis 9:321–330, 1950.

411. Fornasier VL, Littlejohn G, Urowitz MB, et al: Spinal entheseal new bone formation: the early changes of spinal diffuse idiopathic skeletal hyperostosis. J Rheumatol 10:939–947, 1983.

412. Fors B, Stenkvist B: Giant-cell tumor of thoracic vertebra: case report. Acta Orthop Scand 37:191–196, 1966.

413. Forsyth HF: Extension injuries of the cervical spine. J Bone Joint Surg 46A:1792–1797, 1964.

414. Frager DH, Subbarao K: The "bone within a bone." JAMA 249:77–79, 1983.

415. Frame B, Frost HM, Ormond RS, et al: Atypical osteomalacia involving the axial skeleton. Ann Intern Med 55:632–639, 1961.

416. Frame B, Marel GM: Paget disease: a review of current knowledge. Radiology 141:21–24, 1981.

417. Frank DF, Miller JE: Hypoplasia of the lumbar vertebral body simulating spondylolisthesis. Radiology 133:59–60, 1979.

418. Franklin EL, Matheson I: Melorheostosis: report on a case with a review of the literature. Br J Radiol 15:185–191, 1942.

419. Fredickson BE, Baker D, McHolick WJ, et al: The natural history of spondylolysis and spondylolisthesis. J Bone Joint Surg 66A:699–707, 1984.

420. Freehafer AA, Heiser DP, Saunders AP: Infection of the lower lumbar spine with Neisseria meningitidis: a case report. J Bone Joint Surg 60A:1001–1002, 1978.

421. Freiberger RH, Loitman BS, Helpern M, et al: Osteoid osteoma: a report on 80 cases. AJR 82:194–205, 1959.

422. Freiberger RH, Wilson PD Jr, Nicholas JA: Aquired absence of the odontoid process. J Bone Joint Surg 47A:1231–1236, 1965.

423. Freilich M, Virapongse C, Kier EL, et al: Foramen transversarium enlargement due to tortuosity of the vertebral artery: computed tomographic appearance. Spine 11:95–98, 1986.

424. French BN: Midline fusion defects and defects of formation. In Youmans JR (ed): Neurological Surgery, vol 3. Philadelphia: WB Saunders Company, 1982, pp 1236–1380.

425. Fried JA, Athreya B, Gregg JR: The cervical spine in juvenile rheumatoid arthritis. Clin Orthop 179:102–106, 1983.

426. Friedenberg ZB, Edeiken J, Spencer HN, et al: Degenerative changes in the cervical spine. J Bone Joint Surg 41A:61–70, 1959.

427. Friedenberg ZB, Miller WT: Degenerative disc disease of the cervical spine: a comparative study of asymptomatic and symptomatic patients. J Bone Joint Surg 45A:1171–1178, 1963.

428. Friedmann E: Narrowing of the spinal canal due to thickened lamina a cause of low-back pain and sciatica. Clin Orthop 21:190–197, 1961.

429. Friis J, Jensen EM, Karle AK: Calcified periarthritis at multiple sites including lumbar intervertebral discs: report of a case. Acta Radiol [Diagn] 20:928–931, 1979.

430. Fripp AT: Vertebra plana. J Bone Joint Surg 40B:378–384, 1958.

431. Frost HM: The pathomechanics of osteoporosis. Clin Orthop 200:198–225, 1985.

432. Fry VG, Van Dellen JR: Aneurysmal bone cysts of the spine. S Afr Med J 58:211–213, 1980.

433. Frykholm R: Lower cervical vertebrae and intervertebral discs. Surgical anatomy and pathology. Acta Chir Scand 101:345–359, 1951.

434. Frymoyer JW, Newberg A, Pope MH, et al: Spine radiographs in patients with low-back pain: an epidemiological study in men. J Bone Joint Surg 66A:1048–1055, 1984.

435. Frymoyer JW, Pope MH, Clements JH, et al: Risk factors in low-back pain: an epidemiological survey. J Bone Joint Surg 65A:213–218, 1983.

436. Frymoyer JW, Selby DK: Segmental instability: rationale for treatment. Spine 10:280–286, 1985.

437. Fullenlove TM, Williams AJ: Comparative roentgen findings in symptomatic and asymptomatic backs. Radiology 68:572–574, 1957.

438. Furey WW: Fractures of the pelvis: with special reference to associated fractures of the sacrum. AJR 47:89–96, 1942.

439. Galasko CSB: Mechanisms of lytic and blastic metastatic disease of bone. Clin Orthop 169:20–27, 1982.

440. Gamba JL, Martinez S, Apple J, et al: Computed tomography of axial skeletal osteoid osteomas. AJR 142:769–772, 1984.

441. Garfin SR, Rothman RH: Fibrous dysplasia (polyostotic): case report 346. Skeletal Radiol 15:72–76, 1986.

442. Garver P, Resnick D, Haghighi P, et al: Melorheostosis of the axial skeleton with associated fibrolipomatous lesions. Skeletal Radiol 9:41–44, 1982.

443. Gehweiler JA, Capp MP, Chick EW: Observations on the roentgen patterns in blastomycosis of bone. AJR 108:497–519, 1970.

444. Gehweiler JA Jr, Clark WM, Schaff RE, et al: Cervical spine trauma: the common combined conditions. Radiology 130:77–86, 1979.

445. Gehweiler JA Jr, Daffner RH, Osborne RL Jr: Relevant signs of stable and unstable thoracolumbar vertebral column trauma. Skeletal Radiol 7:179–193, 1981.

446. Gehweiler JA Jr, Daffner RH, Roberts L Jr: Malformations of the atlas vertebra simulating the Jefferson fracture. AJR 140:1083–1086, 1983.

447. Gehweiler JA Jr, Duff DE, Martinez S, et al: Fractures of the atlas vertebra. Skeletal Radiol 1:97–102, 1976.

448. Gehweiler JA Jr, Martinez S, Clark WM, et al: Spondylolisthesis of the axis vertebra. AJR 128:682–684, 1977.

449. Gehweiler JA Jr, Osborn RL Jr, Becker RF: The Radiology of Vertebral Trauma. Philadelphia: WB Saunders Company, 1980.

450. Gelbke H: The influence of pressure and tension on growing bone in experiments with animals. J Bone Joint Surg 33A:947–954, 1951.

451. Gelman MI: Cauda equina compression in acromegaly. Radiology 112:357–360, 1974.

452. Gelman MI, Umber JS: Fractures of the thoracolumbar spine in ankylosing spondylitis. AJR 130:485–491, 1978.

453. Genant HK, Baron JM, Straus FH II, et al: Osteosclerosis in primary hyperparathyroidism. Am J Med 59:104–113, 1975.

454. Genant HK, Heck LL, Lanzl LH, et al: Primary hyperparathyroidism: a comprehensive study of clinical, biochemical and radiographic manifestations. Radiology 109:513–524, 1973.

455. George K, Rippstein J: A comparative study of the two popular methods of measuring scoliotic deformity of the spine. J Bone Joint Surg 43A:809–818, 1961.

456. Gershon-Cohen J, Schraer H, Sklaroff DM, et al: Dissolution of the intervertebral disk in the aged normal: the phantom nucleus pulposus. Radiology 62:383–386, 1954.

457. Gertzbein SD, Offierski C: Complete fracture-dislocation of the thoracic spine without spinal cord injury: a case report. J Bone Joint Surg 61A:449–451, 1979.

458. Ghelman B, Freiberger RH: The limbus vertebra: an anterior disc herniation demonstrated by discography. AJR 127:854–855, 1976.

459. Gianturco C: A roentgen analysis of the motion of the lower lumbar vertebrae in normal individuals and in patients with low back pain. AJR 52:261–268, 1944.

460. Giordano GB, Cerisoli M: Diastematomyelia and scoliosis. Usefulness of CT examination. Spine 8:111–112, 1983.

461. Gitelis S, Bertoni F, Picci P, et al: Chondrosarcoma of bone. J Bone Joint Surg 63A:1248–1257, 1981.

462. Gitelis S, Ryan WG, Rosenberg AG, et al: Adult-onset hypophosphatemic osteomalacia secondary to neoplasm: a case report and review of the pathophysiology. J Bone Joint Surg 68A:134–142, 1986.

463. Glasauer FE: Benign osteoblastoma of cervical spine. NY State J Med 79:1424–1427, 1979.

464. Gleason IO, Urist MR: Atlanto-axial dislocation with odontoid separation in rheumatoid disease. Clin Orthop 42:121–129, 1965.

465. Goldberg RP, Vine HS, Sacks BA, et al: The cervical split: a pseudofracture. Skeletal Radiol 7:267–272, 1982.

466. Goldenberg DB, Rienhoff WF III, Rao PS: Osteochondroma with spinal cord compression: report of a case. J Can Assoc Radiol 19:192–194, 1968.

467. Goldenberg RR, Campbell CJ, Bonfiglio M: Giant-cell tumor of bone. J Bone Joint Surg 52A:619–664, 1970.

468. Goldman AB, Abrahams TG: Multiple findings of renal osteodystrophy reflected in the vertebral bodies and apophyseal joints of the cervical spine. Case report 356. Skeletal Radiol 15:308–312, 1986.

469. Goldman AB, Freiberger RH: Localized infectious and neuropathic diseases. Semin Roentgenol 14:19–32, 1979.

470. Goldstein LA, Waugh TR: Classification and terminology of scoliosis. Clin Orthop 93:10–22, 1973.

471. Gondos B: Late clinical and roentgen observations following Thorotrast treatment administration. Clin Radiol 24:195–203, 1973.

472. Gonem MN: Osteoclastoma of the thoracic spine: case report. J Neurosurg 44:748–752, 1976.

473. Gooding CA, Neuhauser EBD: Growth and development of the vertebral body in the presence and absence of normal stress. AJR 93:388–394, 1965.

474. Gooding GA, Ball JH: Idiopathic juvenile osteoporosis. Radiology 93:1349–1350, 1969.

475. Gootnick LT: Solitary myeloma: review of sixty-one cases. Radiology 45:385–391, 1945.

476. Gordan GS: Estrogen and bone: Marshal R. Urist's contributions. Clin Orthop 200:174–180, 1985.

477. Gosling HR, Gilmer WS Jr: Skeletal cryptococcosis (torulosis); report of a case and review of the literature. J Bone Joint Surg 38A:660–668, 1956.

478. Grabias S: The treatment of spinal stenosis. J Bone Joint Surg 62A:308–314, 1980.

479. Granger W, Whitaker R: Hodgkin's disease in bone, with special reference to periosteal reaction. Br J Radiol 40:939–948, 1967.

480. Gray JE, Hoffman AD, Peterson HA: Reduction of radiation exposure during radiography for scoliosis. J Bone Joint Surg 65A:5–12, 1983.

481. Greditzer HG III, McLeod RA, Unni KK, et al: Bone sarcomas in Paget's disease. Radiology 146:327–333, 1983.

482. Green AE Jr, Ellswood WH, Collins JR: Melorheostosis and osteopoikilosis: with a review of the literature. AJR 87:1096–1111, 1962.

483. Green JD, Harle TS, Harris JH Jr: Anterior subluxation of the cervical spine: hyperflexion sprain. AJNR 2:243–250, 1981.

484. Green NE, Robertson WW Jr, Kilroy AW: Eosinophilic granuloma of the spine with associated neural deficit: report of three cases. J Bone Joint Surg 62A:1198–1202, 1980.

485. Greenfield GB: Radiology of Bone Diseases, 4th ed. Philadelphia: JB Lippincott Company, 1986.

486. Griffin JB: Benign osteoblastoma of the thoracic spine: case report with fifteen-year follow-up. J Bone Joint Surg 60A:833–835, 1978.

487. Griffiths HED, Jones DM: Pyogenic infection of the spine: a review of twenty-eight cases. J Bone Joint Surg 53B:383–391, 1971.

488. Griffiths HJ, Ennis JT, Bailey G: Skeletal changes following renal transplantation. Radiology 113:621–626, 1974.

489. Grobovschek M, Scheibelbrandner W: Atlanto-occipital dislocation. Neuroradiology 25:173–174, 1983.

490. Gross RJ, Yelin G: Multiple myeloma complicating Paget's disease. AJR 65:585–589, 1951.

491. Grossman H, Winchester PH, Bragg DG, et al: Roentgenographic changes in childhood Hodgkin's disease. AJR 108:354–364, 1970.

492. Groswasser Z, Reider-Groswasser I: Heterotopic new bone formation in the cervical spine following head injury: case report. J Neurosurg 64:513–515, 1986.

493. Guerra J Jr, Garfin SR, Resnick D: Vertebral burst fractures: CT analysis of the retropulsed fragment. Radiology 153:769–772, 1984.

494. Gulati DR, Rout D: Atlantoaxial dislocation with quadriparesis in achondroplasia: case report. J Neurosurg 40:394–396, 1974.

495. Gumley G, Taylor TKF, Ryan MD: Distraction

fractures of the lumbar spine. J Bone Joint Surg 64B:520–525, 1982.

496. Gunderson CA, Taddonio RF Jr: Congenital atlantoaxial fusion: a case report. Spine 4:9–11, 1979.

497. Gunther SF: Congenital anomaly of the cervical spine: fusion of the occiput, atlas and odontoid process: a case report. J Bone Joint Surg 62A:1377–1378, 1980.

498. Guyer PB: Paget's disease of bone: the anatomical distribution. Metab Bone Dis Rel Res 4:239–242, 1981.

499. Gwinn JL, Smith JL: Acquired and congenital absence of the odontoid process. AJR 81:424–431, 1962.

500. Haas SL: Growth in length of vertebrae. Arch Surg 38:245–249, 1939.

501. Hadden WA, Swanson AJG: Spinal infection caused by acupuncture mimicking a prolapsed intervertebral disc. J Bone Joint Surg 64A:624–626, 1982.

502. Hadley A: Intervertebral joint subluxation, bony impingement and foramen encroachment with nerve root changes. AJR 65:377–402, 1951.

503. Hadley LA: Roentgenographic studies of the cervical spine. AJR 52:173–195, 1944.

504. Hadley LA: Congenital absence of pedicle from the cervical vertebra: report of three cases. AJR 55:193–197, 1946.

505. Hadley LA: Atlanto-occipital fusion, ossiculum terminale and occipital vertebra as related to basilar impression with neurological symptoms. AJR 59:511–524, 1948.

506. Hadley LA: The covertebral articulations and cervical foramen encroachment. J Bone Joint Surg 39A:910–920, 1957.

507. Hadley LA: Anatomico-roentgenographic studies of the posterior spinal articulations. AJR 86:270–276, 1961.

508. Hadley LA: Stress fracture with spondylolysis. AJR 90:1258–1262, 1963.

509. Hadley MN, Browner C, Sonntag VKH: Axis fractures: a comprehensive review of management and treatment in 107 cases. Neurosurgy 17:281–290, 1985.

510. Hall FM: Overutilization of radiological examinations. Radiology 120:443–448, 1976.

511. Hall FM: Back pain and the radiologist. Radiology 137:861–863, 1980.

512. Hall MC, Selin G: Spinal involvement in gout: a case report with autopsy. J Bone Joint Surg 42A:341–343, 1960.

513. Halperin EC, Greenberg MS, Suit HD: Sarcoma of bone and soft tissue following treatment of Hodgkin's disease. Cancer 53:232–236, 1984.

514. Hamsa WR, Campbell LS: Giant-cell tumor of the spine: a report of two cases. J Bone Joint Surg 35A:476–478, 1953.

515. Hanna M, Watt I: Posterior longitudinal ligament calcification of the cervical spine. Br J Radiol 52:901–905, 1979.

516. Hansen GC, Gold RH: Central depression of multiple vertebral end-plates: a "pathognomonic" sign of sickle hemoglobinopathy in Gaucher's disease. AJR 129:343–344, 1977.

517. Hanson R: On the development of spinal vertebrae, as seen on skiagrams, from late foetal life to the age of fourteen. Acta Radiol 5:112–126, 1926.

518. Harding JR, McCall IW, Park WM, et al: Fracture

519. Harris DJ, Fornasier VL: An ivory vertebra: monostotic Paget's disease of bone. Clin Orthop 136:173–175, 1978.

520. Harris JH Jr: Acute injuries of the spine. Semin Roentgenol 13:53–68, 1978.

521. Harris JH Jr: The Radiology of Acute Cervical Spine Trauma. Baltimore: Williams & Wilkins Company, 1978.

522. Harris JH Jr, Burke JT, Ray RD, et al: Low (Type III) odontoid fracture: a new radiographic sign. Radiology 153:353–356, 1984.

523. Harris RI, Macnab I: Structural changes in the lumbar intervertebral discs. Their relationship in low back pain and sciatica. J Bone Joint Surg 36B:304–322, 1954.

524. Harris RI, Wiley JJ: Acquired spondylolysis as a sequel to spine fusion. J Bone Joint Surg 45A:1159–1170, 1963.

525. Harrison RB, Keats TE, Winn HR, et al: Pseudosubluxation of the axis in young adults. J Can Assoc Radiol 31:176–177, 1980.

526. Hart KZ, Brower AC: Unilateral hypertrophy of multiple pedicles. AJR 129:739–740, 1977.

527. Hart LE, Bianchi FA, Banna M: Posterior atlantoaxial subluxation in rheumatoid arthritis. J Can Assoc Radiol 32:240–241, 1981.

528. Harvie JN, Lester RS, Little AH: Sacroiliitis in severe psoriasis. AJR 127:579–584, 1976.

529. Hasenhuttl K: Osteopetrosis: review of the literature and comparative studies on a case with a twenty-four year follow up. J Bone Joint Surg 44A:359–370, 1962.

530. Hashimoto M: The distribution of active marrow in the bones of normal adult. Kyush J Med Sci 11:103–111, 1960.

531. Hashimoto M: Pathology of bone marrow. Acta Haematol 27:193–216, 1962.

532. Hassan I: Cauda equina syndrome in ankylosing spondylitis: a report of six cases. J Neurol Neurosurg Psychiatry 39:1172–1178, 1976.

533. Hassler O: The human intervertebral disc: a micro-angiographical study on its vascular supply at various ages. Acta Orthop Scand 40:765–772, 1970.

534. Hasterlik RJ, Miller CE, Finkel AJ: Radiographic development of skeletal lesions in man many years after acquisition of radium burden. Radiology 93:599–603, 1969.

535. Hastings DE, Macnab I, Lawson V: Neoplasms of the atlas and axis. Can J Surg 11:290–296, 1968.

536. Hasue M, Kikuchi S, Matsui T, et al: Spondylolysis of the axis: report of four cases. Spine 8:901–906, 1983.

537. Hatfield PM, Schulz MD: Postirradiation sarcoma: including five cases after x-ray therapy of breast carcinoma. Radiology 96:593–602, 1970.

538. Hatlinghus S, Sager M: Tuberous sclerosis: bone and lung changes mimicking metastatic malignancy. Eur J Radiol 2:90–91, 1982.

539. Haun CL: Retropharyngeal tendinitis. AJR 130:1137–1140, 1978.

540. Hawkins RJ, Fielding JW, Thompson WJ: Os odontoideum: congenital or acquired: a case report. J Bone Joint Surg 58A:413–414, 1976.

541. Hay MC, Paterson D, Taylor TKF: Aneurysmal bone cysts of the spine. J Bone Joint Surg 60B:406–411, 1978.

542. Hayashi K, Tabuchi K, Yabuki T, et al: The

position of the superior articular process of the cervical spine. Its relationship to cervical spondylotic radiculopathy. Radiology 124:501–503, 1977.

543. Hayashi K, Yabuki T: Origin of the uncus and of Luschka's joint in the cervical spine. J Bone Joint Surg 67A:788–791, 1985.

544. Hayashi S, Suit HD: Effect of fractionation of radiation dose on callus formation at site of fracture. Radiology 101:181–186, 1971.

545. Hayes WS, Berg RA, Dorfman HD, et al: Candida discitis and vertebral osteomyelitis at L1–L2 from hematogenous spread. Case report 291. Skeletal Radiol 12:284–287, 1984.

546. Healey JH, Lane JM: Structural scoliosis in osteoporotic women. Clin Orthop 195:216–223, 1985.

547. Healy M, Herz DA, Pearl L: Spinal hemangiomas. Neurosurgery 13:689–691, 1983.

548. Heard G, Payne EE: Scalloping of the vertebral bodies in von Recklinghausen's disease of the nervous system (neurofibromatosis). J Neurol Neurosurg Psychiatry 25:345–351, 1962.

549. Heaston DK, Libshitz HI, Chan RC: Skeletal effects of megavoltage irradiation in survivors of Wilms' tumor. AJR 133:389–395, 1979.

550. Heckman JD, Keats PK: Fracture of the sacrum in a child: a case report. J Bone Joint Surg 60A:404–405, 1978.

551. Hefti FL, McMaster MJ: The effect of the adolescent growth spurt on early posterior spinal fusion in infantile and juvenile idiopathic scoliosis. J Bone Joint Surg 65B:247–254, 1983.

552. Heiman ML, Cooley CJ, Bradford DS: Osteoid osteoma of a vertebral body. Report of a case with extension across the intervertebral disk. Clin Orthop 118:159–163, 1976.

553. Henderson ED, Dahlin DC: Chondrosarcoma of bone: a study of two hundred and eighty-eight cases. J Bone Joint Surg 45A:1450–1458, 1963.

554. Henkin WA: Collapse of the vertebral bodies in sickle cell anemia. AJR 62:395–401, 1949.

555. Henry MJ, Grimes HA, Lane JW: Intervertebral disk calcification in childhood. Radiology 89:81–84, 1967.

556. Hensinger RN, DeVito PD, Ragsdale CG: Changes in the cervical spine in juvenile rheumatoid arthritis. J Bone Joint Surg 68A:189–198, 1986.

557. Herndon JH, Cohen J: Chondroma of a lumbar vertebral body in a child. J Bone Joint Surg 52A:1241–1247, 1970.

558. Herring JA: The spinal disorders in diastrophic dwarfism. J Bone Joint Surg 60A:177–182, 1978.

559. Herron LD, Williams RC: Fracture-dislocation of the lumbosacral spine: report of a case and review of the literature. Clin Orthop 186:205–211, 1984.

560. Hertzanu Y, Glass RBJ, Mendelsohn DB: Sacrococcygeal chordoma in young adults. Clin Radiol 34:327–329, 1983.

561. Hess WE: Giant-cell tumor of the cervical spine: a case report. J Bone Joint Surg 42A:480–484, 1960.

562. Heywood AWB, Meyers OL: Rheumatoid arthritis of the thoracic and lumbar spine. J Bone Joint Surg 68B:362–368, 1986.

563. Highland TR, Salciccioli GG: Is immobilization adequate treatment of unstable burst fractures of the atlas?: a case report with long term follow-up evaluation. Clin Orthop 201:196–200, 1985.

564. Higinbotham NL, Phillips RF, Farr HW, et al: Chordoma. Thirty-five year study at Memorial Hospital. Cancer 20:1841–1850, 1967.

565. Hilal SK, Marton D, Pollack E: Diastematomyelia in children. Radiology 112:609–621, 1974.

566. Hill RM: Non-specific (eosinophilic) granuloma of bone. Br J Surg 37:69–76, 1949.

567. Hinck VC, Clark WM Jr, Hopkins CE: Normal interpediculate distances (minimum and maximum) in children and adults. AJR 97:141–153, 1966.

568. Hinck VC, Hopkins CE: Measurement of the atlanto-dental interval in the adult. AJR 84:945–951, 1960.

569. Hinck VC, Hopkins CE, Clark WM: Sagittal diameter of the lumbar spinal canal in children and adults. Radiology 85:929–937, 1965.

570. Hinck VC, Hopkins CE, Savara BS: Diagnostic criteria of basilar impression. Radiology 76:572–585, 1961.

571. Hinck VC, Hopkins CE, Savara BS: Sagittal diameter of the cervical spinal canal in children. Radiology 79:97–108, 1962.

572. Hinck VC, Sachdev NS: Developmental stenosis of the cervical spinal canal. Brain 89:27–36, 1966.

573. Hindman BW, Poole CA: Early appearance of the secondary vertebral ossification centers. Radiology 95:359–361, 1970.

574. Hinkel CL: The effect of roentgen rays upon the growing long bones of albino rats: histopathological changes involving endochondral growth centers. AJR 49:321–348, 1943.

575. Hipps HE: Fissure formation in articular facets of the lumbar spine: operative findings in one case. J Bone Joint Surg 21:289–303, 1939.

576. Hipps HE: Changes in the growing spine produced by anterior poliomyelitis. Clin Orthop 21:96–105, 1961.

577. Hiramatsu Y, Nobechi T: Calcification of the posterior longitudinal ligament of the spine among Japanese. Radiology 100:307–312, 1971.

578. Hirsch LF, Thanki A, Spector HB: Primary spinal chondrosarcoma with eighteen-year follow up: case report and literature review. Neurosurgery 14:747–749, 1984.

579. Hirschmann JV, Everett ED: Candida vertebral osteomyelitis: case report and review of the literature. J Bone Joint Surg 58A:573–575, 1976.

580. Hodges FJ, Peck WS: Clinical and roentgenological study of low back pain with sciatic radiation. AJR 37:461–468, 1937.

581. Hohl M: Normal motions in the upper portion of the cervical spine. J Bone Joint Surg 46A: 1777–1779, 1964.

582. Hohl M, Baker HR: The atlanto-axial joint: roentgenographic and anatomic study of normal and abnormal motion. J Bone Joint Surg 46A: 1739–1752, 1964.

583. Holdsworth F: Fractures, dislocations and fracture-dislocations of the spine. J Bone Joint Surg 52A:1534–1551, 1970.

584. Holdsworth FW: Fractures, dislocations and fracture-dislocations of the spine. J Bone Joint Surg 45B:6–20, 1963.

585. Holt JF: Neurofibromatosis in children. AJR 130:615–639, 1978.

586. Hood RW, Riseborough EJ, Nehme A-M, et al: Diastematomyelia and structural spinal deformities. J Bone Joint Surg 62A:520–528, 1980.

587. Hooyman JR, Melton LJ III, Nelson AM, et al:

Fractures after rheumatoid arthritis: a population based study. Arthritis Rheum 27:1353–1361, 1984.

588. Horan FT: Bone involvement in Hodgkin's disease: a survey of 201 cases. Br J Surg 56:277–281, 1969.

589. Houang MTW, Brenton DP, Renton P, et al: Idiopathic juvenile osteoporosis. Skeletal Radiol 3:17–23, 1978.

590. Howland WJ, Curry JL, Buffington CB: Fulcrum fractures of the lumbar spine: transverse fracture induced by an improperly placed seat belt. JAMA 193:240–241, 1965.

591. Howland WJ, Loeffler RK, Starchman DE, et al: Postirradiation atrophic changes of bone and related complications. Radiology 117:677–685, 1975.

592. Hsu LCS, Leong JCY: Tuberculosis of the lower cervical spine (C2 to C7): a report on 40 cases. J Bone Joint Surg 66B:1–5, 1984.

593. Hubbard DD, Gunn DR: Secondary carcinoma of the spine with destruction of the intervertebral disk. Clin Orthop 88:86–88, 1972.

594. Huggins C, Blocksom BH Jr, Noonan WJ: Temperature conditions in the bone marrow of rabbit, pigeon and albino rat. Am J Physiol 115:395–401, 1936.

595. Huggins C, Noonan WJ: An increase in reticuloendothelial cells in outlying bone marrow consequent upon a local increase in temperature. J Exp Med 64:275–280, 1936.

596. Hughes RG, Kay HEM: Major bone lesions in acute lymphoblastic leukemia. Med Pediatr Oncol 10:67–70, 1982.

597. Hulth A, Olerud S: The reaction of bone to experimental cancer. Acta Orthop Scand 36:230–240, 1965.

598. Hungerford GD, Akkaraju V, Rawe SE, et al: Atlanto-occipital and atlanto-axial dislocations with spinal cord compression in Down's syndrome: a case report and review of the literature. Br J Radiol 54:758–761, 1981.

599. Hunter T: Solitary eosinophilic granuloma of bone. J Bone Joint Surg 38B:545–557, 1956.

600. Hunter T, Dubo HIC: Spinal fractures complicating ankylosing spondylitis. A long-term followup study. Arthritis Rheum 26:751–759, 1983.

601. Hurxthal LM: Measurement of anterior vertebral compressions and biconcave vertebrae. AJR 103:635–644, 1968.

602. Hutter RVP, Foote FW Jr, Frazell EL, et al: Giant cell tumors complicating Paget's disease of bone. Cancer 16:1044–1056, 1963.

603. Hutter VP, Worcester JN Jr, Francis KC, et al: Benign and malignant giant cell tumors of bone. Cancer 15:653–690, 1962.

604. Hutton WC, Stott JRR, Cyron BM: Is spondylolysis a fatigue fracture? Spine 2:202–209, 1977.

605. Huvos AG, Butler A, Bretsky SS: Osteogenic sarcoma associated with Paget's disease of bone: a clinicopathologic study of 65 patients. Cancer 52:1489–1495, 1983.

606. Huvos AG, Woodard HQ, Cahan WG, et al: Postradiation osteogenic sarcoma of bone and soft tissues: a clinicopathologic study of 66 patients. Cancer 55:1244–1255, 1985.

607. Imler AE, Meilstrup DB, Bogart FB: Primary Ewing's sarcoma of the spine. Radiology 46:597–600, 1946.

608. Ippolito E, Farsetti P, Tudisco C: Vertebra plana: long-term follow-up in five patients. J Bone Joint Surg 66A:1364–1368, 1984.

609. Ippolito E, Ponseti IV: Juvenile kyphosis: histological and histochemical studies. J Bone Joint Surg 63A:175–182, 1981.

610. Irwin GAL: Benign osteoblastoma of spine. NY State J Med 70:687–689, 1970.

611. Iwasaki Y, Akino M, Abe H, et al: Calcification of the ligamentum flavum of the cervical spine: report of four cases. J Neurosurg 59:531–534, 1983.

612. Jackson RP, Reckling FW, Mantz FA: Osteoid osteoma and osteoblastoma. Similar histologic lesions with different natural histories. Clin Orthop 128:303–313, 1977.

613. Jacobs LG: Roentgenography of the second cervical vertebra by Ottonello's method. Radiology 31:412–413, 1938.

614. Jacobs P: Osteolytic Paget's disease. Clin Radiol 25:137–144, 1974.

615. Jacobs SC, Pikna D, Lawson RK: Prostatic osteoblastic factor. Invest Urol 17:195–198, 1979.

616. Jacobson G, Bleecker HH: Pseudosubluxation of the axis in children. AJR 82:472–481, 1959.

617. Jacobson HG: Dense bone—too much bone: radiological considerations and differential diagnosis. Part I. Skeletal Radiol 13:1–20, 1985.

618. Jacobson HG, Poppel MH, Shapiro JH, et al: The vertebral pedicle sign. A roentgen finding to differentiate metastatic carcinoma from multiple myeloma. AJR 80:817–821, 1958.

619. Jacobson HG, Siegelman SS: Some miscellaneous solitary bone lesions. Semin Roentgenol 1:314–335, 1966.

620. Jaffe HL: Benign osteoblastoma. Bull Hosp Joint Dis 17:141–151, 1956.

621. Jaffe HL: Metabolic, Degenerative, and Inflammatory Diseases of Bones and Joints. Philadelphia: Lea & Febiger, 1972.

622. Jaffe HL, Lichtenstein L, Portis RB: Giant cell tumor of bone: its pathologic appearance, grading, supposed variants and treatment. Arch Pathol 30:993–1031, 1940.

623. Jájic I: Gout in the spine and sacro-iliac joints: radiological manifestations. Skeletal Radiol 8:209–212, 1982.

624. Jájic I, Furst Z, Vuksic B: Spondylitis erosiva: report on 9 patients. Ann Rheum Dis 41:237–241, 1982.

625. Jájic I, Kerhin V, Kastelan A: Ankylosing spondylitis syndrome in patients without HLA-B27. Br J Rheumatol (Suppl. 2) 22:136, 1983.

625a. James AE Jr, Merz T, Janower ML, et al: Radiological features of the most common autosomal disorders: trisomy 21–22 (mongolism or Down's syndrome), trisomy 18, trisomy 13–15, and the cri du chat syndrome. Clin Radiol 22:417–433, 1971.

626. Janetos GP: Paget's disease in the cervical spine. AJR 97:655–657, 1966.

627. Janin Y, Epstein JA, Carras R, et al: Osteoid osteomas and osteoblastomas of the spine. Neurosurgery 8:31–38, 1981.

628. Jeanneret B, Magerl F, Stanisic M: Thrombosis of the vertebral artery: a rare complication following traumatic spondylolisthesis of the second cervical vertebra. Spine 11:179–182, 1986.

629. Jefferson A: Localized enlargement of the spinal

canal in the absence of tumour: a congenital abnormality. J Neurol Neurosurg Psychiatry 18:305–309, 1955.

630. Jefferson G: Fracture of the atlas vertebra: report of four cases, and a review of those previously recorded. Br J Surg 7:407–422, 1920.

631. Jelsma RK, Kirsch PT, Rice JF, et al: The radiographic description of thoracolumbar fractures. Surg Neurol 18:230–236, 1982.

632. Jenkins P, Davies GR, Harper PS: Morquio-Brailsford disease: a report of four affected sisters with absence of excessive keratan sulphate in the urine. Br J Radiol 46:668–675, 1973.

633. Joffe N: Some radiological aspects of scurvy in the adult. Br J Radiol 34:429–437, 1961.

634. Johnson AD: Pathology of metastatic tumors in bone. Clin Orthop 73:8–32, 1970.

635. Johnson LC, Meador GE: The nature of benign "solitary myeloma" of bone. Bull Hosp Joint Dis 12:298–313, 1951.

636. Johnsson K-E, Willner S, Johnsson K: Postoperative instability after decompression for lumbar spinal stenosis. Spine 11:107–110, 1986.

637. Johnston CE II, Happel LT Jr, Norris R, et al: Delayed paraplegia complicating sublaminar segmental spinal instrumentation. J Bone Joint Surg 68A:556–563, 1986.

638. Jones MW, Kaufmann JCE: Vertebrobasilar artery insufficiency in rheumatoid atlantoaxial subluxation. J Neurol Neurosurg Psychiatry 39:122–128, 1976.

639. Jones RAC, Thomas JLG: The narrow lumbar canal: a clinical and radiological review. J Bone Joint Surg 50B:595–605, 1968.

640. Juhl JH, Miller SM, Roberts GW: Roentgenographic variations in the normal cervical spine. Radiology 78:591–597, 1962.

641. Jumshyd A, Khan MA: Ankylosing hyperostosis in American blacks: a longitudinal study. Clin Rheumatol 2:123–126, 1983.

642. Kahanovitz N, Rimoin DL, Sillence DO: The clinical spectrum of lumbar spine disease in achondroplasia. Spine 7:137–140, 1982.

643. Kaibara N, Takagishi K, Katsuki I, et al: Spondyloepiphyseal dysplasia tarda with progressive arthropathy. Skeletal Radiol 10:13–16, 1983.

644. Kam J, Funston MR: Venous collaterals causing vertebral body notching. Br J Radiol 53:491, 1980.

644a. Kaplan P, Resnick D, Murphey M, et al: Destructive noninfectious spondyloarthropathy in hemodialysis patients: a report of four cases. Radiology 162:241–244, 1987.

645. Kapur P, Banna M: Spinal osseous angioma: Gelfoam embolization. J Can Assoc Radiol 31:271–272, 1980.

646. Karasick D, Karasick S: Calcific retropharyngeal tendinitis. Skeletal Radiol 7:203–205, 1981.

647. Karasick S, Karasick D, Schilling J: Acute megakaryoblastic leukemia (acute "malignant" myelofibrosis): an unusual cause of osteosclerosis. Skeletal Radiol 9:45–46, 1982.

648. Karian JM, DeFilipp G, Buchheit WA, et al: Vertebral osteochondroma causing spinal cord compression: case report. Neurosurgery 14:483–484, 1984.

649. Karparov M, Kitov D: Aneurysmal bone cyst of the spine. Acta Neurochir 39:101–113, 1977.

650. Kassel EE, Cooper PW, Rubenstein JD: Radiology of spinal trauma: practical experience in a trauma unit. J Can Assoc Radiol 34:189–203, 1983.

651. Kattan KR: Backward "displacement" of the spinolaminar line at C2: a normal variation. AJR 129:289–290, 1977.

652. Kattan KR, Pais MJ: The spinous process: the forgotten appendage. Skeletal Radiol 6:199–204, 1981.

653. Kattan KR, Pais MJ: Some borderlands of the cervical spine. Part I: the normal (and nearly normal) that may appear pathologic. Skeletal Radiol 8:1–6, 1982.

654. Kattan KR, Pais MJ: Some borderlands of the cervical spine. Part II: the subtle and the hidden abnormal. Skeletal Radiol 8:7–12, 1982.

655. Katz JF: Back disorders in children. Clin Orthop 21:62–77, 1961.

656. Kaufman RA, Dunbar JS, Botsford JA, et al: Traumatic longitudinal atlanto-occipital distraction injuries in children. AJNR 3:415–419, 1982.

657. Kaye JJ, Freiberger RH: Eosinophilic granuloma of the spine without vertebra plana: a report of two unusual cases. Radiology 92:1188–1191, 1969.

658. Keats TE: The inferior accessory ossicle of the anterior arch of the atlas. AJR 101:834–836, 1967.

659. Keats TE, Riddervold HO, Michaelis LL: Thanatophoric dwarfism. AJR 108:473–480, 1970.

660. Keats TE, Burns TW: The radiographic manifestations of gonadal dysgenesis. Radiol Clin North Am 2:297–313, 1964.

661. Keene JS, Goletz TH, Lilleas F, et al: Diagnosis of vertebral fractures: a comparison of conventional radiography, conventional tomography and computed axial tomography. J Bone Joint Surg 64A:586–595, 1982.

661a. Kehl DK, Alonso JE, Lovell WW: Scoliosis secondary to an osteoid-osteoma of the rib. J Bone Joint Surg 65A:701–703, 1983.

662. Keim HA, Keagy RD: Congenital absence of lumbar articular facets: a report of three cases. J Bone Joint Surg 49A:523–526, 1967.

663. Keim HA, Reina EG: Osteoid-osteoma as a cause of scoliosis. J Bone Joint Surg 57A:159–163, 1975.

664. Kelsey JL, Hardy RJ: Driving of motor vehicles as a risk factor for acute herniated lumbar intervertebral disc. Am J Epidemiol 102:63–73, 1975.

665. Kemp HBS, Jackson JW, Jeremiah JD, et al: Pyogenic infections occurring primarily in intervertebral discs. J Bone Joint Surg 55B:698–714, 1973.

666. Keplinger JE, Bucy PC: Giant-cell tumors of the spine. Ann Surg 154:648–661, 1961.

667. Khan MA, van der Linden SM, Kushner I, et al: Spondylitic disease without radiologic evidence of sacroiliitis in relatives of HLA-B27 positive ankylosing spondylitis patients. Arthritis Rheum 28:40–43, 1985.

668. Killebrew K, Gold RH, Sholkoff SD: Psoriatic spondylitis. Radiology 108:9–16, 1973.

669. King HA, Bradford DS: Fracture-dislocation of the spine after spine fusion and Harrington instrumentation for idiopathic scoliosis: a case report. J Bone Joint Surg 62A:1374–1376, 1980.

670. Kirchmer NA, Sarwar M: Absent arch and hypoplastic pedicle: another confusing cervical spine anomaly. AJR 129:154–155, 1977.

671. Kirkaldy-Willis WH, Farfan HF: Instability of the lumbar spine. Clin Orthop 165:110–123, 1982.

672. Kirkaldy-Willis WH, Paine KWE, Cauchoix J, et

al: Lumbar spinal stenosis. Clin Orthop 99: 30–50, 1974.

673. Kirkaldy-Willis WH, Wedge JH, Yong-Hing K, et al: Pathology and pathogenesis of lumbar spondylosis and stenosis. Spine 3:319–328, 1978.

674. Kirwan EO'G, Hutton PAN, Pozo JL, et al: Osteoid osteoma and benign osteoblastoma of the spine. J Bone Joint Surg 66B:21–26, 1984.

675. Kittleson AC, Lim LW: Measurement of scoliosis. AJR 108:775–777, 1970.

675a. Klein DM, Weiss RL, Allen JE: Scheuermann's dorsal kyphosis and spinal cord compression: case report. Neurosurgery 18:628–631, 1986.

675b. Kleinman P, Rivelis M, Schneider R, et al: Juvenile ankylosing spondylitis. Radiology 125: 775–780, 1977.

676. Kleinman PK: Down syndrome (trisomy 21). Case report 244. Skeletal Radiol 10:192–195, 1983.

677. Klinghoffer L, Murdock MG: Spondylolysis following trauma: a case report and review of the literature. Clin Orthop 166:72–74, 1982.

678. Klinghoffer L, Murdock MG, Hermel MB: Congenital absence of lumbar articular facets: report of two cases. Clin Orthop 106:151–154, 1975.

679. Klippel M, Feil A: A case of absence of cervical vertebrae with the thoracic cage rising to the base of the cranium (cervical thoracic cage): the classic. Clin Orthop 109:3–8, 1975.

680. Knutsson F: The instability associated with disk degeneration in the lumbar spine. Acta Radiol 25:593–609, 1944.

681. Knutsson F: Growth and differentiation of the postnatal vertebra. Acta Radiol 55:401–408, 1961.

682. Kobori M, Takahashi H, Mikawa Y: Atlantoaxial dislocation in Down's syndrome: report of two cases requiring surgical correction. Spine 11: 195–200, 1986.

683. Koontz WW Jr, Prout GR Jr: Agenesis of the sacrum and the neurogenic bladder. JAMA 203:481–486, 1968.

684. Kornberg M: Primary Ewing's sarcoma of the spine: a review and case report. Spine 11:54–57, 1986.

685. Kornberg M, Rechtine GR, Dupuy TE: Unusual presentation of spinal osteomyelitis in a patient taking propylthiouracil. Spine 10:104–107, 1985.

686. Korobkin M, Novick HP, Palubinskas AJ: Asymptomatic sacral agenesis with neurogenic bladder in a 42 year old man. AJR 115:611–613, 1972.

687. Korsten J, Grossman H, Winchester PH, et al: Extramedullary hematopoiesis in patients with thalassemia anemia. Radiology 95:257–263, 1970.

688. Koss JC, Dalinka MA: Atlantoaxial subluxation in Behçet's syndrome. AJR 134:392–393, 1980.

689. Kovarik J, Küster W, Seidl G, et al: Clinical relevance of radiologic examination of the skeleton and bone density measurements in osteoporosis of old age. Skeletal Radiol 7:37–41, 1981.

690. Kozlowski K, Beluffi G, Masel J, et al: Primary vertebral tumors in children: report of 20 cases with brief literature review. Pediatr Radiol 14:129–139, 1984.

691. Kricun ME: Radiographic evaluation of solitary bone lesions. Orthop Clin North Am 14:39–64, 1983.

692. Kricun ME: Red-yellow marrow conversion: its effects on the location of some solitary bone lesions. Skeletal Radiol 14:10–19, 1985.

693. Kricun ME: Radiographic approach to the arthritides. In Katz WA (ed): Diagnosis and Management of Rheumatoid Disorders. Philadelphia: JB Lippincott Company, 1987.

694. Kricun R, Kricun ME: Computed Tomography of the Spine: Diagnostic Exercises. Rockville, Maryland: Aspen Publishers, Inc, 1987.

695. Krol G, Sundaresan N, Deck M: Computed tomography of axial chordomas. J Comput Assist Tomogr 7:286–289, 1983.

696. Krølner B, Berthelsen B, Nielsen SP: Assessment of vertebral osteopenia: comparison of spinal radiography and dual-photon absorptiometry. Acta Radiol [Diagn] 23:517–521, 1982.

697. Krook L, Whalen JP, Dorfman HD, et al: Osteopetrosis: an interpretation of its pathogenesis. Skeletal Radiol 7:185–189, 1981.

698. Kudo S, Ono M, Russell WJ: Ossification of thoracic ligamenta flava. AJR 141:117–121, 1983.

699. Laasonen EM, Riska EB: Preoperative radiological assessment of fractures of the thoracolumbar spine causing traumatic paraplegia. Skeletal Radiol 1:231–234, 1977.

700. Lachman E: Osteoporosis: the potentialities and limitations of its roentgenologic diagnosis. AJR 74:712–715, 1955.

701. Lachmann M, Kricun ME, Schwartz EE: Primary hyperparathyroidism (HPR), with patchy diffuse osteosclerosis at multiple skeletal sites. Case report 310. Skeletal Radiol 13:248–252, 1985.

702. Ladd JR, Cassidy JT, Martel W: Juvenile ankylosing spondylitis. Arthritis Rheum 14:579–590, 1971.

703. Lagier R, MacGee W: Spondylodiscal erosions due to gout: anatomico-radiological study of a case. Ann Rheum Dis 42:350–353, 1983.

704. Lagier R, Mbakop A, Bigler A: Osteopoikilosis: a radiological and pathological study. Skeletal Radiol 11:161–168, 1984.

705. Lagier R, Sit'aj S: Vertebral changes in ochronosis. Anatomical and radiological study of one case. Ann Rheum Dis 33:86–92, 1974.

706. Lander PH, Hadjipavlou AG: A dynamic classification of Paget's disease. J Bone Joint Surg 68B:431–438, 1986.

707. Lane JM, Vigorita VJ: Osteoporosis. J Bone Joint Surg 65A:274–278, 1983.

708. Lang EK, Bessler WT: The roentgenologic features of acromegaly. AJR 86:321–328, 1961.

709. Lange TA, Zoltan D, Hafez GR: Simultaneous occurrence in the spine of osteoblastoma and hemangioendothelioma: a case report. Spine 11:92–95, 1986.

710. Langer LO Jr: Spondyloepiphyseal dysplasia tarda: hereditary chondrodysplasia with characteristic vertebral configuration in the adult. Radiology 82:833–839, 1964.

711. Langer LO Jr: Diastrophic dwarfism in early infancy. AJR 93:399–404, 1965.

712. Langer LO Jr, Baumann PA, Gorlin RJ: Achondroplasia. AJR 100:12–26, 1967.

713. Langer LO Jr, Carey LS: The roentgenographic features of the KS mucopolysaccharidosis of Morquio (Morquio-Brailsford's) disease. AJR 97: 1–20, 1966.

714. Larsen JL: The posterior surface of the lumbar vertebral bodies. Part I. Spine 10:50–58, 1985.

714a. Larsson S-E, Lorentzon R, Boquist L: Giant-cell tumors of the spine and sacrum causing neurological symptoms. Clin Orthop 111:201–211, 1975.

715. Latchaw RE, Meyer GW: Reiter disease with atlanto-axial subluxation. Radiology 126:303–304, 1978.

716. Lauten GJ, Wehunt WD: Computed tomography in absent cervical pedicle. AJNR 1:201–203, 1980.

717. Lavellee G, Lemarbre L, Bouchard R, et al: Ewing's sarcoma in adults. J Can Assoc Radiol 30:223–227, 1979.

718. Lederman HM, Kaufman RA: Congenital absence and hypoplasia of pedicle in the thoracic spine. Skeletal Radiol 15:219–233, 1986.

719. Lee C, Kim KS, Rogers LF: Sagittal fracture of the cervical vertebral body. AJR 139:55–60, 1982.

720. Lee C, Kim KS, Rogers LF: Triangular cervical vertebral body fractures: diagnostic significance. AJR 138:1123–1132, 1982.

721. Lee CK, Weiss AB: Isolated congenital cervical block vertebrae below the axis with neurological symptoms. Spine 6:118–124, 1981.

722. Leeds NE, Jacobson HG: Plain film examination of the spinal canal. Semin Roentgenol 7:179–196, 1972.

723. Leeds NE, Jacobson HG: Spinal neurofibromatosis. AJR 126:617–623, 1976.

724. Leehey P, Naseem M, Every P, et al: Vertebral hemangioma with compression myelopathy: metrizamide CT demonstration. J Comput Assist Tomogr 9:985–986, 1985.

725. Leeson MC, Rechtine GR, Makley JT, et al: Primary amyloidoma of the spine: a case report and review of the literature. Spine 10:303–306, 1985.

726. Legant O, Ball, RP: Sickle-cell anemia in adults: roentgenographic findings. Radiology 51:665–675, 1948.

727. Lehman TJA, Hanson V, Kornreich H, et al: HLA-B27–negative sacroiliitis: a manifestation of familial Mediterranean fever in childhood. Pediatrics 61:423–426, 1978.

728. Lehtinen K, Kaarela K, Anttila P, et al: Sacroiliitis in inflammatory joint diseases. Scand J Rheumatol 52:19–22, 1984.

729. LeMay M, Blunt JW JR: A factor determining the location of pseudofractures in osteomalacia. J Clin Invest 28:521–525, 1949.

730. Leune JSM, Mok CK, Leong JCY, et al: Syphilitic aortic aneurysm with spinal erosion. J Bone Joint Surg 59B:89–92, 1977.

731. Lewin H, Stein JM: Solitary plasma cell myeloma with new bone formation. AJR 79:630–637, 1958.

732. Lewinnek GE, Peterson SE: A calcified fibrocartilaginous nodule in the ligamentum nuchae: presenting as a tumor. Clin Orthop 136:163–165, 1978.

733. Libshitz HI, Hortobagyi GN: Radiographic evaluation of therapeutic response in bony metastases of breast cancer. Skeletal Radiol 7:159–165, 1981.

734. Libson E, Bloom RA: Anteroposterior angulated view. A new radiographic technique for the evaluation of spondylolysis. Radiology 149:315–316, 1983.

735. Libson E, Bloom RA, Rinari G, et al: Oblique lumbar spine radiographs: importance in young patients. Radiology 151:89–90, 1984.

736. Lichtenstein BW: "Spinal dysraphism." Spina bifida and myelodysplasia. Arch Neurol Psychiatr 44:792–810, 1940.

737. Lichtenstein L: Aneurysmal bone cyst: observation on fifty cases. J Bone Joint Surg 39A:873–882, 1957.

738. Lichtenstein L: Bone Tumors, 4th ed. St. Louis: CV Mosby Company, 1972, p 169.

739. Lichtenstein L, Sawyer WR: Benign osteoblastoma. Further observations and report of twenty additional cases. J Bone Joint Surg 46A:755–765, 1964.

740. Lichtenstein L, Scott HW, Levin MH: Pathologic changes in gout: survey of 11 necropsied cases. Am J Pathol 32:871–895, 1956.

741. Lifeso RM, Harder E, McCorkell SJ: Spinal brucellosis. J Boint Joint Surg 67B:345–351, 1985.

742. Lifeso RM, Weaver P, Harder EH: Tuberculous spondylitis in adults. J Bone Joint Surg 67A:1405–1413, 1985.

743. Lifeso RM, Younge D: Aneurysmal bone cysts of the spine. Int Orthop 8:281–285, 1985.

744. Lindholm TS, Snellman O, Österman K: Scoliosis caused by benign osteoblastoma of the lumbar spine: a report of three patients. Spine 2:276–281, 1977.

745. Lindsey RW, Piepmeier J, Burkus JK: Tortuosity of the vertebral artery: an adventitious finding after cervical trauma. J Bone Joint Surg 67A:806–808, 1985.

746. Lindvall N: Early x-ray diagnosis and spondylitis. Scand J Rheum (Suppl 32) 9:115–119, 1980.

747. Lindvall N: Early x-ray diagnosis of sacro-iliitis. Scand J Rheum (Suppl 32) 9:98–102, 1980.

748. Linkowski GD, Tsai FY, Recher L, et al: Solitary osteochondroma with spinal cord compression. Surg Neurol 23:388–390, 1985.

748a. Linquist PR, McDonnell DE: Rheumatoid cyst causing extradural compression: a case report. J Bone Joint Surg 52A:1235–1240, 1970.

749. Lippitt AB: The facet joint and its role in spine pain; management with facet joint injections. Spine 9:746–750, 1984.

750. Lipson SJ: Rheumatoid arthritis of the cervical spine. Clin Orthop 182:143–149, 1984.

751. Lipson SJ: Cervical myelopathy and posterior atlanto-axial subluxation in patients with rheumatoid arthritis. J Bone Joint Surg 67A:593–597, 1985.

752. Lloyd HM, Aitken RE, Ferrier TM: Primary hyperparathyroidism resembling rickets of late onset. Br Med J 2:853–856, 1965.

753. Lloyd-Roberts GC, Pincott JR, McMeniman P, et al: Progression in idiopathic scoliosis: a preliminary report of a possible mechanism. J Bone Joint Surg 60B:451–460, 1978.

754. Locke GR, Gardner JI, Van Epps EF: Atlas-dens interval (ADI) in children—a survey based on 200 normal cervical spines. AJR 97:135–140, 1966.

755. Lodwick GS: The radiologic diagnosis of metastatic cancer in bone. In M.D. Anderson Hospital and Tumor Institute (ed): Tumors of Bone and Soft Tissues. Chicago: Year Book Medical Publishers, Inc, 1965, pp 253–277.

756. Loftus CM, Michelsen CB, Rapoport F, et al: Management of plasmacytomas of the spine. Neurosurgery 13:30–36, 1983.

757. Lombardi G: The occipital vertebra. AJR 86:260–269, 1961.

758. Lonstein JE, Carlson M: The prediction of curve

progression in untreated idiopathic scoliosis during growth. J Bone Joint Surg 66A:1061–1071, 1984.

759. Lott G, Klein E: Osteopetrosis: a case presentation. AJR 94:616–620, 1965.

760. Lott IT, Richardson EP Jr: Neuropathological findings and the biology of neurofibromatosis. Adv Neurol 29:23–32, 1981.

760a. Lowe RW, Hayes TD, Kaye J, et al: Standing roentgenograms in spondylolisthesis. Clin Orthop 117:80–84, 1976.

761. Lubert M: Actinomycosis of the vertebrae. AJR 51:669–676, 1944.

762. Ludwig H, Kumpan W, Sinzinger H: Radiography and bone scintigraphy in multiple myeloma: a comparative analysis. Br J Radiol 55:173–181, 1982.

763. Lundeen MA, Herring JA: Osteoid-osteoma of the spine: sclerosis in two levels. J Bone Joint Surg 62A:476–478, 1980.

764. Luyendijk W, Matricali B, Thomeer RTWM: Basilar impression in an achondroplastic dwarf: causative role in tetraparesis. Acta Neurochir 41:243–253, 1978.

765. Lyon E: Uncovertebral osteophytes and osteochondrosis of the cervical spine. J Bone Joint Surg 27:248–253, 1945.

766. MacCarthy JMT, Carey MC: Bone changes in homocystinuria. Clin Radiol 19:128–134, 1968.

767. MacEwen GD: Experimental scoliosis. Clin Orthop 93:69–74, 1973.

768. MacEwen GD, Winter RB, Hardy JH: Evaluation of kidney anomalies in congenital scoliosis. J Bone Joint Surg 54A:1451–1454, 1972.

769. MacLellan DI, Wilson FC Jr: Osteoid osteoma of the spine. A review of the literature and report of six new cases. J Bone Joint Surg 49A:111–121, 1967.

770. Macnab I: The traction spur: an indicator of segmental instability. J Bone Joint Surg 53A:663–670, 1971.

771. Macnab I: Cervical spondylosis. Clin Orthop 109:69–77, 1975.

772. MacNeil P, Long NG: Ewing's sarcoma of the cervical spine: with a case report. Am J Surg 88:928–932, 1954.

773. Macpherson RI: Aneurysmal bone cyst of spine diagnosed by percutaneous opacification. J Can Assoc Radiol 31:210–212, 1980.

774. Madigan R, Worrall T, McClain EJ: Cervical cord compression in hereditary multiple exostosis: review of the literature and report of a case. J Bone Joint Surg 56A:401–404, 1974.

775. Maeyama I: Bone tumors in Japan. Clin Orthop 184:65–70, 1984.

776. Maiman DJ, Larson SJ: Management of odontoid fractures. Neurosurgery 11:471–476, 1982.

777. Mainzer F: Herniation of the nucleus pulposus: a rare complication of intervertebral-disk calcification in children. Radiology 107:167–170, 1973.

778. Major P, Resnick D, Dalinka M, et al: Coexisting rheumatoid arthritis and ankylosing spondylitis. AJR 134:1076–1979, 1980.

779. Malawista SE, Seegmiller JE, Hathaway BE, et al: Sacroiliac gout. JAMA 194:106–108, 1965.

780. Malcolm BW: Spinal deformity secondary to spinal injury. Orthop Clin North Am 10:943–952, 1979.

781. Maldague BE, Malghem JJ: Unilateral arch hypertrophy with spinous process tilt: a sign of arch deficiency. Radiology 121:567–574, 1976.

782. Maldague BE, Noel HM, Malghem JJ: The intravertebral vacuum cleft: a sign of ischemic vertebral collapse. Radiology 129:23–29, 1978.

783. Manaster BJ, Norman A: CT diagnosis of thoracic pedicle aplasia: case report. J Comput Assist Tomogr 7:1090–1091, 1983.

784. Mandell GA: The pedicle in neurofibromatosis. AJR 130:675–678, 1978.

785. Mandell GA, Kricun ME: Exaggerated anterior vertebral notching. Radiology 131:367–369, 1979.

786. Manning HJ: Symptomatic hemangioma of the spine. Radiology 56:58–65, 1951.

786a. Mansfield CM: A vertical fracture of the fifth cervical vertebra without neurologic symptoms. AJR 86:277–280, 1961.

787. Marklund T: Relative width of the lower spinal cord in children. Acta Radiol [Diagn] 23:313–321, 1982.

788. Marklund T: Predictive value of interpeduncular distance measurement in children. Acta Radiol [Diagn] 26:599–602, 1985.

789. Marks SC Jr: Congenital osteopetrotic mutations as probes of the origin, structure and function of osteoclasts. Clin Orthop 189:239–263, 1984.

790. Markuske H: Sagittal diameter measurements of the bony cervical spinal canal in children. Pediatr Radiol 6:129–131, 1977.

791. Marr JT: Gas in intervertebral discs. AJR 70:804–809, 1953.

792. Marsh BW, Bonfiglio M, Brady LP, et al: Benign osteoblastoma: range of manifestations. J Bone Joint Surg 57A:1–9, 1975.

793. Marsh HO, Choi C-B: Primary osteogenic sarcoma of the cervical spine originally mistaken for benign osteoblastoma: a case report. J Bone Joint Surg 52A:1467–1471, 1970.

794. Martel W: The occipito-atlanto-axial joints in rheumatoid arthritis and ankylosing spondylitis. AJR 86:223–240, 1961.

795. Martel W: The occipito-atlanto-axial joints in rheumatoid arthritis. Proceedings of the international symposium organized by ISRA. Amsterdam, 1963.

796. Martel W, Braunstein EM, Borlaza G, et al: Radiologic features of Reiter disease. Radiology 132:1–10, 1979.

797. Martel W, Holt JF, Cassidy JT: Roentgenologic manifestations of juvenile rheumatoid arthritis. AJR 88:400–423, 1962.

798. Martel W, McCarter DK, Solsky MA, et al: Further observations on the arthropathy of calcium pyrophosphate crystal deposition disease. Radiology 141:1–15, 1981.

799. Martel W, Seeger JF, Wicks JD, et al: Traumatic lesions of the discovertebral junction in the lumbar spine. AJR 127:457–464, 1976.

800. Martel W, Tishler JM: Observations on the spine in mongoloidism. AJR 97:630–638, 1966.

801. Martel W, Uyhman R, Stimson CW: Subluxation of the atlas causing spinal cord compression in a case of Down's syndrome with a "manifestation of an occipital vertebra." Radiology 93:839–840, 1969.

802. Martinez S, Morgan CL, Gehweiler JA Jr, et al: Unusual fractures and dislocations of the axis vertebra. Skeletal Radiol 3:206–212, 1979.

803. Mason RC, Kozlowski K: Chondrodysplasia

punctata: report of ten cases. Radiology 109: 145–150, 1973.

804. Matozzi F, Moreau JJ, Jiddane M, et al: Correlative anatomic and CT study of the lumbar lateral recess. AJNR 4:650–652, 1983.
805. Matsushita T, Suzuki K: Spastic paraparesis due to cryptococcal osteomyelitis. Clin Orthop 196:279–284, 1985.
806. Mawhinney R, Jones R, Worthington BS: Spinal cord compression secondary to Paget's disease of the axis: case reports. Br J Radiol 58: 1203–1206, 1985.
807. Mawk JR, Erickson DL, Chou SN, et al: Aspergillus infections of the lumbar disc spaces: report of three cases. J Neurosurg 58:270–274, 1983.
808. Mayer BS: Chondromyxoid fibroma of lumbar spine. J Can Assoc Radiol 29:271–272, 1978.
809. Mayer L: Malignant degeneration of so-called benign osteoblastoma. Bull Hosp Joint Dis 28:4–13, 1967.
810. Mayfield JK, Erkkila JC, Winter RB: Spine deformity subsequent to acquired childhood spinal cord injury. J Bone Joint Surg 63A:1401–1411, 1981.
811. Mayfield JK, Riseborough EJ, Jaffe N, et al: Spinal deformity in children treated for neuroblastoma: the effect of radiation and other forms of treatment. J Bone Joint Surg 63A:183–193, 1981.
812. Mayfield JK, Winter RB, Bradford DS, et al: Congenital kyphosis due to defects of anterior augmentation. J Bone Joint Surg 62A:1291–1301, 1980.
813. Mazess RB: On aging bone loss. Clin Orthop 165:239–252, 1982.
814. McAfee PC, Bohlman HH: Complications following Harrington instrumentation for fractures of the thoracolumbar spine. J Bone Joint Surg 67A:672–686, 1985.
815. McAlister WH, Shackelford GD: Classification of spinal curvatures. Radiol Clin North Am 13:93–112, 1975.
816. McAlister WH, Shackelford GD: Measurement of spinal curvatures. Rad Clin North Am 13:113–121, 1975.
817. McBryde AM Jr, McCollum DE: Ankylosing spondylitis in women. The disease and its prognosis. NC Med J 34:34–37, 1973.
818. McCall IW, Park WM, McSweeney T: The radiological demonstration of acute lower cervical injury. Clin Radiol 24:235–240, 1973.
819. McCarthy EF, Dorfman HD: Idiopathic segmental sclerosis of vertebral bodies. Skeletal Radiol 9:88–91, 1982.
820. McCarty DJ Jr, Haskin ME: The roentgenographic aspects of pseudogout (articular chondrocalcinosis): an analysis of 20 cases. AJR 90: 1248–1257, 1963.
821. McClelland RR, Marsh DG: Double diastematomyelia. Radiology 123:378, 1977.
822. McClenahan JL: Wasted x-rays. Radiology 96:453–456, 1970.
823. McCook TA, Felman AH, Ayoub E: Streptococcal skeletal infections: observations in four infants. AJR 130:465–467, 1978.
824. McDonald DJ, Sim FH, McLeod RA, et al: Giant-cell tumor of bone. J Bone Joint Surg 68A: 235–242, 1986.
825. McEwen C: Arthritis accompanying ulcerative colitis. Clin Orthop 57:9–17, 1968.
826. McGahan JP, Graves DS, Palmer PES: Coccidioidal spondylitis. Usual and unusual radiographic manifestations. Radiology 136:5–9, 1980.
827. McGregor M: The significance of certain measurements of the skull in the diagnosis of basilar impression. Br J Radiol 21:171–181, 1948.
828. McKee DF, Barr WM, Bryan CS, et al: Primary aspergillosis of the spine mimicking Pott's paraplegia. J Bone Joint Surg 66A:1481–1483, 1984.
829. McLaurin RL, Vernal R, Salmon JH: Treatment of fractures of the atlas and axis by wiring without fusion. J Neurosurg 36:773–780, 1972.
830. McLeod RA, Beabout JW: The roentgenographic features of chondroblastoma. AJR 118:464–471, 1973.
831. McLeod RA, Dahlin DC, Beabout JW: The spectrum of osteoblastoma. AJR 126:321–335, 1976.
832. McLoughlin DP, Wortzman G: Congenital absence of a cervical vertebral pedicle. J Can Assoc Radiol 23:195–200, 1972.
833. McManners T: Odontoid hypoplasia. Br J Radiol 56:907–910, 1983.
834. McMaster MJ: Infantile idiopathic scoliosis: Can it be prevented? J Bone Joint Surg 65B:612–617, 1983.
834a. McMaster MJ: Occult intraspinal anomalies and congenital scoliosis. J Bone Joint Surg 66A: 588–601, 1984.
835. McPhee IB: Spinal fractures and dislocations in children and adolescents. Spine 6:533–537, 1981.
836. McPhee IB, O'Brien JP: Scoliosis in symptomatic spondylolisthesis. J Bone Joint Surg 62B: 155–157, 1980.
837. McRae DL: Bony abnormalities in the region of the foramen magnum: correlation of the anatomic and neurologic findings. Acta Radiol 40:335–354, 1953.
838. McRae DL: The significance of abnormalities of the cervical spine. AJR 84:3–25, 1960.
839. McRae DL, Barnum AS: Occipitalization of the atlas. AJR 70:23–46, 1953.
840. Meema ME: Cortical bone atrophy and osteoporosis as a manifestation of aging. AJR 89: 1287–1295, 1963.
841. Meema HE, Meema S: Improved roentgenologic diagnosis of osteomalacia by microradioscopy of hand bones. AJR 125:925–935, 1975.
842. Meema HE, Oreopoulos DG, Meema S: A roentgenologic study of cortical bone resorption in chronic renal failure. Radiology 126:67–74, 1978.
843. Mehta MH: Radiographic estimate of vertebral rotation in scoliosis. J Bone Joint Surg 55B:513–520, 1973.
844. Mehta MH, Murray RO: Scoliosis provoked by painful vertebral lesions. Skeletal Radiol 1:223–230, 1977.
845. Melnick JC: Osteopathia condensans disseminata (osteopoikilosis). AJR 82:229–238, 1959.
846. Melnick JC, Silverman FN: Intervertebral disk calcification in childhood. Radiology 80: 399–408, 1963.
847. Menelaus MB: Discitis: an inflammation affecting the intervertebral discs in children. J Bone Joint Surg 46B:16–23, 1964.
848. Menezes AH, Van Gilder JC, Clark CR, et al: Odontoid upward migration in rheumatoid arthritis: an analysis of 45 patients with "cranial settling." J Neurosurg 63:500–509, 1985.
849. Meredith SC, Simon MA, Laros GS, et al: Pycnodysostosis: a clinical, pathological and ultra-

microscopic study of a case. J Bone Joint Surg 60A:1122–1127, 1968.

850. Merrick MV, Merrick JM: Observations on the natural history of Paget's disease. Clin Radiol 36:169–174, 1985.

851. Merrill V: Atlas of roentgenographic positions and standard radiologic procedures, vol. 1. St. Louis: CV Mosby Company, 1975, pp 207–269.

852. Merryweather R, Middlemiss JH, Sanerkin NG: Malignant transformation of osteoblastoma. J Bone Joint Surg 62B:381–384, 1980.

853. Meszaros WT: The many facets of multiple myeloma. Semin Roentgenol 9:219–228, 1974.

854. Meyer JE, Lepke RA, Lindfors KK, et al: Chordomas: their CT appearance in the cervical, thoracic and lumbar spine. Radiology 153:693–696, 1984.

855. Meyerding HW: Spondylolisthesis. Surg Gynecol Obstet 54:371–377, 1932.

856. Middlemass IBD: Bone changes in adult cretins. Br J Radiol 32:685–688, 1959.

857. Middlemiss JH, Raper AB: Skeletal changes in the haemoglobinopathies. J Bone Joint Surg 48B:693–702, 1956.

858. Mikhael MA, Ciric I, Tarkington JA, et al: Neurological evaluation of lateral recess syndrome. Radiology 140:97–107, 1981.

859. Milch RA, Changus GW: Response of bone to tumor invasion. Cancer 9:340–351, 1956.

860. Milgram JW, Jasty M: Osteopetrosis: a morphological study of twenty-one cases. J Bone Joint Surg 64A:912–929, 1982.

861. Milgram JW, Romine JS: Spontaneous osteomyelitis complicating a compression fracture of the lumbar spine: a case report. Spine 7:179–182, 1982.

862. Millard DG: Displacement of the linear thoracic paraspinal shadow of Brailsford: an early sign in osteomyelitis of the thoracic spine. AJR 90:1231–1235, 1963.

863. Miller F, Whitehill R: Carcinoma of the breast metastatic to the skeleton. Clin Orthop 184:121–127, 1984.

863a. Miller JDR, Capusten BM, Lampard R: Changes at the base of skull and cervical spine in Down syndrome. J Can Assoc Radiol 37:85–89, 1986.

864. Miller MD, Gehweiler JA, Martinez S, et al: Significant new observations on cervical spine trauma. AJR 130:659–663, 1978.

865. Miller TR, Nicholson JT: End results in reticulum cell sarcoma of bone treated by bacterial toxin therapy alone or combined with surgery and/or radiotherapy (47 cases) or with concurrent infection (5 cases). Cancer 27:524–548, 1971.

866. Mindell ER, Shah NK, Webster JH: Postradiation sarcoma of bone and soft tissue. Orthop Clin North Am 8:821–834, 1977.

867. Minderhoud JM, Braakman R, Penning L: Os odontoideum: clinical radiological and therapeutic aspects. J Neurol Sci 8:521–544, 1969.

868. Mitchell GE, Lourie H, Berne AS: The various causes of scalloped vertebrae with notes on their pathogenesis. Radiology 89:67–74, 1967.

869. Mitchell ML, Ackerman LV: Metastatic and pseudomalignant osteoblastoma: a report of two unusual cases. Skeletal Radiol 15:213–218, 1986.

870. Mnaymneh W, Brown M, Tejada F, et al: Primary osteogenic sarcoma of the second cervical vertebra. Case report. J Bone Joint Surg 61A:460–462, 1979.

871. Modena V, Maiocco I, Bosio A, et al: Intravertebral vacuum cleft: notes on five cases. Clin Exp Rheumatol 3:23–27, 1985.

872. Moës CAF: Spondylarthritis in childhood. AJR 91:578–587, 1964.

873. Mohan V, Gupta SK, Tuli SM, et al: Symptomatic vertebral hemangiomas. Clin Radiol 31:575–579, 1980.

874. Moilanen A, Kokko M-L, Pitkänen M: Gonadal dose reduction in lumbar spine radiography. Skeletal Radiol 9:153–156, 1983.

875. Moll JMH: Inflammatory bowel disease. Clin Rheum Dis 11:87–111, 1985.

876. Moreton RD, Winston JR, Bibby DE, et al: Radiologic considerations in placement examinations of the lumbar spine. Radiology 63:667–672, 1954.

877. Morgan DF, Young RF: Spinal neurological complications of achondroplasia: results of surgical treatment. J Neurosurg 52:463–472, 1980.

878. Morin ME, Palacios E: The aplastic hypoplastic lumbar pedicle. AJR 122:639–642, 1974.

879. Morreels CL Jr, Fletcher BD, Weilbaecher RG, et al: The roentgenographic features of homocystinuria. Radiology 90:1150–1158, 1968.

880. Morris JM, Samilson RL, Corley CL: Melorheostosis: review of the literature and report of an interesting case with a nineteen year follow-up. J Bone Joint Surg 45A:1191–1206, 1963.

881. Morris JW: Skeletal fluorosis among Indians of the American Southwest. AJR 94:608–615, 1965.

882. Moseley JE: Skeletal changes in the anemias. Semin Roentgenol 9:169–184, 1974.

883. Mueller CE, Seeger JF, Martel W: Ankylosing spondylitis and regional enteritis. Radiology 112:579–581, 1974.

884. Mundy GR, Raisz LG, Cooper RA, et al: Evidence for the secretion of an osteoclast stimulating factor in myeloma. N Engl J Med 291:1041–1046, 1974.

885. Murali R, Rovit RL, Benjamin MW: Chordoma of the cervical spine. Neurosurgery 9:253–256, 1981.

886. Murone I: The importance of the sagittal diameters of the cervical spinal canal in relation to spondylosis and myelopathy. J Bone Joint Surg 56B:30–36, 1974.

887. Murphy FD Jr, Blount WP: Cartilaginous exostoses following irradiation. J Bone Joint Surg 44A:662–668, 1962.

888. Murphy WA, Seligman PA, Tillack T, et al: Osteosclerosis, osteomalacia and bone marrow aplasia: a combined late complication of Thorotrast administration. Skeletal Radiol 3:234–238, 1979.

889. Murray RO: Radiological bone changes in Cushing's syndrome and steroid therapy. Br J Radiol 33:1–19, 1960.

889a. Murray RO, Jacobson HJ: The Radiology of Skeletal Disorders: Exercises in Diagnosis, 2nd ed. London: Churchill Livingstone, 1977, 633.

890. Murray RO, McCredie J: Melorheostosis and the sclerotomes: a radiological correlation. Skeleton Radiol 4:57–71, 1979.

891. Muthukrishnan N, Shetty MVK: Pycnodysostosis: report of a case. AJR 114:247–252, 1972.

892. Nachemson A: Lumbar spine instability: a critical update and symposium summary. Spine 10:290–292, 1985.

893. Nachemson AL: The lumbar spine: an orthopaedic challenge. Spine 1:59–71, 1976.

894. Nachemson AL, Sahlstrand T: Etiologic factors in adolescent idiopathic scoliosis. Spine 2:176–184, 1977.

895. Naidich JB, Naidich TP, Garfein C, et al: The widened interspinous distance: a useful sign of anterior cervical dislocation in the supine frontal projection. Radiology 123:113–116, 1977.

896. Naidich TP, McLone DG, Harwood-Nash DC: Spinal dysraphism. In Newton TH, Potts DG (eds): Computed Tomography of the Spine and Spinal Cord. San Anselmo: Clavadel Press, 1983, pp 299–353.

897. Naim-ur-Rahman: Atypical forms of spinal tuberculosis. J Bone Joint Surg 62B:162–165, 1980.

898. Nance EP Jr, Lams P, Gerlock AJ Jr: The opisthion on the lateral radiograph of the cervical spine. AJR 133:905–908, 1979.

899. Nanni G, Hudson TM: Posterior ring apophyses of the cervical spine. AJR 139:383–384, 1982.

900. Nash CL Jr, Gregg EC, Brown RH, et al: Risks of exposure to x-rays in patients undergoing long-term treatment for scoliosis. J Bone Joint Surg 61A:371–374, 1979.

901. Nash CL, Moe JH: A study of vertebral rotation. J Bone Joint Surg 51A:223–229, 1969.

902. Nassonova VA, Alekberova ZS, Folomeyev MY, et al: Sacroiliitis in male systemic lupus erythematosus. Scand J Rheumatol (Suppl) 52:23–29, 1984.

903. Nathan H: Osteophytes of the vertebral column: an anatomical study of their development according to age, race and sex with considerations as to their etiology and significance. J Bone Joint Surg 44A:243–268, 1962.

904. Nelson JD: The Marfan syndrome, with special reference to congenital enlargement of the spinal canal. Br J Radiol 31:561–564, 1958.

905. Nelson OA, Greer RB III: Localization of osteoid osteoma of the spine using computerized tomography. J Bone Joint Surg 65A:263–264, 1983.

906. Neugut AI, Casper ES, Godwin TA, et al: Osteoblastic metastases in renal cell carcinoma. Br J Radiol 54:1002–1004, 1981.

907. Neuhauser EBD, Wittenborg MH, Berman CZ, et al: Irradiation effects of roentgen therapy on the growing spine. Radiology 59:637–650, 1952.

908. Newmark H III, Forrester DM, Brown JC, et al: Calcific tendinitis of the neck. Radiology 128:355–358, 1978.

909. Newmark H III, Zee CS, Frankel P, et al: Chronic calcific tendinitis of the neck. Skeletal Radiol 7:207–208, 1981.

910. Nicholas JA, Saville PD, Bronner F: Osteoporosis, osteomalacia and the skeletal system. J Bone Joint Surg 45A:391–404, 1963.

911. Nicolet V, Chalaoui J, Vezina JL, et al: C2 "target": composite shadow. AJNR 5:331–332, 1984.

912. Niemeyer T, Penning L: Functional roentgenographic examination in a case of cervical spondylolisthesis. J Bone Joint Surg 45A:1671–1678, 1963.

913. Nixon GW: Hematogenous osteomyelitis of metaphyseal-equivalent locations. AJR 130:123–129, 1978.

914. Nixon GW, Gwinn JL: The roentgen manifestations of leukemia in infancy. Radiology 107:603–609, 1973.

915. Norman WJ, Johnson C: Congenital absence of a pedicle of a lumbar vertebra. Br J Radiol 46:631–633, 1973.

916. Northfield DWC: The Surgery of the Central Nervous System. London: Blackwell Scientific Publications, 1973.

917. Nottage WM, Waugh TR, McMaster WC: Radiation exposure during scoliosis screening radiography. Spine 6:456–459, 1981.

918. Novick GS, Pavlov H, Bullough PG: Osteochondroma of the cervical spine: report of two cases in preadolescent males. Skeletal Radiol 8:13–15, 1982.

919. Numaguchi Y: Osteitis condensans ilii, including its resolution. Radiology 98:1–8, 1971.

920. Nunez C, Bennett T, Bohlman HH: Chondromyxoid fibroma of the thoracic spine: case report and review of the literature. Spine 7:436–439, 1982.

921. O'Hara AE: Roentgenographic osseous manifestations of the anemias and the leukemias. Clin Orthop 52:63–82, 1967.

922. Ochsner HC, Moser RH: Ivory vertebra. AJR 29:635–637, 1933.

922a. Oestreich AE: The stylohyoid ligament in Hurler syndrome and related conditions: comparison with normal children. Radiology 154:665–666, 1985.

923. Oestreich AE, Young LW: The absent cervical pedicle syndrome: a case in childhood. AJR 107:505–510, 1969.

924. Ogata M, Ishikawa K, Ohira T: Cervical myelopathy in pseudogout: case report. J Bone Joint Surg 66A:1301–1303, 1984.

925. Ogden JA, Conlogue GJ, Phillips SB, et al: Sprengel's deformity. Radiology of the pathologic deformation. Skeletal Radiol 4:204–211, 1979.

926. Ogihara Y, Sekiguchi K, Tsuruta T: Osteogenic sarcoma of the fourth thoracic vertebra: long-term survival by chemotherapy only. Cancer 53:2615–2618, 1984.

927. Olbrantz K, Bohrer SP: Fusion of the anterior arch of the atlas and dens. Skeletal Radiol 12:21–22, 1984.

928. Omojola MF, Cockshott WP, Beatty EG: Osteoid osteoma: an evaluation of diagnostic modalities. Clin Radiol 32:199–204, 1981.

929. Omojola MF, Fox AJ, Viñuela FV: Computed tomographic metrizamide myelography in the evaluation of thoracic spinal osteoblastoma. AJNR 3:670–673, 1982.

930. Omojola MF, Vas W, Banna M: Plain film assessment of spinal canal stenosis. J Can Assoc Radiol 32:95–96, 1981.

931. Onitsuka H: Roentgenologic aspects of bone islands. Radiology 123:607–612, 1977.

932. Ono K, Ota H, Tada K, et al: Ossified posterior longitudinal ligament. A clinicopathologic study. Spine 2:126–138, 1977.

933. Oppenheimer A: The apophyseal intervertebral articulations, roengenologically considered. Radiology 30:724–740, 1938.

934. Ores R, Rosen P, Ortiz J: Localization of acid phosphatase activity in a giant cell tumor of bone. Arch Pathol 88:54–57, 1969.

935. Orofino C, Sherman MS, Schechter D: Luschka's joint—a degenerative phenomenon. J Bone Joint Surg 42A:853–858, 1960.

936. Palacios E, Brackett CE, Leary DJ: Ossification of

the posterior longitudinal ligament associated with a herniated intervertebral disk. Radiology 100:313–314, 1971.

937. Paling MR, Herdt JR: Radiation osteitis: a problem of recognition. Radiology 137:339–342, 1980.

938. Park EA: The imprinting of nutritional disturbances on the growing bone. Pediatrics 33:815–862, 1964.

939. Park WM, O'Neill M, McCall IW: The radiology of rheumatoid involvement of the cervical spine. Skeletal Radiol 4:1–7, 1979.

940. Parker F Jr, Jackson H Jr: Primary reticulum cell sarcoma of bone. Surg Gynecol Obstet 68:45–53, 1939.

941. Pastershank SP, Resnick D: Pseudoarthrosis in ankylosing spondylitis. J Can Assoc Radiol 31:234–235, 1980.

942. Pate D, Katz A: Clostridia discitis: a case report. Arthritis Rheum 22:1039–1040, 1979.

943. Patel DV, Ferguson RJL, Schey WL: Enlargement of the intervertebral foramina: an unusual cause. AJR 131:911–913, 1978.

944. Patel DV, Hammer RA, Levin B, et al: Primary osteogenic sarcoma of the spine. Skeletal Radiol 12:276–279, 1984.

945. Patriquin HB, Beauregard G, Dunbar JS: The right pleuromediastinal reflections in children. J Can Assoc Radiol 27:9–15, 1976.

946. Patton JT: Differential diagnosis of inflammatory spondylitis. Skeletal Radiol 1:77–85, 1976.

947. Paul LW, Moir WW: Non-pathologic variations in relationship of the upper cervical vertebrae. AJR 62:519–524, 1949.

948. Paul LW, Pohle EA: Solitary myeloma of bone. Radiology 35:651–666, 1940.

949. Payne EE, Spillane JD: The cervical spine. An anatomico-pathological study of 70 specimens (using a special technique) with particular reference to the problem of cervical spondylosis. Brain 80:571–596, 1957.

950. Pear BL: Skeletal manifestations of the lymphomas and leukemias. Semin Roentgenol 9:229–240, 1974.

951. Pearchy M, Shepherd J: Is there instability in spondylolisthesis? Spine 10:175–177, 1985.

952. Pearlman AW, Friedman M: Radiation therapy of benign giant cell tumor arising in Paget's disease of bone: iso-effective recovery study. AJR 102:645–651, 1968.

953. Peck FC Jr: A calcified thoracic intervertebral disk with herniation and spinal cord compression in a child: case report. J Neurosurg 14:105–109, 1957.

954. Peison B, Benisch B: Malignant myelosclerosis simulating metastatic bone disease. Radiology 125:62, 1977.

955. Pellicci PM, Ranawat CS, Tsairis P, et al: A prospective study of the progression of rheumatoid arthritis of the cervical spine. J Bone Joint Surg 63A:342–350, 1981.

956. Penfil RL, Brown ML: Genetically significant dose to the United States population from diagnostic medical roentgenology, 1964. Radiology 90:209–216, 1968.

957. Pennes DR, Martel W, Ellis CN: Retinoid-induced ossification of the posterior londitudinal ligament. Skeletal Radiol 14:191–193, 1985.

958. Penning L: Some aspects of plain radiography of the cervical spine in chronic myelopathy. Neurology 12:513–519, 1962.

959. Penning L: Prevertebral hematoma in cervical spine injury: incidence and etiologic significance. AJR 136:553–561, 1981.

960. Penning L, Blickman JR: Instability in lumbar spondylolisthesis: a radiologic study of several concepts. AJR 134:293–301, 1980.

961. Perovic MN, Kopits SE, Thompson RC: Radiological evaluation of the spinal cord in congenital atlanto-axial dislocation. Radiology 109:713–716, 1973.

962. Pettine KA, Klassen RA: Osteoid-osteoma and osteoblastoma of the spine. J Bone Joint Surg 68A:354–361, 1986.

963. Phillipe J, Sheybani E, Hirschel B, et al: Air in the bones: multifocal anaerobic osteomyelitis associated with oat cell carcinoma. Br Med J 290:969, 1985.

964. Pinckney LE, Currarino G, Highgenboten CL: Osteomyelitis of the cervical spine following dental extraction. Radiology 135:335–337, 1980.

965. Piney A: The anatomy of the bone marrow: with special reference to the distribution of the red marrow. Br Med J 2:792–795, 1922.

966. Pinto RS, Lin JP, Firooznia H, et al: The osseous and angiographic features of vertebral chordomas. Neuroradiology 9:231–241, 1975.

967. Pitt M: Osteopenic bone disease. Orthop Clin North Am 14:65–80, 1983.

968. Pitt MJ: Rachitic and osteomalacic syndromes. Radiol Clin North Am 19:581–599, 1981.

969. Pitt MJ: Rickets and osteomalacia. In Resnick D, Niwayama G (eds): Diagnosis of Bone and Joint Disorders: With Emphasis on Articular Abnormalities, vol 2. Philadelphia: WB Saunders Company, 1981, pp 1682–1720.

970. Pitt MJ, Haussler MR: Vitamin D: biochemistry and clinical applications. Skeletal Radiol 1: 191–208, 1977.

971. Pochaczevsky R, Yen YM, Sherman RS: The roentgen appearance of benign osteoblastoma. Radiology 75:429–437, 1960.

972. Poker N, Finby N, Archibald RM: Spondyloepiphysial dysplasia tarda: four cases in childhood and adolescence and some considerations regarding platyspondyly. Radiology 85:474–480, 1965.

973. Polga JP, Cramer GG: Cleft anterior arch of atlas simulating odontoid fracture. Radiology 113:341, 1974.

974. Pollen JJ, Shlaer WJ: Osteoblastic response to successful treatment of metastatic cancer of the prostate. AJR 132:927–931, 1979.

975. Pool RD: Congenital scoliosis in monozygotic twins: genetically determined or acquired in utero? J Bone Joint Surg 68B:194–196, 1986.

976. Pope MH, Hanley EN, Matteri RE, et al: Measurement of intervertebral disc space height. Spine 2:282–286, 1977.

977. Poppel MH, Jacobson HG, Duff BK, et al: Basilar impression and platybasia in Paget's disease. Radiology 61:639–644, 1953.

978. Poppel MH, Lawrence LR, Jacobson HG, et al: Skeletal tuberculosis: a roentgenographic survey with reconsideration of diagnostic criteria. AJR 70:936–963, 1953.

979. Porter RW, Park W: Unilateral spondylolysis. J Bone Joint Surg 64B:344–348, 1982.

980. Postacchini F, Massobrio M, Ferro L: Familial lumbar stenosis: case report of three siblings. J Bone Joint Surg 67A:321–323, 1985.

981. Potdar GG: Ewing's Tumor. Clin Radiol 22:528–533, 1971.

982. Powers B, Miller MD, Kramer RS, et al: Traumatic anterior atlanto-occipital dislocation. Neurosurgery 4:12–17, 1979.

983. Pozo JL, Crockard HA, Ransford AO: Basilar impression in osteogenesis imperfecta: a report of three cases in one family. J Bone Joint Surg 66B:233–238, 1984.

984. Prager PJ: Differential diagnosis and radiological work-up in bilateral lateral atlantoaxial offset. Eur J Radiol 3:309–313, 1983.

985. Present AJ: Radiography of the lower back in pre-employment physical examinations. Radiology 112:229–230, 1974.

986. Price CHG: Myeloma occurring with Paget's disease of bone. Skeletal Radiol 1:15–19, 1976.

987. Prusick VR, Samberg LC, Wesolowski DP: Klippel-Feil syndrome associated with spinal stenosis: a case report. J Bone Joint Surg 67A:161–164, 1985.

988. Pueschel SM, Herndon JH, Gelch MM, et al: Symptomatic atlantoaxial subluxation in persons with Down syndrome. J Pediatr Orthop 4:682–688, 1984.

989. Puite RH, Tesluk H: Whipple's disease. Am J Med 19:383–400, 1955.

990. Rabinowitz JG, Moseley JE: The lateral lumbar spine in Down's syndrome: a new roentgen feature. Radiology 83:74–79, 1964.

991. Rahimi A, Beabout JW, Ivins JC, et al: Chondromyxoid fibroma: a clinicopathologic study of 76 cases. Cancer 30:726–736, 1972.

992. Ramani PS: Chondromyxoid fibroma: a rare cause of spinal cord compression: case report. J Neurosurg 40:107–109, 1974.

993. Ramirez H Jr, Navarro JE, Bennett WF: "Cupid's bow" contour of the lumbar vertebral end plates detected by computed tomography. J Comput Assist Tomogr 8:121–124, 1984.

994. Ramsey J, Bliznak J: Klippel-Feil syndrome with renal agenesis and other anomalies. AJR 113:460–463, 1971.

995. Ransford AO, Pozo JL, Hutton PAN, et al: The behavior pattern of the scoliosis associated with osteoid osteoma or osteoblastoma of the spine. J Bone Joint Surg 66B:16–20, 1984.

996. Rappoport MS: Solitary collapsed vertebra. Semin Roentgenol 14:3, 1979.

997. Rasmussen TB, Kernohan JW, Adson AW: Pathologic classification, with surgical consideration, of intraspinal tumors. Ann Surg 111:513–530, 1940.

998. Ratcliffe JF: The arterial anatomy of the adult human lumbar vertebral body: a microarteriographic study. J Anat 131:57–79, 1980.

999. Ratcliffe JF: The arterial anatomy of the developing human dorsal and lumbar vertebral body: a microarteriographic study. J Anat 133:625–638, 1981.

1000. Ratcliffe JF: An evaluation of the intra-osseous arterial anastomoses in the human vertebral body at different ages. A microarteriographic study. J Anat 134:373–382, 1982.

1001. Ratcliffe JF: Anatomic basis for the pathogenesis and radiologic features of vertebral osteomyelitis and its differentiation from childhood discitis: a microarteriographic investigation. Acta Radiolog [Diagn] 26:137–143, 1985.

1002. Ravichandran G: A radiologic sign in spondylolisthesis. AJR 134:113–117, 1980.

1003. Ravichandran G: Multiple lumbar spondylolyses. Spine 5:552–557, 1980.

1004. Ravichandran G: Spinous process deviation: predictive value of a radiologic sign in lumbar disc surgery. Spine 8:342–344, 1983.

1005. Rawlings CE III, Wilkins RH, Gallis HA, et al: Postoperative intervertebral disc space infection. Neurosurgery 13:371–376, 1983.

1005a. Rechtine GR, Hassan MO, Bohlman HH: Malignant fibrous histiocytoma of the cervical spine: report of an unusual case and description of light and electron microscopy. Spine 9:824–830, 1984.

1006. Redlund-Johnell I: Subaxial caudal dislocation of the cervical spine in rheumatoid arthritis. Neuroradiology 26:407–410, 1984.

1007. Redlund-Johnell I, Pettersson H: Radiographic measurements of the cranio-vertebral region: designed for evaluation of abnormalities in rheumatoid arthritis. Acta Radiol [Diagn] 25:23–28, 1984.

1008. Redlund-Johnell I, Pettersson H: Vertical dislocation of the C1 and C2 vertebrae in rheumatoid arthritis. Acta Radiol [Diagn] 25:133–141, 1984.

1009. Regen EM, Haber A: Giant-cell tumor of cervical vertebra with unusual symptoms. J Bone Joint Surg 39A:196–200, 1957.

1010. Reilly BJ, Davidson JW, Bain H: Lymphangiectasis of the skeleton. A case report. Radiology 103:385–386, 1972.

1011. Renshaw TS: Sacral agenesis: a classification and review of twenty-three cases. J Bone Joint Surg 60A:373–383, 1978.

1012. Resnik CS, Scheer CE, Adelaar RS: Lumbosacral dislocation. J Can Assoc Radiol 36:259–261, 1985.

1013. Resnick D: Abnormalities of bone and soft tissue following renal transplantation. Semin Roentgenol 13:329–340, 1978.

1014. Resnick D: Radiology of seronegative spondyloarthropathies. Clin Orthop 143:38–45, 1979.

1015. Resnick D: The "rugger jersey" vertebral body. Arthritis Rheum 24:1191–1194, 1981.

1016. Resnick D: The sclerotic vertebral body. JAMA 249:1761–1763, 1983.

1017. Resnick D: Hyperostosis and ossification in the cervical spine. Arthritis Rheum 27:564–569, 1984.

1018. Resnick D: Degenerative diseases of the vertebral column. Radiology 156:3–14, 1985.

1019. Resnick D, Durd J, Shapiro RF, et al: Radiographic abnormalities of rheumatoid arthritis in patients with diffuse idiopathic skeletal hyperostosis. Arthritis Rheum 21:1–5, 1978.

1020. Resnick D, Dwosh IL, Goergen TG, et al: Clinical and radiographic abnormalities in ankylosing spondylitis: a comparison of men and women. Radiology 119:293–297, 1976.

1021. Resnick D, Greenway GD, Bardwick PA, et al: Plasma-cell dyscrasia with polyneuropathy, organomegaly, endocrinopathy, M-protein and skin changes: the POEMS syndrome. Radiology 140:17–22, 1981.

1022. Resnick D, Guerra J Jr, Robinson CA, et al: Association of diffuse idiopathic skeletal hyperostosis (DISH) and calcification and ossification of the posterior longitudinal ligament. AJR 131:1049–1053, 1978.

1023. Resnick D, Nemcek AA Jr, Haghighi P: Spinal enostoses (bone islands). Radiology 147: 373–376, 1983.

1024. Resnick D, Niwayama G: Subchondral resorption of bone in renal osteodystrophy. Radiology 118:315–321, 1976.

1025. Resnick D, Niwayama G: Radiographic and pathologic features of spinal involvement in diffuse idiopathic skeletal hyperostosis (DISH). Radiology 119:559–568, 1976.

1026. Resnick D, Niwayama G: Intravertebral disk herniations: cartilaginous (Schmorl's) nodes. Radiology 126:57–65, 1978.

1027. Resnick D, Niwayama G: Intervertebral disc abnormalities associated with vertebral metastasis: observation in patients and cadavers with prostatic cancer. Invest Radiol 13:182–190, 1978.

1028. Resnick D, Niwayama G: Diagnosis of Bone and Joint Disorders: With Emphasis on Articular Abnormalities. Philadelphia: WB Saunders Company, 1981.

1029. Resnick D, Niwayama G: Entheses and enthesopathy: anatomical, pathological and radiological correlation. Radiology 146:1–9, 1983.

1030. Resnick D, Niwayama G, Goergen TG: Degenerative disease of the sacroiliac joint. Invest Radiol 10:608–621, 1975.

1031. Resnick D, Niwayama G, Goergen TG: Comparison of radiographic abnormalities of the sacroiliac joint in degenerative disease and ankylosing spondylitis. AJR 128:189–196, 1977.

1032. Resnick D, Niwayama G, Goergen TG, et al: Clinical, radiographic and pathologic abnormalities in calcium pyrophosphate dihydrate deposition disease (CPPD): pseudogout. Radiology 122:1–15, 1977.

1033. Resnick D, Niwayama G, Guerra J Jr, et al: Spinal vacuum phenomena: anatomical study and review. Radiology 139:341–348, 1981.

1034. Resnick D, Pineda C: Vertebral involvement in calcium pyrophosphate dihydrate crystal deposition disease: radiographic-pathological correlation. Radiology 153:55–60, 1984.

1035. Resnick DL: Fish vertebrae. Arthritis Rheum 25:1073–1077, 1982.

1036. Resnik CS, Resnick D: Crystal deposition disease. Semin Arthritis Rheum 12:390–403, 1983.

1037. Resnik CS, Resnick D: Radiology of disorders of the sacroiliac joints. JAMA 253:2863–2866, 1985.

1038. Resnik CS, Smithson LV, Bradshaw JA, et al: The two-eyed Scotty dog: a normal anatomic variant. Radiology 149:680, 1983.

1039. Reymond RD, Wheeler PS, Perovic M, et al: The lucent cleft, a new radiographic sign of cervical disc injury or disease. Clin Radiol 23:188–192, 1972.

1040. Reynolds J: Roentgenographic and clinical appraisal of sickle cell–hemoglobin C disease. AJR 88:512–522, 1962.

1041. Reynolds J: A re-evaluation of the "fish vertebra" sign in sickle cell hemoglobinopathy. AJR 97: 693–707, 1966.

1042. Reynolds J, Pritchard JA, Ludders D, et al: Roentgenographic and clinical appraisal of sickle cell beta-thalassemia disease. AJR 118:378–400, 1973.

1043. Rezaian SM: The incidence of scoliosis due to

neurofibromatosis. Acta Orthop Scand 47: 534–539, 1976.

1044. Rhangos WC, Chick EW: Mycotic infections of bone. South Med J 57:664–674, 1964.

1045. Rhea JT, Deluca SA, Llewellyn HJ, et al: The oblique view: an unnecessary component of the initial adult lumbar spine examination. Radiology 134:45–47, 1980.

1046. Ricciardi JE, Kaufer H, Louis DS: Acquired os odontoideum following acute ligament injury: report of a case. J Bone Joint Surg 58A:410–412, 1976.

1047. Rich TA, Schiller A, Suit HD, et al: Clinical and pathologic review of 48 cases of chordoma. Cancer 56:182–187, 1985.

1048. Richards AJ, Hamilton EBD: Spinal changes in idiopathic chondrocalcinosis articularis. Rheumatol Rehabil 15:138–142, 1976.

1049. Richardson ML, Pozzi-Mucelli RS, Kanter AS, et al: Bone mineral changes in primary hyperparathyroidism. Skeletal Radiol 15:85–95, 1986.

1050. Richman S, Friedman RL: Vertical fracture of cervical vertebral bodies. Radiology 62:536–543, 1954.

1051. Richter DE, Nash CL Jr, Moskowitz RW, et al: Idiopathic adolescent scoliosis—a prototype of degenerative joint disease. Clin Orthop 193: 221–229, 1985.

1052. Riggs W Jr, Rockett JF: Roentgen chest findings in childhood sickle cell anemia. A new vertebral body finding. AJR 104:838–845, 1968.

1053. Riggs W Jr, Wilroy RS Jr, Etteldorf JN: Neonatal hyperthyroidism with accelerated skeletal maturation, craniosynostosis, and brachydactyly. Radiology 105:621–625, 1972.

1054. Rigler LG: Is this radiograph really necessary? Radiology 120:449–450, 1976.

1055. Riseborough EJ: Irradiation induced kyphosis. Clin Orthop 128:101–106, 1977.

1056. Riseborough EJ, Grabias SL, Burton RI, et al: Skeletal alterations following irradiation for Wilms' tumor: with particular reference to scoliosis and kyphosis. J Bone Joint Surg 58A:526–536, 1976.

1057. Ritz E, Krempien B, Mehls O, et al: Skeletal abnormalities in chronic renal insufficiency before and during maintenance hemodialysis. Kidney Int 4:116–127, 1973.

1058. Roaf R: A study of the mechanics of spinal injuries. J Bone Joint Surg 42B:810–823, 1960.

1059. Roberts FF, Kishore PRS, Cunningham ME: Routine oblique radiography of the pediatric lumbar spine: Is it necessary? AJR 131:297–298, 1978.

1060. Roberts M, Rinaudo PA, Vilinskas J, et al: Solitary sclerosing plasma-cell myeloma of the spine. J Neurosurg 40:125–128, 1974.

1061. Robinson RA: Anterior and posterior cervical spine fusions. Clin Orthop 35:34–62, 1964.

1062. Roche MB: The pathology of neural-arch defects. A dissection study. J Bone Joint Surg 31A: 529–537, 1949.

1063. Roche MB, Rowe GG: The incidence of separate neural arch and coincident bone variations: a survey of 4200 skeletons. Anat Rec 109:233–252, 1951.

1064. Roche MB, Rowe GG: Anomalous centers of ossification for inferior articular processes of the lumbar vertebrae. Anat Rec 109:253–259, 1951.

1065. Roche MB, Rowe GG: The incidence of separate

neural arch and coincident bone variations: a summary. J Bone Joint Surg 34A:491–494, 1952.

1066. Rogala EF, Drummond DS, Gurr J: Scoliosis: incidence and natural history. A prospective epidemiologic study. J Bone Joint Surg 60A: 173–176, 1978.

1067. Rogalsky RJ, Black B, Reed MH: Orthopaedic manifestations of leukemia in children. J Bone Joint Surg 68A:494–501, 1986.

1068. Rogers LF: The roentgenographic appearance of transverse or Chance fractures of the spine: the seat belt fracture. AJR 111:844–849, 1971.

1069. Rogers LF: Radiology of Skeletal Trauma, vol 1. New York: Churchill Livingstone, 1982.

1070. Rogers LF, Thayer C, Weinberg PE, et al: Acute injuries of the upper thoracic spine associated with paraplegia. AJR 134:67–73, 1980.

1071. Rogers WA: Fractures and dislocation of the cervical spine. An end-result study. J Bone Joint Surg 39A:341–376, 1957.

1072. Rohlfing BM: Vertebral end-plate depression: report of two patients without hemoglobinopathy. AJR 128:599–600, 1977.

1073. Roman G: Hereditary multiple exostoses. A rare cause of spinal cord compression. Spine 3:230–233, 1978.

1074. Rose GA: The radiological diagnosis of osteoporosis, osteomalacia and hyperparathyroidism. Clin Radiol 15:75–83, 1964.

1075. Rosen RA, Deshmukh SM: Growth arrest recovery lines in hypoparathyroidism. Radiology 155:61–62, 1985.

1076. Rosenbaum DM, Blumhagen JD, King HA: Atlantooccipital instability in Down syndrome. AJR 146:1269–1272, 1986.

1077. Rosendahl-Jensen SV: Fibrous dysplasia of the vertebral column. Acta Chir Scand 111:490–494, 1956.

1078. Rosenkranz W: Ankylosing spondylitis: cauda equina syndrome with multiple spinal arachnoid cysts: case report. J Neurosurg 34:241–243, 1971.

1078a. Ross FGM: Osteogenic sarcoma. Br J Radiol 37:259–276, 1964.

1079. Ross P, Logan W: Roentgen findings in extramedullary hematopoiesis. AJR 106:604–613, 1969.

1080. Roth A, Rosenthal A, Hall JE, et al: Scoliosis and congenital heart disease. Clin Orthop 93:95–102, 1973.

1081. Roth M: Idiopathic scoliosis from the point of view of the neuroradiologist. Neuroradiology 21:133–138, 1981.

1082. Rothman SLG, Glenn WV Jr, Kerber CW: Postoperative fractures of lumbar articular facets: occult cause of radiculopathy. AJR 145:779–784, 1985.

1083. Rothschild BM, Cohn L, Aviza A, et al: Aortic aneurysm producing back pain, bone destruction and paraplegia. Clin Orthop 164:123–125, 1982.

1084. Rowe GG, Roche MB: The lumbar neural arch. Roentgenographic study of ossification. J Bone Joint Surg 32A:554–557, 1950.

1085. Rubin, P: Dynamic Classification of Bone Dysplasias. Chicago: Year Book Medical Publishers, Inc, 1972.

1085a. Rubinstein JD, Gertzbein S: Radiographic assessment of Harrington rod instrumentation for spinal fractures. J Can Assoc Radiol 35:159–163, 1984.

1086. Ruff ME, Weis LD, Kean JR: Acute thoracic kyphosis in Gaucher's disease. Spine 9:835–837, 1984.

1086a. Ruiter DJ, vanRijssel TG, van der Velde EA: Aneurysmal bone cysts: a clinicopathological study of 105 cases. Cancer 39:2231–2239, 1977.

1087. Rusnak SL, Driscoll SG: Congenital spinal anomalies in infants of diabetic mothers. Pediatrics 35:989–995, 1965.

1088. Russell DS: Malignant osteoclastoma and the association of malignant osteoclastoma with Paget's osteitis deformans. J Bone Joint Surg 31B:281–290, 1949.

1089. Russell DS, Rubinstein LJ: Pathology of Tumours of the Nervous System, 4th ed. Baltimore: Williams & Wilkins Company, 1977.

1090. Russell JGB: Cost and effectiveness of methods of radiation protection in x-ray diagnosis. Clin Radiol 36:37–40, 1985.

1091. Russin LA, Robinson MJ, Engle HA, et al: Ewing's sarcoma of the lumbar spine: a case report of long-term survival. Clin Orthop 164:126–129, 1982.

1092. Rutherford H, Dodd GD: Complications of radiation therapy: growing bone. Semin Roentgenol 9:15–27, 1974.

1093. Sabanas AO, Dahlin DC, Childs DS Jr, et al: Postradiation sarcoma of bone. Cancer 9:528–542, 1956.

1094. Sackler JP, Liu L: Heparin-induced osteoporosis. Br J Radiol 46:548–550, 1973.

1095. Sakkas L, Thouas B, Kotsou S, et al: Cervical myelopathy with ankylosing hyperostosis of the spine. Surg Neurol 24:43–46, 1985.

1096. Salerno NR, Edeiken J: Vertebral scalloping in neurofibromatosis. Radiology 97:509–510, 1970.

1097. Samra Y, Hertz M, Shaked Y, et al: Brucellosis of the spine: a report of three cases. J Bone Joint Surg 64B:429–431, 1982.

1098. Sanchez RL, Llovet J, Moreno A, et al: Symptomatic eosinophilic granuloma of the spine: report of two cases and review of the literature. Orthopaedics 7:1721–1726, 1984.

1099. Sartoris DJ, Clopton P, Nemcek A, et al: Vertebral-body collapse in focal and diffuse disease: patterns of pathologic processes. Radiology 160:479–493, 1986.

1100. Sartoris DJ, Luzzatti L, Weaver DD, et al: Type IX Ehlers-Danlos syndrome. A new variant with pathognomonic radiographic features. Radiology 152:665–670, 1984.

1101. Sartoris DJ, Parker BR: Histiocytosis X: rate and pattern of resolution of osseous lesions. Radiology 152:679–684, 1984.

1102. Sartoris DJ, Resnick D, Resnik C, et al: Musculoskeletal manifestations of sarcoidosis. Semin Roentgenol 20:376–386, 1985.

1103. Sartoris DJ, Resnick D, Tyson R, et al: Age-related alterations in the vertebral spinous processes and intervening soft tissues: radiologic pathologic correlation. AJR 145:1025–1030, 1985.

1104. Sarwar M, Kelly PJ: Adult diastematomyelia. Spine 2:60–64, 1977.

1105. Saunders AJS: Diffuse infection of the spine by pseudomonas pyocyaneus. Br J Radiol 52:325–326, 1979.

1106. Saunders WW: Basilar impression: the position of the normal odontoid. Radiology 41:589–590, 1943.

1107. Sauser DD, Goldman AB, Kaye JJ: Discogenic vertebral sclerosis. J Can Assoc Radiol 29:44–50, 1978.

1108. Scatliff JH, Till K, Hoare RD: Incomplete, false and true diastematomyelia. Radiology 116: 349–354, 1975.

1109. Scavone JG, Latshaw RF, Rohrer GV: Use of lumbar spine films. Statistical evaluation at a university teaching hospital. JAMA 246: 1105–1108, 1981.

1110. Scavone JG, Latshaw RF, Weidner WA: Anteroposterior and lateral radiographs: an adequate lumbar spine examination. AJR 136:715–717, 1981.

1111. Schaad UB, McCracken GH Jr, Nelson JD: Pyogenic arthritis of the sacroiliac joint in pediatric patients. Pediatrics 66:375–379, 1980.

1112. Schaaf RE, Gehweiler JA Jr, Miller MD, et al: Lateral hyperflexion injuries of the cervical spine. Skeletal Radiol 3:73–78, 1978.

1113. Schabel SI, Moore TE, Rittenberg GM, et al: Vertebral vacuum, phenomenon. A radiographic manifestation of metastatic malignancy. Skeletal Radiol 4:154–156, 1979.

1114. Schabel SI, Tyminski L, Holland D, et al: The skeletal manifestations of chronic myelogenous leukemia. Skeletal Radiol 5:145–149, 1980.

1115. Schaffer L, Kranzler LI, Siqueira EB: Aneurysmal bone cyst of the spine: a case report. Spine 10:390–393, 1985.

1116. Schajowicz F: Giant-cell tumors of bone (osteoclastoma). J Bone Joint Surg 43A:1–29, 1961.

1117. Schajowicz F, Araujo ES, Berenstein M: Sarcoma complicating Paget's disease of bone: a clinicopathological study of 62 cases. J Bone Joint Surg 65B:299–307, 1983.

1118. Schajowicz F, Gallardo H: Epiphyseal chondroblastoma of bone: a clinico-pathological study of sixty-nine cases. J Bone Joint Surg 52B:205–226, 1970.

1119. Schajowicz F, Gallardo H: Chondromyxoid fibroma (fibromyxoid chondroma) of bone: a clinico-pathological study of thirty-two cases. J Bone Joint Surg 53B:198–216, 1971.

1120. Schajowicz F, Lemos C: Osteoid osteoma and osteoblastoma: closely related entities of osteoblastic derivation. Acta Orthop Scand 41: 272–291, 1970.

1121. Schajowicz F, Lemos C: Malignant osteoblastoma. J Bone Joint Surg 58B:202–211, 1976.

1122. Schajowicz F, Slullitel I: Giant-cell tumor associated with Paget's disease of bone. J Bone Joint Surg 48A:1340–1349, 1966.

1123. Schajowicz F, Slullitel J: Eosinophilic granuloma of bone and its relationship to Hand-Schüller-Christian and Letterer-Siwe syndromes. J Bone Joint Surg 55B:545–565, 1973.

1124. Schajowicz F, Ubios AM, Araujo ES, et al: Virus-like intranuclear inclusions in giant cell tumor of bone. Clin Orthop 201:247–250, 1985,

1125. Scher A, Vambeck V: An approach to the radiological examination of the cervico-dorsal junction following injury. Clin Radiol 28:243–246, 1977.

1126. Scher AT: Unilateral locked facet in cervical spine injuries. AJR 129:45–48, 1977.

1127. Schiff DCM, Park WW: The arterial supply of the odontoid process. J Bone Joint Surg 55A:1450–1456, 1973.

1128. Schlezinger NS, Ungar H: Hemangioma of the vertebra with compression myelopathy. AJR 42:192–216, 1939.

1129. Schmidek HH, Smith DA, Kristiansen TK: Sacral fractures. Neurosurgery 15:735–746, 1984.

1129a. Schmorl G, Junghanns H: The Human Spine in Health and Disease. New York: Grune & Stratton, 1971.

1130. Schneck CD: The anatomy of lumbar spondylosis. Clin Orthop 193:20–37, 1985.

1131. Schneider R: Radiologic methods of evaluating generalized osteopenia. Orthop Clin North Am 15:631–651, 1984.

1132. Schneider RC, Kahn EA: Chronic neurological sequelae of acute trauma to the spine and spinal cord. Part I: the significance of the acute-flexion or "teardrop" fracture-dislocation of the cervical spine. J Bone Joint Surg 38A:985–997, 1956.

1133. Schnier BR: Pseudotumor of the hypopharynx and larynx due to anterior cervical osteophytes. AJR 115:544–546, 1972.

1133a. Schnyder P, Fankhauser H, Mansouri B: Computed tomography in spinal hemangioma with cord compression: report of two cases. Skeletal Radiol 15:372–375, 1986.

1134. Schorr S, Adler E: Calcified intervertebral disc in children and adults. Acta Radiol 41:498–504, 1954.

1135. Schulman L, Dorfman HD: Nerve fibers in osteoid osteoma. J Bone Joint Surg 52A:1351–1356, 1970.

1136. Schulz EE, Engstrom H, Sauser DD, et al: Osteoporosis: radiographic detection of fluoride-induced extra-axial bone formation. Radiology 159:457–462, 1986.

1137. Schumacher TM, Genant HK, Kellet MJ, et al: HLA-B27 associated arthropathies. Radiology 126:289–297, 1978.

1138. Schwartz AM, Homer MJ, McCauley RGK: "Step-off" vertebral body: Gaucher's disease versus sickle cell hemoglobinopathy. AJR 132:81–85, 1979.

1139. Schwartz AM, Wechsler RJ, Landy MD, et al: Posterior arch defects of the cervical spine. Skeletal Radiol 8:135–139, 1982.

1139a. Schwarz GS: The width of the spinal canal in the growing vertebra with special reference to the sacrum: maximum interpediculate distances in adults and children. AJR 76:476–481, 1956.

1140. Schwarz SS, Fisher WS III, Pulliam MW, et al: Thoracic chordoma in a patient with paraparesis and ivory vertebral body. Neurosurgery 16:100–112, 1985.

1141. Schwimer SR, Bassett LW, Mancuso AA, et al: Giant cell tumor of the cervicothoracic spine. AJR 136:63–67, 1981.

1142. Scoles PV, Quinn TP: Intervertebral discitis in children and adolescents. Clin Orthop 162: 31–36, 1982.

1143. Seamen WB, Wells J: Destructive lesions of the vertebral bodies in rheumatoid disease. AJR 86:241–250, 1961.

1144. Sebes JI, Nasrallah NS, Rabinowitz JG, et al: The relationship between HLA-B27 positive peripheral arthritis and sacroiliitis. Radiology 126:299–302, 1978.

1144a. Sebes JI, Niell HB, Palmieri GMA, et al: Skeletal surveys in multiple myeloma: radiologic-clinical correlation. Skeletal Radiol 15:354–359, 1986.

1145. Segal D, Franchi AV: Congenital absence of lumbar facets as a cause of lower-back pain. Spine 11:78–80, 1986.

1146. Seifert MJ: The biology of macrophages in osteopetrosis: structure and function. Clin Orthop 182:270–277, 1984.

1147. Seimon LP: Eosinophil granuloma of the spine. J Pediatr Orthop 1:371–376, 1981.

1147a. Seki T, Fukuda H, Ishii Y, et al: Malignant transformation of benign osteoblastoma: a case report. J Bone Joint Surg 57A:424–426, 1975.

1148. Seljeskog EL, Chou SN: Spectrum of the hangman's fracture. J Neurosurg 45:3–8, 1976.

1149. Selye H: Action of parathyroid hormone on the epihyseal junction of the young rat. Arch Pathol 14:60–65, 1932.

1150. Semine AA, Ertel AN, Goldberg MJ, et al: Cervical-spine instability in children with Down syndrome (trisomy 21). J Bone Joint Surg 60A:649–652, 1978.

1151. Shacked I, Tadmor R, Wolpin G, et al: Aneurysmal bone cyst of a vertebral body with acute paraplegia. Paraplegia 19:294–298, 1981.

1152. Shahriaree H, Sajadi K, Rooholamini SA: A family with spondylolisthesis. J Bone Joint Surg 61A:1256–1258, 1979.

1153. Shallat RF, Taekman MS, Nagle RC: Unusual presentation of cervical chordoma with long-term survival: case report. J Neurosurg 57:716–718, 1982.

1154. Shanahan MDG, Ackroyd CE: Pyogenic infection of the sacro-iliac joint: a report of 11 cases. J Bone Joint Surg 67B:605–608, 1985.

1155. Shands AR Jr, Budens WD: Congenital deformities of the spine. Analysis of the roentgenograms of 700 children. Bull Hosp Joint Dis 17:110–133, 1956.

1156. Shapiro F, Glimcher MJ, Holtrop ME, et al: Human osteopetrosis: a histological, ultrastructural, and biochemical study. J Bone Joint Surg 62A:384–399, 1980.

1157. Shapiro R: Radiologic aspects of renal osteodystrophy. Radiol Clin North Am 10:557–568, 1972.

1158. Shapiro R, Youngberg AS, Rothman SLG: The differential diagnosis of traumatic lesions of the occipito-atlanto-axial segment. Radiol Clin North Am 11:505–526, 1973.

1159. Shaw MT, Davies M: Primary hyperparathyroidism presenting as spinal cord compression. Br Med J 4:230–231, 1968.

1160. Shealy CN, Lemay M, Haddad FS: Posterior scalloping of vertebral bodies in uncontrolled hydrocephalus. J Neurol Neurosurg Psychiatry 27:567–573, 1964.

1161. Sheehan S, Bauer RB, Meyer JS: Vertebral artery compression in cervical spondylosis. Neurology 10:968–986, 1960.

1162. Sheikholeslamzadeh S, Aalami-Harandi B, Fateh H, et al: Spondylolisthesis of the cervical spine: report of a case. J Bone Joint Surg 59B:95–96, 1977.

1163. Sherk HH, Dawoud S: Congenital os odontoideum with Klippel-Feil anomaly and fatal atlanto-axial instability: a case report. Spine 6:42–45, 1981.

1164. Sherk HH, Nicholson JT, Nixon JE: Vertebra plana and eosinophilic granuloma of the cervical spine in children. Spine 3:116–121, 1978.

1165. Sherk HH, Pasquariello PS, Watters WC: Multiple dislocations of the cervical spine in a patient with juvenile rheumatoid arthritis and Down's syndrome. Clin Orthop 162:37–40, 1982.

1166. Sherman FC, Wilkinson RH, Hall JE: Reactive sclerosis of a pedicle and spondylolysis in the lumbar spine. J Bone Joint Surg 59A:49–54, 1977.

1167. Shikata J, Mikawa Y, Ikeda T, et al: Atlanto-axial subluxation with spondyloschisis in Down syndrome: case report. J Bone Joint Surg 67A:1414–1417, 1985.

1168. Shirakuni T, Tamaki N, Matsumoto, S, et al: Giant cell tumor in cervical spine. Surg Neurol 23:148–152, 1985.

1169. Shirkhoda A, Brashear HR, Zelenik ME, et al: Sacral abnormalities—computed tomography versus conventional radiography. CT: J Comput Tomog 8:41–51, 1984.

1170. Shives TC, Dahlin DC, Sim FH, et al: Osteosarcoma of the spine. J Bone Joint Surg 68A:660–668, 1986.

1171. Sholkoff SD, Glickman MG, Steinbach HL: Roentgenology of Reiter's syndrome. Radiology 97:497–503, 1970.

1172. Sim FH, Cupps RE, Dahlin DC, et al: Postradiation sarcoma of bone. J Bone Joint Surg 54A:1479–1489, 1972.

1173. Sim FH, Dahlin DC, Beabout JW: Osteoid-osteoma: diagnostic problems. J Bone Joint Surg 57A:154–159, 1975.

1174. Simon K, Mulligan ME: Growing bone islands revisited: a case report. J Bone Joint Surg 67A:809–811, 1985.

1175. Simril WA, Thurston D: The normal interpediculate space in the spines of infants and children. Radiology 64:340–347, 1955.

1176. Sindelar WF, Costa J, Ketcham AS: Osteosarcoma associated with Thorotrast administration: report of two cases and literature review. Cancer 42:2604–2608, 1978.

1177. Singh A, Dass R, Hayreh SS, et al: Skeletal changes in endemic fluorosis. J Bone Joint Surg 44B:806–815, 1962.

1178. Singleton EB, Rosenberg HS, Dodd GD: Sclerosing osteogenic sarcomatosis. AJR 88:483–490, 1962.

1179. Singson RD, Dee G, Quader MA: Scalloping and destruction of pedicles of lumbar vertebral bodies on the right side secondary to venous collaterals associated with thrombosis of the inferior vena cava. Case report 265. Skeletal Radiol 11:293–295, 1984.

1180. Slabaugh PB, Smith TK: Neuropathic spine after spinal cord injury: a case report. J Bone Joint Surg 60A:1005–1006, 1978.

1181. Sloat JI, Peterson LT: Ewing's tumor of the sacrum: five year survival after irradiation. JAMA 119:1499–1500, 1942.

1182. Slover WP, Kiley RF: Cervical vertebral erosion caused by tortuous vertebral artery. Radiology 84:112–114, 1965.

1183. Slowik T, Bittner-Manioka M, Grochowski W: Chondroma of the cervical spine: case report. J Neurosurg 29:276–279, 1968.

1184. Smith GR, Abel MS, Cone L: Visualization of the posterolateral elements of the upper cervical vertebrae in the anteroposterior projection. Radiology 115:219–220, 1975.

1185. Smith GR, Northrop CH, Loop JW: Jumpers' fractures: patterns of thoracolumbar spine injuries associated with vertical plunges: a review of 38 cases. Radiology 122:657–663, 1977.

1186. Smith GW, Robinson RA: The treatment of certain cervical spine disorders by anterior removal of the intervertebral disk and interbody fusion. J Bone Joint Surg 40A:607–623, 1958.

1187. Smith J: Radiation—induced sarcoma of bone: clinical and radiographic findings in 43 patients irradiated for soft tissue neoplasms. Clin Radiol 33:205–221, 1982.

1188. Smith J, Botet JF, Veh SDJ: Bone sarcomas in Paget disease: a study of 85 patients. Radiology 152:583–590, 1984.

1189. Smith J, O'Connell RS, Huvos AG, et al: Hodgkin's disease complicated by radiation sarcoma in bone. Br J Radiol 53:314–321, 1980.

1190. Smith J, Wixon D, Watson RC: Giant-cell tumor of the sacrum. J Can Assoc Radiol 30:34–39, 1979.

1191. Smith NR: The intervertebral discs. Br J Surg 18:358–375, 1931.

1192. Smith R: Idiopathic osteoporosis in the young. J Bone Joint Surg 62B:417–427, 1980.

1193. Smith RF, Taylor TKF: Inflammatory lesions of intervertebral discs in children. J Bone Joint Surg 49A:1508–1520, 1967.

1194. Smith SW: Roentgen findings in homocystinuria. AJR 100:147–154, 1967.

1195. Smith TK, Livermore NB III: Hoarseness accompanying Pott's paraplegia: a case report. J Bone Joint Surg 63A:159–161, 1981.

1196. Smith WS, Kaufer H: Patterns and mechanisms of lumbar injuries associated with lap seat belts. J Bone Joint Surg 51A:239–254, 1969.

1197. Smyrnis PN, Valavanis J, Alexopoulos A, et al: School screening for scoliosis in Athens. J Bone Joint Surg 61B:215–217, 1979.

1198. Sobel JW, Bohlman HH, Freehafer AA: Charcot's arthropathy of the spine following spinal cord injury. J Bone Joint Surg 67A:771–776, 1985.

1199. Soholt ST: Tuberculosis of the sacro-iliac joint. A review of seventy-five cases. J Bone Joint Surg 33A:119–130, 1951.

1200. Sonnabend DH, Taylor TKF, Chapman GK: Intervertebral disc calcification syndromes in children. J Bone Joint Surg 64B:25–31, 1982.

1201. Soren A, Waugh TR: Spondylolisthesis and related disorders: a correlative study of 105 patients. Clin Orthop 193:171–177, 1985.

1202. Southwell RB, Reynolds AF, Badger VM, et al: Klippel-Feil syndrome with cervical cord compression resulting from cervical subluxation in association with an omo-vertebral bone. Spine 5:480–482, 1980.

1203. Southwick WO: Management of fractures of the dens (odontoid process). J Bone Joint Surg 62A:482–486, 1980.

1204. Southworth JD, Bersack SR: Anomalies of the lumbosacral vertebrae in five hundred and fifty individuals without symptoms referable to the low back. AJR 64:624–634, 1950.

1205. Spagnoli I, Gattoni F, Viganotti G: Roentgenographic aspects of non-Hodgkin's lymphomas presenting with osseous lesions. Skeletal Radiol 8:39–41, 1982.

1206. Speck GR, McCall IW, O'Brien JP, et al: Spondylolisthesis: the angle of kyphosis. Spine 9:659–660, 1984.

1207. Spence KF Jr, Decker S, Sell KW: Bursting atlantal fracture associated with rupture of the transverse ligament. J Bone Joint Surg 52A:543–549, 1970.

1208. Spencer JD: Bone and joint infection in a renal unit. J Bone Joint Surg 68B:489–493, 1986.

1209. Spiegel PG, Kengla KW, Isaacson AS, et al: Intervertebral disc–space inflammation in children. J Bone Joint Surg 54A:284–296, 1972.

1210. Spillane JD, Pallis C, Jones AM: Developmental abnormalities in the region of the foramen magnum. Brain 80:11–48, 1957.

1211. Splithoff CA: Lumbosacral junction. Roentgenographic comparison of patients with and without backaches. JAMA 152:1610–1613, 1953.

1212. Spranger JW, Langer LO Jr: Spondyloepiphyseal dysplasia congenita. Radiology 94:313–322, 1970.

1213. Springfield DS, Capanna R, Gherlinzoni F, et al: Chondroblastoma: a review of seventy cases. J Bone Joint Surg 67A:748–755, 1985.

1214. Standefer M, Hardy RW Jr, Marks K, et al: Chondromyxoid fibroma of the cervical spine: a case report with a review of the literature and a description of an operative approach to the lower anterior cervical spine. Neurosurgery 11:288–292, 1982.

1215. Stanley JK, Owen R, Koff S: Congenital sacral anomalies. J Bone Joint Surg 61B:401–409, 1979.

1216. Stanley P, Duncan AW, Isaacson J, et al: Radiology of fracture-dislocation of the cervical spine during delivery. AJR 145:621–625, 1985.

1217. Steinbach HL: Some roentgen features of Paget's disease. AJR 86:950–964, 1961.

1218. Steinbach HL: The roentgen appearances of osteoporosis. Radiol Clin North Am 2:191–207, 1964.

1219. Steinbach HL: Infections of bones. Semin Roentgenol 1:337–369, 1966.

1220. Steinbach HL, Boldrey EB, Sooy FA: Congenital absence of the pedicle and superior facet from a cervical vertebra. Radiology 59:838–840, 1952.

1221. Steinbach HL, Feldman R, Goldberg MB: Acromegaly. Radiology 72:535–549, 1959.

1222. Steinbach HL, Gordon GS, Eisenberg E, et al: Primary hyperparathyroidism: a correlation of roentgen, clinical and pathologic features. AJR 86:329–343, 1961.

1223. Steinbach HL, Noetzli M: Roentgen appearance of the skeleton in osteomalacia and rickets. AJR 91:955–972, 1964.

1224. Steinberg H, Waldron BR: Idiopathic hypoparathyroidism: analysis of 52 cases including the report of a new case. Medicine 31:133–154, 1952.

1225. Steinberg VL, Storey G: Ankylosing spondylitis and chronic inflammatory lesions of the intestines. Br Med J 2:1157–1159, 1957.

1226. Stewart GC Jr, Gehweiler JA Jr, Laib RH, et al: Horizontal fracture of the anterior arch of the atlas. Radiology 122:349–352, 1977.

1227. Stewart TD: Pathologic changes in aging sacroiliac joints: a study of dissecting-room skeletons. Clin Orthop 183:188–196, 1984.

1228. Stillwell WT, Fielding JW: Aneurysmal bone cyst of the cervicodorsal spine. Clin Orthop 187:144–146, 1984.

1229. Stilwell DL Jr: Structural deformities of vertebrae: bone adaptation and modeling in experimental scoliosis and kyphosis. J Bone Joint Surg 44A:611–634, 1962.

1230. Stoddard A, Osborn JF: Scheuermann's disease or spinal osteochondrosis. Its frequency and relationship with spondylosis. J Bone Joint Surg 61B:56–58, 1979.

1231. Stokes IAF, Bigalow LC, Moreland MS: Measurement of axial rotation of vertebrae in scoliosis. Spine 11:213–218, 1986.

1232. Stoltmann HF, Blackwood W: The role of the ligamenta flava in the pathogenesis of myelopathy in cervical spondylosis. Brain 87:45–50, 1964.

1233. Stover CN, Hayes JT, Holt JF: Diastrophic dwarfism. AJR 89:914–922, 1963.

1234. Stratemeier PH, Jensen SR: Partial regressive occipital vertebra. Neuroradiology 19:47–49, 1980.

1235. Strauss L: The pathology of gargoylism. Report of a case and review of the literature. Am J Pathol 24:855–887, 1948.

1236. Stuber JL, Palacios E: Vertebral scalloping in acromegaly. AJR 112:397–400, 1971.

1237. Stulberg BN, Licata AA, Bauer TW, et al: Hyperparathyroidism, hyperthyroidism and Cushing's disease. Orthop Clin North Am 15:697–710, 1984.

1238. Stump D, Spock A, Grossman H: Vertebral sarcoidosis in adolescents. Radiology 121:153–155, 1976.

1239. Subbarao K, Jacobson HG: Primary malignant neoplasms. Semin Roentgenol 14:44–57, 1979.

1240. Sullivan AW: Subluxation of the atlanto-axial joint: sequel to inflammatory processes of the neck. J Pediatr 35:451–464, 1949.

1241. Sundaram M, Scholz C: Primary hyperparathyroidism presenting with acute paraplegia. AJR 128:674–676, 1977.

1242. Sundaresan N, Galicich JH, Chu FCH, et al: Spinal chordomas. J Neurosurg 50:312–319, 1979.

1243. Sundaresan N, Huvos AG, Rosen G, et al: Postradiation osteosarcoma of the spine following treatment of Hodgkin's disease. Spine 11:90–92, 1986.

1244. Suomalainen O, Pääkkönen M: Fracture dislocation of the lumbar spine without paraplegia: a case report. Acta Orthop Scand 55:466–468, 1984.

1245. Suss RA, Zimmerman RD, Leeds NE: Pseudospread of the atlas: false sign of Jefferson fracture in young children. AJR 140:1079–1082, 1983.

1246. Swee RG, McLeod RA, Beabout JW: Osteoid osteoma. Detection, diagnosis and localization. Radiology 130:117–123, 1979.

1247. Swischuck LE: Spine and spinal cord trauma in the battered child syndrome. Radiology 92:733–738, 1969.

1248. Swischuk LE: The beaked, notched or hooked vertebra. Radiology 95:661–664, 1970.

1249. Swischuk LE: Anterior displacement of C2 in children: physiologic or pathologic? A helpful differentiating line. Radiology 122:759–763, 1977.

1250. Swischuk LE, Fagan CJ, Sarwar M: Persistence of the dens as the body of C1. A case report of a rare anomaly. Radiology 127:330, 1978.

1251. Swischuk LE, Hayden CK Jr, Sarwar M: The posteriorly tilted dens—a normal variation mimicking a fractured dens. Pediatr Radiol 8:27–28, 1979.

1252. Tabb JL, Tucker JT: Actinomycosis of the spine. AJR 29:628–634, 1933.

1253. Taybi H: Diastrophic dwarfism. Radiology 80:1–10, 1963.

1254. Taybi H, Keele D: Hypoparathyroidism: a review of the literature and report of two cases in sisters, one with steatorrhea and intestinal pseudo-obstruction. AJR 88:432–442, 1962.

1255. Taylor MM, Moore TM, Harvey JP Jr: Pycnodysostosis: a case report. J Bone Joint Surg 60A:1128–1130, 1968.

1256. Teitelbaum SL, Coccia PF, Brown DM, et al: Malignant osteopetrosis: a disease of abnormal osteoclast proliferation. Metab Bone Dis Rel Res 3:99–105, 1981.

1257. Templeton AW, Jaconett JR, Ormond RS: Localized osteosclerosis in hyperparathyroidism. Radiology 78:955–958, 1962.

1258. Teng P: Spondylosis of the cervical spine with compression of the spinal cord and nerve roots. J Bone Joint Surg 42A:392–407, 1960.

1259. Tenney RF, Kerekes ES: Cervical spine lateral horizontal beam technique. Radiology 124:520, 1977.

1260. Teplick JG: Tuberous sclerosis: extensive roentgen findings without the usual clinical picture: a case report. Radiology 93:53–55, 1969.

1261. Teplick JG, Head GL, Kricun ME, et al: Ghost infantile vertebrae and hemipelves within adult skeleton from Thorotrast administration in childhood. Radiology 129:657–660, 1978.

1262. Thickman D, Bonakdar-pour A, Clancy M, et al: Fibrodysplasia ossificans progressiva. AJR 139:935–941, 1982.

1263. Thompson GH, Khan MA, Bilenker RM: Spontaneous atlantoaxial subluxation as a presenting manifestation of juvenile ankylosing spondylitis: a case report. Spine 7:78–79, 1982.

1264. Tillman BP, Dahlin DC, Lipscomb PR, et al: Aneurysmal bone cyst: an analysis of ninety-five cases. Mayo Clin Proc 43:478–495, 1968.

1265. Ting YM: Osteomyelitis of the spine. Radiology 76:27–31, 1961.

1266. Tini PG, Wieser C, Zinn WM: The transitional vertebra of the lumbosacral spine: its radiological classification, incidence, prevalence and clinical significance. Rheum Rehab 16:180–185, 1977.

1267. Tomita K, Nomura S, Nanri Y: Thoracic cord compression from the chondroma of rib: a case report. Spine 9:535–538, 1984.

1268. Tompsett AC Jr, Donaldson SW: The anterior tubercle of the first cervical vertebra and the hyoid bone: their occurrence in newborn infants. AJR 65:582–589, 1951.

1269. Tomsick TA, Lebowitz ME, Campbell C: The congenital absence of the pedicles in the thoracic spine: report of two cases. Radiology 111:587–589, 1974.

1270. Tong D, Griffin TW, Laramore GE, et al: Solitary plasmacytoma of bone and soft tissues. Radiology 135:195–198, 1980.

1271. Torgerson WR, Dotter WE: Comparative roentgenographic study of the asymptomatic and symptomatic lumbar spine. J Bone Joint Surg 58A:850–853, 1976.

1272. Trueta J: The three types of acute haematogenous osteomyelitis: a clinical and vascular study. J Bone Joint Surg 41B:671–680, 1959.

1273. Tsou PM: Embryology of congenital kyphosis. Clin Orthop 128:18–25, 1977.

1274. Tsukamoto Y, Onitsuka H, Lee K: Radiologic aspects of diffuse idiopathic skeletal hyperostosis in the spine. AJR 129:913–918, 1977.

1275. Tsusi H, Tsutomu Y, Sainoh H: Developmental balloon disc of the lumbar spine in healthy subjects. Spine 10:907–911, 1985.

1276. Tsuyama N: Ossification of the posterior longitudinal ligament of the spine. Clin Orthop 184:71–84, 1984.

1277. Tuddenham WJ: Quality assurance in diagnostic radiology: an irreverent view of a sacred cow. Radiology 131:579–588, 1979.

1278. United States Department of Health, Education and Welfare, Public Health Service, Food and Drug Administration, Bureau of Radiological Health, Division of Training and Medical Applications: Gonadal doses and genetically significant dose from diagnostic radiology: U.S. 1964, 1970 and 1976. Rockville, Maryland: Public Health Service.

1279. Unni KK, Ivins JC, Beabout JW, et al: Hemangioma, hemangiopericytoma, and hemangioendothelioma (angiosarcoma) of bone. Cancer 27:1403–1414, 1971.

1280. Utne JR, Pugh DG: The roentgenologic aspects of chordoma. AJR 74:593–608, 1955.

1281. Valderrama JAF, Bullough PG: Solitary myeloma of the spine. J Bone Joint Surg 50B:82–90, 1968.

1282. van Ameyden, van Duym FC, van Wiechen PJ: Herniation of calcified nucleus pulposus in the thoracic spine. J Comput Assist Tomogr 7:1122–1123, 1983.

1283. Vanel D, Contesso G, Couanet D, et al: Computed tomography in the evaluation of 41 cases of Ewing's sarcoma. Skeletal Radiol 9:8–13, 1982.

1283a. Vanel D, Hagay C, Rebibo G, et al: Study of three radio-induced malignant fibrohistiocytomas of bone. Skeletal Radiol 9:174–178, 1983.

1284. VanSchaik JPJ, Verbiest H, Van Schaik FDJ: The orientation of laminae and facet joints in the lower lumbar spine. Spine 10:59–63, 1985.

1285. Verbiest H: Giant-cell tumours and aneurysmal bone cysts of the spine. J Bone Joint Surg 47B:699–713, 1965.

1286. Verbiest H: Pathomorphologic aspects of developmental lumbar stenosis. Orthop Clin North Am 6:177–196, 1975.

1287. Verbiest H: Fallacies of the present definition, nomenclature and classification of the stenosis of the lumbar vertebral canal. Spine 1:217–225, 1976.

1288. Verjaal A, Harder NC: Backward luxation of the atlas: report of a case. Acta Radiolog 3:173–176, 1965.

1289. Vines FS: The significance of "occult" fractures of the cervical spine. AJR 107:493–504, 1969.

1290. Vinstein AL, Cockerill EM: Involvement of the spine in gout. A case report. Radiology 103:311–312, 1972.

1291. Vinstein AL, Franken EA Jr: Hereditary multiple exostoses: report of a case with spinal cord compression. AJR 112:405–407, 1971.

1292. Vohra VG: Roentgen manifestations in Ewing's sarcoma. A study of 156 cases. Cancer 20:727–733, 1967.

1293. Volpe R, Mazabraud A: A clinicopathologic review of 25 cases of chordoma (a pleomorphic and metastasizing neoplasm). Am J Surg Pathol 7:161–170, 1983.

1294. von Torklus D, Gehle W: The Upper Cervical Spine. New York: Grune & Stratton, 1972.

1295. Waggener RG, Kereiakes JG, Shalek RJ: CRC Handbook of Medical Physics, vol 2. Boca Raton, Florida: CRC Press, 1984.

1296. Wagner AC: "Spurious" defect of the lumbar vertebral body. AJR 135:1095–1096, 1980.

1297. Wagoner G, Pendergrass EP: Intrinsic circulation of the vertebral body with roentgenologic considerations. AJR 27:818–826, 1932.

1298. Wagoner G, Pendergrass EP: The anterior and posterior "notch" shadows seen in lateral roentgenograms of the vertebrae of infants. An anatomic explanation. AJR 42:663–670, 1939.

1299. Wagoner GW, Hunt AD Jr, Pendergrass EP: A study of the relative importance of the cortex and spongiosa in the production of the roentgenogram of the normal vertebral body. AJR 53:40–48, 1945.

1300. Waine H, Bennett GA, Bauer W: Joint disease associated with acromegaly. Am J Med Sci 209:671–687, 1945.

1301. Wald SL, Roland TA: Intradural spinal metastasis in Ewing's sarcoma: case report and review of the literature. Neurosurgery 15:873–877, 1984.

1302. Walker BA, Scott CI, Hall JG, et al: Diastrophic dwarfism. Medicine 51:41–59, 1972.

1303. Wang AM, Joachim CL, Shillito JR, et al: Cervical chordoma presenting with intervertebral foramen enlargement mimicking neurofibroma: CT findings. J Comput Assist Tomogr 8:529–532, 1984.

1304. Wang AM, Lipson SJ, Haykal HA, et al: Computed tomography of aneurysmal bone cyst of the L1 vertebral body. J Comput Assist Tomogr 8:1186–1189, 1984.

1305. Wang CC, Schulz MD: Ewing's sarcoma: A study of fifty cases treated at the Massachusetts General Hospital, 1930–1952 inclusive. N Engl J Med 248:571–576, 1953.

1306. Wang GJ, Mabie KN, Whitehall R, et al: The nonsurgical management of odontoid fractures in adults. Spine 9:229–230, 1984.

1307. Wasner C, Kraines RG, Kaye RL: Oblique view radiographs in the diagnosis of sacroiliitis. Arthritis Rheum 22:671, 1979.

1308. Wear JE, Baylin GJ, Martin TL: Pyogenic osteomyelitis of the spine. AJR 67:90–94, 1952.

1309. Weatherley CR, Jaffray D, O'Brien JP: Radical excision of an osteoblastoma of the cervical spine. J Bone Joint Surg 68B:325–328, 1986.

1310. Weaver EN Jr, England GD, Richardson DE: Sacral fracture: case presentation and review. Neurosurgery 9:725–728, 1981.

1311. Weaver P, Lifeso RM: The radiological diagnosis of tuberculosis of the adult spine. Skeletal Radiol 12:178–186, 1984.

1312. Webster EW, Merrill OE: Radiation hazards. II. Measurements of gonadal dose in radiographic examinations. N Engl J Med 257:811–819, 1957.

1313. Wedge JH, Tchang S, MacFadyen DJ: Computed tomography in localization of spinal osteoid osteoma. Spine 6:423–427, 1981.

1314. Weens HS: Calcification of the intervertebral discs in childhood. J Pediatr 26:178–188, 1945.

1315. Weinberger A, Myers AR: Intervertebral disc calcification in adults: a review. Semin Arthritis Rheum 8:69–75, 1978.

1316. Weinfeld A, Ross MW, Sarasohn SH: Spondyloepiphyseal dysplasia tarda: a cause of premature osteoarthritis. AJR 101:851–859, 1967.

1317. Weinstein JB, Siegel MJ, Griffith RC: Spinal Ewing sarcoma: misleading appearances. Skeletal Radiol 11:262–265, 1984.

1318. Weinstein PR, Karpman RR, Gall EP, et al: Spinal cord injury, spinal fracture and spinal stenosis in ankylosing spondylitis. J Neurosurg 57:609–616, 1982.

1319. Weinstein SL, Ponseti IV: Curve progression in idiopathic scoliosis. J Bone Joint Surg 65A:447–455, 1983.

1320. Weinstein SL, Zavala DC, Ponseti IV: Idiopathic scoliosis: long-term follow-up and prognosis in untreated patients. J Bone Joint Surg 63A:702–712, 1981.

1321. Weir DC: Roentgenographic signs of cervical injury. Clin Orthop 109:9–17, 1975.

1322. Weissman BNW, Aliabadi P, Weinfeld MS, et al: Prognostic features of atlantoaxial subluxation in rheumatoid arthritis patients. Radiology 144:745–751, 1982.

1323. Weisz GM, Lee P: Spinal canal stenosis. Concept of spinal reserve capacity: radiologic measurements and clinical applications. Clin Orthop 179:134–140, 1983.

1324. Weller M, Edeiken J, Hodes PJ: Renal osteodystrophy. AJR 104:354–363, 1968.

1325. Wells F, Thomas TL, Matthewson MH, et al: Neurilemmoma of the thoracic spine: a case report. Spine 7:66, 1982.

1326. Wenger DR, Bobechko WP, Gilday DL: The spectrum of intervertebral disc–space infection in children. J Bone Joint Surg 60A:100–108, 1978.

1327. Wertzberger KL, Peterson HA: Acquired spondylolysis and spondylolisthesis in the young child. Spine 5:437–442, 1980.

1328. Wesselius LJ, Brooks RJ, Gall EP: Vertebral coccidioidomycosis presenting as Pott's disease. JAMA 238:1397–1398, 1977.

1329. Westerman MP, Greenfield GB, Wong PWK: "Fish vertebrae," homocystinuria and sickle cell anemia. JAMA 230:261–262, 1974.

1330. Weston WJ, Goodson GM: Vertebra plana (calve). J Bone Joint Surg 41B:477–485, 1959.

1331. Whalen JP, Woodruff CL: The cervical prevertebral fat stripe. A new aid in evaluating the prevertebral soft tissue space. AJR 109:445–451, 1970.

1332. Whelan MA, Feldman F: The variant lumbar pedicle. Neuroradiology 22:235–242, 1982.

1333. White AA III, Johnson RM, Panjabi MM, et al: Biomechanical analysis of clinical stability in the cervical spine. Clin Orthop 109:85–96, 1975.

1334. White AA III, Moss HL: Hangman's fracture with non-union and late cord compression. J Bone Joint Surg 60A:839–840, 1978.

1335. Whitehouse GH, Griffiths GJ: Roentgenologic aspects of spinal involvement by primary and metastatic Ewing's tumor. J Can Assoc Radiol 27:290–297, 1976.

1336. Whitesides TE Jr: Traumatic kyphosis of the thoracolumbar spine. Clin Orthop 128:78–92, 1977.

1337. Wholey MH, Bruwer AJ, Baker HL Jr: The lateral roentgenogram of the neck (with comments on the atlanto-odontoid-basion relationship). Radiology 71:350–356, 1958.

1338. Wholey MH, Pugh DG, Bickel WH: Localized destructive lesions in rheumatoid spondylitis. Radiology 74:54–56, 1960.

1339. Wickbom GI, Williamson MR: Anomalous foramen transversarium of C2 simulating erosion of bone. Neuroradiology 19:43–45, 1980.

1340. Wiesseman GJ, Wood VE, Kroll LL: Pseudomonas vertebral osteomyelitis in heroin addicts: report of five cases. J Bone Joint Surg 55A:1416–1424, 1973.

1340a. Wilber RG, Thompson GH, Shaffer JW, et al: Postoperative neurological deficits in segmental spinal instrumentation: a study using spinal cord monitoring. J Bone Joint Surg 66A:1178–1187, 1984.

1341. Wiley AM, Trueta J: The vascular anatomy of the spine and its relationship to pyogenic vertebral osteomyelitis. J Bone Joint Surg 41B:796–809, 1959.

1342. Wilkinson RH, Hall JE: The sclerotic pedicle: tumor or pseudotumor? Radiology 111:683–688, 1974.

1343. Wilkinson RH, Strand RD: Congenital anomalies and normal variants. Semin Roentgenol 14:7–18, 1979.

1344. Wilkinson RH, Willi UV, Gilsanz V, et al: Radiographic evaluation of the spine after surgical correction of scoliosis. AJR 133:703–709, 1979.

1345. Willems MHA, Braakman R, Linge BV: Bilateral locked facets in the thoracic spine. Acta Orthop Scand 55:300–303, 1984.

1346. Willis RA: Solitary plasmocytoma of bone. J Pathol Bacteriol 53:77–85, 1941.

1347. Willis TA: Lumbosacral retrodisplacement. AJR 90:1263–1266, 1963.

1348. Wilson CB, Norrell HA Jr: Congenital absence of a pedicle in the cervical spine. AJR 97:639–647, 1966.

1349. Wilson TW, Pugh DG: Primary reticulum-cell sarcoma of bone, with emphasis on roentgen aspects. Radiology 65:343–351, 1955.

1350. Wiltse LL: The etiology of spondylolisthesis. J Bone Joint Surg 44A:539–560, 1962.

1351. Wiltse LL, Newman PH, Macnab I: Classification of spondylolysis and spondylolisthesis. Clin Orthop 117:23–29, 1976.

1352. Wiltse LL, Widell EH Jr, Jackson DW: Fatigue fracture: the basic lesion in isthmic spondylolisthesis. J Bone Joint Surg 57A:17–22, 1975.

1353. Wiltse LL, Winter RB: Terminology and measurement of spondylolisthesis. J Bone Joint Surg 65A:768–772, 1983.

1354. Winter RB: Congenital scoliosis. Clin Orthop 93:75–94, 1973.

1355. Winter RB: Severe spondylolisthesis in Marfan's syndrome: report of two cases. Pediatr Orthop 2:51–55, 1982.

1356. Winter RB, Hall JE: Kyphosis in childhood and adolescence. Spine 3:285–308, 1978.

1357. Winter RB, Moe JH, Eilers VE: Congenital scoliosis: a study of 234 patients treated and untreated. Part I: natural history. J Bone Joint Surg 50A:1–15, 1968.

1358. Winter RB, Moe JH, Lonstein JE: The incidence of Klippel-Feil syndrome in patients with congenital scoliosis and kyphosis. Spine 9:363–366, 1984.

1359. Winter WG Jr, Larson RK, Zettas JP, et al: Coccidioidal spondylitis. J Bone Joint Surg 60A:240–244, 1978.

1360. Wirth CR, Jacobs RL, Rolander SD: Neuropathic spinal arthropathy: a review of the Charcot spine. Spine 5:558–567, 1980.

1361. Witt I, Vestergaard A, Rosenklint A: A comparative analysis of x-ray findings of the lumbar spine in patients with and without lumbar pain. Spine 9:298–300, 1984.

1362. Wodarski KH: Orthotopic and ectopic chondrogenesis and osteogenesis mediated by neoplastic cells. Clin Orthop 200:248–265, 1985.

1363. Wolf BS, Khilnani M, Malis L: The sagittal diameter of the bony cervical spinal canal and its significance in cervical spondylosis. J Mt Sinai Hosp 23:283–292, 1956.

1364. Wollin DG: The os odontoideum. J Bone Joint Surg 45A:1459–1471, 1484, 1963.

1365. Wong DF, Bobechko PE, Becker EJ, et al: Coexistent multiple myeloma and Paget's disease of bone. J Can Assoc Radiol 32:251–253, 1981.

1366. Woodring JH, Goldstein SJ: Fractures of the articular processes of the cervical spine. AJR 139:341–344, 1982.

1367. Woodring JH, Selke AC Jr, Duff DE: Traumatic atlantooccipital dislocation with survival. AJNR 2:251–254, 1981.

1368. Woodruff RK, Malpas JS, White EF: Solitary plasmacytoma: II. Solitary plasmacytoma of bone. Cancer 43:2344–2347, 1979.

1369. Woodward HR, Chan DPK, Lee J: Massive osteolysis of the cervical spine: a case report of bone graft failure. Spine 6:545–549, 1981.

1370. Woolfenden JM, Pitt MJ, Durie BGM, et al: Comparison of bone scintigraphy and radiography in multiple myeloma. Radiology 134:723–728, 1980.

1371. Wortzman G, Steinhardt MI: Congenitally absent lumbar pedicle: a reappraisal. Radiology 152:713–718, 1984.

1372. Wu KK, Guise ER: Osteochondroma of the atlas: a case report. Clin Orthop 136:160–162, 1978.

1373. Wu KK, Guise ER: Unicameral bone cyst of the spine. A case report. J Bone Joint Surg 63A:324–326, 1981.

1374. Wu KK, Mitchell DC, Guise ER: Chordoma of the atlas: a case report. J Bone Surg 61A:140–141, 1979.

1375. Wynne-Davies R, Gormley J: The prevalence of skeletal dysplasias: an estimate of their minimum frequency and the number of patients requiring orthopaedic care. J Bone Joint Surg 67B:133–137, 1985.

1376. Wynne-Davies R, Scott JHS: Inheritance and spondylolisthesis: a radiographic family survey. J Bone Joint Surg 61B:301–305, 1979.

1377. Yagan R: CT diagnosis of limbus vertebra: case report. J Comput Assist Tomogr 8:149–151, 1984.

1378. Young DA, Laman ML: Radiodense skeletal lesions in Boeck's sarcoid. AJR 114:553–558, 1972.

1379. Young LW, Oestreich AE, Goldstein LA: Roentgenology in scoliosis: contribution to evaluation and management. AJR 108:778–795, 1970.

1379a. Yousefzadeh DK, El-Khory GY, Lupetin AR: Congenital aplastic-hypoplastic lumbar pedicle in infants and young children. Skeletal Radiol 7:259–265, 1982.

1380. Yousefzadeh DK, El-Khoury GY, Smith WL: Normal sagittal diameter and variation in the pediatric cervical spine. Radiology 144:319–325, 1982.

1381. Yu R, Brunner DR, Rao KCVG: Role of computed tomography in symptomatic vertebral hemangiomas. J Comput Tomogr 8:311–315, 1984.

1382. Zimmerman HB: Osteosclerosis in chronic renal disease: report of 4 cases associated with secondary hyperparathyroidism. AJR 88:1152–1169, 1962.

1383. Zimmerman HB, Farrell WJ: Cervical vertebral erosion caused by vertebral artery tortuosity. AJR 108:767–770, 1970.

1384. Ziter FMH Jr: Central vertebral end-plate depression in chronic renal disease: report of two cases. AJR 132:809–811, 1979.

1385. Zoltan JD, Gilula LA, Murphy WA: Unilateral facet dislocation between the fifth lumbar and first sacral vertebrae: case report. J Bone Joint Surg 61A:767–769, 1979.

1386. Zvaifler NJ, Martel W: Spondylitis in chronic ulcerative colitis. Arthritis Rheum 3:76–87, 1960.

1387. Zvetina JR, Demos TC, Rubinstein H: *Mycobacterium intracellulare* infection of the shoulder and spine in a patient with steroid-treated systemic lupus erythematosus. Skeletal Radiol 8:111–113, 1982.

5

Jesse Littleton III, M.D.

Conventional Pluridirectional Tomography

Conventional pluridirectional tomography (CPT) is an imaging modality that can produce sectional radiographic images in multiple projections. Historically, conventional pluridirectional tomography represented the first major improvement in roentgen imagery of the spine.[1, 3, 5] With the advent of computed tomography (CT) and, more recently, magnetic resonance imaging (MRI), imaging capabilities have been extended. However, CPT still plays an important role in the evaluation and work-up of many spinal disorders, and in some clinical practices, it may be the only sectional imaging modality available. The purpose of this chapter is to demonstrate the comprehensive imaging capabilities of CPT and to assess the ability of the CPT image to demonstrate spinal pathology.

INDICATIONS

If the plain film review of the spine is diagnostic and clinically directive, there is no need for sectional imaging. If the plain film is not clinically directive, CPT may be indicated. The utilization of CPT in certain clinical settings is determined by whether or not CT or MRI is available. Even though CT or MRI might be available, CPT still plays an important role in sectional evaluation for the following situations:

1. When longitudinal assessment is desired in:
   a. complex congenital anomalies extending through several spinal segments, particularly in the upper cervical spine.
   b. evaluation of flexion and extension.
   c. evaluation of subluxation.
   d. postoperative fusion.
2. When fine bone detail is required.
3. When subtle fractures are suspected.
4. When a fracture is suspected to be parallel to the plane of CT section (base of the odontoid process, some facet fractures, and others).
5. To monitor the progress of postoperative fusion and to assess healing of spinal fractures.

When CT and MRI are not available, CPT becomes the major sectional imaging modality. In addition to the indications just listed, conventional pluridirectional tomography may define cortical margins not well visualized on the plain film. It becomes the main sectional imaging modality for spinal trauma. CPT may be utilized when the plain radiograph is abnormal but not diagnostic or clinically directive, or when the plain radiograph and the CT image are normal and there is clinical evidence to suggest a pathologic process.

LIMITATIONS

The limitations of CPT of the spine are principally the inability to visualize soft-tissue structures and difficulty in evaluating some areas of the spine.

Soft-tissue structures such as intervertebral discs, ligaments, spinal cord, nerve roots, epidural space, thecal sac, and paravertebral muscles cannot be differentiated, because contrast discrimination in the CPT system is lower than that in CT and MRI. The resolving capability of a satisfactory CPT system is approximately five line pairs per mm, which is less than that of a plain radiograph but significantly better than the reconstructed images of CT and MRI.

Some residual blur is present even in the most optimal conventional tomogram. Complex motion tomography keeps artifacts to a minimum, and they are seldom confusing if only sharply defined structures in the tomograms are interpreted. Serious errors in diagnosis occur when unsharp portions of the tomogram are considered in the diagnostic evaluation.

Some areas of the spine are more difficult to visualize than others—particularly the

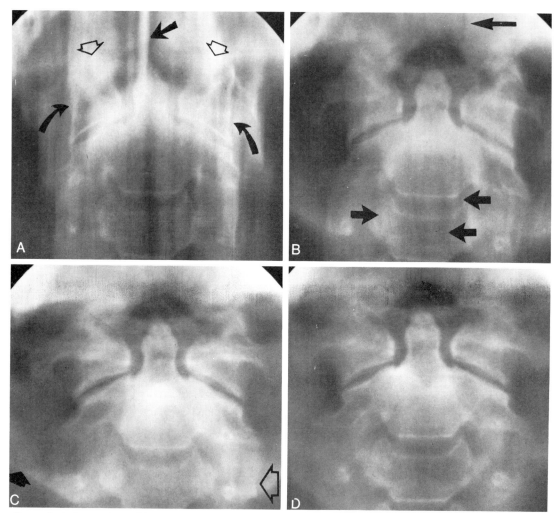

Figure 5–1. Comparison of four tomographic movements to visualize upper cervical segments. *A,* Linear longitudinal movement. Note retained image of the nasal septum (straight black arrow) with poor visualization of the lateral masses of C1 (curved black arrows) and false impression of degenerative arthritic change at the atlantoaxial joint (open arrows). *B,* Elliptic movement shows improved visualization, but linear characteristics are retained. Note false shadow suggesting fracture into the margin of the foramen magnum (large arrow) and retained linear streaking (small arrows). *C,* In the 36 degree circular movement the image is improved, but false shadows of a tooth (open arrow) and the margin of the mandible (black arrow) are present. *D,* Further improvement of marginal detail is noted with hypocycloid movement; false shadows are less prominent. The trispiral movement (not pictured) presents an image similar to that of the hypocycloid movement. (From Littleton JT: Tomography: Physical Principles and Clinical Applications. © 1976, the Williams & Wilkins Company, Baltimore.)

cervicothoracic junction and the lumbosacral junction—but with technical persistence diagnostic studies can generally be obtained.

EQUIPMENT AND TECHNIQUE

Equipment

The principle of producing a tomographic image consists of an x-ray source moving in one direction and a receptor moving synchronously in the opposite direction.

A linear obscuring movement does not result in a sectional image.[5, 7] Attempts to use this method in tomographic studies of the spine may result in serious omissions of imaging or the development of false shadows, which may yield an erroneous diagnosis (Fig. 5–1). A dedicated tomographic device with a compound obscuring movement is a requirement for satisfactory conventional tomography of the spine.

In the author's experience, only devices that have the capability of producing thin section images, approximately 1 mm thick, with either a hypocycloid or a trispiral movement produce the best images. The 48 degree/24 degree hypocycloid movement is preferred to the smaller 34 degree/17degree hypocycloid movement. Trispiral movements should have a total angular displacement of approximately 12 to 45 degrees. Elliptic and circular movements are less effective throughout the spine.

The capability for erect tomography is occasionally helpful. The tomographic device should be mechanically stable. Films of the highest quality will result when a 0.3 mm focal spot tube, oil or water cooled, and a 3 phase, 12 pulse generator are employed.

Technique

In addition to specialized equipment, an experienced or interested radiologist and a dedicated technologist are equally essential. The technologist must be conversant with the clinical problem, have a working knowledge of sectional anatomy of the spine to orient anatomic structures correctly, and communicate closely with the radiologist during the tomographic procedure.

Technical aspects of tomography of the spine have been lucidly described elsewhere.[4] Three special techniques are worthy of mention. The first is laser localization, in which projection of a laser beam to the long axis of the spine aids in attaining proper alignment in the lateral and oblique views (Fig. 5–2). A laser localizer is equally helpful in the identification of section levels. A second technique that will improve the image when the entire cervical spine is being examined is use of bolus or collimator filters to balance the extreme density differences between the upper and lower cervical spine (Fig. 5–3). Third, marked improvement of contrast in lateral projections of the lower lumbar spine and of the cervicothoracic

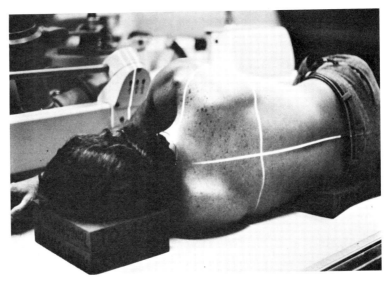

Figure 5–2. Laser light localizing system.

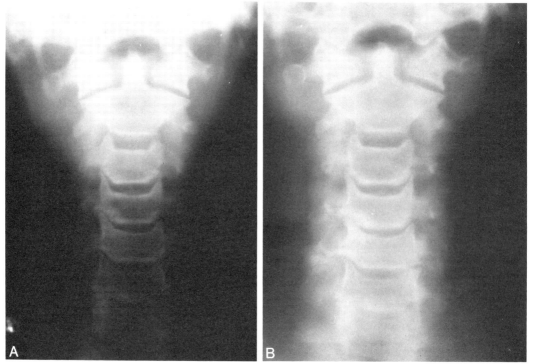

Figure 5–3. Density balanced with bolus. *A*, Anteroposterior (AP) tomogram without bolus, extending from the first cervical vertebra to the seventh. Note the change in radiographic density between the upper and lower cervical vertebrae. *B*, Addition of bolus (flour sacks or aluminum collimator filter or both) to the upper cervical spine balances the density throughout the cervical segments.

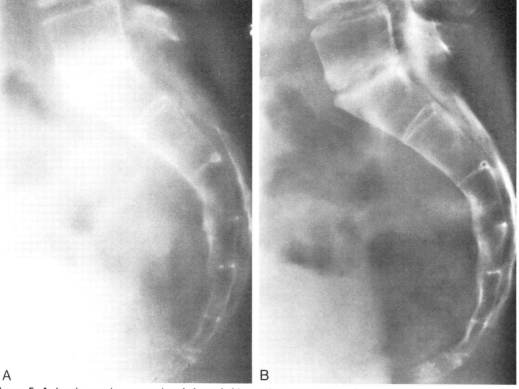

Figure 5–4. Lumbosacral zonography. *A*, Lateral thin section tomograms of the lower lumbar spine in an obese patient. Note the low contrast and poor detail. *B*, Lateral zonogram, 8 degree circular movement. Because the section is thicker, detail and contrast are improved in the lumbosacral spine of this large patient. (From Littleton JT: Tomography: Physical Principles and Clinical Applications. © 1976, the Williams & Wilkins Company, Baltimore.)

292

junction can be obtained by using small-angle circular movements. In general, an 8 degree circular movement providing a thick section of approximately 0.5 cm⁴ is satisfactory. These are the only areas of the spine where "thick sections" may be preferred (Fig. 5–4).

NORMAL TOMOGRAM

Interpretation of CPT studies of the spine requires a working familiarity with three-dimensional anatomy of the spine. Variations in the appearance of the spine exist between vertebrae throughout the axial skel-

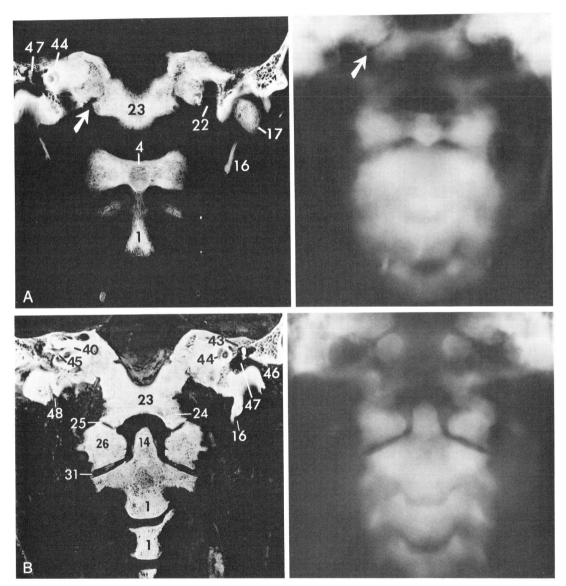

Figure 5–5. Craniovertebral junction, coronal sections. *A* through *F* show anatomic specimens (left) and tomograms (right) through the craniovertebral junction. *G* and *H* show anatomic specimens. The anatomic sections and tomograms from *A* to *H* are at 3 mm intervals from anterior to posterior, beginning at the level of the anterior arch of C1 (*A*). *A, B, Key*: **1** = body; **4** = anterior arch, C1; **14** = odontoid process; **16** = styloid process; **17** = mandibular condyle; **22** = carotid foramen; **23** = basilar part, occipital bone; **24** = occipital condyle; **25** = atlanto-occipital joint; **26** = lateral mass, C1; **31** = atlantoaxial joint; **40** = internal auditory canal; **43** = ossicular chain; **44** = cochlea; **45** = vestibule and semicircular canals; **46** = external auditory canal; **47** = tympanic cavity; **48** = stylomastoid foramen; **arrows** = suture between basilar part of occipital bone and petrous apex.

Illustration continued on following page

eton, and subtle differences are present within each anatomic area. Tomographic anatomy also varies as the result of the malalignment of the spine that occurs in scoliosis, lordosis, or kyphosis.

Correlation of anatomic specimens and conventional tomography of the cran/over-tebral region is presented at several slice levels (Figs. 5–5 and 5–6). Anatomic correlation of C2 through the sacrum, as well as

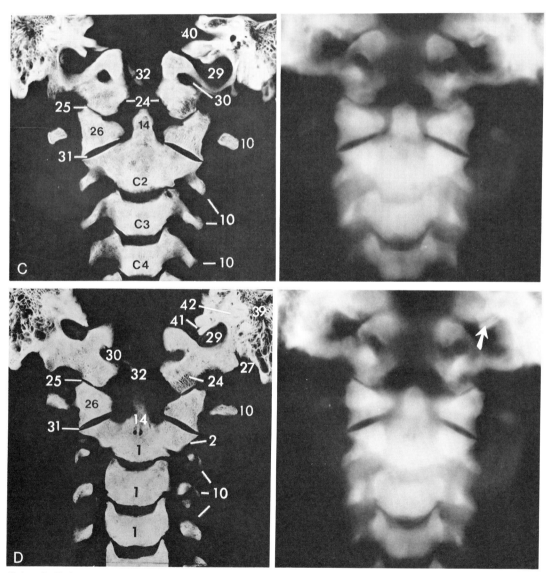

Figure 5–5 *Continued C–H, Key:* **1** = body; **2** = pedicle; **3** = posterior arch, C1; **7** = vertebral foramen (spinal canal); **10** = transverse process; **11** = lamina; **12** = spinous process; **13** = intervertebral foramina; **14** = odontoid process; **24** = occipital condyle; **25** = atlanto-occipital joint; **26** = lateral mass, C1; **27** = digastric notch; **28** = floor of posterior fossa (occipital bone); **29** = jugular foramen and fossa; **30** = hypoglossal canal; **31** = atlantoaxial joint; **32** = foramen magnum; **33** = petrous pyramid; **39** = mastoid; **40** = internal auditory canal; **41** = cochlea canaliculus; **42** = semicircular canals; **arrow** = cochlea canaliculus.

Illustration continued on opposite page

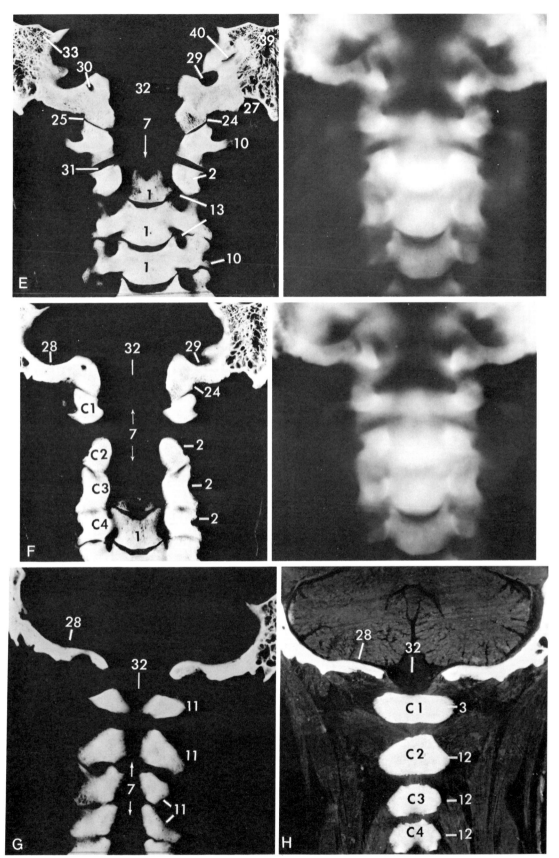

Figure 5–5 *See legend on opposite page*

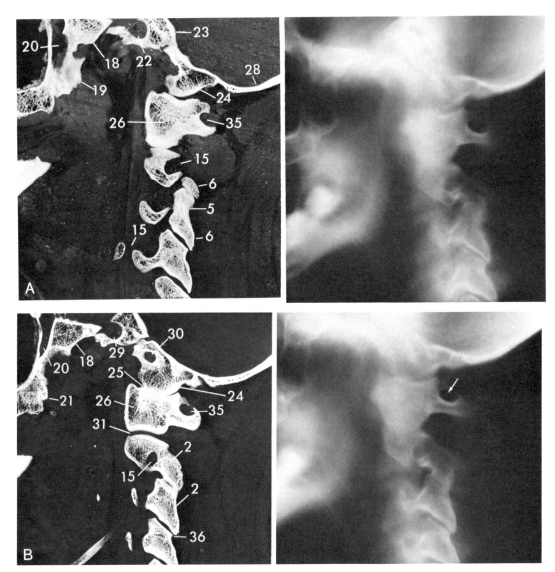

Figure 5–6. Craniovertebral junction, sagittal sections. A through G show anatomic specimens (left) and tomograms (right) through the craniovertebral junction. The anatomic sections and tomograms from *A* to *G* are at 3 mm intervals, beginning at the right parasagittal region (*A*). *A–E, Key:* **1** = body; **2** = pedicle; **4** =anterior arch, C1; **5** = superior articular process; **6** = inferior articular process; **7** = vertebral foramen (spinal canal); **8** = superior vertebral notch (incisure); **9** = inferior vertebral notch (incisure); **11** = lamina; **12** = spinous process; **13** = intervertebral foramina; **15** = foramen transversarium; **18** = pterygoid body; **19** = pterygoid wing; **20** = pterygoid fossa; **21** = alveolar ridge; **22** = carotid foramen; **23** = basilar part, occipital bone; **24** = occipital condyle; **25** = atlanto-occipital joint; **26** = lateral mass, C1; **28** = floor of posterior fossa (occipital bone); **29** = jugular foramen and fossa; **30** = hypoglossal canal; **31** = atlantoaxial joint; **32** = foramen magnum; **35** = foramen arcuate (groove, or foramen, for vertebral artery); **36** = apophyseal joint; **38** = sphenoid; **arrow** in *B* = foramen arcuate; **arrows** in *D* = atlanto-occipital joint (medial aspect).

Illustration continued on opposite page

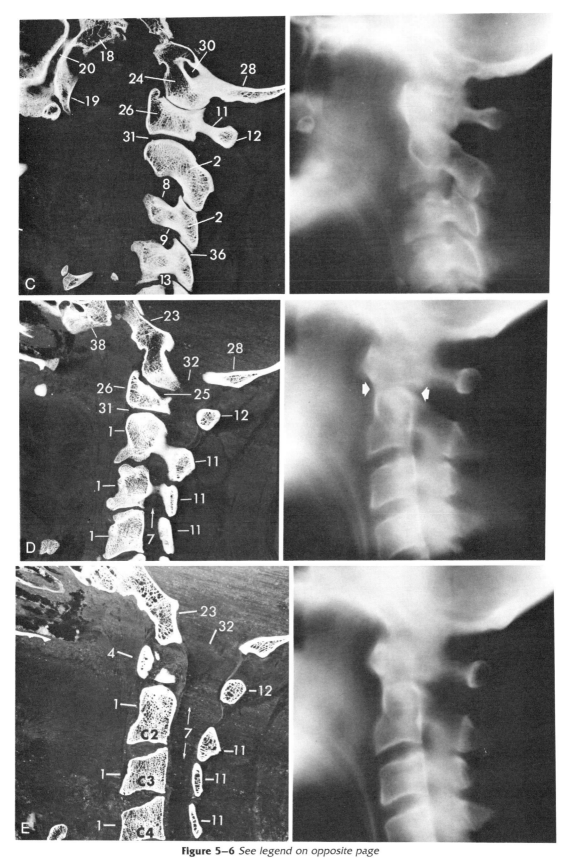

Figure 5–6 See legend on opposite page

Illustration continued on following page

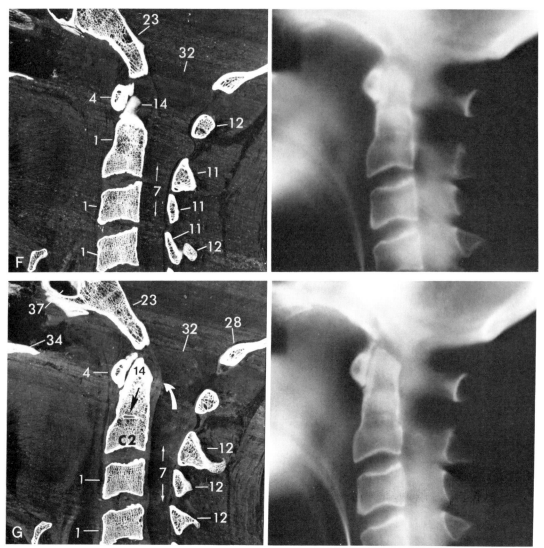

Figure 5–6 *Continued F, G, Key:* **1** = body; **4** = anterior arch, C1; **7** vertebral foramen (spinal canal); **11** = lamina; **12** = spinous process; **14** = odontoid process; **23** = basilar part, occipital bone; **28** = floor of posterior fossa (occipital bone); **32** = foramen magnum; **34** = hard palate; **37** = sphenoid sinus; **white arrow** = transverse ligament; **black arrow** = subdental synchondrosis.

technique for specimen preparation, is discussed elsewhere.[5, 6]

As serial sections are viewed, one should note the gradual transition of detail throughout the tomographic sections. It is essential that *only those anatomic sections that are sharply in focus be interpreted.* The marginal blur of adjacent levels carries through several sections and may be interpreted erroneously. The reader should note that the image of the odontoid process persists in

Figures 5–5D and 5–5E, whereas it has disappeared from the anatomic section. Nevertheless, there is excellent correlation between those elements that are sharply in focus in the tomogram and the similar segment of anatomic specimen. Anatomic landmarks of the base of the skull are identified in detail, because some of these structures, particularly sutures, may be confused with pathologic changes such as fracture.

Figures 5–7 through 5–11, showing thin-

Text continued on page 303

Figure 5–7. Tomograms of a normal cervical spine. *A,* Coronal section of the upper cervical vertebrae. The odontoid process and atlanto-occipital joints are well seen. *B* Lower cervical segments through midplane vertebral bodies. *C,* Lateral view through the midsagittal plane. Vertebral bodies and spinous processes are in sharp focus outlining the spinal canal. *D,* Oblique section through the articular processes and intervertebral foramina (arrows). *E,* Axial view of C1 shows the anterior arch (large white arrow), lateral masses (small white arrows), posterior arch (small black arrows), and the tip of the odontoid process (open arrow). *F,* Axial section through the midplane of C2. The body (large white arrow), foramina transversarium (small white arrows), lamina, and spinous process (small black arrows) are clearly demonstrated. *G,* Lateral masses, anterior arch, and foramen transversarium (large black arrow) of C1 shown in axial projection in another patient. Note the soft tissues of the hypopharynx, including the tonsils (white arrows). (Parts *E, F, G* from Littleton JT: Tomography: Physical Principles and Clinical Applications. © 1976, the Williams & Wilkins Company, Baltimore.)

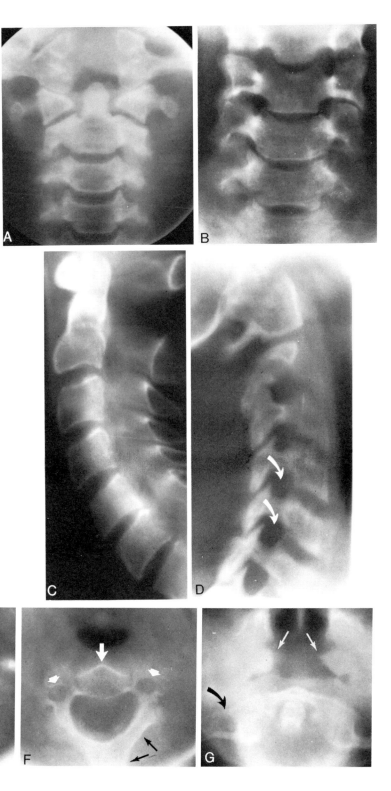

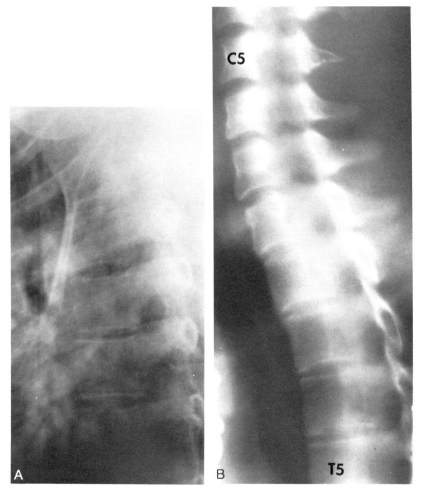

Figure 5–8. Normal cervicothoracic junction; sagittal view. *A*, Cervicothoracic area poorly imaged in routine radiograph. *B*, Midplane tomogram section through bodies and spinous processes of C5, C6, C7, and T1; also lateral portion of bodies and apophyseal joints of T2–T5. Radiographic density has been balanced by the addition of bolus to the lower cervical area.

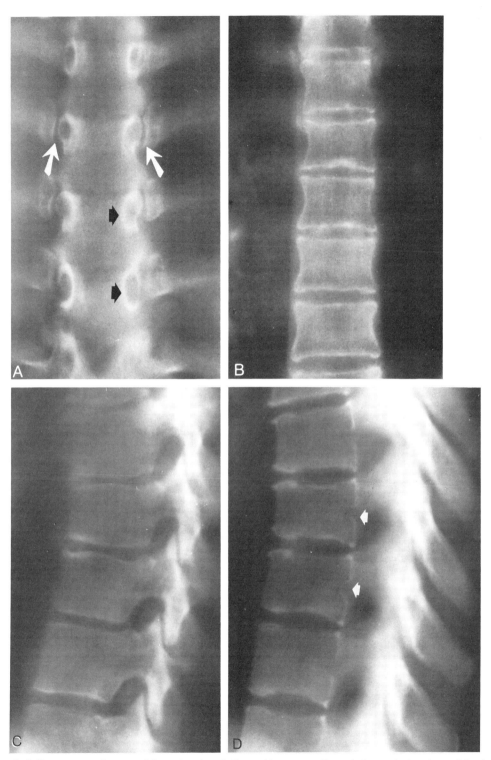

Figure 5–9. Tomograms of a normal thoracic spine. *A,* Coronal tomogram through the posterior plane of the thoracic spine. Pedicles (black arrows) and costovertebral joints (white arrows) are in focus. *B,* More anterior coronal section through the midplane of vertebral bodies. *C,* Parasagittal tomogram visualizing the lateral portion of vertebral bodies, pedicles, and articular facets. *D,* Sagittal section through midplane vertebral bodies and vertebral foramina. Note nutrient foramina in the posterior portion of vertebral bodies (arrows). (Parts *A* and *B* from Littleton JT: Tomography: Physical Principles and Clinical Applications. © 1976, the Williams & Wilkins Company, Baltimore.)

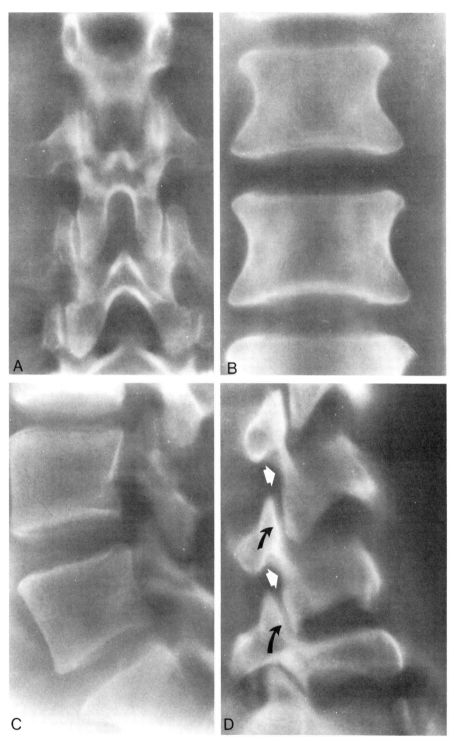

Figure 5–10. Tomograms of a normal lumbar spine. *A,* Coronal tomogram at a level through posterior elements of L2 and L3. *B,* More anterior section through bodies of the same vertebrae. *C,* Sagittal section through L4 and L5. *D,* Tomogram in oblique projection demonstrating pars interarticularis (white arrows) and apophyseal joints (black arrows). (Parts *A, B, D* from Littleton JT: Tomography: Physical Principles and Clinical Applications. © 1976, the Williams & Wilkins Company, Baltimore.)

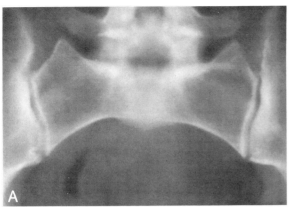
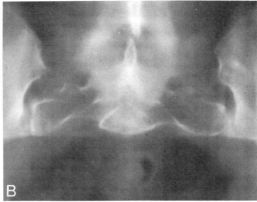

Figure 5–11. Normal sacrum. *A*, Tomogram through the midplane of the body of the sacrum, with crisp detail of the sacroiliac joints. *B*, A more posterior section identifies posterior contours of the sacrum.

section pluridirectional tomograms at various levels of the cervical through lumbosacral spine, are presented for reference.

CONGENITAL ABNORMALITIES

Conventional pluridirectional tomography is ideal for evaluating complex congenital abnormalities, particularly in the craniovertebral region. The modality delineates anatomic structures in the longitudinal plane, and in that respect it is preferable to CT. CPT is superior to the plain film in the evaluation of this area, owing to overlying bony structures encountered on the plain film. It can help differentiate congenital anomalies from fracture when an abnormal-

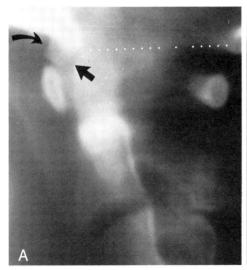
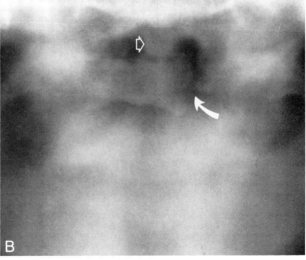

Figure 5–12. Congenital anomalies of the upper cervical spine. *A*, The third condyle. Sagittal tomogram (acute trauma patient) identifies a congenital anomaly of the anterior margin of the foramen magnum, with formation of a third condyle (curved arrow) and a pseudojoint between the tip of the odontoid process and this bony projection (straight arrow). An early pseudobasilar impression is noted, with the tip of the odontoid process at Chamberlain's line (not shown completely) (dotted line). The latter results from spreading of the lateral masses of C1 secondary to other congenital anomalies of the arch of C1. *B*, Suspected fracture of the anterior arch of C1 (curved arrow) proves to be congenital failure of fusion of the anterior arch. Asymmetry of opposing ends of the unfused fragments differentiates congenital anomaly from acute fracture. Third condyle (open arrow) is seen in coronal projection. Though not shown, a congenital defect of the posterior arch of C1 (right) is present. The summation of congenital arch defects simulates the elements of a Jefferson fracture of C1, permitting the spreading of the lateral masses and the pseudoplatybasia.

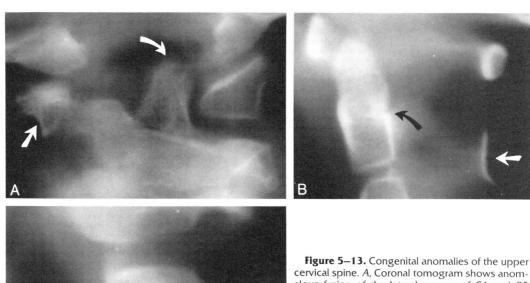

Figure 5–13. Congenital anomalies of the upper cervical spine. *A,* Coronal tomogram shows anomalous fusion of the lateral masses of C1 and C2 (straight arrow). Unfused tip of the odontoid process is incidentally noted (curved arrow). *B,* Sagittal midplane section shows persistent subchondral synchondrosis (black arrow) and fusions of the spinous processes of C2 and C3 (white arrow). *C,* Sagittal tomogram shows congenital fusion of the left laminae of C2 and C3 (arrow).

ity is discovered in a patient being evaluated for trauma.

Cervical Spine

Anomalies and malformations of the cervical spine are most common in the upper cervical region.[8, 9] Numerous variations in segmentation occur in the craniovertebral junction (Fig. 5–12) and upper three cervical segments (Figs. 5–13, 5–14). Because many of the congenital variations may involve one or more vertebral elements and occur in more than one vertebral level, a complete assessment of the anomaly is best appreciated with multiple CPT projections in coronal, sagittal, and, occasionally, oblique projections. Congenital anomalies may result in malalignment of the cervical spine, which may be misinterpreted as occurring secondary to trauma (Fig. 5–15). Anomalies

of the arch of C1 are frequent and also may simulate a fracture on the plain film. CT can delineate neural arch defects, but detail on CT sometimes may not permit a reasonable differentiation between fracture and congenital defect.

The author has encountered a large number of congenital anomalies of the upper cervical segments and feels confident that CPT is the best technique to solve these complex anatomic problems. Anomalies in the lower cervical segments are less common (Fig. 5–16) and may extend across the cervicothoracic junction. Some congenital anomalies may become symptomatic as the result of late sequelae from remodeling and the development of degenerative arthritis (Fig. 5–17). In other cases, such as a hypoplastic or absent odontoid process, it may be difficult on the plain radiograph to determine whether the defect is congenital or acquired.

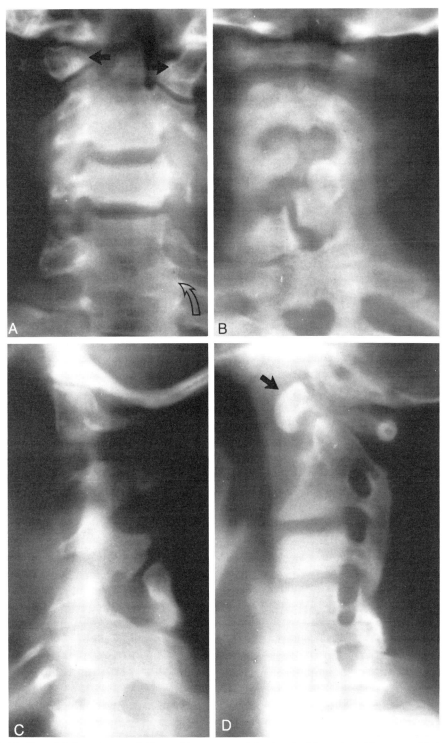

Figure 5–14. Klippel-Feil syndrome. *A*, Coronal tomogram at the level of the odontoid process. Note asymmetric lateral masses of C1 (straight arrows) and partial fusion of C2 and C3. Also note hemivertebrae and fused lower cervical segments (curved arrow). *B*, Posterior coronal section shows defects of the posterior segments of the mid and lower cervical spine. *C*, Sagittal tomogram (right) shows absence and deformity of apophyseal joints. *D*, Sagittal tomogram (left) shows multiple fusions and abnormal apophyseal joints throughout cervical segments. Anterior arch of C1 (arrow) is unusual.

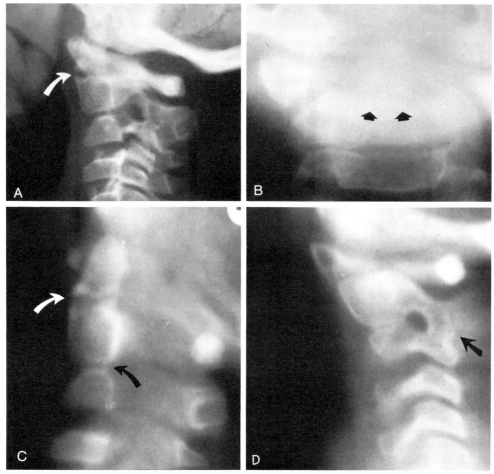

Figure 5–15 *See legend on opposite page*

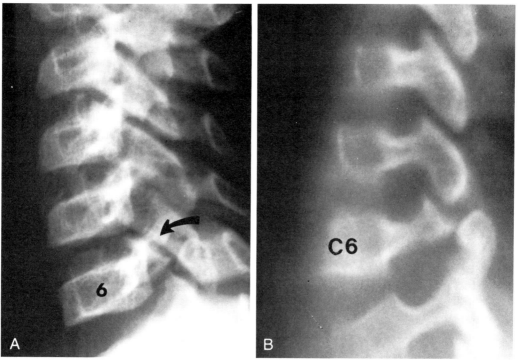

Figure 5–16 *See legend on opposite page*

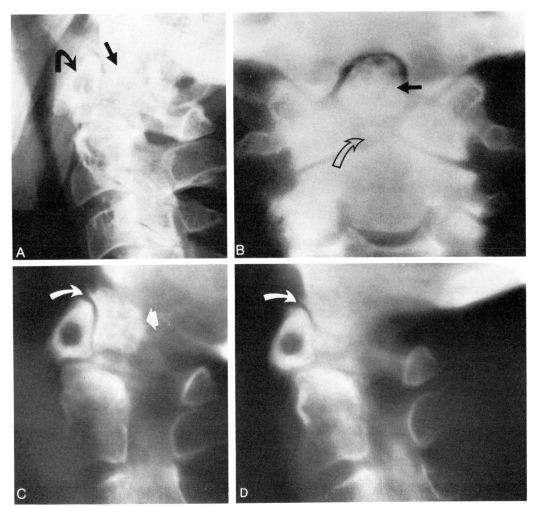

Figure 5–17. Os odontoideum. *A*, Lateral plain film shows apparent os odontoideum (straight arrow) and hypertrophy of the anterior arch of C1 (curved arrow). *B*, Coronal tomogram shows the large os odontoideum (straight arrow) in the anterior arch of the foramen magnum. A small fragment at the expected position of the base of the odontoid process is also visualized (curved arrow). *C*, Section near the midsagittal plane shows hypertrophied os odontoideum (straight arrow) with unusual pseudoarticulation (curved arrow) with a hypertrophied anterior arch of C1 and relative anterior displacement and hypertrophy of the body of C2. Anteroposterior diameter of the spinal canal has narrowed to 15.5 mm at the level of C2. *D*, Midsagittal tomogram shows an anomalous articulation of the hypertrophied anterior arch of C1 with the occipital condyle (arrow). Additional flexion and extension views, not shown, exhibit excessive mobility at the atlanto-occipital and atlantoaxial joints. A complex problem such as this is difficult to assess adequately with computed tomography.

Figure 5–15. Synchondrosis mimicking a fracture. Six year old female. *A*, Lateral plain film suggests fracture at the base of the odontoid process (arrow). There is also abnormal angulation between C3 and C4. *B*, Coronal tomogram shows unfused subdental synchondrosis (arrows). *C*, Midplane sagittal tomogram shows ancient unfused subdental synchondrosis at C2 (white arrow) and narrowed intervertebral space between C2 and C3 (black arrow). *D*, Sagittal tomogram, left, shows fusion of the lateral elements of C2 and C3 (arrow). Suspected fracture proves to be congenital anomalies.

Figure 5–16. Hypoplastic articular process, C6. *A*, Lateral plain film demonstrates possible fracture of the pars interarticularis of C6 (arrow). *B*, Lateral tomogram shows a congenital anomaly of C6 on the left, consisting of a hypoplastic pedicle that forms an unusual articulation with the inferior facet of C5. The superior articular process of C7 is also abnormally developed.

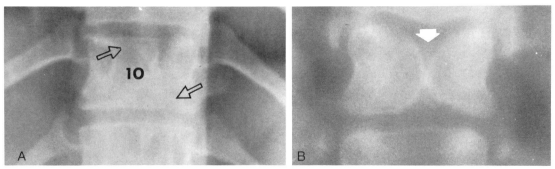

Figure 5–18. Butterfly vertebra. *A,* Anteroposterior plain film of the lower thoracic spine suggests fractures of the superior and inferior articular plates of T10 (arrows). *B,* Anteroposterior tomogram demonstrates typical vertical cleft of a butterfly vertebra (arrow). (From Littleton JT: Tomography: Physical Principles and Clinical Applications. © 1976, the Williams & Wilkins Company, Baltimore.)

Thoracic Spine

Congenital anomalies of the thoracic spine are less common and may occasionally be confused with a traumatic event. The plain film may suggest a vertebral body fracture, and CPT can clarify this diagnostic dilemma (Fig. 5–18). Butterfly vertebra, hemivertebra, and complex anomalous developments can be defined with CPT.

Lumbosacral Spine

A narrow spina bifida, common in the lower lumbar and upper sacral segments, is not usually of any clinical significance but may be encountered on a lumbosacral tomogram. Wide spina bifida with splaying of the laminae may be a manifestation of spinal dysraphism and may be associated with other congenital anomalies. CPT can define bony abnormalities and may give a clue to the location of other dysraphic conditions. Ossified bony midline spur can give the location of underlying diastematomyelia. These skeletal anomalies are better defined with CPT than with conventional radiography. CT, on the other hand, is more sensitive than CPT in the detection of a bony spur in diastematomyelia and the evaluation of in-

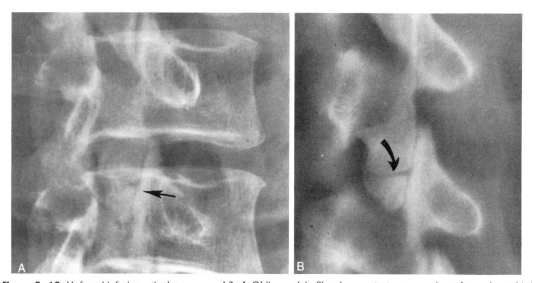

Figure 5–19. Unfused inferior articular process, L3. *A,* Oblique plain film demonstrates narrowing of apophyseal joint space without other definite finding (arrow). *B,* Oblique tomogram reveals unfused tip of the inferior facet of L3 (arrow), with resulting degenerative arthritis of this apophyseal joint. (From Littleton JT: Tomography: Physical Principles and Clinical Applications. © 1976, the Williams & Wilkins Company, Baltimore.)

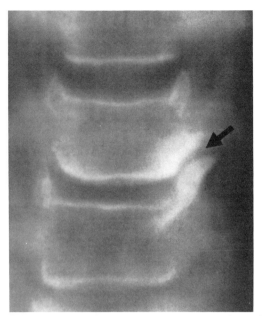

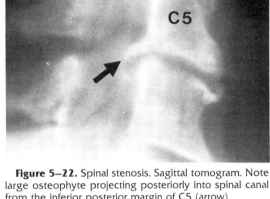

Figure 5–22. Spinal stenosis. Sagittal tomogram. Note large osteophyte projecting posteriorly into spinal canal from the inferior posterior margin of C5 (arrow).

Figure 5–20. Localized degenerative arthritis. Coronal tomogram shows localized degnerative changes, left, between C5 and C6 (arrow).

traspinal soft-tissue structures. CPT is better than reformatted CT, however, in the longitudinal evaluation of dysraphic changes in the bony spine.

Multiple ossification centers that have failed to fuse may be associated with clinical symptoms (Fig. 5–19). These defects are

most usually asymptomatic but must be differentiated from fracture in the traumatized patient.

DEGENERATIVE DISORDERS

Conventional pluridirectional tomography adequately demonstrates the osseous abnormalities of degenerative disorders of the spine. Alterations in the uncovertebral joints and osteophytes encroaching on the neural foramen and spinal canal can be identified (Figs. 5–20 to 5–22). Central spinal stenosis

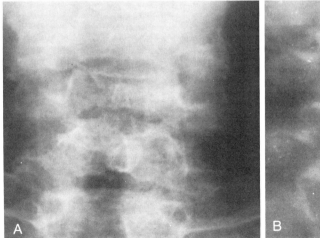

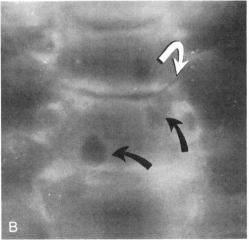

Figure 5–21. Osteoarthritis with fracture. *A,* Anteroposterior plain film of the lower cervical spine. Note the marginal changes caused by osteoarthritis. *B,* Anteroposterior tomogram demonstrates typical degenerative changes with cystic areas of absorption (black arrows) that should not be mistaken for metastases. Small chip fracture is seen at superolateral margin of C7 (white arrow). (From Littleton JT: Current Problems in Radiology. Chicago: Year Book Medical Publishers, 1974.)

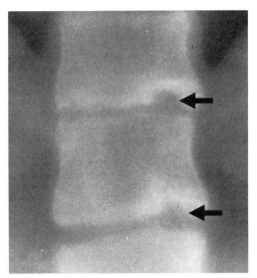

Figure 5–23. Schmorl's nodes. Tomogram showing typical Schmorl's nodes with marginal sclerosis in the lower thoracic spine (arrows). These should not be mistaken for metastases. (From Littleton JT: Tomography: Physical Principles and Clinical Applications. © 1976, the Williams & Wilkins Company, Baltimore.)

can be precisely diagnosed using CPT in the sagittal plane. The longitudinal extent of spinal stenosis can be evaluated more accurately than on the reformatted sagittal CT image. Schmorl's nodes, representing protrusion of disc material into the vertebral body, should not be mistaken for infection or trauma (Fig. 5–23). Soft-tissue structures such as the intervertebral disc and spinal ligaments are not demonstrated by CPT unless calcified (Fig. 5–24).

ARTHRITIDES

CPT is helpful in assessing the spectrum of changes of rheumatoid arthritis, which may be as minimal as ligamentous laxity or as advanced as spinal fusion. Subluxation of the C1–C2 relationship due to disruption of the transverse ligament can be accurately measured on the sagittal tomogram (Fig. 5–25). Erosions and resorption of the odontoid process as well as inflammatory changes of the atlanto-occipital and atlantoaxial articulations may be delineated much better with CPT than with conventional radiography (Fig. 5–26). Cranial settling, with the odontoid process protruding cephalad into the foramen magnum, is another complication of long-standing advanced rheumatoid arthritis (Fig. 5–27). In the lower cervical spine, narrowing of the intervertebral disc or apophyseal joint may be identified (Fig. 5–28). When the inflammatory process is more diffuse, longitudinal assessment is helpful. The degree of spinal motion can also be evaluated in advanced disease.

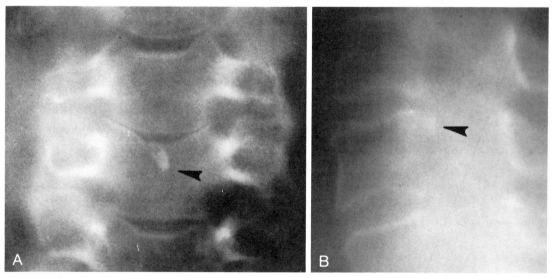

Figure 5–24. Calcification of the posterior longitudinal ligament. Coronal (A) and sagittal (B) tomograms of the cervical spine demonstrate focal calcification of the posterior ligament (arrowheads). Calcification of the ligament was difficult to appreciate on the routine radiographs.

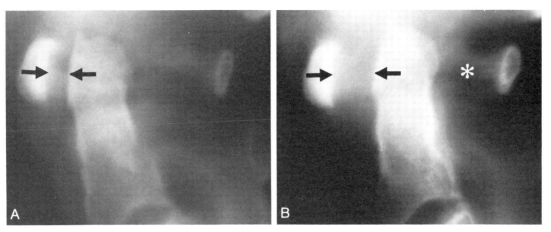

Figure 5–25. Laxity of the transverse ligament (C2) caused by rheumatoid arthritis. *A*, Sagittal midplane tomogram made during flexion. Note widening of the joint space between the anterior arch of C1 and the dens (arrows). *B*, The increase in subluxation of C1–C2 (arrows) indicates marked laxity of the transverse ligament. Anterior space measures 9.5 mm (corrected). Notice the concomitant narrowing of the spinal canal (asterisk).

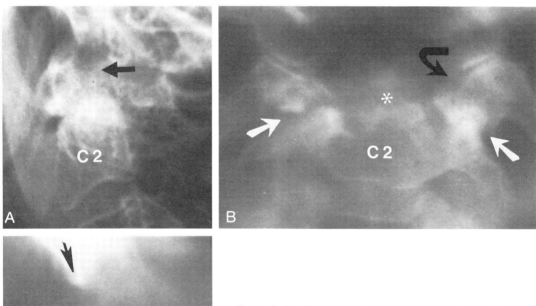

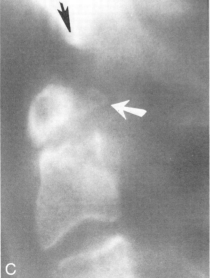

Figure 5–26. Rheumatoid arthritis. Resorption of the odontoid process. *A*, Sagittal plain film of the cervical spine shows poor detail of the odontoid process (arrow). *B*, Coronal tomogram shows extensive erosion and resorption of the odontoid process (asterisk) and erosions and joint destruction of the C1–C2 articulations (straight arrows). Small erosions are present in the left atlanto-occipital joint (curved arrow). *C*, Sagittal midplane tomogram shows almost complete resorption of the odontoid process, with a small fragment (white arrow) remaining posterior to the anterior arch of C1. Note that the tip of the clivus (black arrow) points to the posterior margin of C2, indicating marked anterior subluxation of C2. In addition, there is mild subluxation of C3 on C4 and C4 on C5 (not shown).

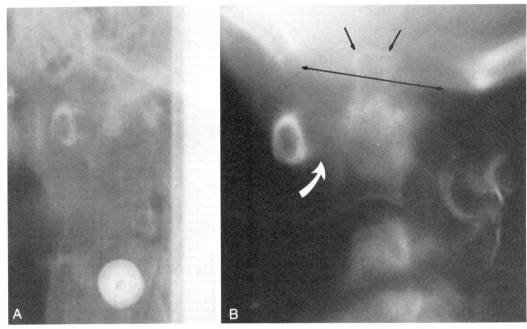

Figure 5–27. Advanced rheumatoid arthritis. *A,* Lateral plain film of the cervical spine of a patient with advanced rheumatoid arthritis. The odontoid is difficult to visualize due to extensive osteopenia. Patient is unable to support her head, requiring continuous use of a cervical collar. *B,* Sagittal midplane tomogram. There is cranial settling, with the upward displacement of the odontoid process (small arrows) above the plane of Chamberlain's line (not shown completely) (long arrow) into the foramen magnum (pseudoplatybasia). Widening of the joint space between the anterior arch of C1 and the body of C2 indicates subluxation (white arrow).

Erosions and subchondral cysts of the sacroiliac joints are more accurately delineated with CPT than with conventional radiography.

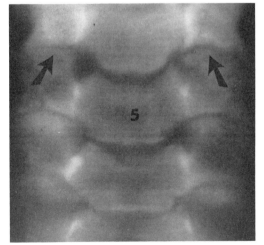

Figure 5–28. Rheumatoid arthritis. Coronal tomogram of the cervical spine demonstrates erosions of the apophyseal joints (arrows) from rheumatoid arthritis. The plain radiograph was unremarkable.

TUMOR

Tumors and tumorlike conditions may be evaluated with conventional pluridirectional tomography, for it is usually superior to the plain radiograph in detecting cortical destruction. Patients who have a positive radionuclide scan and a normal-appearing plain film and who are suspected clinically of having bony metastasis or myeloma may be further studied with CPT, which may detect destruction of cortex or define an osteolytic or osteoblastic lesion within cancellous bone (Figs. 5–29 to 5–31). Conventional longitudinal tomography examines multiple vertebrae simultaneously—a process that is time consuming when CT is utilized. In patients with lesions of the posterior elements (osteoid osteoma, osteoblastoma, aneurysmal bone cyst), CPT detects the presence and extent of destruction in osseous structures but cannot determine the extent of intraspinal or paraspinal involvement. It may delineate the nidus of osteoid osteoma but not as accurately as CT.

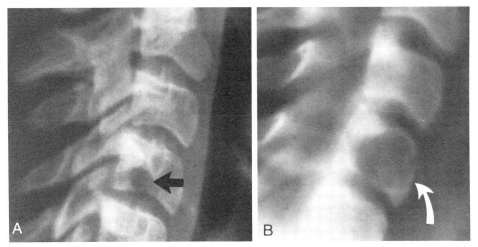

Figure 5–29. Eosinophilic granuloma, C4. *A*, Lateral plain film showing questionable loss of density of C4 (arrow). *B*, Lateral tomogram clearly demonstrates a lytic lesion involving a major portion of the body of C4 (arrow). Biopsy disclosed eosinophilic granuloma. (From Littleton JT: Tomography: Physical Principles and Clinical Applications. © 1976, the Williams & Wilkins Company, Baltimore.)

Medial erosion of pedicles from intraspinal masses can also be demonstrated.

Metastasis and other lesions of the sacrum may go undetected on the plain film because of the curved nature of this bone and the presence of overlying bowel gas. CPT is better than the plain film in demonstrating bony lesions of the sacrum.

INFECTION

CPT demonstrates cortical destruction of vertebral end-plates and disc narrowing in patients with osteomyelitis (Fig. 5–32). Osteolytic bone destruction may be present alone or may be associated with reactive sclerosis (Fig. 5–33). Osteomyelitis and disc involvement may progress to complete fusion. This modality is also helpful in evaluating the postoperative patient for suspected infection and for follow-up of patients with osteomyelitis.

TRAUMA

Conventional pluridirectional tomography may play an important role in the evaluation

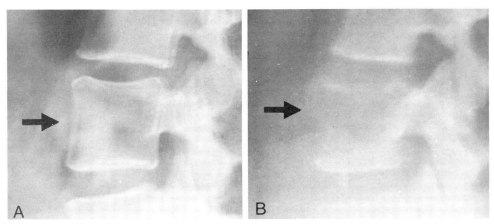

Figure 5–30. Metastasis. *A*, Plain film in lateral projection does not reveal any bone destruction (arrow). *B*, Extensive destruction from metastatic carcinoma of the cervix is visualized in sagittal tomogram (arrow). (From Littleton JT: Current Problems in Radiology. Chicago: Year Book Medical Publishers, 1974.)

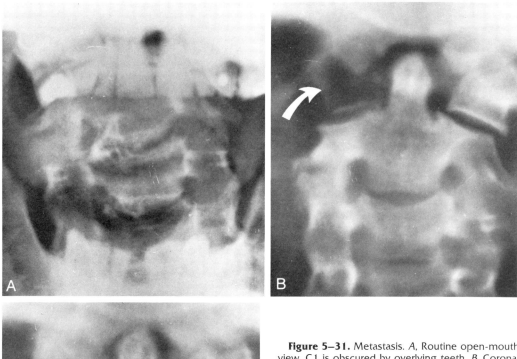

Figure 5–31. Metastasis. *A*, Routine open-mouth view. C1 is obscured by overlying teeth. *B*, Coronal tomogram demonstrates extensive destruction of the right lateral mass of C1 (arrow). *C*, Excellent therapeutic response with ossification followed chemotherapy (arrow). (From Littleton JT: Tomography: Physical Principles and Clinical Applications. © 1976, the Williams & Wilkins Company, Baltimore.)

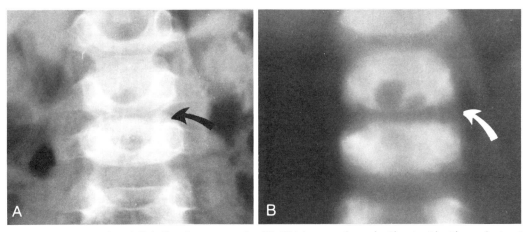

Figure 5–32. Osteomyelitis. *A*, Plain film shows narrowing L2–L3 interspace (arrow) without evident bone destruction. *B*, Tomogram reveals bone destruction from osteomyelitis (arrow). (From Littleton JT: Current Problems in Radiology. Chicago: Year Book Medical Publishers, 1975.)

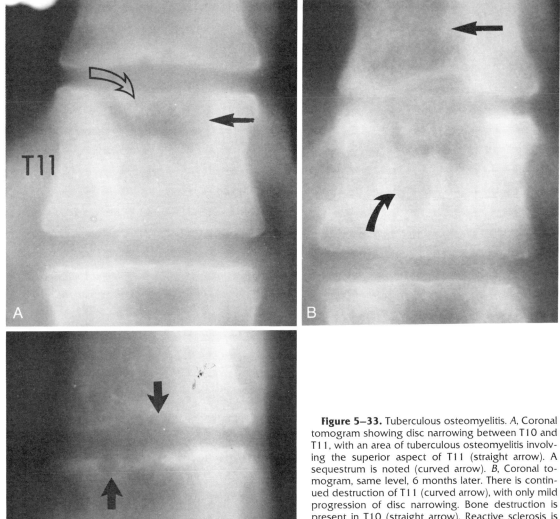

Figure 5–33. Tuberculous osteomyelitis. *A*, Coronal tomogram showing disc narrowing between T10 and T11, with an area of tuberculous osteomyelitis involving the superior aspect of T11 (straight arrow). A sequestrum is noted (curved arrow). *B*, Coronal tomogram, same level, 6 months later. There is continued destruction of T11 (curved arrow), with only mild progression of disc narrowing. Bone destruction is present in T10 (straight arrow). Reactive sclerosis is present. *C*, Coronal tomogram, same level, 12 months later. There is now complete resolution of the tuberculous osteomyelitis, with residual disc narrowing and irregularity of the end plates (arrows).

of patients with spinal trauma and in some settings may be the only sectional imaging modality available. Although CT may be the preferred sectional imaging modality in some patients with spinal trauma, CPT may be more effective in others. For example, CPT can better delineate a fracture of the odontoid process, since the plane of the fracture is usually in the same plane as the CT slice, on which it may go undiagnosed. In addition, CPT may be preferred to CT if a fracture is suspected but the clinical and conventional radiographic examinations fail to localize the fracture. In this clinical setting, one is able to evaluate multiple vertebral levels of the spine easily with CPT.

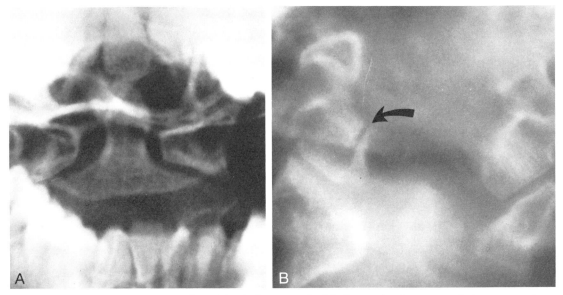

Figure 5–34. Fracture of the occipital condyle. *A,* Open-mouth plain film study of upper cervical segments shows no evidence of recent fracture. *B,* Fracture of the right occipital condyle (arrow) is clearly seen in this coronal tomogram.

CPT has distinct advantages over conventional radiography, for it can readily demonstrate fractures not visible on the plain radiograph. Approximately 50% of fractures of the cervical spine may not be identified on the conventional radiograph.[2] CPT aids in diagnosing fractures of the upper cervical spine and of the posterior elements. Fractures of the upper cervical spine segments may cause very few acute clinical symptoms.

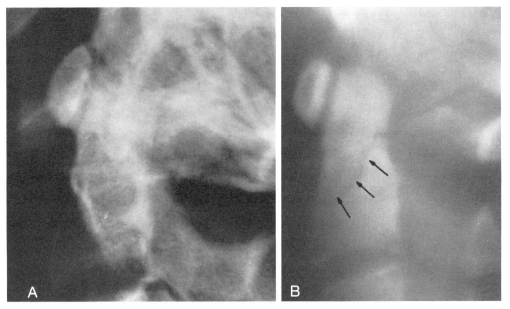

Figure 5–35. Fracture of the base of the odontoid process. *A,* Lateral plain film appears normal and has no evidence of fracture. Plain film in anteroposterior projection and coronal tomogram (not shown) also appeared normal. *B,* Only on sagittal tomogram is the oblique fracture through the base of the odontoid process readily visible (arrows).

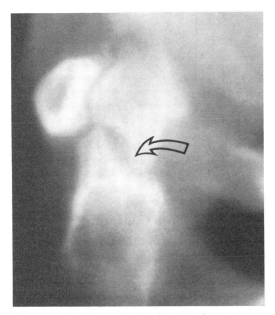

Figure 5–36. Nonunion of a fracture of the odontoid process. Sagittal midplane tomogram shows nonunion of a fracture of the odontoid process (arrow). The margins of the fracture are sclerotic. There is remodeling of the articular surface of the anterior arch of C1. Flexion and extension views 6 months later demonstrated no change. There was no motion of fragments, indicating a stable fibrous union.

CPT can also define congenital abnormalities that may be suspected to be fracture on the conventional radiograph.

There are several criteria for the utilization of CPT in patients with spinal trauma when CT is unavailable; they are as follows:

1. Suspicious radiographic findings, including indirect signs of underlying fracture (subluxation, malalignment, soft-tissue swelling, etc.).

2. Areas not well visualized following repeated attempts with conventional radiography (i.e., C7 region).

3. Known fracture. CPT is performed to evaluate the extent of the fracture diagnosed on the conventional radiograph as well as to detect the presence of additional fractures.

4. High index of suspicion for fracture with neurologic signs and symptoms of spinal cord or nerve root injury in spite of a normal conventional radiographic examination.

Tomography is performed with sections taken at 5 mm intervals in both AP and if possible lateral projections. Thin sections of 2 mm are also obtained when one is examining the region of interest and when additional, finer detail is desired.[4] Sometimes patients are too severely injured to allow examination in the lateral projection.

In the craniovertebral region, CPT can be used to detect fractures of the occipital condyles not visible on the plain film (Fig. 5–34), differentiate fractures from normal variants such as the synchondrosis of C2 in children, delineate fractures of the odontoid process (Fig. 5–35), and assess fracture healing and nonunion (Fig. 5–36). Mach bands occasionally may escape diagnosis on conventional radiography, and fracture can be ruled out in such cases with CPT (Fig. 5–37).

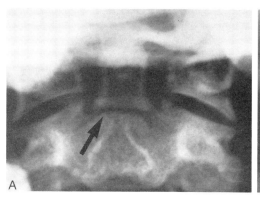
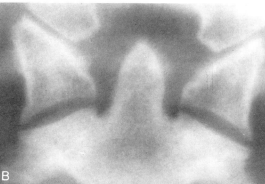

Figure 5–37. Mach band at the base of the odontoid process. *A*, Anteroposterior plain film study of upper cervical segments suggests fracture of base of odontoid process (arrow). *B*, Coronal tomograms show no evidence of fracture. Lateral tomogram (not shown) also produced negative findings. The questionable fracture in the plain film study proved to be a Mach band.

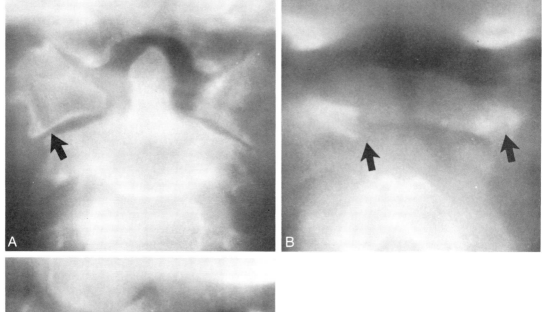

Figure 5–38. Complex fracture, C1. *A*, Coronal tomogram shows fracture of the lateral mass of C1 (arrow). *B*, Coronal tomogram through the level of posterior elements shows bilateral fracture of the posterior arch of C1 (arrows). *C*, The fracture of the lateral mass involves the inferior articular surface of C1 (black arrow), and fractures of the posterior arch are evident (white arrows).

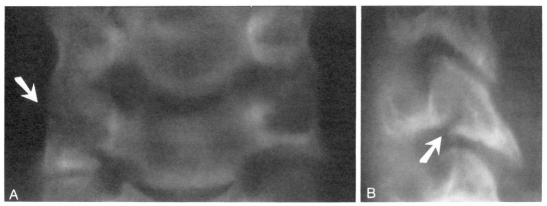

Figure 5–39. Fracture of facet, C5. Coronal (*A*) and oblique (*B*) tomograms show fracture of the lateral mass of C5 (arrows). Fracture shows to better advantage in the oblique projection.

If CT is unavailable, complex fractures of the ring of C1 can be imaged satisfactorily with conventional tomography (Fig. 5–38). Subluxation, particularly at C1–C2, is well demonstrated by tomography. In the lower cervical segments, CPT adequately demonstrates fractures and fracture fragment displacement into the spinal canal, as well as malalignment. Fractures of cervical articular facets may be difficult to visualize in the coronal plane; however, they are well demonstrated in the sagittal and, if necessary, oblique projections (Fig. 5–39).

CPT is superior to conventional radiography in the evaluation of fractures of the thoracic and lumbosacral segments of the spine, particularly those of the posterior elements. Fractures may be stable (Fig. 5–40) or unstable (Figs. 5–41, 5–42). A locked facet can be detected as well (Fig. 5–43). In the lumbar spine, fractures of the pars interarticularis are often diagnosed on the plain radiograph. However, when the conventional radiograph is normal and clinical suspicion is high or the radionuclide scan is positive, CPT can be used to demonstrate the pars fracture (Fig. 5–44) and can show any degree of slippage of one vertebra on another. Congenital defects in the pars interarticularis and limbus vertebra should not be mistaken for fractures. Fractures of the sacrum and disruption of the sacroiliac joints can also be detected on CPT (Fig. 5–45).

Fractures associated with gunshot wounds may be difficult to assess with CT when major bullet fragments remain within the spine, because metal fragments cause artifact defects on the CT image. Metal fragments do not adversely affect the CPT image, which

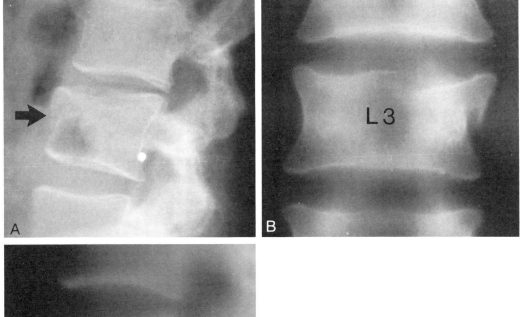

Figure 5–40. Stable fracture, L3. *A*, Plain film (lateral view) shows a simple anterior compression fracture of L3 (arrow). Coronal (*B*) and sagittal (*C*) tomograms confirm acute compression fracture of the left lateral superior surface of L3, with mild depression of the fragment. Posterior elements were intact, confirming the impression of a stable fracture.

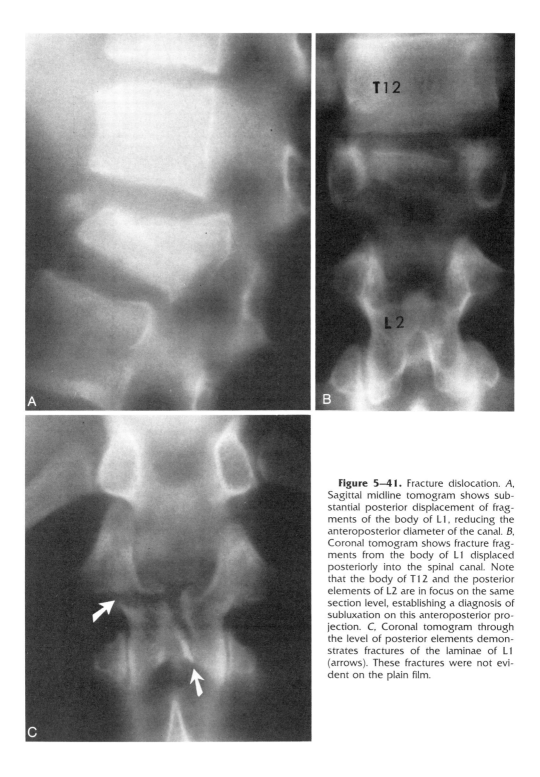

Figure 5–41. Fracture dislocation. *A,* Sagittal midline tomogram shows substantial posterior displacement of fragments of the body of L1, reducing the anteroposterior diameter of the canal. *B,* Coronal tomogram shows fracture fragments from the body of L1 displaced posteriorly into the spinal canal. Note that the body of T12 and the posterior elements of L2 are in focus on the same section level, establishing a diagnosis of subluxation on this anteroposterior projection. *C,* Coronal tomogram through the level of posterior elements demonstrates fractures of the laminae of L1 (arrows). These fractures were not evident on the plain film.

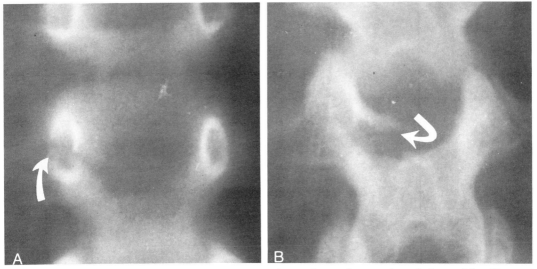

Figure 5–42. Chance fracture, L1. *A,* Coronal tomogram shows obvious fracture through the pedicle of L1 on the right (arrow). *B,* A more posterior section shows the fracture extending into the base of the lamina of L1 (arrow).

can show the location of the fracture and the level of the bullet. Although the blurred bullet fragment may be disturbing to the viewer at some levels, it will appear sharply in focus in the appropriate section (Fig. 5–46).

POSTOPERATIVE SPINE

Conventional pluridirectional tomography aids in the postoperative evaluation of spinal fusion (Figs. 5–47, 5–48). Stability of fusion can be further assessed with lateral tomog-

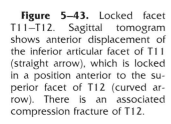

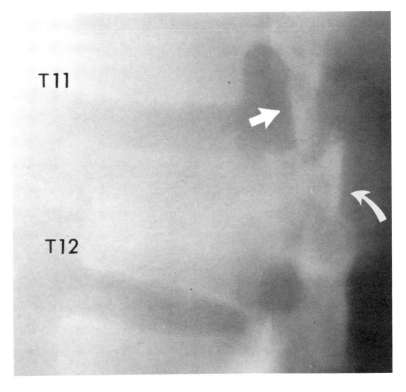

Figure 5–43. Locked facet T11–T12. Sagittal tomogram shows anterior displacement of the inferior articular facet of T11 (straight arrow), which is locked in a position anterior to the superior facet of T12 (curved arrow). There is an associated compression fracture of T12.

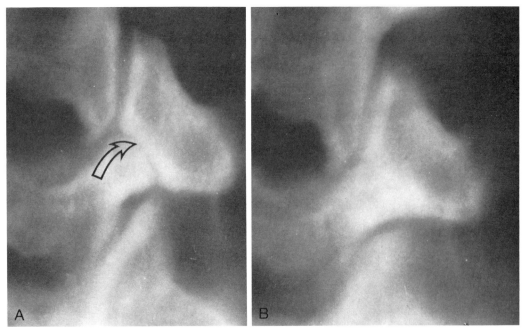

Figure 5–44. Fracture of the pars interarticularis; 15 year old female who sustained a lumbar spine injury. Results of the initial plain film study were interpreted as normal. Persistence of symptoms prompted a tomographic study. A, Oblique tomogram, right, shows a healing fracture of the pars interarticularis of L4 (arrow). The margins are sclerotic. B, A 6 month follow-up tomogram shows solid bony union. An identical fracture with complete fusion was also present on the opposite side.

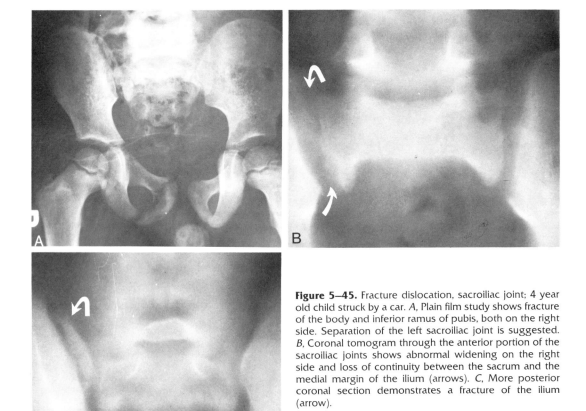

Figure 5–45. Fracture dislocation, sacroiliac joint; 4 year old child struck by a car. A, Plain film study shows fracture of the body and inferior ramus of pubis, both on the right side. Separation of the left sacroiliac joint is suggested. B, Coronal tomogram through the anterior portion of the sacroiliac joints shows abnormal widening on the right side and loss of continuity between the sacrum and the medial margin of the ilium (arrows). C, More posterior coronal section demonstrates a fracture of the ilium (arrow).

322

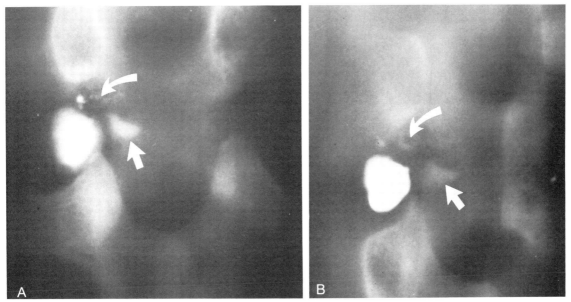

Figure 5–46. Gunshot fracture, lumbar spine. Coronal (*A*) and sagittal (*B*) tomograms show a large bullet fragment in the intervertebral foramen between L1 and L2. A bone fragment is clearly seen projecting posteromedially into the spinal canal (straight arrows), and several other tiny fractures are present (curved arrows).

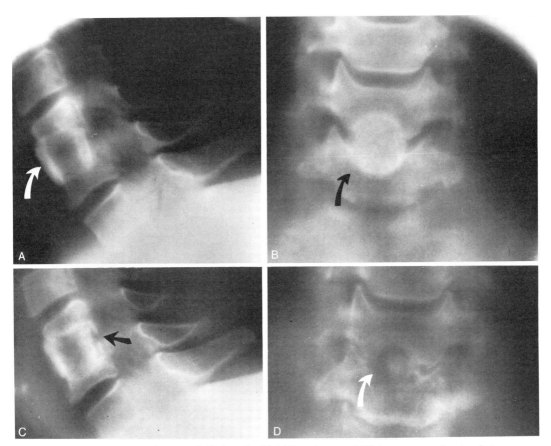

Figure 5–47. Heterogeneous bone graft Fusion. Sagittal (*A*) and coronal (*B*) tomograms showing heterogeneous bone graft in good position (arrows). *C*, Lateral tomogram taken 3 months later shows resorption of the posterior margin of the plug graft (arrow). *D*, Anteroposterior tomogram shows partial resorption of the graft (arrow). (Modified from Littleton JT: Tomography: Physical Principles and Clinical Applications. © 1976, the Williams & Wilkins Company, Baltimore.)

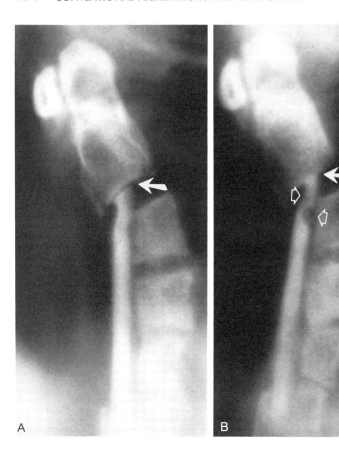

Figure 5–48. Spinal fusion, cervical spine. Late rheumatoid arthritis with fusion of the cervical spines *A,* Sagittal tomogram shows position of graft. Note gap between graft and C2 (arrow). *B,* Taken 3 months after fusion, lateral tomogram shows strut fused to the inferior margin of C2 (closed arrow); focal resorption (open arrow) is apparent.

raphy obtained during extremes of flexion and extension.

ACKNOWLEDGMENTS

The author is indebted to William Callahan, Ph.D., for his generous assistance in labeling the anatomic sections and for his helpful advice in the preparation of the anatomic sections.

M. L. Durizch, R.T., M.B.A., should more properly be listed as coauthor of this chapter. In her capacity as Research Associate she has participated actively in all phases of this project. The quality of the clinical tomograms laud her technical expertise.

A special thanks to Mrs. Pat DeWitt for typing the manuscript.

References

1. Andersen PE: Relative effectiveness of computed and conventional tomography in lesions of the spine. In Littleton JT, Durizch ML (eds): Sectional Imaging Methods: A Comparison. Baltimore: University Park Press, 1983, pp 235–243.
2. Anderson LD, Smith BL, DeTorre J, et al: The role of polytomography in the diagnosis and treatment of cervical spine injuries. In Urist MR (ed): Clin Orthop 165:64–67, 1982.
3. Bokstrom I: Principles of vertebral tomography. Acta Radiol [Suppl 103], 1953.
4. Durizch ML: Technical Aspects of Tomography. Baltimore: Williams & Wilkins Company, 1978, pp 195–209.
5. Littleton JT: The Spine. In Littleton JT (ed): Tomography: Physical Principles and Clinical Applications. Baltimore: Williams & Wilkins Company, 1976, pp 324–429.
6. Littleton JT, Shaffer KA, Callahan WP, et al: Temporal bone: Comparison of pluridirectional tomography and high resolution computed tomography. AJR 137:835–845, 1981.
7. Littleton JT, Vannier MW: The linear "tomogram." In Littleton JT, Durizch ML (eds): Sectional Imaging Methods: A comparison. Baltimore: University Park Press, 1983, pp 3–16.
8. Torklus D, Gehle W: The Upper Cervical Spine: Regional Anatomy, Pathology and Traumatology. New York: Grune & Stratton, 1972.
9. Wackenheim A: Roentgen Diagnosis of the Craniovertebral Region. New York: Springer-Verlag, 1974.

Norman E. Leeds, M.D.
Charles M. Elkin, M.D.
Eduardo Leon, M.D.
Stephen Kieffer, M.D.
Steven Schonfeld, M.D.

6

Myelography

The examination of the spinal cord and its contents may be performed to advantage by the introduction of an opaque contrast medium into the spinal subarachnoid space to outline and therefore identify the spinal cord and the nerve roots. Abnormalities affecting the dura mater or arachnoid mater may then also be appreciated. A complementary examination that can be performed at the same time, if water-soluble contrast is utilized, is computed tomographic myelography (CTM). In the past, myelography was performed with oily contrast, iophendyhlate (Pantopaque) and, occasionally, air.

Oil-based contrast medium was first introduced in 1921.[79] Iophendylate (Pantopaque, 1944)[63] was used until a nonionic water-soluble contrast agent (metrizamide) was introduced in 1975. Air myelography was first utilized in 1921.[34] Air myelography had been used in selective cases until the introduction of the nonionic iodide contrast material. Air myelography, like oil-based contrast myelography, has almost disappeared as a contrast modality since the introduction of nonionic contrast material. Today, in our department, only water-soluble contrast myelography is performed.

The examination of the spinal canal contents with water-soluble contrast material has enlarged the value of the examination by making it possible to visualize the nerve roots in detail, thus extending the diagnostic capability of the examiner.

The purpose of this chapter is to demonstrate the use of myelography in the investigation of lesions affecting the spinal canal, including bony margins and contents. The advantages and disadvantages of water-soluble contrast media will be emphasized. The complementary value of computed tomographic myelography (CTM) will be discussed.

CONTRAST AGENTS

Ideal Agent

The suggested requirements of the ideal contrast agent for myelography are as follows:[12]

1. The agent should be nontoxic and nonirritating to spinal cord, nerves, and meninges—no scarring or neurotoxicity.
2. The agent should be absorbable.
3. Side effects should be minimal.
4. Its use should result in satisfactory studies.

Nonionic Water-Soluble Agents

Nonionic water-soluble contrast material best satisfies the preceding requirements for the ideal agent. This type of agent is preferred today because it is easy to use, does not need to be removed, and defines anatomy. Table 6–1 lists the advantages and disadvantages of nonionic water-soluble agents.

Metrizamide (Amipaque) is, at present, the agent most often in use. Recently, however, a group of new nonionic water-soluble agents has been developed. These agents seem to have all of the advantages of metrizamide, with fewer and less intense adverse effects. The new agents are iohexol,[25a] iopamidol,[17a, 17b] iopromide,[48a] ioglucomide,[33a]

325

Table 6–1. ADVANTAGES AND DISADVANTAGES OF NONIONIC
WATER-SOLUBLE CONTRAST MATERIAL FOR MYELOGRAPHY

Advantages		Disadvantages	
	Lower viscosity permits excellent filling of the nerve root		Contrast material may become diluted if bolus is not maintained in prolonged examination
	Decreased density allows better visualization of spinal contents, including cord and roots.		Often only two of three regions (cervical, dorsal, and lumbar) can be examined
	The contrast material need not be removed		May cause seizures
	The needle used is 22 gauge and may be removed after introduction of the contrast medium, reducing the opportunity of CSF leakage		Intracranial complications, including psychologic effects, stroke, and blindness, may result from cerebral penetration of contrast material
	Computed tomography may be used to provide new or additional information and to substantiate findings		Causes headaches, nausea, and vomiting
	Rarely causes arachnoiditis		Should not be used in patients with seizures or on phenothiazine medications
	Patient may sit up after examination and have bathroom privileges		
	It may be used even if spinal tap is bloody		

and iotrol.[35a] Iohexol and iopamidol have recently been approved for clinical use by the FDA, after extensive study. Because of their newness, it seems useful to summarize comparisons of these two agents with metrizamide.

Metrizamide is only mildly hyperosmolar at concentrations utilized in myelography and has a lower osmolality than iohexol or iopamidol.[17a, 25a] The osmolality of iohexol is greater than that of iopamidol at equivalent concentrations of iodine.

Iohexol and iopamidol, although they do not contain the glucosamine residue and are only mildly hyperosmolar, occasionally cause adverse reactions—a result of the reaction of all contrast media with CSF macromolecules. This interaction changes the extracellular milieu in which the neurons function. Iopamidol and iohexol appear to be safer than metrizamide for lumbar and cervical myelography in terms of total incidence of adverse reactions while yielding roentgenograms of equivalent diagnostic quality.[17a, 17b, 25a]

The reported incidence of adverse reactions following lumbar myelography with iopamidol is 37%, slightly greater than that with iohexol (27%). It has been determined that raising the concentration of contrast material may not result in more adverse effects.[83a] There are variations in iodine (I) utilized: 180 mg I per ml of iohexol and 200 mg I per ml of iopamidol. These concentrations should be considered equivalent because their osmolalities are similar. There-

fore the data suggesting that lumbar myelography with iohexol is safer than that with iopamidol are only preliminary, because precise definition of adverse reactions has not been presented. A prospective, double-blind comparison between the two media is necessary to determine which contrast agent results in fewer adverse effects.

Seizures were not demonstrated in any patient following myelography with iohexol or iopamidol, but changes in mental status were noted. Psychic impairment has been observed following the use of both metrizamide and iohexol in lumbar myelography.[16a] The impairment was more severe with metrizamide, especially with the subjective questionnaire. Psychologic tests demonstrated that iopamidol and iohexol were much less neurotoxic than metrizamide used in both lumbar and cervical myelography.[16a, 25b]

Arachnoiditis, which has not been demonstrated following myelography in clinical trials in humans with metrizamide, appears also to be absent with iopamidol and iohexol during experimental studies.[30a, 30b]

Careful analysis and study of potential adverse effects of iopamidol and iohexol should be made in view of their current widespread use following recent approval by the FDA.

Iophendylate

Iophendylate (Pantopaque) has only limited use because of the availability of non-

Table 6–2. ADVANTAGES AND DISADVANTAGES
OF IOPHENDYLATE (PANTOPAQUE) FOR MYELOGRAPHY

Advantages		Disadvantages	
Advantages	All three spinal regions may be examined	Disadvantages	Lack of filling of nerve roots
	Intracranial complications are uncommon		Too dense
	Contrast not absorbed, so the length of study is not an issue and delayed examination may be performed		Arachnoiditis occurs in at least 25% of cases
			Needs to be removed
			Cannot be used with CT
			Patient must be flat for 8 hours
			18 gauge needle used, increasing possibility of cerebrospinal fluid (CSF) leakage
			Headaches are frequent and of long duration
			Removal, although essential, may be difficult and painful
			Should not be injected if spinal tap is bloody

ionic water-soluble contrast material. The problems with iophendylate are the high incidence of arachnoiditis and the density of the material. It may be used in the evaluation of the cervical region or in patients with suspected spinal block. Table 6–2 lists the advantages and disadvantages of iophendylate.

Air

Air myelography is used rarely, and then only in patients with congenital lesions or allergies to contrast media. Air is a poor contrast agent, and large volumes must be injected and the patient examined with tomography. The duration of the study and maintenance of the position are difficult for many patients, particularly older ones. Table 6–3 lists the advantages and disadvantages of air as a contrast agent for myelography.

INDICATIONS FOR MYELOGRAPHY

Myelography using nonionic water-soluble agents is useful for the investigations of spinal canal lesions and is most effective to examine the patient with narrow canal syndrome and to differentiate between bulging discs and extruded discs by demonstrating alterations in the thecal sac and nerve roots. This modality is of value in studying abnormalities of the cauda equina and arachnoiditis, because nerve roots are seen to advantage. In the cervical region, degenerative disease as well as disc disease may be clearly delineated. The spinal cord subarachnoid space or surrounding dura may be clearly distinguished. Congenital lesions may be visualized, particularly the tethered cord, because the contrast medium used is less dense than iophendylate.

The indications for oil-based contrast agents are similar to those for nonionic ma-

Table 6–3. ADVANTAGES AND DISADVANTAGES OF AIR FOR MYELOGRAPHY

Advantages		Disadvantages	
Advantages	Entire spinal canal and intracranial contents may be examined	Disadvantages	Requires use of tomographic equipment, since air is a poor contrast agent
	Causes no allergic reaction		Nerve roots are not well seen
	Readily available		Large volumes of air may be required, so headaches, nausea, and vomiting may develop
	Does not cause arachnoiditis		The head-down (Trendelenburg) position, which must be maintained for 6 to 8 hours to prevent entry of air into the cranial cavity, is difficult and uncomfortable for older patients
			Hypotension may develop as a result of the volume of air introduced
			Necessitates a lengthy examination

terials, except that nerve root pouches are poorly filled and therefore incompletely evaluated, and the contrast material is more dense radiographically.

Air has been used as a contrast agent, particularly in patients with congenital spinal lesions and in those with a history of allergy to other agents.

THE MYELOGRAPHIC EXAMINATION

Varying volumes and concentrations of water-soluble contrast agent may be used, depending upon the site of the examination. The scope of the examination can be extended by using computed tomography. It is always advantageous to puncture near the site to be examined, that is, C1–C2 puncture for cervical examinations and lumbar puncture for lumbar examinations. Techniques of cervical examination from the lumbar route have been devised by various authors.[24, 36] The object is to maintain the contrast pool in a continuous bolus and thereby reduce dilution. This can be done effectively with reproducibly excellent examinations in almost all cases.

The first advantage of water-soluble contrast material is that, because of its solubility, a smaller needle (22 gauge) may be used instead of the 18 gauge needle required with iophendylate. The needle may also be removed after the introduction of contrast material, since the current water-soluble contrast agents are diluted, absorbed, and finally excreted, therefore not requiring removal. The small-caliber needle and the short time the needle is in place mean that there is less chance of dural leakage after the examination; thus, patients may sit up after the examination, ambulate, and have bathroom privileges, instead of being restricted to bed in a flat position for 8 to 12 hours, as with iophendylate myelography. The upright position after use of a water-soluble agent aids in the dilution of the agent and in reduction of adverse effects.

It is important to review all the data available prior to beginning the myelogram: clinical history, physical findings, plain roentgenograms, the diagnosis suspected, previous myelograms, and CT examination. The examiner should know what information can be obtained from the examination to be performed. An appropriate plan should

be decided upon before the examination is begun, although one should be prepared for any eventuality.

If only a single area is to be examined, cervical or lumbar, a small vial of 3.75 g metrizamide, as opposed to the larger vial of 6.75 g, may suffice.[82] The significant advantage of using the smaller dose is a reduction in side effects (nausea, vomiting, and headache). One may also improve technique, because the smaller dose allows a small focal spot, low kilovoltage, optimized film-screen combination, and tight coning. We usually prefer to use 190 mg per 100 ml for examining the cervical region.

Lumbar Approach

After needle puncture at L3–L4. and collection of cerebrospinal fluid (CSF) for specimens, a small amount of contrast material is introduced under fluoroscopic control to be sure the needle is within the subarachnoid space. The contrast material should occupy the thecal sac so that one may observe nerve roots, the caudal sac, or a fluid level. Any unusual or bizarre configuration, lack of movement, or unusual increased density of contrast material or nonvisualization of spinal cord and nerve roots should alert the examiner to the need for roentgenograms in two projections to confirm the location of the needle. If all is well, one may proceed. If the needle is in the wrong space, change in position or repuncture may be performed if only a small amount of contrast has been used, or C1–C2 puncture may be attempted. One may also discontinue the procedure. Remember, there is always another day!

If iophendylate is used, subdural collections of the agent will lie dorsally. This is not necessarily the case with metrizamide and other water-soluble contrast agents, which surround and outline the thecal sac (Fig. 6–1). Epidural contrast lies ventral and extends along nerve roots (Fig. 6–1). Contrast material outside the thecal sac tends to move sluggishly, although on occasion it may move quickly, similar to contrast material in the subarachnoid space. In extradural injection, the spinal cord will not be visualized (Fig. 6–2). If the contrast is within the thecal sac, continue the injection slowly.

In almost all examinations, at least two of the three regions (cervical, dorsal, and lum-

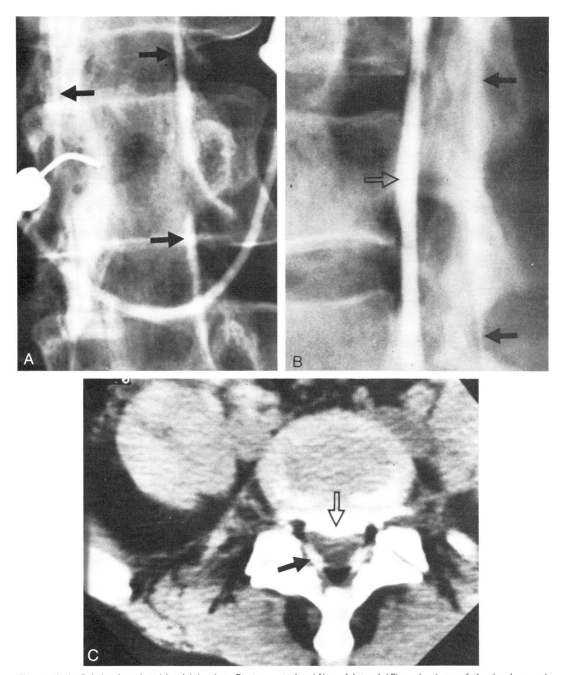

Figure 6–1. Subdural and epidural injection. Posteroanterior (A) and lateral (B) projections of the lumbar region demonstrate metrizamide in the subdural space posteriorly and laterally (closed arrows). Metrizamide noted ventrally is within the epidural space (open arrow), since subarachnoid metrizamide is not really seen on the posteroanterior projection. The lack of definition of nerve roots and the absence of a fluid level establish the diagnosis of an extra-arachnoidal injection. C, An axial CT scan in the lumbar region in this case confirms the extra-arachnoidal injection of metrizamide, with the subdural collection noted laterally (closed arrow) and the epidural contrast noted ventrally (open arrow). Note the absence of circumferential contrast outlining the thecal sac, which excludes the presence of subarachnoid contrast material.

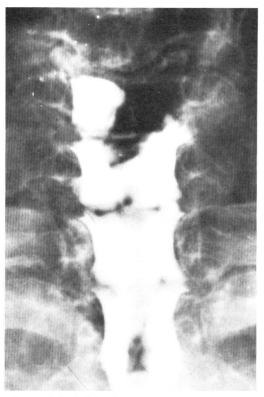

Figure 6–2. Subdural injection. Iophendylate (Pantopaque) is noted in the posteroanterior projection of the cervicothoracic region. The contrast medium has a slightly conglomerate appearance, and the spinal cord and nerve roots are not identified.

bar) are examined; a lumbar examination is not complete without the study of the conus medullaris. Since this is best examined in supine projection,[72] one should also visualize the remainder of the dorsal region. If the metrizamide becomes too diluted, the study may be extended by utilizing multidirectional tomography or CT to evaluate areas inadequately visualized.

The water-soluble material should be injected slowly (over 3 to 5 minutes) to reduce dilution. The patient should not move, and all motion should be passive to reduce mixing of contrast. A plan should be conceived at the outset so that the least motion is utilized to obtain the optimum number of films in the appropriate position; speed is of the essence.

Lumbar Examination

For the lumbar examination, a posteroanterior projection of L3–L4, L4–L5, and L5–S1 is made with the patient semierect at 30 to 60 degrees so that the caudal sac is filled out (Fig. 6–3). A more erect image may be required for distention of the caudal sac.

The patient is then rotated to a 15 to 20 degree oblique angle for visualization of the nerve roots in profile from L3 through the sacrum, and comparative paired right and left oblique views should be obtained with one or two roentgenograms, depending upon the area covered (Fig. 6–4). A cross-table lateral is then obtained from L3 through the sacrum (Fig. 6–5). All the roentgenograms are scrutinized at this time for completeness. Additional films may then be obtained, including horizontal beam (decubitus) or supine oblique projections for improved opacification of nerve roots.

With the horizontal beam oblique view, the nerve roots occupy a more dependent position, permitting better filling by gravity (Fig. 6–6).

Supine oblique views often result in improved visualization of the nerve roots, because in this position the nerve roots are dependent[48] (Fig. 6–7). Metrizamide has a higher specific gravity than cerebrospinal

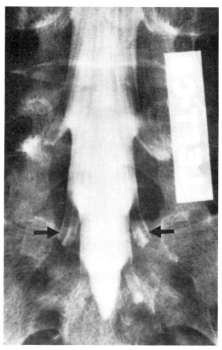

Figure 6–3. Normal lumbar myelogram. Posteroanterior projection. A myelographic spot film in the lumbar region demonstrates the nerve roots as well as the intrinsic rootlets at each level (arrows).

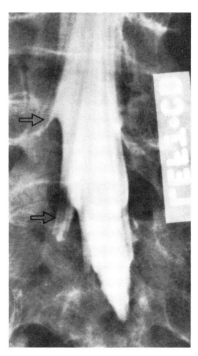

Figure 6–4. Normal lumbar myelogram. Right prone oblique spot film demonstrates the nerve roots in profile, with multiple roots within each sleeve (arrows).

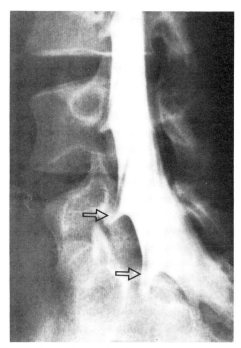

Figure 6–6. Normal lumbar myelogram. Horizontal beam, oblique projection. Oblique cross-table view also demonstrates excellent visualization of the nerve root sheaths and intrinsic nerve roots (arrows).

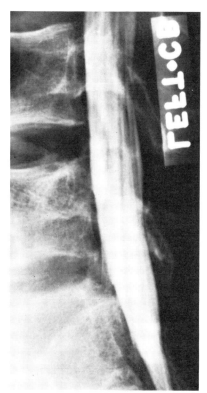

Figure 6–5. Normal lumbar myelogram. Cross-table lateral projection. The thecal sac and nerve roots are easily identified.

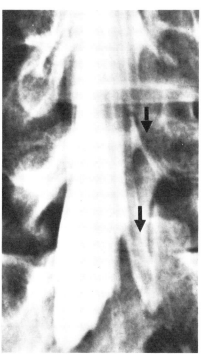

Figure 6–7. Compared with Figure 6–4, this oblique film, taken with patient in the supine position, demonstrates even better the individual nerve root sheaths filled with rootlets (arrows).

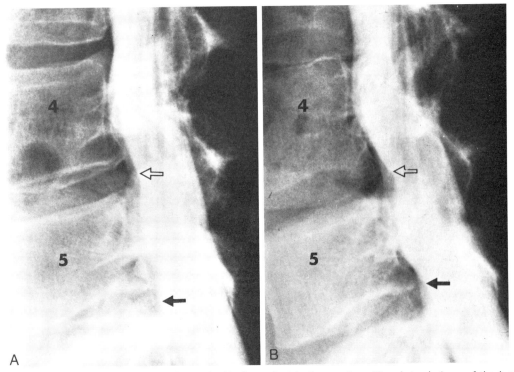

Figure 6–8. Value of the myelogram obtained with the patient in the erect position. Lateral views of the lumbar region were obtained following the injection of metrizamide with the patient (*A*) partially erect and (*B*) fully erect. On the film taken with the patient in the partially erect position, a minimal bulge is seen at the level of L4–L5 in the midline (open arrow), and no bulge is seen at the L5–S1 level (closed arrow). On the view with the patient in the fully erect position, accentuation of the bulge is apparent, with the midline defect at the L4–L5 level (open arrow). In addition, a midline defect is now seen at L5–S1 level (closed arrow).

fluid, and thus the nerve roots lying in the dependent position are filled to greater advantage. An erect lateral view may be necessary in the patient with the wide epidural space in order to reduce this space and to better visualize the relation of the ventral aspect of the subarachnoid space to the spinal canal (Fig. 6–8). A sitting lateral projection may also be used to distend the thecal sac and reduce the size of the epidural space.

The patient is then tilted into a 15 degree head-down (Trendelenburg) position slowly to opacify the upper lumbar and perhaps the lower dorsal regions. The patient is then slowly brought to the horizontal position and passively turned supine with the head elevated and the neck flexed. Fluoroscopic spot films of the conus medullaris (Fig. 6–9) and dorsal region may then be obtained. Overhead horizontal and vertical beam films are then obtained (Fig. 6–10). These roentgenograms are carefully reviewed.

The patient is brought to the upright po-

sition to pool the contrast material in the caudal sac. The patient is then returned to the horizontal position and transferred to a stretcher in the sitting position. The patient is told to remain in an upright or sitting position with the head elevated for 6 to 8 hours. In addition, the patient is advised to drink as much liquid as possible in order to facilitate dilution of contrast agent and thus to reduce risks and complications.[93] Bathroom privileges are permitted, but the patient should remain in bed otherwise, in the sitting position or with head elevated.

Cervical Examination

The examination of the cervical region may be performed using injection of the lumbar region,[24, 36] although the C1–C2 puncture is advised because of its proximity to the area of interest.[54, 67, 83]

In the examination of the cervical region from the lumbar route, 10 ml of 250 mg of I

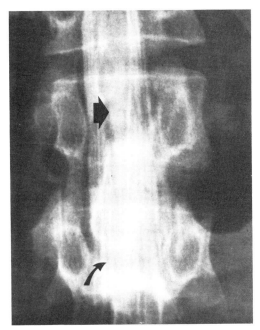

Figure 6–9. Normal lumbar myelogram. Conus medullaris. A supine film of the distal aspect of the spinal cord demonstrates the conus medullaris (straight arrow) and the multiple nerve roots (curved arrow) of the cauda equina. The filum terminale is not easily identified.

per 100 ml is injected at L2–L3 or L3–L4 with the patient 10 degrees above the horizontal in the prone position. The contrast agent is injected slowly.

After injection, the patient is passively turned 45 degrees to an oblique position, and the head is rotated into a lateral position with the neck extended and elevated. The table is then slowly tilted 30 degrees downward so that the patient is in the Trendelenburg position. The pooled contrast agent will then flow cephalad and pool in the cervical region as a bolus. The movement of the contrast agent should be followed fluoroscopically. The first roentgenogram may be an oblique lateral view obtained when the contrast agent is identified in the upper cervical region. The patient is then turned passively to the prone position in the posteroanterior position with the neck extended, so that the mandible is at the level of the foramen magnum. This allows visualization of the cervical spine from C2–C3 to the cervicothoracic junction. If too much extension is utilized, the upper cervical spine is hidden and foreshortened so that visualization is from C3–C4 caudad. The patient is then tilted down slowly under fluoroscopic control, to visualize the foramen magnum region. The foramen magnum has been opacified when one or more of the following observations are made: (1) the central filling defect of the odontoid process is observed; (2) the negative shadow of the vertebral artery and basilar artery is noted; and (3) lateral indentations of the metriza-

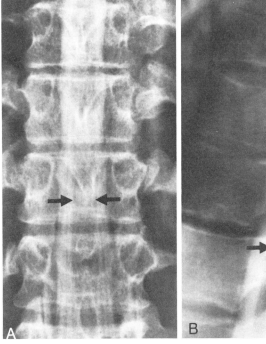
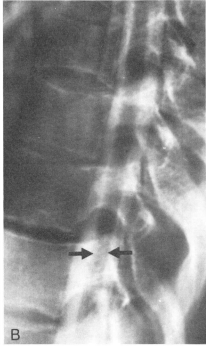

Figure 6–10. Normal thoracic myelogram. Anteroposterior supine (A) and lateral (B) views of the thoracic spine with metrizamide demonstrate the size and position of the spinal cord within the thecal sac (arrows).

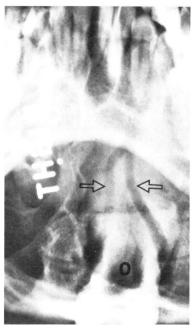

Figure 6–11. Normal cervical myelogram. Foramen magnum. A radiograph taken through the region of the foramen magnum during myelography demonstrates the odontoid process (*O*) and the vertebral arteries (arrows). Defects seen adjacent and lateral to the odontoid process represent deformation of the metrizamide column as it enters the foramen magnum.

mide column are present bilaterally, representing an impression on the contrast column by the rim of the foramen magnum (Fig. 6–11).

Immediately after the foramen magnum projections are obtained, the table is elevated 10 to 15 degrees to minimize any intracranial spill. Then at least two to four postero-anterior projections of the cervical region are obtained (Fig. 6–12). Oblique films may then be made, if required, to visualize the nerve roots. Cross-table lateral roentgenograms are obtained for the upper cervical region (Fig. 6–13), and a swimmer's projection is performed to visualize the cervicothoracic junction (Fig. 6–14). The roentgenograms are then scrutinized for completeness and to determine whether additional roentgenograms are necessary. The patient is passively turned supine with the head elevated and now flexed while the table is elevated 10 to 15 degrees above the horizontal. A cross-table lateral view in the supine projection is obtained. The table is then slowly elevated until the contrast material pools in

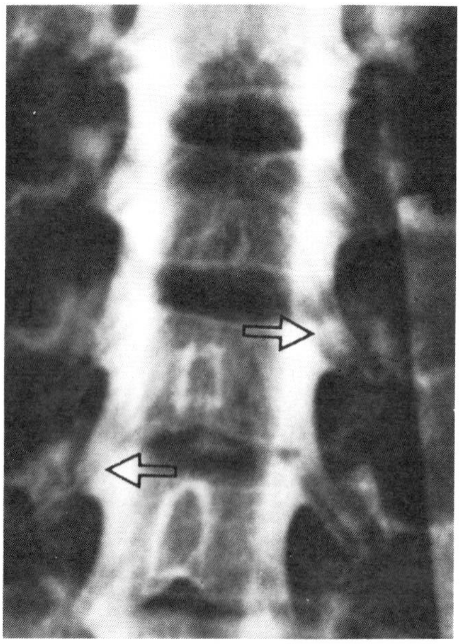

Figure 6–12. Normal cervical myelogram. A normal posteroanterior projection of the cervical region demonstrates the normal-appearing cord outlined by metrizamide, with contrast material filling the nerve root sleeves. The multiple nerve rootlets in a sleeve can be seen at several levels (arrows).

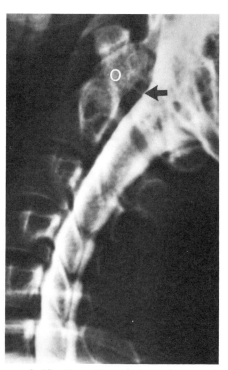

Figure 6–13. Normal cervical myelogram. Lateral roentgenogram of the cervical region demonstrates the position and size of the cervical cord. The space between the anterior margin of the thecal sac (arrow) and the odontoid process (**O**) represents the transverse ligament.

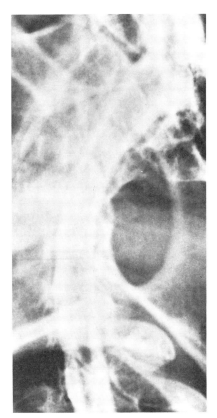

Figure 6–14. Normal cervical myelogram. Swimmer's lateral projection. The lower cervical and upper dorsal regions are visualized to advantage.

the thoracic spine. Roentgenograms of the thoracic spine may then be taken in the antero-posterior and lateral projections (see Fig. 6–10). One could then continue to elevate the table and turn the patient prone, enabling roentgenograms of the lumbar region to be obtained.

In our department, the majority of complete and cervical myelograms are performed by the lumbar route. The cervical examination, when performed from the lumbar route and adhering to the technique described, results in diagnostic roentgenograms in 95% of cases. Two of three regions are almost always observed satisfactorily, but the third region, either cervical or lumbar, depending upon which site one begins the examination with, may be seen well in only 50% to 60% of cases, fairly in 20% to 30% of cases, and poorly in 10% to 20% of cases. One may always raise these figures to almost 100% by utilizing adjunctive studies, such as computed tomography or complex

motion tomography, in those regions that are inadequately opacified.

Cervical Approach

The lateral C1–C2 puncture is selected as the primary site of injection of contrast media in the following cases: (1) cervical trauma, (2) inability of the patient to adequately extend the neck, (3) severe scoliosis, (4) abnormalities of the lumbar region (narrow canal, severe spondylosis, infection, neoplasm, prior surgery, tethered cord), (5) inability to perform lumbar puncture, and (6) complete block in the lumbar or dorsal subarachnoid space during lumbar myelography. In some institutions, C1–C2 puncture is the preferred approach for all patients undergoing cervical myelography.

The technique used in our department is the lateral approach to C1–C2 in the prone position with C-arm or biplane available. If a fluoroscopic spot film device in vertical beam technique only is available, the patient is placed in the prone position and the neck is rotated to the lateral projection on sponges with no angulation (neutral). Under fluoroscopic control, the head is aligned to proper lateral position so that a satisfactory space at C1–C2 can be obtained for the puncture. Since only one plane is visualized by fluoroscopy in this technique, horizontal beam films may be obtained at appropriate levels to observe depth of puncture on the antero-posterior plane.

The technique may be performed with 18 or 22 gauge needles. In our department, 22 gauge needles are used. Once the patient is properly aligned under fluoroscopic control, a small amount of anesthetic is injected posteriorly between C1 and C2 and just anterior to the spinolaminar line. The needle is left in place to be sure it is in proper anatomic position. If the position is satisfactory, then more anesthetic is injected at greater depth to increase the zone of anesthesia. The anesthetic needle is left in place as a guide for the spinal needle. The 22 gauge spinal needle is then introduced. The original monitoring is performed in the lateral plane to observe the posterior position of the needle and its relationship to the spinolaminar line. The patient is cautioned concerning neck movement, coughing, and swallowing while the needle is in place. The needle is slowly advanced under fluoro-scopic control, and the stylet is removed after short movements to check for fluid or blood. Once the needle is fixed by surround-ing tissue, depth should be checked in the anteroposterior plane by horizontal beam films. The needle is slowly advanced, and fluid is checked for every 1 to 2 mm. Two signs may indicate that the needle is close to or within subarachnoid space. One may feel a pop or give as the dura is penetrated and the subarachnoid space entered, or one may observe droplets of blood at the hub as the epidural space is crossed.[54]

With the tenting effect on the dura,[54] the needle may appear to cross the midline be-fore cerebrospinal fluid is encountered. Therefore, one should pass the midline be-fore considering that the puncture is too posterior and repuncturing with a slightly more anterior track. *Unlike* in lumbar spinal punctures, once the dura has been pene-trated and cerebrospinal fluid (CSF) ob-tained, the needle should not be advanced another 1 to 2 mm; otherwise the needle would be within the subdural space.[54] Once the puncture has been accomplished, the needle should be withdrawn 1 to 2 mm, because as a result of dural tenting, it is usually well beyond the midline.

COMPLICATIONS OF MYELOGRAPHY

Complications may occur with myelogra-phy, and the type of complication and inci-dence vary depending upon the contrast agent.

The use of iophendylate (Pantopaque) may result in arachnoiditis.[28] This complication has been observed in up to 25% of cases.

The complications observed after the in-troduction of metrizamide are the result of four different pathophysiologic changes:

1. Meningeal irritation, which may ac-count for the headache, nausea, vomiting, and dizziness.[30]

2. Spinoradicular symptoms, consisting of radicular pain, hyperesthesia, hyper-re-flexia, and urinary retention.[30]

3. Cerebral and spinocerebral symptoms, including seizures, visual and auditory dis-turbances, ischemic symptoms, stroke, con-fusion, psychologic reactions (e.g., anxiety and confusion), and hypertension.[30, 38, 93]

4. Miscellaneous symptoms such as those observed with introduction of any agents into CSF: fever, leukocytosis, and CSF pleo-cytosis.

Headache, the most common adverse re-action, has been observed 6 to 24 hours after conclusion of the examination in 29% to 67% of cases. Various causes have been invoked, from lumbar puncture to type of contrast material used, patient position, and needle gauge and size. Because children in-frequently develop headache, the stress of the procedure may be a contributing factor.

Nausea, dizziness, and vomiting are the next most common occurrences in adults but the most common reactions in children. These symptoms occur 8 to 24 hours after conclusion of the examination. Dizziness, which may last for several days, occurs in 12% to 37% of patients. Early ambulation and standing may reduce these complica-tions.

Thirty percent of patients experience nau-sea and radicular pain. The pain, developing predominantly in the lower back and legs, is often transitory and appears to be the consequence of nerve root irritation.

Urinary retention, hyperesthesia, hyper-reflexia and areflexia are observed when there is prolonged contact between contrast material and conus medullaris and proximal cauda equina, in which reduced dilution occurs.

Seizures, hyper-reflexia, visual and audi-tory disturbances, psychologic reactions, strokelike patterns, and confusion are the result of cerebral penetration by the metri-zamide and the irritating effect on the brain, as well as abnormalities in cerebral autore-gulation due to the blood-brain barrier ab-erration.[93] Electroencephalography abnor-malities have been observed in 34% of patients after myelography, although EEG has not proved useful in predicting which patients may develop seizures as a result of the aberration in electrical activity. Pretreat-ment with phenobarbital and diazepam has been recommended.

Patients who have been on phenothiazines and other antidepressants should discon-tinue medication at least 48 hours prior to myelography, since these medications in-crease the risks of adverse reactions.

The reasons for the brain penetration are that no barrier exists to the CSF and simple diffusion occurs into extracellular space.[92] There are gaps in the pial and ependymal membranes that permit solutes to pass easily, in contradistinction to limitations in diffusion imposed by choroid plexus capillary endothelium and arachnoid.

Noncontrast CT scans performed 20 hours after installation of metrizamide reveal diffuse enhancement of cortex and adjacent white matter in patients with seizures, confirming the cerebral penetration of these water-soluble contrast materials.[16a]

Another mechanism invoked to explain toxic cerebral complications of metrizamide is the inhibition of hexokinase,[19] which results in interference in glucose utilization by the brain. Metrizamide may also interfere with acetycholine and cholinesterase activity,[41] which also may play a role in adverse reactions.

INTERVERTEBRAL DISCS

Normal Discs

The intervertebral discs are interspersed between adjacent vertebral bodies from the axis to the sacrum. Disc thickness varies in different parts of the same disc and at varying levels within the spine. The discs make up one fifth of the length of the spine. In the cervical and lumbar segments of the spine, the anterior half is thicker than the posterior half, accounting for the cervical and lumbar lordosis. The discs are nearly uniform in thickness and are thinnest in the thoracic spine. In the cervical region, the discs are constricted laterally by the uncinate processes.

In the lumbar region, the discs become slightly thicker (8 to 12 mm) as one descends caudad, to the disc space at the L5–S1 level. This level may vary, usually being decreased in size.

The intervertebral disc adheres to hyaline cartilage lining the vertebral end-plates above and below. The disc is also attached to the anterior and posterior longitudinal ligaments. In the thoracic region, in addition, there is a lateral attachment to the intra-articular ligaments encompassing the heads of the ribs.

The intervertebral disc is divided into the nucleus pulposus and annulus fibrosus. The annulus fibrosus forms the laminated outer portion of the disc and consists of fibrocartilage. The nucleus pulposus lies within the annulus fibrosus and tends to be closer to the posterior than to the anterior surface.

At birth, the disc tends to be soft and elastic, with a high water content. Biochemical changes occur in the mucopolysaccharide segment of the proteoglycan complex as a person ages, resulting in a loss of water content within the disc, with a concomitant reduction in elasticity. As a consequence, it is often difficult to distinguish the nucleus pulposus from the annulus fibrosus in the adult, because they appear as a fibrous mass.[15] With aging, the disc is less resistant to stress, and fissuring develops.

Disc Abnormalities

It is important to understand terminology to avoid the confusion that often occurs

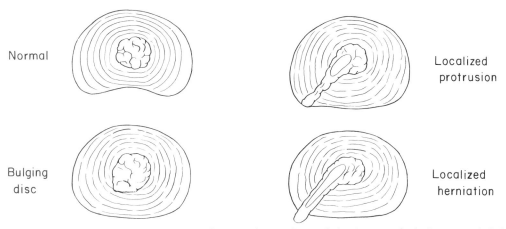

Figure 6–15. Diagrammatic representation of some abnormalities of the intervertebral disc—normal, bulging, protrusion, and herniation. Sequestration (not shown) involves a separation of all or part of the herniated fragment.

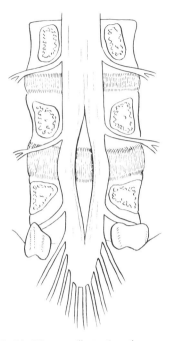

Figure 6–16. Diagram illustrating the appearance of central disc bulge. Note that the nerve roots exit below the pedicle and above the disc level.

because of misunderstanding and misuse of terms, with a resultant lack of communication.

Basically, four terms may be used commonly in the diagnosis of the abnormal disc during myelographic examination: bulge, protrusion, herniation (HNP), and sequestration or extrusion (Fig. 6–15).

As noted previously, there are biomechanical factors that affect the mucopolysaccharide content of the disc, with resultant loss of water content. Concurrently, elasticity is diminished, and fissuring results from the repeated mechanical stresses upon the disc. The multiple fissures cause disc bulges and reduction in disc space.[91] The other disc abnormalities listed previously may also occur.

The disc bulge occurs as part of the aging process and is diffuse (Fig. 6–16). The bulges are seen as extensions beyond the vertebral body and are most pronounced in the midline at the level of the disc space. Disc bulge is often recognized as a midline smooth indentation of the thecal sac on the lateral

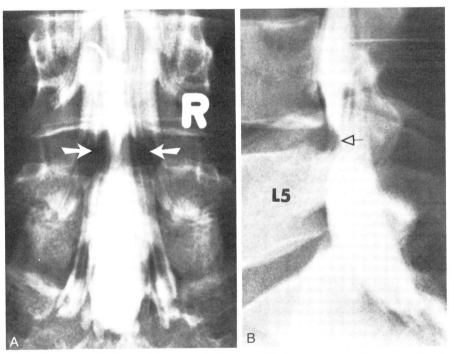

Figure 6–17. Midline lumbar disc bulge. *A,* Posteroanterior view of the lumbar region with metrizamide demonstrates a central constriction (arrows) with nerve roots unaffected. *B,* Lateral projection. A ventral bulge is seen at the L4–L5 level, accounting for the central constriction (arrow).

projection without nerve root defects on the anteroposterior or oblique projection. In the patient with a large, diffuse bulge at myelography, in addition to a large ventral defect at the level of the disc space, a waistlike defect is seen bilaterally on the anteroposterior and oblique projections without nerve root cutoff[37] (Fig. 6–17). Some authors have reported an accuracy of 97% in distinguishing disc bulge from disc herniation using water-soluble contrast myelography.[37] A protrusion develops if a localized rather than diffuse bulge develops, causing localized expansion of the disc with only outer fibers of the annulus surrounding the bulge. These are more common laterally, since the annulus and posterior longitudinal ligament are weakest at this site. Herniation occurs when the annulus is ruptured and disc material extends under the posterior longitudinal ligament. This subligamentous herniation occurs posterolaterally, where the ligament is weakest. Sequestration or extrusion occurs when a portion of herniated disc separates from the remainder and migrates cephalad or caudad.

The myelographic criteria used for disc bulge are a waistlike defect of the thecal sac, usually greater on anteroposterior than oblique projections, and no nerve root cutoff at the level of the disc space (see Fig. 6–17).

In contradistinction, in disc herniation, the findings include a unilateral angular defect and nerve root cutoff.[37] In addition, the affected nerve root in disc herniation is widened distally over a short segment, and the abnormality may extend above or below the disc space[37] (Fig. 6–18). A fragment may separate from the remainder of the disc and extend through or around the posterior longitudinal ligament in the epidural space. This fragment, which may migrate above or below the disc space, is called an extruded, sequestered, or free fragment.[25]

Lumbar Discs

The majority of disc herniations are anterolateral, although the incidence of central disc herniation (Fig. 6–19) varies from 5% to 12%. One group has reported an incidence of 31% in central discs.[25] The higher incidence these authors observed may be accounted for by the fact that they included in their data central discs with lateral extension. They also noted that the majority (78%) of free fragments migrated superiorly but

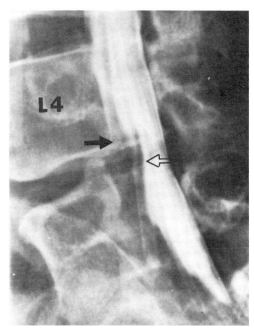

Figure 6–18. Anterolateral disc herniation. Metrizamide myelogram, oblique view. On the right oblique projection there is evidence of a cutoff of the L5 nerve root at the L4–L5 level, with slight expansion distally at the site of the cutoff (closed arrow). There is displacement of the S1 nerve root (open arrow), with slight edema a little more distally.

only 6% extended inferiorly. The remainder were mixed. The most common sites of disc herniation are L4–L5 (54%) and L5–S1 (38%), with 8% at L3–L4 and only rare occurrences at other levels.[25]

Calcified discs occasionally herniate, as do vacuum discs, with air remaining within the fragment. An important point concerning nerve root involvement with disc herniation is to remember that the L4 nerve root emerges under the pedicle of L4, so it is spared by an L4–L5 HNP unless disc migration occurs. In such a case, the L5 root is compressed. CT best demonstrates the extruded disc fragment.

There is a high degree of concurrence between CT and myelography. The only limitations of myelography are at L5–S1, because of the wide epidural space, and in the evaluation of the patient with a lateral disc.[3, 65, 85, 90] CT, however, would be diagnostic at these sites.

Thoracic Discs

In the dorsal region, disc bulging or herniation with cord compression is much less

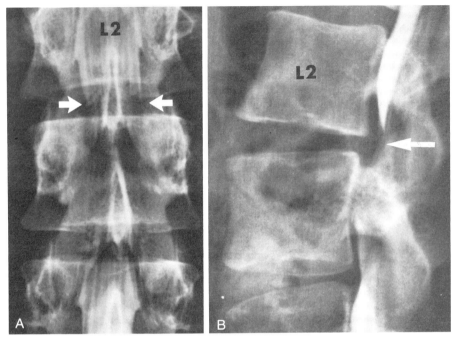

Figure 6–19. Central disc herniation. *A,* Posteroanterior projection during lumbar myelography demonstrates an incomplete block at the level of L2–L3 (arrows). *B,* Lateral projection. A ventral defect is noted (arrow). The midline central defect seen on 6–19*A* and the ventral defect seen on 6–19*B* are evidence of a central disc herniation.

common than in the lumbar region. When it does occur, it tends to affect the lower dorsal spine more commonly, at T9–T10, T10–T11, or T11–T12. The degenerative disc changes in the thoracic region seem to occur more slowly, although disc space calcification is often observed. CT myelography shows these lesions to advantage.

Cervical Discs

In the cervical region, lateral discs may be soft (disc protrusion or herniation) or hard (bony). The CT scan, because of its spatial and contrast resolution, permits accurate differentiation between soft and hard discs. Central disc herniation or bulge is more significant in the cervical than in the lumbar region, because of the potential for cord compression. Cervical disc herniations are most common at C6–C7 (75%) and C5–C6 (20%). In males between 20 and 40 years of age, trauma may result in disc herniation, particularly centrally (Fig. 6–20).

In the cervical region, the nerve root sheath is composed of several rootlets (see Fig. 6–12). A large, smooth defect of the nerve root sheath with obliteration of root-

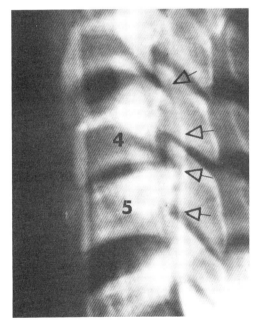

Figure 6–20. Herniated cervical disc secondary to trauma. There is a ventral defect adjacent to C4–C5 (arrows), with the greatest defect juxtaposed to the body of C4. Disc space narrowing at the C4–C5 level is also present. The facet joint is widened at C4–C5 owing to tearing of the interfacetal ligament. Widening between the spinous processes (not shown) was also observed. These changes are due to ligamentous damage resulting from a flexion injury.

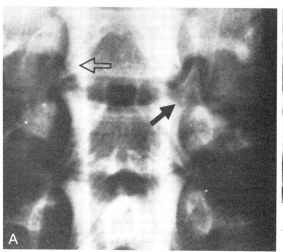

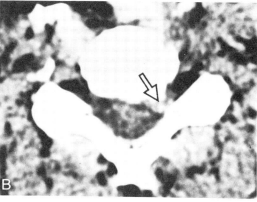

Figure 6–21. Lateral disc herniation. *A,* Posteroanterior myelogram in the cervical region reveals normal cervical nerve roots on the right (open arrow) as compared with the cutoff of the nerve root on the left and the sharply defined defect (closed arrow). *B,* A noncontrast axial CT scan through the same disc space confirms the presence of a left lateral soft tissue extrathecal mass in the neural foramen (arrow).

lets is characteristic of herniation on the anteroposterior projection (Fig. 6–21). High-resolution CT with or without contrast infusion may reveal the presence of a herniated disc.[5, 72] Some irregularity or tenting of these root sheaths is more characteristic of spondylosis and is common after age 40.

Spondylosis and Spinal Stenosis

The narrow canal is usually developmentally characterized by broad, short pedicles and heavy, convergent laminae[21, 22] (Fig. 6–22). The intervertebral foramina become elongated and narrowed dorsoventrally. Any

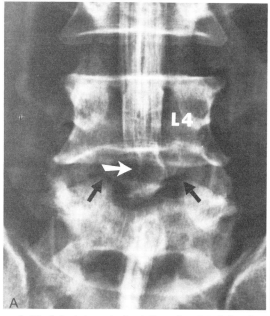

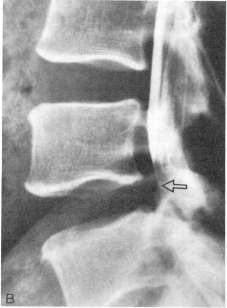

Figure 6–22. Spinal stenosis simulating a herniated disc. Posteroanterior (*A*) and lateral (*B*) projections of the lumbar region on metrizamide myelography demonstrate a narrow thecal sac. A ventral defect is seen at the level of L4–L5 on the lateral view (open arrow). On the posteroanterior projection, compression of the thecal sac can be seen at the L4–L5 disc space (white arrow). The deformation is the result of hypertrophied facets (black arrows). An incomplete block is present, with a small amount of metrizamide below the deformity at the L4–L5 level.

intrusion by osseous structures, ligaments, or disc bulge or herniation may compromise an already borderline thecal sac and nerve roots.

Localized narrowing is more often acquired than developmental and tends to occur more commonly at L3–L4 and L4–L5 and uncommonly at L5–S1.[22]

As the disc space narrows because of disc degeneration, the supporting ligaments are strained, and, consequently, ligamentous laxity and thickening occur. In addition, the supporting osseous structures, the facets, are affected, resulting in arthrosis, facet overriding, and malalignment. These spondylotic changes further strain the ligamentous structures, so that the process of degenerative changes affecting the ligamentous and osseous support structures is continuous.

In spinal stenosis, the disc abnormalities, nerve root changes, and narrow canal are clearly delineated. The presence of lateral recess stenosis, however, cannot be demonstrated with myelography (Fig. 6–23). This inability to demonstrate these anatomic alterations has been one of the causes of failure of back surgery.[13]

Lateral Recess Syndrome

In the patient with the lateral recess syndrome, the nerve roots are compressed at

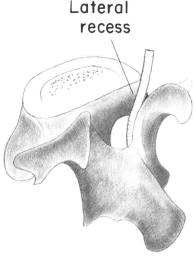

Lateral recess

Figure 6–23. Lateral recess. Diagrammatic representation of the lateral recess. The nerve root lies between the vertebral body anteriorly and the superior facet posteriorly.

the superior border of the pedicle by the superior articular facet.[45] The recess is narrowed by the overgrowth of the superior articular facet. In addition to lateral recess narrowing as a cause of back pain, it has been pointed out that the neural foramen narrows when overriding of the vertebral bodies occurs.[43] Others have reported finding nerve root entrapment in 25 of 400 patients with normal myelograms and positive CT scans that demonstrated narrowed neural foramina and lateral recess syndrome.[68] The normal recess measures 5 mm or more; 3 mm may cause or contribute to symptoms, and 2 mm or less accounts for the patient's symptoms.[14, 45] The symptom complex described is disabling intermittent pain in one or both legs brought on by standing 5 to 10 minutes and relieved by squatting or sitting.[45] Objective neurologic findings are often absent. In the patient with a herniated disc, symptoms progress and objective neurologic findings are present. Unfortunately, patients rarely have pure disc or nerve entrapment syndromes, since the pathoanatomic features often cause a mixture of anatomic aberrations.

Central Canal Stenosis

The narrow canal syndrome as described is either developmental on an anatomic basis or acquired from spondylotic changes, which occur most commonly at L3–L4 and L4–L5.[22] In either case, any intrusion into an already compromised spinal canal will cause symptomatology through compression of nerve roots. Incomplete or complete blocks may be demonstrated (Fig. 6–24); they are exacerbated by disc bulge or protrusion and/or ligamentous thickening. The narrow canal may be demonstrated on myelography by the thin, reduced size of the thecal sac, which may be signified by a larger number of disc spaces covered by the usual volume of contrast material injected (see Fig. 6–22). Almost the entire region is covered. A washboard configuration of the thecal sac is observed, owing to anterior disc bulges and posterior facet overgrowth and ligamentous thickening on lateral projection[21] (see Fig. 6–24).

On posteroanterior projection, in addition to the thin column with the increased number of disc spaces covered by contrast media, an hourglass deformity is observed; it is caused by lateral defects also resulting from disc bulge, facet changes, and ligamentous thickening. The soft tissue, osseous, and disc intrusions into the thecal sac result in partial or complete blocks. In some cases, the nerve roots of the cauda equina are noted to be thickened and coiled, causing serpiginous filling defects (Figs. 6–24, 6–25). A partial or complete block is also present. Affected nerves may be distinguished from dilated veins, because nerve root involvement is above the stenosis or block and veins are below.[27] Extension causes accentuation of the nerve root changes, whereas flexion reduces or obliterates the observed defects.[22, 27, 92] These nerve root appearances are probably accounted for by intermittent nerve root entrapment with postural changes noted previously, which result in stretching and elongation of nerve roots.[27, 89] The differential diagnosis of these filling defects consists of the following: dilated tortuous arteries, veins due to vascular malformations, vascular compression by a mass, hypertrophic interstitial neuropathy of Dejerine and Sottas,

arachnoiditis, and inflammatory or carcinomatous meningitis.

In the cervical region, as in the lumbar region, developmental and acquired stenosis occurs. In developmental stenosis, the occurrence of degenerative changes contributes to the alterations that relate to the occurrence of symptoms as well. The pathologic changes are similar to those in the lumbar region, with fissuring of the disc resulting in disc bulging or thinning of the disc space and bony overgrowth of the vertebral bodies. In addition, stability is reduced, and motion of the vertebral bodies results in malalignment, with overriding of the facets and ligamentous thickening. These combined changes compromise the spinal canal and compress the cord as well as nerve roots, so there are root, myelopathic, and long tract findings. The sites of involvement are most commonly C4–C5 and C5–C6 and then C6–C7.[20]

A spinal canal with a sagittal measurement of less than 11 mm almost always results in symptoms. Thirteen mm is the

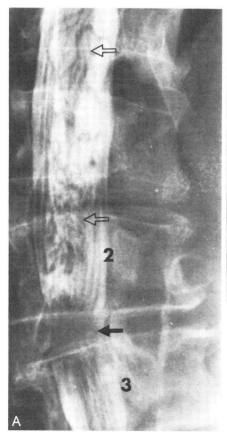

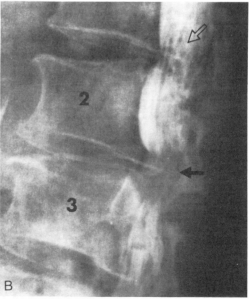

Figure 6–24. Spinal stenosis. Posteroanterior (A) and lateral (B) projections obtained during metrizamide myelography demonstrate the presence of an incomplete block at the L2–L3 level (closed arrows). Metrizamide of lesser density is also noted caudad to the block. Tortuosity and elongation of nerve roots can be seen in the dorsolumbar region and just above the level of the incomplete block (open arrows).

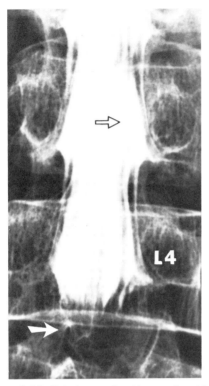

Figure 6–25. Spinal stenosis with complete block. A posteroanterior projection of the lumbar spine during metrizamide myelography demonstrates a complete block of the metrizamide column at the L4–L5 level (white arrow). In addition, tortuosity and secondary elongation of nerve roots are noted (open arrow).

lowest level that is considered normal, and more than 15 mm is considered normal.[6, 20, 94]

During myelography from below, an incomplete or partial block may be encountered in the lower cervical region, owing to a combination of disc bulge, ligamentous thickening, and bony overgrowth accentuated by the hyperextended position of the neck. To overcome these obstacles and to prove whether a block is present, the patient is brought to the neutral position. The apparent obstruction will be overcome with this change in position and filling of the remainder of the cervical region. An important clue demonstrating that this is an apparent, rather than a true, obstruction is that the defect observed is adjacent to a disc space with bilateral lateral indentations of the contrast column, without deviation or enlargement of the spinal cord. On lateral projection, the thecal sac has a washboard configuration, with ventral and dorsal indentations due to intrusion by disc, bone, and

ligaments[20] (Fig. 6–26). Cord widening is seen on the posteroanterior projection as a consequence of ventral compression by osseous structures or dorsal compression by ligamentous structures. Nerve root defects are common at C4–C5, C5–C6, and C6–C7.

A more recently described entity, first seen in Japanese people but now encountered in all groups, that may account for extradural cord compression and may simulate disc disease or spondylosis is ossification of the posterior longitudinal ligament (OPLL).[47, 53] This finding is most common in the cervical spine, although it is seen also in the thoracic spine, where it is more likely asymptomatic. The cervical ligamentous changes are encountered in patients with other forms of ligamentous calcification, such as diffuse idiopathic skeletal hyperostosis (DISH; Forestier's disease).[2, 66] OPLL may be focal or diffuse. Diffuse forms are easy to recognize, but the focal lesion, when adjacent to the disc space, may simulate a calcified disc. Calcification or ossification of the ligamentum flavum may also occur.

Differential Diagnosis

In the patient with suspected disc herniation, one must exclude disc bulge,[37, 91] spondylosis[22] or spondylolisthesis,[37, 88] other extradural lesions such as postoperative scarring,[9, 23] extradural metastases,[90] lymphoma, narrow canal, infection, and extradural neurofibroma. During CT one must exclude, in addition to the lesions just listed, conjoined nerve roots,[32] synovial cysts, perineural cysts, and spondylolisthesis.

Postoperative Patient

An accurate diagnosis may be difficult in the patient with persistent symptoms, new onset of low back pain, or radiculopathy following surgery. The patient should be examined with the following possible causes of the symptoms in mind: (1) new disc herniation, (2) recurrent disc herniation, (3) operative scar, (4) arachnoiditis, (5) infection, (6) overlooked pathology such as nerve root entrapment due to foraminal or lateral recess encroachment, (7) spinal stenosis, (8) postoperative cyst, (9) mechanical instability or meningocele, (10) a lesion at a higher level, (11) spinal canal encroachment, and (12) pseudarthrosis after a spinal fusion.[10]

The procedure for the examination of such a patient should begin with a postoperative CT scan with pre-scan intravenous administration of contrast agent. A noncontrast scan is performed to re-evaluate the region.

If an abnormality is observed and there is question of scar or epidural fibrosis, repeat sections at the exact levels may be performed again following contrast infusion.[10, 74, 75] It is important to scan while the contrast is running. Scar enhancement following intravenous contrast infusion enables one to distin-

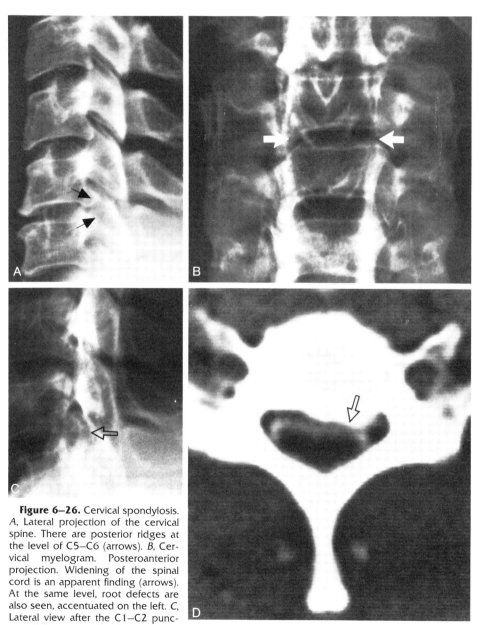

Figure 6–26. Cervical spondylosis. A, Lateral projection of the cervical spine. There are posterior ridges at the level of C5–C6 (arrows). B, Cervical myelogram. Posteroanterior projection. Widening of the spinal cord is an apparent finding (arrows). At the same level, root defects are also seen, accentuated on the left. C, Lateral view after the C1–C2 puncture. A large ventral defect is seen protruding into the thecal sac, causing compression of the cord (arrow). This ventral defect is due to spurs seen in 6–26A and accounts for the apparent cord widening observed in the posteroanterior projection. D, Computed tomographic myelography (CTM) performed at the level of C5 following the metrizamide myelogram demonstrates the presence of the large spur ventrally and to the left (arrow). It is compressing the thecal sac on the left. Compare the compressed thecal sac on the left with the normal thecal sac on the right.

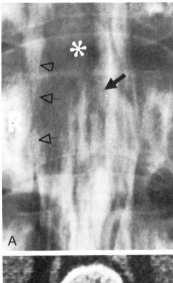

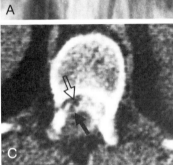

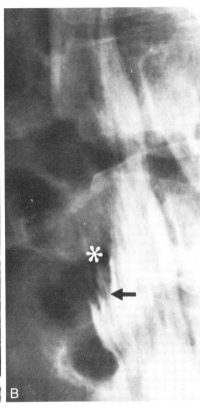

Figure 6–27. Postoperative arachnoiditis. Posteroanterior (*A*) and oblique (*B*) projections of the thoracolumbar region at the level of the conus medullaris demonstrate the presence of a long, slightly irregular filling defect (asterisk) within the subarachnoid space. On the posteroanterior projection, the presence of an intradural lesion is suspected because of the lateral deviation of the contrast material on the right (open arrows) compared with the left. Obliteration of the nerve roots on the right, with some irregularity of nerve roots of the conus medullaris (closed arrow), demonstrates an intrinsic lesion with nerve root deformation. Irregularity and slight widening suggest the presence of an intrinsic lesion. In view of the history and the findings, the diagnosis of localized arachnoiditis was made. *C,* Axial CT scan demonstrates a lesion affecting the thecal sac and confirms the localization suggested. Extradural defect (open arrow) and an intradural lesion (closed arrow) are seen.

guish the scar from disc material that does not opacify. The enhancement is considered to be related to the vascularity of the granulation tissue forming the scar. A measurement of the density on CT may aid in differential diagnosis also. Scar measures 40 to 90 Hounsfield units (HU) and a disc measures 80 to 120 HU. Another factor adding to difficulty of postoperative CT is the decrease or loss of epidural fat. The presence of epidural fat contributes to the advantage of CT in the diagnosis of disc disease in the lumbar region.[31] CT is more effective in the lumbar region than in the thoracic or cervical region because of the difference in epidural fat content.

If CT with or without contrast agent is not revealing, then myelography should be considered as the next step. Following the myelogram, CT myelography (CTM) should be performed. This latter procedure often provides additional information.[3]

Epidural scar or fibrosis occurs postoperatively in the majority of cases. The scar is limited to the operative site (Fig. 6–27). In some cases, arachnoiditis may account for the recurrent symptoms in up to 16% of patients with failed back surgery. Arachnoiditis is actually a misnomer, because all three dural layers are affected by the inflammatory process.

A variety of patterns may be observed after scar formation during myelography, depending upon the extent of involvement: (1) root sleeve blunting, (2) irregular lateral defects of the thecal sac, (3) angular defects, (4) band or web, (5) spreading out of contrast in streak or droplets, and (6) clumping of contrast agent.[61]

The characteristic patterns should be recognized so they will not be confused with other abnormalities. The so-called branchless tree pattern refers to obliteration of nerve roots during myelography. In these instances, one or more roots may be obliterated (Fig. 6–28). These changes may be distinguished from those of disc herniation. Disc herniation causes root sleeve cutoff with distal swelling and an angular defect of the thecal sac.[37] On CT, displacement of the sac toward rather than away from the lesion is another valuable sign of epidural scarring. On myelography, marked deformity with bands or webs makes it difficult to

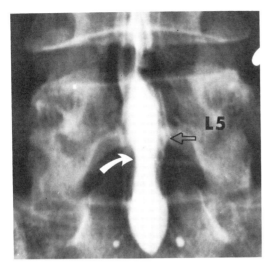

Figure 6–28. Arachnoiditis and recurrent disc herniation. Posteroanterior projection. A branchless tree pattern exists, with obliteration and reduction of nerve roots. On the left at the L5–S1 level, a cutoff of the swollen nerve root (open arrow) indicates disc herniation. A defect on the metrizamide column just caudad (white arrow) is from compression of the thecal sac.

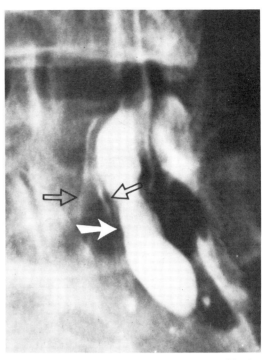

Figure 6–30. Postoperative herniated disc. Metrizamide myelogram in the oblique projection. There is deformity of the thecal sac distally (white arrow) as well as some deformity more proximally as a result of epidural fibrosis. In addition, there is evidence of recurrent herniated disc manifested by expansion and cutoff of the S1 nerve root (open arrows).

distinguish between disc herniation and scar (Fig. 6–29).

When a disc herniation is also present, the findings are characteristic of a disc herniation (Fig. 6–30). The findings that aid in

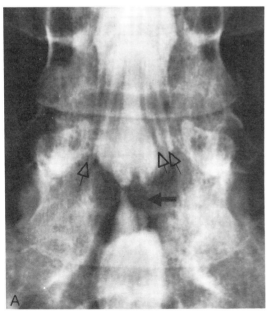

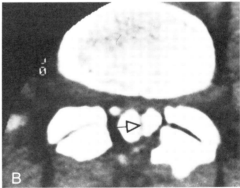

Figure 6–29. Arachnoiditis. Postoperative patient treated for disc disease. *A*, Posteroanterior projection demonstrates a localized constriction of the thecal sac overlying L5 (solid arrow). Slight irregularity of the metrizamide column above and below the constriction is noted without focal mass, so the diagnosis contemplated on this examination with a high degree of certainty is postoperative arachnoiditis, not recurrent disc disease. Nerve roots are obliterated (open arrows), not cut off. *B*, Axial CTM. A vertical band crossing the thecal sac represents a scar (arrow). In addition, some irregularity of the metrizamide margins is identified.

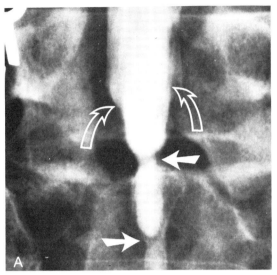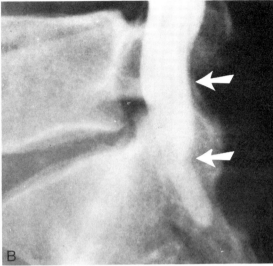

Figure 6–31. Postoperative scarring. Posteroanterior (A) and lateral (B) projections of the lumbar region. Myelographic examination reveals irregularity and deformity affecting the caudal thecal sac (straight arrows). In addition, obliteration of the nerve roots over the L5 region is observed (curved arrows).

confirming the presence of scar on CTM are deformity, ipsilateral displacement of thecal sac, obliteration of epidural fat, no evidence of ventral or ventrolateral mass, and lack of root cutoff, edema, and displacement.[87]

In the postoperative patient, the presence of a long lesion will aid in distinguishing scar from recurrent disc herniation, which is more focal[16] (Fig. 6–31).

Postoperative pseudomeningocele occurs when the dura and arachnoid inadvertently are cut during surgery, with a leakage of CSF into the paraventricular tissue. It represents a collection of CSF outside the spinal canal surrounded by fibrous tissue. Only rarely does the arachnoid herniate through the defect forming the border. In some instances, the lesion may communicate with the thecal sac (Fig. 6–32), but in others it becomes walled off and separate from the thecal sac.

CT MYELOGRAPHY (CTM) EXAMINATION

CTM may be performed at the conclusion of a myelogram as a supplementary examination or as a separate procedure with small amounts (3 to 5 ml) of dilute water-soluble contrast material (160 to 170 mg per 100 ml). When this examination is performed as a separate procedure, the contrast material is introduced following a lumbar puncture. The patient is rotated into the position for an oblique projection and slowly turned 20 degrees head-down for examination of the dorsal region and 30 degrees head-down for examination of the cervical region. The patient is then turned in the supine position, and the examination begins.

In the patient who has had a water-soluble myelogram, CTM should be delayed 2 to 4 hours to reduce the density of the contrast material by dilution effect.[18] In addition, the patient should be turned over at least two times to obtain an even distribution of the contrast material and to reduce layering effects.[18] A high-resolution scanner is preferred, utilizing a preliminary radiograph on which are annotated the sections required so that the slices obtained may be accurately correlated with the anatomy.

The number of sections and the slice thickness are determined by the information to be obtained. In the cervical or dorsal region, for evaluation of the disc space, 1.5 to 2 mm consecutive sections over the disc space are required. In the lumbar region, 3 mm consecutive sections are satisfactory.

In the evaluation of the spinal cord, accurate assessment of the cord size may be made only with proper windowing. According to some authors, an appropriate window

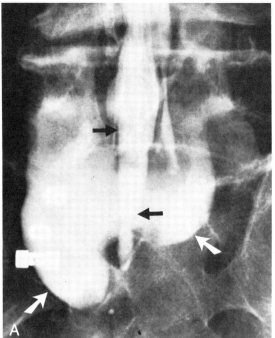

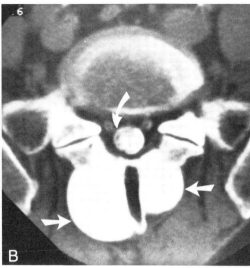

Figure 6–32. Postoperative pseudomeningocele. A, Metrizamide myelography. There is deformity of the distal thecal sac, with constriction and irregularity (black arrows). This represents epidural fibrosis. In addition, nerve root cutoff is seen at the levels of L4–L5 and L5–S1 on the right. Large, bilateral, well-demarcated, contrast-filled sacs are seen surrounding the thecal sac, slightly larger on the right than on the left. These represent an extradural collection of contrast material (white arrows). B, Axial CTM demonstrates minimal irregularity of the thecal sac, with epidural fibrosis posteriorly on the right. There is also a clumping of nerve roots on the right (curved arrow). Extradural posterior collections of contrast material indicate that the pseudomeningocele (straight arrows) is communicating with the thecal sac, although not at this level.

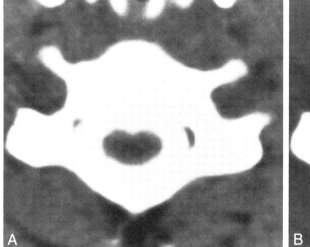

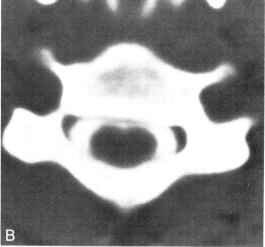

Figure 6–33. Accurate cord visualization with appropriate center settings on metrizamide myelography. A, Axial CTM at a window setting of 300 and a center setting of 70. The true cord dimensions are not appreciated, as it is difficult to separate cord from surrounding metrizamide because of the poor boundary zone. B, Same level as that of part A, with a higher window setting of 500 and a center setting of 100. The true cord is now seen, because a sharp delineation occurs between spinal cord and metrizamide in the thecal sac.

center is important in determination of cord size, but window width is not as important.[68, 76] Window width has been considered effective only for aesthetics; it does not alter cord size (Fig. 6–33).

The advantages of CTM are as follows:

1. The axial projection provides optimal visualization of the relationships of the spinal canal and its contents.

2. CTM is more sensitive than radiographic myelography to contrast difference, so that tissue variation may be visualized (e.g., fat, calcium, bone, or contrast material entering a cyst or a cavity within cord). In a block, small amounts of contrast agent extending above the block may be detected, defining the upper extent of the lesion and obviating the need for a C1–C2 puncture.

3. Extradural involvement, as well as paraspinal pathology, may be appreciated.

4. The entire extent of the pathologic process may be appreciated, with precise localization.

The advantage of the preliminary myelographic examination is that the lesion may be identified, but then, as noted previously, precise additional information may be obtained through the use of complementary CT. In addition, CT will be of value in areas where visualization is poor or contrast is dilute, since CT is sensitive even to small amounts of contrast material. In these instances, CT will add significantly to the study and substantiate the presence or absence of a lesion.[86] In one study of patients with a demonstrated abnormality, CTM was shown to provide more significant information than myelography in 40% of cases and to provide no advantage in 59%.[18] The advantage of CTM was supported by others.[3, 86]

INTRASPINAL AND SPINAL LESIONS

The examination of the intraspinal contents in patients with suspected mass lesions begins with assessment of the patient's history and physical findings, which provides an indication of lesion location. Plain roentgenograms should be examined for osseous abnormalities, spinal canal enlargement, or calcification.

One may then proceed to myelography with 3 to 5 ml of water-soluble contrast media in a concentration of 190 mg per 100 ml. The needle is left in position and the

patient is tilted downward with the neck hyperextended slowly so that the flow of contrast can be examined for any abnormalities such as partial or complete block. If no abnormality is seen or the findings are uncertain or questionable, the remainder of contrast agent (7 to 9 ml) is injected, and one continues the study to examine more fully the spinal canal to the level of the foramen magnum, in order to determine whether an insidious abnormality is present. It is imperative that roentgenograms be obtained at right angles so that, at best, posteroanterior or anteroposterior and lateral projections are obtained. When a complete block is identified, the contrast agent should be placed above the lesion via a C1–C2 puncture to demonstrate the length of the lesion or whether the patient may have more than one lesion.

In examining the abnormality, it is important to determine which compartment is affected by the lesion. The three major com-

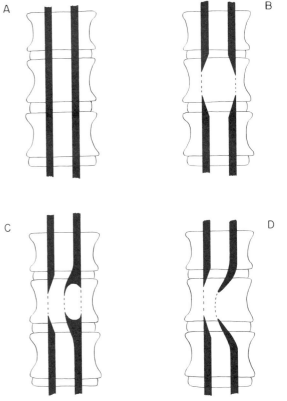

Figure 6–34. Diagram of compartments with spinal canal lesions. *A,* Normal. *B,* Intradural-intramedullary. *C,* Intradural-extramedullary. *D,* Extradural.

partments are as follows: (1) intradural-intramedullary, (2) intradural-extramedullary, and (3) extradural (Fig. 6–34).

Intradural-Intramedullary Lesions

Intradural-intramedullary lesions are located within the spinal cord; gliomas (astrocytomas and ependymomas) and syringomyelia or hydromyelia are the most common lesions. Other less common lesions include hemangioblastoma, lipoma, epidermoid, myelitis, and post-traumatic cysts or hematomyelia. Ependymomas occur more commonly in the conus medullaris and filum terminale and next in frequency in the cervical region. Cystic degeneration is common and occurs in one third to one half of cases. Astrocytomas occur most commonly in the thoracic cord and next in the cervical cord; up to one third are cystic.

Myelographic Findings With Intradural-Intramedullary Lesions

These lesions are characterized on myelography by cord expansion, with narrowing of the surrounding subarachnoid space. The cord widening is confirmed by being observed in both anteroposterior and lateral projections (Fig. 6–35). In the cervical region, the contrast material is observed ventral to the cord, with the cord maintained in a dorsal position. The presence of such a lesion expanding the spinal cord will result in expansion of the cord into the ventral subarachnoid space (the dipping sign) (Fig. 6–35).

In patients with syringohydromyelia, the expanded cord may diminish in size when the patient is erect, CSF is removed, and air is introduced—the "collapsing cord sign."[8] If no change in cord size occurs with this technique, a diagnosis of intramedullary neoplasm may be suspected (Fig. 6–36).

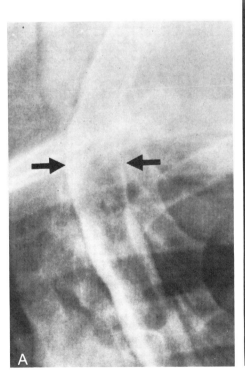
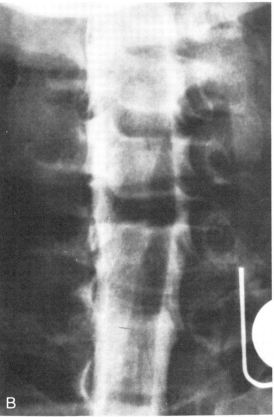

Figure 6–35. Intramedullary astrocytoma. *A*, A lateral projection from a cervical myelogram demonstrates a localized intramedullary lesion expanding the cervical spinal cord and indenting the thecal sac (arrows). The lesion is localized to this region. *B*, Posteroanterior projection in the cervical region shows the localized intramedullary tumor thinning the contrast-filled subarachnoid space.

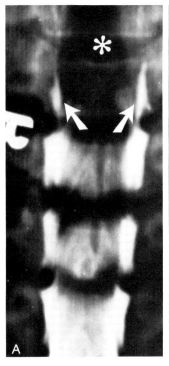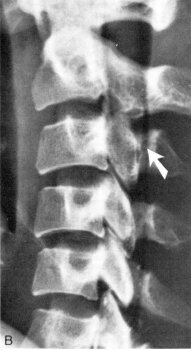

Figure 6–36. Astrocytoma. *A,* Posteroanterior myelogram performed with iophendylate (Pantopaque) demonstrates expansion of the spinal cord (arrows), which causes an almost complete obstruction in the upper cervical region (asterisk). This represents an intramedullary lesion. *B,* Lateral projection during air myelography again demonstrates the expanded cervical cord, which is partially obliterating the circumferential air in the subarachnoid space (arrow). No change in this large mass occurred with change in position or following cerebrospinal fluid drainage. This mass is an astrocytoma.

CTM Findings With Intradural-Intramedullary Lesions

CTM may be used as a complementary examination to demonstrate the occurrence of cysts or syringohydromyelia on immediate or delayed scans, as well as to confirm the presence and location of the intramedullary lesion.[35]

Cord widening is characteristic of intradural-intramedullary lesions. Collections within the cord are observed in some neoplasms immediately or after delays of up to 24 hours[35] (Fig. 6–37). The important finding differentiating the intraspinal collections in tumors from syringohydromyelia is the localized extent of the pooled contrast within the cord. In tumors, the collection does not

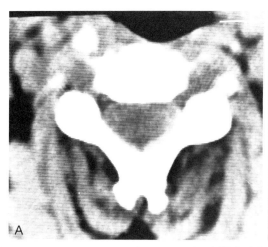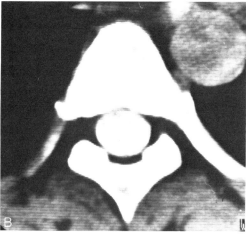

Figure 6–37. Astrocytoma with syrinx. *A,* Axial CTM of the cervical spine. Intramedullary lesion with thinning of the subarachnoid space. *B,* Axial CTM of the thoracic cord. Delay of four hours reveals opacification of a cyst within the spinal cord.

extend over the entire lesion, as it does in syringohydromyelia.[35] The opacification of the cystic cavity in tumors supports the theory of transneural passage of fluid as the etiology of the cyst or cavity.[35] In such cases, syringohydromyelia can be differentiated from tumor only if the opacified cavity occupies the entire extent of the enlarged cord.

In patients with syringohydromyelia, cord enlargement is seen only in a minority of cases (6/64), and in the remainder of cases cord size is either normal or small.[4] In 67 of 75 cases in one series, a central low-density cavity was seen without metrizamide.[4] Cavity opacification with metrizamide was seen by 4 hours in these cases (Fig. 6–38), and 79% of their patients had a Chiari I malformation.[4]

Myelography (Fig. 6–39) or the combined use of myelography and CTM to assess fully lesions seen on myelography with the presence of subarachnoid seeding has been demonstrated in patients with intramedullary tumors. The tumor extension is presumed to occur as a consequence of exophytic growth of the neoplasm to the pia mater and then seeding within the subarachnoid space.

Cord atrophy, which may be focal or diffuse, may also be seen[42] (Figs. 6–40, 6–41).

Intravenous contrast enhancement has been observed in gliomas of the cord as well as in vascular neoplasms or malformations[49] (Fig. 6–42). Spinal cord angiography then aids in visualization of the full extent of vascular lesions.

Intradural-Extramedullary Lesions

An intradural-extramedullary lesion is located in the subarachnoid space situated between the pia mater surrounding the cord and the arachnoid mater (see Fig. 6–34). The abnormality may be dorsal, ventral, lateral, or a combination of these. The most common lesions are meningiomas and neurofibromas. Meningiomas are the most common tumor in this location, composing about one fourth to one half of spinal neoplasms. Meningiomas occur in middle-aged females (50 to 80 years of age) in the dorsal region, although they may reside anywhere in the spinal canal. Neurofibromas make up 10% of spinal tumors and may be located in any portion of the spinal cord. The majority, so-called dumbbell tumors, have an extradural component in addition to the intradural tumor; one fourth are intradural, one sixth are

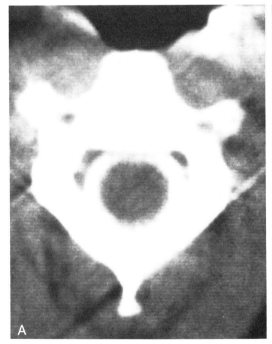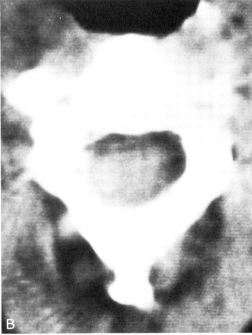

Figure 6–38. Syringohydromyelia. *A*, Axial CTM. The cord has increased dimensions within an enlarged thecal sac in the cervical region. *B*, A 6 hour delayed scan of the same region shows a central opacification, indicating a syrinx.

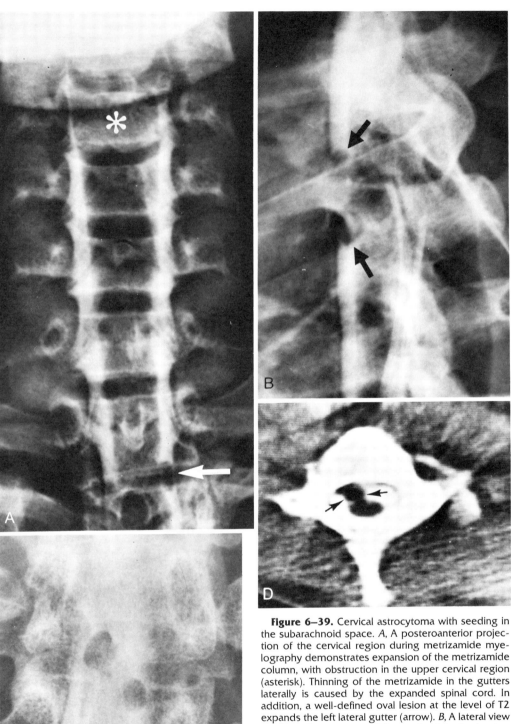

Figure 6–39. Cervical astrocytoma with seeding in the subarachnoid space. *A,* A posteroanterior projection of the cervical region during metrizamide myelography demonstrates expansion of the metrizamide column, with obstruction in the upper cervical region (asterisk). Thinning of the metrizamide in the gutters laterally is caused by the expanded spinal cord. In addition, a well-defined oval lesion at the level of T2 expands the left lateral gutter (arrow). *B,* A lateral view confirms the presence of the ventral intradural-extramedullary lesion (arrows). *C,* An examination at the same time in a posteroanterior projection of the lower thoracolumbar region reveals two well-defined intradural-extramedullary lesions representing subarachnoid seeding. *D,* CTM at the level of the lesion at T2. There is a sharply demarcated intradural-extramedullary lesion situated anterolaterally (arrows) within the subarachnoid space.

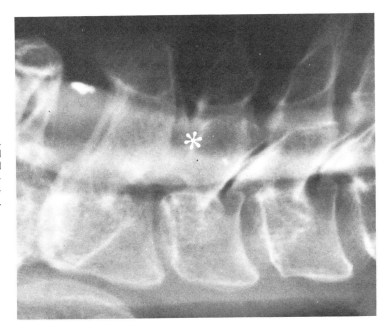

Figure 6–40. Spinal cord atrophy. A lateral projection during cervical myelography demonstrates the small spinal cord within the thecal sac (asterisk). This patient had subacute combined degeneration of the spinal cord.

extradural, and approximately 5% are observed as multiple lesions. Other tumors in this location are uncommon; they consist of metastases arising from the posterior fossa or other spinal neoplasms or from seeding from lung and breast, arachnoid cysts, and vascular malformations.

Myelographic Findings With Intradural-Extramedullary Lesions

In the patient with intradural-extramedullary tumors, the spinal cord is compressed and displaced either dorsally, ventrally, or laterally. The subarachnoid space at the site of the mass is widened, and the opposite side is constricted by the displaced spinal cord, with the overall thecal sac being widened (see Fig. 6–34). Another feature is that the lesion may be sharply etched, with well-defined borders (Figs. 6–43 to 6–45). Tomography may add information by providing greater detail,[33] particularly in the smaller lesion (Fig. 6–43). Calcification may be seen in 45% of meningiomas (Fig. 6–44), and although seen on plain roentgenograms, it is observed with greater clarity during CT.

CTM Findings With Intradural-Extramedullary Lesions

On CTM, the calcification may be obscured by the metrizamide. In many cases,

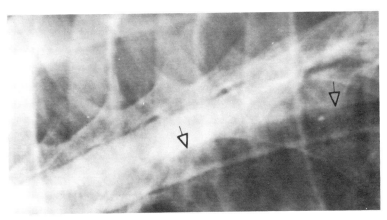

Figure 6–41. Cord atrophy. A single lateral projection of the thoracic region during myelography demonstrates a small, ventrally situated thoracic cord in the spinal canal (arrows).

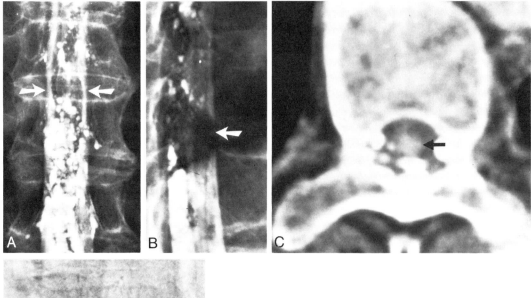

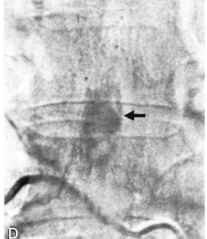

Figure 6–42. Hemangioblastoma. Posteroanterior (*A*) and lateral (*B*) views obtained during metrizamide thoracic myelography reveal a localized intramedullary lesion at the T8–T9 level (arrows). The overlying density is iophendylate (Pantopaque) from a previous myelogram. *C*, Axial CT scan through T9 following intravenous administration of contrast demonstrates contrast enhancement of the lesion (arrow). *D*, Spinal arteriography demonstrates focal nodular contrast enhancement of the tumor (arrow).

Figure 6–43. Meningioma. Postero-anterior (*A*) and lateral (*B*) tomographic projections during metrizamide myelography in the thoracic region demonstrate a well-defined intradural-extramedullary lesion on the left (arrows). Note the widening of the subarachnoid space on the left (asterisk) and the constriction of the contralateral gutter. This is characteristic of an intradural-extramedullary lesion.

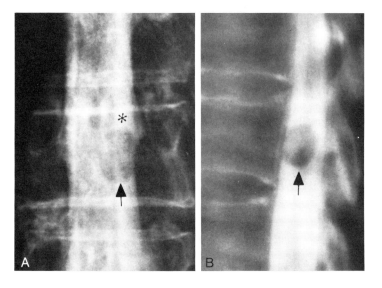

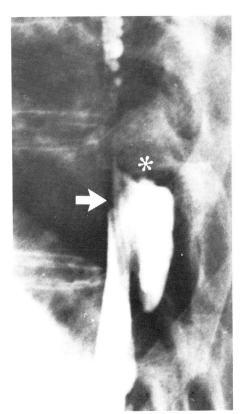

Figure 6–44. Meningioma. Lateral projection during thoracic myelography. A large intradural-extramedullary lesion is arising dorsally but extending toward the ventral surface (asterisk). The lesion itself is partially calcified. Note the forward displacement of the spinal cord by this lesion (arrow).

the appearance of neurofibroma is similar to that of meningiomas (Fig. 6–44, 6–45). Neurofibromas rarely calcify, but they are characterized by dumbbell lesions. These are mass lesions with combined intradural-extramedullary and extradural-extramedullary components (Fig. 6–46). These tumors may affect multiple nerve roots (Fig. 6–46) or may cause abnormalities of the spinal canal, such as enlargement of a neural foramen, scalloping of the vertebral bodies, and erosion or flattening of a pedicle.

The exact location of the lesion, as well as the torsion, rotation, or compression of the spinal cord, will be demonstrated on CTM. If a complete block is present, the upper level is usually visualized because of the sensitivity of CT scanning to contrast material. Any extradural component will be identified (see Fig. 6–44). Calcification, fat, and other soft tissue changes may be appre-

ciated. A dumbbell lesion as well as purely extradural neuromas may be seen.

Extradural Lesions

Those lesions that arise lateral to the thecal sac compose what are called extradural lesions (see Fig. 6–34). The most common lesions in this compartment are spondylotic changes and disc herniations. The most common tumor is metastasis. In 90% of the patients with extradural metastasis, the site of origin is adjacent axial skeleton.[12] The most common metastatic tumors originate from breast, lung, or prostate tumors.

Myelographic Findings With Extradural Lesions

The critical finding is the displacement of the myelographic thecal sac away from adjacent bone in either the posteroanterior or lateral projection. In addition, the circumferential subarachnoid space is constricted bilaterally, but particularly on the side of the lesion (Fig. 6–47). Wrap-around lesions that circumscribe the thecal sac may occur (Fig. 6–48). Metastatic lesions arising in the pelvis may disseminate to involve the lumbosacral region. These lesions may cause constriction of the terminal caudal sac (Fig. 6–49). Lymphoma also produces extradural lesions with bone involvement, but this is less common than metastases. A characteristic of the patient with lymphoma is the extent of the lesion. The lesions are often long. In addition, extensive involvement of paraspinal soft tissues may be present (Fig. 6–50).

Neurofibromas rarely are purely extradural. In some instances, however, this location does occur. Extradural neurofibromas may be distinguished from other extradural lesions by the observation of osseous changes occurring concurrently with the extradural component (Fig. 6–51). These include enlargement of the neural foramen, pedicle erosion, and vertebral body erosion.

Metastatic lesions or lymphoma may extend via hematogenous spread to seed the meninges and cause carcinomatous or lymphomatous meningitis.[39] The inflammation results from diffuse involvement of the meninges or the nerve roots. Enlarged nerve roots

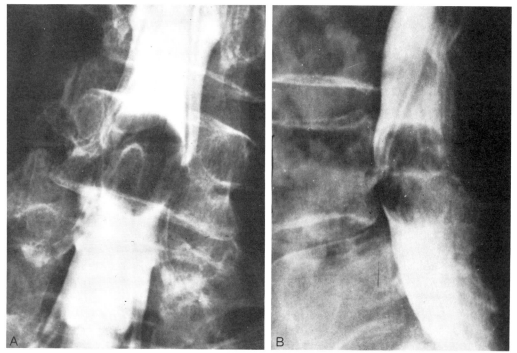

Figure 6–45. Neurofibroma. Posteroanterior *(A)* and lateral *(B)* projections of the lumbar spine after metrizamide myelography demonstrate a large, well-defined, round lesion that is intradural and extramedullary. It displaces nerve roots laterally on the posteroanterior projection and anteriorly on the lateral projection.

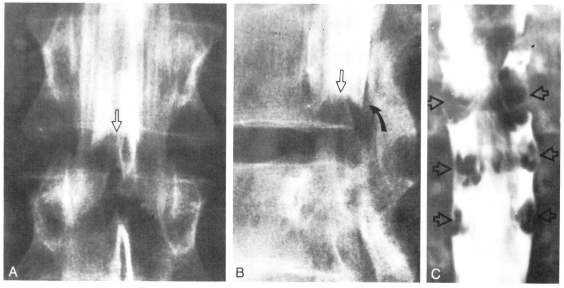

Figure 6–46. Dumbbell neurofibroma and multiple neurofibromas. Posteroanterior *(A)* and lateral *(B)* projections during myelography demonstrate a sharply defined intradural-extramedullary lesion in the lumbar region (straight arrows). In *B*, an extradural component is also present, displacing the thecal sac anteriorly (curved arrow). *C*, Posteroanterior projection of the cervical region reveals multiple neurofibromas of nerve roots (arrows).

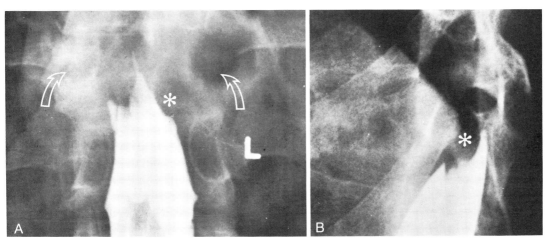

Figure 6–47. Metastasis. Posteroanterior (*A*) and lateral (*B*) projections in the thoracic region of an iophendylate (Pantopaque) myelogram demonstrate the presence of a ventrolateral extradural mass (asterisks). There is vertebral body destruction, sclerosis of the right pedicle and destruction of left pedicle (arrows), and decrease in height of the vertebral body. On both views there is displacement of the thecal sac and spinal cord away from the bone, with thinning of the subarachnoid space. The patient had a primary carcinoma of the kidney.

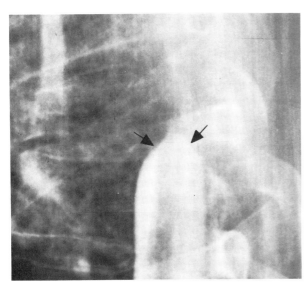

Figure 6–48. Metastasis. A single lateral projection of an iophendylate myelogram demonstrates a circumferential lesion that is causing a complete block in the dorsal region (arrows). Note the destruction of a vertebral body just anterior to the obstruction.

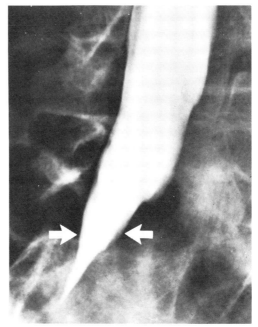

Figure 6–49. Metastasis. A lumbar myelogram in oblique projection demonstrates a tapered, constricted caudal sac due to a circumferential metastatic neoplasm (arrows).

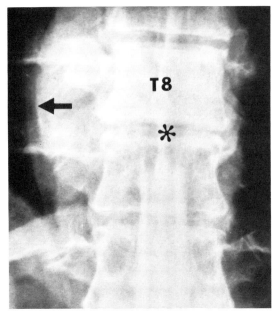

Figure 6–50. Epidural lymphoma. A complete block of the metrizamide column is observed at the upper level of T9 (asterisk). In addition, there is an adjacent paraspinal mass on the right (arrow) and sclerosis of T8.

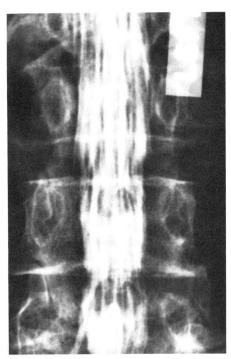

Figure 6–52. Lymphomatous meningitis. A posteroanterior projection of the lumbar region on a metrizamide myelogram demonstrates enlarged, irregular nerve roots caused by lymphoma surrounding the nerve roots.

may be observed with metastatic seeding. The nerve roots are enlarged, thickened, nodular, and irregular (Fig. 6–52). In addition, the clumping of cells within the CSF

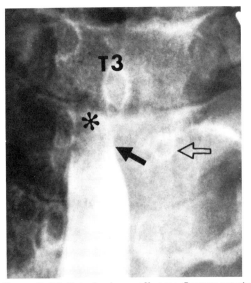

Figure 6–51. Extradural neurofibroma. Posteroanterior myelogram with metrizamide demonstrates a complete block at the upper level of T4 (asterisk), with an extrinsic mass laterally on the left compressing the thecal sac (closed arrow). Note the left pedicle of T4 is hypoplastic (open arrow). The left pedicle of T3 is absent.

may cause a partial block. Delayed studies may demonstrate the slow caudal extension of the contrast material to outline the affected nerve roots of the cauda equina (Fig. 6–53).

Metastases, in addition to being solitary or showing meningeal involvement, may reveal multiple lesions. These lesions may affect various sites or compartments (Fig. 6–54).

Although metastases and lymphoma are the most common tumors in this compartment, other lesions that may occur include neurofibromas (see Fig. 6–51), epidural hematoma, extradural abscess, and lesions arising in bone, such as osteoblastoma, aneurysmal bone cyst, plasmacytoma or myeloma, giant cell tumor, chordoma, Paget's disease, and eosinophilic granuloma (Fig. 6–55).

Vascular Malformations of the Spinal Cord

These lesions arise within the subarachnoid space or, less often, in the extradural compartment. The characteristic myelo-

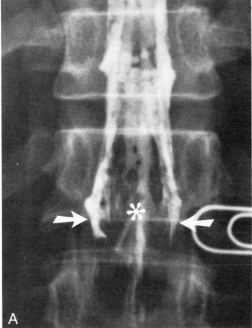

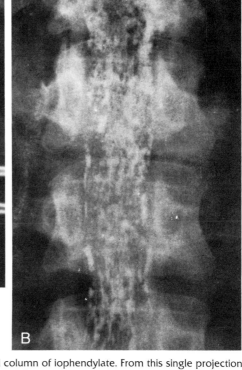

Figure 6–53. Carcinomatous meningitis with complete block. *A,* Posteroanterior projection demonstrates a complete block of the iophendylate (Pantopaque) column at the level of T12–L1 (asterisk). The distal sac is slightly dilated at the level of the block (arrows), with slight irregularity of the distal column of iophendylate. From this single projection one could not be sure whether this was an intramedullary or extradural lesion. *B,* A delayed study demonstrates slow seepage of irregular-appearing iophendylate distally. This is due to tumor occupying the subarachnoid space and surrounding nerve roots. It fills the subarachnoid space predominantly, resembling meningitis. This patient had carcinoma of the lung.

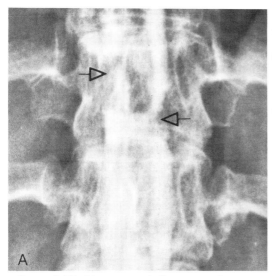

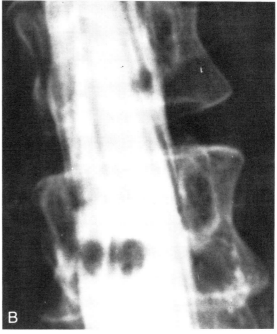

Figure 6–54. Metastases. *A,* Posteroanterior projection in the thoracic region demonstrates extradural lesions indenting the subarachnoid space bilaterally (arrows). *B,* A posteroanterior projection through the upper lumbar region reveals multiple, sharply demarcated, intradural-extramedullary filling defects within the subarachnoid space and along nerve roots. This patient had carcinoma of the breast.

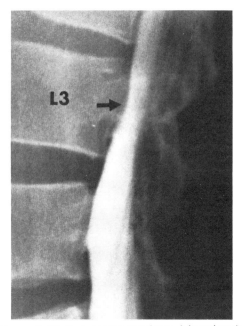

Figure 6–55. Eosinophilic granuloma. A lateral projection from a metrizamide myelogram demonstrates evidence of an extradural ventral defect indenting the thecal sac at the level of L3 (arrow). Note also the destruction of the posterior margin of this vertebral body, compared with the vertebral body below. The destruction was due to eosinophilic granuloma.

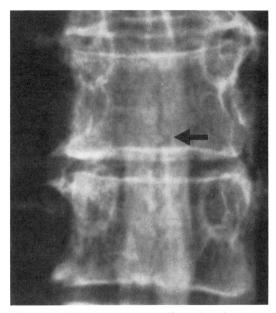

Figure 6–56. Arteriovenous malformation. A posteroanterior projection of the thoracic region obtained during metrizamide myelography demonstrates an enlargement of the artery of Adamkiewicz (arrow).

graphic patterns described are one or two vessels over several segments, a localized nodular component, and a large conglomerate lesion with many feeding and draining vessels over many segments (Figs. 6–56, 6–57).[17] The myelographic examination reveals minimal or marked vascular accentuation. The presence of a vascular malformation and its morphologic configuration are characterized by vascular opacification studies (see Fig. 6–40).

Arachnoiditis

The patterns of abnormalities observed in patients with arachnoiditis do not conform to those found in the previously described three compartments but rather to what has been designated as a fourth compartment. The radiographic appearance is a bizarre lesion or abnormality that may be confused with extra-arachnoidal injection. Obliteration of some or many nerve roots may be observed (the "branchless tree") (Fig. 6–58). In addition, no cord displacement occurs,

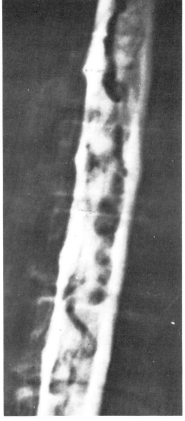

Figure 6–57. Arteriovenous malformation. A posteroanterior projection of the thoracic region obtained during metrizamide myelography demonstrates marked enlargement and tortuosity of arteries and veins.

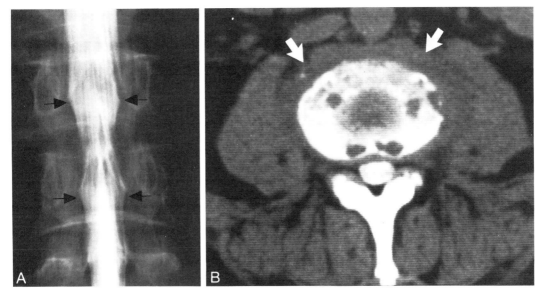

Figure 6–58. Osteomyelitis with arachnoiditis. *A*, Lumbar metrizamide myelogram in posteroanterior projection reveals a branchless tree pattern, paucity of nerve roots (arrows), and a constricted thecal sac. *B*, Axial CTM shows vertebral body osteomyelitis, with lytic defects in the vertebral end-plate and erosions of the osseous margin. A paraspinal mass reflecting infected tissue is also seen (arrows).

although an obstruction may be present. In lesions affecting the three major compartments, the cord is enlarged or displaced.

TRAUMA

The results of trauma may be fully assessed by CT myelography. Following acute cervical trauma, the major abnormalities occur in the osseous structures and the ligaments. The spinal cord nerve roots and meninges are then affected secondarily as a result of these disruptions and distortions.

Traumatic disc rupture may occur, particularly in the cervical region, as a consequence of flexion injuries, with disruption of the interspinous, intralaminar, and posterior longitudinal ligaments. The disc enters the spinal canal because of the traumatic rupture of the posterior longitudinal ligament, particularly at C5–C6 and C6–C7 (see Fig. 6–20).

The occurrence of cystic degeneration within the spinal cord has been reported in patients months to years following a severe spinal cord injury. The patients usually present with new or progressively worsening neurologic symptoms.[60] The majority of lesions occur in the cervical region.[60, 70, 77]

As in syringohydromyelia, although the cord may enlarge, it is often normal in size or occasionally diminished. The cavity or cyst is secondary to hematomyelia, cord hemorrhage, or myelomalacia.[60] The cavity or cyst, which is dorsal in location, fills with contrast up to 4 hours after the myelogram. Traumatic dural tears may be identified on either myelography or CTM, with leakage of contrast into and opacifying the avulsed nerve root sleeve (Fig. 6–59). The compres-

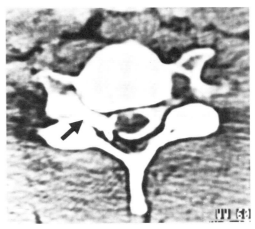

Figure 6–59. Avulsion of the nerve root. Axial CTM reveals disruption of the dura on the right, with avulsion of the nerve root. Metrizamide outlines the nerve and extends into the neural foramen (arrow) and beyond.

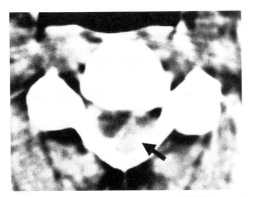

Figure 6–60. Epidural hematoma. Axial CTM reveals a compressed thecal sac displaced by a dense extradural mass, an epidural hematoma (arrow).

sion of the thecal sac may be visualized. These lesions are most commonly seen after motorcycle injuries with trauma to the brachial plexus.

In the acute trauma patient with fracture and neurologic symptoms, CTM may demonstrate the abnormality affecting the thecal sac with presence of extradural lesion as well as any osseous abnormality. Site of a fracture, compromise of spinal canal, presence of bony fragments within the spinal canal, and malalignment may be appreciated using axial CT with reconstruction or reformatting in the coronal and sagittal planes.[95]

The presence and extent of extradural hematoma may be identified (Fig. 6–60). In these cases, an extradural lesion is identified with displacement of the spinal cord. Affected patients present with severe pain that feels like a tearing in the chest and is similar to the pain that develops in a patient with a dissecting aneurysm. The patient often has underlying hypertension and displays acute neurologic deficits.

INFECTION

Inflammatory osteomyelitis of the axial skeleton occurs most commonly in the lumbar spine, and the offending organism is often *Staphylococcus aureus*.[11, 26] The inflammatory changes are the result of hematogenous spread from an inflammatory focus elsewhere or via pelvic veins from inflammatory processes within the pelvis. Drug abusers are often affected. The site of involvement is the vertebral end-plate, with eventual erosion of the cortical bone and involvement of the disc space. Progressive

destruction of the vertebra occurs, with later compression or collapse. Although the diagnosis may be made with nuclear scan, plain roentgenograms, and myelography, the CT scan provides precise anatomic information. An accurate image of the entire process, including the vertebral body, the paraspinal tissues, and the epidural space, is possible only with CT (see Fig. 6–58). Myelography is nonspecific, in that either a pattern similar to arachnoiditis (the "branchless tree"; see Figs. 6–28, 6–58) or occasionally an epidural abscess is seen (Fig. 6–61). These myelographic patterns, in addition to the bony abnormalities, permit an accurate diagnosis.

Discitis or spondylitis, although not an uncommon process, is confined to the vertebral end-plate or disc space or both and is often not diagnosed. Thinning of the disc space occurs, as well as erosion with or without sclerosis of the vertebral end-plate with sparing of the vertebral body. These lesions are also often accompanied by paraspinal mass that is detected only on CT.

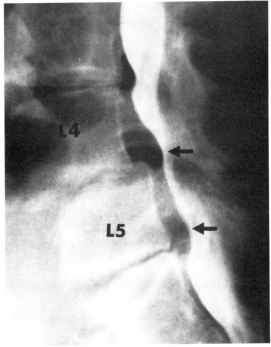

Figure 6–61. Epidural abscess. Lateral projection during metrizamide myelography demonstrates a large, ventral, extradural lesion adjacent to L4 and L5, displacing the thecal sac posteriorly (arrows). There is obliteration of the L4–L5 disc space, with destruction of the apposing vertebral margins. First degree spondylolisthesis is also noted at the L4–L5 level.

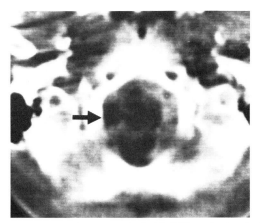

Figure 6–62. Cysticercosis. Axial CTM at the level of the foramen magnum. Numerous large and small oval, sharply defined, intradural-extramedullary cysts are seen (arrow).

The most likely diagnosis is infection, but recovery of organisms with biopsy is uncommon. In some instances the changes may be secondary to trauma and reflect aseptic necrosis.

Tuberculous spondylitis or osteomyelitis occurs more commonly in the thoracic and lumbar portions of the spine. In affected patients, the anterior portion of the body and disc space are involved, sparing the posterior elements. There is often significant paraspinal disease with psoas abscesses that may calcify. Lytic destructive changes in the vertebral body are common, but sclerosis is unusual. Accompanying kyphosis and scoliosis reflect the loss in vertical height of single or multiple vertebral bodies.

In patients with cysticerosis, subarachnoid lesions are observed in the spinal canal. These may cause well-defined defects within the subarachnoid space (Fig. 6–62) that are identical to other processes that may seed within the subarachnoid space, such as inflammatory, granulomatous, and metastatic processes.

In patients with acquired immune deficiency syndrome (AIDS) and in other immunocompromised patients, a variety of unusual inflammatory lesions of the spinal canal are observed, much like observations elsewhere in the body.

PEDIATRIC MYELOGRAPHY

Although the myelographic appearance of lesions in children corresponds to that in adults, the diseases affecting the pediatric spine differ. In the majority of cases, myelography is required for investigation of the lumbar region for dysraphism, with possible tethered cord. Lumbar puncture in these cases entails a risk of damaging the low-lying spinal cord (Fig. 6–63); therefore, the needle should be positioned laterally in the thecal sac.[56] The thecal sac is often wide in the dysraphic spine, facilitating lateral puncture.[52] Even when the spinal cord is inadvertently punctured, injury is uncommon,[29] or perhaps it is masked by any neurologic deficit that is present.[56] The frequent association of the various anomalies with tonsillar herniation (Fig. 6–64) precludes routine use of lateral C1–C2 puncture for contrast injection.[57]

General anesthesia is mandatory for all children age 6 years or younger and for most children up to age 12.[57] If the study can be limited to a specific level, CTM may be performed following sedation without gen-

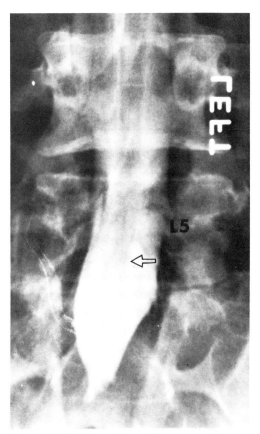

Figure 6–63. Tethered cord. A metrizamide myelogram in posteroanterior projection demonstrates the low position of the spinal cord (arrow) in the subarachnoid space.

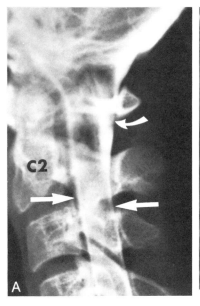
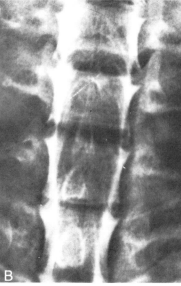

Figure 6–64. Chiari malformation and hydromyelia. *A,* A lateral projection during metrizamide myelography demonstrates evidence of tonsillar ectopia to the level of C2 (curved arrow). It is manifested by a posterior soft tissue mass that is intradural and extramedullary. In addition, there is marked expansion of the spinal cord, with thinning of anterior and posterior gutters from syringohydromyelia (straight arrows). *B,* A posteroanterior projection confirms the expansion of the spinal cord within the thecal sac, with thinning of lateral gutters.

eral anesthesia.[57] In the child small enough for proper orientation in the scanner gantry, direct coronal or sagittal computed tomographic metrizamide scanning may demonstrate large areas of the spinal column, obviating the need for full-dose myelography.

Dysraphism

The dysraphic disorders studied constitute a spectrum of abnormalities relating to fusion defects of the embryologic neural tube. Endoderm, mesoderm, and ectoderm interact to form the cord and its coverings, giving rise to many pathologic permutations. Ultrasonography should be the first radiographic study after plain films in patients suspected of dysraphism,[46, 50, 62, 73] because the lack of bone reduces the interference to ultrasonography noted in the intact spine. Metrizamide myelography and CTM are then performed for full preoperative anatomic definition.[50]

Extensive reviews[51, 57] form the basis for the following discussion. In 110 cases of dysraphism studied by CTM,[57] 10% demonstrated only the vertebral body fusion defects. In 2% of cases, findings were limited to a widened thecal sac and spinal canal. The remaining 88% included vertebral body fusion defects, a widened thecal sac, and combinations of the following (in order of frequency): tethered cord with thick filum

terminale, lipomatous tissue (Fig. 6–65), myelomeningocele, diastematomyelia (Fig. 6–66), syringohydromyelia (Fig. 6–64), and Chiari malformation (Figs. 6–64, 6–67). Rare events included neurenteric cysts, lipoma, dermoid, teratoma, and arachnoid cyst. The severity of the osseous abnormality did not correlate with the neurologic defect.

The vertebral body defects seen in dysraphism can be suspected at an earlier age than fusion would normally occur because the vertebral arches are everted, not encircling the canal.

The distal end of the conus is at or above the L2–L3 level in infants, and at or above the L1–L2 level by age 12. A cord extending lower may be tethered by a thick (greater than 2 mm) filum terminale or by a lipomyelomeningocele.

A meningocele contains only dura and arachnoid that herniates dorsally into the subcutaneous tissue. In myelocele, neural elements (the placode) are exposed on the skin, whereas in myelomeningocele the dilated subarachnoid space pushes the exposed neural tissue above the surface of the skin.

Lipomatous tissue is frequently associated with a myelomeningocele, resulting in a lipomyelomeningocele. Incorrect fusion of the fetal neural tube induces adjacent mesenchyme to form fat. This occurs most often at the level of the tethered conus. CTM demonstrates the relationship of the neural elements in the placode to the adjacent lipo-

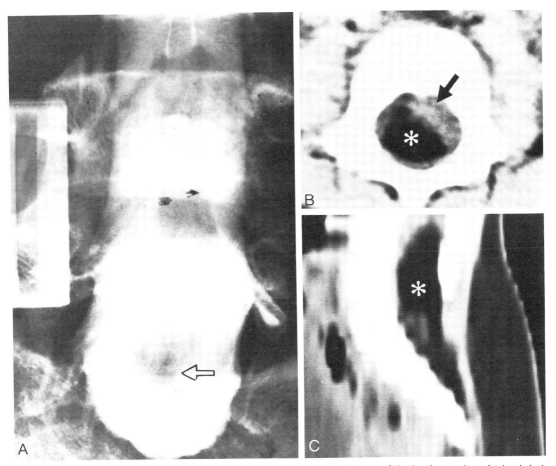

Figure 6–65. Tethered spinal cord with lipoma. *A*, Posteroanterior projection of the lumbar region obtained during myelography demonstrates the presence of a spinal cord extending caudally to the sacral region (arrow). In addition, the spinal cord appears to be slightly thicker than one would expect. The thecal sac is enlarged. *B*, A noncontrast axial CT section through the lower lumbar region demonstrates a large low-density area representing a lipoma (asterisk). This accounts for the apparent partial enlargement of the spinal cord on myelography. Along the left side of this lipoma is a slightly hyperdense, half-moon–shaped conus (arrow). *C*, A reformatted image in the sagittal plane demonstrates the low-density lipoma occupying a large portion of the lumbar spinal canal (asterisk).

matous tissue. The most cephalic, widely bifid vertebral lamina is at the level of the fibrous band tethering the placode. This band also notches the superior surface of the meningocele. Preoperative radiographic dissection of this anatomy is essential to proper resection of the fibrous band and lipomatous tissue without injury to the placode and the associated nerve roots.[52]

Lipomas also occur intradurally, usually at thoracic or cervical levels. They are intimately attached to the cord, with extramedullary extension at the upper or lower pole. Only mild dysraphic osseous changes are present.

Diastematomyelia indicates a sagittal division of the cord into two unequal halves separated by fibrous material or an osteocartilaginous spur (see Fig. 6–66).

Cyst formation in the cord and dilatation of the central canal cannot be easily distinguished even with pathologic examination; therefore syringohydromyelia is the appropriate descriptive term.

CTM demonstrates entry of contrast agent into the cyst, either directly through a patent obex or by diffusion through the cyst wall. This is best seen with scanning 4 or 5 hours after contrast injection (see Fig. 6–38). The cyst commonly occurs in the cervical or thoracic region but may extend the entire length of the cord. Scanning must include the cervico-occipital junction if one is searching for the ectopic tonsils of a Chiari I malformation (see Figs. 6–64, 6–67).

The rare split notochord syndrome results from a persistent connection through the notochord between the gut and the skin. Parts of the connection disappear, but cysts may remain adjacent to the bowel (enteric duplications), between bowel and spine (neurenteric cysts), or between spine and skin (postvertebral enteric cysts). A fistulous connection may occur between gut and the dorsal skin that is rarely complicated by herniation of bowel.

Uncommon persistent connection between ectoderm and neurectoderm leads to dermal sinuses, varying from the innocuous pilonidal cyst to an intradural dermoid or epidermoid mass.

In all the lesions just described, metrizamide myelography combined with CTM will delineate the relationship between abnormalities of the cord, thecal sac, vertebral bodies, and adjacent cutaneous or deep lesions that may be present in the dysraphic spine.

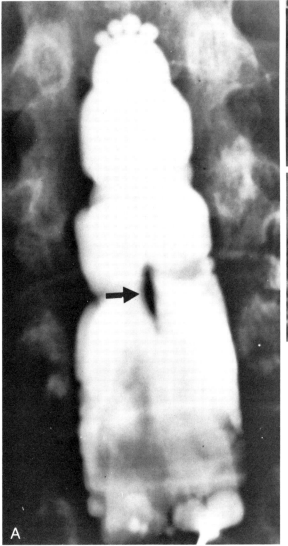

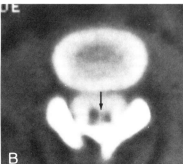

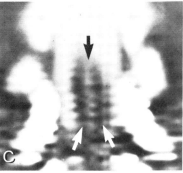

Figure 6–66. Diastematomyelia. *A,* A posteroanterior projection during myelography demonstrates a defect (septum) within the center of the opacified thecal sac (arrow). The subarachnoid space is dilated. *B,* Axial CTM demonstrates the presence of the septum (arrow), with two adjacent hemicords within the thecal sac. *C,* A reformatted coronal CTM projection demonstrates the central septum (black arrow) with the two adjacent hemicords (white arrows).

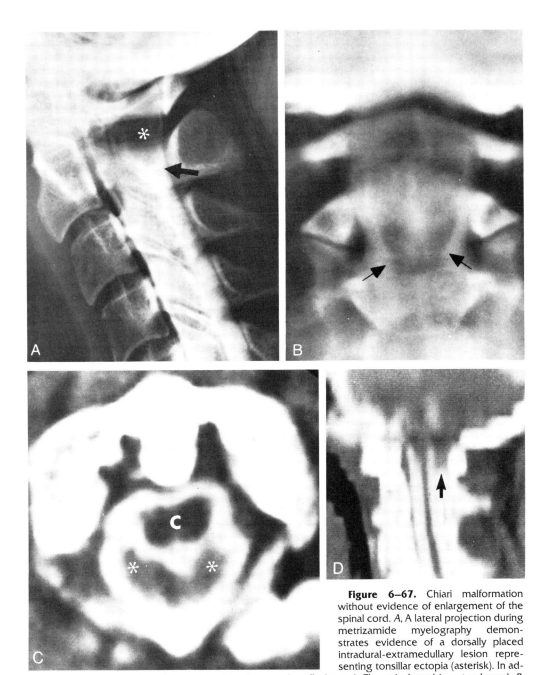

Figure 6–67. Chiari malformation without evidence of enlargement of the spinal cord. *A,* A lateral projection during metrizamide myelography demonstrates evidence of a dorsally placed intradural-extramedullary lesion representing tonsillar ectopia (asterisk). In addition, note the expansion of the subarachnoid space dorsally (arrow). The spinal cord is not enlarged. *B,* A tomographic section in posteroanterior projection obtained at the same time demonstrates local expansion of the thecal sac and the bi-lobed tonsillar ectopia (arrows). *C,* Axial CTM at the level of the odontoid process reveals tonsillar ectopia (asterisks) lying within the subarachnoid space posterior to the cervical cord (**c**). *D,* A reformatted sagittal image shows the extent of the tonsillar ectopia (arrow) below the foramen magnum.

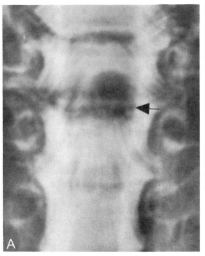

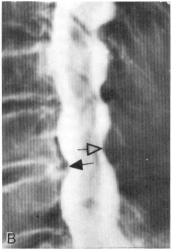

Figure 6–68. Spurious defect. Spondylosis and ligament hypertrophy. *A,* On the posteroanterior projection of the cervical region, a sharply demarcated, oval intradural-extramedullary lesion is apparent (arrow). *B,* On lateral projection of the same area, no intradural-extramedullary lesion is seen, but spurs arising from the vertebral body posteriorly (closed arrow) as well as ligamentous hypertrophy posteriorly (open arrow) indent the subarachnoid space, producing the spurious defect seen in part *A.*

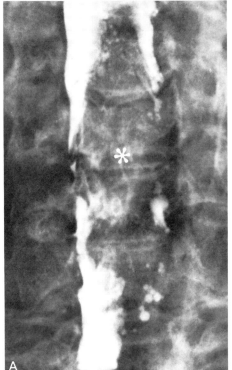

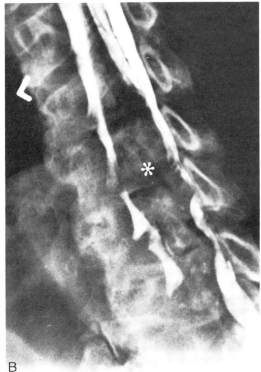

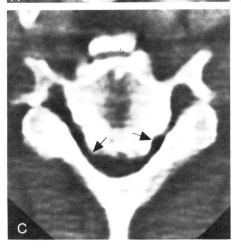

Figure 6–69. Spurious defect. Hypertrophy of the posterior longitudinal ligament. Anteroposterior (*A*) and oblique (*B*) views of the cervical region taken during an iophendylate (Pantopaque) myelogram demonstrate what appears to be a long intramedullary lesion, with marked expansion of the spinal cord in both the anterior and oblique planes (asterisks). Examination of a lateral projection was not entirely satisfactory, though it raised the question of an extradural lesion. *C,* Axial computed tomographic section through the cervical region at the site of the apparent cord widening demonstrates the presence of a narrow canal caused by extensive hypertrophy of the posterior longitudinal ligament (arrows). The apparent cord widening seen in parts *A* and *B* resulted from compression of the spinal cord by the long extradural lesion.

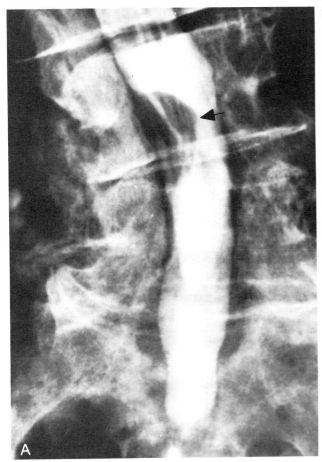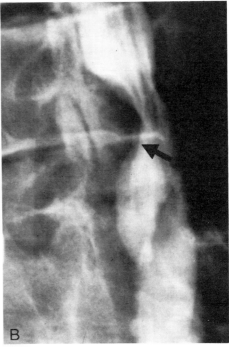

Figure 6–70. Spurious defect. Herniated disc simulating a subarachnoid lesion. *A*, Posteroanterior projection during lumbar myelography demonstrates a sharply demarcated lesion overlying L4 (arrow) but extending over the disc space on the right on this projection. It certainly looks like an intradural extramedullary lesion situated to the right. *B*, On the oblique projection, the profile view, one can observe that the lesion is purely extradural, displacing the thecal sac away from the bone (arrow), and is not an intradural-extramedullary lesion. This actually represents an extruded disc that has extended cephalad.

TECHNICAL ERRORS, MISINTERPRETATIONS, AND SPURIOUS DEFECTS

The spinal canal is in fact a small space, and consequently a variety of spurious lesions, as well as technical errors and misinterpretations, may occur.

The technical artifact may be the result of improper placement of the contrast material[12, 55] (see Figs. 6–1, 6–2).

A spurious defect may occur because of indentation of the thecal sac by ligamentous thickening and vertebral body spurs that may simulate an intradural-extramedullary lesion (Fig. 6–68). A similar problem may occur from an extradural process that is quite extensive and that, without good profile roentgenograms, may simulate a lesion in another compartment (Figs. 6–69, 6–70).

Lesions may be misinterpreted if details that are present on the roentgenograms are overlooked. In one instance in our experience, a long ventral epidural metastatic lesion resulted in constriction of the thecal sac, thus simulating a narrow spinal canal (Fig. 6–71); in another instance, a ventrolateral metastasis simulated a herniated disc (Fig. 6–72). The distinguishing features in the latter case were the length of the lesion, the shape, and particularly the sparing of the nerve root by an extradural mass.

Finally, conjoined nerve roots on CT may simulate a lateral disc[32] (Fig. 6–73). The differential features include the difference in densities of root and disc, the presence of slight enlargement of the subarticular gutter with slight posterolateral erosion or compression of the vertebral body, the absence of the nerve root at the level above the

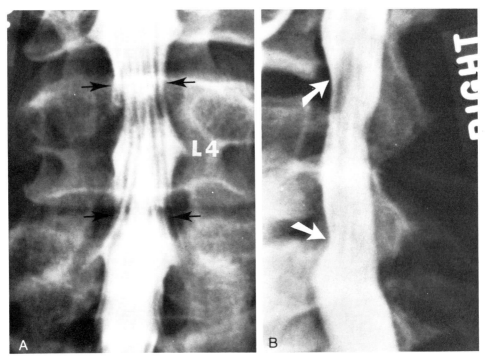

Figure 6–71. Spurious defect. Epidural metastasis simulating a narrow canal. *A,* Anteroposterior projection demonstrates evidence of localized narrowing of the thecal sac from the lower level of L3 though the upper level of L5 (arrows). No nerve root cutoff is seen, though the nerve roots appear to be slightly swollen. *B,* The lateral projection reveals a large extradural ventral defect (arrows) with shelflike defects noted superiorly and inferiorly. In this case, the extradural lesion compressed the thecal sac and gave an appearance of spinal stenosis, although the actual constriction was caused by an epidural metastasis.

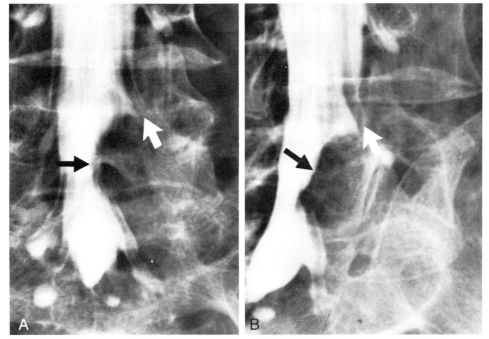

Figure 6–72. Spurious lesion. Metastatic lesion that appears similar to a disc. *A,* On the posteroanterior projection, a left lateral defect indents the thecal sac (black arrow). There is elevation and cutoff of the L5 nerve root (white arrow). The defect was thought to be due to an extruded disc. *B,* On the oblique projection, the defect (black arrow) and the cutoff of the nerve root (white arrow) are again noted. The slight irregularity and length of the lesion suggest that it is more likely an extradural neoplasm than a true extradural sequestered disc.

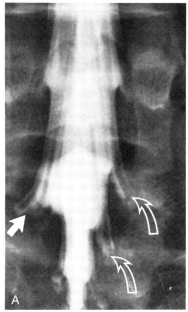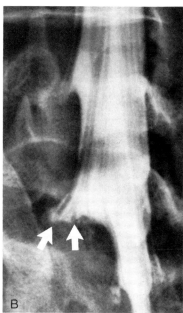

Figure 6–73. Conjoined nerve roots. *A,* Metrizamide myelogram, posteroanterior projection. On the right, the S1 and S2 roots emerge at the same site (straight arrow). On the contralateral side, one can see the separate roots at two levels (curved arrows). *B,* An oblique projection to the right demonstrates the two roots in the same sleeve (arrows).

conjoined nerve root, and the ability with thin slices from high-resolution scanners to observe nerve roots in greater detail to avoid this error.

References

1. Ahn HS, Rosenbaum AE: Lumbar myelography with metrizamide. Supplementary technique. AJR 136:547–551, 1981.
2. Alenghat JP, Hallett M, Kido DK: Spinal cord compression in diffuse idiopathic skeletal hyperostosis. Radiology 142:119–120, 1982.
3. Anand AK, Lee BC: Plain and metrizamide CT of lumbar disc disease: Comparison with myelography. AJNR 3:567–571, 1982.
4. Aubin ML, Vignaud J, Jardin C, et al: Computed tomography in 75 clinical cases of syringomyelia. AJNR 2:199–204, 1981.
5. Balériaux D, Noterman J, Ticket L: Recognition of cervical soft disc herniation by contrast-enhanced CT. AJNR 4:607–608, 1983.
6. Boijsen E: The cervical spinal canal in intraspinal expansive processes. Acta Radiol 42:101–115, 1954.
7. Bonafé A, Ethier R, Melacon D, et al: High-resolution computed tomography in cervical syringomyelia. J Comput Assist Tomogr 4:42–47, 1980.
8. Bradac GB: The value of gas myelography in the diagnosis of syringomyelia. Neuroradiology 4:41–45, 1972.
9. Braun IF, Hoffman JC, Davis PC, et al: Contrast enhancement in CT differentiation between recurrent disc herniation and prospective post-operative scar: Prospective study. AJNR 6:607–612, 1985.
10. Braun IF, Lin JP, Benjamin MV, et al: Computed tomography of the asymptomatic post surgical lumbar spine. Analysis of the physiological scar. AJR 142:149–152, 1984.
11. Burke DR, Brant-Zawadzki M: CT of pyogenic spine infection. Neuroradiology 27:131–137, 1985.
12. Burrows E, Leeds NE: Neuroradiology. New York: Churchill Livingstone, 1981.
13. Burton CL, Kirkaldy-Willis WH, Yong-Hing K, et al: Causes of failure of surgery on the lumbar spine. Clin Orthop 157:191–199, 1981.
14. Ciric I, Mikhael MA, Tarkington JA, et al: The lateral recess syndrome: A variant of spinal stenosis. J Neurosurg 53:433–443, 1980.
15. Coventry MB, Ghormley RK, Kernohan JW: The intervertebral disc: Its microscopic anatomy and pathology: II. Changes in the intervertebral disc concomitant with age. J Bone Joint Surg 27:233–247, 1945.
16. Cronquist S: The post-operative myelogram. Acta Radiol 52:45–51, 1959.
16a. Cronqvist SE, Holtas SL, Laike T, et al: Psychic changes following myelography with metrizamide and iohexol. Acta Radiol [Diagn] 25:369–373, 1984.
17. DiChiro G, Wener L: Angiography of the spinal cord. A review of contemporary techniques and applications. J Neurosurg 39:1–29, 1973.
17a. Drayer BP, Vassallo C, Sudilovsky A, et al: A double-blind clinical trial of iopamidol versus metrizamide for lumbosacral myelography. J Neurosurg 58:531–537, 1983.
17b. Drayer BP, Warner MA, Sudilovsky A, et al: Iopamidol versus metrizamide: A double-blind study for cervical myelography. Neuroradiology 24:77–84, 1982.
18. Dublin AB, McGahan JP, Reid MH: The value of computed tomographic metrizamide myelography in the neuroradiological evaluation of the spine. Radiology 146:79–86, 1983.
19. Ekholm SE, Reece K, Coleman JR, et al: Metrizamide. A potential in vivo inhibitor of glucose metabolism. Radiology 147:119–121, 1983.

20. Epstein BS, Epstein JA, Jones MD: Cervical spinal stenosis. Radiol Clin North Am. 15:215–226, 1977.
21. Epstein BS, Epstein JA, Jones MD: Lumbar spinal stenosis. Radiol Clin North Am 15:227–239, 1977.
22. Epstein JA: Spondylosis in the elderly. Contemp Neurosurg 5(19):1–6, 1983.
23. Firooznia H, Benjamin V, Kricheff II, et al: CT of lumbar spine disc herniation: Correlation with surgical findings. AJNR 5:91–96, 1984.
24. Fox AJ, Viñuela FV, Debrun GM: Complete myelography with metrizamide. AJNR 2:79–84, 1981.
25. Fries JW, Abodeely DA, Vijungco JG, et al: Computed tomography of herniated and extruded nucleus pulposus. J Comput Assist Tomogr 6:874–887, 1982.
25a. Gabrielsen TO, Gebarski SS, Knake JE, et al: Iohexol versus metrizamide for lumbar myelography: Double-blind trial. AJNR 5:181–183, 1984.
25b. Galle G, Huk W, Arnold K: Psychopathometric demonstration and quantification of mental disturbances following myelography with metrizamide and iopamidol. Neuroradiology 26:229–233, 1984.
26. Golimbu C, Firooznia H, Rafii M: CT of osteomyelitis of the spine. AJNR 4:1207–1211, 1983.
27. Hacker DA, Latchaw RE, Yock DH Jr, et al: Redundant lumbar nerve root syndrome: Myelographic features. Radiology 143:457–461, 1982.
28. Hansen EB, Fahrenkrug A, Praestholm J: Late meningeal effects of myelographic contrast media with special reference to metrizamide. Br J Radiol 5:321–327, 1978.
29. Harwood-Nash DCF, Fitz CR: Neuroradiological techniques and indications in infancy and childhood. In Kaufman HJ (ed): Progress in Pediatric Radiology. Vol. 5: Skull, Spine, and Contents. Basel: S. Karger, 1976, pp 2–85.
30. Hauge O, Falkenberg H: Neuropsychologic reactions and other side effects after metrizamide myelography. AJNR 3:229–232, 1982.
30a. Haughton VM, Ho KC: Arachnoiditis from myelography with iopamidol, metrizamide and iocarmate compared in the animal model. Invest Radiol 15:S267–S269, 1980.
30b. Haughton VM, Ho KC, Lipman BT: Experimental study of arachnoiditis from iohexol, an investigational nonionic aqueous contrast medium. AJNR 3:375–377, 1982.
31. Haughton VM, Syvertsen A, Williams AL: Soft tissue anatomy within the spinal canal as seen on computed tomography. Radiology 134:649–655, 1980.
32. Helms CA, Dorwart RH, Gray M: The CT appearance of conjoined nerve roots and differentiation for a herniated nucleus pulposus. Radiology 144:803–807, 1982.
33. Holder JC, Binet EF: Metrizamide myelography with complex-motion tomography. Radiology 145:201–202, 1982.
33a. Hopkins RM, Adams MD, Lau DHM, et al: Ioglucomide: A new nonionic myelographic agent: Preclinical studies. Radiology 140:713, 1981.
34. Jacobaeus HC: On insufflation of air into the spinal canal for diagnostic purposes in cases of tumor of the spinal canal. Acta Med Scand 55:555–564, 1921.
35. Kan S, Fox AJ, Viñuela F, et al: Delayed CT metrizamide enhancement of syringomyelia secondary to tumor. AJNR 4:73–78, 1983.
35a. Kerber CW, Sovak M, Ranganathan RS, et al: Iotrol,

a new myelographic agent: 1. Radiography, CT, CSF clearance, and brain penetration. AJNR 4:317–318, 1983.
36. Khan A, Marc JA, Cher M, et al: Total myelography with metrizamide through the lumbar route. AJR 136:771–776, 1981.
37. Kieffer SA, Sherry RG, Wellerstein DE, et al: Bulging lumbar intervertebral disk: Myelographic differentiation for herniated disk with nerve root compression. AJNR 3:51–58, 1982.
38. Killebrew K, Whaley RA, Hayward JN, et al: Complications of metrizamide myelography. Arch Neurol 40:78–80, 1983.
39. Kim KS, Ho SU, Weinberg PE, et al: Spinal leptomeningeal infiltration by systemic cancer: Myelographic features. AJR 139:361–365, 1982.
40. Lee YY, Glass JP, Wallace S.: Myelography in cancer patients: Modified technique. AJNR 6:617–621, 1985.
41. Marder E, O'Neil M, Grossman RI, et al: Cholinergic actions of metrizamide. AJNR 4:61–65, 1983.
42. Mawad ME, Hilal SK, Fetell MR, et al: Patterns of spinal cord atrophy by metrizamide CT. AJNR 4:611–613, 1983.
43. McNab I: Negative disc exploration. J Bone Joint Surg 53:892–903, 1971.
44. Meyer JD, Latchaw RE, Roppolo HM, et al: Computed tomography and myelography of the postoperative lumbar spine. AJNR 3:223–228, 1982.
45. Mikhael MA, Ciric I, Tarkington JA, et al: Neuroradiological evaluation of lateral recess syndrome. Radiology 140:97–107, 1981.
46. Miller JH, Reid BS, Kemberling CR: Utilization of ultrasound in the evaluation of spinal dysraphism in children. Radiology 143:737–740, 1982.
47. Miyasake K, Karede K, Ito T, et al: Ossification of spinal ligaments causing thoracic radiculomyelopathy. Radiology 143:463–468, 1982.
48. Monajati A, Spitzer RM, Weinstein MA: Supine oblique metrizamide lumbar radiculography. Radiology 145:540–541, 1982.
48a. Muetzel W, Speck W: Pharmacochemical profile of iopromide. AJNR 4:350–352, 1983.
49. Nagagawa H, Huang YP, Malis LI, et al: Computed tomography of intraspinal and paraspinal neoplasms. J Comput Assist Tomogr 1:377–390, 1977.
50. Naidich TP: Evaluation of spinal dysraphism. Syllabus for the Categorical Course of Neuroradiology 1983. American College of Radiology, 1983, pp 174–183.
51. Naidich TP, McLone DG, Harwood-Nash DCF: Spinal dysraphism. Newton TH, Potts DG (eds): In Computed Tomography of the Spine and Spinal Cord. San Anselmo, CA: Clavadel Press, 1983, pp 299–353.
52. Naidich TP, McLone DG, Mutluer S: A new understanding of dorsal dysraphism with lipoma (lipomyeloschisis). AJNR 4:103–116, 1983.
53. Ono M, Russell WJ, Kudo S, et al: Ossification of the thoracic posterior longitudinal ligament in a fixed population. Radiology 143:469–474, 1982.
54. Orrison WW, Eldevik OP, Sackett JF: Lateral C1–2 puncture for cervical myelography. Part III: Historical, anatomical and technical considerations. Radiology 146:401–408, 1983.
55. Orrison WW, Sackett JF, Amundsen P: Lateral C1–2 puncture for cervical myelography. Part II. Recognition of improper injection of contrast material. Radiology 146:395–400, 1983.
56. Pettersson H, Fitz CR, Harwood-Nash DCF, et al:

Adverse reactions to myelography with metrizamide in infants, children and adolescents. Acta Radiol [Diagn] 23(3B):331–335, 1982.

57. Pettersson H, Harwood-Nash DCF: CT and Myelography of the Spine and Cord. Techniques, Anatomy and Pathology in Children. Berlin: Springer-Verlag, 1982.

58. Pettersson H, Harwood-Nash DCF, Fitz CR, et al: Conventional myelography (MM) and computed tomographic metrizamide myelography (CTMM) in scoliosis. Radiology 142:111–114, 1982.

59. Poser CM: The relationship between syringomyelia and neoplasm. In American Lecture Series No. 262. American Lectures in Neurology. Springfield, Illinois: Charles C Thomas, 1956.

60. Quencer RM, Green BA, Eismont FJ: Post-traumatic spinal cord cysts: Clinical features and characterization with metrizamide computed tomography. Radiology 146:415–423, 1983.

61. Quencer RM, Tenner M, Rothman L: The Postoperative myelogram. Radiology 123:667–679, 1977.

62. Raghavendra BN, Epstein FJ, Pinto RS, et al: The tethered spinal cord: Diagnosis by high-resolution real-time ultrasound. Radiology 149:123–128, 1983.

63. Ramsey GH, French JD, Strain WH: Iodinated organic compounds as contrast media for radiographic diagnoses: Pantopaque myelography. Radiology 43:226–240, 1944.

64. Ramsey RG, Penn RD: Computed tomography of a false post-operative meningocele. AJNR 5:326–328, 1984.

65. Raskin SP, Keating JW: Recognition of lumbar disc disease: Comparison of myelography and computed tomography. AJNR 3:215–221, 1982.

66. Resnick D, Guerra J Jr, Robinson CA, et al: Association of diffuse idiopathic skeletal hyperostosis (DISH) and calcification and ossification of the posterior longitudinal ligament. AJR 131:1049–1053, 1978.

67. Rice JF, Bathia AL: Lateral C1–2 puncture for myelography: Posterior approach. Radiology 132:760–762, 1979.

68. Risius B, Modic MT, Hardy RW Jr, et al: Sector computed tomographic spine scanning in the diagnosis of lumbar nerve root entrapment. Radiology 143:109–114, 1982.

69. Rosenbloom S, Cohen WA, Marshall C, et al: Imaging factors influencing spine and cord measurements by CT: A phantom study. AJNR 4:646–649, 1983.

70. Rossier AB, Foo D, Naheedy MH, et al: Radiography of posttraumatic syringomyelia. AJNR 4:637–640, 1983.

71. Russell EJ, D'Angelo CM, Zimmerman RD, et al: Cervical disk herniation: CT demonstration after contrast enhancement. Radiology 152:703–712, 1984.

72. Russell EJ, Pinto RS, Kricheff II: Supine metrizamide myelography: Technique for achieving excellent visualization of the thoracic cord and conus medullaris. Radiology 135:227–228, 1980.

73. Scheible W, James HE, Leopold GR, et al: Occult spinal dysraphism in infants: Screening with high-resolution real-time ultrasound. Radiology 146:743–746, 1983.

74. Schubiger O, Valavaris A: CT differentiation between recurrent disc herniation and post-operative scar formation: The value of contrast enhancement. Neuroradiology 22:251–254, 1980.

75. Schubiger O, Valavaris A: A post-operative lumbar CT: Technique, results, and indications. AJNR 4:595–597, 1983.

76. Seibert CE, Barnes JE, Driesbach JN: Accurate CT measurement of the spinal cord using metrizamide: Physical factors. AJR 136:777–780, 1981.

77. Seibert CE, Driesbach JN, Swanson WB, et al: Progressive post traumatic cystic myelopathy: Neuroradiologic evaluation. AJNR 2:115–120, 1981.

78. Shapiro, R: Myelography. 3rd ed. Chicago: Year Book Medical Publishers, 1975.

79. Sicard JA, Forestier JE: Méthode générale d'exploration radiologique par l'huile iodée (Lipiodol). Bull Mem Soc Med Paris 46:463–469, 1922.

80. Skalpe IO: Adhesive arachnoiditis following lumbar radiculography with water soluble contrast agents. Radiology 121:647–651, 1976.

81. Skalpe IO, Amundsen P: Lumbar radiculography with metrizamide, a non-ionic water soluble contrast medium. Radiology 115:91–95, 1975.

82. Solti-Bohman L, Bentson JR: Comparative advantages of small- and large-dose metrizamide myelograph. AJR 141:825–828, 1983.

83. Sortland O, Skalpe IO: Cervical myelography by lateral cervical and lumbar injection of metrizamide. A comparison. Acta Radiol [Suppl] 335:154, 1977.

83a. Stoddart PGP, Watt I: The symptomatic complications of iopamidol (Niopam) and metrizamide (Amipaque) following lumbar radiculography. Br J Radiol 57:349–350, 1984.

84. Stovring J, Saksoner SJ, Fernando LT, et al: Successful myelography after dry spinal puncture. Radiology 143:265–266, 1982.

85. Stratemeier PH: Evaluation of the lumbar spine: A comparison between computed tomography and myelography. Radiol Clin North Am 21:221–257, 1983.

86. Tadmor R, Cacayorin ED, Kieffer SA: Advantages of supplementary CT in myelography of intraspinal masses. AJNR 4:618–621, 1983.

87. Teplick JG, Haskin ME: Review: Computed tomography of the post-operative lumbar spine. AJNR 4:1053–1072, 1983.

88. Teplick JG, Teplick SK, Goodman L, et al: Pitfalls and unusual findings in CT of the lumbar spine. J Comput Assist Tomogr 6:888–893, 1982.

89. Verbiest H: Radicular syndrome from developmental narrowing of lumbar vertebral canal. J Bone Joint Surg 36:230–237, 1954.

90. Williams AL, Haughton VM, Daniels DL, et al: CT recognition of lateral lumbar disk herniation. AJNR 3:211–213, 1982.

91. Williams AL, Haughton VM, Meyer GA, et al: Computed tomographic appearance of the bulging annulus. Radiology 142:403–408, 1982.

92. Wilmink JT, Penning L, Van der Burg W: Role of stenosis of spinal canal in L4–L5 nerve root compression assessed by flexion-extension myelography. Neuroradiology 26:173–181, 1984.

93. Winkler SS, Sackett JF: Explanation of metrizamide brain penetration: A review. J Comput Assist Tomogr 4:191–193, 1980.

94. Wolf BS, Khilani M, Malis L: The sagittal diameter of the bony cervical spinal canal and its significance in cervical spondylosis. J Mt Sinai Hosp 23:283–292, 1956.

95. Zilkha A, Irwin GA, Fagelman D: Computed tomography of spinal epidural hematoma. AJNR 4:1073–1076, 1983.

7

Robert Kricun, M.D.
Morrie E. Kricun, M.D.

Computed Tomography

INDICATIONS

Computed tomography (CT) is a noninvasive imaging modality that utilizes x-rays to produce radiographic images in the axial, coronal, or sagittal plane.

It has gained increased importance in the diagnostic evaluation of patients with disorders of the spine. The ability of high resolution CT scanners to demonstrate detailed normal anatomy and pathologic processes of the spine has made CT the primary imaging modality in many clinical situations. Thus CT is valuable in the evaluation of patients with spinal disorders such as disc disease, spinal stenosis, tumors and tumorlike conditions, infection, and inflammation. CT is also of great importance in the study of patients with congenital, post-traumatic, and postoperative abnormalities. It is the purpose of this chapter to explore the use of CT in the evaluation of these various spinal disorders.

LIMITATIONS

In the evaluation of the spine, images are best obtained in the axial plane. Coronal and sagittal images are usually produced by a process called reformatting (reconstruction), and the images do not demonstrate the high resolution obtained with axial scans. Another limitation is the inability to evaluate lesions of the spinal cord and dura adequately without introduction of intrathecal contrast agent. The CT images of obese patients may be unsatisfactory. Additionally, metal artifacts may degrade the CT image.

TECHNIQUE

The evaluation of the lumbar spine is usually performed with the patient in the supine position. A lateral digital radiograph is obtained, which permits accurate localization of subsequent axial images. The examiner determines the plane of section and the number of sections to be obtained. For patients with low back pain or radiculopathy or both, two general methods of scanning have been recommended.[54, 158, 187] In one method, scans are obtained parallel to the disc being examined, with images produced from the pedicle above to the pedicle below the disc. Individualized gantry angulation is used at each level studied (Fig. 7–1). Scanning parallel to the disc provides excellent visualization of the disc and the relationship of the posterior disc margin to the thecal sac and nerve roots. Most studies include L3–L4, L4–L5, and L5–S1 unless clinical findings suggest otherwise. It should be noted that the maximum gantry angle (which varies from 15 to 25 degrees depending on the particular CT unit being used) is frequently less than the angle of the L5–S1 disc. Thus, parallel scanning cannot always be obtained at this level.

In the second general method of scanning, no attempt is made to scan parallel to the intervertebral disc. Instead, contiguous scans are obtained at 0 degrees of gantry angulation from the level of the L3 pedicle to the superior aspect of the sacrum (Fig. 7–2). This method has the advantage of allowing one to study the spine in an uninterrupted manner, thus preventing a pathologic process at a midvertebral body level from

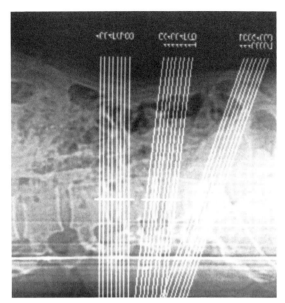

Figure 7–1. Technique of scanning parallel to the intervertebral disc. The lateral digital radiograph demonstrates the plane of scanning obtained parallel to the L3–L4, L4–L5, and L5–S1 intervertebral disc spaces. Individual gantry angulation is utilized at each level.

going unexamined. In addition, computer software packages permit reformatting of the axial images into the sagittal, coronal, and oblique planes. With the contiguous method of scanning, all spinal levels are examined in the axial plane at the same gantry angulation and can thus be reformatted together in these additional planes. Some CT software enables one to use a sagittally reformatted image to generate an axial image parallel to the disc.[200]

For most lumbar spine examinations, axial CT scans are obtained at a slice thickness of 3, 4, or 5 mm, depending on the CT equipment available. The interval of scanning corresponds to the scan slice thickness, although in some cases an overlapping technique may be chosen (for example, a 5 mm slice thickness at 4 mm intervals). In cases in which sagittal or coronal reconstruction views are considered particularly important, small scan slice thickness or the overlapping technique or both are particularly useful. Scanning technique either parallel to the disc or contiguous at 0 degrees of CT gantry angulation are both satisfactory. We prefer, as do others,[54] to scan parallel to the disc when there is clinical suspicion of disc herniation, especially in younger age groups in which osseous abnormalities are less likely

to play an important role. On the other hand, we prefer contiguous scanning at 0 degrees of angulation when there is clinical suspicion of spinal stenosis or when reconstruction views are thought to play an important diagnostic role.

The technique used for examination of the cervical spine varies with the type of disorder being evaluated. Cervical disc herniation can be studied with 1.5 to 2 mm sections. The spinal cord is better studied with thicker 4 or 5 mm sections. Cervical disc herniation is evaluated with the scans obtained parallel to the disc. Contiguous scanning can be performed in patients with suspected fracture or tumor and in the evaluation of long segments of the spinal cord.

It is very important that the patient remain still while a CT examination of the spine is being performed. Patient movement detracts from the image and may inadvertently cause some spinal levels to be left unexamined. In addition, patient motion leads to poor quality reconstruction studies. During cervical examinations the patient is asked not to breathe or swallow. CT of the spine requires high resolution scanners capable of producing necessary spatial and contrast resolution. Magnification technique is utilized, and all

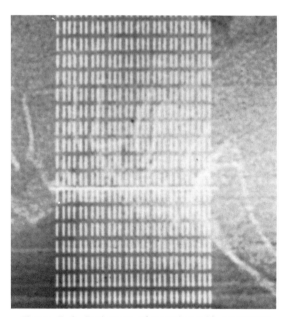

Figure 7–2. Technique of scanning with contiguous sections. The lateral digital radiograph demonstrates the plane of CT sections obtained in a contiguous fashion. In this method no attempt is made to scan parallel to the intervertebral disc space.

studies are examined at "soft tissue" and "bone" window settings. For example, in the lumbar spine the sections may be viewed at a window width of approximately 350 to 500 Hounsfield units (HU) and a window level of 25 to 50 HU ("soft tissue windows"), as well as at a window width of 1000 to 2000 HU and a window level of 200 to 350 HU ("bone windows"). In the cervical spine, a window width of 250 HU is satisfactory for evaluation of the soft tissue structures.

CT examination of the sacrum is best performed with the gantry angled as parallel to the plane of the sacrum as possible (Fig. 7–3). This usually requires maximum gantry angulation opposite the direction used to study the L5–S1 disc. In this way the sacrum and the sacroiliac joints can be ideally studied.

Computed tomographic myelography (CTM) is performed after the intrathecal introduction of water-soluble contrast agent. The intrathecal contrast material may be introduced for conventional myelography preceding the CTM study, or it may be used in low dose for CTM alone (without conventional myelography). The initial CTM studies utilized metrizamide contrast. A CTM scan of the lumbar spine could be obtained 2 to 6 hours after myelography performed with 15 ml of 190 mg iodine per ml metrizamide, or immediately after introduction of 3 ml of 150 mg iodine per ml metrizamide. More recently, newer nonionic water-soluble contrast agents such as iopamidol and iohexol have been introduced and are preferable to metrizamide because they are associated with less patient morbidity. CTM of the lumbar spine may follow within the first few hours of conventional myelography performed with 10 to 15 ml of 200 mg iodine per ml iopamidol or with 10 to 17 ml of 180 mg iodine per ml iohexol. Immediate low dose scanning can be achieved with these contrast agents. Doses vary for cervical examinations as directed by the manufacturers. CTM is particularly useful in the evaluation of intraspinal tumors, dysraphism, and arachnoiditis, and it may be used in some cases of trauma, disc herniation, spinal stenosis, and postoperative disorders.

Intravenous contrast material plays a role in the CT examination of some patients with spinal disorders. For example, intravenous contrast agent can enhance some intraspinal tumors, thus further delineating and char-

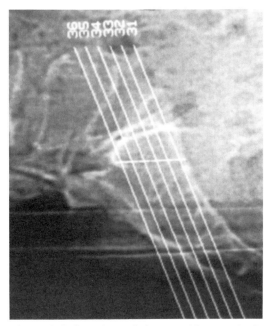

Figure 7–3. Scanning technique used for examination of the sacrum. The lateral digital radiograph demonstrates the plane of CT sections, which are obtained with the gantry angled as parallel to the plane of the sacrum as possible.

acterizing them. Enhancement of fibrotic scar may permit differentiation from disc herniation in the postoperative patient. Intravenous contrast agent enhances the appearance of the epidural veins and dura and consequently has been recommended by some authors in the evaluation of cervical disc herniation.

RADIATION BURDEN

The amount of gonadal radiation received during a CT examination of the lumbosacral spine is variable and in part dependent upon the number of images obtained and the level of the lumbosacral spine scanned. It has been estimated that CT delivers about 5.5 to 7 rad per examination.[134] In the United States, approximately 10% of all CT examinations are of the spine, but the percentage is increasing.[134] Those CT scanners that have a 360 degree rotational exposure motion demonstrate a more uniform surface dose. However, even with newer scanners, the absorbed dose has not decreased.[134] Patient dose may differ with various CT scanners that produce images of the same quality.[295]

COMPLICATIONS

There are no known complications of conventional computed tomography of the spine. The complications associated with CTM and intravenous contrast enhanced CT are those of myelography and the contrast agents utilized.

ANATOMY

Anatomy of the spine has been described in Chapter 2 and will not be discussed in detail at this time. However, the ability of high resolution CT scanners to demonstrate anatomic detail clearly in the axial plane is of considerable importance. For this reason, we present representative CT scans of the spine and sacrum for the purpose of review (Figs. 7–4 through 7–10).

Differences in CT attenuation values permit differentiation of various tissues and structures. The intervertebral disc measures approximately 50 to 100 HU and thus appears "lighter" than the thecal sac, whose measurement, because of the presence of cerebrospinal fluid and nerve roots, ranges from 0 to 30 HU. Fat has negative attenuation values, whereas bone and metal have very high CT attenuation levels. Most density differences are visible to the eye; however, the CT cursor can be placed on a region of interest, and numerical values can be recorded. In addition, CT software allows the "highlighting" of those density measurements that fall within a range specified by the examiner. This gives the interpreter an enhanced pictorial representation of density measurements, which may increase diagnostic certainty.

PITFALLS OF CT DIAGNOSIS

Normal and Variants of Normal

The CT appearance of several nonpathologic processes may simulate a pathologic process. Familiarity with normal structures

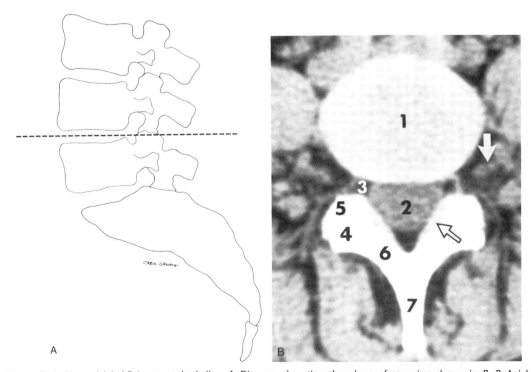

Figure 7–4. Normal L4–L5 intervertebral disc. *A,* Diagram denoting the plane of scanning shown in *B. B,* Axial CT scan at the level of the L4–L5 intervertebral disc. At this level, the L4 nerve has emerged from the neural foramen above. The disc margin is slightly flattened posteriorly and is normal. *Key:* **1** = intervertebral disc; **2** = thecal sac; **3** = epidural fat; **4** = inferior articular process of L4; **5** = superior articular process of L5; **6** = lamina of L4; **7** = spinous process of L4; **closed arrow** = L4 nerve root; **open arrow** = ligamentum flavum.

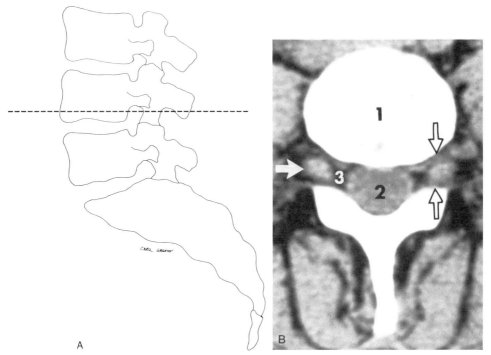

Figure 7–5. Normal neural foramen (intervertebral canal). *A*, Diagram denoting the plane of scanning shown in *B*. *B*, Axial CT scan through the neural foramen cephalad to the L4–L5 intervertebral disc space. The L4 dorsal nerve root ganglion is within the neural foramen. *Key:* **1** = vertebral body; **2** = thecal sac; **3** = epidural fat; **closed arrow** = dorsal root ganglion; **open arrows** = neural foramen.

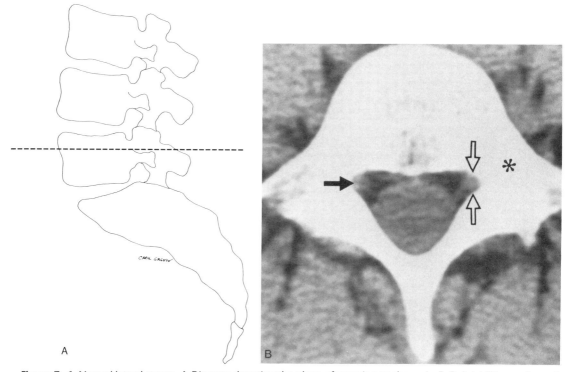

Figure 7–6. Normal lateral recess. *A*, Diagram denoting the plane of scanning as shown in *B*. *B*, Axial CT scan through the lateral recess of L5. *Key:* **asterisk** = pedicle of L5; **open arrows** = height of lateral recess; **closed arrow** = nerve root within lateral recess.

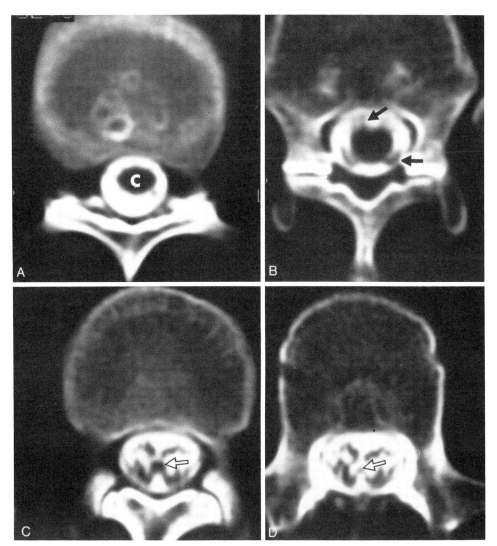

Figure 7–7. Axial CTM scans through different levels of the distal spinal cord, conus medullaris, and filum terminale. *A,* Distal spinal cord at T11. **C** = Spinal cord. *B,* Lumbosacral plexus just caudal to *A* at T12. The spinal cord has widened owing to the large nerve roots of the lumbosacral plexus. Note the emerging nerve roots (arrows). *C,* Conus medullaris (arrow) at L1. The spinal cord has tapered at this level. Notice the spiderlike configuration of the emerging dorsal and ventral nerve roots that make up the cauda equina. *D,* Filum terminale (arrow) surrounded by nerve roots of the cauda equina caudal to *C.* (From Kricun R, Kricun ME: Computed Tomography of the Spine: Diagnostic Exercises. Rockville, Maryland: Aspen Publishers, Inc, 1987. Reprinted with permission of Aspen Publishers, Inc.)

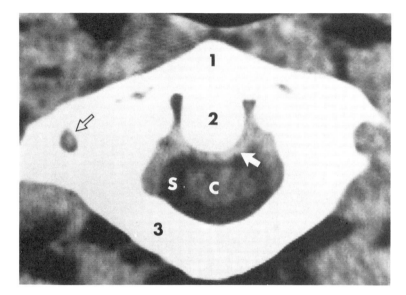

Figure 7–8. Atlantoaxial articulation. Axial CT scan. *Key:* **1** = anterior arch of C1; **2** = odontoid process; **3** = posterior arch of C1; **C** = spinal cord; **S** = subarachnoid space; **white arrow** = transverse ligament; **open arrow** = vertebral artery in foramen transversarium. (From Kricun R, Kricun ME: Computed Tomography of the Spine: Diagnostic Exercises. Rockville, Maryland: Aspen Publishers, Inc, 1987. Reprinted with permission of Aspen Publishers, Inc.)

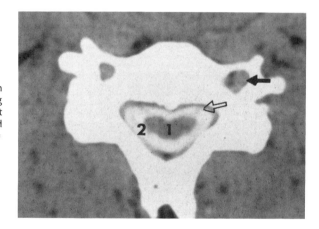

Figure 7–9. Midcervical spine. Axial CT scan through the level of a cervical vertebral body following introduction of intrathecal water-soluble contrast agent (CTM). *Key:* **1** = spinal cord; **2** = subarachnoid space; **open arrow** = nerve root; **closed arrow** = vertebral artery in the foramen transversarium.

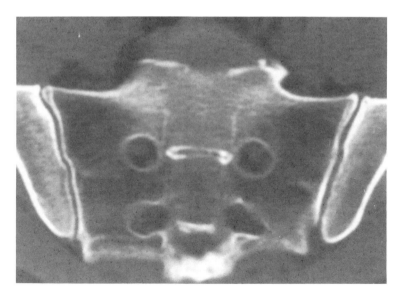

Figure 7–10. Sacrum and sacroiliac joints. Coronal CT scan through the sacroiliac joints. The margins of the sacroiliac joints are smooth and sclerotic. The nerve roots within the neural foramina are surrounded by fat.

and their variants is necessary to prevent misdiagnosis in these cases. A list of many of these pitfalls is presented in Table 7–1. These structures may be of disc, neural, vascular, or osseous origin and may simulate disc herniation, fracture, mass lesion, destructive lesion of bone, or osteophyte formation.

Pseudoherniation of the Disc

Pseudoherniation of the disc is frequently encountered at the L5–S1 level. This occurs when there is nonparallel scanning through the plane of the disc. At the L5–S1 level, the angle of the intervertebral disc space often exceeds the maximum gantry angle of the CT scanner. The posterior margin of the L5–S1 disc will therefore appear on the axial CT scan to lie posterior to the L5 vertebral body (Fig. 7–11). This simulates disc herniation; however, there is a lack of compression of the thecal sac or obliteration of the epidural fat. At the level of the next, more caudad scan, the sacrum is seen having the same configuration as the posteriorly projected pseudoherniation of the disc.

Other causes of pseudoherniation of the

Table 7–1. NORMAL OR VARIANTS OF NORMAL SIMULATING PATHOLOGY ON CT

Normal or Variant of Normal	Simulated Pathology
Disc	
Pseudoherniation of disc	Disc herniation
Neural	
Conjoined nerve roots	Disc herniation
Cystic nerve root sleeve dilatation and Tarlov's cyst	Disc herniation or mass
Vascular	
Anterior internal vertebral veins	Disc herniation
Bony septum of basivertebral venous groove	Osteophyte
Groove of basivertebral vein	Fracture
Osseous	
Butterfly vertebra	Fracture
Limbus vertebra	Fracture
Os odontoideum	Fracture
Congenital cleft of C1	Fracture
Aplasia and hemiaplasia of arch of C1	Fracture
Congenital absence of pedicle	Destructive lesion of bone
Schmorl's node	Metastasis
Cupid's bow	Metastasis

disc include spondylolisthesis and scoliosis. Patients with spondylolisthesis may again have disc material projecting beyond the margin of the next superior vertebral body.

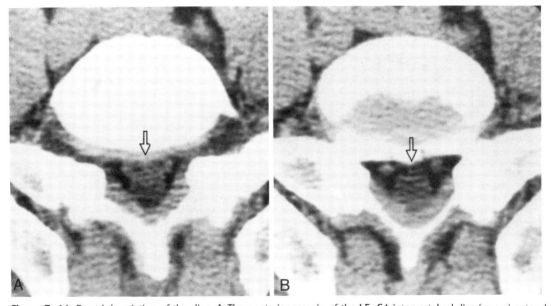

Figure 7–11. Pseudoherniation of the disc. *A*, The posterior margin of the L5–S1 intervertebral disc (arrow) extends symmetrically posterior to the L5 vertebral body. This occurs owing to nonparallel scanning through the plane of the intervertebral disc. Note that the epidural fat is preserved. *B*, Axial CT section obtained 4 mm caudad to *A*. The posterior margin of the sacrum (arrow) is now seen posterior to the anterior and middle portions of the intervertebral disc. The posterior aspect of the sacrum has the same general configuration as the posterior margin of the disc seen in *A*.

The diagnosis of disc herniation must be made with caution in this clinical setting. Asymmetric compression of the thecal sac, nerve root, or epidural fat may suggest actual disc herniation. Sagittal reconstruction of the images may be helpful in determining the degree of disc protrusion. Patients with scoliosis may appear to have disc protruding posterolaterally or far laterally because of the asymmetric scanning of the left and right sides of the vertebral bodies and intervertebral disc.

Conjoined Nerve Roots

Neural processes such as conjoined nerve roots and cystic nerve root sleeve dilatation may simulate disc herniation or mass lesion on the CT study.[194, 330, 350, 426, 483] Conjoined nerve roots are congenital anomalies in

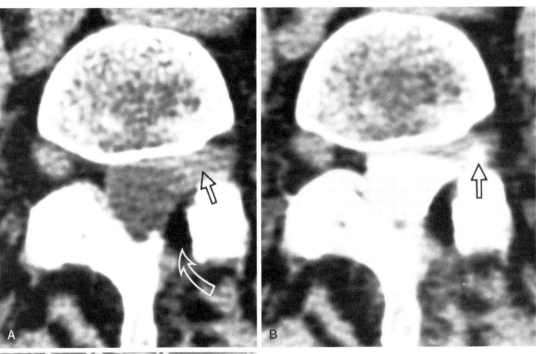

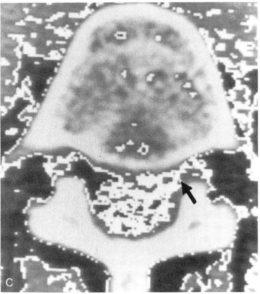

Figure 7–12. Conjoined nerve roots. *A,* Axial CT scan 9 mm cephalad to the L5–S1 intervertebral disc space. Conjoined nerve roots are present on the left (straight arrow) and are the cause of increased CT attenuation within the neural foramen compared with the perineural fat seen on the right. Note the laminectomy defect and surgical fat graft (curved arrow). *B,* CT scan performed after introduction of intrathecal water-soluble contrast agent. Contrast material is seen within the conjoined nerve root sleeve (arrow) in the neural foramen on the left. *C,* Axial CT scan in another patient with conjoined L5 and S1 nerve roots on the left. The technique of "highlighting" was used to accentuate structures with CT attenuation values between 0 and 30 HU. Note the highlighting of the conjoined nerve roots (arrow) and thecal sac. (Part *C* from Kricun R, Kricun ME: Computed Tomography of the Spine: Diagnostic Exercises. Rockville, Maryland: Aspen Publishers, Inc, 1987. Reprinted with permission of Aspen Publishers, Inc.)

which two nerve roots emerge from a common dural sheath. L5 and S1 nerve roots are most frequently conjoined. Conjoined nerve roots have been reported in 1% of lumbar disc operations[88, 476] and 8% of anatomic specimens.[215] The nerve roots may exit from the same foramen or may exit separately, with the bifurcation of the conjoined nerve roots in close approximation to the intervening pedicle.[476] As an isolated finding, conjoined nerve roots are usually asymptomatic.[194] However, sciatica may occur when conjoined nerve roots are compressed by neural canal stenosis. In some cases, disc herniation may be present at the site of conjoined nerve roots, with symptoms occurring at more than one nerve root level. Myelographic and CT correlation may be required to diagnose coexistent disc herniation and conjoined nerve roots.[154]

Conjoined nerve roots appear on the CT scan as a soft tissue density in the anterior epidural space, neural foramen, and lateral recess and cause obliteration of the epidural and perineural fat (Fig. 7–12). The soft tissue density may superficially simulate a disc herniation with lateral extension; however, density measurements are much less than disc measurements and are similar to or only slightly greater than the density measurement of the thecal sac.[194, 350] Highlighting a predetermined range of density measurements can give a pictorial representation of the CT attenuation values (Fig. 7–12C). Studying the sequential scans may also reveal asymmetry of the nerve root origins, further suggesting the diagnosis of conjoined nerve roots. Some patients with conjoined nerve roots have slight dilatation of the ipsilateral lateral recess, which may serve as another diagnostic clue.[202]

Cystic Nerve Root Sleeve Dilatation and Tarlov's Cyst

Cystic nerve root sleeve dilatation occurs from enlargement of the subarachnoid space that surrounds the exiting nerve root. The dilatation of the nerve root sleeve occurs proximal to the dorsal root ganglion. The etiology is not known but may be related to increased hydrostatic pressure of the cerebrospinal fluid. A Tarlov or perineurial cyst differs in that it occurs at the level of the dorsal root ganglion and contains neural

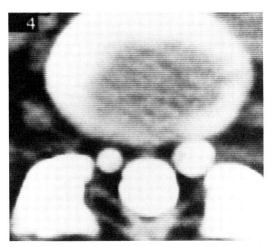

Figure 7–13. Cystic nerve root sleeve dilatation. Axial CTM scan demonstrates cystic nerve root sleeve dilatation most prominent on the left.

elements in its wall.[441] The CT appearance of cystic nerve root sleeve dilatation is similar to that of perineurial cyst, although the latter may fill less readily with intrathecal contrast agent. Both appear as a round mass in the region of the neural foramen. The mass is isodense with the thecal sac and causes asymmetry of the perineural fat (Fig. 7–13). In addition there may be enlargement of the neural foramen and scalloping of the adjacent vertebral body and pedicle.[118, 324, 330, 483] Dural ectasia and multilevel involvement are other associated features.[257, 330] The CT appearance may simulate a lateral or an extruded disc herniation; however, the presence of low CT attenuation measurements should exclude those diagnoses. A neurofibroma is another diagnostic consideration. It may appear as a mass in the neural foramen, causing widening of the foramen and vertebral scalloping. Density measurements of a neurofibroma are usually slightly greater than those of cystic nerve root sleeve dilatation. If further evaluation is needed, CTM can be performed. Water-soluble contrast agent that fills a dilated nerve root sleeve clearly distinguishes cystic nerve root sleeve dilatation from a mass such as a neurofibroma.

Normal Vascular Structures

Several normal vascular structures may simulate a pathologic process on axial CT study. At the midvertebral body level, vertebral venous drainage courses in part posteriorly through the basivertebral veins and empties into the retrovertebral plexus of veins,[90–92, 289] which resides in the space between the vertebral body and the overlying posterior longitudinal ligament. These plexuses are joined by longitudinally oriented anterior internal vertebral veins, which are also in the epidural space and are located posterior to the vertebral bodies and intervertebral discs. In the lower lumbar spine, abundant epidural fat surrounds the anterior internal vertebral veins and retrovertebral plexus of veins, making them clearly visible. The anterior internal veins appear on CT study as several round soft tissue densities in the anterior epidural space[186] (Fig. 7–14). Confluence of these vascular structures should not be confused with disc herniation.[300] The anterior vertebral veins and retrovertebral plexus of veins are not well visualized in the cervical, thoracic, or upper lumbar spine owing to the paucity of epidural fat in these locations.

Radicular (intervertebral, pedicular) veins join the anterior internal vertebral veins of the internal venous system with the ascending lumbar veins of the external venous system. They course along the intervertebral

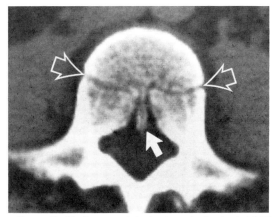

Figure 7–15. Groove of the basivertebral vein. Axial CT scan demonstrates a Y-shaped radiolucency (open arrows) that represents vascular grooves. The bony septum (closed arrow) separates the paired posterior venous channels of the basivertebral veins. (From Kricun R, Kricun ME: Computed Tomography of the Spine: Diagnostic Exercises. Rockville, Maryland: Aspen Publishers, Inc, 1987. Reprinted with permission of Aspen Publishers, Inc.)

canal and exit via the neural foramen. They are more horizontal in direction and are thinner than nerve roots that also course through the intervertebral canal.

The groove of the basivertebral vein can be seen on axial CT scans as Y- or V-shaped channels at the midvertebral level[401] (Fig. 7–15) and should not be confused with fracture. The groove is always visualized in the midvertebral body level, whereas fracture lines can be viewed on consecutive scans.[401] In addition, the margins of the vascular groove are sclerotic. Posteriorly, the basivertebral groove empties as a single channel or as paired channels with an interposed osseous septum. The septum may project slightly into the spinal canal at this midvertebral level and should not be mistaken for an osteophyte, which typically occurs at the vertebral margin.

Butterfly Vertebra

Butterfly vertebra is a developmental abnormality caused by failure of fusion of the lateral halves of the vertebral body due to persistence of notochord tissue.[406] Disc tissue protrudes into the cleft, causing depression of the vertebral surfaces centrally. The CT study readily identifies the cleft, which may have sclerotic margins. Irregular-shaped bands of soft tissue density, which represent

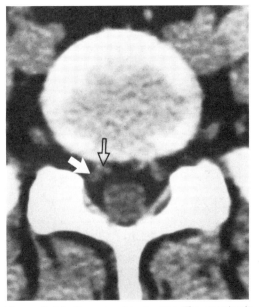

Figure 7–14. Normal epidural veins. The anterior internal vertebral veins (open arrow) appear in the axial plane as small, rounded densities within the anterior epidural space. Confluence of these vascular structures should not be confused with protrusion of the disc. Note the larger nerve root (closed arrow).

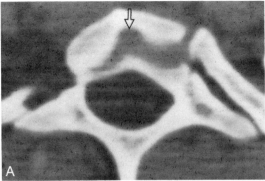

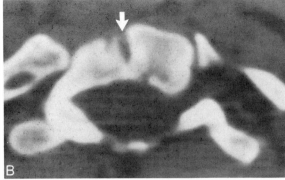

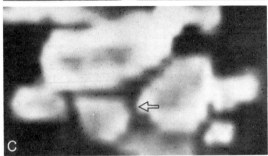

Figure 7–16. Butterfly vertebra. *A,* Axial CT scan at the level of a midvertebral body demonstrates inwardly protruding disc tissue (arrow). *B,* A sagittally oriented cleft (arrow) is seen on the scan obtained adjacent to part *A.* Note the sclerotic margins of the cleft. *C,* Reformatted images in the coronal plane demonstrate the characteristic features of the butterfly vertebra with its sagittal cleft (arrow). Reconstructed images are useful in clarifying complex anatomic features. (From Kricun R, Kricun ME: Computed Tomography of the Spine: Diagnostic Exercises. Rockville, Maryland: Aspen Publishers, Inc, 1987. Reprinted with permission of Aspen Publishers, Inc.)

the inwardly protruding disc tissue, may be seen both above and below the midportion of the vertebral body (Fig. 7–16). The cleft should not be confused with a fracture. Coronal reconstruction of the axial images and review of the conventional radiographs will resolve diagnostic difficulties.

Limbus Vertebra

Limbus vertebra is another abnormality that may be confused with vertebral body fracture. A limbus vertebra occurs when disc tissue herniates anteriorly, penetrating vertebral trabeculae at the junction of the cartilaginous end-plate and the bony vertebral rim.[378, 406] A small bone fragment (or fragments) thus separates from the vertebral body most frequently in the lumbar spine at the anterosuperior margin of the vertebral body. The axial CT examination demonstrates a triangular or rounded, well-corticated bony fragment adjacent to the anterosuperior margin of the vertebral body. There is sclerosis of the posterior margin of the fragment and of the anterior margin of the adjacent vertebral body[488] (Fig. 7–17). Herniated disc tissue separates the fragment from the vertebral body and appears as a radiolucent band.

Os Odontoideum

Os odontoideum is another anomaly that may present a confusing picture when viewed with axial CT. It appears as a small, round or oval, corticated ossicle that is lo-

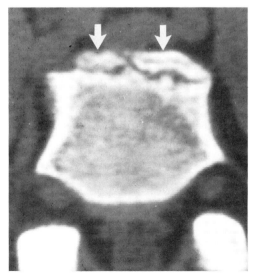

Figure 7–17. Limbus vertebra. Axial CT scan through superior aspect of L5. Irregular bone fragments are seen anteriorly (arrows). There is sclerosis of the posterior margin of the fragments and of the anterior margin of the vertebral body. This should not be mistaken for fracture.

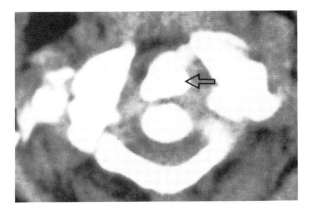

Figure 7–18. Os odontoideum. Axial CT scan at the level of the atlas demonstrates an os odontoideum (arrow) anterior to the odontoid process, which is displaced posteriorly and is compromising the spinal canal.

cated cranial to a hypoplastic odontoid process (Fig. 7–18). This most likely represents a congenital anomaly,[299, 485] although some authors believe that it occurs secondary to childhood trauma.[136] Hypoplasia of the posterior arch of C1 and hypertrophy of the anterior arch of C1 are associated findings.[485] Awareness of this entity should prevent confusion with a fracture fragment.

Congenital Abnormalities of the Arch of C1

Congenital abnormalities of the arch of C1, such as clefts, aplasia, and hemiaplasia, should be differentiated from fracture. Congenital clefts are rare, with posterior clefts occurring more frequently than anterior clefts.[155] Characteristically a posterior cleft has smooth, well-corticated margins compared with a fracture, which has a more jagged, irregular appearance.[106] A cleft may be associated with lateral offset of C1–C2; however, this offset is limited to 1 to 2 mm, unlike a Jefferson fracture, which usually has lateral offset greater than 3 mm.[155] Congenital aplasia or hemiaplasia of the arch of C1 more frequently involves the posterior arch.[106] A persistent posterior tubercle may be present.

Congenital Absence of Pedicle

Congenital absence of the pedicle is rare and should not be mistaken for a pedicle destroyed by tumor[95] or infection[261] (Fig. 7–19). Usually there are other associated osseous changes, such as hypertrophy and sclerosis of the contralateral pedicle and vertebral arch, which occur secondary to

added bony stress.[282, 451] In addition there is frequently hypoplasia or absence of the ipsilateral superior articular process, hypoplasia of the ipsilateral lamina, and widening of the intervertebral foramen.*

Schmorl's Node and "Cupid's Bow"

The CT appearance of Schmorl's node and "Cupid's bow" should not be confused with metastatic disease to the vertebral body. A Schmorl's node is an intraosseous herniation of the nucleus pulposus. Axial CT scan reveals a round, low density lesion of the vertebral end-plate with a sclerotic rim (Fig. 7–20). Extensive sclerosis may sometimes be present. The vertebral end-plate location and sclerotic rim help differentiate a Schmorl's

---

*Reference numbers 89, 95, 109, 282, 451, 493.

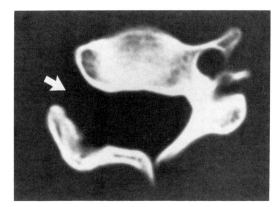

Figure 7–19. Congenital absence of the pedicle. Congenital absence of the right pedicle at C5 (arrow) is demonstrated on this axial CT section as well as on adjacent sections. This should not be confused with a destructive lesion of the pedicle. Dysplasia of the right lamina is also noted.

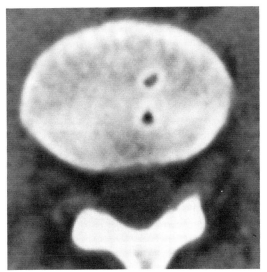

Figure 7–20. Schmorl's nodes. Axial CT scan at the inferior aspect of a lumbar vertebra. Schmorl's nodes (intraosseous herniations of the nucleus pulposus) are seen in this patient as two areas of low density within the vertebral body. A typical rim of sclerosis is noted.

node from a metastatic lesion. "Cupid's bow" contour is a normal variant. It gains its name from the appearance of paired parasagittal concavities on the inferior end-plates of lumbar vertebrae as visualized on AP radiographs.[101] The etiology of this anatomic deformity is not clear but is thought to be related to the turgor of the nucleus pulposus as it expands against the cartilaginous end-plate.[378] Axial CT demonstrates paired parasagittal areas of disc density located posteriorly within 5 to 7 mm of the inferior cartilaginous end-plate.[143] Apparent sclerosis surrounding the radiolucencies is due to depressed subchondral bone and creates an "owl's eyes" appearance on the axial CT scan[363] (Fig. 7–21). At the apex of the "Cupid's bow" there is frequently additional sclerosis, which may be exuberant and should not be mistaken for osteosclerotic metastasis.

CT Artifact

Artifacts may sometimes degrade the CT image. In some cases this may make interpretation of the study suboptimal, and in other cases it may entirely prevent interpretation of the pathology. The most common types of artifact encountered in everyday practice are listed in Table 7–2. Metallic substances present in the scanning field may cause a flaring, streaking artifact. Surgical clips, screws, and rods are sources of artifact

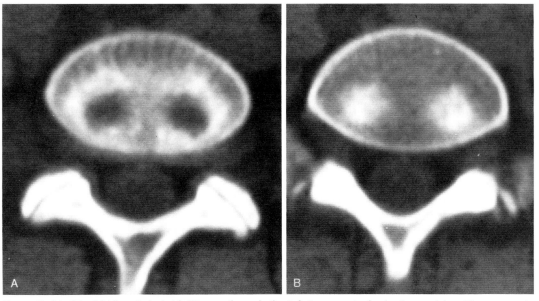

Figure 7–21. "Cupid's bow." *A*, Axial CT scan through the inferior aspect of a lumbar vertebra. There are paired parasagittal regions of decreased CT attenuation within the vertebral body. Surrounding sclerosis creates an "owl's eyes" appearance typical of the "Cupid's bow" contour. *B*, Axial CT scan 4 mm above *A*. Considerable sclerosis is present cephalad to the parasagittal areas of low CT attenuation. The appearance of "Cupid's bow" contour should not be confused with osteolytic or osteoblastic metastatic disease.

Table 7–2. SOURCES OF CT ARTIFACT

Metallic substance in CT field
   Dental filling
   Surgical clips, screws, and rods
   Bullet fragments
   Pantopaque myelographic contrast
     agent
Obese patient
"Shoulder" artifact
"Facet" artifact
"Ring" artifact

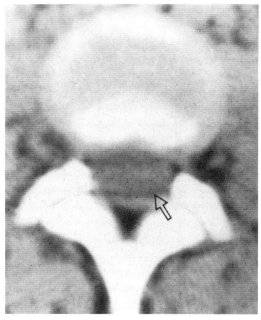

(Fig. 7–22). In particular, large Harrington rods may make soft tissue evaluation difficult; however, in·most cases "bone window" settings provide adequate visualization of the osseous structures. Bullet fragments and iophendylate (Pantopaque) myelographic contrast agent within the spinal canal are other sources of metallic artifact. On images of the upper cervical spine, a dental filling may cause a streaking artifact through the spinal canal, degrading the image to an unacceptable level. In order to correct this problem, a lateral digital radiograph is generated, and a scan slice angulation that avoids the dental filling is chosen.

The "facet" artifact is a horizontal, low density line that may be seen within the spinal canal (Fig. 7–23). The line appears to extend between the anterior medial aspect of both facet joints and is caused by the edge effect resulting from the sudden change in

Figure 7–23. Facet artifact. There is a horizontal band of low CT attenuation within the spinal canal between the facet joints (arrow). This facet artifact is caused by the change in CT attenuation values of the osseous articular processes and the facet joints as measured by the CT scanner.

density between the bone of the articular processes and the intervening joint space. The low density "facet" artifact creates the appearance of higher density anteriorly,

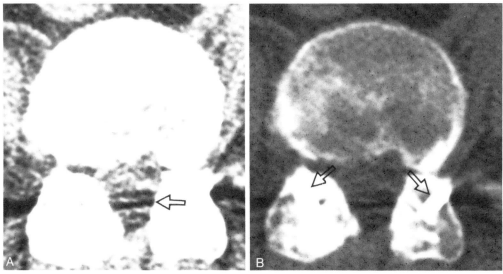

Figure 7–22. Artifact created by the presence of metallic surgical screws. *A,* Axial CT scan viewed at soft tissue window settings demonstrates a radiolucent band between the facets (arrow). This degrades the image of the structures within the spinal canal. *B,* Scan section similar to that of part *A* but photographed at bone window settings reveals the surgical screws (arrows) that produced the artifact.

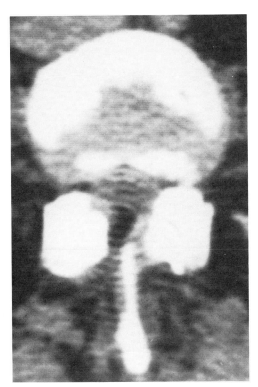

Figure 7–24. Ring artifact. Axial CT scan at L4–L5 demonstrates a ring artifact degrading the image within the spinal canal.

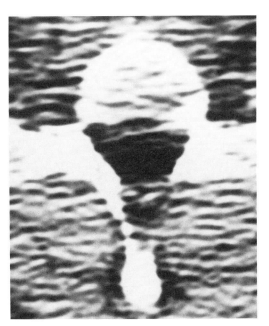

Figure 7–25. Shoulder artifact. Axial CT scan at C7–T1 demonstrates degradation of image due to artifact created by scanning through the plane of the shoulders.

which should not be confused with a disc herniation. The so-called ring artifact is a CT artifact not limited to spinal examinations (Fig. 7–24).

Each CT examining table has a weight limitation beyond which patients cannot be studied. Some patients fall within the weight guidelines but are still too obese for optimal study. The CT image of the obese patient is frequently grainy, thus diminishing diagnostic accuracy. Scanning through the plane of the shoulders creates another difficulty for CT study. Thus, when studying the region of C7–T1, "shoulder" artifact may be present, with low density streaks traversing the spinal canal (Fig. 7–25). This artifact may occur despite the use of shoulder and cervical traction with the patient stretching the arms downward as far as possible.

DISORDERS OF THE LUMBAR DISC

With the advent of high resolution scanning, CT has become an important imaging modality in the evaluation of disorders of the lumbar disc. In many institutions, CT scanning is the primary imaging method for evaluating disc herniation. Disorders of the lumbar disc can be studied with the contiguous method with zero degree gantry angulation or with angulation of the CT gantry parallel to the plane of the disc. The CT examination usually includes the L3–L4, L4–L5, and L5–S1 intervertebral disc spaces. These disc spaces account for almost all lumbar disc herniations (Table 7–3). The CT examination permits differentiation of bulging of the annulus fibrosus from herniation of the nucleus pulposus. In some cases extrusion of a free disc fragment can be diagnosed with CT. Disc herniations can be further characterized with CT as central, posterolateral, or lateral. Furthermore, displacement of disc material from the intervertebral disc space (that is, cephalad or caudad) can be determined.

Table 7–3. FREQUENCY OF LUMBAR DISC HERNIATION BY DISC LEVEL

L5–S1	= 35%–40%
L4–L5	= 50%–60%
L3–L4	= 5%–10%
L1–L2, L2–L3	= <1%

Bulging Annulus Fibrosus

There are several biochemical and biomechanical factors that may lead to generalized bulging of the annulus fibrosus with aging.[478, 481] The nucleus pulposus may lose turgor, with subsequent decreased disc space height. The annulus fibrosus develops fissuring, hyalin degeneration, and increased pigmentation. The annulus loses elasticity and bulges in a generalized fashion beyond the vertebral body margins.[478, 481] Tears may develop in the inner fibers of the annulus; however, the outer fibers remain intact, thus preventing any nuclear material from herniating.[481] Patients with generalized bulging of the disc may have back pain; however, findings of a radiculopathy are usually absent.

Although CT cannot distinguish the annulus fibrosus from the nucleus pulposus, generalized bulging of the annulus fibrosus can nevertheless be accurately diagnosed and differentiated from disc herniation by virtue of its CT appearance.[185, 478, 481] Bulging of the annulus fibrosus appears as a generalized, usually symmetric extension of the disc beyond the vertebral body margins (Fig. 7–26). This occurs posteriorly, laterally, and anteriorly. There is no focal protrusion of the disc margin such as occurs with herniation of the nucleus pulposus. Typically a

bulging annulus has a convex posterior margin, although occasionally this margin may remain concave owing to reinforcement of the central portion of the annulus by the posterior longitudinal ligament.[478, 481] Gas within the disc (vacuum disc phenomenon) is another common feature of degenerative disc disease and may be found in association with bulging of the annulus. Calcification of the outer fibers of the annulus fibrosus may also be detected in some cases.

Disc Herniation

Herniation of the nucleus pulposus occurs when the nucleus protrudes through a tear in the annulus fibrosus. The disc most often remains anterior to the posterior longitudinal ligament and is then referred to as a subligamentous herniation. CT is a highly accurate, noninvasive method of diagnosing disc herniation.* The major advantages and disadvantages of CT in diagnosing disc herniations are listed in Tables 7–4 and 7–5.

Posterolateral Disc Herniation

The most common type of disc herniation occurs posterolaterally (60–85%).[149, 482] This frequently causes nerve root compression

---

*Reference numbers 8, 47, 73, 185, 365, 442, 444, 482.

Table 7–4. ADVANTAGES OF CT IN DIAGNOSING LUMBAR DISC HERNIATION

Accurate method of diagnosis (92% to 94%)
More accurate than myelography at L5–S1
Accurate method of diagnosing lateral disc herniation
Detects accompanying central or lateral spinal stenosis
Noninvasive
No hospitalization required

Table 7–5. DISADVANTAGES OF CT IN DIAGNOSING LUMBAR DISC HERNIATION

False negative study when pathologic level not examined (e.g., conus lesion)
Obese patients may have suboptimal study
Postoperative fibrotic scan may be difficult to differentiate from disc herniation (but CT still more accurate than myelography in this diagnosis)
Radiation exposure (unlike magnetic resonance imaging)

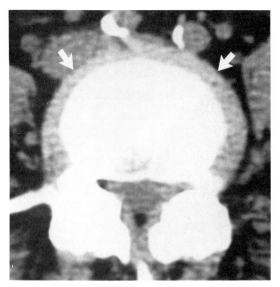

Figure 7–26. Bulging annulus. The L4–L5 intervertebral disc is bulging symmetrically and concentrically (arrows) beyond the vertebral body margin.

Table 7–6. EFFECT OF POSTEROLATERAL AND FAR LATERAL DISC HERNIATION ON LUMBAR NERVE ROOT

Nerve Root	Posterolateral Disc Herniation	Far Lateral Disc Herniation	Decreased or Absent Reflex*	Pain and Paresthesias*
L3	L2–L3	L3–L4	Knee	Anterior thigh and knee
L4	L3–L4	L4–L5	Knee	Anterior thigh and knee, medial leg
L5	L4–L5	L5–S1	± Ankle	Hip, posterolateral thigh, lateral calf, dorsal foot, first or second and third toes
S1	L5–S1	—	Ankle	Midgluteal, posterior thigh, posterior calf to heel, outer plantar foot, fourth and fifth toes

*Data from Adams RD, Victor M: Principles of Neurology, 3rd ed. New York: McGraw-Hill, 1985.

From Kricun R, Kricun ME: Computed Tomography of the Spine: Diagnostic Exercises. Rockville, Maryland: Aspen Publishers, Inc, 1987. Reprinted with permission of Aspen Publishers, Inc.

leading to a radiculopathy in the distribution of the involved nerve root (Table 7–6). Normally, the posterior margin of the L5–S1 disc is flat or slightly convex, whereas the posterior margin at L4–L5 and at the lumbar disc spaces above is flat or slightly concave.[149] The most important CT features of a posterolateral disc herniation have been described[73, 137, 149, 239, 365, 482] and are listed in Table 7–7. At the L5–S1 level, the S1 nerve root is usually visualized because of surrounding epidural fat. Compression of this nerve root by disc herniation is readily detected (Fig. 7–27). At L4–L5, the L5 nerve root is often not visualized unless intrathecal contrast agent is utilized. Nevertheless, the diagnosis of herniation of the nucleus pulposus can be made with confidence owing to the focal alteration of the posterior disc margin, obliteration of the anterior epidural fat, and compression of the thecal sac[73, 137, 149, 239, 365, 482] (Fig. 7–28). CT can differentiate the "soft" disc herniation from the less common "hard" disc, which represents either calcified disc herniation or osteophyte formation (Fig. 7–29). The hard disc may cause compression of the thecal sac and nerve root

Table 7–7. CT FEATURES OF DISC HERNIATION

Focal alteration of disc margin due to protrusion of disc
Displacement or compression of nerve root
Displacement or compression of thecal sac
Displacement or obliteration of epidural fat
Calcification or gas occasionally within disc herniation

similar to a "soft" or noncalcified disc herniation.

Central Disc Herniation

Central disc herniation accounts for 5% to 35% of disc herniations.[149, 482] Typically, a central disc herniation compresses the thecal sac while sparing individual nerve roots. This leads to low back pain due to sensory innervation of the meninges, posterior lon-

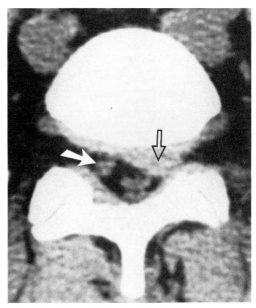

Figure 7–27. Posterolateral disc herniation. A posterolateral disc herniation at L5–S1 on the left (open arrow) is encroaching on epidural fat and compressing the S1 nerve root. Notice the uninvolved S1 nerve root on the right (closed arrow), which is surrounded by epidural fat.

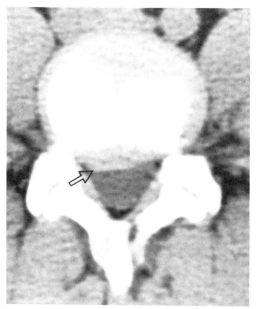

Figure 7–28. Posterolateral disc herniation at L4–L5. There is asymmetric protrusion of the disc (arrow) encroaching on the less dense thecal sac. This represents posterolateral disc herniation. The nerve roots are not well visualized because of the absence of abundant epidural fat at this level compared with that found at the L5–S1 level.

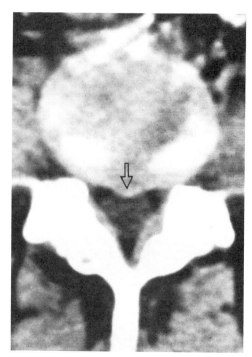

Figure 7–30. Central disc herniation. On this axial CT scan at L4–L5, there is a small, central, focal protrusion of the disc (arrow).

gitudinal ligament, and outer layers of the annulus fibrosus. Radiculopathy is usually absent unless the disc herniation is large

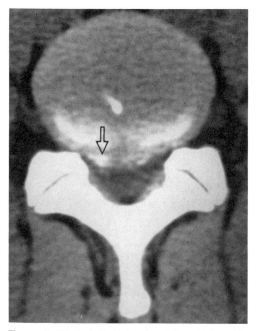

Figure 7–29. Calcified disc herniation. This axial CT scan at L4–L5 demonstrates a calcified disc (arrow) compressing the thecal sac.

enough to cause compression of the cauda equina. The CT examination demonstrates a midline focal protrusion of the disc (Fig. 7–30). At L5–S1 CT may demonstrate a central disc herniation that is not identified myelographically because of the large amount of epidural fat at this level.

Lateral Disc Herniation

Herniation of the nucleus pulposus laterally into or beyond the neural foramen is termed a lateral disc herniation. This accounts for approximately 5% of disc herniations.[149, 334, 479] The CT diagnosis of lateral disc herniation is extremely important because the myelographic study is frequently unremarkable.[164, 420, 436] Myelography performed with water-soluble contrast agent demonstrates the nerve root sheath to the termination near the dorsal root ganglion within the neural foramen. Disc herniation that is located lateral to the ganglion may therefore go undetected with myelography. In addition, the preoperative diagnosis of lateral disc herniation alters the surgical approach. Failure to appreciate the lateral location of the disc herniation preoperatively may lead to a negative surgical exploration.[278]

The CT examination of lateral disc herniation demonstrates focal protrusion of the disc within or lateral to the neural foramen, displacement of fat within the foramen, and absence of dural sac deformity[479] (Fig. 7–31). Occasionally the disc herniation is large enough to appear as a soft tissue mass in the foramen. The lateral disc herniation has CT density measurements that are similar to or slightly less than those of the intervertebral disc and are almost always greater than the CT density measurement of the thecal sac.[151, 412]

The nerve root exits the neural foramen approximately 1 to 1.5 cm above the next lower intervertebral disc. A lateral disc herniation that extends cephalad may thus compromise the nerve root in the foramen. This is the same nerve root that would be compressed by the more common posterolateral disc herniation occurring at the next higher level. Thus, a patient with a clinical L5 radiculopathy is likely to have a posterolateral disc herniation at L4–L5 but may instead have a far lateral disc herniation at L5–S1 (see Table 7–6). CT can be used to diagnose these clinical problems and to aid in the surgical planning.

The differential diagnosis of lateral disc

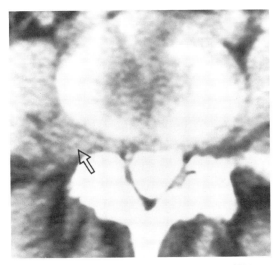

Figure 7–31. Far lateral disc herniation. This CTM examination is at the L4–L5 level. There is a soft tissue "mass" obliterating perineural fat within the neural foramen on the right (arrow). This mass has CT attenuation values similar to those of the intervertebral disc and represents a far lateral disc herniation. (From Kricun R, Kricun ME: Computed Tomography of the Spine: Diagnostic Exercises. Rockville, Maryland: Aspen Publishers, Inc, 1987. Reprinted with permission of Aspen Publishers, Inc.)

herniation by CT includes schwannoma, soft tissue involvement by lymphoma or metastatic disease, infection, cystic nerve root sleeve dilatation, and conjoined nerve root sheath anomaly.[151, 412, 479] A schwannoma located in the neural foramen may simulate a lateral disc herniation; however, widening of the neural foramen may be noticed, and enhancement after intravenous injection of contrast has been described.[151] Metastasis and lymphoma typically have irregular, indistinct margins, with an infiltrative appearance, and may have widening of the paraspinal soft tissues.[151, 412] Destruction of an adjacent pedicle or vertebral body is often associated with metastasis. Soft tissue infection also has indistinct margins and is usually associated with adjacent bone destruction. Cystic dilatation of the nerve root sleeve is isodense with the thecal sac and thus of lower density than lateral disc herniation. Conjoined nerve roots are also less dense than disc herniation and have CT attenuation values similar to or only slightly greater than those of the thecal sac. The study of serial scans may demonstrate the asymmetric derivation of the nerve roots from the thecal sac.[194]

Extruded Disc

Nucleus pulposus that protrudes through a tear in the annulus fibrosus and then extends through or around the posterior longitudinal ligament is termed an extruded disc.[73, 480] In one series of patients with disc herniation, 35% had an extruded disc at surgery.[149] The portion of the nucleus pulposus that extends beyond the posterior longitudinal ligament may remain attached to the parent disc or may be separated from the parent disc and lie as a free fragment in the canal. Rarely, a free fragment may tear the dura and have an intradural location, with compression of the cauda equina.[78, 103]

It is not always possible to distinguish a subligamentous herniation from an extruded disc by CT. However, several CT features of extruded disc may suggest this diagnosis (Table 7–8). A free disc fragment displaced posteriorly into the canal may be separated from the posterior margin of the intervertebral disc by epidural fat. A separation of the free fragment by fat is noted in approximately 50% of cases[103, 480] (Fig. 7–32). In other cases, the free fragment may be dis-

Table 7–8. DIFFERENTIAL FEATURES OF EXTRUDED DISC AND SUBLIGAMENTOUS DISC HERNIATION

	Extruded Disc	Subligamentous Disc Herniation
Separation from posterior disc	50% are separated from disc margin by fat[94, 477]	Contiguous with remainder of disc
Cephalad or caudad displacement	85% >6 mm from mid-disc[94]	Most prominent at disc space level
Size	Often large	Usually not large
Shape	Irregular, polypoid	Smooth, curvilinear

From Kricun R, Kricun ME: Computed Tomography of the Spine: Diagnostic Exercises. Rockville, Maryland: Aspen Publishers, Inc, 1987. Reprinted with permission of Aspen Publishers, Inc.

placed cephalad or caudad and may be found as far as 15 to 30 mm from the intervertebral disc space. The extruded fragment is found 6 mm or more from the center of the disc space in 85% of cases of disc extrusion.[103] The extruded disc fragment may appear larger in the cephalad or caudad direction than at the disc level. This finding is not present in patients with subligamentous herniation.[103] Extruded discs tend to be larger than subligamentous disc herniations. In one study, the maximum AP diameter of the herniated disc was compared with the anticipated normal sagittal diameter of the dural sac.[149] Only 10% of those patients with a ratio of less than one half had an extruded disc at surgery. On the other hand, 90% of patients with a ratio of one half or more were found to have an extruded disc.

The CT diagnosis of a free fragment is important clinically in preoperative planning. It also suggests that chymopapain chemonucleolysis would likely have a less favorable result.[32, 160]

DISORDERS OF THE CERVICAL DISC

CT is an accurate method of diagnosing cervical disorders such as disc herniation and spondylosis (Figs. 7–33 and 7–34). Patients with a cervical radiculopathy and a well-defined clinical level can be evaluated with CT at least as accurately as with conventional myelography, and with less morbidity to the patient.[15, 81, 82, 96] Patients with cervical myelopathy are best studied initially by magnetic resonance imaging or myelography because of the large extent of the cervical canal that must be examined.[94, 395, 417] After myelographic localization, CTM can be performed to better define the pathology and to differentiate soft disc herniation from spondylosis. Good correlation has been found between the degree of spinal cord deformity demonstrated by CTM and the results of surgery. In one study, all pa-

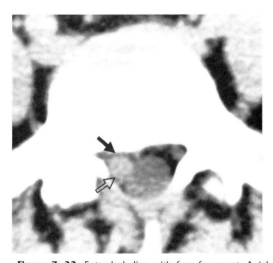

Figure 7–32. Extruded disc with free fragment. Axial CT scan obtained 8 mm caudad to the L5–S1 intervertebral disc. There is a free disc fragment (open arrow) causing slight compression of the thecal sac and partial obliteration of the anterior epidural fat on the right. Note the presence of a thin layer of epidural fat (closed arrow) between the posterior margin of the vertebral body and the free fragment. (From Kricun R, Kricun ME: Computed Tomography of the Spine: Diagnostic Exercises. Rockville, Maryland: Aspen Publishers, Inc, 1987. Reprinted with permission of Aspen Publishers, Inc.)

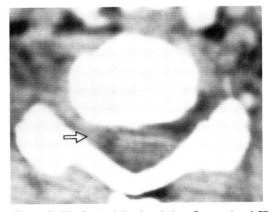

Figure 7–33. Cervical disc herniation. Conventional CT scan without contrast at the C5–C6 level demonstrates a disc herniation (arrow) extending laterally into the right neural foramen. Asymmetry of the fat within the foramina is noted.

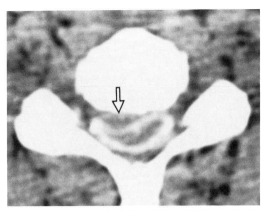

Figure 7–34. Cervical disc herniation. CTM examination demonstrates herniation of the disc (arrow) at the C5–C6 level. The disc herniation is compressing the contrast-filled subarachnoid space and the spinal cord.

tients with severe deformity of the spinal cord and most patients with moderate deformity of the spinal cord had substantial improvement in their clinical findings after surgery.[495]

Several technical factors in the cervical spine examination differ from those of the lumbar study.[187] The cervical spine lacks the abundant epidural fat that is present in the lumbar region. Although disc is of higher density than the thecal sac and the cerebrospinal fluid, the difference in CT attenuation is not as great as that between disc and epidural fat. For this reason, identifying the disc margin may be more difficult in the cervical region than in the lumbar spine. In addition, thin scan slices are required for cervical evaluation owing to the narrower disc spaces. The thin scan slices lead to decreased contrast resolution. Another factor that must be considered is the presence of artifact, particularly when scanning through the plane of the shoulders at the C7–T1 level.

The CT study is performed by angling the gantry parallel to the intervertebral disc space. Scan slice thickness varies with the scanner available, but it is usually 1.5 or 2 mm thick. Approximately 7 sections are obtained at each disc level, with sections obtained above, through, and below the intervertebral disc space. The patient is asked to extend the arms downward as far as possible in an attempt to avoid shoulder artifact. The patient is asked not to breathe, move, or swallow during the CT exposure. Magnification is utilized, and scans are photo-

graphed at both soft tissue and bone window settings.

Although some authors prefer conventional CT scans of the cervical spine,[81, 82] others perform the CT study after the introduction of intrathecal contrast agent,[15, 94, 239, 347] and still others utilize intravenous contrast agent.[19, 489] One study suggests that conventional CT produces suboptimal visualization of the disc space in 50% of cases.[110] CT performed with intrathecal water-soluble contrast agent permits better visualization of the subarachnoid space, spinal cord, and nerve roots and permits better appreciation of spinal cord and nerve root compression.[417] Intravenous contrast agent, on the other hand, enhances the CT appearance of the epidural veins and dura and thus accentuates the interface between the subarachnoid space and the disc, permitting increased diagnostic accuracy of disc herniation.[395] The cervical nerve roots can also be visualized in this manner because of opacification of the surrounding intervertebral venous plexus.[190] Some cervical disc herniations that are not visualized with unenhanced CT may be seen after intravenous contrast enhancement of the dura and venous structures.[395]

DISORDERS OF THE THORACIC DISC

Thoracic disc herniation is a much rarer disorder than are lumbar and cervical disc herniations. Clinically they can present with a confusing picture, and the exact anatomic level of involvement may be difficult to determine. Most thoracic disc herniations occur in the lower thoracic spine, with approximately 75% occurring below T8.[10] Conventional radiographs demonstrate calcification within the spinal canal at the level of intervertebral disc space narrowing in approximately 55% of cases.[292] CT can be utilized to diagnose thoracic disc herniation[10, 35, 201, 404, 454] (Fig. 7–35). Calcified disc herniation is readily demonstrated by unenhanced CT; however, noncalcified thoracic disc herniations are more difficult to demonstrate because of the lack of abundant epidural fat in the thoracic spine and because of the difficulty in determining the exact clinical level of involvement. Myelography or MRI may be used to evaluate for thoracic disc herniation. CTM can follow the myelogram

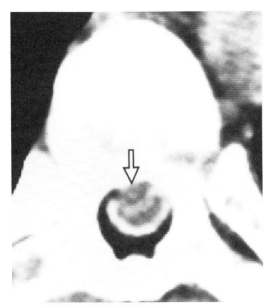

Figure 7–35. Thoracic disc herniation. Axial CTM scan at T6–T7 demonstrates a disc herniation to the right of the midline (arrow), causing compression and displacement of the contrast-filled subarachnoid space and spinal cord.

and further delineate the abnormality. On occasion, CTM can be utilized to demonstrate a disc herniation that was not identified by conventional myelography.[10] Multiple thoracic disc herniations have also been demonstrated by CTM.[35]

SPINAL STENOSIS

Spinal stenosis can be classified as either congenital-developmental stenosis or acquired stenosis[11] (Table 7–9). The congenital-developmental form of spinal stenosis includes the idiopathic and achondroplastic stenoses. Acquired spinal stenosis includes degenerative, spondylolisthetic, iatrogenic (postsurgical fibrosis, postsurgical fusion, postchemonucleolysis), and post-traumatic. Paget's disease,[287, 472] acromegaly and giantism,[116, 130] steroid-induced epidural lipomatosis,[162] fluorosis, and ligamentous ossification are also acquired forms of spinal stenosis. Some patients with congenital stenosis may develop degenerative changes and are then classified as having a combined form of stenosis.

CT is particularly helpful in classifying spinal stenosis anatomically. In this classification, spinal stenosis can be divided into central stenosis and lateral stenosis (Table 7–10). The central form leads to narrowing of the thecal sac, with impingement on the spinal cord or cauda equina, depending on the spinal level of involvement. Lateral stenosis can be divided into lateral recess (subarticular) stenosis and neural foraminal (intervertebral canal) stenosis.[284]

Central Spinal Stenosis (Congenital-Developmental)

Developmental stenosis is typically uniform throughout several or all lumbar segments. The pedicles and laminae are thickened, and the pedicles are short, leading to decreased AP diameter of the canal. The interpedicular distance is decreased in approximately 20% of vertebrae of patients with idiopathic spinal stenosis.[356]

The CT features of congenital-developmental stenosis are presented in Table 7–11. The CT examination of the lumbar spine typically demonstrates thick, short pedicles, decreased AP diameter of the spinal canal,

Table 7–9. ETIOLOGIC CLASSIFICATION OF SPINAL STENOSIS

Congenital-Developmental
Idiopathic
Achondroplastic
Morquio's disease

Acquired
Degenerative
Spondylolisthetic
Iatrogenic (postsurgical fibrosis, fusion, postchemonucleolysis)
Post-traumatic
Paget's disease
Acromegaly and giantism
Steroid-induced epidural lipomatosis
Fluorosis
Ossification of posterior longitudinal ligament and ligamentum flavum

Combined

Table 7–10. ANATOMIC CLASSIFICATION OF SPINAL STENOSIS

Central
Impingement on cauda equina or spinal cord

Lateral
Impingement on nerve root
   Lateral recess stenosis (subarticular)
   Neural foraminal stenosis (intervertebral canal)

Table 7–11. CHARACTERISTIC CT FEATURES OF CONGENITAL-DEVELOPMENT CENTRAL STENOSIS

Uniform narrowing over several or all lumbar segments
Decreased AP diameter of canal (absolute stenosis ≤ 10 mm; relative stenosis 10 to 12 mm)
Short thick pedicles and thickened laminae
Interpedicular distance decreased progressively from L1 to L5 in achondroplasia
Interpedicular distance decreased in 20% of lumbar vertebrae in patients with idiopathic stenosis

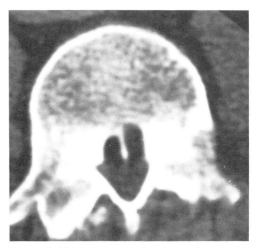

Figure 7–37. Spinal stenosis with widening of the basivertebral grooves (same patient as in Fig. 7–36). Axial CT scan demonstrates widening of the basivertebral grooves that is most likely due to increase in epidural venous pressure secondary to severe spinal stenosis. Again note the short, broad pedicles in this patient with achondroplasia.

small subarachnoid space, and diminished epidural fat (Figs. 7–36 and 7–37). Some attempts have been made to correlate AP diameters of the spinal canal in the midsagittal plane with the degree of spinal stenosis. One CT study suggests that a midsagittal diameter of 10 mm or less indicates absolute stenosis, which may cause compression of the cauda equina.[457] An AP diameter of 10 mm to 12 mm represents relative stenosis and may lead to symptoms when minimal degenerative changes occur. It is necessary, however, to evaluate the relative size of the spinal canal and the thecal sac, since a small

bony canal may not be associated with symptoms when the thecal sac is also small.

Achondroplasia represents a classic example of congenital spinal stenosis. It is a congenital disorder of endochondral bone formation that leads to the development of short pedicles.[5, 169, 312] Early fusion of the neurocentral synchondroses occurs, leading to central stenosis, which is most severe in the AP dimension.[127] Classically, the interpedicular distance is narrowed progressively from L1 to L5. This is the opposite of that found in normal individuals. Although the spinal cord and nerve roots are normal, they are contained within a small bony canal.

Although the thoracolumbar spine is the most frequent symptomatic region in patients with achondroplasia,[312] neurologic symptoms referable to the thoracolumbar spine are usually not found in childhood or early adulthood. These symptoms usually develop after age 40 years, when degenerative changes occur leading to further decrease in the effective space of the central canal.[5, 169] Bulging of the annulus fibrosus may occur at multiple levels, especially in the upper and midlumbar regions.[325] Patients with achondroplasia may also have scoliosis, thoracolumbar kyphosis, lumbar lordosis, or severe gibbous deformity.[276, 325] Spinal cord atrophy and degenerative changes of the lower cervical spine have

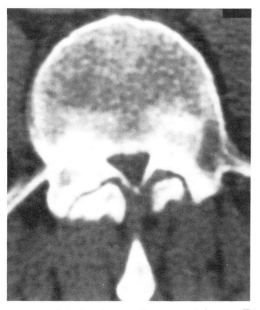

Figure 7–36. Spinal stenosis—congenital type. This patient has achondroplasia, a characteristic form of congenital spinal stenosis. The spinal canal is small, and the pedicles are short and broad. The spinal canal was small through all levels examined.

also been demonstrated with CT.[439] Abnormalities in the cervical or occipitocervical region are especially significant in neonates and infants with achondroplasia, in whom a small foramen magnum and basilar impression may be demonstrated.[312, 325] Marked dilatation of epidural veins due to venous stasis may be a sign of significant spinal stenosis[217] and may be reflected in widening of the basivertebral groove (Fig. 7–37).

Central Spinal Stenosis (Degenerative)

Osseous or soft tissue encroachment on the central spinal canal may lead to degenerative spinal stenosis. Unlike developmental stenosis, which is typically uniform, degenerative stenosis is typically segmental.[229] In degenerative stenosis the narrowed portion of the canal is typically at the level of the disc and facet joints. One or more vertebral levels of involvement may be present; however, the canal diameter between the levels of stenosis may be normal. Hypertrophy of the inferior and superior articular processes leads to central spinal stenosis with decrease in the transverse diameter of the canal. Vertebral osteophytes are another osseous cause of spinal stenosis. A normal osseous canal may still be associated with degenerative spinal stenosis, since the soft tissues may be abnormal. Thus, hypertrophy of the ligamentum flavum, either isolated or in association with osseous changes, is an important cause of spinal stenosis. Generalized bulging of the disc may cause additional stenosis in the patient with osseous and ligamentous hypertrophy.

Table 7–12. CHARACTERISTIC CT FEATURES OF DEGENERATIVE CENTRAL STENOSIS

Segmental rather than uniform—
   stenosis occurs at level of disc and
   facet joints
Hypertrophy and osteophytes from
   articular processes of facets with
   decrease in transverse diameter of
   canal
Thickening of ligamentum flavum
Generalized bulging of annulus fibrosus
Posterior vertebral body osteophytes
Decreased cross-sectional area of
   thecal sac
Decreased AP diameter of canal in only
   20%
Obliteration of epidural fat

The characteristic CT features of degenerative central spinal stenosis are presented in Table 7–12. CT is a reliable method of identifying hypertrophy of the articular processes and vertebral margins as well as hypertrophy of the ligamentum flavum and bulging of the annulus fibrosus (Figs. 7–38 and 7–39). Measurements of the AP diameter of the osseous canal are not as valuable in the evaluation of degenerative spinal stenosis as they are in developmental spinal stenosis. CT study of patients with degenerative central stenosis demonstrates decreased AP diameter of the spinal canal (less than 13 mm) in only 20% of patients.[40] For this reason, some authors suggest that measurement of the cross-sectional area of the thecal sac is a more reliable method of evaluating degenerative stenosis. In one study, the cross-sectional area of the thecal sac was determined by CT, and a cross-sectional area of 180 mm^2 ± 50 mm^2 was considered normal.[40] Measurements of 100 to 130 mm^2 are considered likely to represent early stenosis, whereas those of 100 mm^2 or less are thought to represent absolute lumbar stenosis.

Most often, measurements of canal or thecal sac size are not required for the CT diagnosis of spinal stenosis. The presence of ligamentous hypertrophy, articular process hypertrophy, and bulging of the annulus fibrosus associated with compression of the

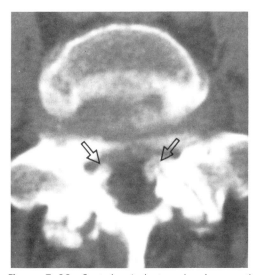

Figure 7–38. Central spinal stenosis—degenerative type. The decrease in the transverse diameter of the spinal canal is caused by osteophytes derived from the articular processes (arrows).

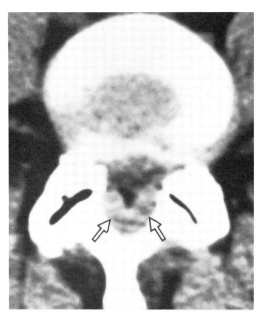

Figure 7–39. Spinal stenosis. The size of the thecal sac is diminished owing to thickening of the ligamenta flava (arrows). Gas within the facet joints (vacuum facet) is evident.

canal size measurements.[388] Although attempts are usually made to scan perpendicular to the spinal canal, the gantry angle does not have a significant effect on the spinal canal measurement when scan slice thickness is 5 mm or less.[113] When a scan slice thickness of 10 mm is used, gantry angulation exceeding 15 degrees from the transverse plane of the canal may lead to underestimation of canal size.[113]

Clinically, patients with spinal stenosis have back pain that may be accompanied by sciatica or claudication in the legs.[484] Typically the pain occurs when the patient is walking or standing and is relieved by lying down or sitting. Pain is also accentuated with hyperextension and relieved by flexion. Chronic back pain precedes radicular pain more often in patients with central spinal stenosis than in those with disc herniation. In addition, the pain is more frequently bilateral, and physical examination less often uncovers reduced straight leg raising.[342]

thecal sac is sufficient to make the diagnosis of degenerative spinal stenosis. In patients who have not had previous surgery, the absence of epidural fat is thought to represent another CT finding of spinal stenosis, indicating a decrease in the effective canal space.[196, 289] In some patients with spinal stenosis, a myelographic block may be demonstrated. In these patients, CTM may follow the conventional myelogram to better delineate the cause of the block and to permit evaluation of the levels beyond the block. Spinal stenosis is frequently multilevel, and the information gained by means of CT or CTM study in a patient with a myelographic block is therefore of considerable importance in the preoperative evaluation.

From a technical point of view, it should be noted that the CT determination of spinal canal size varies with window width, window levels, and the density of the intrathecal contents.[388] The most accurate measurements are obtained at a wide window width (1000 to 4000 HU). The window level is set at approximately the Hounsfield unit measurement that represents the average between the CT measurement of the object being studied and that of the surrounding structures.[388] Intrathecal water-soluble contrast agent is also useful in obtaining reproducible

Central Spinal Stenosis (Combined)

The patient with combined developmental and degenerative spinal stenosis typically becomes symptomatic earlier in life than the patient with pure degenerative stenosis. The patient with combined stenosis has a congenitally small spinal canal, which can then be further compromised by even minor degenerative changes (Fig. 7–40). In this situation, the CT findings will again show short, thick pedicles and thick laminae, with decreased AP diameter of the canal and possible decreased interpedicular distance. In addition, degenerative changes may be identified, such as hypertrophy of the articular processes and marginal vertebral body osteophytes.

Lateral Recess Stenosis

As the lower lumbar and lumbosacral nerve roots leave the thecal sac, they course obliquely in a caudal and lateral direction to exit through their respective neural foramina. Along this path, they traverse a region referred to as the lateral recess. The boundaries of the lateral recess are listed in Table 7–13.[79, 305] Bony or soft tissue encroachment

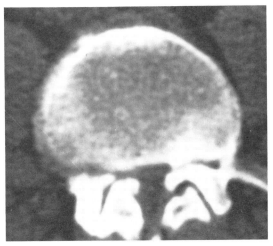

Figure 7–40. Combined degenerative and congenital spinal stenosis (same patient as in Figs. 7–36 and 7–37). The patient, a 47 year old man with achondroplasia, has developed secondary degenerative changes of the articular processes, which are encroaching on the thecal sac.

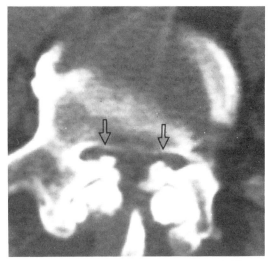

Figure 7–41. Lateral recess stenosis. Axial CT scan demonstrates narrowing of the lateral recesses (arrows) that is caused by osteophytes of the articular processes. In addition, there is central spinal stenosis.

upon the lateral recess may lead to lateral recess stenosis (subarticular stenosis). This encroachment is most often due to medial hypertrophy of the superior articular process, an abnormality that can be identified readily with CT[79, 305] (Fig. 7–41). Other causes of lateral recess stenosis include vertebral body osteophytes and subluxation of the facet joints. Bulging of the annulus fibrosus usually does not by itself cause nerve root compression but may be seen in association with other hypertrophic changes and thus lead to additional nerve root compromise.[191]

The lateral recess can be measured on transaxial CT scans. A CT measurement of 5 mm or more is normal, 4 mm is borderline, and less than 3 mm is stenotic[230] (Table 7–14). It should be noted that approximately 15% of skeletons examined have a trefoil-shaped spinal canal at one or more levels, most frequently at L5.[119] The trefoil shape of the canal does not by itself represent stenosis

but may predispose one to acquired lateral recess stenosis, with associated osteophytes and bulging of the annulus fibrosus.

CT is a more sensitive and more accurate method of studying the lateral recess than are the other modalities available, such as myelography.[64, 289, 384] This has clinical importance because patients operated upon for disc herniation frequently have coexistent lateral stenosis or central stenosis or both. Unrecognized or inadequately treated lateral stenosis (lateral recess or neural foraminal) is considered a major cause of the failed back surgery syndrome.[64, 230, 278, 360] In one study, more than 50% of patients with the failed back surgery syndrome who had been operated on for disc herniation had lateral spinal stenosis either alone or in combination with disc herniation.[64] Patients with lateral recess stenosis may have neurogenic claudication with unilateral or bilateral leg pain that is accentuated by standing and walking and relieved by squatting, sitting in a flexed position, or lying down with hips flexed.[79, 305]

Table 7–13. BOUNDARIES OF LATERAL RECESS

Anterior
Posterolateral margin of vertebral body and disc

Posterior
Superior articular process

Lateral
Pedicle

Table 7–14. MEASUREMENT OF LATERAL RECESS IN AXIAL PLANE

≥ 5 mm = Normal
4 mm = Borderline
< 3 mm = Stenotic

Table 7–15. BOUNDARIES OF NEURAL FORAMEN (INTERVERTEBRAL CANAL)

Superior
   Pedicle of vertebra above

Inferior
   Pedicle of vertebra below

Anterior
   Posterior aspect of vertebral bodies and intervertebral disc

Posterior
   Pars interarticularis and apex of superior articular process of inferior vertebral body

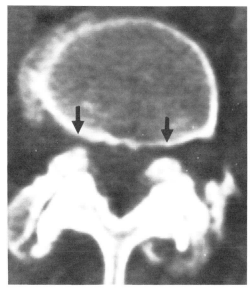

Figure 7–42. Neural foraminal stenosis. Axial CT scan at L4 demonstrates narrowing of the neural foramina (arrows) that is caused by osteophyte formation of the superior articular processes at this level. Mild central stenosis can also be observed.

Stenosis of the Neural Foramen

As the lumbosacral nerve roots pass beyond the lateral recess, they traverse the intervertebral canal and exit through their respective neural foramina. The boundaries of the neural foramen are listed in Table 7–15.[228] The nerve root courses through the upper portion of the neural foramen, approximately 1 to 1.5 cm cephalad to the next lower intervertebral disc. Bony or soft tissue encroachment upon the foramen leads to neural foraminal stenosis.

CT is a more accurate method of evaluating the intervertebral canal than are conventional radiography and myelography.[289, 341, 384] Hypertrophy of the superior articular process or osteophyte derived from the pos-

terolateral vertebral body margin may cause osseous encroachment upon the neural foramen, leading to flattening or enlargement of the dorsal root ganglion and obliteration of the perineural fat within the foramen[192] (Figs. 7–42 and 7–43). Several factors influence the measurement of the neural fora-

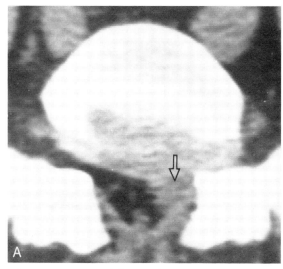
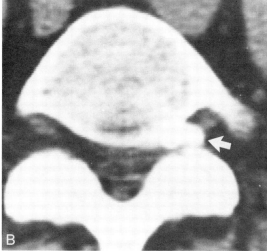

Figure 7–43. Neural foraminal stenosis and disc herniation. *A,* Axial CT scan through L5–S1 intervertebral disc demonstrates posterolateral disc herniation on left (arrow). *B,* CT scan through neural foramina above L5–S1 disc reveals large vertebral body osteophyte causing stenosis of the neural foramen (arrow). The CT recognition of combined disc herniation and spinal stenosis is important for preoperative planning.

minal width on transaxial CT scans and may lead to interobserver discrepancies.[30] These factors include the CT window settings utilized and the reference points used for measurement. Increased diagnostic accuracy is achieved with the use of parasagittal and oblique reconstruction of the axial images.[192] In addition to osseous stenosis, neural foraminal nerve root entrapment may also be caused by lateral disc herniation, postoperative fibrotic scarring, spondylolisthesis, and tumor.[196, 341]

LIGAMENTOUS OSSIFICATION

The posterior longitudinal liagment and the ligamentum flavum may ossify and cause spinal stenosis, with symptoms of myelopathy and radiculopathy. CT is useful in diagnosing these entities and in evaluating the extent of the process.

Ossification of the posterior longitudinal ligament (OPLL) is more prevalent in Japan and eastern Asian countries, where it occurs in 1% to 3% of the population with cervical symptoms.[317, 453] The incidence among Caucasians is only 0.2%.[317, 453] The most frequent site of involvement is the cervical spine, with more than one cervical level usually involved. Clinically there may be numbness of the hands, weakness of the legs, spastic gait, pain in the neck and arms, and urinary or intestinal symptoms.[178, 182] Some patients may be asymptomatic despite severe spinal stenosis.

OPLL may be segmental (behind each vertibral body); continuous (involving multiple vertebrae without interruption); mixed (segmental and continuous); or localized (limited to the intervertebral disc level).[453] The localized form is the least frequent type and may be difficult to distinguish from spondylosis. OPLL is seen as a midline ossified mass just posterior to the vertebral bodies. This mass typically has an ovoid or oblong shape on the axial CT scan[317] (Fig. 7–44A). In some CT sections, the ossification may appear attached to the vertebral body, whereas at other levels it may appear unattached.[182, 317] Interposed between the ossified ligament and the posterior aspect of the vertebral body may be an unossified deep layer of the posterior longitudinal ligament[182, 377] or venous structures. In some cases, a tandem type of ossification is seen, with two layers of ossification present.[317] This phenomenon may be due to a mixed segmental and continuous type of ossification, with the continuous layer of ossification located posterior to a separate segmental layer of ossification.[317] Severe myelopathy in patients with OPLL is most likely to occur when the stenosis demonstrated by axial CT

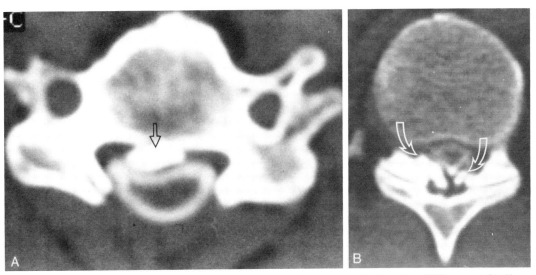

Figure 7–44. Ligamentous ossification. *A*, Posterior longitudinal ligament ossification. Axial CTM scan at C5. There is thick ossification in the epidural space (arrow) that is encroaching on the contrast-filled subarachnoid space. This represents ossification of the posterior longitudinal ligament. *B*, Ossification of the ligamenta flava in another patient. Axial CTM scan demonstrates moderate encroachment on the thecal sac caused by ossification of the ligamenta flava (arrows) in the lower thoracic spine.

exceeds 30%.[178] Sagittal reconstruction of the axial images further defines the longitudinal extent of the ossification and helps delineate the degree of stenosis. CT can also be used in the follow-up examination of surgically treated patients. Surgery may include partial resection of the vertebrae, release or removal of the ossified mass, and insertion of an iliac bone graft.[179] Ossification or calcification of the posterior longitudinal liagment has also been found in 50% of patients with diffuse idiopathic skeletal hyperostosis (DISH).[377]

Ossification of the ligamentum flavum (OLF) most commonly occurs in the lower thoracic spine, particularly at T9–T10 and T10–T11.[309] OLF has been found on conventional radiographs of the thoracic spine in approximately 5% of an asymptomatic Japanese population.[242] These ossifications are described as hook-type and are located on the lateral portion of the ligamentum flavum, adjacent to the articular processes. Patients with myelopathy secondary to OLF more frequently have extensive nodular or masslike ossification along the anterior margin of the laminae bilaterally[309] (Fig. 7–44B). CTM can be utilized to delineate the degree of spinal cord compression. OLF may occur separately or in association with OPLL.

FACET JOINTS

The facet joints are lined by synovial membrane and are formed by the articulation of the inferior articular process of the vertebra above and the superior articular process of the vertebra below. CT is an ideal method for evaluating the facet joints of the lumbar spine because of the oblique orientation of the joints. Bone window settings (window width of 1000 to 2000 HU and window level of 200 to 350 HU) are utilized.

The normal facet joint has smooth, regular cortical margins, with a joint space width of 2 to 4 mm (Fig. 7–45). The orientation of the facet joints varies with the level examined. The joints tend to have a more sagittal orientation at L3–L4, a more coronal orientation at L5–S1, and an intermediate position at L4–L5.[455] Abnormalities of facet joints are frequently discovered by CT, being found in 43% of patients studied for low back pain or sciatica or both.[72] The types of facet joint abnormalities identified by CT are listed in

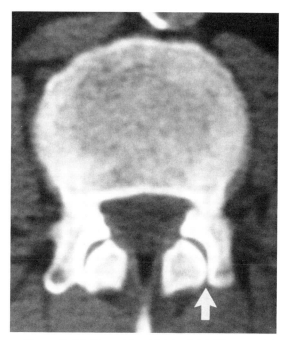

Figure 7–45. Normal facet joints. Axial CT scan at L4. The facet joints (arrow) are normal in width, and the cortical margins are smooth and regular.

Table 7–16. Of these abnormalities, the most frequent are osteophytes and articular facet hypertrophy. An osteophyte is an outgrowth of cortical bone that is derived from the articular margin, and it therefore lacks a medullary space (Fig. 7–46). Hypertrophy is an enlargement of the articular process with normal medullary and cortical proportions[71, 72] (Fig. 7–47). Osteophytes and hypertrophic changes of the articular processes may lead to central or lateral spinal stenosis. Other CT findings, such as joint space narrowing, subchondral sclerosis, and subchondral erosions and cysts, are abnormalities of

Table 7–16. ABNORMALITIES OF FACET JOINTS IDENTIFIED BY CT

Osteophyte of articular process
Hypertrophy of articular process
Joint space narrowing (< 2 mm)
Subchondral sclerosis
Subchondral erosions and cysts
Gas within joint (vacuum facet)
Calcification in periarticular region
Subluxation (i.e., associated with degenerative spondylolisthesis or retrospondylolisthesis)
Synovial cyst

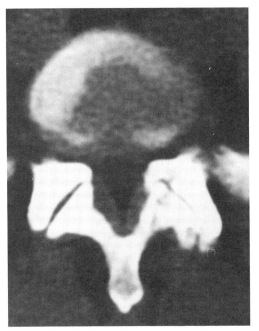

Figure 7–46. Degenerative osteoarthritis. The left facet joint is markedly narrowed. Cysts, erosions, and osteophytes are present.

evaluated for back pain[71] (see Fig. 7–39). The significance of this finding is uncertain; however, it has been seen along with other changes of severe osteoarthritis of the facet joints[255] and has been described in association with degenerative spondylolisthesis.[265] Subluxation of the facet joints may be identified. This may be associated with degenerative spondylolisthesis (anterior subluxation of inferior articular processes) or retrospondylolisthesis (posterior subluxation of inferior articular processes). CT is helpful in differentiating those patients with erosive and cystic changes of the facet joints from those with osteophytes and hypertrophic changes. This differentiation may be useful in treatment planning. Patients with the facet joint syndrome may benefit from intra-articular injection of local anesthetic and steroid suspension,[69, 72, 100, 311] percutaneous radio frequency facet denervation,[422] or surgical fusion.[369] On the other hand, large osteophytes of the articular processes may cause spinal stenosis with symptoms that

osteoarthritis[71, 72] (see Fig. 7–46). Gas within a facet joint (vacuum facet) appears as a linear or elliptic low-attenuation area within the joint and is noted in 20% of patients

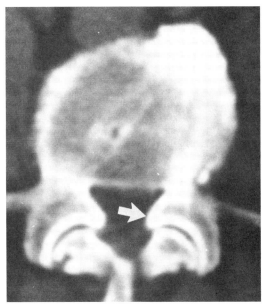

Figure 7–47. Hypertrophy of the facet joints. Hypertrophy of the superior articular processes is causing moderate encroachment on the central spinal canal (arrow).

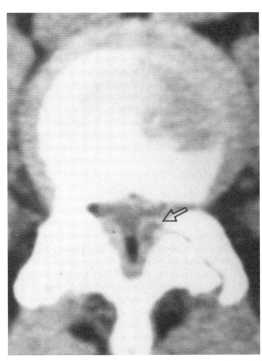

Figure 7–48. Synovial cyst. A synovial cyst (arrow) is seen adjacent to the left facet joint. It has a dense rim and a lucent center. A bulging annulus is also noted. (From Kricun R, Kricun ME: Computed Tomography of the Spine: Diagnostic Exercises. Rockville, Maryland: Aspen Publishers, Inc, 1987. Reprinted with permission of Aspen Publishers, Inc.)

might instead be successfully treated by foraminotomy.

Synovial cysts may occur adjacent to a lumbar facet joint, most commonly at the L4–L5 level.[36, 197, 244] These cysts are thought to occur in response to degenerative changes of the synovial membrane–lined facet joints. Typically, a synovial cyst has a low density center surrounded by a rim of calcification[74, 197, 244, 302] (Fig. 7–48). Gas may be present within the cyst, having dissected from an adjacent facet joint with a vacuum phenomenon.[413, 433]

SPONDYLOLYSIS AND SPONDYLOLISTHESIS

Spondylolysis

Spondylolysis is a break in the pars interarticularis. This abnormality can be identified readily on CT examination, even in the absence of confirmation by conventional radiographs.[172, 251, 447] Characteristic axial CT scan features of spondylolysis should help prevent mistaking this abnormality for a facet joint.[172] For example, the pars defect is located approximately 10 to 15 mm above the intervertebral disc space level. The pars defect has jagged, irregular, noncorticated margins (Fig. 7–49). In comparison, facet

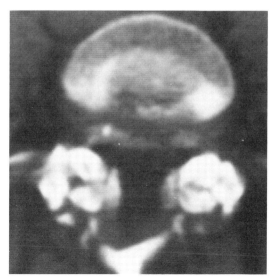

Figure 7–50. Spondylolysis with fragmentation. In this patient with bilateral pars defects, osseous fragmentation and callus formation are present, causing encroachment on the central spinal canal. (From Kricun R, Kricun ME: Computed Tomography of the Spine: Diagnostic Exercises. Rockville, Maryland: Aspen Publishers, Inc, 1987. Reprinted with permission of Aspen Publishers, Inc.)

joints are located at and adjacent to the intervertebral disc space and typically have smooth, straight, or slightly curved cortical margins (see Fig. 7–45). In addition, the pars defect frequently is in a coronal plane and is located anterior to the facet joint. The diagnosis of spondylolysis can be excluded if a complete, intact cortical ring outlining the bony spinal canal is demonstrated above the level of the neural foramen.[251] The AP diameter of the spinal canal appears elongated in patients with spondylolysis, usually but not always in association with spondylolisthesis.

CT can also demonstrate callus or granulation tissue adjacent to the pars defect in approximately 20% of cases[391] (Fig. 7–50). This may be a cause of compression of the thecal sac or nerve root. Fragmentation of the laminae is seen in approximately 15% of conventional radiographs of patients with spondylolysis.[6] This finding is readily appreciated on the axial CT scan.[239] In some cases, the pars interarticularis may appear narrow or sclerotic. Unilateral spondylolysis is less common than bilateral spondylolysis and may be associated with contralateral neural arch sclerosis and hypertrophy.

The axial CT examination is studied at bone window settings. In most cases, the axial scans are sufficient for diagnosis of

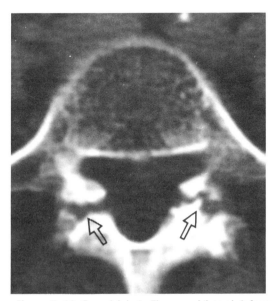

Figure 7–49. Spondylolysis. There are bilateral defects in the pars articularis with irregular, jagged margins (arrows).

spondylolysis.[172, 447] Parasagittal reconstruction views can also be obtained to further delineate a defect in the pars interarticularis.

Spondylolisthesis

Spondylolisthesis refers to slippage of one vertebral body upon the adjacent vertebra. There are several categories in the classification of spondylolisthesis, and a few are discussed at this time.

Isthmic Spondylolisthesis

Isthmic spondylolisthesis is an anterior slippage of one vertebral body upon the adjacent caudad vertebra, with an associated break in the pars interarticularis of the superior vertebra. This most frequently occurs at L5–S1. The slippage can be identified on conventional radiographs and on the lateral digital radiograph obtained with the CT study. Axial CT examination demonstrates two vertebrae and their interposed disc or elongation of the AP diameter of the spinal canal. A pseudoherniation of the disc is seen, with disc material noted posterior to the L5 vertebral body (Fig. 7–51). It is unusual for a disc herniation to occur at the level of isthmic spondylolisthesis. Disc herniation is more likely to occur at the next superior disc level.[123, 391] However, at the level of spondylolisthesis, disc herniation may be suspected if there is asymmetric compression of the epidural fat, thecal sac, or nerve root.[54] Sagittal reconstruction has been used to determine whether the disc extends significantly beyond the posterior aspect of the sacrum.[123, 391]

CT is also useful in evaluating additional structural abnormalities that are associated with isthmic spondylolisthesis. The most common associated finding is stenosis of the intervertebral canal (neural foraminal stenosis), which occurs in approximately 25% of symptomatic patients with isthmic spondylolisthesis.[123] Central and lateral recess stenoses occur less often. Sagittal recon-

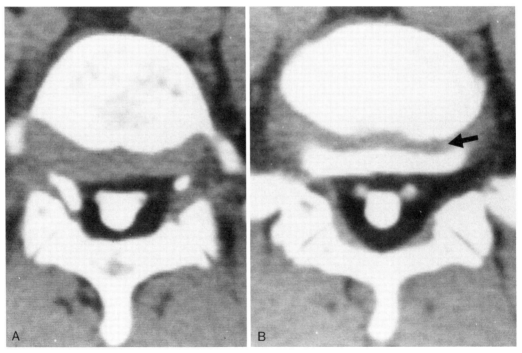

Figure 7–51. Spondylolisthesis with pseudoherniation of the disc. *A,* Axial CTM scan obtained through the plane of the posterior aspect of the L5–S1 disc. The posterior margin of the disc extends beyond the vertebral margin of L5. In this patient, pseudoherniation occurred because of grade II spondylolisthesis. Note preservation of the epidural fat. *B,* Axial CTM scan obtained 4 mm caudad to *A.* The posterior aspect of S1 can be seen posterior to a portion of L5–S1 disc (arrow) and has the same configuration as the previously described pseudoherniation of the disc. (From Kricun R, Kricun ME: Computed Tomography of the Spine: Diagnostic Exercises. Rockville, Maryland: Aspen Publishers, Inc, 1987. Reprinted with permission of Aspen Publishers, Inc.)

struction views may be helpful in the evaluation of these stenotic changes.[123, 391]

Degenerative Spondylolisthesis

Degenerative spondylolisthesis is an anterior slippage of one vertebra upon the next caudad vertebra with an intact neural arch. Over 90% of cases of degenerative spondylolisthesis occur at L4–L5.[447] The lateral digital radiograph reveals the anterior slippage, which is usually limited to grade I/IV. Axial CT examination reveals abnormality of the facet joints, which frequently have a sagittal orientation. Subluxation of the facet joints may be demonstrated, with posterior displacement of the superior articular process of the vertebra below. Osteoarthritic changes of the facet joints, such as joint space narrowing, sclerosis, osteophytes, and vacuum phenomenon, are common. Approximately 75% of symptomatic patients with degenerative spondylolisthesis have an additional structural abnormality.[123] These secondary changes include neural foraminal stenosis, central spinal stenosis, and disc herniation. It should be noted that the disc herniation occurring in patients with degenerative spondylolisthesis most often occurs at the level of slippage rather than at the next higher level, as is most often seen in patients

with isthmic spondylolisthesis.[123] In the evaluation of the secondary changes, multiplanar reconstruction may be helpful.[123, 392]

Retrospondylolisthesis

Retrospondylolisthesis is an uncommon abnormality in which there is posterior slippage of one vertebra on the adjacent caudad vertebra. This occurs most commonly at L2–L3 and L3–L4 and less often at L4–L5.[447] The slippage is usually limited to 2 to 3 mm. The axial CT scan demonstrates anterior subluxation of the superior articular process of the vertebra below. The facet joints usually have a sagittal orientation; however, osteoarthritic changes are most often absent.[447]

OSSEOUS TUMORS AND TUMORLIKE CONDITIONS

Metastasis

Metastasis is the most common tumor of the spine, occurring with increasing frequency after age 40.[237] It most often develops from hematogenous spread secondary to carcinoma of the breast, prostate, and lung in adults and from neuroblastoma in the infant

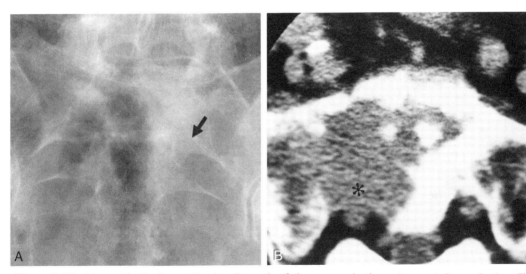

Figure 7–52. Metastasis. *A*, Conventional radiograph of the sacrum in the anteroposterior projection. There is suggestion of focal bone destruction involving the most proximal arcuate line on the left (arrow). The arcuate lines on the right appear normal and are sharp and distinct. *B*, Axial CT scan taken 2 days following *A* demonstrates extensive bone destruction due to metastatic disease. The margin of the right sacral foramen (asterisk) is destroyed by tumor, and the sacral nerve is displaced. CT can detect bone destruction better than conventional radiographs can.

and child. Direct extension from paravertebral tumor can occur, causing osseous destruction or scalloping of the vertebral body margin. Rectal carcinoma may invade the sacrum directly, causing bone destruction.

Evaluation of patients suspected of having metastatic disease begins with radionuclide bone scanning and conventional radiography. The radionuclide bone scan is highly sensitive to the presence of metastasis but is nonspecific, since benign conditions such as Paget's disease, healing fracture, and degenerative disorders also demonstrate increased isotope uptake. The conventional radiograph lacks sensitivity, since approximately 50% of cancellous bone must be destroyed before spinal metastasis can be detected.[115] Because of its superior resolution, CT demonstrates osseous metastatic disease more readily than conventional radiography[316, 371] (Fig. 7–52). CT is useful in the evaluation of patients at high risk for osseous metastasis (with carcinoma of the breast, lung, prostate) who have a positive radionuclide bone scan and normal conventional radiographs.[183, 193, 316, 371] Patients with metastatic disease can be separated from those with a positive bone scan secondary to degenerative disease or other benign disorders.

The CT appearance of metastatic disease

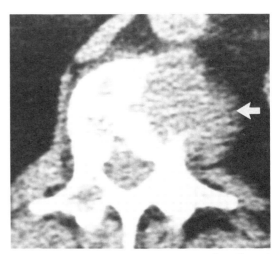

Figure 7–54. Metastasis to lumbar vertebra. There is destruction of the left side of the lumbar vertebral body. Tumor has extended into the paravertebral soft tissues (arrow). CT affords excellent visualization of soft tissue structures, permitting diagnosis of paravertebral extension of tumor that might be difficult to detect by other diagnostic measures.

is usually that of single or multiple destructive osteolytic lesions of the vertebral body or sacrum (Figs. 7–53 through 7–56). The pedicles are another frequent site of metastasis. Metastatic lesions usually do not have a sclerotic rim or calcification within the matrix. Reactive osseous sclerosis may occur following radiation therapy or chemotherapy. Osteosclerotic metastatic disease is typ-

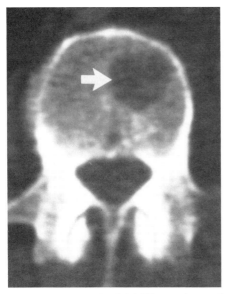

Figure 7–53. Metastasis. Axial CT scan demonstrates a single osteolytic lesion of the cancellous portion of the vertebral body (arrow). The cortical margin of the vertebral body is intact. A lesion of this size in cancellous bone may not be detected on the conventional radiograph.

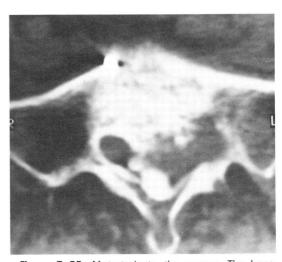

Figure 7–55. Metastasis to the sacrum. The bone destruction in the left portion of the sacrum is displacing the contrast-filled thecal sac and obliterating the left nerve root sleeve.

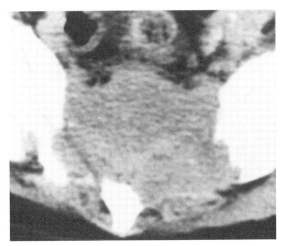

Figure 7–56. Metastasis. Axial CT scan of the sacrum demonstrates almost complete destruction of the sacrum at this scan level. The mass extends anteriorly into the pelvis and posteriorly into the buttocks. Such extensive metastasis resembles a primary bone tumor.

ical of carcinoma of the prostate gland and lymphoma and may occasionally occur secondary to carcinoma of the breast (Fig. 7–57). The sclerosis is not due to the tumor itself but rather to reactive changes secondary to the presence of underlying tumor.[237] Importantly, CT can detect epidural and paravertebral extension of osseous metastatic disease (see Figs. 7–54 and 7–55).

CT is useful in the early detection of metastatic disease to the spine. It delineates

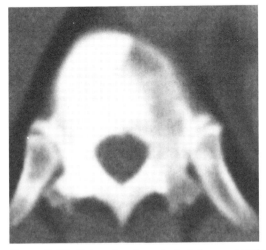

Figure 7–57. Osteosclerotic metastasis from prostatic carcinoma. Extensive osteosclerosis of the vertebra and posterior elements is noted on this axial CT scan and represents reactive bone formation from underlying metastasis.

the extent of tumor, which aids in delivering appropriate therapy. This may prevent vertebral fracture or epidural extension of the tumor, which in turn could lead to compression of the spinal cord or cauda equina.[371] CT can be used to guide closed needle biopsy, and this procedure has less risk of complication than biopsy performed under conventional radiographic guidance.[4] CT is also helpful in the evaluation of tumor both before and after radiotherapy.

Myeloma

Although the radionuclide bone scan is sensitive to the detection of metastatic disease, it is rather insensitive to the detection of myeloma, appearing normal in 27% of patients with radiographically proven myeloma.[51] The conventional radiograph is not highly sensitive to the detection of early myeloma because, as stated previously, approximately 50% of cancellous bone must be destroyed before a lesion is radiographically visible.[115] The CT scan is more sensitive than conventional radiography in demonstrating vertebral myeloma, and the CT scan may demonstrate lesions in cases in which conventional radiographs and radionuclide bone scans are unrewarding.[195, 408, 430] CT can be used to evaluate patients who are clinically suspected of having myeloma but have normal conventional radiographs and radionuclide bone scans. The CT scan is performed to include the vertebrae in the symptomatic regions. CT can also be used to further evaluate questionable conventional radiographic findings. Those patients known to have multiple myeloma may have bone pain and normal spinal radiographs. In this clinical situation, CT evidence of bony involvement at the symptomatic site often indicates a need to initiate therapy.[408] CTM may be utilized when there is clinical evidence of spinal cord or cauda equina compression suggesting epidural extension.

The CT appearance of myeloma may consist of multiple small osteolytic foci measuring 1 to 5 mm; however, lesions greater than 10 mm may also occur frequently[408, 430] (Fig. 7–58). The vertebral bodies are most frequently involved because of the presence of red marrow.[238] The pedicles possess little red marrow and are infrequently involved early in the course of disease. With more

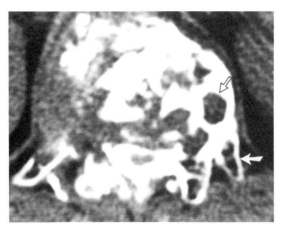

Figure 7–58. Multiple myeloma. Axial CTM scan demonstrates marked fragmentation of the vertebral body caused by pathologic fracture from underlying myeloma. Focal destructive lesions are noted (arrows).

advanced disease, fat marrow in the pedicles changes to red marrow, thus subjecting the pedicles to the development of myeloma.[238]

With advancing disease, vertebral collapse may occur secondary to marked vertebral body destruction. Tumor or hemorrhage may extend into the paravertebral and epidural spaces, causing spinal cord or cauda equina compression. Sagittal reconstruction of axial CT images can be useful in evaluating these patients. In some cases, myeloma may produce an expansile lesion of bone that may encroach on the spinal canal and neural elements. Rarely, myeloma may appear osteosclerotic either in untreated patients or following radiation therapy or chemotherapy.[114, 400] Osteosclerotic myeloma may also be associated with a syndrome of polyneuropathy, organomegaly, endocrinopathy, M-protein, and skin changes (the POEMS syndrome).[376, 400]

Other Primary Osseous Lesions of the Spine and Sacrum

Primary bone lesions of the spine and sacrum may in some cases be evaluated adequately by radionuclide bone scans and conventional radiographs. However, CT frequently provides additional information, such as soft tissue extension into the paravertebral and epidural regions, presence of posterior element involvement, increased sensitivity to the presence of calcification, and detection of an important diagnostic clue (e.g., the presence of a nidus in osteoid osteoma). Sacral lesions in general are difficult to evaluate by conventional radiography, and CT is useful in demonstration of these lesions.

Chondrosarcoma. Chondrosacroma is a malignant tumor of cartilage matrix that occurs rarely in the spine and sacrum. It may arise de novo or secondary to malignant degeneration of an osteochondroma or secondary to radiation.[438] CT demonstrates an osteolytic lesion with punctate calcifications of tumor matrix (Fig. 7–59). Occasionally, the calcifications may appear partly amorphous when they are extensive.

Osteosarcoma. Osteosarcoma is a highly malignant bone tumor that rarely involves the spine. This tumor may arise de novo or may occur secondary to Paget's disease or radiation therapy.[423, 438] Approximately 70% of patients with spinal osteosarcoma present with neurologic symptoms.[423] CT demonstrates radiodense amorphous bone tumor that may extend into the paravertebral soft tissues and epidural space (Fig. 7–60). Osteosarcoma may appear osteosclerotic, osteolytic, or as a mixed lesion.

Ewing's Sarcoma. Ewing's sarcoma is a malignant bone tumor that usually occurs during the first 2 decades of life. About 3.5% of Ewing's sarcomas involve the axial skeleton.[234] The sacrum is the most frequent site of Ewing's sarcoma in the axial skeleton, accounting for approximately 60% of such

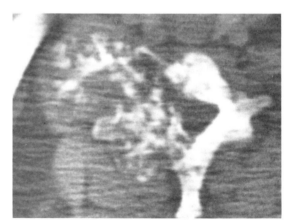

Figure 7–59. Chondrosarcoma. Axial CT scan of C7. There is marked destruction of the right aspect of the vertebral body, pedicle, and lamina, with encroachment into the spinal canal. The mass extends into the paravertebral soft tissue structures and contains punctate calcifications suggestive of cartilage matrix. (Courtesy of Dr. J. G. Teplick, Philadelphia, Pennsylvania.)

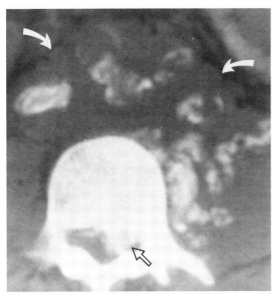

Figure 7–60. Osteosarcoma. There is osteosclerosis of the left half of the vertebral body, and ossific density extends into the spinal canal (straight arrow). Punctate and amorphous densities are present in the large paravertebral soft tissue mass (curved arrows). (Courtesy of Dr. D. Vanel, France.)

lesions.[477] CT demonstrates aggressive osteolytic bone destruction, often with a large presacral mass. In some cases, there may be reactive sclerosis, and occasionally an entirely osteoblastic lesion may be found. CT is useful in treatment planning and for follow-up evaluation of patients with Ewing's sarcoma.[456]

Giant Cell Tumor. Giant cell tumor is the second most frequent primary tumor of the sacrum, second only to chordoma.[428] The sacrum is the most common site of giant cell tumor within the axial skeleton.[428] The CT examination may demonstrate an osteolytic lesion surrounded by a thin sclerotic margin.[267] With advancing disease, the bone may appear to expand symmetrically, and eventually the cortex is destroyed. Giant cell tumor may be associated with a large mass that may extend anteriorly into the presacral region or posteriorly into the buttock.[267]

Chordoma. Chordoma, a tumor that arises from notochord rests, most frequently occurs in the sacrococcygeal region (50%), followed by the clivus (35%) and the vertebral column (15%).[437] Within the spine, the cervical and lumbar regions are more involved than the thoracic levels.[304, 437] CT demonstrates an osteolytic or mixed osteolytic and osteoblastic

lesion of the vertebral body or sacrum (Fig. 7–61). Rarely, vertebral chordoma may appear as an entirely osteoblastic lesion resembling an "ivory" vertebra.[415] The presence of vertebral or sacral destruction is more readily detected by CT than by conventional radiography.[140] Although the posterior elements are not commonly involved initially, there is frequent posterior involvement with recurrent disease.[304] A large paravertebral or presacral mass is frequently found with chordoma and is often much larger than might be expected from the amount of bone involvement.[240, 304] CT is more sensitive than conventional radiography in the detection of calcification. CT demonstrates calcification within the soft tissue mass of 40% of vertebral chordomas[304] and of an even greater percentage of sacral chordomas.[240] The calcifications are usually amorphous and tend to be more extensive at the periphery of the tumor.[240] Areas of low attenuation may be found within the tumor mass in 30% to over 50% of vertebral chordomas,[140, 304] most likely representing myxomatous or gelatinous tissue.[437] Chordoma may involve two contiguous vertebral bodies, a feature that is unusual in other tumors of the spine.[141] CT is useful in demonstrating epidural extension of tumor. Soft tissue extension of tumor into the sacral canal may be detected by CT even in areas that are below the level of the thecal sac and thus inaccessible to myelographic evaluation.[240] Rarely, a cervical chordoma may cause enlargement

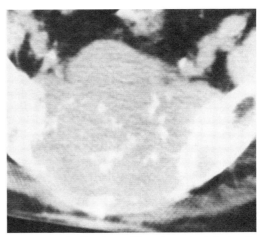

Figure 7–61. Chordoma. There is marked destruction of the sacrum. Tumor mass extends anteriorly into the soft tissues. Calcifications are evident within the mass. (Courtesy of Dr. W. Murphy, St. Louis, Missouri.)

of the intervertebral foramen, which simulates the findings of a neurofibroma.[460]

Osteoblastoma. Osteoblastoma is a rare primary bone tumor; however, approximately 35% of osteoblastomas arise in the spine or sacrum.[209] Osteoblastoma of the spine is usually detected by conventional radiography; however, CT is useful in determining the exact anatomic location, the extent of the tumor, and its relationship to surrounding structures[129, 213, 231, 463] (Fig. 7–62). The CT study reveals an osteolytic, frequently expansile lesion of the posterior elements. The margin of the lesion is typically sclerotic and sharply defined, although occasionally the margin may suggest an aggressive lesion.[1] Typically an osteoblastoma is larger than 1 cm and usually larger than 2 cm in diameter when initially discovered.[213, 296] The ossified matrix of an osteoblastoma is more readily demonstrated by CT than by conventional radiography, and ossified tumor extending into the spinal canal can be identified.[181]

Osteoid Osteoma. Osteoid osteoma most frequently involves the posterior elements. There is usually a radiolucent nidus measuring 1 cm or less that is surrounded by exuberant sclerosis. The nidus may be difficult to detect by conventional radiography.[152, 213] The highly sensitive radionuclide bone scan is almost always positive in cases of osteoid osteoma;[152] however, this study

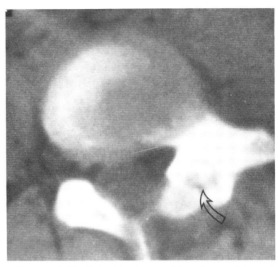

Figure 7–63. Osteoid osteoma. There is a radiolucent nidus in the left lamina (arrow), within which is a rounded area of sclerosis. There is extensive sclerosis in the surrounding bone and in the pedicle and transverse process. (Courtesy of Dr. J. Mall, San Francisco, California.)

lacks specificity. CT can demonstrate the characteristic radiolucent nidus and the surrounding reactive sclerosis[152, 209, 281] (Fig. 7–63). CT may be the only imaging modality to demonstrate the nidus.[152, 281] The nidus typically has a smooth inner surface.[281] Occasionally, ossification may occur within the nidus and is more readily detected by CT than by conventional radiography.[18, 213] The ossified center is round, smooth, and centrally located within the nidus.[281] CT identifies the precise location of the nidus, which is important in preoperative planning and helps eliminate unnecessary surgical resection that might otherwise lead to compromise of spinal stability.* Some patients may present with an osteosclerotic lesion of the pedicle identified on conventional radiography. CT detection of the nidus differentiates an osteoid osteoma from other causes of an osteosclerotic pedicle.[466] Occasionally the nidus is not visualized on CT owing to partial volume averaging.

Aneurysmal Bone Cyst. Aneurysmal bone cyst is a tumorlike condition that appears on CT as a highly expansile osteolytic lesion (Fig. 7–64). A thin rim of bone is present and is more readily detected by CT than by conventional radiography.[181] The matrix does not calcify. Aneurysmal bone cyst usu-

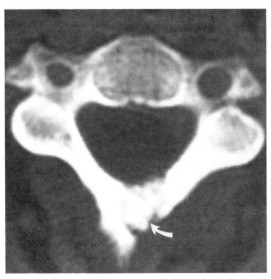

Figure 7–62. Osteoblastoma. There is destruction of the left lamina and spinous process of C4. The matrix of the mass is partially ossified (arrow).

---

*Reference numbers 152, 209, 213, 331, 338, 466.

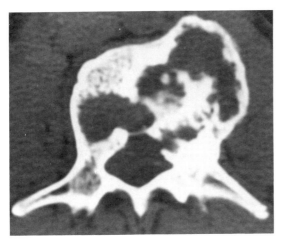

Figure 7–64. Aneurysmal bone cyst. Axial CT scan through the L3 vertebra demonstrates an expansile osteolytic lesion involving most of the vertebral body and left pedicle.

Hemangioma. On conventional radiography, hemangioma has a typical appearance that is diagnostic. Similarly, the CT appearance of hemangioma is readily identifiable. CT demonstrates a well-defined osteolytic lesion, with multiple round densities present within the matrix owing to thickened trabeculae. This gives a characteristic "polka dot" appearance (Fig. 7–65). Hemangiomas are known to contain fat within the matrix,[318] and we have observed negative CT attenuation values, indicating fat tissue.[239] Rarely patients may be symptomatic beause of compression of the spinal cord, cauda equina, or nerve root.* These patients can be evaluated by CT or CTM (Fig. 7–66). Because of its marked vascularity, visualization of hemangioma is enhanced after the administration of intravenous contrast agent.[494]

ally involves the lamina or pedicle and may extend into the vertebral body. The lesion may extend to involve two adjacent vertebrae.[7] Paravertebral and intraspinal extension of the aneurysmal bone cyst can be detected by CT.[459, 462]

*Reference numbers 16, 264, 310, 407, 494.

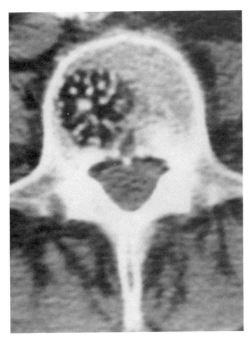

Figure 7–65. Hemangioma. There is a large radiolucent lesion within the vertebral body. The multiple rounded densities present within the lesion are caused by thickening of the remaining trabeculae. Their presence creates the characteristic "polka dot" appearance of hemangioma. The cortex remains intact. Within the matrix is fat, which is identified by its negative CT attenuation values.

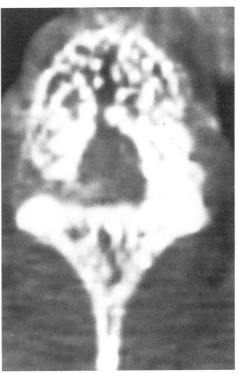

Figure 7–66. Hemangioma. This patient presented clinically with signs of spinal cord compression. Axial CTM scan at T4 demonstrates extensive hemangioma in the vertebral body and posterior elements. The characteristic "polka dot" appearance is noted. Contrast material is not visualized in the thecal sac, owing to compression of the sac; however, contrast material was visualized both above and below this level.

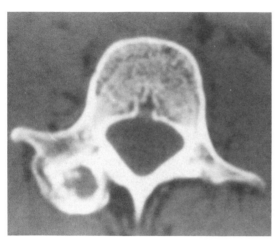

Figure 7–67. Osteochondroma. Axial CT scan of L3. There is an osteochondroma arising from the posterior margin of the right transverse process. The cortex of the osteochondroma is intact. Punctate calcification within the lesion indicates cartilage matrix. (Courtesy of Dr. R. Kerr, Los Angeles, California.)

Osteochondroma. Osteochondroma (exostosis) is a benign bone lesion that rarely involves the spine. It may occur singly or as part of hereditary multiple exostoses.[132, 222, 253, 279] Spinal osteochondromas usually involve either the cervical or the thoracic level. On CT, osteochondroma may appear as an irregularly shaped bony protrusion (Fig. 7–67), which most commonly develops in the vertebral arch or spinous process[273, 335] and less commonly from the transverse process.[132] The cartilaginous cap of an osteochondroma is not visible unless calcified. Compression of the spinal cord or nerve root may occur when the lesion involves the neural arch.[222, 253]

Paget's Disease. Paget's disease may involve the spine or sacrum (Fig. 7–68). The appearance of Paget's disease is related to disturbances of osseous remodeling and modeling. Remodeling is described as bone renewal and turnover without change in size or shape.[497] In Paget's disease, remodeling is classified as osteolytic, osteosclerotic, or mixed. There is excellent correlation between CT and conventional radiography in determining the phases of remodeling.[497] Modeling determines size or shape of bone, and in Paget's disease, disturbances of modeling lead to enlargement of the vertebral bodies and posterior elements.[497] This results in spinal stenosis, which is best studied by CT. Thickening of trabeculae, thickening of the cortex, and facet arthropathy may also be found in Paget's disease.

INTRASPINAL TUMORS

Epidural

Epidural tumor usually arises from direct extension of vertebral tumor into the epidural compartment. This can be identified with CT or CTM study. With conventional CT, epidural extension of osseous tumor may be identified as increased soft tissue density within the spinal canal causing obliteration of epidural fat. The bony cortex of the spinal canal is destroyed at the site of tumor extension. In this manner, CT can demonstrate epidural extension of osseous lesions, such as metastatic disease, myeloma, or other primary lesions of bone (see Fig. 7–55). In some cases epidural extension of tumor may be subtle and difficult to identify with conventional CT. In this situation CTM is quite helpful in determining the presence and extent of epidural tumor (Fig. 7–69). Occasionally, metastatic disease may occur within the epidural space without

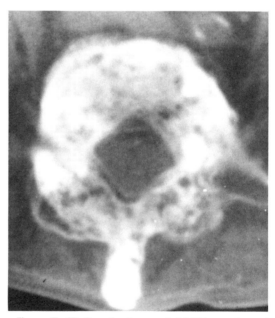

Figure 7–68. Paget's disease. Axial CT scan through the L5 vertebral body. Extensive sclerosis as well as prominence of trabeculae and thickening of cortical margins, laminae, and the spinous process are noted. This patient also has ankylosing spondylitis.

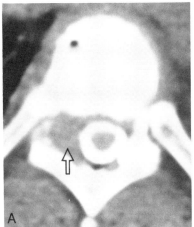

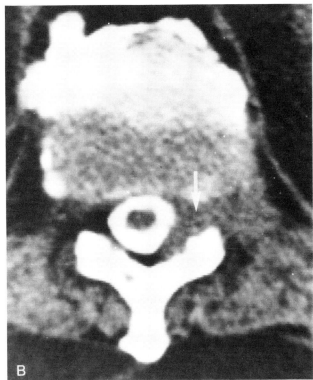

Figure 7–69. Epidural metastasis. *A,* Axial CTM scan of thoracic vertebra demonstrates slight displacement of the contrast-filled subarachnoid space by epidural tumor (arrow). Destruction of the right pedicle is noted. *B,* Another patient with epidural metastasis. Axial CTM scan at T11–T12 demonstrates epidural extension of tumor (arrow), causing slight compression on the contrast-filled subarachnoid space. Adjacent scan sections revealed osseous metastasis of T11 secondary to bronchogenic carcinoma.

involvement of the osseous structures. Again, CTM is helpful in delineating this abnormality.

Intradural-Extramedullary

The most frequent intradural-extramedullary tumors include meningiomas and tumors of nerve root or peripheral nerve origin (neurofibromas) and those of nerve sheath origin (schwannomas). Neurofibromas usually occur at multiple sites in association with neurofibromatosis. Schwannomas are usually solitary but may be multiple, sometimes occurring in patients with neurofibromatosis.[275, 394]

Conventional myelography can be utilized to determine the presence of intraspinal tumor and to evaluate the compartment involved (i.e., extradural, intradural-extramedullary, intramedullary). CTM can also be used to determine the compartment involved, the morphology of the tumor, and the alterations of surrounding bony structures. It is especially helpful in the presence of a "complete" myelographic block, since intrathecal contrast may be identified be-

yond the block owing to the superior contrast resolution of CT compared with conventional radiography.[440]

Neurofibromas typically appear on the CT scan as homogeneous, smooth masses of soft tissue density[84] (Fig. 7–70). Some authors have suggested that in patients with neurofibromatosis, the CT demonstration of an inhomogeneous mass with low density areas accentuated by intravenous contrast agent strongly suggests malignant transformation of a neurofibroma.[84] Others, however, have found similar inhomogeneity with benign schwannomas,[80] although they too are most often homogeneous masses of soft tissue density. Neurofibromas and schwannomas are frequently grouped together, and for the purpose of the following discussion the term *neurofibroma* is used.

Several characteristic features of neurofibroma and meningioma can be used to help differentiate these two tumors. Meningiomas frequently occur in the thoracic spine of middle-aged women. Punctate or globular calcification is frequent and is readily identified by CT[329] (Fig. 7–71). Reactive sclerosis of the adjacent vertebral body may be present. On the other hand, neurofibromas usu-

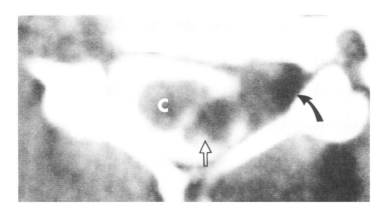

Figure 7–70. Neurofibroma in a patient with neurofibromatosis. Axial CTM scan in the cervical region demonstrates a lobulated mass involving both the intradural-extramedullary compartment (straight arrow) and the epidural compartment (curved arrow). The tumor is causing displacement and compression of the spinal cord (*C*). (Courtesy of Dr. S. Borden, IV, Philadelphia, Pennsylvania.)

ally do not calcify or cause vertebral body sclerosis. However, neurofibromas may be associated with widening of the neural foramen and scalloping of the vertebral body. While neurofibromas occur more frequently than meningiomas in the spine, meningiomas are the most frequent tumor confined to the intradural-extramedullary compartment. This is because approximately one third of neurofibromas involve the extradural compartment. Thus, a dumbbell-shaped tumor (i.e., an intradural tumor that extends into or beyond the neural foramen) is more likely to represent a neurofibroma than a meningioma. Both meningioma and neurofibroma may occur as single or multiple lesions.

Intramedullary

Most intramedullary tumors are gliomas (ependymomas and astrocytomas). Ependymoma is the most frequent intramedullary tumor, accounting for approximately 50% of such lesions.[366] Astrocytoma is the second most frequent intramedullary tumor[366] and in some series is the most frequent intramedullary tumor in children.[99] These lesions may be focal or quite extensive and involve the entire cord (holocord).[22, 128] Less frequent intramedullary tumors include hemangioblastoma, metastasis, and lipoma.

Myelography performed with water-soluble contrast agent and CTM are used to evaluate intramedullary tumors. CTM helps establish the extent of the lesion, especially when a "complete" myelographic block is present. In addition, CTM can be used to demonstrate a coexistent syrinx. The CTM study of intramedullary tumor demonstrates enlargement of the spinal cord with thinning of the surrounding contrast-filled subarachnoid space (Fig. 7–72). This is the characteristic appearance of an intramedullary lesion. A syrinx cavity may be demonstrated on delayed CTM obtained 6 to 24 hours after the introduction of intrathecal contrast agent.[219] Approximately 30% of intramedullary tumors are associated with coexistent syrinx at autopsy.[219] Cystic cavities may be found rostral and caudal to the solid component of holocord astrocytomas in children. CTM demonstration of contrast within the cystic cavity may be used to localize the cystic component of these tumors. Differen-

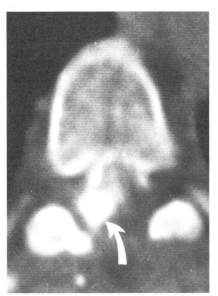

Figure 7–71. Meningioma. Conventional CT of the thoracic spine performed without intrathecal contrast demonstrates a mass with amorphous calcification (arrow). This represents a meningioma.

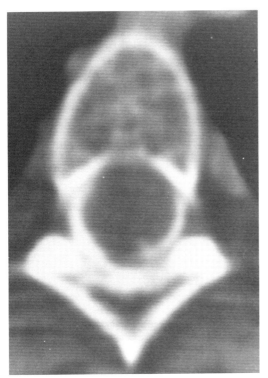

Figure 7–72. Ependymoma. Axial CTM scan through T4 demonstrates marked thinning of the subarachnoid space due to an intramedullary mass. (From Kricun R, Kricun ME: Computed Tomography of the Spine: Diagnostic Exercises. Rockville, Maryland: Aspen Publishers, Inc, 1987. Reprinted with permission of Aspen Publishers, Inc.)

tiation of cystic and solid components of a tumor may be helpful in surgical treatment, since some authors have recommended surgical removal of the solid tumor and drainage of the associated cysts.[128] Delayed CTM examination has also demonstrated contrast filling of a rare solitary intramedullary metastasis.[370]

Intravenous contrast-enhanced CT has been used to demonstrate intramedullary tumors and to help differentiate the solid and cystic components[126, 180, 254] (Fig. 7–73). Astrocytoma and ependymoma may show mild to marked enhancement, which may be solid, patchy, or ringlike. The solid component of the tumor may appear as an enhancing nodular mass.[180, 254] After intravenous contrast enhancement of tumor, several rounded low density regions may be demonstrated within the tumor and are due to multilocular cysts.[126, 254] The use of intravenous contrast agent may be particularly helpful in a patient who has had surgical removal of intramedullary tumor with clin-

ical suspicion of recurrent tumor. In this clinical situation, the level of suspected tumor is known, and the intravenous contrast may enhance a recurrent tumor, clearly delineating its extent.

Other intramedullary tumors are much less frequent than ependymoma and astrocytoma. Hemangioblastoma may be multiple and associated with von Hippel-Lindau disease. These tumors demonstrate marked intravenous enhancement owing to their highly vascular nature.[254] Lipoma is an intramedullary tumor that can be clearly distinguished by CT study because of its negative CT attenuation.[107]

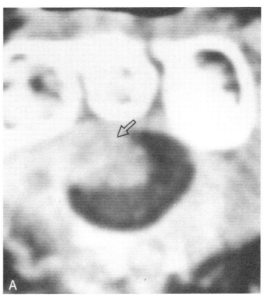

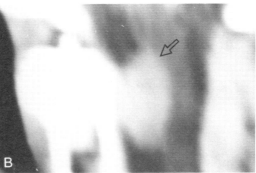

Figure 7–73. Intravenous contrast-enhanced melanoma. *A,* Axial CT scan at level of the axis after intravenous injection of iodinated contrast material. Melanoma (arrow) is present within the spinal canal and demonstrates increased CT attenuation after administration of intravenous contrast material. *B,* Reformatted images in the parasagittal plane reveal the extent of the tumor (arrow). This intraspinal tumor was the only clinical evidence of melanoma in this patient.

Tumors of the Cauda Equina, Conus Medullaris, and Filum Terminale

The most frequent tumors to involve the cauda equina are ependymoma and neurofibroma.[225] Approximately 45% to 75% of spinal ependymomas are found in the cauda equina, conus medullaris, or filum terminale,[23, 314, 366] whereas about 20% of spinal neurofibromas occur in the cauda equina.[270] Ependymomas are frequently large bulky lesions that cause a complete myelographic block. The tumors are usually isodense or of slightly increased CT attenuation when compared with normal thecal sac. The tumor may therefore be imperceptible on conventional CT performed without intrathecal or intravenous contrast agent. CTM examination may demonstrate contrast beyond the myelographic block; however, these tumors are frequently so large that contrast is not seen beyond the block, even with CT. Myelographic introduction of contrast agent on both sides of the block can delineate the extent of the tumor. In some cases, intravenous contrast enhancement of the tumor may demonstrate the full extent of the tumor, obviating the need for a second mye-

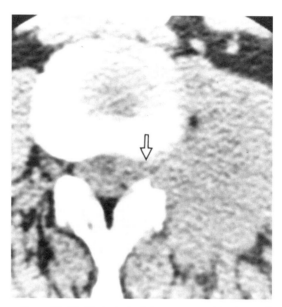

Figure 7–75. Metastasis. A large paravertebral mass is invading the neural foramen (arrow). Note the lack of epidural fat on the left.

lographic approach.[239] Ependymomas may cause scalloping of the vertebral bodies and laminae at multiple levels. Demonstration of tumor extension into the neural foramina and posterior paraspinal musculature is readily accomplished by CT and provides useful information in treatment planning (Fig. 7–74).

Neurofibromas and schwannomas may be quite extensive and have a CT appearance similar to that of ependymoma.[340] Osseous erosion and foraminal extension of tumor may be demonstrated by CT. Neurofibrosarcoma is an unusual tumor that may involve this region.

PARASPINAL ABNORMALITIES

Conventional radiography can demonstrate paraspinal abnormalities in the thoracic region but is less sensitive to paraspinal abnormalities of the cervical and lumbar regions. CT, on the other hand, can clearly delineate the paraspinal soft tissues throughout the spine. Paraspinal soft tissue extension of tumor or infection is clearly demonstrated by CT (Figs. 7–75 through 7–77). In addition, CT can be utilized to evaluate and help differentiate the paraspinal mass of neurofibroma and lateral thoracic meningocele.

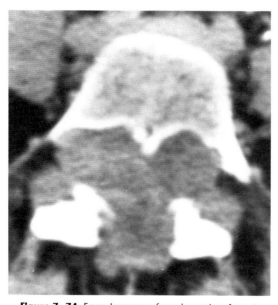

Figure 7–74. Ependymoma of cauda equina. An extensive ependymoma is present within the spinal canal and extends lateral and posterior to the canal. The tumor is causing posterior scalloping of the vertebral body. (From Kricun R, Kricun ME: Computed Tomography of the Spine: Diagnostic Exercises. Rockville, Maryland: Aspen Publishers, Inc, 1987. Reprinted with permission of Aspen Publishers, Inc.)

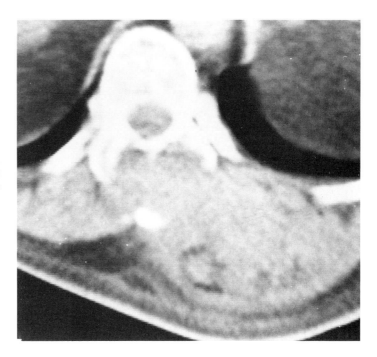

Figure 7–76. Malignant fibrous histiocytoma. A large posterior paravertebral mass is present and has destroyed the spinous process and laminae.

OSTEOMYELITIS

CT plays an important role in the evaluation of the patient with suspected or known osteomyelitis of the spine. Although radionuclide bone scanning is sensitive in the

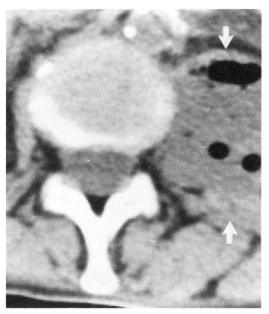

Figure 7–77. Abscess. A large paravertebral abscess containing gas is noted on the left (arrows).

early detection of osteomyelitis, it is nevertheless nonspecific. Conventional radiography is useful in the diagnosis of osteomyelitis and typically demonstrates osteolysis of the vertebral end-plates, with narrowing of the intervening disc space. However, conventional radiographs may appear normal early in the course of the disease.

The most frequent CT findings of spinal osteomyelitis include osteolysis and fragmentation of the vertebral body end-plates and paravertebral soft tissue mass[198] (Fig. 7–78). Rarely the pedicle may be destroyed, with sparing of the vertebral body.[261] Bone destruction secondary to osteomyelitis appears more marked on CT study than on conventional radiographs.[165] In some cases the conventional radiographs may be interpreted as normal despite the presence of CT evidence of osteolysis.[165, 185, 357] CT is particularly useful in evaluating soft tissue extension of infection. The paravertebral soft tissues are poorly visualized in the lumbar region on conventional radiographs but are well seen on CT.

Less common CT findings include protrusion of osseous fragments into the spinal canal, sagittal pathologic fracture of the vertebral body, and destruction of the posterior elements.[165, 198] Atlantoaxial subluxation may occur when infection involves this region.[108] Some authors have noted hypoden-

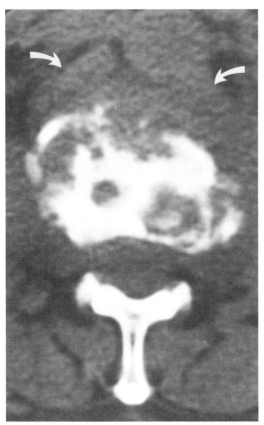

Figure 7–78. Osteomyelitis. Axial CT scan of the inferior end-plate of the L1 vertebral body. There is osteolytic destruction of the vertebral body end-plate as well as paravertebral soft tissue extension (arrows). Adjacent CT sections demonstrated destruction of the superior end-plate of L2.

sity of the disc in patients with lumbar osteomyelitis;[256] however, this finding has not been observed by other investigators.[233] Rarely, intradiscal or intraosseous gas may accompany osteomyelitis.[37]

Typically, osteomyelitis leads to decreased bone density owing to bone destruction and purulent reaction in the marrow, as well as decreased paravertebral soft tissue density, caused by edema and inflammatory exudate in infected granulation tissue.[223] After appropriate antibiotic treatment, bone density increases because of osteoblastic activity and new bone formation.[223] In addition, the adequately treated patient demonstrates decrease in size of the paravertebral soft tissue mass caused by decrease in edema and inflammatory exudate.

CT is also useful in the detection of epi-

dural extension of infection, with soft tissue mass obliterating epidural fat. The epidural inflammatory process may be chronic and represent granulation tissue associated with adjacent osteomyelitis or may represent an acute epidural abscess, which can occur with or without osseous involvement. An epidural abscess may appear on CT as a low density collection that demonstrates rim enhancement after injection of intravenous contrast agent.[475] Intravenous contrast agent has been used to enhance the rim of the inflammatory mass, thus providing additional accuracy in the diagnosis of epidural infection and further delineating the degree of compression of the spinal cord or thecal sac.[475] When an epidural abscess is suspected, myelography an be used to determine the level and extent of the epidural mass. CTM with low volume and low concentration technique can be used to obtain similar information and may replace conventional myelography in the evaluation of these patients.[49]

CT is useful in the evaluation of patients with tuberculous osteomyelitis of the spine and demonstrates osteolysis, disc space narrowing, paravertebral soft tissue mass, multilevel involvement, and kyphosis.[173, 248, 285, 465, 474] Early findings are typically osteolysis of the anteroinferior end-plate or the presence of a paravertebral soft tissue abscess.[465] The posterior elements are rarely involved.[248, 465] The adjacent vertebral body is affected as the infectious process spreads beneath the anterior longitudinal ligament.[465, 474] Two adjacent vertebral bodies are involved in 50% of cases of tuberculous osteomyelitis, and three or more adjacent vertebral bodies are involved in 25%.[465] In the remaining 25% of cases, the disease is either confined to one vertebral body or has spread to involve two or more noncontiguous vertebral bodies. The disc space is maintained longer in tuberculous osteomyelitis than in pyogenic infection.[474] A paravertebral or psoas abscess is readily demonstrated with CT, and calcification within the abscess reflects the chronicity of the tuberculous process.[285] The rim of the tuberculous abscess is thick and nodular and may become enhanced after the injection of intravenous contrast agent.[474] Compared with a pyogenic abscess, a tuberculous paraspinal abscess is more likely to be multilocular and calcified, to spread to superficial dorsal soft tissues, and to have a thick, irregular rim.[474]

In both pyogenic and tuberculous osteomyelitis, CT can be used to guide abscess aspiration and to plan surgical intervention.[61, 165, 198] CT is also helpful in the follow-up examination for evaluation of therapeutic results.

INFECTIOUS SACROILIITIS

Patients with pyogenic sacroiliitis have a wide spectrum of clinical presentation, making early diagnosis difficult. Radionuclide bone scanning is a useful screening procedure for infectious disease of the sacroiliac joint; however, it is a nonspecific examination and has occasional false negative and false positive results.[21, 313] During the first 2 to 3 weeks of the illness, conventional radiographs are usually normal.[21, 167] CT is a more sensitive method of detecting the changes of pyogenic sacroiliitis. The abnormalities are usually unilateral and include widening of the sacroiliac joint, cortical irregularity and destruction, and bone fragmentation within the joint[21, 313, 387] (Fig. 7–79). In addition, soft tissue extension of infection is best demonstrated by CT. Para-articular soft tissue mass or thickening of the iliac and gluteal muscles may be seen. Gas present within a soft tissue abscess is readily appreciated with CT.

Tuberculous sacroiliitis may resemble pyogenic infection; however, tuberculosis is more indolent, has a more protracted course, and demonstrates more extensive sclerosis.

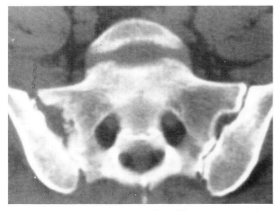

Figure 7–79. Pyogenic sacroiliitis. There is destruction on both sides of the right sacroiliac joint, with small bony fragments noted within the joint.

ARACHNOIDITIS

Arachnoiditis is a noninfectious inflammation of the meningeal layers: the pia, arachnoid, and dura. It almost invariably leads to low back and leg pain, which is increased by activity. There are often motor, sensory, and reflex deficits, which may be bilateral and multilevel.[31, 63] Some patients have urinary and bowel sphincter dysfunction. Patients with arachnoiditis frequently have a previous history of disc herniation, Pantopaque myelography, and spinal surgery.[31, 361, 421] Other causes of arachnoiditis include spinal trauma, infection, tumor, hemorrhage, spinal anesthesia, and intrathecal serum injection.[31, 361] Some cases are idiopathic. Arachnoiditis is thought to be the primary pathologic process in 6% to 16% of all patients with the failed back surgery syndrome.[64]

The CT and CTM features of arachnoiditis and its sequelae are listed in Table 7–17. The diagnosis of arachnoiditis by computed tomography requires the use of intrathecal water-soluble contrast agent. The CTM examination demonstrates clumping of the nerve roots of the cauda equina (Fig. 7–80) or peripheral adherence of the nerve roots to the dural margins, leading to an "empty sac" appearance.[424, 490] A large tubular mass of nerve roots may be identified within the

Table 7–17. CT AND CTM FEATURES OF ARACHNOIDITIS AND ITS SEQUELAE

Arachnoiditis
  Study with CTM
  Thickening of nerve roots of cauda equina
  Peripheral adherence of nerve roots of cauda equina ("empty thecal sac")
  Clumping of cauda equina into single tubular mass

Postarachnoiditis intradural cysts and intramedullary cavities
  Study with CTM
  Filling of cystic structure 6 to 24 hours after introduction of intrathecal contrast agent

Arachnoiditis ossificans
  CT study without intrathecal contrast agent
  Thin circumferential ring of ossification or calcification surrounding the arachnoid
  Large ossified tubular mass

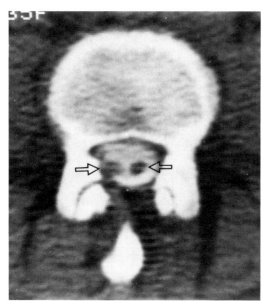

Figure 7–80. Arachnoiditis. Axial CTM scan at L4 demonstrates clumping of the nerve roots (arrows) of the cauda equina due to arachnoiditis.

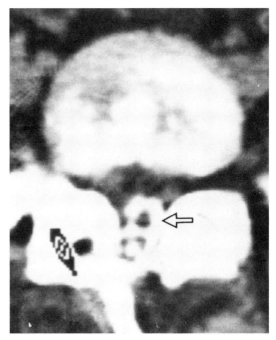

Figure 7–81. Arachnoiditis ossificans. Conventional CT without intrathecal contrast agent demonstrates an ossified mass within the spinal canal (arrow) that is caused by arachnoiditis ossificans. Within the mass are rounded areas of decreased CT attenuation that are due to entrapped nerve roots of the cauda equina. A surgical screw is noted on the right.

thecal sac. CTM is helpful when the myelographic study is inconclusive or when a myelographic block is demonstrated. CTM can also identify coexistent pathologies such as spinal stenosis and disc herniation, which are possible correctable causes of the patient's symptoms.[58]

Sequelae of arachnoiditis such as intradural arachnoid cyst or intramedullary cavities can also be evaluated with CTM.[361] The CTM scan obtained 6 to 24 hours after introduction of intrathecal water-soluble contrast agent may demonstrate filling of the cystic structure. Arachnoiditis ossificans is a sequela of arachnoiditis that can be diagnosed on CT performed without intrathecal water-soluble contrast agent. It is a proliferative bony metaplasia of the arachnoid that closely envelops the spinal cord and nerve roots.[328] Unenhanced CT may reveal a thin circumferential ring of calcification or ossification surrounding the arachnoid or a large, thick, tubular ossified mass[25, 97, 418] (Fig. 7–81).

SPONDYLITIS AND SACROILIITIS

Rheumatoid Arthritis

The cervical spine is a common site of involvement in rheumatoid arthritis. CT can

provide the anatomic detail necessary to evaluate various pathologic conditions of the cervical spine and the craniocervical junction that are found in this disorder. The pathologic alterations that can be demonstrated by CT or CTM are listed in Table 7–18.

Table 7–18. CT AND CTM FINDINGS IN CERVICAL RHEUMATOID ARTHRITIS

Atlantoaxial subluxation
  Anterior subluxation is most common
    (> 3 mm in adults, > 5 mm in
    children)
  Posterior, lateral, and rotational
    subluxation are less common
Cranial settling
Odontoid process erosion
Spinal cord compression
Pannus formation
Transverse ligament alterations
  Thinning, thickening, or rupture
Pathologic fracture of odontoid process
Subaxial subluxation
Low attenuation zone between
  odontoid and transverse ligament
  may represent edema or
  inflammatory change in synovial
  cavity

Atlantoaxial subluxation is the most common spinal manifestation of rheumatoid arthritis.[274] The most common atlantoaxial subluxation is anterior, with widening of the space between the anterior arch of C1 and the odontoid process. Subluxation is present when this distance is greater than 3 mm in the adult or greater than 5 mm in the child[344] (Fig. 7–82). In normal individuals, the strong transverse ligament helps prevent posterior displacement of the odontoid process. However, patients with rheumatoid arthritis may develop laxity or rupture of the transverse ligament, with subsequent subluxation. Other nontraumatic causes of anterior atlantoaxial subluxation include psoriatic arthritis, juvenile rheumatoid arthritis, ankylosing spondylitis,[431] Marfan's syndrome,[266] and Down's syndrome.[206, 307] Patients with rheumatoid arthritis may also have posterior, lateral, or rotational subluxation at C1–C2. Cranial settling is a serious complication that occurs in 5% to 8% of patients with rheumatoid arthritis.[121] This occurs when pannus from the inflamed synovial joints leads to erosion and collapse of the lateral masses of C1.[121, 301] The occipital condyles and articular facets of C2 may also be eroded to a lesser extent. These pathologic changes permit the skull to settle at a lower level on the cervical spine. CT demonstrates the odontoid process above the level of the foramen magnum when axial scans are obtained parallel to a line connecting the anterior and posterior arches of C1.[55, 75] In this situation, the base of the odontoid process

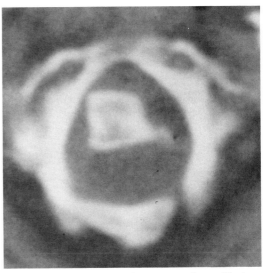

Figure 7–83. Cranial settling in a patient with rheumatoid arthritis. This axial CT scan was taken through the atlas. The base of the odontoid process is at the level of the ring of C1 owing to cranial settling.

or the body of the axis may be within the ring of the atlas (Fig. 7–83).

Erosions of the odontoid process are readily identified by CT (see Fig. 7–82) The odontoid process may have a stellate appearance owing to the erosions and proliferative changes, or the odontoid may have a flat or teardrop configuration in advanced disease.[75] These erosive changes are more readily identified by CT than by conventional radiography.[55, 75] Erosive changes of the lateral masses of C1, occipital condyles, and articular facets of C2 are also well demonstrated by CT.

The demonstration of spinal cord compression is an important finding on CT examination. In the craniocervical region, the spinal cord can be well delineated without intrathecal contrast agent because of the presence of surrounding low density cerebrospinal fluid in a large subarachnoid space. Some authors, however, prefer CTM study because it can provide the best delineation of deformity and displacement of the subarachnoid space and spinal cord.[247, 452] Clinically, spinal cord compression with myelopathy most frequently occurs secondary to anterior C1–C2 subluxation exceeding 9 mm or secondary to cranial settling.[471]

Other CT findings that have been observed in the cervical spine of patients with rheumatoid arthritis include pannus formation, thinning or thickening of the transverse lig-

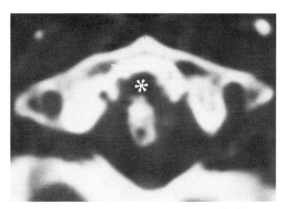

Figure 7–82. Rheumatoid arthritis. Axial CT scan through the atlantoaxial articulation. There is widening of the atlantoaxial space (asterisk), indicating anterior subluxation. The rheumatoid process has produced erosions of the anterior ring of C1 and the odontoid process.

ament, and a low attenuation zone between the odontoid process and the transverse ligament.[55][75] This low attenuation zone is thought to represent edema or inflammatory change in the synovial cavity.[75] A pathologic fracture of the odontoid process occurs rarely. Subaxial subluxation can also be evaluated by CT.

Conventional radiography with additional lateral views during flexion and extension of the neck remains the screening procedure of choice in patients with rheumatoid arthritis. Some authors suggest that CT should be reserved for the evaluation of patients in whom clinical findings are not explained by conventional radiography or conventional tomography and for those patients for whom surgical intervention is considered.[55] Other authors recommend using CTM to evaluate patients with cervical rheumatoid arthritis and neurologic symptoms, especially when anterior atlantoaxial subluxation exceeds 8 mm, cranial settling is progressive, or subaxial subluxation is suspected.[247]

Ankylosing Spondylitis

Ankylosing spondylitis is a spondyloarthropathy that involves the spine and sacroiliac joints. The CT and CTM features of ankylosing spondylitis are listed in Table 7–19. Other abnormalities, such as the presence of spondylitis with thin, bilateral, symmetric syndesmophytes and squaring of the vertebrae, are more readily demonstrated with conventional radiography.

The sacroiliitis found in ankylosing spondylitis is almost always bilateral when first discovered. Diagnostic findings at any age include uniform joint space narrowing ($<$ 2

Table 7–19. CT AND CTM FINDINGS IN ANKYLOSING SPONDYLITIS

Sacroiliitis
Scalloping of laminae
Dural ectasia
Multiple dorsal diverticulae
Fusion of apophyseal joints
Calcification or ossification of
  interspinous and supraspinous
  ligaments
Disc calcification
Atlantoaxial subluxation
Fracture dislocations
Fatty replacement of paraspinal
  musculature

mm), erosions, and intra-articular ankylosis.[70][235][458] Several CT findings often observed in asymptomatic older patients would be suggestive of sacroiliitis if found in younger age groups. These include focal joint space narrowing, focal increased sacral subchondral sclerosis, and overall asymmetry of the joints.[458] Sclerosis that is isolated to the iliac bone is not considered a diagnostic finding of sacroiliitis.[70]

The diagnosis of noninfectious sacroiliitis is usually made by careful examination of fine quality conventional radiographs.[46][398] However, 10% of patients with sacroiliitis who are evaluated with a complete series of radiographs have equivocal results and benefit from a CT examination.[398] In addition, CT may be used when there is a high level of clinical suspicion despite normal conventional radiographs.[398] Other causes of noninfectious sacroiliitis can be evaluated by CT and include Reiter's syndrome, psoriatic arthritis, ulcerative colitis, Crohn's disease, and gout.

Ankylosing spondylitis may cause the cauda equina syndrome, with slowly progressive leg or buttock pain, sensory or motor impairment, and bowel or bladder dysfunction.[396] In this clinical setting, the CT examination may reveal scalloping of the laminae and spinous processes at multiple lumbar levels[174][196][236] (Fig. 7–84). This is due to pressure erosion from dural ectasia and multiple dorsal diverticulae.[389][396] CTM examination can be performed if needed to exclude the possibility of tumor causing the erosive changes. The posterior diverticulae fill with intrathecal contrast agent on CTM study.

Fractures and dislocations of the spine may occur secondary to minor trauma in patients with ankylosing spondylitis. The spine is rigid, and it fractures like a long bone, with through and through fractures that may extend beyond the intervertebral disc space to involve adjacent vertebrae. The fractures frequently involve the posterior elements and are associated with high morbidity and mortality. These fractures are frequently unstable and have associated dislocation, neural arch displacement, or complete transection.[171][469] In one series, 12% of patients with ankylosing spondylitis had had a spinal fracture, and 8% of this group had paralytic spinal cord injury.[469] CT can be used to demonstrate fracture of the

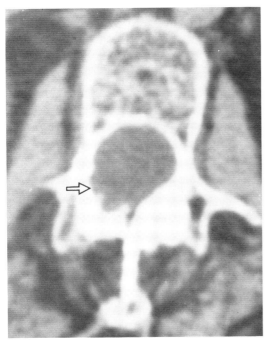

Figure 7–84. Ankylosing spondylitis. Axial CT scan at L2. There is scalloping of the lamina on the right (arrow). Moderate fatty replacement of the posterior paraspinal musculature is noted.

posterior elements, fracture fragment displacement, and compression of the spinal cord or nerve roots. Spinal cord contusion without evidence of fracture has also been described.[469]

Fatty replacement of the paraspinal musculature may be noted in some patients with ankylosing spondylitis.[399] Very severe fatty replacement of the paraspinal musculature has been demonstrated in patients with neuromuscular disorders such as poliomyelitis and muscular dystrophy.[177] Other reports have described varying degrees of fatty replacement of the sacrospinal muscle group in patients who have had previous lumbar surgery[246] and in otherwise normal individuals, especially elderly females.[177]

DISORDERS OF CRYSTAL DEPOSITION

Disorders of crystal deposition that may involve the spine include calcium hydroxyapatite deposition disease (HADD), calcium pyrophosphate dihydrate crystal deposition disease (CPPD/CDD [pseudogout]), and gout. HADD may occur as a primary disorder or may be found in patients with secondary

hyperparathyroidism who are on dialysis, in those with scleroderma, and in those with other disorders.[43] This crystal deposition most commonly occurs in the appendicular skeleton in periarticular locations such as tendons, bursae, and ligaments. Less often, intra-articular deposits are found. Abnormalities may range from periarticular calcification to joint destruction.[43] Massive calcifications may occur about the shoulders, hips, elbows, and knees. Massive intraspinal and paraspinal calcifications have been demonstrated by CT in the upper cervical spine.[239] In this rare situation, CT can be used to determine the presence and extent of the calcific mass as well as the presence of neural foraminal or spinal cord compression (Fig. 7–85). HADD may lead to calcification in the longus colli muscle and its tendon anterior to the upper cervical vertebrae.[33, 379] Hydroxyapatite crystals have also been noted in extensively calcified discs of patients with ochronosis.[379]

CPPD/CDD may occur as a primary disorder or in association with hyperparathyroidism or hemochromatosis.[379] It most commonly involves the appendicular skeleton, especially the knees, wrists, and hands. Within the spine, CPPD/CDD may involve the intervertebral disc, apophyseal joints, sacroiliac joints, posterior median atlantoaxial joint, and intraspinal and extraspinal ligaments.[380] Crystal deposition within the

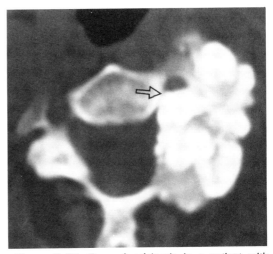

Figure 7–85. Tumoral calcinosis in a patient with scleroderma. Axial CT scan at the level of C2. There are large amorphous masses of calcification extending into the spinal canal, neural foramen, and foramen transversarium (arrow).

discs begins in the outer layers of the annulus fibrosus but may involve the entire disc.[380] Disc narrowing, vacuum disc phenomenon, and vertebral sclerosis may develop. Calcification of articular cartilage within the apophyseal joint occurs, along with joint space narrowing and osteophyte formation. Atlantoaxial subluxation may be present. Massive tumorous deposition of CPPD crystal is rare. When it occurs in the spine, it may be associated with spinal cord displacement and pressure erosions of bone.[120] Spinal ligamentous involvement with CPPD/CDD includes the posterior longitudinal ligaments, intraspinal and supraspinous ligaments, ligamentum flavum, and transverse atlas ligament.[104, 380] Deposition of calcium pyrophosphate dihydrate crystal in the ligamentum flavum may cause spinal cord compression and myelopathy.[337] The calcifications may appear mottled or linear on CT.[104]

Tophaceous deposits of gout in the spine are rare. They may produce vertebral erosions, atlantoaxial erosions and subluxation, or spinal cord compression.[280] Calcification of tophi is unusual.

Other disorders may cause osseous encroachment on the spinal canal. Extensive heterotopic new bone formation may occur in the cervical spine in patients with fibrodysplasia ossificans progressiva (myositis ossificans progressiva)[373] and in patients who have sustained previous head injury.[175] Rarely, synovial osteochondromatosis may develop about the posterior elements, forming a calcified or ossified paraspinal mass that may extend into the neural foramen.[86] CT demonstrates the calcified or ossified masses earlier and with more anatomic detail than conventional radiography.[373] Information provided by CT can be used in treatment planning when surgical intervention is contemplated.

DYSRAPHISM

Spinal dysraphism indicates a failure of complete fusion of tissues in the dorsal median plane of the developing embryo that leads to anomalies of the skin, bones, dura, spinal cord, and nerves.[271] Dysraphism is a complex clinical state that is associated with a broad spectrum of abnormalities, which may occur alone or in combination and which vary in severity. Dysraphic disorders may be categorized as overt or occult. The overt dysraphic disorders are clearly visible, usually diagnosed on physical examination, and include myelocele, myelomeningocele, and most meningoceles. The occult dysraphic disorders are not visible on physical examination and include lipomyelomeningocele, diastematomyelia, tethered cord, some meningoceles, and associated intraspinal masses such as lipomas and cysts. Occult forms of spinal dysraphism are suspected when various cutaneous and/or neurologic, orthopedic, or urologic abnormalities are evident.[414] The diagnosis is usually established during childhood or early adolescence,[148] but occasionally occult spinal dysraphism is not diagnosed until adult life.[432]

The cutaneous abnormalities that offer a clue to the possible presence of occult spinal dysraphism are usually located in the low back and include a patch of hair, nevus, subcutaneous lipoma, skin tags, telangiectasia, and dermal sinus.[62, 148, 211] Cutaneous markers are present in 83% of cases of occult spinal dysraphism, although in some forms, the percentage may be lower.[148] The absence of a cutaneous marker should not rule out occult spinal dysraphism.[62, 148] Spina bifida is present in virtually all cases of occult spinal dysraphism.[211] Neurologic and orthopedic abnormalities occur in about two thirds of patients and include foot or ankle deformity, muscle atrophy, abnormal reflexes, leg weakness, and sensory loss.[148] Neurologic dysfunction may occur from normal flexion and extension motion, which causes stretching and chronic repetitive trauma to the fixed spinal cord.[148] Urinary bladder dysfunction occurs in about 30% of patients.

Although conventional CT can be utilized to diagnose certain aspects of dysraphic disorders such as bony defects, the spur of diastematomyelia, meningocele sacs, and lipomas,[212, 486] CTM is preferred to conventional CT because of the additional information obtained in the evaluation of intraspinal contents. CTM is particularly helpful in the evaluation of patients with occult dysraphism. The position and abnormalities of the spinal cord, the presence and extent of the intraspinal masses and their relationship to the spinal cord, and the presence and extent of the syringohydromelia and Chiari malformation can be assessed.[144] The CTM findings of various forms of spinal dysraphism are included subsequently under each disorder.

Spina Bifida

Spina bifida (bifid spine) is a skeletal dysraphism in which there is failure of fusion of the vertebral arch or, rarely, failure of fusion of the vertebral body.[324] The defect varies from a narrow cleft in the lamina to wide splaying or absence of the laminae at several levels. A narrow posterior spina bifida, particularly at L5–S1, is often discovered in asymptomatic patients and is termed spina bifida occulta.[44] This term is not synonymous with occult spinal dysraphism. It is of no clinical significance and occurs in 20% of the population.

Meningocele

A meningocele is a herniation of skin-covered arachnoid and dura through a localized and relatively mild spina bifida.[148] It is most common in the lumbosacral region. There is no neural tissue present within the protruding sac,[333] and there is no association with syringohydromyelia, Chiari malformation, or hydrocephalus. Most meningoceles are easily diagnosed at birth and, in healthy infants, may be repaired during the first week of life.[148] Surgery is relatively uncomplicated, and since these patients do not have a tethered cord or Chiari malformation, imaging other than conventional radiography or sonography is usually not performed even though the thecal sac is easily accessible.[144, 148] On CT, the thecal sac extends through a spina bifida into the subcutaneous tissues. On CTM, the subarachnoid continuation of the sac is confirmed, and no neural tissue is noted in the sac. CT and CTM are helpful in those cases in which a fluctuant mass in the low back may not be a meningocele but rather a lipoma, cystic tumor, or other cystic lesion[148] (Fig. 7–86).

Myelocele and Myelomeningocele

Myelocele and myelomeningocele are severe forms of spinal dysraphism. A myelocele is a plaque of neural tissue that represents malformed spinal cord and lies exposed and flush with the surface of the skin.[324, 333] Dorsal and ventral nerve roots arise from the neural plaque and traverse the subarachnoid space to exit their respective neural foramina.[324]

A myelomeningocele is a myelocele that is elevated above the skin's surface by a protruding subarachnoid space (meningocele).[148, 324] The term myelomeningocele is often used to express both myelomeningocele and myelocele (myelomeningocele with or without a sac) and will be employed

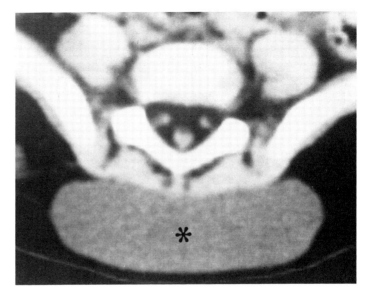

Figure 7–86. Lymphangioma. Axial CT scan through the lumbosacral region in this six month old demonstrates a mass of fluid density (asterisk) in the subcutaneous tissues. The laminae are intact, and the mass does not communicate with the subarachnoid space, thus excluding a dysraphic condition. (Courtesy of Dr. S. Borden, IV, Philadelphia, Pennsylvania.)

similarly in this chapter. Myelomeningoceles are most frequent in the lumbosacral and thoracolumbar regions.[148] They are clinically more devastating than simple meningoceles (especially if the myelomeningocele is not limited to the sacrum or the lower two lumbar segments) and almost invariably are associated with a tethered cord and Chiari II malformation.[324, 333] Hydrocephalus occurs in 75% to 90% of cases.[66, 148, 333] Spina bifida occurs in all cases of myelomeningocele and is much more extensive than that found in patients with simple meningocele. There is often fusiform widening of the spinal canal. The widest interpedicular distance is at the site of maximum spina bifida.[324] Syringohydromyelia occurs in approximately 30% to 75% of patients with myelomeningocele, and diastematomyelia is observed in about 30% to 45% of cases.[66, 125, 324]

Myelomeningocele is easily diagnosed at birth, and since most viable patients are treated surgically as soon as possible (within 30 to 36 hours after birth),[148] imaging is not performed preoperatively. Injecting contrast agent intrathecally is difficult, and it is known that these patients have a tethered cord and Chiari malformation. Through CTM the physician can, however, delineate the neural plaque and nerve roots within the sac (Fig. 7–87), evaluate the spinal cord for hydromyelia and diastematomyelia, and evaluate for Chiari malformation and compression of the brain stem. Following surgical repair of myelomeningocele, the neural plaque may be identified within the thecal sac.[144] CTM is helpful in the evaluation of patients who develop complications after surgery. Retethering of the spinal cord may develop following surgical repair of myelomeningocele.[144]

Lipomyelomeningocele

Lipomyelomeningocele is a skin-covered myelomeningocele associated with a subcutaneous lipomatous connective tissue mass (lipoma). The meningocele and spinal cord herniate posteriorly into the subcutaneous lipomatous tissue.[326] The lipoma is attached to the dorsal surface of the neural plaque by fibroareolar tissue and thus tethers the cord.[326] At the site of attachment, the lipomatous mass lies outside the subarachnoid space but within the central canal and epen-

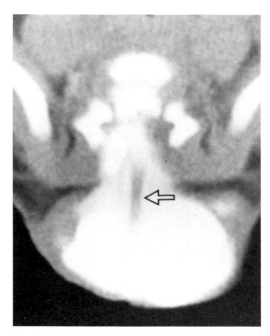

Figure 7–87. Myelomeningocele. Axial CTM scan of the lumbosacral region in a six day old infant. There is posterior protrusion of the contrast-filled subarachnoid space through a wide spina bifida. Neural tissue (arrow) is noted within the contrast-filled sac. (Courtesy of Dr. D. Armstrong, Toronto, Ontario.)

dymal surface of the neural plaque;[297] thus the mass is actually extradural in location. The nerve roots leave the neural plaque and course through the subarachnoid space to exit via their corresponding neural foramina. The meningocele herniates to the side opposite the lipoma. The lipoma may extend into the spinal canal through the spina bifida.[326] Rarely, two discontinuous lipomyelomeningoceles may occur.[168]

Patients with lipomyelomeningocele usually have a neuromuscular syndrome that is evident at birth;[148] however, Chiari malformation, syringohydromyelia, hydrocephalus, and diastematomyelia usually are not associated features of lipomyelomeningocele.[324] Skeletal manifestations of dysraphism are evident, including focal spina bifida and widening of the spinal canal.[326] Occasionally an anomalous bone articulates with the ilium posteriorly at the sacroiliac joint.[291, 326]

Lumbosacral Lipomas

Subcutaneous lipomas in the lumbosacral region consisting mainly of normal fat and excessive connective tissue stroma[117, 124] may be associated with dorsal dysraphism without a meningocele.[326] The subcutaneous mass may extend intraspinally through a spina bifida[148] to merge with a low lying conus medullaris or filum terminale,[298] or sometimes it may attach more proximally on the spinal cord[148] (Fig. 7–88). Those lipomas that affect the spinal cord, particularly the conus medullaris, demonstrate variable limited involvement of the filum terminale; whereas those of the filum terminale demonstrate variable limited involvement of the lower aspect of the conus medullaris.[298] Intraspinal lipomas thus tether the spinal cord dorsally within the spinal canal. The intraspinal component may fuse focally with the neural elements or may form a large mass that embeds into neural tissue.[148] Certain forms of lipomatous masses are partially encapsulated.[124] Even though these lipomatous masses are not true neoplasms, they may compress neural tissue by their mass effect.[449]

About one half of the cases of lumbosacral lipomas do not demonstrate cutaneous markers of occult spinal dysraphism.[148] Patients with subcutaneous lipomas usually present clinically in infancy or childhood. Occasionally, however, they present in young adult life. Some intraspinal lipomas remain almost completely within a normal or mildly bifid spinal canal.[324, 449] Some lipomas do not extend into the spinal canal but remain within the subcutaneous space. They may be associated with other forms of occult spinal dysraphism such as diastematomyelia, congenital dermal sinus, or a thickened filum terminale.[148]

Although the spina bifida and lipomatous tissue are easily detected with conventional CT,[409, 487] CTM is preferred for preoperative evaluation of intraspinal lipomas.[326] The size and extent of the lipomatous mass, its relationship to neural tissue, and the position of the spinal cord can be adequately delineated. The lipomas reside in the dorsal aspect of the spinal canal. CT images can be obtained at fixed intervals (for instance 5 mm) from above the last intact vertebral arch caudally through the sacrum.[326] Reformatted images can be obtained in the coronal and sagittal planes.

Rarely, an extradural-intraspinal lipoma may extend into the mediastinum and present as a mediastinal mass.[362] CT can outline the full extent of the mass. Excessive fat may develop in the epidural space of otherwise normal patients treated with glucocorticoids.[397] On the CT scan, an epidural mass of fat surrounds the thecal sac and may cause compression.

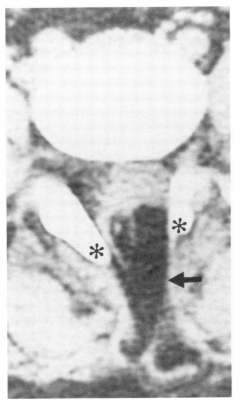

Figure 7–88. Lipoma. There is a lipoma (arrow) extending from the spinal canal to the subcutaneous tissues through a spina bifida (asterisks). The lipoma is readily demonstrated owing to its negative attenuation values. CTM could better delineate the relationship of a lipoma to a tethered cord.

Diastematomyelia

Diastematomyelia is a form of occult spinal dysraphism in which the spinal cord, conus medullaris, and/or filum terminale are partially or completely divided in the sagittal plane into two nearly equal hemicords.[320] Each hemicord has a central canal and an ipsilateral dorsal and ventral horn.[199] In about 50% to 80% of cases, the two hemicords are within a common subarachnoid space surrounded by a single arachnoid and dura.[320, 349, 416] A fibrous septum or osseous cartilaginous spur is not present in this form of diastematomyelia[320] (Fig. 7–89). In the remaining 20% to 50% of cases, the two hemicords lie within their own separate subarachnoid spaces covered by their own separate arachnoid and dura.[320, 349, 416] In this form of diastematomyelia, a fibrous septum or osseous cartilaginous spur separates the two dural tubes, each containing a hemicord[320] (Fig. 7–90). The spinal cord may be tethered by the septum or bony spur.

Diastematomyelia is most common in the lumbar spine and is rare in the cervical spine.[241, 268, 386] Rarely, double diastematomyelia may be observed.[294] Like other forms of occult spinal dysraphism, diastematomyelia is usually discovered in children and is rare in adults.[34, 77] Of those children with spinal dysraphism examined by CTM, 28% demonstrated diastematomyelia.[349] Diastematomyelia is present in 5% of patients with congenital scoliosis.[163] On the other hand, scoliosis is present in 60%[205] to 80%[28] of patients with diastematomyelia.

Diplomyelia has been described as a dysraphic disorder in which there is a perfect duplication of the spinal cord, with each hemicord containing one central canal, two dorsal horns, two ventral horns, and four segmental nerve roots at each level.[320] The cases reported to date are probably varying degrees of diastematomyelia.[148]

CTM can adequately demonstrate diaste-

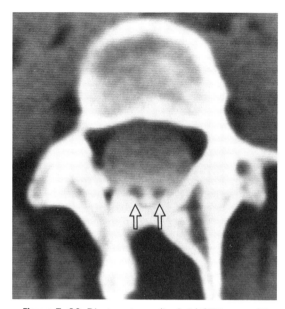

Figure 7–90. Diastematomyelia. Axial CTM scan of the lumbar spine. The two round densities represent the divided spinal cord (arrows). In this form, both hemicords are within a common thecal sac, and there is no fibro-osseous septum. Spina bifida is noted. (From Kricun R, Kricun ME: Computed Tomography of the Spine: Diagnostic Exercises. Rockville, Maryland: Aspen Publishers, Inc, 1987. Reprinted with permission of Aspen Publishers, Inc.)

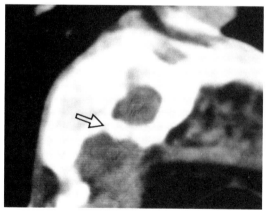

Figure 7–89. Diastematomyelia. Unenhanced axial CT scan at a thoracic level. Scoliosis distorts the spinal image. A bony septum (arrow) is noted dividing the spinal canal. The contents within the canal cannot be delineated; however, further CTM study demonstrated that the bony septum divided the cord into two hemicords, each contained within its own thecal sac. (Courtesy of Dr. G. Mandell, Wilmington, Delaware.)

matomyelia as well as its frequently associated disorders.[12, 320, 416, 468] The location and extent of the split spinal cord and bony spur as well as the associated skeletal abnormalities can be assessed. Myelography performed prior to CTM can detect a second diastematomyelia.[294]

Tethered Cord (Conus)

The spinal cord is considered low lying if the conus medullaris is caudad to the level of the L2–L3 intervertebral disc after the age of 5 years.[145] It should be recalled that during gestation, the vertebral column develops more rapidly than the spinal cord, so that the distal cord (conus) is carried along with the spine and assumes a more cephalad position compared with its position in the lower end of the spinal canal early in gestation.[24] During the 9- to 16-week gestational period, the spinal cord rapidly "ascends" and, by birth, is at the lower border of the L2 vertebra.[24] Two months after birth the conus reaches the "adult" level, which is usually opposite the L1 or L2 vertebra. However, it may lie anywhere from T12 to the L2–L3 disc level.[24]

The spinal cord may be tethered (fixed) by one or several abnormalities, such as a short, thickened filum terminale, a lipomatous mass, fibrous adhesions, the fibrous or osseous cartilaginous septum of diastematomyelia, the neural plaque of myelomeningocele, or by adhesions that develop following repair of a myelomeningocele.[189, 343] A filum terminale is considered thickened if it measures more than 2 mm in diameter.[145, 402] The various abnormalities that cause tethering cause longitudinal traction or compression on the spinal cord,[221, 402] and the traction may produce ischemia, a possible cause of symptoms.[145] Clinically the tethered cord syndrome may consist of unexplained spastic gait, scoliosis, lower extremity weakness, foot deformity, neurogenic bladder or bowel dysfunction, and other symptoms.[145] The symptoms are usually manifested during childhood but may go undetected until adult years.[17, 221, 343] Cutaneous manifestations of occult spinal dysraphism occur in about one half of the cases.[145, 343] Spina bifida is always present, usually mild, and involves at least one level.[189, 343]

With CTM, the location of the spinal cord can be accurately determined, and the exact

nature of cord tethering may be discovered (Fig. 7–91). In the case of intraspinal lipoma, the junction between normal spinal cord and lipomatous infiltration can be assessed. The thickness of the filum terminale can be measured.

Reformatted images can be obtained in the sagittal plane.

Chiari Malformation

The Chiari malformation is a congenital abnormality in which there are varying degrees of protrusion of the hindbrain through the foramen magnum and into the cervical spinal canal. In the Chiari I malformation, cerebellar tonsils, the only structures to protrude through the foramen magnum, usually extend to the C1–C2 level and lie dorsal and lateral to the cervical spinal cord[323, 333] (Fig. 7–92). Tonsils are at the level of C1 in one half of the cases and at C2 or slightly below in the remaining half.[351] (It should be recalled that cerebellar tonsils are usually at or above the foramen magnum in normal individuals.[2]) The medulla and fourth ventricle remain in their normal positions.[39, 323] Hydromyelia is common and hydrocephalus is rare in patients with Chiari I malforma-

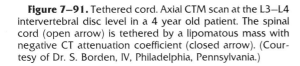
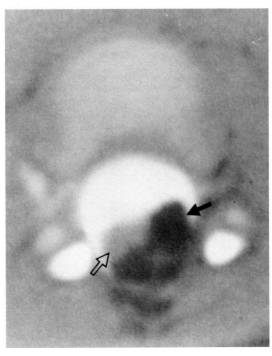

Figure 7–91. Tethered cord. Axial CTM scan at the L3–L4 intervertebral disc level in a 4 year old patient. The spinal cord (open arrow) is tethered by a lipomatous mass with negative CT attenuation coefficient (closed arrow). (Courtesy of Dr. S. Borden, IV, Philadelphia, Pennsylvania.)

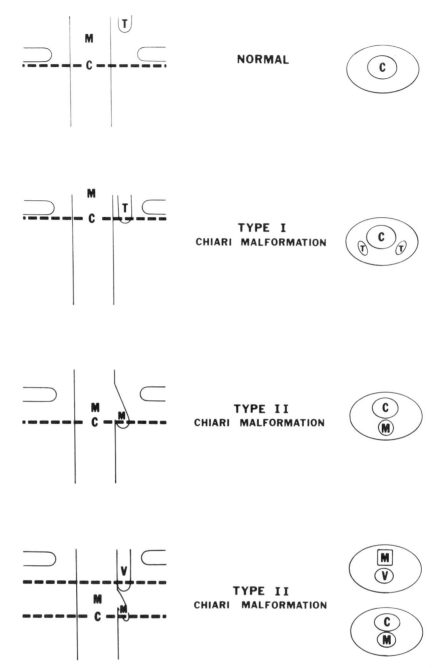

Figure 7–92. Chiari malformation. Diagrammatic representation demonstrating the relationships of the medulla, cerebellar tonsils, and spinal cord to the foramen magnum as found in normal individuals, those with Chiari I malformation, and those with Chiari II malformation. Sagittal drawings are on the left and axial drawings are on the right. (From Kricun R, Kricun ME: Computed Tomography of the Spine: Diagnostic Exercises. Rockville, Maryland: Aspen Publishers, Inc, 1987. Reprinted with permission of Aspen Publishers, Inc.)

tion.[111, 381] Severe spina bifida and myelomeningocele do not occur with this disorder.

The Chiari II malformation is almost always associated with myelomeningocele[321] and is much more extensive and clinically more severe compared with Chiari I malformation (Fig. 7–93). The medulla, pons, fourth ventricle, and cerebellar vermis protrude in varying degrees through the foramen magnum into the cervical spinal canal[39, 323] (see Fig. 7–92). The small cerebellar hemispheres and cerebellar tonsils

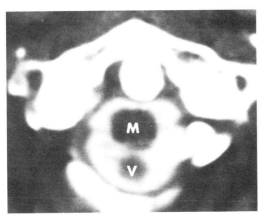

Figure 7–93. Chiari II malformation. CTM scan at the level of C1 demonstrates the cerebellar vermis (**V**) posterior to the low-lying medulla (**M**), forming a "figure of 8" configuration. Compare with Figure 7–92.

may or may not herniate through the foramen magnum,[323] and the relatively large cerebellar vermis may be dorsal to the medulla. The medulla may be displaced downward into the cervical spinal canal.[321] The upper cervical segments of the spinal cord reside at a lower level than normal, and their nerve roots exit in an upward direction to enter their respective neural foramina.[333] More commonly, the medulla protrudes even more caudad, causing a "kink" at the medulla-cord junction,[321, 333] which is usually located around the level of C2–C4[321] (see Fig. 7–92). As the medulla is displaced downward, it may take with it the upper cervical cord. The kink allows the medulla to lie posterior to the cervical cord. Protruding cerebellum and medulla may cause compression of the spinal cord.[321] Hydromyelia and, to a lesser extent, diastematomyelia are common associated findings with Chiari II malformation.[66]

CTM is more accurate than conventional myelography or unenhanced CT in establishing the diagnosis of Chiari malformation.[147] It is helpful in determining the nature and position of protruding structures, their relationship to the spinal cord, and the degree of spinal cord compression. Scans obtained in the region of the foramen magnum should be parallel to the foramen magnum. Sagittal reconstruction aids in determining the full extent of the protruding structures. Utilizing CTM in the axial plane, the Chiari I malformation demonstrates protruding cerebellar tonsils that appear as crescent-shaped, often

asymmetric filling defects in the contrast-filled subarachnoid space.[323] They often reside at different levels posterolateral to the spinal cord. It should be mentioned that, rarely, a brain stem neoplasm may mimic a Chiari malformation clinically early in its course as well as on CTM.[351] However, displacement of neural structures and enhancement following injection of intravenous contrast agent can establish the correct diagnosis of tumor.

The CTM appearance of patients with Chiari II malformation is variable depending on the nature and extent of the protruding intracerebral structures. On the axial CTM scan, the spinal cord, cerebellar vermis, and medulla are central structures. The spinal cord and cerebellar vermis demonstrate rounded lateral margins, whereas the lateral margins of the medulla may be rounded or compressed and indented.[323] Cerebellar hemispheres appear as large masses posterolaterally in the spinal canal that may compress the medulla at or just below the foramen magnum. A "figure of 8" configuration on axial scan is noted when there is, according to the level scanned, overlapping of the cerebellar vermis dorsally on the medulla or overlapping of the medulla dorsally on the cervical cord[321] (see Fig. 7–93). The overlapping medulla may compress and flatten the spinal cord. The fourth ventricle is usually not visualized or appears small. The lateral ventricles are dilated as a manifestation of hydrocephalus.[327] In Chiari II malformation, CTM can also detect hydromyelia on delayed scans. Myelomeningoceles and other forms of dysraphism can be evaluated as well. The foramen magnum and the upper cervical canal are commonly widened, and the posterior arch of C1 demonstrates a defect in 70% of cases.[321]

Syringohydromyelia

Hydromyelia is a cystic dilatation of the central canal of the spinal cord that is lined by ependymal cells.[333] It is of congenital origin and is commonly associated with hindbrain abnormalities such as the Chiari malformation.[153] Hydrocephalus may be present in about 10% to 30% of patients.[14, 65, 111, 147]

Syringomyelia is a cavity within the spinal cord lined by glial cells and is extrinsic to the central canal of the spinal cord. It may develop secondary to hydromyelia[153] as well as other disorders. Syringomyelia that develops secondary to hydromyelia has been termed "true"[20] or "primary"[333] syringomyelia. It usually involves the dorsal aspect of the cervical cord; however, the cavity may extend into the thoracic region and sometimes involve the entire spinal cord as far caudad as the conus medullaris.[93, 461] There may be single or multiple cavities that may communicate.[333] Since hydromyelia and syringomyelia are closely associated developmentally, clinically, and even radiographically, they are frequently combined and referred to as syringohydromyelia.[20]

The etiology of congenital hydromyelia and syringomyelia is controversial, and several theories have been reviewed by others.[65] For example in the Gardner theory,[153] it is felt that hydromyelia may develop as a result of the impermeabiliy of the foramina of the fourth ventricle during fetal life, thus preventing cerebrospinal fluid (CSF) from escaping from the cerebral ventricles into the subarachnoid space. Increased pressure within the ventricles causes ventricular dilatation (hydrocephalus), which decompresses into the communicating central canal, causing dilatation of the canal (hydromyelia). Hydrocephalus also causes inferior displacement of the cerebellar tonsils, re-sulting in the Chiari malformation. To relieve the pressure of hydrocephalus further, the dilated central canal may rupture, allowing CSF to escape into the spinal cord parenchyma, forming a paracentral cavitation or communicating intramedullary cyst (syringomyelia). The limitation of this theory is that the patients examined all had myelomeningocele and hydrocephalus.[14]

Syringohydromyelia may sometimes be diagnosed with conventional CT[383] by virtue of its low attenuation value, which is that of cerebrospinal fluid (about 15 HU less than that of spinal cord).[358] However, cysts that are isodense with the spinal cord or are small or collapsed may not be detected on plain CT.[14] CTM is an excellent imaging modality for the diagnosis and localization and evaluation of syringohydromyelia.* Only a small percentage of cysts are opacified immediately following intrathecal injection of contrast agent. However, most cysts become opacified on scans obtained 6 to 10 hours later[14] (Fig. 7–94). The size and shape of the spinal cord can be evaluated by means of CTM, thus possibly giving clues to the presence of syringohydromyelia. In one series of adults, spinal cord size was usually normal (45%) or small (45%), being enlarged

---

*Reference numbers 14, 26, 41, 42, 93, 147, 461.

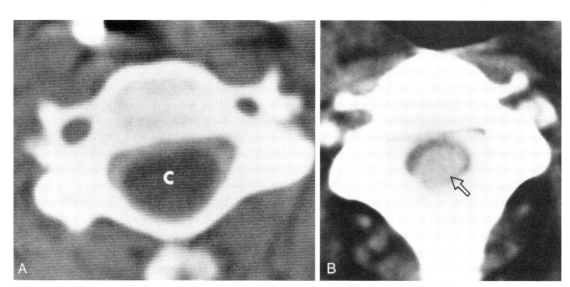

Figure 7–94. Syringomyelia. *A*, CTM scan performed immediately after myelography with water-soluble contrast agent. The spinal cord (**C**) is enlarged and is encroaching on the faintly visualized contrast-filled thecal sac. *B*, Same patient as in part *A*. This CTM scan was delayed 6 hours after the intrathecal administration of water-soluble contrast agent. The contrast material is now noted within the spinal cord, indicating a large syrinx cavity (arrow). (Courtesy of Dr. N. Komer, Tucson, Arizona.)

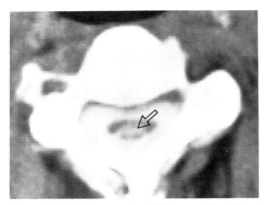

Figure 7–95. Syringomyelia. CTM scan at the C3 level demonstrates contrast material within a syrinx cavity (arrow). The spinal cord is small and flattened. (Courtesy of Dr. R. Wachter, Tucson, Arizona.)

in only 10% of cases.[14] In children with syringohydromyelia, cord size is usually enlarged.[349] The spinal cord may appear round, oval, or flat (collapsed, flaccid). A flattened cord that changes shape with change in patient position is diagnostic of syringohydromyelia[220, 374] (Fig. 7–95), but this feature is more easily diagnosed with air myelography. In addition to the previously mentioned features of syringohydromyelia, CTM can detect a Chiari malformation associated with hydromyelia,[14] thus confirming the congenital nature of this lesion. The fourth ventricle may be opacified in about 85% of cases but only if the head is tilted downward.[14] Hydrocephalus can be diagnosed by either CT or CTM, whereas other associated intraspinal congenital disorders are better evaluated with CTM. Additionally, CTM can easily assess the status of the syringohydromyelia and any change in its size following surgery.[218] Patients with Chiari I malformation demonstrate filling of the syrinx cavity with contrast material after posterior fossa decompression and plugging of the obex. This suggests that the syrinx cavities are maintained not only by flow of CSF through the obex but also by CSF that passes through the spinal cord tissue from the subarachnoid space.[218]

Syringomyelia cavities may develop within the parenchyma of the spinal cord as neural tissue is replaced by gliosis and cavitation, which may occur in association with spinal cord trauma and hematomyelia,[359, 390, 419] spinal cord tumors,[20, 153, 219] and arachnoiditis.[425] Less commonly, syringomyelia

has been noted in patients with sarcoidosis[367] and multiple sclerosis.[245] These forms of syringomyelia are called "acquired"[20] or "secondary"[333] forms of syringomyelia, and CTM is preferred to conventional CT for their evaluation.

Syringomyelia may develop in the presence of intramedullary tumors. Transudate from tumor capillaries may be responsible for cavity formation.[20, 153] Ependymomas originating in the vestigial central canal may form fluid that may redistend the canal or form a syrinx parallel to the canal.[153] Clinically, the onset of symptoms is more rapid than with congenital syringohydromyelia.[13] It is interesting that around 15% of patients with a clinical diagnosis of syringomyelia have an unexpected intramedullary tumor and about 30% of patients with intramedullary tumor have an associated syrinx.[219] Thus, intramedullary tumor should be searched for in those patients who present with a clinical syringomyelia syndrome and who do not have evidence of a congenital, post-traumatic, or postinflammatory etiology to account for the cyst formation. Differentiating syringohydromyelia from cystic tumor or cysts associated with tumor may be difficult.[358] Intramedullary tumors usually demonstrate enlarged spinal cords. CT density of an associated syrinx may be isodense (due to elevated protein in the CSF), low, or occasionally elevated (dermoid cyst) relative to the spinal cord.[358] The presence of low CT attenuation within an enlarged tumor may or may not indicate a cyst, since there may be edema, gliosis, or fatty elements within the tumor. In most cases, an enlarged spinal cord of normal density will be an intramedullary tumor.[358]

Intramedullary tumors associated with syringomyelia may be suspected on a CTM scan if the syrinx cannot be demonstrated at all levels of spinal cord enlargement,[219] if the syrinx extends over a short segment, if the syrinx has a nodular irregular wall, or if it does not involve the upper to midcervical cord (the characteristic location of "true" syringohydromyelia).[358] The most common location of tumors associated with the syrinx is in the lower cervical or upper thoracic cord.[319, 427] Some authors have noted that a syrinx associated with an intramedullary tumor uncommonly opacifies immediately following injection of intrathecal water-soluble contrast agent.[254, 358] Others have demonstrated opacification of the cyst on a delayed scan, 7 to 24 hours after similar administration of contrast material.[219] This delayed filling of the syrinx cavity is most likely due to transneural passage of contrast material from the subarachnoid space to the syrinx cavity.[219]

Cystic degeneration of the spinal cord is an uncommon complication of spinal cord injury,[390] occurring in 1% to 2% of spinal cord injuries.[359, 419] It may develop from hematomyelia that breaks down and becomes cystic. However, cord trauma without hemorrhage may produce a cyst as well—probably owing to tissue ischemia.[359] Adhesions may form and cause tethering of the cord, subjecting the cord to unusual stresses caused by normal pressure changes of a Valsalva maneuver.[419] This may elevate spinal venous pressure, causing extension of the syrinx. Clinically, there is a period of 3 months to 13 years from the time of spinal cord injury to the development of new symptoms.[359] Less frequently, there is either a progressive deterioration in the neurologic status from the onset of injury or a failure of development of newer progressive symptoms. CTM can adequately demonstrate the presence and extent of the cysts, which may be single or multiple. Cysts vary from 0.5 cm in length to those that involve the entire spinal cord.[359] Most cysts involve the dorsal cord, extend cranially,[419] and usually fill with contrast agent on the delayed scan. However, some cysts do not fill with contrast agent.[390, 419] The spinal cord is normal in size in about 70%, atrophic in about 20%, and enlarged in about 10% of cases.[119a] Opacification of the syrinx is more commonly observed when the spinal cord is enlarged. CTM is helpful in the postoperative management of the patient. The size of the cyst and position of the shunt may be determined.[390]

A syrinx cavity may rarely develop secondary to arachnoiditis and is caused either by vascular compromise from inflammatory arachnoid adhesions that lead to ischemia and cavitation or by alterations in CSF flow that cause spinal cord edema and cavitation.[425] CTM can demonstrate the syrinx cavity and the findings of adhesive arachnoiditis. In the lumbar region, nerve roots appear clumped together or located peripherally adjacent to the dura. Arachnoid cysts may also occur with arachnoiditis and can be detected by CTM.

NEUROFIBROMATOSIS

Neurofibromatosis is a hereditary hamartomatous disorder, probably of neural crest origin, involving neuroectodermal, mesodermal, and endodermal tissues.[204] Spinal abnormalities occur frequently in neurofibromatosis and are most often due to mesodermal dysplasia (bone, dura) but may also be caused by neural tumors and lateral thoracic meningoceles.[204, 263] The CT and CTM features of neurofibromatosis are listed in Table 7–20 (Figs. 7–96 and 7–97).

Neurofibromatosis is the most frequent cause of posterior scalloping of one or more vertebral bodies.[263] Posterior scalloping is found in approximately 14% of patients with neurofibromatosis and is most often due to dural ectasia, although neurofibromatosis may sometimes be a cause of this scalloping. CTM and conventional myelography may be used to differentiate dural ectasia from tumor as a cause of vertebral scalloping.[9]

Another use of CT in patients with neurofibromatosis is in the differentiation of a paraspinal mass due to a neurofibroma from a paraspinal mass due to a lateral thoracic meningocele. A lateral thoracic meningocele is formed by protrusion of the dura and arachnoid through an enlarged neural foramen.[131, 339] A patient with a lateral thoracic meningocele has associated neurofibromatosis in 65% to 85% of cases.[131, 306, 467] Lateral thoracic meningoceles are multiple in 11% of cases and are bilateral in 7%.[306] The etiology of lateral thoracic meningocele is uncertain; however, causes that have been advanced include dural ectasia, faulty

Table 7–20. CT AND CTM FEATURES OF NEUROFIBROMATOSIS

Dural ectasia
Neural tumors (schwannoma, neurofibroma)
Lateral thoracic meningocele
Vertebral body scalloping
  Posterior vertebral body scalloping most common
  Lateral and anterior vertebral body scalloping less common
Kyphoscoliosis
Abnormal pedicle
  Aplasia, hypoplasia, mesial erosions
Neural foraminal widening
Spinal canal widening
Transverse process hypoplasia
Spina bifida
Thinning of ribs

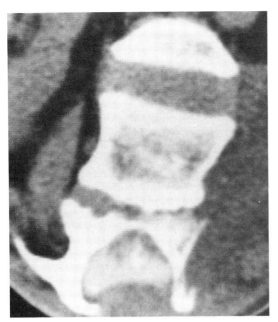

Figure 7–96. Neurofibromatosis. Axial CTM scan of thoracolumbar spine. Multiple vertebrae are visualized on single scan section owing to severe kyphosis. Dural ectasia, posterior scalloping of the vertebral body, and mesial scalloping of hypoplastic pedicles are demonstrated in this patient with neurofibromatosis. (From Kricun R, Kricun ME: Computed Tomography of the Spine: Diagnostic Exercises. Rockville, Maryland: Aspen Publishers, Inc, 1987. Reprinted with permission of Aspen Publishers, Inc.)

attachment of the dura in the intervertebral foramen, elongated nerve root sleeves, and bone dysplasia.[45, 131, 306] Conventional CT demonstrates a paravertebral mass that protrudes through a wide neural foramen and is isodense with the cerebrospinal fluid (Fig. 7–98). Neural tumors such as neurofibroma and schwannoma (see Figs. 7–96 and 7–97) may be of slightly higher density;[35, 84] however, relatively low attenuation values (20 to 30 HU) are not infrequent.[84, 243] CTM may be useful in the further evaluation of these paraspinal masses. A lateral thoracic meningocele fills readily with water-soluble contrast material, thus distinguishing it from a neurofibroma.[9, 467] Should intravenous contrast agent be administered, a neurofibroma may demonstrate homogeneous increase of attenuation values, whereas a lateral thoracic meningocele demonstrates no enhancement.[84]

TRAUMA

CT has become an integral part of the evaluation of the victim of spinal trauma. These patients are sometimes faced with unstable injuries that can lead to severe neurologic deficit and therefore require accurate and safe imaging assessment. CT provides this diagnostic ability and, along with conventional radiography, alleviates the need for conventional tomography in most patients.[51, 277, 353]

The patient is examined in the supine position without the need for turning, a procedure that is frequently required with conventional tomography. In the cervical region, scan slice thickness of 1.5 to 3 mm can be used when scanning a field limited to three or fewer vertebral bodies. This technique has the advantage of detecting subtle fractures and permitting optimal reconstruc-

Figure 7–97. Neurofibromatosis. Axial CT scan at L3–L4 intervertebral disc demonstrates multiple neurofibromas in a patient with neurofibromatosis. Neurofibromas are present within both neural foramina (open arrows) and extend laterally. Note a neurofibroma along the lateral aspect of the psoas muscle (closed arrow). Neurofibromas were demonstrated at multiple levels and measured between 13 and 44 HU.

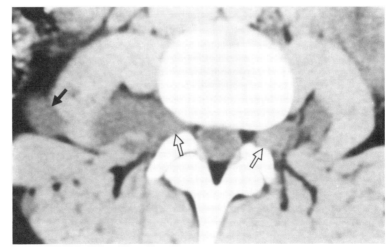

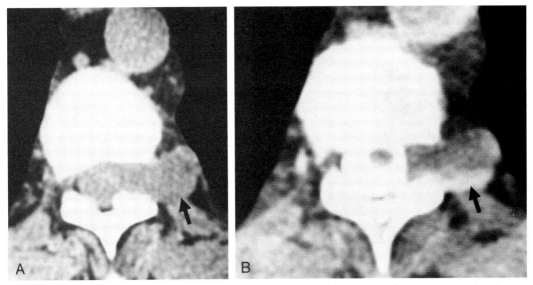

Figure 7–98. Lateral thoracic meningocele. *A*, Conventional CT scan of thoracic vertebra without intrathecal contrast. The mass in the left neural foramen extends into the paravertebral region (arrow). This mass measured 26 HU. *B*, CTM scan demonstrates contrast agent (arrow) layered posteriorly within a lateral thoracic meningocele. A smaller meningocele was noted at another thoracic level.

tion of the axial images into additional planes. When evaluation requires examining longer segments of the cervical spine or when the thoracolumbar spine is studied, a scan slice thickness of 3 to 5 mm can be utilized. An overlapping method is useful (e.g., 5 mm scan slice thickness obtained at 3 or 4 mm intervals) and improves the reconstructed image in the sagittal, coronal, and oblique planes. CTM performed after myelography or independently utilizing low dose technique is helpful in diagnosing nonosseous abnormalities such as spinal cord edema, post-traumatic disc herniation, nerve root avulsion, and post-traumatic syrinx.

Osseous Trauma to Cervical Spine

Atlas

CT is ideally suited for the evaluation of fractures of C1. The atlas is a ring with an anterior and posterior arch. Fractures through this ring most often occur perpendicular to the plane of CT scanning and are thus readily appreciated by CT (Fig. 7–99). The most frequent fractures of C1 are fractures of the posterior arch and the Jefferson fracture.[156] Less common fractures include horizontal fracture of the anterior arch, frac-

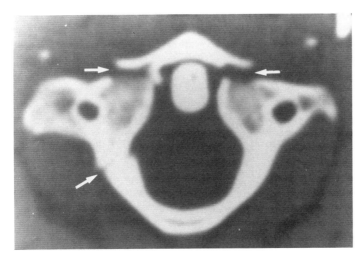

Figure 7–99. Fractures of atlas. Axial CT scan through the atlas demonstrates bilateral fractures of the anterior arch and a fracture of the right posterior arch (arrows).

ture of the transverse process, and isolated fracture of the lateral mass.

The Jefferson fracture, for example, can be readily identified by CT. Classically, the Jefferson fracture includes bilateral fractures of the posterior and anterior arches of C1, with bilateral lateral offset of C1.[214] When conventional radiographs are inadequate, CT can differentiate isolated posterior arch fracture from the Jefferson burst fracture.[27] In addition to being the optimal method of identifying the fractures, CT also permits identification of the presence of a bone fragment within the spinal canal—one of the few indications for surgery in the Jefferson fracture.[226] Reconstruction of the axial images into the coronal plane can be used to demonstrate the lateral displacement of the lateral masses of C1.

Other more subtle findings may be identified with CT, such as fracture of the medial tubercle of the lateral mass of C1 or linear fracture through the lateral mass. In addition, CT may be used to demonstrate C1–C2 rotatory subluxation when conventional radiographs are not definitive.[27]

Axis

The most frequent fracture of C2 is a fracture of the odontoid process, which accounts for 13% of cervical spine fractures or dislocations or both.[286] Fracture through the odontoid process may be difficult to identify with conventional radiography. CT is also somewhat limited in its ability to evaluate odontoid fractures when the fracture occurs horizontal to the plane of scanning. In this setting, thin axial sections (1.5 mm or 2.0 mm) are needed to obtain the most satisfactory reconstruction images. Reconstruction in the sagittal plane may be required to establish the diagnosis of odontoid fracture in some cases. Sagittal reconstruction images are also helpful in determining the presence and degree of fracture displacement and spinal cord compression.

The second most frequent fracture of C2 is the "hangman's fracture." In this hyperextension injury there are bilateral fractures of the pedicles of C2 that may or may not be associated with anterior displacement of the C2 vertebral body on C3 (traumatic spondylolisthesis of the axis) (Fig. 7–100). Avulsion fracture of the anteroinferior aspect of the

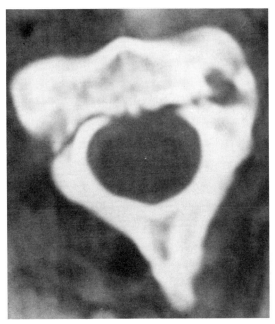

Figure 7–100. Fracture of axis (hangman's fracture). CT scan of axis reveals fracture of both pedicles. Traumatic spondylolisthesis of C2–C3 was present on sagittal reconstruction.

C2 vertebral body or the anterosuperior margin of C3 may also be present.[122]

Atypical fractures of the neural arch of C2 occur less frequently and include fractures of both laminae of C2 or fracture of one pedicle and the opposite lamina. Bilateral symmetric fractures of C2 are usually readily identified by conventional radiographs, so that CT adds little to the diagnostic evaluation. However, when fractures occur asymmetrically at different sites of the vertebral arch, they may be more difficult to detect with conventional radiographs because the fracture may be obscured by supraimposition of solid bone from the opposite side.[385] When the conventional radiographs leave diagnostic uncertainty, CT can readily identify fracture through the neural arch of C2.

Mid- and Lower Cervical Spine (C3–C7)

Fracture of the vertebral arch is found in 50% of patients with cervical spine fracture or dislocation or both and is the most frequent fracture in cervical spine injury.[308] From C3 to C7, the pillar fracture is the most frequent type of vertebral arch fracture[308] (Fig. 7–101). The superior and inferior articular processes of each vertebra fuse to form

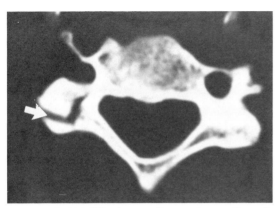

Figure 7–101. Pillar fracture. Fracture is seen through the pillar of C5 on the right (arrow).

the rhomboid-shaped pillar. CT can demonstrate fractures of the pillar even when these structures appear normal with conventional radiography.[83, 354, 434] However, some pillar fractures may be difficult to detect with CT when they occur in the horizontal plane and superficially resemble a normal or distracted facet joint.[346, 491] The CT demonstration of a distracted uncovertebral joint or facet joint without other identified abnormalities suggests the need for additional evaluation, such as CT reconstruction views or conventional tomography.[491]

A hyperflexion fracture dislocation ("teardrop") of the cervical spine can be evaluated by CT. A sagittal vertical fracture, which is frequently associated with this injury, can be identified.[262] Fracture fragments displaced into the spinal canal can be evaluated, and the degree of spinal cord compression can be determined. Sagittal reconstruction aids in the evaluation of these patients.

Bilateral locked facets have a typical CT appearance. Normally, the inferior articular processes of the vertebra above lie posterior to the superior articular processes of the vertebra below and have rounded posterior margins. When locking of the facets occurs, the half-moon–shaped superior articular processes lie posterior to the inferior articular processes and have flat posterior margins.[491] Reconstruction of the axial images in the parasagittal and oblique planes can further demonstrate the locked facets. Bilateral locking of the facets requires at least 50% anterior displacement of one vertebra on the next lower vertebra.[29, 184] This can be demonstrated by conventional radiography or midsagittal reconstruction of the axial images.

The diagnosis of unilateral locked facet is overlooked on the initial radiographic examination in approximately 50% of cases.[48] CT or conventional tomography can be used to clarify difficult diagnostic problems. Unilateral locked facet is found in 16% of patients with trauma to the cervical spinal cord, and approximately 80% of these injuries occur at C4–C5 or C5–C6.[403] The CT examination demonstrates the superior process of the vertebral below lying posterior to the inferior articular process of the vertebra above on one side, while the normal articulation is seen on the opposite side (Fig. 7–102). Patients with unilateral locked facet may have associated distraction of the uncovertebral joint or fractures of the vertebral body and the vertebral arch.[491] Rotation of the spinous process toward the abnormal side is noted in one third of cases.[403]

In addition to being locked and subluxated (Fig. 7–103), the facet may be "perched" (see Fig. 7–102C). This occurs when the tip of the inferior articular process above rests on the tip of the superior articular process below. The axial CT examination demonstrates a "naked" facet, with the superior and inferior articular process imaged at different levels.[491] This injury may be bilateral or unilateral.

Osseous Trauma to Thoracolumbar Spine

The evaluation of patients with trauma to the thoracolumbar spine begins with conventional radiography in the AP and lateral projections. When significant radiographic or neurologic findings are present, the preliminary radiographs are followed by CT examination. The use of CT eliminates the need for conventional tomography in most cases.[50, 51, 113, 224, 227] In the evaluation of thoracolumbar fractures, a three column approach has been used.[96, 135, 290] The anterior column includes the anterior longitudinal ligament and the anterior two thirds of the vertebral body and disc. The middle column includes the posterior longitudinal ligament and the posterior third of the vertebral body and disc. The posterior column includes the laminae, spinous process, articular processes, facet joint capsules, ligamenta flava,

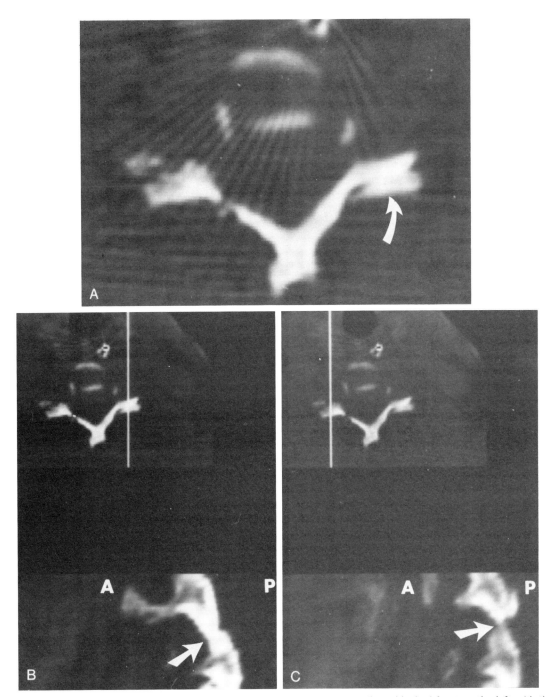

Figure 7–102. Facet injuries. *A*, Axial CT scan at C6–C7 demonstrates a unilateral locked facet on the left, with the superior articular process of C7 (arrow) lying posterior to the inferior articular process of C6. Fractures of the right articular processes are present. *B*, Parasagittal reconstruction through the plane of the left facet joint. The unilateral locked facet is seen (arrow). *C*, Parasagittal reconstruction through the plane of the right facet joint. There is perching of the inferior articular process of C6 on the superior articular process of C7 (arrow). *Key:* **A** = anterior; **P** = posterior.

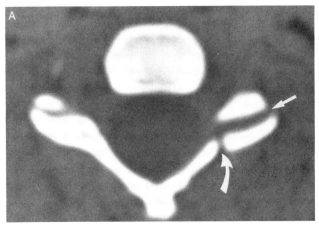

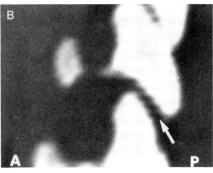

Figure 7–103. Subluxation of facet joint. A, Axial CT scan demonstrates widening of the C5–C6 facet joint on the left (straight arrow). A fracture of the left lamina is noted (curved arrow). B, Parasagittal reconstruction of the axial images through the plane of the left facet joint again reveals widening of the facet joint (arrow). *Key:* **A** = anterior; **P** = posterior.

and supraspinous and interspinous ligaments. CT can be used to determine the integrity of these three columns. This information in turn is useful in the evaluation of spinal stability.

The simple anterior wedge fracture of the thoracolumbar spine involves the anterior column only and has a characteristic CT appearance with a crescentic arch of bone displaced from the anterior portion of the vertebral body.[227] Typically these injuries involve compression of less than 50% of the height of the anterior column; however, more than 50% compression suggests the possibility of additional injury to the posterior elements and possible progression of spinal deformity and neurologic compromise.[135]

Burst fracture of the thoracolumbar spine is a more significant injury caused by axial compression, with fracture of the inferior vertebral end-plate of sufficient force to cause the nucleus pulposus to be thrust into the vertebral body, producing comminution of the body[203] (Fig. 7–104). This leads to failure of the anterior and middle columns under compression.[96] A sagittally oriented fracture of the inferior end-plate is seen, along with broadening and comminution of the fracture more superiorly.[227, 272] CT adds additional information to the conventional radiographs by permitting evaluation of the retropulsed fracture fragments and determining the presence of injury to the posterior elements[50, 277] (Table 7–21). The posteriorly displaced fracture fragment is usually derived from the superior aspect of the ver-

tebral body and may have intrafragment fracture, anterior rotation, and/or cephalad or caudad displacement. These findings suggest preoperatively that adequate reduction of the fragment may be difficult to obtain.[176] The degree of spinal canal narrowing can be evaluated in both the transaxial and sagittal planes. The information gained by the CT study, along with the clinical assessment of

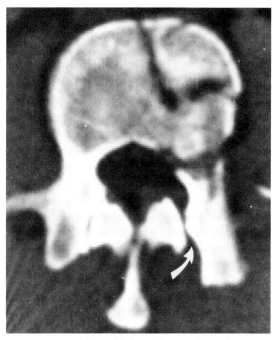

Figure 7–104. Unstable burst fracture. There is a comminuted fracture of the lumbar vertebral body and left pedicle, with subluxation of the left facet joint (arrow).

Table 7–21. USE OF CT IN EVALUATION OF THORACOLUMBAR BURST FRACTURE

Evaluation of fracture fragments in canal
Evaluation of spinal stenosis
Evaluation of fracture and/or dislocation of posterior elements
Characterization of retropulsed fracture fragments (e.g., intrafragmental fracture, anterior rotation, cephalad or caudad displacement)
Providing information for evaluation of instability

the patient, is useful in determining the therapeutic approach, which in some cases may require stabilization or decompression.

A fracture is considered unstable if it may lead to progressive increased spinal deformity or increased neurologic deficit. There is some controversy as to which injuries are stable and which are unstable. Clearly, however, a burst fracture is unstable if it is associated with subluxation or dislocation of the articular processes or fracture dislocation of the articular processes[96, 135] (see Fig. 7–104). Some authors feel that a burst fracture is unstable when the middle column has been disrupted and bone has been displaced into the canal.[96, 135] Disruption of the posterior elements is another indication of potential instability; however, a minimally displaced vertical fracture of the laminae, for example, may not necessarily indicate instability.[210]

CT is also useful in the postoperative evaluation of patients with burst fracture injury. The most common abnormality found in patients who have failed to recover after Harrington rod distraction instrumentation is the presence of residual bone fragments within the canal.[166] Symptomatic patients in the late recovery stage may have abundant callus compromising the spinal canal. In some cases, a lack of osseous fusion of the anterior vertebral body bone grafts can be demonstrated.[166]

Flexion compression injury of the thoracolumbar spine is another injury that can be evaluated by CT. This injury may lead to osseous, ligamentous, or combined osseous and ligamentous abnormalities. These injuries may occur secondary to forced flexion about a fulcrum point centered at the abdominal wall, such as occurs with a lap-type seat belt injury.[429] The Chance fracture, for

example, is a horizontal fracture through the spinous process and neural arch.[76] This may be associated with additional fracture of the posterosuperior aspect of the vertebral body. A combined osseous and ligamentous injury has been termed a Smith fracture and consists of horizontal fracture through the pedicles, laminae, and transverse processes, along with disruption of the posterior ligamentous complex.[157, 429] Associated fractures may occur, such as fractures of the superior articular processes and avulsion of the superior or inferior aspect of the posterior portion of the vertebral body.[157, 429] The presence of diastasis at the site of horizontal fracture through the laminae may lead to the CT appearance of a "disappearing laminae" sign, with laminae identified both above and below the site of diastasis.[239] Oblique and parasagittal reconstruction views through the posterior elements help clarify these fractures. Another type of injury is the facet distraction injury in which the pedicles, laminae, and spinous process remain intact while the forces are directed through the posterior ligamentous complex, resulting in vertical distraction of the articular processes.[336, 429] Axial CT demonstrates the "naked facet" sign, with the inferior articular processes of the vertebra above lying "naked" without their companion superior articular processes of the vertebra below[336] (Fig. 7–105). Sagittal reconstruction can be useful in delineating the relationship of the articular processes, the wide separation of the spinous processes, and additional vertebral body compression and subluxation.

Osseous Trauma to Sacrum

Fractures of the sacrum are difficult to visualize with conventional radiography owing to the curved orientation of the sacrum and the presence of overlying bowel gas and fecal material. CT has been used successfully to diagnose sacral fractures, determine their extent, and visualize soft tissue abnormalities such as pelvic hematoma[210, 464] (Fig. 7–106). Approximately 90% of sacral fractures occur in association with fractures of the anterior arch of the pelvis, and, consequently, sacral fractures should be carefully sought when such fractures are present.[405] During the initial radiographic examination of patients with multiple fractures of the

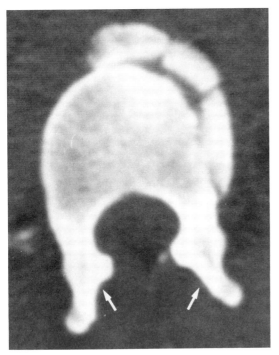

Figure 7–105. Facet distraction injury with "naked facet" sign. The superior articular processes (arrows) lie "naked" without their companion inferior articular processes. This is caused by disruption of the posterior ligamentous complex. Fracture of the vertebral body is seen anteriorly. (From Kricun R, Kricun ME: Computed Tomography of the Spine: Diagnostic Exercises. Rockville, Maryland: Aspen Publishers, Inc, 1987. Reprinted with permission of Aspen Publishers, Inc.)

pelvic ring, more than 60% of sacral fractures are overlooked.[208] In one report, CT of the pelvis was performed in patients with multiple injuries, including the pelvic fractures.[112] This study revealed that CT was "extremely helpful" in 65% of cases.[112] In this group of patients, additional fractures of the sacrum or diastasis of the sacroiliac joint was found, although neither had been identified by conventional radiography.

Other investigators, however, believe that although CT may be of value in evaluating the deformity of the sacral canals and posterior elements, it is not essential in diagnosing sacral fractures if careful attention is paid to the conventional radiograph.[208]

Insufficiency fractures of the sacrum may occur in elderly patients with osteopenia or in patients who have received radiation therapy to the pelvis. These patients may have normal conventional radiographs and a positive bone scan. In this setting, CT is useful in diagnosing an insufficiency fracture and excluding other disorders such as metastasis, which might be a diagnostic consideration in an elderly patient with pain and a positive bone scan.[150] The fracture usually has a vertical orientation with marginal reactive sclerosis, is located in the sacral ala, and lies parallel to the sacroiliac joint.[85, 98]

Widening of the sacroiliac joint can be demonstrated by CT, although it may be difficult to detect on the AP radiograph of the pelvis. Normally, the sacroiliac joint measures 2.5 to 4 mm.[260] CT is useful in the evaluation of children with subchondral fractures of the iliac bone. Initially the conventional radiographs and CT scan of this type of injury may suggest sacroiliac widening.[105] However, CT scans obtained several days after the injury demonstrate a normal sacroiliac joint and subchondral new bone at the fracture site, indicating the true nature of the injury.[105]

Nonosseous Post-Traumatic Abnormalities

CT and CTM can be used to evaluate the nonosseous abnormalities that occur secondary to trauma. For example, CT can clearly

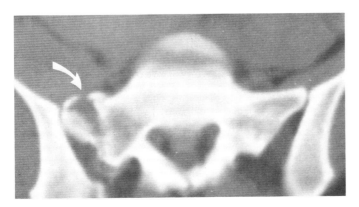

Figure 7–106. Fracture of the sacrum. Axial CT scan demonstrates a comminuted fracture of the right side of the sacrum (arrow). The sacroiliac joints appear normal.

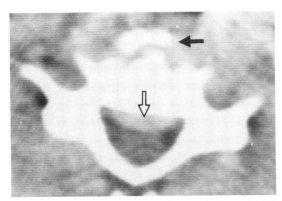

Figure 7–107. Post-traumatic disc herniation. Axial CT scan demonstrates acute herniation of the C5–C6 disc (open arrow). Fracture of the C5 vertebral body is noted anteriorly (closed arrow).

delineate a paravertebral or a presacral hematoma that might go undiagnosed by conventional radiography. Acute epidural hematoma may be a post-traumatic finding and can be studied by CT. Patients with bullet injuries to the spine may benefit from CT study. CT is more accurate than conventional radiography or conventional tomography in determining the presence and location of metallic or bony fragments within the spinal canal.[51, 352, 354]

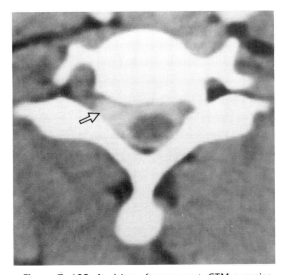

Figure 7–108. Avulsion of nerve root. CTM examination of the lower cervical vertebra demonstrates an outpouching of contrast agent within the right neural foramen (arrow) due to avulsion of the nerve root. (From Kricun R, Kricun ME: Computed Tomography of the Spine: Diagnostic Exercises. Rockville, Maryland: Aspen Publishers, Inc, 1987. Reprinted with permission of Aspen Publishers, Inc.)

Acute traumatic disc herniation is not common but may occur in association with severe flexion or extension injury to the cervical spine. This is an important entity to recognize because it is a surgically correctable cause of cord compression. Both CT and CTM are useful in evaluating post-traumatic disc herniation (Fig. 7–107). CTM is preferable to CT in the evaluation of spinal cord edema, cervical nerve root avulsion, and dural tear. After the introduction of intrathecal water-soluble contrast material, a cervical nerve root avulsion appears as an expanded outpouching of contrast agent extending ventrolaterally from the thecal sac into the neural foramen[315, 348] (Fig. 7–108). The collection of contrast material is sometimes separated from the thecal sac by a thin dural plane.[348] Evaluation of a dural tear reveals contrast material escaping beyond the subarachnoid space. In some cases, this is more readily appreciated by CTM than by conventional myelography.[315]

In the chronic stages following spinal trauma, CTM can be used in the diagnosis of post-traumatic arachnoiditis and post-traumatic syrinx. Arachnoiditis is seen as clumping of nerve roots. A post-traumatic syrinx usually fills with contrast agent on delayed CTM study.[390, 419] It forms by liquefaction of the hemorrhagic necrosis at the site of injury and from extension of the necrosis into adjacent normal cord.[435] Cysts may be single or multiple and may be small or involve the entire cord.[359]

EVALUATION OF THE POSTOPERATIVE PATIENT

The postoperative patient may be difficult to evaluate from both a clinical and an imaging standpoint. Many abnormalities found in the postoperative state are well demonstrated by CT and CTM and are discussed subsequently.

Postoperative Disc Herniation Versus Fibrotic Scar

Myelography has not been a reliable method of evaluating postoperative fibrotic scar and differentiating it from disc herniation.[207] This diagnostic problem is not easily solved by CT,[53, 185] although in many cases the correct diagnosis can be made.[52, 303, 410, 411, 445]

Both disc herniation and scar appear as increased soft tissue density that obliterates epidural fat and obscures the margins of the thecal sac and nerve root. Typically, a scar appears linear or strandlike, contours itself around the thecal sac, and retracts the thecal sac.[445] In comparison, a disc herniation is more often nodular and acts as a mass compressing the nerve root or thecal sac. It should be noted, however, that there is overlap in the CT appearance of disc herniation and fibrotic scar. For example, whereas fibrotic scar tends to occur throughout a longer segment and disc herniation is usually limited to the disc space level, an extruded disc may extend well beyond the intervertebral disc space. Similarly, although the disc is usually of higher density than scar, some overlap does occur in the CT attenuation values.

In cases of diagnostic difficulty, some authors have recommended the use of intrathecal water-soluble contrast agent,[303] whereas others have preferred using intravenous contrast enhancement.* When normal anatomic landmarks of fat and thecal sac are obliterated by scar, CTM is useful in determining the size and configuration of the sac and position of the nerve roots. Some authors have successfully differentiated disc herniation from postoperative scar by the use of intravenous contrast injection. Initially, an unenhanced CT scan is obtained, and the area of interest is then restudied after rapid drip[446] or bolus[411] injection of intravenous contrast agent. Typically, fibrotic scar is enhanced after injection of intravenous contrast agent, whereas disc herniation is not enhanced† (Fig. 7–109). In one study, scar was enhanced 26 ± 16 HU, whereas disc did not demonstrate significant increase in density (9 ± 4 HU [mean ± standard deviation]).[470] Nevertheless, some difficulties in this technique remain. For example, scar and disc herniation may coexist. The enhancement of scar surrounding a nonenhanced area might suggest the presence of both scar

*Reference numbers 52, 410, 411, 443, 446, 470.
†Reference numbers 52, 410, 411, 443, 446, 470, 473.

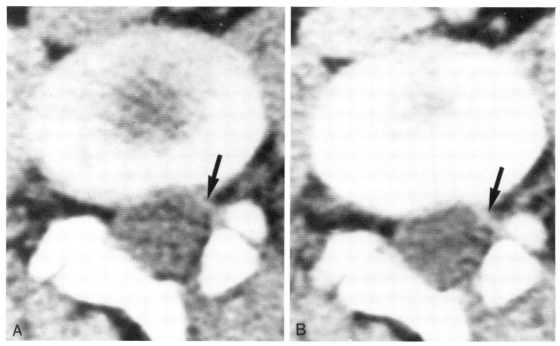

Figure 7–109. Postoperative scar. *A,* Unenhanced CT scan at L4–L5 level. There is soft tissue density partially obliterating the epidural fat on the left (arrow). This patient had a partial left laminectomy. *B,* Following intravenous administration of iodinated contrast material, there is marked enhancement of a linear fibrotic scar (arrow). (From Kricun R, Kricun ME: Computed Tomography of the Spine: Diagnostic Exercises. Rockville, Maryland: Aspen Publishers, Inc, 1987. Reprinted with permission of Aspen Publishers, Inc.)

and disc herniation; however, scar could be surrounding a nonenhanced nerve root, and a definitive diagnosis may not always be possible.[52] It is believed, however, that the use of intravenous contrast material increases diagnostic confidence and accuracy.[470]

Spinal Stenosis

Patients with disc herniation frequently also have lateral or central spinal stenosis. Failure to alleviate the stenosis adequately is one of the major causes of the failed back surgery syndrome in patients who undergo surgery for disc herniation.[64, 230, 278, 360] CT affords an opportunity to diagnose coexistent disc herniation and spinal stenosis in the preoperative state. In the postoperative patient, CT demonstration of lateral recess stenosis, neural foraminal stenosis, or central spinal stenosis may explain postoperative symptoms.

Postoperative Arachnoiditis

Arachnoiditis is discussed separately in this chapter (pp. 423–424). However, it should be noted that this is thought to represent the primary pathologic process in 6% to 16% of all patients with the failed back surgery syndrome.[64] Disc herniation is thought to act as a primary inflammatory focus, which is potentiated by an extrinsic process such as surgery or Pantopaque myelography.[64] Although myelography is the primary method of diagnostic imaging for arachnoiditis, CTM may also be useful in diagnosing this disorder and its complications. CTM demonstrates thickening and clumping of the nerve roots in patients with arachnoiditis (see Fig. 7–80). Syringomyelia, a complication of arachnoiditis, can also be demonstrated with CTM study. Ultrasound CT is useful in diagnosing arachnoiditis ossificans, another complication of arachnoiditis (see Fig. 7–81).

Postoperative Osteomyelitis

Approximately 0.2% to 3% of patients with lumbar disc surgery develop disc space infection.[368] Usually symptoms begin between the first and fourth postoperative weeks, but they may be delayed for several months.[368] The CT findings have been described elsewhere in this chapter (pp. 421–423) and include disc space narrowing, osteolysis of the vertebral end-plates on either side of the disc, and paravertebral and/or epidural soft tissue extension of the infection. Some pitfalls in the diagnosis of osteomyelitis in the postoperative patient should be mentioned. A postdiskectomy patient may have paravertebral edema or hemorrhage that may have an appearance similar to that of infection.[233] In addition, aggressive curettage of the vertebral end-plates during diskectomy may have an appearance similar to the vertebral erosions of osteomyelitis.[233] Careful examination of the CT findings in conjunction with the clinical presentation should lead to the correct diagnosis.

Epidural Hematoma

Epidural hematoma is a potentially life-threatening complication of surgery found in approximately 0.2% of patients who have undergone surgery for lumbar disc herniation.[102] A symptom-free postoperative period lasting approximately 1 day may be followed by persistent paresthesias over the dermatome of the exposed nerve root.[102] This may progress to weakness and urinary retention and can lead to paraplegia or quadriplegia.[335]

CT examination may demonstrate either a peripheral, sharply defined biconvex mass measuring approximately 60 to 80 HU or an area of similar increased CT attenuation filling the entire canal.[188, 269, 355, 496] The epidural hematoma may extend well beyond a single vertebral level. If there is diagnostic uncertainty, myelography with water-soluble contrast material can be performed, followed by CTM examination. CTM demonstrates the epidural hematoma as a lenticular mass compressing the subarachnoid space and displacing the spinal cord or cauda equina.[216, 252, 355, 496] Subacute or chronic epidural hematomas may appear isodense with the thecal sac but may be delineated by CTM.[269, 496]

Pseudomeningocele

A pseudomeningocele is a posterior localized collection of cerebrospinal fluid that usually occurs from inadequate closure or inadvertent tear of the dura following laminectomy.[345, 364, 448] Leakage of cerebrospinal fluid occurs and eventually becomes surrounded by a fibrous capsule. Less frequently, intact arachnoid herniates through the dural tear, with formation of an arachnoid-lined true meningocele.[448] Although approximately 2% of symptomatic postoperative patients have a pseudomeningocele, the degree to which the pseudomeningocele is related to postoperative symptoms is uncertain.

CT demonstrates a round homogeneous mass with CT attenuation similar to that of cerebrospinal fluid. Pseudomeningoceles are usually unilocular and develop posterior to the sac at the laminectomy site[249, 448] (Fig. 7–110). A higher density capsule may be present and occasionally calcifies.[68, 364, 448] In some cases, CTM may demonstrate a pseudomeningocele that is not visualized with conventional myelography, owing to the superior contrast resolution of CT.[345, 364] CTM performed with the patient in both the supine and the prone positions may delineate the exact site of communication of the sub-

arachnoid space, thus providing information that may be useful to the surgeon contemplating repair of the dural tear.[345]

Fat Graft

Free and pedicle fat grafts have been utilized in patients treated for spinal stenosis as a means of preventing postoperative fibrosis.[60, 192, 250, 492] The fat may act as a mechanical barrier preventing serous fluid and blood from collecting at the surgical site, thus inhibiting formation of epidural and perineural fibrosis.[192, 492] The presence and extent of a fat graft are readily determined by CT owing to the negative attenuation values of fat (see Fig. 7–12A). In the early postoperative period, the fat graft compresses the thecal sac but does not appear to be a cause of symptoms. After more than 6 months have passed from the time of surgery, the fat volume decreases by approximately 30% to 50%, and compression of the thecal sac abates.[60, 192] CT demonstrates the presence of fat in approximately 60% of patients who have had a free fat graft.[60] The CT demonstration of fat indicates that revascularization of the fat graft has occurred. It is possible that the lack of CT demonstration of fat in these patients may suggest that revascularization has not taken place.[60]

Surgical Fusion

Surgical fusion may be posterior, lateral, or interbody and is performed to correct instability that may develop in various pathologic conditions, such as trauma, infection, tumor, spondylolisthesis, and arthritis.

Posterior lumbar fusion is performed with bone graft placed between the laminae and spinous processes of adjacent vertebrae. Lateral fusion occurs when bone graft is placed between transverse processes. CT can be used to evaluate the solidity of a posterior or lateral fusion and to evaluate complications related to the fusion. Immediately after surgical fusion, discrete, isolated bone can be visualized; however, in time, solid fusion occurs, with increased bone mass encompassing the laminae, spinous processes, and articular processes (Fig. 7–111). In some cases, ankylosis of the facet joints may occur. CT can demonstrate failure of fusion, with

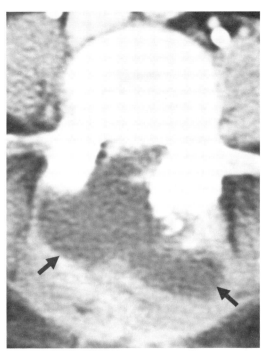

Figure 7–110. Pseudomeningocele. Axial CT scan at a lumbar level demonstrates a fluid collection within the subcutaneous tissues (arrows). This represents a postoperative pseudomeningocele. Note the bilateral laminectomy.

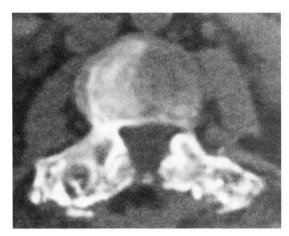

Figure 7–111. Bone fusion. Solid fusion is noted posterolaterally. This is the normal postoperative appearance following spinal fusion.

incomplete bony coalescence, pseudarthrosis, and incomplete facet joint fusion (Fig. 7–112). Spinal stenosis is a complication of surgical fusion that can be evaluated by CT. This occurs most frequently after posterior fusion, with the stenosis located at the disc space level immediately above the superior extent of the fusion. The stenosis is due to a combination of disc herniation, thickening and infolding of the ligamentum flavum, medial hypertrophy of articular processes, and ventral projection of the upper margin of the fusion mass.[57, 169] Less often, the stenosis occurs at the level of fusion and is due to hypertrophy of the midline fusion mass.

Lumbar interbody fusion is performed with removal of disc tissue and positioning of bone plugs in the intervertebral disc space extending from one vertebral body to the next. During the first weeks after surgery, the interbody graft has a discrete margin that is separate from the host bone and is well visualized with sagittal and coronal reformatted images.[393] As solid fusion occurs, there is obliteration of the host-graft interface. The most significant complications of interbody fusion are failure of osseous fusion with pseudarthrosis, graft displacement, and degenerative disc disease at the level above solid fusion.[87, 166, 393] Failure of osseous fusion may be best visualized with reformatted images in the sagittal and coronal planes. CT demonstrates a lack of callus and fusion between the vertebral body and the bone graft, disintegration of the graft, radiolucency of the involved vertebral body endplate, and loss of disc height.[166, 393] Bone plug displacement may be a potentially serious complication of interbody fusion and can be demonstrated on both axial images and sagittal reconstruction[87] (Fig. 7–113).

Cervical fusion can also be studied by CT. The CT appearance varies depending on the procedure used (bone graft, bone dowel, or strut graft). The complication rate is high with anterior cervical fusions (21%).[146] This high rate is thought to be in part related to the performance of an anterior fusion in the presence of unrecognized posterior instability.[146] The most frequent complications include extrusion of the bone graft and kypho-

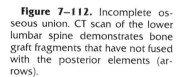

Figure 7–112. Incomplete osseous union. CT scan of the lower lumbar spine demonstrates bone graft fragments that have not fused with the posterior elements (arrows).

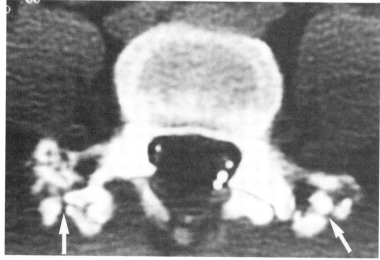

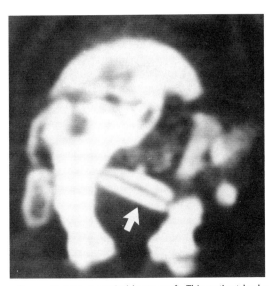

Figure 7–113. Extruded bone graft. This patient had a bone graft inserted for stabilization. The graft, however, became displaced posteriorly into the spinal canal (arrow). It is easily detected by CT. (From Kricun R, Kricun ME: Computed Tomography of the Spine: Diagnostic Exercises. Rockville, Maryland: Aspen Publishers, Inc, 1987. Reprinted with permission of Aspen Publishers, Inc.)

sis.[146] Posterior cervical fusion may be accomplished with metallic wiring and the use of cortical onlay bone grafts and has a lower complication rate than anterior fusion.[146] Combined anterior and posterior fusions may be performed.

CHEMONUCLEOLYSIS

Chymopapain chemonucleolysis has been used as a method of treating intractable sciatica caused by lumbar disc herniation. Chymopapain causes an enzymatic hydrolysis of the chondromucoprotein portion of the nucleus pulposus, leading to loss of its water-binding capacity and thus decreased pressure of the herniated disc on adjacent nerve roots.[59, 161, 283] Chymopapain chemonucleolysis is not without risk, and complications have been described.

CT is useful in the selection of patients for chemonucleolysis therapy.[59, 160, 232] Patients treated with chymopapain chemonucleolysis are more likely to have favorable results when there is evidence of a focal disc herniation causing nerve root compression. Unfavorable results have been reported when the underlying pathology is bulging of the annulus fibrosus, central spinal stenosis,

lateral recess stenosis, or neural foraminal stenosis.[160, 161, 283] The presence of a free disc fragment suggests that treatment with chymopapain chemonucleolysis may be unsuccessful,[59] although some patients have responded favorably.[160, 161]

CT is also used to evaluate the results of chemonucleolysis.[59, 161, 232, 283] The most frequent findings after chemonucleolysis therapy are disc space narrowing and the presence of a vacuum disc phenomenon.[16, 283] Decrease in size of the herniated disc has been demonstrated with CT (Fig. 7–114); however, this is frequently a subtle change, which may at first go unrecognized.[59] In one study, only 8% of patients treated with chymopapain chemonucleolysis had CT demonstration of decreased disc protrusion 6 weeks after therapy, although 76% had a successful clinical response.[161] The investigators suggested that early improvement in sciatica after chemonucleolysis may be due to intervertebral disc space narrowing, with subsequent reduction in nerve root tension and compression, rather than actual decrease in size of the disc protrusion. Reduction of the inflammatory reaction may also play a role in early clinical improvement, although this theory is speculative.[232, 283] Follow-up examination 6 months after therapy reveals decrease in size of the disc protrusion in approximately 60% of patients.[161]

BONE MINERAL CONTENT

Osteoporosis is a major health care problem that is responsible for about 2.3 million fractures in the United States yearly. Almost one half of the fractures involve vertebral bodies.[382] The spine is composed of about two thirds cancellous (trabecular) bone and one third compact (cortical) bone,[159] with the vertebral body composed mainly of cancellous bone.

It has been estimated that trabecular bone mineral content (BMC) begins to diminish in young adulthood (20 to 40 years of age) in both sexes[288] and proceeds at a rate of about 6% to 8% per decade. In patients who demonstrate onset of trabecular bone loss after the age of 40 or 50 years, the rate of loss is about 10% per decade in both sexes. Other authors feel that trabecular bone loss begins at around 40 to 45 years of age in women and at about 60 years of age in

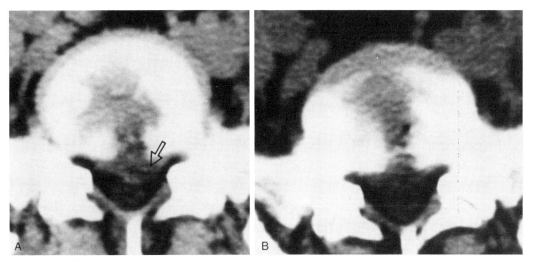

Figure 7–114. Chemonucleolysis. *A*, Axial CT scan at S1 demonstrates disc herniation (arrow) in a patient with left sciatica. *B*, Axial CT scan at S1 41 days after chymopapain injection. The disc herniation has resolved. (From Mall JC, Kaiser JC: Post-chymopapain [chemonucleolysis]—clinical and computed tomography correlation: preliminary results. Skeletal Radiol 12:270–275, 1984.)

men.[332] Cancellous bone, having a greater surface area, is more active metabolically than cortical bone and therefore is more responsive to alterations in BMC.[382]

Quantitative computed tomography (QCT) has become an important noninvasive method of evaluating BMC.* It has definite advantages over other imaging modalities, for it allows measurement of trabecular or cortical bone alone or in combination, with

---

*Reference numbers 67, 138, 139, 142, 159, 170, 258, 259, 288, 293, 372.

a high degree of accuracy, sensitivity, and precision.[138, 170, 372] The examination takes 10 to 15 minutes, and the radiation burden to the upper abdomen is relatively low, being in the range of 100 to 200 mrem.[67, 159] However, a radiation burden of 500 to 1000 mrem has been reported.[382] One of the limitations of QCT is difficulty in positioning the patient, which may lead to errors in attenuation measurements.[56] In addition, factors such as intrinsic drift and beam hardening may affect reproducibility. However, current scanners are capable of precise and repro-

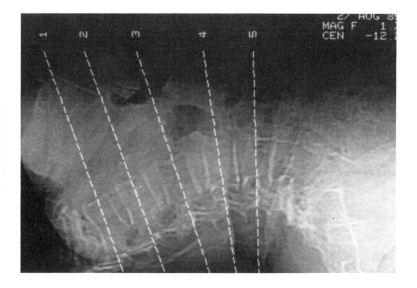

Figure 7–115. Bone mineral determination. Lateral digital radiograph of the lumbar spine. The cursor lines indicate the spinal levels and plane of scanning obtained from T12 to L4.

ducible positioning, so that the same point can be measured on serial examinations.[138]

The patient is placed supine on a phantom that contains five equivalent densities: mineral (aqueous solution of dipotassium hydrogen phosphate at 200 mg per cc, 100 mg per cc and 50 mg per cc), water, and fat. A lateral localizing image of the lower thoracic and lumbar regions of the spine is obtained, and the cursor is placed at the midplane of vertebrae T12–L4, parallel to the end-plates (Fig. 7–115). The lumbosacral region is avoided owing to the frequent association of degenerative changes and sclerosis in verte-brae that may alter bone mineral measurements. Single, 1 cm thick images are obtained at each level, with scanning performed at either 80 or 85 kVp. When viewing the axial images, a round or oval region of interest is determined in the anterior aspect of the vertebral body (Fig. 7–116). Care should be taken to obtain a similar region of interest at all levels and to assure that the size and shape of the circle of interest are similar. The vertebral cortex and the basivertebral groove should not be included within the circle of interest. Scanning the cortex will elevate the measured

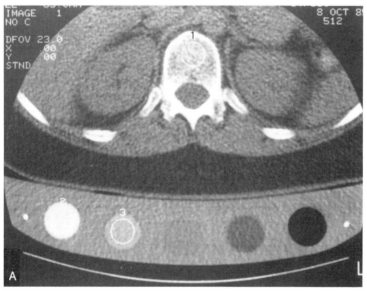

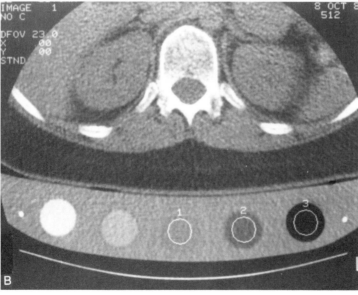

Figure 7–116. Axial CT scan obtained for bone mineralization, with the patient lying on the phantom. *A,* Circles of interest for densitometry are indicated. *Key:* **1** = cancellous bone in the midvertebral body; **2** and **3** = bone mineral equivalent densities. *B,* Same scan section as that shown in part *A.* Circles of interest for equivalent densities are noted. *Key:* **1** = bone mineral equivalent; **2** = water; **3** = fat.

result, and scanning the basivertebral groove will lower the result. The phantom is scanned simultaneously at each vertebral level, and the results are then used to calculate bone mineral equivalent (see Fig. 7–116). Calculation of bone mineral density can be performed using a linear regression method of calculation, or currently, software packages can be obtained that calculate the results. Vertebral bodies that demonstrate compression fractures are eliminated from the calculation, since the presence of callous formation and condensation of trabeculae elevates bone mineral measurements (Fig. 7–117).

The normal mean value of vertebral BMC for men and women in the age range of 20 to 40 years is 175 mg per cc.[159] By the age of 70 years, it is about 110 mg per cc in men and 90 mg per cc in women. It is estimated that patients are at risk for vertebral compression fractures when the BMC becomes less than 105 mg per cc[159]—the fracture threshold below which a great majority of fractures occur. Some authors consider the fifth percentile value of spinal trabecular BMC of normal postmenopausal women (45 years of age) as the threshold below which 85% of spontaneous spinal fractures occur.[139, 142] This is slightly less than 90 mg per cc and encompasses about 85% of women with spinal fractures.

Single-energy (80 or 85 kVp) QCT underestimates the actual density measurement of bone by about 25 mg per cc in men and 40 mg per cc in women.[264] This is probably due to the increase in vertebral fat marrow associated with aging.[238] Vertebral fat content also increases with immobilization osteoporosis.[259] Fat, which has a low CT attenuation, diminishes the calculated density of trabecular bone. The distribution of fat within vertebrae is unpredictable, unequal, and varies at different vertebral levels.[259] Some authors, however, feel that the inaccuracy of measurement produced by fat accumulation is insignificant,[293] particularly in postmenopausal women.[372]

Dual-energy QCT, that is, scanning at 80 or 85 kVp and at 130 or 140 kVp, corrects for errors caused by the presence of vertebral fat by simultaneously calibrating bone and soft tissue (which includes fat) at the two scanning energies[258, 259, 372] and, by means of calculations, arriving at a more accurate measurement. Thus, the results of dual-energy CT are closer to the true bone density and less influenced by the presence of fat than are single-energy calculations. However, the accuracy achieved by dual-energy QCT is offset by loss in reproducibility.[138, 293] This method may not be necessary in all clinical settings.[159]

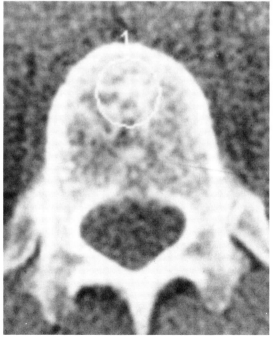

Figure 7–117. Axial CT scan for bone mineralization, with the circle of interest over an area of callous formation, giving an elevated measurement. Care should be taken to avoid taking measurements over areas of callous, cortex, or the basivertebral groove.

ACKNOWLEDGMENTS

We are extremely grateful to Carol Gagnon for preparation of the manuscript and for her medical illustrations. We thank Eastman Kodak Company for technical assistance with radiographic reproductions. Ronald Pecoul was particularly helpful in this regard. Steve Strommer, G. Douglas Thayer, and Juanita James provided additional photographic assistance. We wish to thank the Dorothy Rider Pool Health Care Trust for generously funding this project.

References

1. Abdelwahab IF, Frankel VH, Klein MJ: Aggressive osteoblastoma of the third lumbar vertebra: case report 351. Skeletal Radiol 15:164–169, 1986.
2. Aboulezz AO, Sartor K, Geyer CA, et al: Position of cerebellar tonsils in the normal population and in patients with Chiari malformation: a quantita-

tive approach with MR imaging. J Comput Assist Tomogr 9:1033–1036, 1985.

3. Adams RD, Victor M: Principles of Neurology, 3rd ed. New York: McGraw-Hill, 1985.

4. Adapon BD, Legada BD Jr, Lim EVA, et al: CT-guided closed biopsy of the spine. J Comput Assist Tomogr 5:73–78, 1981.

5. Alexander E Jr: Significance of the small lumbar spinal canal: cauda equina compression syndromes due to spondylosis: achondroplasia. J Neurosurg 31:513–519, 1969.

6. Amato M, Totty WG, Gilula LA: Spondylolysis of the lumbar spine: demonstration of defects and laminal fragmentation. Radiology 153:627–629, 1984.

7. Ameli NO, Abbassioun K, Saleh H: Aneurysmal bone cysts of the spine: report of 17 cases. J Neurosurg 63:685–690, 1985.

8. Anand AK, Lee BCP: Plain and metrizamide CT of lumbar disk disease: comparison with myelography. AJNR 3:567–571, 1982.

9. Angtuaco EJC, Binet EF, Flanigan S: Value of computed tomographic myelography in neurofibromatosis. Neurosurgery 13:666–671, 1983.

10. Arce CA, Dohrmann GJ: Thoracic disc herniation: improved diagnosis with computed tomographic scanning and a review of the literature. Surg Neurol 23:356–361, 1985.

11. Arnoldi CC, Brodsky AE, Cauchoix J, et al: Lumbar spinal stenosis and nerve root entrapment syndromes: Definition and classification. Clin Orthop 115:4–5, 1976.

12. Arredondo F, Haughton VM, Hemmy DC, et al: The computed tomographic appearance of the spinal cord in diastematomyelia. Radiology 136:685–688, 1980.

13. Aubin ML, Vignaud J: Syringomyelia and Arnold-Chiari malformation. In Post MJD (ed): Computed Tomography of the Spine. Baltimore: Williams & Wilkins, 1984, pp 298–306.

14. Aubin ML, Vignaud J, Jardin C, et al: Computed tomography in 75 clinical cases of syringomyelia. AJNR 2:199–204, 1981.

15. Badami JP, Norman D, Barbaro NM, et al: Metrizamide CT myelography in cervical myelopathy and radiculopathy: correlation with conventional myelography and surgical findings. AJR 144:675–680, 1985.

16. Baker ND, Greenspan A, Neuwirth M: Symptomatic vertebral hemangioma: a report of four cases. Skeletal Radiol 15:458–463, 1986.

17. Balagura S: Late neurological dysfunction in adult lumbosacral lipoma with tethered cord. Neurosurgery 15:724–726, 1984.

18. Balasubramanian E, Keim HA, Hajdu M: Osteoid osteoma of the thoracic spine with surgical decompression aided by somatosensory evoked potentials. Spine 10:396–398, 1985.

19. Balériaux D, Noterman J, Ticket L: Recognition of cervical soft disk herniation by contrast-enhanced CT. AJNR 4:607–608, 1983.

20. Ballantine HT Jr, Ojemann RG, Drew JH: Syringohydromyelia. Prog Neurol Surg 4:227–245, 1971.

21. Bankoff MS, Sarno RC, Carter BL: CT scanning in septic sacroiliac arthritis or periarticular osteomyelitis. Comput Radiol 8:165–170, 1984.

22. Banna M, Gryspeerdt GL: Intraspinal tumors in children (excluding dysraphism). Clin Radiol 22:17–32, 1971.

23. Barone BM, Elvidge AR: Ependymomas: a clinical survey. J Neurosurg 33:428–438, 1970.

24. Barson AJ: The vertebral level of termination of the spinal cord during normal and abnormal development. J Anat 106:489–497, 1970.

25. Barthelemy CR: Case report: arachnoiditis ossificans. J Comput Assist Tomogr 6:809–811, 1982.

26. Batnitzky S, Hall PV, Lindseth RE, et al: Meningomyelocele and syringomyelia. some radiological aspects. Radiology 120:351–357, 1976.

27. Baumgarten M, Mouradian W, Boger D, et al: Computed axial tomography in C1–C2 trauma. Spine 10:187–192, 1985.

28. Beals RK: Nosologic and genetic aspects of scoliosis. Clin Orthop 93:23–32, 1973.

29. Beatson TR: Fractures and dislocations of the cervical spine. J Bone Joint Surg 45B:21–35, 1963.

30. Beers GJ, Carter AP, Leiter BE, et al: Interobserver discrepancies in distance measurements from lumbar spine CT scans. AJR 144:395–398, 1985.

31. Benner B, Ehni G: Spinal arachnoiditis: the postoperative variety in particular. Spine 3:40–44, 1978.

32. Benoist M, Deburge A, Busson J, et al: Treatment of lumbar disc herniation by chymopapain chemonucleolysis. Spine 7:613–617, 1982.

33. Bernstein SA: Acute cervical pain associated with soft-tissue calcium deposition anterior to the interspace of the first and second cervical vertebrae. J Bone Joint Surg 57A:426–428, 1975.

34. Beyerl BD, Ojemann RG, Davis KR, et al: Cervical diastematomyelia presenting in adulthood. J Neurosurg 62:449–453, 1985.

35. Bhole R, Gilmer RE: Two-level thoracic disc herniation. Clin Orthop 190:129–131, 1984.

36. Bhushan C, Hodges FJ III, Wityk JJ: Synovial cyst (ganglion) of the lumbar spine simulating extradural mass. Neuroradiology 18:263–268, 1979.

37. Bielecki DK, Sartoris D, Resnick D, et al: Intraosseous and intradiscal gas in association with spinal infection: report of three cases. AJR 147:83–86, 1986.

38. Biondetti PR, Vigo M, Fiore D, et al: CT appearance of generalized von Recklinghausen neurofibromatosis. J Comput Assist Tomogr 7:866–869, 1983.

39. Bloch S, Van Rensburg MJ, Danziger J: The Arnold-Chiari malformation. Clin Radiol 25:335–341, 1974.

40. Bolender NF, Schönström NSR, Spengler DM: Role of computed tomography and myelography in the diagnosis of central spinal stenosis. J Bone Joint Surg 67A:240–246, 1985.

41. Bonafé A, Ethier R, Melançon D, et al: High resolution computed tomography in cervical syringomyelia. J Comput Assist Tomogr 4:42–47, 1980.

42. Bonafé A, Manelfe C, Espagno J, et al: Evaluation of syringomyelia with metrizamide computed tomographic myelography. J Comput Assist Tomogr 4:797–802, 1980.

43. Bonavita JA, Dalinka MK, Schumacher HR Jr: Hydroxyapatite deposition disease. Radiology 134:621–625, 1980.

44. Boone D, Parsons D, Lachmann SM, et al: Spina bifida occulta: lesion of anomaly? Clin Radiol 36:159–161, 1985.

45. Booth AE: Lateral thoracic meningocele. J Neurol Neurosurg Psychiatry 32:111–115, 1969.

46. Borlaza GS, Seigel R, Kuhns LR, et al: Computed tomography in the evaluation of sacroiliac arthritis. Radiology 139:437–440, 1981.

47. Bosacco SJ, Berman AT, Garbarino JL, et al: A comparison of CT scanning and myelography in the diagnosis of lumbar disc herniation. Clin Orthop 190:124–128, 1984.

48. Braakman R, Vinken PJ: Old luxations of the lower cervical spine. J Bone Joint Surg 50B:52–60, 1968.

49. Brandt-Zawadzki M, Burke VD, Jeffrey RB: CT in the evaluation of spine infection. Spine 8:358–364, 1983.

50. Brandt-Zawadzki M, Jeffrey RB Jr, Minagi H, et al: High resolution CT of thoracolumbar fractures. AJR 138:699–704, 1982.

51. Brandt-Zawadzki M, Miller EM, Federle MP: CT in the evaluation of spine trauma. AJR 136:369–375, 1981.

52. Braun IF, Hoffman JC Jr, Davis PC, et al: Contrast enhancement in CT differentiation between recurrent disk herniation and postoperative scar: prospective study. AJR 145:785–790, 1985.

53. Braun IF, Lin JP, Benjamin MV, et al: Computed tomography of the asymptomatic postsurgical lumbar spine: analysis of the physiologic scar. AJR 142:149–152, 1984.

54. Braun IF, Lin JP, George AE, et al: Pitfalls in the computed tomographic evaluation of the lumbar spine in disc disease. Neuroradiology 26:15–20, 1984.

55. Braunstein EM, Weissman BN, Seltzer SE, et al: Computed tomography and conventional radiographs of the craniocervical region in rheumatoid arthritis: a comparison. Arthritis Rheum 27:26–31, 1984.

56. Breatnach E, Robinson PJ: Repositioning errors in measurement of vertebral attenuation values by computed tomography. Br J Radiol 56:299–305, 1983.

57. Brodsky AE: Post-laminectomy and post-fusion stenosis of the lumbar spine. Clin Orthop 115:130–139, 1976.

58. Brodsky AE: Cauda equina arachnoiditis: a correlative clinical and roentgenologic study. Spine 3:51–60, 1978.

59. Brown BM, Stark EH, Dion G, et al: Computed tomography and chymopapain chemonucleolysis: preliminary findings. AJR 144:667–670, 1985.

60. Bryant MS, Bremer AM, Nguyen TQ: Autogenic fat transplants in the epidural space in routine lumbar spine surgery. Neurosurgery 13:367–370, 1983.

61. Burke DR, Brandt-Zawadzki M: CT of pyogenic spine infection. Neuroradiology 27:131–137, 1985.

62. Burrows FGO: Some aspects of occult spinal dysraphism: a study of 90 cases. Br J Radiol 41:496–507, 1968.

63. Burton CV: Lumbosacral arachnoiditis. Spine 3:24–30, 1978.

64. Burton CV, Kirkaldy-Willis WH, Yong-Hing K, et al: Causes of failure of surgery on the lumbar spine. Clin Orthop 157:191–199, 1981.

65. Cahan LD, Bentson JR: Considerations in the diagnosis and treatment of syringomyelia and the Chiari malformation. J Neurosurg 57:24–31, 1982.

66. Cameron AH: The Arnold-Chiari and other neuroanatomical malformations associated with spina bifida. J Pathol 73:195–211, 1957.

67. Cann CE: Low-dose CT scanning for quantitative spinal mineral analysis. Radiology 140:812–815, 1981.

68. Carollo C, Rigobello L, Carteri A, et al: Postsurgical calcified pseudocyst of the lumbar spine. J Comput Assist Tomogr 6:627–629, 1982.

69. Carrera GF: Lumbar facet joint injection in low back pain and sciatica: preliminary results. Radiology 137:665–667, 1980.

70. Carrera GF, Foley WD, Kozin F, et al: CT of sacroiliitis. AJR 136:41–46, 1981.

71. Carrera GF, Haughton VM, Syvertsen A, et al: Computed tomography of the lumbar facet joints. Radiology 134:145–148, 1980.

72. Carrera GF, Williams AL: Current concepts in evaluation of the lumbar facet joints. CRC Crit Rev Diagn Imaging 21:85–104, 1985.

73. Carrera GF, Williams AL, Haughton VM: Computed tomography in sciatica. Radiology 137:433–437, 1980.

74. Casselman ES: Radiologic recognition of symptomatic spinal synovial cysts. AJNR 6:971–973, 1985.

75. Castor, WR, Miller JDR, Russell AS, et al: Computed tomography of the craniocervical junction in rheumatoid arthritis. J Comput Assist Tomogr 7:31–36, 1983.

76. Chance GQ: Note on a type of flexion fracture of the spine. Br J Radiol 21:452–453, 1948.

77. Chehrazi B, Haldeman S: Adult onset of tethered spinal cord syndrome due to fibrous diastematomyelia: case report. Neurosurgery 16:681–685, 1985.

78. Ciappetta P, Delfini R, Cantore GP: Intradural lumbar disc hernia: Description of three cases. Neurosurgery 8:104–107, 1981.

79. Ciric I, Mikhael MA, Tarkington JA, et al: The lateral recess syndrome: a variant of spinal stenosis. J Neurosurg 53:433–443, 1980.

80. Cohen LM, Schwartz AM, Rockoff SD: Benign schwannomas: pathologic basis for CT inhomogeneities. AJR 147:141–143, 1986.

81. Coin CG: Computed tomography of cervical disc disease (herniation and degeneration). In Post MJD (ed): Computed Tomography of the Spine. Baltimore: Williams & Wilkins, 1984, pp 387–405.

82. Coin CG, Coin JT: Computed tomography of cervical disk disease: technical considerations with representative case reports. J Comput Assist Tomogr 5:275–280, 1981.

83. Coin CG, Pennink M, Ahmad WD, et al: Diving-type injury of the cervical spine: contribution of computed tomography to management. J Comput Assist Tomogr 3:362–372, 1979.

84. Coleman BG, Arger PH, Dalinka MK, et al: CT of sarcomatous degeneration in neurofibromatosis. AJR 140:383–387, 1983.

85. Cooper KL, Beabout JW, Swee RG: Insufficiency fractures of the sacrum. Radiology 156:15–20, 1985.

86. Coscia MF, Edmonson AS, Pitcock JA: Paravertebral synovial osteochondromatosis: a case report. Spine 11:82–87, 1986.

87. Coughlin JD: Extrusion of bone graft after lumbar fusion: CT appearance. J Comput Assist Tomogr 10:399–400, 1986.

88. Coughlin JR, Miller JDR: Metrizamide myelography in conjoined lumbosacral nerve roots. J Can Assoc Radiol 34:23–25, 1983.

89. Cox HE, Bennett WF: Computed tomography of absent cervical pedicle: case report. J Comput Assist Tomogr 8:537–539, 1984.

90. Crock HV, Goldwasser M: Anatomic studies of the circulation in the region of the vertebral end-plate in adult Greyhound dogs. Spine 9:702–706, 1984.

91. Crock HV, Yoshizawa H: The blood supply of the lumbar vertebral column. Clin Orthop 115:6–21, 1976.

92. Crock HV, Yoshizawa H, Kame SK: Observations on the venous drainage of the human vertebral body. J Bone Joint Surg 55B:528–533, 1973.

93. Crolla D, Hens L, Wilms G, et al: Metrizamide enhanced CT in hydrosyringomyelia. Neuroradiology 19:34–41, 1980.

94. Daniels DL, Grogan JP, Johansen JG, et al: Cervical radiculopathy: computed tomography and myelography compared. Radiology 151:109–113, 1984.

95. Degesys GE, Miller GA, Newman GE, et al: Absence of a pedicle in the spine: metastatic disease versus aplasia. Spine 11:76–77, 1986.

96. Denis F: Spinal instability as defined by the three-column spine concept in acute spinal trauma. Clin Orthop 189:65–76, 1984.

97. Dennis MD, Altschuler E, Glenn W, et al: Arachnoiditis ossificans: a report diagnosed with computerized axial tomography. Spine 8:115–117, 1983.

98. DeSmet AA, Neff JR: Pubic and sacral insufficiency fractures: clinical course and radiologic findings. AJR 145:601–606, 1985.

99. DeSousa AL, Kalsbeck JE, Mealey J Jr, et al: Intraspinal tumors in children. J Neurosurg 51:437–445, 1979.

100. Destouet JM, Gilula LA, Murphy WA, et al: Lumbar facet joint injection, technique, clinical correlation, and preliminary results. Radiology 145:321–325, 1982.

101. Dietz GW, Christensen EE: Normal "Cupid's bow" contour of the lower lumbar vertebrae. Radiology 121:577–579, 1976.

102. DiLauro L, Poli R, Bortoluzzi M, et al: Paresthesias after lumbar disc removal and their relationship to epidural hematoma. J Neurosurg 57:135–136, 1982.

103. Dillon WP, Kaseff LG, Knackstedt VE, et al: Computed tomography and differential diagnosis of the extruded lumbar disc. J Comput Assist Tomogr 7:969–975, 1983.

104. Dirheimer Y, Bensimon C, Christmann D, et al: Syndesmo-odontoid joint and calcium pyrophosphate dihydrate deposition disease (CPPD). Neuroradiology 25:319–321, 1983.

105. Donoghue V, Daneman A, Krajbich I, et al: CT appearance of sacroiliac joint trauma in children. J Comput Assist Tomogr 9:352–356, 1985.

106. Dorne HL, Just N, Lander PH: CT recognition of anomalies of the posterior arch of the atlas vertebra: Differentiation from fracture. AJNR 7:176–177, 1986.

107. Dossetor RS, Kaiser M, Veiga-Pires JA: CT scanning in two cases of lipoma of the spinal cord. Clin Radiol 30:227–231, 1979.

108. Dowd CF, Sartoris DJ, Haghighi P, et al: Tuberculous spondylitis resulting in atlanto-axial dislocation: case report 344. Skeletal Radiol 15:65–68, 1986.

109. Downey EF Jr, Whiddon SM, Brower AC: Computed tomography of congenital absence of posterior elements in the thoracolumbar spine. Spine 11:68–71, 1986.

110. Dublin AB, McGahan JP, Reid MH: The value of computed tomographic metrizamide myelography in the neuroradiological evaluation of the spine. Radiology 146:79–86, 1983.

111. duBoulay G, Shah SH, Currie JC, et al: The mechanism of hydromyelia in Chiari type 1 malformation. Br J Radiol 47:579–587, 1974.

112. Dunn EL, Berry PH, Connally JD: Computed tomography of the pelvis in patients with multiple injuries. J Trauma 23:378–382, 1983.

113. Durward QJ, Schweigel JF, Harrison P: Management of fractures of the thoracolumbar and lumbar spine. Neurosurgery 8:555–560, 1981.

114. Edelman RR, Kaufman H, Kolodny GM: Multiple myeloma-blastic type: case report 350. Skeletal Radiol 15:160–163, 1986.

115. Edelstyn GA, Gillespie PJ, Grebbell FS: The radiological demonstration of osseous metastases: experimental observations. Clin Radiol 18:158–162, 1967.

116. Efird TA, Genant HK, Wilson CB: Pituitary giantism with cervical spinal stenosis. AJR 134:171–173, 1980.

117. Ehni G, Love JG: Intraspinal lipomas: report of cases; review of the literature, and clinical and pathologic study. Arch Neurol Psychiatr 53:1–28, 1945.

118. Eisenberg D, Gomori JM, Findler G, et al: Symptomatic diverticulum of the sacral nerve root sheath: case note. Neuroradiology 27:183, 1985.

119. Eisenstein S: The trefoil configuration of the lumbar vertebral canal: a study of South African skeletal material. J Bone Joint Surg 62B:73–77, 1980.

119a. Eismont FJ, Green BA, Quencer RM: Post-traumatic spinal cord cyst: a case report. J Bone Joint Surg 66A:614–618, 1984.

120. El-Khoury GY, Tozzi JE, Clark CR, et al: Massive calcium pyrophosphate crystal deposition at the craniovertebral junction. AJR 145:777–778, 1985.

121. El-Khoury GY, Wener MH, Menezes AH, et al: Cranial settling in rheumatoid arthritis. Radiology 137:637–642, 1980.

122. Elliott JM, Rogers LF, Wissinger JP, et al: The hangman's fracture: fractures of the neural arch of the axis. Radiology 104:303–307, 1972.

123. Elster AD, Jensen KM: Computed tomography of spondylolisthesis: patterns of associated pathology. J Comput Assist Tomogr 9:867–874, 1985.

124. Emery JL, Lendon RG: Lipomas of the cauda equina and other fatty tumours related to neurospinal dysraphism. Dev Med Child Neurol 11:62–70, 1969.

125. Emery JL, Lendon RG: The local cord lesion in neurospinal dysraphism (meningomyelocele). J Pathol 110:83–96, 1973.

126. Enzmann DR, Murphy-Irwin K, Silverberg GD, et al: Spinal cord tumor imaging with CT and sonography. AJNR 6:95–97, 1985.

127. Epstein BS: The Spine. A Radiological Text and Atlas. Philadelphia: Lea & Febiger, 1976.

128. Epstein F, Epstein N: Surgical treatment of spinal cord astrocytomas of childhood: a series of 19 patients. J Neurosurg 57:685–689, 1982.

129. Epstein N, Benjamin V, Pinto R, et al: Benign

osteoblastoma of the thoracic vertebra. J Neurosurg 53:710–713, 1980.

130. Epstein N, Whelan M, Benjamin V: Acromegaly and spinal stenosis. J Neurosurg 56:145–147, 1982.

131. Erkulvrawatr S, Gammal TE, Hawkins J, et al: Intrathoracic meningoceles and neurofibromatosis. Arch Neurol 36:557–559, 1979.

132. Esposito PW, Crawford AH, Vogler C: Solitary osteochondroma occurring on the transverse process of the lumbar spine: a case report. Spine 10:398–400, 1985.

133. Eubanks BA, Cann CE, Brandt-Zawadzki M: CT measurement of the diameter of spinal and other bony canals: effects of section angle and thickness. Radiology 157:243–246, 1985.

134. Evens RJ, Mettler FA: National CT use and radiation exposure: United States 1983. AJR 144:1077–1081, 1985.

135. Ferguson RL, Allen BL Jr: A mechanistic classification of thoracolumbar spine fractures. Clin Orthop 189:77–88, 1984.

136. Fielding JW, Griffin PP: Os odontoideum: an acquired lesion. J Bone Joint Surg 56A:187–190, 1974.

137. Firooznia H, Benjamin V, Kricheff II, et al: CT of lumbar spine disk herniation: correlation with surgical findings. AJR 142:587–592, 1984.

138. Firooznia H, Golimbu C, Rafii M, et al: Quantitative computed tomography assessment of spinal trabecular bone. I. Age-related regression in normal men and women. J Comput Assist Tomogr 8:91–97, 1984.

139. Firooznia H, Golimbu C, Rafii M, et al: Quantitative computed tomography assessment of spinal trabecular bone. II. In osteoporotic women with and without vertebral fractures. J Comput Assist Tomogr 8:99–103, 1984.

140. Firooznia H, Golimbu C, Rafii M, et al: Computed tomography of spinal chordomas. J Comput Tomogr 10:45–50, 1986.

141. Firooznia H, Pinto RS, Lin JP, et al: Chordoma: radiologic evaluation of 20 cases. AJR 127:797–805, 1976.

142. Firooznia H, Rafii M, Golimbu C, et al: Trabecular mineral content of the spine in women with hip fracture: CT measurement. Radiology 157:737–740, 1986.

143. Firooznia H, Tyler I, Golimbu C, et al: Computerized tomography of the Cupid's bow contour of the lumbar spine. Comput Radiol 7:347–350, 1983.

144. Fitz CR: Midline anomalies of the brain and spine. Radiol Clin North Am 20:95–104, 1982.

145. Fitz CR, Harwood-Nash DC: The tethered conus. AJR 125:515–523, 1975.

146. Foley MJ, Lee C, Calenoff L, et al: Radiologic evaluation of surgical cervical spine fusion. AJR 138:79–89, 1982.

147. Forbes WS, Isherwood I: Computed tomography in syringomyelia and the associated Arnold-Chiari type I malformation. Neuroradiology 15:73–78, 1978.

148. French BN: Midline fusion defects and defects of formation. In Youmans JR (ed): Neurological Surgery, vol 3. Philadelphia: WB Saunders Company, 1982, pp 1236–1380.

149. Fries JW, Abodeely DA, Vijungco JG, et al: Computed tomography of herniated and extruded nucleus pulposus. J Comput Assist Tomogr 6:874–887, 1982.

150. Gacetta DJ, Yandow DR: Computed tomography of spontaneous osteoporotic sacral fractures: case report. J Comput Assist Tomogr 8:1190–1191, 1984.

151. Gado M, Patel J, Hodges FJ III: Lateral disc herniation into the lumbar intervertebral foramen: differential diagnosis. AJNR 4:598–600, 1983.

152. Gamba JL, Martinez S, Apple J, et al: Computed tomography of axial skeletal osteoid osteomas. AJR 142:769–772, 1984.

153. Gardner WJ: Hydrodynamic mechanism of syringomyelia: its relationship to myelocele. J Neurol Neurosurg Psychiatry 28:247–259, 1965.

154. Gebarski SS, McGillicuddy JE: "Conjoined" nerve roots: a requirement for computed tomographic and myelographic correlation for diagnosis. Neurosurgery 14:66–68, 1984.

155. Gehweiler JA Jr, Daffner RH, Roberts L Jr: Malformations of the atlas vertebra simulating the Jefferson fracture. AJR 140:1083–1086, 1983.

156. Gehweiler JA Jr, Duff DE, Martinez S, et al: Fractures of the atlas vertebra. Skeletal Radiol 1:97–102, 1976.

157. Gehweiler JA Jr, Osborne RL Jr, Becker RF: The radiology of vertebral trauma. Philadelphia: WB Saunders Company, 1980.

158. Genant HK: Computed tomography of the lumbar spine: technical considerations. In Genant HK, Chafetz N, Helms CA (eds): Computed Tomography of the Lumbar Spine. San Francisco: University of California, 1982, pp 23–52.

159. Genant HK, Cann CE: Spinal osteoporosis: advanced assessment using quantitative computed tomography. In Genant HK, et al (eds): Spine Update 1984: Perspective in Radiology, Orthopedic Surgery, and Neurosurgery. San Francisco: Radiology Research and Education Foundation, 1983.

160. Gentry LR, Strother CM, Turski PA, et al: Chymopapain chemonucleolysis: correlation of diagnostic radiographic factors and clinical outcome. AJR 145:351–360, 1985.

161. Gentry LR, Turski PA, Strother CM, et al: Chymopapain chemonucleolysis: CT changes after treatment. AJR 145:361–369, 1985.

162. George WE Jr, Wilmot M, Greenhouse A, et al: Medical management of steroid induced epidural lipomatosis. N Engl J Med 308:316–319, 1983.

163. Giordano GB, Cerisoli M: Diastematomyelia and scoliosis. Usefulness of CT examination. Spine 8:111–112, 1983.

164. Godersky JC, Erickson DL, Seljeskog EL: Extreme lateral disc herniation: diagnosis by computed tomographic scanning. Neurosurgery 14:549–552, 1984.

165. Golimbu C, Firooznia H, Rafii M: CT of osteomyelitis of the spine. AJR 142:159–163, 1984.

166. Golimbu C, Firooznia H, Rafii M, et al: Computed tomography of thoracic and lumbar spine fractures that have been treated with Harrington instrumentation. Radiology 151:731–733, 1984.

167. Gordon G, Kabins SA: Pyogenic sacroiliitis. Am J Med 69:50–56, 1980.

168. Gorey MT, Naidich TP, McLone DG: Double discontinuous lipomyelomeningocele: CT findings. J Comput Assist Tomogr 9:584–591, 1985.

169. Grabias S: The treatment of spinal stenosis. J Bone Joint Surg 62A:308–313, 1980.

170. Graves VB, Wimmer R: Long-term reproducibility of quantitative computed tomography vertebral mineral measurements. J Comput Tomogr 9:73–76, 1985.

171. Grisolia A, Bell RL, Peltier LF: Fractures and dislocations of the spine complicating ankylosing spondylitis. J Bone Joint Surg 49A:339–344, 386, 1967.

172. Grogan JP, Hemminghytt S, Williams AL, et al: Spondylolysis studied with computed tomography. Radiology 145:737–742, 1982.

173. Gropper GR, Acker JD, Robertson JH: Computed tomography in Pott's disease. Neurosurgery 10:506–508, 1982.

174. Grosman H, Gray R, St Louis EL: CT of long-standing ankylosing spondylitis with cauda equina syndrome. AJNR 4:1077–1080, 1983.

175. Groswasser Z, Reider-Groswasser I: Heterotopic new bone formation in the cervical spine following head injury: Case report. J Neurosurg 64:513–515, 1986.

176. Guerra J Jr, Garfin SR, Resnick D: Vertebral burst fractures: CT analysis of the retropulsed fragment. Radiology 153:769–772, 1984.

177. Hadar H, Gadoth N, Heifetz M: Fatty replacement of lower paraspinal muscles: normal and neuro-muscular disorders. AJR 141:895–898, 1983.

178. Hanai K, Adachi H, Ogasawara H: Axial transverse tomography of the cervical spine narrowed by ossification of the posterior longitudinal ligament. J Bone Joint Surg 59A:481–484, 1977.

179. Hanai K, Inouye Y, Kawai K, et al: Anterior decompression for myelopathy resulting from ossification of the posterior longitudinal ligament. J Bone Joint Surg 64B:561–564, 1982.

180. Handel S, Grossman R, Sarwar M: Computed tomography in the diagnosis of spinal cord astrocytoma. J Comput Assist Tomogr 2:226–228, 1978.

181. Haney P, Gellad F, Swartz J: Aneurysmal bone cyst of the spine. Computed tomographic appearance. J Comput Tomogr 7:319–322, 1983.

182. Hanna M, Watt I: Posterior longitudinal ligament calcification of the cervical spine. Br J Radiol 52:901–905, 1979.

183. Harbin WP: Metastatic disease and the nonspecific bone scan: value of spinal computed tomography. Radiology 145:105–107, 1982.

184. Harris JH Jr: Acute injuries of the spine. Semin Roentgenol 13:53–68, 1978.

185. Haughton VM, Eldevik OP, Magnaes B, et al: A prospective comparison of computed tomography and myelography in the diagnosis of herniated lumbar disks. Radiology 142:103–110, 1982.

186. Haughton VM, Syvertsen A, Williams AL: Soft-tissue anatomy within the spinal canal as seen on computed tomography. Radiology 134:649–655, 1980.

187. Haughton VM, Williams AL: Computed tomography of the spine. St. Louis: CV Mosby Company, 1982.

188. Haykal HA, Wang A-M, Zamani AA, et al: Computed tomography of spontaneous acute cervical epidural hematoma. J Comput Assist Tomogr 8:229–231, 1984.

189. Heinz ER, Rosenbaum AE, Scarff TB, et al: Tethered spinal cord following meningomyelocele repair. Radiology 131:153–160, 1979.

190. Heinz ER, Yeates A, Burger P, et al: Opacification of epidural venous plexus and dura in evaluation of cervical nerve roots: CT technique. AJNR 5:621–624, 1984.

191. Heithoff KB: High-resolution computed tomography of the lumbar spine. Postgrad Med 70:193–213, 1981.

192. Heithoff KB: High-resolution computed tomography and stenosis: an evaluation of the causes and cures of the failed back surgery syndrome. In Post MDJ (ed): Computed Tomography of the Spine. Baltimore: Williams & Wilkins, 1984, pp 506–545.

193. Helms CA, Cann CE, Brunelle FO, et al: Detection of bone-marrow metastases using quantitative computed tomography. Radiology 140:745–750, 1981.

194. Helms CA, Dorwart RH, Gray MG: The CT appearance of conjoined nerve roots and differentiation from a herniated nucleus pulposus. Radiology 144:803–807, 1982.

195. Helms CA, Genant HK: Computed tomography in the early detection of skeletal involvement with multiple myeloma. JAMA 248:2886–2887, 1982.

196. Helms CA, Vogler JB: Computed tomography of spinal stenoses and arthroses. Clin Rheum Dis 9:417–441, 1983.

197. Hemminghytt S, Daniels DL, Williams AL, et al: Intraspinal synovial cysts: natural history and diagnosis by CT. Radiology 145:375–376, 1982.

198. Hermann G, Mendelson DS, Cohen BA, et al: Role of computed tomography in the diagnosis of infectious spondylitis. J Comput Assist Tomogr 7:961–968, 1983.

199. Hilal SK, Marton D, Pollack E: Diastematomyelia in children. Radiology 112:609–621, 1974.

200. Hirschy JC, Leue WM, Berninger WH, et al: CT of the lumbosacral spine: Importance of tomographic planes parallel to vertebral end plate. AJR 136:47–52, 1981.

201. Hochman MS, Pena C, Ramirez R: Calcified herniated thoracic-disc diagnosed by computerized tomography: case report. J Neurosurg 52:722–723, 1980.

202. Hoddick WK, Helms CA: Bony spinal canal changes that differentiate conjoined nerve roots from herniated nucleus pulposus. Radiology 154:119–120, 1985.

203. Holdsworth F: Fractures, dislocations, and fracture-dislocations of the spine. J Bone Joint Surg 52A:1534–1551, 1970.

204. Holt JF: Neurofibromatosis in children. AJR 130:615–639, 1978.

205. Hood RW, Riseborough EJ, Nehme A-M, et al: Diastematomyelia and structural spinal deformities. J Bone Joint Surg 62A:520–528, 1980.

206. Hungerford GD, Akkaraju V, Rawe SE, et al: Atlanto-occipital and atlanto-axial dislocations with spinal cord compression in Down's syndrome: a case report and review of the literature. Br J Radiol 54:758–761, 1981.

207. Irstam L: Differential diagnosis of recurrent lumbar disc herniation and postoperative deformation by myelography: an impossible task. Spine 9:759–763, 1984.

208. Jackson H, Kam J, Harris JH Jr, et al: The sacral arcuate lines in upper sacral fractures. Radiology 145:35–39, 1982.

209. Jackson RP, Reckling FW, Mantz FA: Osteoid osteoma and osteoblastoma: similar histologic lesions with different natural histories. Clin Orthop 128:303–313, 1977.

210. Jacobs RR, Casey MP: Surgical management of thoracolumbar spinal injuries: general principles and controversial considerations. Clin Orthop 189:22–35, 1984.

211. James CCM, Lassman LP: Spinal dysraphism: the diagnosis and treatment of progressive lesions in spina bifida occulta. J Bone Joint Surg 44B: 828–840, 1962.

212. James HE, Oliff M: Computed tomography in spinal dysraphism. J Comput Assist Tomogr 1:391–397, 1977.

213. Janin Y, Epstein JA, Carras R, et al: Osteoid osteomas and osteoblastomas of the spine. Neurosurgery 8:31–38, 1981.

214. Jefferson G: Fracture of the atlas vertebra: report of four cases, and a review of those previously recorded. Br J Surg 7:407–422, 1920.

215. Kadish LJ, Simmons EH: Anomalies of the lumbosacral nerve roots: an anatomical investigation and myelographic study. J Bone Joint Surg 66B:411–416, 1984.

216. Kaiser MC, Capesius P, Ohanna F, et al: Computed tomography of acute spinal epidural hematoma associated with cervical root avulsion. J Comput Assist Tomogr 8:322–323, 1984.

217. Kaiser MC, Capesius P, Roilgen A, et al: Epidural venous stasis in spinal stenosis: CT appearance. Neuroradiology 26:435–438, 1984.

218. Kan S, Fox AJ, Viñuela F: Delayed metrizamide CT enhancement of syringomyelia: postoperative observations. AJNR 6:613–616, 1985.

219. Kan S, Fox AJ, Viñuela F, et al: Delayed CT metrizamide enhancement of syringomyelia secondary to tumor. AJNR 4:73–78, 1983.

220. Kan S, Fox AJ, Viñuela F, et al: Spinal cord size in syringomyelia: change with position on metrizamide myelography. Radiology 146:409–414, 1983.

221. Kaplan JO, Quencer RM: The occult tethered conus syndrome in the adult. Radiology 137: 387–391, 1980.

222. Karian JM, DeFilipp G, Buchheit WA, et al: Vertebral osteochondroma causing spinal cord compression: case report. Neurosurgery 14:483–484, 1984.

223. Kattapuram SV, Phillips WC, Boyd R: CT in pyogenic osteomyelitis of the spine. AJR 140:1199–1201, 1983.

224. Keene JS, Goletz TH, Lilleas F, et al: Diagnosis of vertebral fractures: a comparison of conventional radiography, conventional tomography, and computed axial tomography. J Bone Joint Surg 64A: 586–595, 1982.

225. Ker NB, Jones CB: Tumours of the cauda equina: the problem of differential diagnosis. J Bone Joint Surg 67B:358–361, 1985.

226. Kershner MS, Goodman GA, Perlmutter GS: Computed tomography in the diagnosis of an atlas fracture. AJR 128:688–689, 1977.

227. Kilcoyne RF, Mack LA, King HA, et al: Thoracolumbar spine injuries associated with vertical plunges: reappraisal with computed tomography. Radiology 146:137–140, 1983.

228. Kirkaldy-Willis WH, McIvor GWD: Editorial comment: lumbar spinal stenosis. Clin Orthop 115:2–3, 1976.

229. Kirkaldy-Willis WH, Paine KWE, Cauchoix J, et al: Lumbar spinal stenosis. Clin Orthop 99:30–50, 1974.

230. Kirkaldy-Willis WH, Wedge JH, Yong-Hing K, et

231. Kirwan EO, Hutton PAN, Pozo JL, et al: Osteoid osteoma and benign osteoblastoma of the spine. J Bone Joint Surg 66B:21–26, 1984.

232. Konings JG, Williams FJB, Deutman R: The effects of chemonucleolysis as demonstrated by computerised tomography. J Bone Joint Surg 66B:417–421, 1984.

233. Kopecky KK, Gilmor RL, Scott JA, et al: Pitfalls of computed tomography in diagnosis of discitis. Neuroradiology 27:57–66, 1985.

234. Kornberg M: Primary Ewing's sarcoma of the spine: a review and case report. Spine 11:54–57, 1986.

235. Kozin F, Carrera GF, Ryan LM, et al: Computed tomography in the diagnosis of sacroiliitis. Arthritis Rheum 24:1479–1485, 1981.

236. Kramer LD, Krouth GJ: Computerized tomography: an adjunct to early diagnosis in the cauda equina syndrome of ankylosing spondylitis. Arch Neurol 35:116–118, 1978.

237. Kricun ME: Radiographic evaluation of solitary bone lesions. Orthop Clin North Am 14:39–63, 1983.

238. Kricun ME: Red-yellow marrow conversion: its effect on the location of some solitary bone lesions. Skeletal Radiol 14:10–19, 1985.

239. Kricun R, Kricun ME: Computed Tomography of the Spine: Diagnostic Exercises. Rockville, Maryland: Aspen Publishers, Inc, 1987.

240. Krol G, Sundaresan N, Deck M: Computed tomography of axial chordomas. J Comput Assist Tomogr 7:286–289, 1983.

241. Kuchner EF, Anand AK, Kaufman BM: Cervical diastematomyelia: a case report with operative management. Neurosurgery 16:538–542, 1985.

242. Kudo S, Ono M, Russell WJ: Ossification of thoracic ligamenta flava. AJR 141:117–121, 1983.

243. Kumar AJ, Kuhajda FP, Martinez CR, et al: Computed tomography of extracranial nerve sheath tumors with pathological correlation. J Comput Assist Tomogr 7:857–865, 1983.

244. Kurz LT, Garfin SR, Unger AS, et al: Intraspinal synovial cyst causing sciatica. J Bone Joint Surg 67A:865–871, 1985.

245. Kwee IL, Nakada T: Syrinx formation in multiple sclerosis. Br J Radiol 58:1206–1208, 1985.

246. Laasonen EM: Atrophy of sacrospinal muscle groups in patients with chronic, diffusely radiating lumbar back pain. Neuroradiology 26:9–13, 1984.

247. Laasonen EM, Kankaanpää U, Paukku P, et al: Computed tomographic myelography (CTM) in atlanto-axial rheumatoid arthritis. Neuroradiology 27:119–122, 1985.

248. LaBerge JM, Brandt-Zawadzki M: Evaluation of Pott's disease with computed tomography. Neuroradiology 26:429–434, 1984.

249. Laffey PA, Kricun ME: Sonographic recognition of postoperative meningocele. AJR 143:177–178, 1984.

250. Langenskiöld A, Kiviluoto O: Prevention of epidural scar formation after operations on the lumbar spine by means of free fat transplants: a preliminary report. Clin Orthop 115:92–95, 1976.

251. Langston JW, Gavant ML: "Incomplete ring" sign: a simple method for CT detection of spondylolysis. J Comput Assist Tomogr 9:728–729, 1985.

252. Lanzieri CF, Sacher M, Solodnik P, et al: CT

myelography of spontaneous spinal epidural hematoma: case report. J Comput Assist Tomogr 9:393–394, 1985.

253. Lanzieri CF, Solodnik P, Sacher M, et al: Computed tomography of solitary spinal osteochondromas. J Comput Assist Tomogr 9:1042–1044, 1985.

254. Lapointe JS, Graeb DA, Nugent RA, et al: Value of intravenous contrast enhancement in the CT evaluation of intraspinal tumors. AJR 146:103–107, 1986.

255. Lardé D, Mathieu D, Frija J, et al: Spinal vacuum phenomenon: CT diagnosis and significance. J Comput Assist Tomogr 6:671–676, 1982.

256. Lardé D, Mathieu D, Frija J, et al: Vertebral osteomyelitis: disk hypodensity on CT. AJR 139:963–967, 1982.

257. Larsen JL, Smith D, Fossan G: Arachnoidal diverticula and cystlike dilatations of the nerve-root sheaths in lumbar myelography. Acta Radiol [Diagn] 21:141–145, 1980.

258. Laval-Jeantet AM, Cann CE, Roger B, et al: A postprocessing dual energy technique for vertebral CT densitometry. J Comput Assist Tomogr 8:1164–1167, 1984.

259. Laval-Jeantet AM, Roger B, Bouysse S, et al: Influence of vertebral fat content on quantitative CT density. Radiology 159:463–466, 1986.

260. Lawson TL, Foley WD, Carrera GF, et al: The sacroiliac joints: anatomic, plain roentgenographic, and computed tomographic analysis. J Comput Assist Tomogr 6:307–314, 1982.

261. Lecklitner ML, Potter JL, Growcock G: Computed tomography in acquired absence of thoracic pedicle: case report. J Comput Assist Tomogr 9:395–397, 1985.

262. Lee C, Kim KS, Rogers LF: Sagittal fracture of the cervical vertebral body. AJR 139:55–60, 1982.

263. Leeds NE, Jacobson HG: Spinal neurofibromatosis. AJR 126:617–623, 1976.

264. Leehey P, Naseem M, Every P, et al: Vertebral hemangioma with compression myelopathy: metrizamide CT demonstration. J Comput Assist Tomogr 9:985–986, 1985.

265. Lefkowitz DM, Quencer RM: Vacuum facet phenomenon: a computed tomographic sign of degenerative spondylolisthesis. Radiology 144:562, 1985.

266. Levander B, Mellstrom A, Grepe A: Atlantoaxial instability in Marfan's syndrome. Diagnosis and treatment: a case report. Neuroradiology 21:43–46, 1981.

267. Levine E, Batnitzky S: Computed tomography of sacral and presacral lesions. CRC Crit Rev Diagn Imaging 21:307–374, 1984.

268. Levine RS, Geremia GK, McNeill TW: CT demonstration of cervical diastematomyelia. J Comput Assist Tomogr 9:592–594, 1985.

269. Levitan LH, Wiens CW: Chronic lumbar extradural hematoma: CT findings. Radiology 148:707–708, 1983.

270. Levy WJ Jr, Bay J, Dohn D: Spinal cord meningioma. J Neurosurg 57:804–812, 1982.

271. Lichtenstein BW: "Spinal dysraphism:" Spina bifida and myelodysplasia. Arch Neurol Psychiatr 44:792–810, 1940.

272. Lindahl S, Willen J, Nordwall A, et al: The crush-cleavage fracture: a new thoracolumbar unstable fracture. Spine 8:559–569, 1983.

273. Linkowski GD, Tsai FY, Recher L, et al: Solitary osteochondroma with spinal cord compression. Surg Neurol 23:388–390, 1985.

274. Lipson SJ: Rheumatoid arthritis of the cervical spine. Clin Orthop 182:143–149, 1984.

275. Lott IT, Richardson EP Jr: Neuropathological findings and the biology of neurofibromatosis. Adv Neurol 29:23–32, 1981.

276. Lutter LD, Lonstein JE, Winter RB, et al: Anatomy of the achondroplastic lumbar canal. Clin Orthop 126:139–142, 1977.

277. Lynch D, McManus F, Ennis JT: Computed tomography in spinal trauma. Clin Radiol 37:71–76, 1986.

278. Macnab I: Negative disc exploration: an analysis of the causes of nerve-root involvement in sixty-eight patients. J Bone Joint Surg 53A:891–903, 1971.

279. Madigan R, Worrall T, McClain EJ: Cervical cord compression in hereditary multiple exostosis: review of the literature and report of a case. J Bone Joint Surg 56A:401–404, 1974.

280. Magid SK, Gray GE, Anand A: Spinal cord compression by tophi in a patient with chronic polyarthritis: case report and literature review. Arthritis Rheum 24:1431–1434, 1981.

281. Mahboubi S: CT appearance of nidus in osteoid osteoma versus sequestration in osteomyelitis. J Comput Assist Tomogr 10:457–459, 1986.

282. Maldague BE, Malghem JJ: Unilateral arch hypertrophy with spinous process tilt: a sign of arch deficiency. Radiology 121:567–574, 1976.

283. Mall JC, Kaiser JC: Post-chymopapain (chemonucleolysis)—clinical and computed tomography correlation: preliminary results. Skeletal Radiol 12:270–275, 1984.

284. Mall JC, Kaiser JA, Heithoff KB: Postoperative spine. In Newton TH, Potts DG (eds): Computed Tomography of the Spine and Spinal Cord. San Anselmo, California: Clavadel Press, 1983, pp 187–204.

285. Maritz NGJ, deVilliers JFK, van Castricum OQS: Computed tomography in tuberculosis of the spine. Comput Radiol 6:1–5, 1982.

286. Martinez S, Morgan CL, Gehweiler JA Jr, et al: Unusual fractures and dislocations of the axis vertebra. Skeletal Radiol 3:206–212, 1979.

287. Mawhinney R, Jones R, Worthington BS: Spinal cord compression secondary to Paget's disease of the axis: case reports. Br J Radiol 58:1203–1206, 1985.

288. Mazess RB: On aging bone loss. Clin Orthop 165:239–252, 1982.

289. McAfee PC, Ullrich CG, Yuan HA, et al: Computed tomography in degenerative spinal stenosis. Clin Orthop 161:221–234, 1981.

290. McAfee PC, Yuan HA, Fredrickson BE, et al: The value of computed tomography in thoracolumbar fractures: an analysis of one hundred consecutive cases and a new classification. J Bone Joint Surg 65A:461–473, 1983.

291. McAlister WH, Siegel MJ, Shackelford GD: A congenital iliac anomaly often associated with sacral lipoma and ipsilateral extremity weakness. Skeletal Radiol 3:161–166, 1978.

292. McAllister VL, Sage MR: The radiology of thoracic disc protrusion. Clin Radiol 27:291–299, 1976.

293. McBroom RJ, Hayes WC, Edwards WT, et al: Prediction of vertebral body compressive fracture

using quantitative computed tomography. J Bone Joint Surg 67A:1206–1214, 1985.

294. McClelland RR, Marsh DG: Double diastematomyelia. Radiology 123:378, 1977.

295. McCullough EC, Payne JT: Patient dosage in computed tomography. Radiology 129:457–463, 1978.

296. McLeod RA, Dahlin DC, Beabout JW: The spectrum of osteoblastoma. AJR 126:321–335, 1976.

297. McLone DG, Mutluer S, Naidich TP: Lipomeningoceles of the conus medullaris. In Raimondi AJ (ed): Concepts in Pediatric Neurosurgery. Basel: S. Karger, 1983, pp 170–177.

298. McLone DG, Naidich TP: Laser resection of fifty spinal lipomas. Neurosurgery 18:611–615, 1986.

299. McRae DL: The significance of abnormalities of the cervical spine. AJR 84:3–25, 1960.

300. Meijenhorst GCH: Computed tomography of the lumbar epidural veins Radiology 145:687–691, 1982.

301. Menezes AH, VanGilder JC, Clark CR, et al: Odontoid upward migration in rheumatoid arthritis: an analysis of 45 patients with "cranial settling." J Neurosurg 63:500–509, 1985.

302. Mercader J, Muñoz Gomez J, Cardenal C: Intraspinal synovial cyst: diagnosis by CT: follow-up and spontaneous remission. Neuroradiology 27:346–348, 1985.

303. Meyer JD, Latchaw RE, Roppolo HM, et al: Computed tomography and myelography of the postoperative lumbar spine. AJNR 3:223–228, 1982.

304. Meyer JE, Lepke RA, Lindfors KK, et al: Chordomas: their CT appearance in the cervical, thoracic and lumbar spine. Radiology 153:693–696, 1984.

305. Mikhael MA, Ciric I, Tarkington JA, et al: Neuroradiological evaluation of lateral recess syndrome. Radiology 140:97–107, 1981.

306. Miles J, Pennybacker J, Sheldon P: Intrathoracic meningocele: its development and association with neurofibromatosis. J Neurol Neurosurg Psychiatry 32:99–110, 1969.

307. Miller JDR, Grace MGA, Lampard R: Computed tomography of the upper cervical spine in Down syndrome. J Comput Assist Tomogr 10:589–592, 1986.

308. Miller MD, Gehweiler JA, Martinez S, et al: Significant new observations on cervical spine trauma. AJR 130:659–663, 1978.

309. Miyasaka K, Kaneda K, Sato S, et al: Myelopathy due to ossification or calcification of the ligamentum flavum: radiologic and histologic evaluations. AJNR 4:629–632, 1983.

310. Mohan V, Gupta SK, Tuli SM, et al: Symptomatic vertebral hemangiomas. Clin Radiol 31:575–579, 1980.

311. Mooney V, Robertson J: The facet syndrome. Clin Orthop 115:149–156, 1976.

312. Morgan DF, Young RF: Spinal neurological complications of achondroplasia: results of surgical treatment. J Neurosurg 52:463–472, 1980.

313. Morgan GJ Jr, Schlegelmilch JG, Spiegel PK: Early diagnosis of septic arthritis of the sacroiliac joint by use of computed tomography. J Rheumatol 8:979–982, 1981.

314. Mørk SJ, Løken AC: Ependymoma: a follow-up study of 101 cases. Cancer 40:907–915, 1977.

315. Morris RE, Hasso AN, Thompson JR, et al: Traumatic dural tears: CT diagnosis using metrizamide. Radiology 152:443–446, 1984.

316. Muindi J, Coombes RC, Golding S, et al: The role of computed tomography in the detection of bone metastases in breast cancer patients. Br J Radiol 56:233–236, 1983.

317. Murakami J, Russell WJ, Hayabuchi N, et al: Computed tomography of posterior longitudinal ligament ossification: its appearance and diagnostic value with special reference to thoracic lesions. J Comput Assist Tomogr 6:41–50, 1982.

318. Murray RO, Jacobson HG: The Radiology of Skeletal Disorders: Exercises in Diagnosis. Edinburgh: Churchill Livingstone, 1977.

319. Nagahiro S, Matsukado Y, Kuratsu J, et al: Syringomyelia and syringobulbia associated with an ependymoma of the cauda equina involving the conus medullaris: case report. Neurosurgery 18:357–360, 1986.

320. Naidich TP, Harwood-Nash DC: Diastematomyelia: hemicord and meningeal sheaths; single and double arachnoid and dural tubes. AJNR 4:633–636, 1983.

321. Naidich TP, McLone DG, Fulling KH: The Chiari II malformation: part IV: the hindbrain deformity. Neuroradiology 25:179–197, 1983.

322. Naidich TP, McLone DG, Harwood-Nash DC: Arachnoid cysts, paravertebral meningoceles, and perineural cysts. In Newton TH, Potts DG (eds): Computed Tomography of the Spine and Spinal Cord. San Anselmo, California: Clavadel Press, 1983, pp 383–396.

323. Naidich TP, McLone DG, Harwood-Nash DC: Malformations of the craniocervical junction. In Newton TH, Potts DG (eds): Computed Tomography of the Spine and Spinal Cord. San Anselmo, California: Clavadel Press, 1983, pp 355–366.

324. Naidich TP, McLone DG, Harwood-Nash DC: Spinal dysraphism. In Newton TH, Potts DG (eds): Computed Tomography of the Spine and Spinal Cord. San Anselmo, California: Clavadel Press, 1983, pp 299–353.

325. Naidich TP, McLone DG, Harwood-Nash DC: Systemic malformations. In Newton TH, Potts DG (eds): Computed Tomography of the Spine and Spinal Cord. San Anselmo, California: Clavadel Press, 1983, pp 367–381.

326. Naidich TP, McLone DG, Mutluer S: A new understanding of dorsal dysraphism with lipoma (lipomyeloschisis): radiologic evaluation and surgical correction. AJR 140:1065–1078, 1983.

327. Naidich TP, Pudlowski RM, Naidich JB: Computed tomographic signs of Chiari II malformation. III: ventricles and cisterns. Radiology 134:657–663, 1980.

328. Nainkin L: Arachnoiditis ossificans: report of a case. Spine 3:83–86, 1978.

329. Nakagawa H, Huang YP, Malis LI, et al: Computed tomography of intraspinal and paraspinal neoplasms. J Comput Assist Tomogr 1:377–390, 1977.

330. Neave VCD, Wycoff RR: Computed tomography of cystic nerve root sleeve dilatation: case report. J Comput Assist Tomogr 7:881–885, 1983.

331. Nelson OA, Greer RB III: Localization of osteoid-osteoma of the spine using computerized tomography. J Bone Joint Surg 65A:263–264, 1983.

332. Newton-John HF, Morgan DB: The loss of bone with age, osteoporosis, and fractures. Clin Orthop 71:229–252, 1970.

333. Northfield DWC: The Surgery of the Central Nervous System. London: Blackwell Scientific Publications, 1973.

334. Novetsky GJ, Berlin L, Epstein AJ, et al: The extraforaminal herniated disk: detection by computed tomography. AJNR 3:653–655, 1982.
335. Novick GS, Pavlov H, Bullough PG: Osteochondroma of the cervical spine: report of two cases in preadolescent males. Skeletal Radiol 8:13–15, 1982.
336. O'Callaghan JP, Ullrich CG, Yuan HA, et al: CT of facet distraction in flexion injuries of the thoracolumbar spine: the naked facet. AJR 134:563–568, 1980.
337. Ogata M, Ishikawa K, Ohira T: Cervical myelopathy in pseudogout: case report. J Bone Joint Surg 66A:1301–1303, 1984.
338. Omojola MF, Cockshott WP, Beatty EG: Osteoid osteoma: an evaluation of diagnostic modalities. Clin Radiol 32:199–204, 1981.
339. O'Neill P, Whatmore WJ, Booth AE: Spinal meningoceles in association with neurofibromatosis. Neurosurgery 13:82–84, 1983.
340. Osborn RE, DeWitt JD: Giant cauda equina schwannoma: CT appearance. AJNR 6:835–836, 1985.
341. Osborne DR, Heinz ER, Bullard D, et al: Role of computed tomography in the radiological evaluation of painful radiculopathy after negative myelography: foraminal neural entrapment. Neurosurgery 14:147–153, 1984.
342. Paine KWE: Clinical features of lumbar spinal stenosis. Clin Orthop 115:77–82, 1976.
343. Pang D, Wilberger JE Jr: Tethered cord syndrome in adults. J Neurosurg 57:32–47, 1982.
344. Park WM, O'Neill M, McCall IW: The radiology of rheumatoid involvement of the cervical spine. Skeletal Radiol 4:1–7, 1979.
345. Patronas NJ, Jafar J, Brown F: Pseudomeningoceles diagnosed by metrizamide myelography and computerized tomography. Surg Neurol 16:188–191, 1981.
346. Pech P, Kilgore DP, Pojunas KW, et al: Cervical spinal fractures: CT detection. Radiology 157:117–120, 1985.
347. Penning L, Wilmink JT, van Woerden HH, et al: CT myelographic findings in degenerative disorders of the cervical spine: clinical significance. AJR 146:793–801, 1986.
348. Petras AF, Sobel DF, Mani JR, et al: CT myelography in cervical nerve root avulsion. J Comput Assist Tomogr 9:275–279, 1985.
349. Pettersson H, Harwood-Nash DCF: CT and Myelography of the Spine and Cord: Techniques, Anatomy and Pathology in Children. Berlin: Springer-Verlag, 1982.
350. Peyster RG, Teplick JG, Haskin ME: Computed tomography of lumbosacral conjoined nerve root anomalies: potential cause of false-positive reading for herniated nucleus pulposus. Spine 10:331–337, 1985.
351. Phillips TW, McGillicuddy JE, Hoff JT, et al: Adult Arnold-Chiari malformation and intrinsic brain stem neoplasm: a difficult differential diagnosis. Neurosurgery 13:345–350, 1983.
352. Plumley TF, Kilcoyne RF, Mack LA: Computed tomography in evaluation of gunshot wounds of the spine. J Comput Assist Tomogr 7:310–312, 1983.
353. Post MJD, Green BA: The use of computed tomography in spinal trauma. Radiol Clin North Am 21:327–375, 1983.
354. Post MJD, Green BA, Quencer RM, et al: The value of computed tomography in spinal trauma. Spine 7:417–431, 1982.
355. Post MJD, Seminer DS, Quencer RM: CT diagnosis of spinal epidural hematoma. AJNR 3:190–192, 1982.
356. Postacchini F, Pezzeri G, Montanaro A, et al: Computerized tomography in lumbar stenosis: a preliminary report. J Bone Joint Surg 62B:78–82, 1980.
357. Price AC, Allen JH, Eggers FM, et al: Intervertebral disk-space infection: CT changes. Radiology 149:725–729, 1983.
358. Pullicino P, Kendall BE: Computed tomography of "cystic" intramedullary lesions. Neuroradiology 23:117–121, 1982.
359. Quencer RM, Green BA, Eismont FJ: Posttraumatic spinal cord cysts: clinical features and characterization with metrizamide computed tomography. Radiology 146:415–423, 1983.
360. Quencer RM, Murtagh FR, Post MJD, et al: Postoperative bony stenosis of the lumbar spinal canal: evaluation of 164 symptomatic patients with axial radiography. AJR 131:1059–1064, 1978.
361. Quencer RM, Tenner M, Rothman L: The postoperative myelogram: radiographic evaluation of arachnoiditis and dural/arachnoidal tears. Radiology 123:667–679, 1977.
362. Quinn SF, Monson M, Paling M: Spinal lipoma presenting as a mediastinal mass: diagnosis by CT. J Comput Assist Tomogr 7:1087–1089, 1983.
363. Ramirez H Jr, Navarro JE, Bennett WF: "Cupid's bow" contour of the lumbar vertebral endplates detected by computed tomography. J Comput Assist Tomogr 8:121–124, 1984.
364. Ramsey RG, Penn RD: Computed tomography of a false postoperative meningocele. AJNR 5:326–328, 1984.
365. Raskin SP, Keating JW: Recognition of lumbar disk disease: comparison of myelography and computed tomography. AJR 139:349–355, 1982.
366. Rasmussen TB, Kernohan JW, Adson AW: Pathologic classification, with surgical consideration, of intraspinal tumors. Ann Surg 111:513–530, 1940.
367. Rawlings CE III, Saris SC, Muraki A, et al: Syringomyelia in a man with sarcoidosis. Neurosurgery 18:805–807, 1986.
368. Rawlings CE III, Wilkins RH, Gallis HA, et al: Postoperative intervertebral disc space infection. Neurosurgery 13:371–375, 1983.
369. Raymond J, Dumas J-M: Intraarticular facet block: diagnostic test or therapeutic procedure? Radiology 151:333–336, 1984.
370. Reddy SC, Vijayamohan G, Gao GR: Delayed CT myelography in spinal intramedullary metastasis: case report. J Comput Assist Tomogr 8:1182–1185, 1984.
371. Redmond J III, Spring DB, Munderloh SH, et al: Spinal computed tomography scanning in the evaluation of metastatic disease. Cancer 54:253–258, 1984.
372. Reinbold W-D, Genant HK, Reiser UJ, et al: Bone mineral content in early postmenopausal and postmenopausal osteoporotic women: comparison of measurement methods. Radiology 160:469–478, 1986.
373. Reinig JW, Hill SC, Fang M, et al: Fibrodysplasia ossificans progressiva: CT appearance. Radiology 159:153–157, 1986.

374. Resjö IM, Harwood-Nash DC, Fitz CR, et al: Computed tomographic metrizamide myelography in spinal dysraphism in infants and children. J Comput Assist Tomogr 2:549–558, 1978.

375. Resjö IM, Harwood-Nash DC, Fitz CR, et al: CT metrizamide myelography for intraspinal and paraspinal neoplasms in infants and children. AJR 132:367–372, 1979.

376. Resnick D, Greenway GD, Bardwick PA, et al: Plasma-cell dyscrasia with polyneuropathy, organomegaly, endocrinopathy, M-protein, and skin changes: the POEMS syndrome. Radiology 140:17–22, 1981.

377. Resnick D, Guerra J Jr, Robinson CA, et al: Association of diffuse idiopathic skeletal hyperostosis (DISH) and calcification and ossification of the posterior longitudinal ligament. AJR 131:1049–1053, 1978.

378. Resnick D, Niwayama G: Intravertebral disk herniations: cartilaginous (Schmorl's) nodes. Radiology 126:57–65, 1978.

379. Resnick D, Niwayama G: Diagnosis of Bone and Joint Disorders: With Emphasis on Articular Abnormalities, vol 2. Philadelphia: WB Saunders Company, 1981.

380. Resnick D, Pineda C: Vertebral involvement in calcium pyrophosphate dihydrate crystal deposition disease: radiographic-pathological correlation. Radiology 153:55–60, 1984.

381. Rhoton AL Jr: Microsurgery of Arnold-Chiari malformation in adults with and without hydromyelia. J Neurosurg 45:473–483, 1976.

382. Riggs BL, Melton LJ III: Involutional osteoporosis. N Engl J Med 314:1676–1686, 1986.

383. Rinaldi I, Kopp JE, Harris WO Jr, et al: Computer assisted tomography in syringomyelia. J Comput Assist Tomogr 2:633–635, 1978.

384. Risius B, Modic MT, Hardy RW Jr, et al: Sector computed tomographic spine scanning in the diagnosis of lumbar nerve root entrapment. Radiology 143:109–114, 1982.

385. Rogers LF: Radiology of Skeletal Trauma. New York: Churchill Livingstone, 1982.

386. Roosen N, DeMoor J: Cervicobrachialgia with congenital vertebral anomalies and diastematomyelia. Surg Neurol 21:493–496, 1984.

387. Rosenberg D, Baskies AM, Deckers PJ, et al: Pyogenic sacroiliitis: an absolute indication for computerized tomographic scanning. Clin Orthop 184:128–132, 1984.

388. Rosenbloom S, Cohen WA, Marshall C, et al: Imaging factors influencing spine and cord measurements by CT: a phantom study. AJNR 4:646–649, 1983.

389. Rosenkranz W: Ankylosing spondylitis: cauda equina syndrome with multiple spinal arachnoid cysts. J Neurosurg 34:241–243, 1971.

390. Rossier AB, Foo D, Naheedy MH, et al: Radiography of posttraumatic syringomyelia. AJNR 4:637–640, 1983.

391. Rothman SLG, Glenn WV Jr: CT multiplanar reconstruction in 253 cases of lumbar spondylolysis. AJNR 5:81–90, 1984.

392. Rothman SLG, Glenn WV Jr: Spondylolysis and spondylolisthesis. In Post MJG (ed): Computed Tomography of the Spine. Baltimore: Williams & Wilkins, 1984, pp 591–615.

393. Rothman SLG, Glenn WV Jr: CT evaluation of interbody fusion. Clin Orthop 193:47–56, 1985.

394. Russell DS, Rubinstein LJ: Pathology of Tumours of the Nervous System, 4th ed. Baltimore: Williams & Wilkins, 1977.

395. Russell EJ, D'Angelo CM, Zimmerman RD, et al: Cervical disk herniation: CT demonstration after contrast enhancement. Radiology 152:703–712, 1984.

396. Russell ML, Gordon DA, Ogryzlo MA, et al: The cauda equina syndrome of ankylosing spondylitis. Ann Intern Med 78:551–554, 1973.

397. Russell NA, Belanger G, Benoit BG, et al: Spinal epidural lipomatosis: a complication of glucocorticoid therapy. Can J Neurol Sci 11:383–386, 1984.

398. Ryan LM, Carrera GF, Lightfoot RW Jr, et al: The radiographic diagnosis of sacroiliitis: a comparison of different views with computed tomograms of the sacroiliac joint. Arthritis Rheum 26:760–763, 1983.

399. Sage MR, Gordon TP: Muscle atrophy in ankylosing spondylitis: CT demonstration. Radiology 149:780, 1983.

400. Sartoris DJ, Pate D, Haghighi P, et al: Plasma cell sclerosis of bone: a spectrum of disease. J Can Assoc Radiol 37:25–34, 1986.

401. Sartoris DJ, Resnick D, Guerra J Jr: Vertebral venous channels: CT appearance and differential considerations. Radiology 155:745–749, 1985.

402. Sarwar M, Virapongse C, Bhimani S: Primary tethered cord syndrome: a new hypothesis of its origin. AJNR 5:235–242, 1984.

403. Scher AT: Unilateral locked facet in cervical spine injuries. AJR 129:45–48, 1977.

404. Schimel S, Deeb ZL: Herniated thoracic intervertebral disks. J Comput Tomogr 9:141–143, 1985.

405. Schmidek HH, Smith DA, Kristiansen TK: Sacral fractures. Neurosurgery 15:735–746, 1984.

406. Schmorl G, Junghanns H: The Human Spine in Health and Disease, 2nd ed. New York: Grune & Stratton, 1971.

407. Schnyder P, Frankhauser H, Mansouri B: Computed tomography of spinal hemangioma with cord compression: report of two cases. Skeletal Radiol 15:372–375, 1986.

408. Schreiman JS, McLeod RA, Kyle RA, et al: Multiple myeloma: evaluation by CT. Radiology 154:483–486, 1985.

409. Schroeder S, Lackner K, Weiand G: Lumbosacral intradural lipoma. J Comput Assist Tomogr 5:274, 1981.

410. Schubiger O, Valavanis A: CT differentiation between recurrent disc herniation and postoperative scar formation: the value of contrast enhancement. Neuroradiology 22:251–254, 1982.

411. Schubiger O, Valavanis A: Postoperative lumbar CT: technique, results and indications. AJNR 4:595–597, 1983.

412. Schubiger O, Valavanis A, Hollmann J: Computed tomography of the intervertebral foramen. Neuroradiology 26:439–444, 1984.

413. Schulz EE, West WL, Hinshaw DB et al: Gas in a lumbar extradural juxtaarticular cyst: sign of synovial origin. AJR 143:875–876, 1984.

414. Schut L, Bruce DC, Sutton LN: The management of the child with a lipomyelomeningocele. Clin Neurosurg 30:464–476, 1983.

415. Schwarz SS, Fisher WS III, Pulliam MW, et al: Thoracic chordoma in a patient with paraparesis and ivory vertebral body. Neurosurgery 16:100–102, 1985.

416. Scotti G, Musgrave MA, Harwood-Nash DC, et al.: Diastematomyelia in children: metrizamide and CT metrizamide myelography. AJR 135:1225–1232, 1980.
417. Scotti G, Scialfa G, Pieralli S, et al: Myelopathy and radiculopathy due to cervical spondylosis: myelographic-CT correlations. AJNR 4:601–603, 1983.
418. Sefczek RJ, Deeb ZL: Case report: computed tomography findings in spinal arachnoiditis ossificans. J Comput Tomogr 7:315–318, 1983.
419. Seibert CE, Dreisbach JN, Swanson WB, et al: Progressive posttraumatic cystic myelopathy: neuroradiologic evaluation. AJNR 2:115–119, 1981.
420. Shapiro R: Myelography, 4th ed. Chicago: Year Book Medical Publishers, 1984.
421. Shaw MDM, Russell JA, Grossart KW: The changing pattern of spinal arachnoiditis. J Neurol Neurosurg Psychiatry 41:97–107, 1978.
422. Shealy CN: Facet denervation in the management of back and sciatic pain. Clin Orthop 115:157–164, 1976.
423. Shives TC, Dahlin DC, Sim FH, et al: Osteosarcoma of the spine. J Bone Joint Surg 68A:660–668, 1986.
424. Simmons JD, Newton TH: Arachnoiditis. In Newton TH, Potts DG (eds): Computed Tomography of the Spine and Spinal Cord. San Anselmo, California: Clavadel Press, 1983, pp 223–229.
425. Simmons JD, Norman D, Newton TH: Preoperative demonstration of post-inflammatory syringomyelia. AJNR 4:625–628, 1983.
426. Siqueira EB, Schaffer L, Kranzler LI, et al: CT characteristics of sacral perineural cysts: report of two cases. J Neurosurg 61:596–598, 1984.
427. Sloof JL, Kernohan JW, MacCarty CS: Primary intramedullary tumors of the spinal cord and filum terminale. Philadelphia: WB Saunders Company, 1964.
428. Smith J, Wixon D, Watson RC: Giant-cell tumor of the sacrum. J Can Assoc Radiol 30:34–39, 1979.
429. Smith WS, Kaufer H: Patterns and mechanisms of lumbar injuries associated with lap seat belts. J Bone Joint Surg 51A:239–254, 1969.
430. Solomon A, Rahamani R, Seligsohn U, et al: Multiple myeloma: early vertebral involvement asessed by computerized tomography. Skeletal Radiol 11:258–261, 1984.
431. Sorin S, Askari A, Moskowitz RW: Atlantoaxial subluxation as a complication of early ankylosing spondylitis: two case reports and a review of the literature. Arthritis Rheum 22:273–276, 1979.
432. Sostrin RD, Thompson JR, Rouhe SA, et al: Occult spinal dysraphism in the geriatric patient. Radiology 125:165–169, 1977.
433. Spencer RR, Jahnke RW, Hardy TL: Dissection of gas into an intraspinal synovial cyst from contiguous vacuum facet. J Comput Assist Tomogr 7:886–888, 1983.
434. Steppé R, Bellemans M, Boven F, et al: The value of computed tomography scanning in elusive fractures of the cervical spine. Skeletal Radiol 6:175–178, 1981.
435. Stevens JM, Olney JS, Kendall BE: Post-traumatic cystic and non-cystic myelopathy. Neuroradiology 27:48–56, 1985.
436. Strother CM: Lumbar examination. In Sackett JF, Strother CM (eds): New Techniques in Myelography. Philadelphia: Harper & Row Publishers, 1979, pp 69–89.
437. Sundaresan N, Galicich JH, Chu FCH, et al: Spinal chordomas. J Neurosurg 50:312–319, 1979.
438. Sundaresan N, Huvos AG, Krol G, et al: Postradiation sarcoma involving the spine. Neurosurgery 18:721–724, 1986.
439. Suss RA, Udvarhelyi GB, Wang H, et al: Myelography in achondroplasia: value of a lateral C1–2 puncture and non-ionic, water-soluble contrast medium. Radiology 149:159–163, 1983.
440. Tadmor R, Cacayorin ED, Kieffer SA: Advantages of supplementary CT in myelography of intraspinal masses. AJNR 4:618–621, 1983.
441. Tarlov IM: Spinal perineurial and meningeal cysts. J Neurol Neurosurg Psychiatry 33:833–843, 1970.
442. Tchang SPK, Howie JL, Kirkaldy-Willis WH, et al: Computed tomography versus myelography in diagnosis of lumbar disc herniation. J Can Assoc Radiol 33:15–20, 1982.
443. Teplick JG, Haskin ME: Computed tomography of the postoperative lumbar spine. AJR 141:865–884, 1983.
444. Teplick JG, Haskin ME: CT and lumbar disc herniation. Radiol Clin North Am 21:259–288, 1983.
445. Teplick JG, Haskin ME: CT of the postoperative lumbar spine. Radiol Clin North Am 21:395–420, 1983.
446. Teplick JG, Haskin ME: Intravenous contrast-enhanced CT of the postoperative lumbar spine: improved identification of recurrent disk herniation, scar, arachnoiditis, and diskitis. AJR 143:845–855, 1984.
447. Teplick JG, Laffey PA, Berman A, et al: Diagnosis and evaluation of spondylolisthesis and/or spondylolysis on axial CT. AJNR 7:479–491, 1986.
448. Teplick JG, Peyster RG, Teplick SK, et al: CT identification of postlaminectomy pseudomeningocele. AJR 140:1203–1206, 1983.
449. Thomas JE, Miller RH: Lipomatous tumors of the spinal canal. Mayo Clin Proc 48:393–400, 1973.
450. Tillman BP, Dahlin DC, Lipscomb PR, et al: Aneurysmal bone cyst: an analysis of ninety-five cases. Mayo Clin Proc 43:478–495, 1968.
451. Tomsick TA, Lebowitz ME, Campbell C: The congenital absence of pedicles in the thoracic spine: report of two cases. Radiology 111:587–589, 1974.
452. Toolanen G, Garsson S-E, Fagerlund M: Medullary compression in rheumatoid atlanto-axial subluxation evaluated by computerized tomography. Spine 11:191–194, 1986.
453. Tsuyama N: Ossification of the posterior longitudinal ligament of the spine. Clin Orthop 184:71–84, 1984.
454. van Ameyden van Duym FC, van Wiechen PJ: Herniation of calcified nucleus pulposus in the thoracic spine: case report. J Comput Assist Tomogr 7:1122–1123, 1983.
455. Van Schaik JPJ, Verbiest H, Van Schaik FDJ: The orientation of the laminae and facet joints in the lower lumbar spine. Spine 10:59–63, 1985.
456. Vanel D, Contesso G, Couanet D, et al: Computed tomography in the evaluation of 41 cases of Ewing's sarcoma. Skeletal Radiol 9:8–13, 1982.
457. Verbiest H: The significance and principles of computerized axial tomography in idiopathic developmental stenosis of the bony lumbar vertebral canal. Spine 4:369–378, 1979.
458. Vogler JB III, Brown WH, Helms CA, et al: The normal sacroiliac joint: a CT study of asymptomatic patients. Radiology 151:433–437, 1984.

459. Volikas Z, Singounas E, Saridakes G, et al: Aneurysmal bone cyst of the spine: report of a case. Acta Radiol [Diagn] 23:643–646, 1982.
460. Wang A-M, Joachim CL, Shillito J Jr, et al: Cervical chordoma presenting with intervertebral foramen enlargement mimicking neurofibroma: CT findings. J Comput Assist Tomogr 8:529–532, 1984.
461. Wang A-M, Jolesz F, Rumbaugh CL, et al: CT assessment of thoracic extension and of concomitant lesions in syringohydromyelia. J Comput Assist Tomogr 7:18–24, 1983.
462. Wang A-M, Lipson SJ, Haykal HA, et al: Computed tomography of aneurysmal bone cyst of the L1 vertebral body: case report. J Comput Assist Tomogr 8:1186–1189, 1984.
463. Weatherly CR, Jaffray D, O'Brien JP: Radical excision of an osteoblastoma of the cervical spine. J Bone Joint Surg 68B:325–328, 1986.
464. Weaver EN Jr, England GD, Richardson DE: Sacral fracture: case presentation and review. Neurosurgery 9:725–728, 1981.
465. Weaver P, Lifeso RM: The radiological diagnosis of tuberculosis of the adult spine. Skeletal Radiol 12:178–186, 1984.
466. Wedge JH, Tchang S, MacFadyen DJ: Computed tomography in localization of spinal osteoid osteoma. Spine 6:423–427, 1981.
467. Weinreb JC, Arger PH, Grossman R, et al: CT metrizamide myelography in multiple bilateral intrathoracic meningoceles. J Comput Assist Tomogr 8:324–326, 1984.
468. Weinstein MA, Rothner AD, Duchesneau P, et al: Computed tomography in diastematomyelia. Radiology 118:609–611, 1975.
469. Weinstein PR, Karpman RR, Gall EP, et al: Spinal cord injury, spinal fracture and spinal stenosis in ankylosing spondylitis. J Neurosurg 57:609–616, 1982.
470. Weiss T, Treisch J, Kazner E, et al: CT of the postoperative lumbar spine: the value of intravenous contrast. Neuroradiology 28:241–245, 1986.
471. Weissman BNW, Aliabadi P, Weinfeld MS, et al: Prognostic features of atlantoaxial subluxation in rheumatoid arthritis patients. Radiology 144:745–751, 1982.
472. Weisz GM: Lumbar spinal canal stenosis in Paget's disease. Spine 8:192–198, 1983.
473. Weisz GM: The value of CT in diagnosing postoperative lumbar conditions. Spine 11:164–166, 1986.
474. Whelan MA, Naidich DP, Post JD, et al: Computed tomography of spinal tuberculosis. J Comput Assist Tomogr 7:25–30, 1983.
475. Whelan MA, Schonfeld S, Post JD, et al: Computed tomography of nontuberculous spinal infection. J Comput Assist Tomogr 9:280–287, 1985.
476 White JG, Strait TA, Binkley JR, et al: Surgical treatment of 63 cases of conjoined nerve roots. J Neurosurg 56:114–117, 1982.
477. Whitehouse GH, Griffiths GJ: Roentgenologic aspects of spinal involvement by primary and metastatic Ewing's tumor. J Can Assoc Radiol 27:290–297, 1976.
478. Williams AL: CT diagnosis of degenerative disc disease: the bulging annulus. Radiol Clin North Am 21:289–300, 1983.
479. Williams AL, Haughton VM, Daniels DL, et al: CT recognition of lateral lumbar disc herniation. AJR 139:345–347, 1982.
480. Williams AL, Haughton VM, Daniels DL, et al: Differential CT diagnosis of extruded nucleus pulposus. Radiology 148:141–148, 1983.
481. Williams AL, Haughton VM, Meyer GA, et al: Computed tomographic appearance of the bulging annulus. Radiology 142:403–408, 1982.
482. Williams AL, Haughton VM, Syvertsen A: Computed tomography in the diagnosis of herniated nucleus pulposus. Radiology 135:95–99, 1980.
483. Willinsky RA, Fazl M: Computed tomography of a sacral perineural cyst: case report. J Comput Assist Tomogr 9:599–601, 1985.
484. Wiltse LL, Kirkaldy-Willis WH, McIvor GWD: The treatment of spinal stenosis. Clin Orthop 115:83–91, 1976.
485. Wollin DG: The os odontoideum. J Bone Joint Surg 45A:1459–1471, 1484, 1963.
486. Wolpert SM, Scott RM, Carter BL: Computed tomography in spinal dysraphism. Surg Neurol 8:199–206, 1977.
487. Wood BP, Harwood-Nash DC, Berger P, et al: Intradural spinal lipoma of the cervical cord. AJNR 6:452–454, 1985.
488. Yagen R: CT diagnosis of limbus vertebra: case report. J Comput Assist Tomogr 8:149–151, 1984.
489. Yeates AE: Computed tomographic evaluation of cervical pain syndromes. In Genant HK (ed): Spine Update 1984: Perspective in Radiology, Orthopaedic Surgery, and Neurosurgery. San Francisco Radiology Research and Education Foundation, 1983, pp 291–307.
490. Yeates AE, Newton TH: Applications of metrizamide in computed tomographic examination of the lumbar spine. In Genant HK, Chafetz N, Helms CA (eds): Computed Tomography of the Lumbar Spine. San Francisco: University of California, 1982, pp 67–86.
491. Yetkin Z, Osborn AG, Giles DS, et al: Uncovertebral and facet joint dislocations in cervical articular pillar fractures: CT evaluation. AJNR 6:633–637, 1985.
492. Yong-Hing K, Reilly J, deKorompay V, et al: Prevention of nerve root adhesions after laminectomy. Spine 5:59–64, 1980.
493. Yousefzadeh DK, El-Khoury GY, Lupetin AR: Congenital aplastic hypoplastic lumbar pedicle in infants and young children. Skeletal Radiol 7:259–265, 1982.
494. Yu R, Brunner DR, Rao KCVG: Role of computed tomography in symptomatic vertebral hemangiomas. J Comput Tomogr 8:311–315, 1984.
495. Yu YL, Stevens JM, Kendall B, et al: Cord shape and measurements in cervical spondylotic myelopathy and radiculopathy. AJNR 4:839–842, 1983.
496. Zilkha A, Irwin GAL, Fagelman D: Computed tomography of spinal epidural hematoma. AJNR 4:1073–1076, 1983.
497. Zlatkin MB, Lander PH, Hadjipavlou AG, et al: Paget's disease in the spine: CT with clinical correlation. Radiology 160:155–159, 1986.

Deborah Pate, D.C.
Donald Resnick, M.D.
Michael André, Ph.D.
David J. Sartoris, M.D.

8

Three-Dimensional Computed Tomography

Computed tomography (CT), which has been successfully applied to the diagnosis and management of spinal lesions, has traditionally been displayed in two dimensions consisting of a dozen or more cross-sectional images. Even now, with the advent and common use of standard reformations of CT data, the images remain two-dimensional. The third dimension is provided through mental integration by the observer, a task that requires considerable experience and expertise. With the advent of sophisticated computer processing, multiplanar reformation (MPR) and three-dimensional (3D) display of cross-sectional imaging data are now available. In the evaluation of 101 spinal cases consisting of neoplasms, trauma, infections, degenerative disease, arthritides, and congenital disorders in which 3D CT displays were utilized, we have found this technique most useful for evaluating osseous, as opposed to soft-tissue, lesions. In special cases, such as complex fractures and regions with marked degenerative changes, plastic models of the region of interest can be generated using a computer-interfaced milling machine.

METHOD

Several computer programs and dedicated instruments for 3D display of CT scans have been developed. Some operate on the CT scanner itself, and others require specialized computer equipment.[4, 14, 18] The 3D images illustrated in this chapter are generated by the Cemax 1000 (Cemax Medical Products, Inc., Mountain View, California), consisting of a high-resolution 1024 × 1250 display system and menu-driven software. Although the Cemax 1000 can analyze the CT data derived from numerous types of scanners, we have primarily used image data obtained with a Technicare 2060 or a General Electric scanner.

A protocol consisting of thin contiguous or overlapping CT slices and minimal patient motion is generally utilized for obtaining the CT image data. These data are acquired with either 2 mm slice thickness and 2 mm table incrementation or with 5 mm slice thickness and 3 mm table incrementation. The image data are then transferred to the computer system by 9-track magnetic tapes. Each voxel is deconvolved into a symmetric cube by a linear interpolation scheme and 3D filter appropriate for the specific type of image and tissue to be studied. The resampling of the voxel provides a uniform spatial interval in all three dimensions. The surface of the desired structure, generally the outer edge of a skeletal bone, is defined by locating the voxel with a CT number value equal to the half-maximum point of the edge gradient. The surface contour is computed for each interpolated slice, stacked according to the separation between interpolated slices, and stored as a contour file.[2, 5, 6, 16, 17]

The interpolation process greatly facilitates the construction of high-quality two-dimensional reformations in arbitrary

468

planes. Pseudo-3D images are generated from the contour files in any desired projection view, using a variety of graphic display options. Images can be rotated in space at near real-time rates to allow viewing of the structure from any angle. The removal of overlying soft tissues or bone can be accomplished by editing the contour files. Subsets of the entire stack of slices can be used to view internal structures as well. Finally, in selected cases, the data can be interfaced with a computer-controlled numerical milling machine to produce solid polyethylene models of the diseased area.[3, 9, 13]

CLINICAL APPLICATIONS

This technique is well suited to the identification of osseous abnormalities accompanying degenerative disease, trauma, infection, and neoplasm as well as those seen in the postoperative lumbar spine.[15, 19] It is of less or no benefit in the investigation of soft-tissue alterations, including disc displacement and hypertrophy of the ligamenta flava.

Trauma

Regarding complex vertebral fractures, 3D CT allows precise delineation of the site and size of osseous fragments within the spinal canal and the extent of disruption of the posterior osseous elements (Fig. 8–1). These latter structures can be removed by appropriate editing of the data, providing an unobstructed view of the posterior portions of the vertebral bodies and intervertebral discs. This can be extremely helpful in surgical planning and analysis (Fig. 8–2).

Neoplasm and Infection

The evaluation of osseous destruction is very well demonstrated with 3D CT (Fig. 8–3). Although not beneficial in the early de-

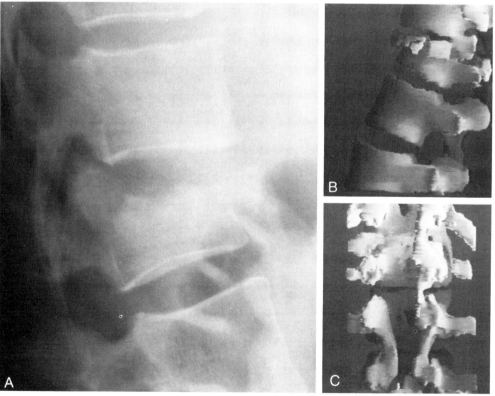

Figure 8–1. Complex fracture of the first lumbar vertebra. *A,* A lateral radiograph reveals a burst-type fracture of the vertebral body with significant involvement of both the anterior and posterior osseous elements. Two 3D CT image displays show the fractured vertebra, in the lateral projection (*B*) and in the posterior projection (*C*), after the laminae and spinous process have been removed by editing the contour files.

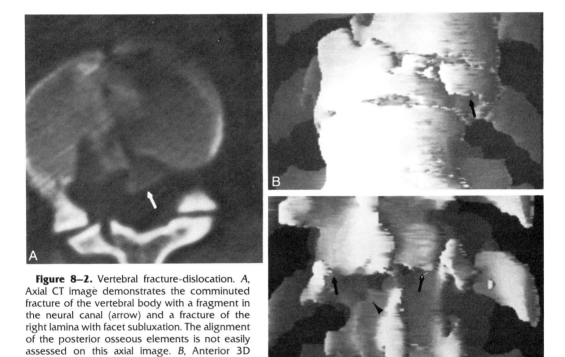

Figure 8–2. Vertebral fracture-dislocation. *A,* Axial CT image demonstrates the comminuted fracture of the vertebral body with a fragment in the neural canal (arrow) and a fracture of the right lamina with facet subluxation. The alignment of the posterior osseous elements is not easily assessed on this axial image. *B,* Anterior 3D surface contour image demonstrates spinal mal-alignment and asymmetric compression of the T12 vertebral body with a large anterolateral fracture fragment (arrow). *C,* Posterior 3D view illustrates offset of spinous processes with facet joint subluxation (arrows) and an oblique fracture of the T12 lamina (arrowhead).

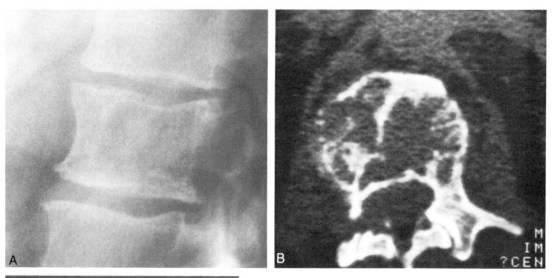

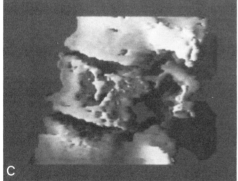

Figure 8–3. Plasmacytoma. *A,* The lateral radiograph reveals osteolysis of a lumbar vertebral body with involvement of the pedicle. *B,* Axial CT image shows marked destruction of the vertebral body. *C,* A lateral 3D CT image display shows the degree of pedicular and laminar involvement.

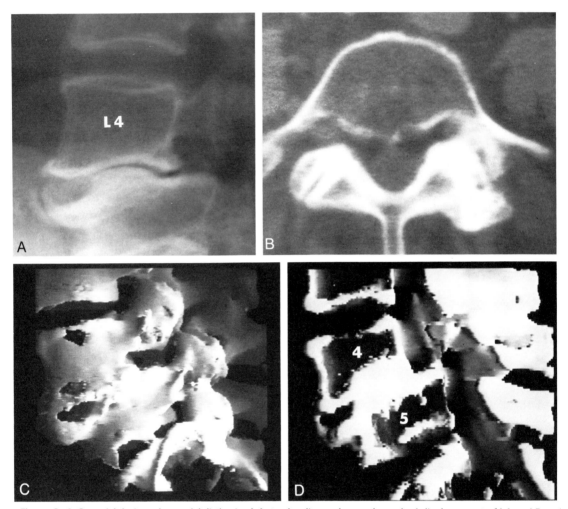

Figure 8–4. Spondylolysis and spondylolisthesis. *A*, Lateral radiograph reveals marked displacement of L4 on L5 and osteophytic formation. *B*, Axial CT demonstrates degenerative changes consisting of joint space narrowing, subchondral sclerosis, and osteophytosis of the apophyseal joints. *C*, A lateral 3D CT image demonstrates the anterolisthesis of L4 on L5. *D*, A 3D CT sagittal section reveals the anterolisthesis and deformity of the central canal caused by the slippage of L4 on L5.

tection of neoplastic processes, this technique is useful in assessing the amount of collapse of a vertebral segment. Similarly, the technique does not allow early detection of an infective process; however, 3D CT can be useful in evaluation of the degree of osseous destruction, which may be difficult to identify on multiple axial CT images.

Degenerative Disorders

Spondylosis deformans and osteoarthritis of the apophyseal joints are the two degenerative processes that are best evaluated with 3D CT. Although both of these processes produce characteristic abnormalities on routine radiographs and axial CT scans, pronounced distortion of the spine related to extensive degenerative changes or accompanying spondylolisthesis, kyphosis, or scoliosis makes interpretation of conventional radiographs and CT scans more difficult in some cases. 3D CT can overcome this difficulty, especially if both surface and sectional image displays are used (Fig. 8–4). The osseous contributions to spinal stenosis, including bone overgrowth and osteophytosis, are readily indentifiable with the 3D technique.

Postoperative Fusion

In the evaluation of posterior and anterior fusions of the spine, 3D CT is able to identify small areas of nonunion when the results of axial and reformatted CT imaging are equivocal (Fig. 8–5).

Spinal Stenosis

The important clinical consequences of spinal stenosis have resulted in increasing interest regarding accurate assessment of the configuration of the spinal canal. Routine radiography and conventional tomography are generally considered to be inadequate or unreliable for this assessment. Although myelography may reveal abnormal impression on the contrast-filled spinal canal or partial or complete obstruction to the flow of the contrast agent, the axial display of computed tomography is considered closer to ideal in defining the extent of spinal

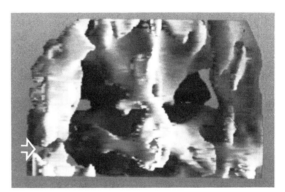

Figure 8–5. Pseudarthrosis following lumbar laminectomy and bone grafting. A posterior 3D surface contour image demonstrates failure of osseous fusion in the lateral onlay bone graft material (arrow).

stenosis and its localization in the central canal, lateral recesses, neural foramina, or combinations of the three. As an extension of this analysis, plastic models of stenotic canals can be constructed directly from computed tomography data.[11] The soft tissues, such as the intervertebral discs and ligamenta flava, that contribute to spinal stenosis are neglected in the creation of such polyethylene models; however, the models allow precise documentation of the dimensions of the spinal canal. This information is more difficult to derive from standard CT (Fig. 8–6). These models also afford the orthopedic surgeon or neurosurgeon a unique three-dimensional look at the narrowed spinal canal and the chance to perform "rehearsal surgery" on those patients who require operative intervention (Fig. 8–7).

FUTURE APPLICATIONS

Quantitative assessment of trabecular bone can be accomplished with three-dimensional histogram analysis. In this technique, the patient is scanned on a calibration phantom containing known concentrations of the mineral equivalent material dipotassium hydrogen phosphate (K_2HPO_4). The CT data are then transferred to the Cemax 1000 system, and the integral trabecular bone volume is obtained by defining the inner cortical contour for each slice using a low-pixel threshold value (approximately 200 Houndsfield units). A histogram plot of pixel values within the volume of interest is generated

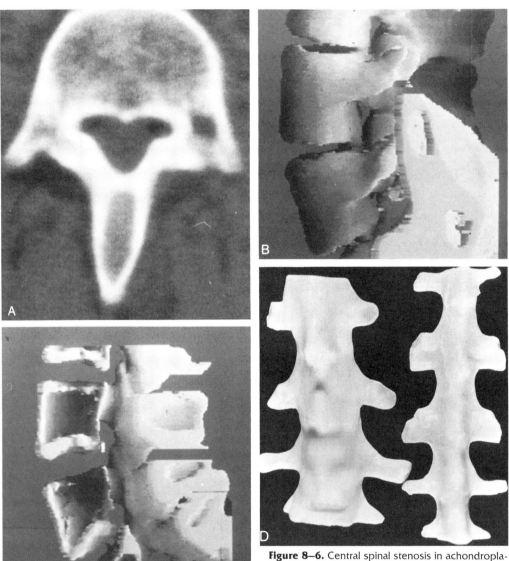

Figure 8–6. Central spinal stenosis in achondroplasia. *A*, An axial CT scan at the level of L4 shows shortening of the pedicles and stenosis of the central spinal canal. A 3D CT image (*B*) of the surface of the lumbar spine and a sagittal section (*C*) of the spine show tall vertebral bodies, narrow intervertebral discs, short pedicles, and central spinal stenosis. *D*, Normal and abnormal spinal canal: plastic models. The normal situation is illustrated on the left, in which the plastic model is viewed from a posterior interosseous position. Note the ample interosseous space in the central canal and within the neural foramina. Spinal stenosis in achondroplasia is illustrated on the right. Central spinal stenosis is more prominent than foraminal stenosis.

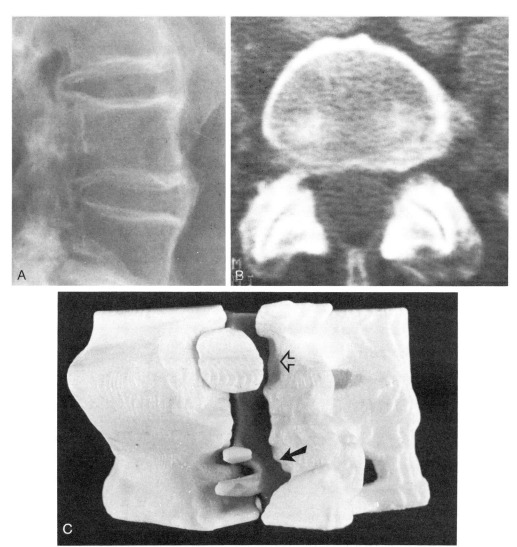

Figure 8–7. Neural foraminal stenosis in a patient with diffuse idiopathic skeletal hyperostosis (DISH). *A*, A lateral radiograph demonstrates classic radiographic features of DISH: flowing ossification of ligaments and relative maintenance of intervertebral disc height. *B*, Axial CT image at the L4–L5 level shows bilateral stenosis of the neural foramina related to osteoarthritis of the apophyseal joints. *C*, A photograph of the left lateral aspect of a plastic model of the spine (the anterior and posterior structures have been separated) and a model of the interosseous spinal canal reveal the features of DISH, including bone ankylosis between vertebral bodies and spinous processes and splitting of the interosseous space within the narrowed left neural foramen (closed arrow). Compare with the normal sized neural foramen above (open arrow).

along with mean, standard deviation, median, and mode. The CT values for cancellous bone are converted to mineral equivalent (mg per ml of K_2HPO_4) by the calibration curve generated from the phantom measurements. Using the same software, this histogram method can be applied to analysis of cortical and cancellous bone either separately or together.[12] Cancellous measurements are most useful in the evaluation of subtle changes in mineral status, whereas cortical and total bone mineral determinations may be more reliable in predicting osseous strength and potential risk of fracture.[7, 8] This technique has been applied to date with regard to the femoral head and neck; however, it is currently being investigated for application in the spine and other sites of orthopedic intervention. Three-dimensional histogram analysis of CT data may be the technique of choice for the assessment of osseous integrity, providing a noninvasive method for estimating bone strength.

ADVANTAGES AND DISADVANTAGES OF 3D TECHNIQUE

Three dimensional CT is best used as an adjunct to other imaging techniques. This method does not provide new data but rather presents standard data in a different manner. The resulting image displays are easier for many clinical colleagues to comprehend and are particularly useful in the preoperative evaluation of a number of disorders. When the images are rotated and viewed from different perspectives, a graphic representation of the morphology of the disease process results. Furthermore, appropriate editing accomplished on the monitor can eliminate overlying or adjacent structures that might otherwise interfere with this representation.[10] The interfacing of the image data with a computerized, numerically controlled milling device further enhances the value of 3D CT by allowing the creation of reasonably accurate polyethylene models of the osseous structures and intraosseous canal. These models can be of aid in the planning of a specific surgical procedure.

As with any new technique, the ultimate value of 3D CT must be determined by comparing its advantages and disadvantages and recognizing its limitations. Specific disad-

vantages of this method include the cost of the software system and the time and effort required to produce the 3D image displays. Several computer systems are available that, with minor differences, can create such displays. The cost of this equipment varies from $30,000 to $200,000 (U.S.). On the basis of our experience with one of these systems, the time required for 3D CT imaging is certainly reasonable. Loading of the magnetic tapes requires approximately 35 minutes, and the subsequent generation of the 3D images takes approximately 40 minutes. Rotation of the displays and projection of any desired view can then be accomplished immediately. The creation of plastic models from the image data is currently accomplished at a single central facility. With regard to radiation exposure to the patient and examination time, we have found these parameters to be identical to those encountered during routine CT imaging.[1] The majority of our images were obtained with a 5 mm slice thickness and 3 mm table incrementation or, less commonly, with a 2 mm slice thickness and 2 mm table incrementation. These are imaging strategies that we routinely employ during CT of the spine. However, patient movement, which can lead to suboptimal standard CT scans, produces marked deterioration of 3D CT displays, so that patient cooperation is mandatory. This method is better applied to tissues of high contrast, such as bone, than to those of lower contrast, such as soft tissues. Adequate 3D CT displays of discal lesions are difficult to obtain.

It is impossible to provide an absolute score for the clinical usefulness of 3D CT of the spine. Generally our clinical colleagues judge this method to be beneficial in the majority of cases and, occasionally, essential in the management of a patient. The further delineation of complex fractures and abnormalities following fusion of the spine represents the situation in which 3D CT is most beneficial.

References

1. Andre MP, Horn RA, Bielecki D, et al: Patient dose considerations for three-dimensional CT displays. Radiology 157:177, 1985.
2. Aretzy E, Frieder G, Herman GT: The theory, design, implementation, and evaluation of a three-dimensional surface detection algorithm. Computer Graphics Image Process 15:1–24, 1981.

3. Dev P, Fellingham LL, Vasiliadis A, et al: 3D graphics for interactive surgical simulation and implant design. Proc SPIE 507:52–57, 1984.

4. Dev P, Wood SL, White DN, et al: An interactive graphics system for planning reconstructive surgery. Proceedings of the National Computer Graphics Association, Chicago, June, 1983.

5. Herman GT, Liu HK: Display of three-dimensional information in computed tomography. J Comput Assist Tomogr 1:155–160, 1977.

6. Jaffey SM, Dutta K, Hesselink L: Digital reconstruction methods for three-dimensional image visualization. Processing and display of three-dimensional data II. Proc SPIE 507:155–163, 1984.

7. Kerr R, Resnick D, Sartoris DJ, et al: Computerized tomography of proximal femoral trabecular patterns. J Orthop Research 4:45–56, 1986.

8. Lafferty C, Sartoris DJ, Resnick D, et al: Acetabular alterations in untreated congenital dysplasia of the hip: Computed tomography with multiplanar reformation and three-dimensional analysis. J Comput Assist Tomogr 10:84–91, 1986.

9. Marsh JL, Vannier MW: The "third" dimension in craniofacial surgery. Plast Reconstr Surg 71:759–767, 1983.

10. Pate D, Resnick D, Andre M, et al: Three-dimensional computed tomographic imaging of the musculoskeletal system: An analysis of 202 patients and a preliminary evaluation of three-dimensional magnetic resonance imaging. AJR 147:545–551, 1986.

11. Resnick D, Pate D, Sartoris DJ, et al: Stenotic spinal canals derived from computed tomographic data: A preliminary investigation. J Comput Tomogr 11:51–55, 1987.

12. Sartoris DJ, Andre M, Resnik C, et al: Work in Progress. Quantitative assessment of trabecular bone density in the proximal femur using computed tomography. Radiology 160:707–712, 1986.

13. Sartoris DJ, Resnick D, Bielecki D, et al: A technique for multiplanar reformation and three-dimensional analysis of computed tomographic data: Application to adult hip disease. J Can Assoc Radiol 37:69–72, 1986.

14. Sunguroff A, Greenberg D: Computer generated images for medical applications. Siggraph 1978 Proceedings, Atlanta, Georgia, 1978, pp 196–202.

15. Totty WG, Vannier MW: Complex musculoskeletal anatomy: Analysis using three-dimensional surface reconstruction. Radiology 150:173–177, 1984.

16. Tuy HK, Tuy LT: Direct 2-D display of 3-D objects. IEEE Comput Graph Appl 4:29–33, 1984.

17. Udupa JK: Display of 3D information in discrete 3D scenes produced by computerized tomography. Proc IEEE 71:420–431, 1983.

18. Vannier MW, Marsh JL, Warren JO: Three-dimensional CT reconstruction images for craniofacial surgical planning and evaluation. Radiology 150:179–184, 1984.

19. Verbout AJ, Falke THM, Tinkelenberg J: A three-dimensional graphic reconstruction method of the vertebral column from CT scans. Eur J Radiol 3:167–170, 1983.

Neil Chafetz, M.D.
Harry K. Genant, M.D.
Thurman Gillespy III, M.D.
Mark Winkler, M.D.

9

Magnetic Resonance Imaging

Magnetic resonance imaging (MRI) is the most recently developed diagnostic imaging modality. The application of MRI to clinical problems has been rapid.[3] The technique affords an opportunity to image the spine without employing ionizing radiation and to visualize the spinal cord without the risks attendant to both the lumbar puncture and the intrathecal introduction of contrast media. Preliminary evaluation of the role of MRI in various diagnostic settings has been performed. MRI has firmly established itself in the evaluation of the contents of the spinal canal. The purpose of this chapter is to provide an overview of MRI in the evaluation of those disorders affecting the spine.

INDICATIONS

A particular imaging modality is indicated when it provides information that is (1) both unique and diagnostically significant, (2) diagnostically significant comparable to that of another imaging modality, and obtained in a less invasive manner, or (3) comparable to that of another imaging modality and obtained at lower cost. MRI of the spine at this time appears to be indicated in those patients suspected of Arnold-Chiari malformation, spinal cord tumor, syringomyelia, bone marrow replacement diseases, spinal osteomyelitis, bone and soft-tissue tumors of the spine including metastatic disease to the bony and soft-tissue structures of the spine, cervical spondylosis deformans, demyelinating disorders, and cervical intervertebral disc disease. The technique may be

helpful but is not the primary imaging modality for C1–C2 subluxation, lumbar spondylosis deformans, and lumbar intervertebral disc disease.

LIMITATIONS

MRI suffers in comparison with CT in that it lacks a digitalized scout image for slice selection. Partial volumes of structures that are not the primary focus of attention may be superimposed upon areas of interest or may make interpretation difficult because slice thickness is relatively wide (compared with CT). A relative limitation of MRI is its high cost.

Although most prostheses commonly used in orthopedics are not ferromagnetic, some less frequently used metallic devices have demonstrated magnetic properties and constitute a contraindication to MRI study. Mayfield and Heifetz aneurysm clips are ferromagnetic and have been shown to undergo significant torquing during MRI. Consequently, MRI is contraindicated in patients with these devices.[2] Federal guidelines exclude patients with cardiac pacemakers from MRI examination. Furthermore, patients with known ocular metallic foreign bodies are not scanned, lest movement of the ferromagnetic object diminish visual acuity.

COMPLICATIONS

Other than the contraindications just described, MRI has no known complications.

478

TECHNIQUE

A complete discussion of the techniques of magnetic resonance imaging is beyond the scope of this chapter; the reader is referred to other sources for a comprehensive approach to this subject.[11a, 15a] A rudimentary introduction follows.

Magnetic resonance images are displayed much like those of CT. Protons (hydrogen nuclei) in the body, when exposed to magnetism, preferentially align themselves with the lines of force from the magnetic field. The application of a radiofrequency pulse at a predefined frequency causes excitation of these protons to a higher energy level (antiparallel to the field). When the radiofrequency pulse is discontinued, the protons return to their original state, emitting energy in the form of radiofrequency waves. The energy is detected as the magnetic resonance signal. This process forms the basis of medical MRI. Spatial resolution of the signal is achieved by the application of magnetic field gradients across the patient; transverse, coronal, and sagittal sections can be selected electronically by manipulation of these gradients. In addition to signal strength, which is proportional to the proton density, the state of motion of the protons and the relaxation times T1 and T2, which represent the behavior of hydrogen protons within tissue placed in a strong magnetic field, play major roles in image formation.[3, 24] Generally speaking, using spin-echo technique, a short relaxation time (TR) will result in a T1-weighted image, and a long TR will result in a T2-weighted image.

Although preliminary investigations have been made,[17] questions regarding the most useful pulse sequences for a given situation and even which type of instrument is best suited for clinical imaging remain unanswered.[2] Consequently, each investigator must attempt to answer these questions in determining the utility of magnetic resonance imaging for assessing clinical problems.

Most of the reported magnetic resonance imaging of the spine has been performed with the spin-echo technique. Although the specifics have not yet been worked out, most investigators would agree that parameters that provide separately both a T1- and a T2-weighted image of the region being scanned are desirable. Table 9–1 lists the structures

Table 9–1. T WEIGHTING RECOMMENDED FOR STRUCTURES AND DISORDERS OF THE SPINE

	T1 Weighting*	T2 Weighting†
Structure to be Observed		
Subarachnoid space		X
Spinal cord	X	
Medullary bone	X	
Intervertebral discs		X
Disorder Suspected		
Intramedullary lesions (solid or cystic)	X	
Cystic cord lesions	X	
Destructive bone lesions	X	
Osteophytic bone spurs		X
Degenerative disc disease (disc and spurs)		X

*Little signal from CSF and cortical bone.
†Strong signal from CSF.

and disorders that have empirically been noted (using spin-echo technique) to be better seen on a T1-weighted image and those better seen on a T2-weighted image. Spinal canal imaging has been markedly improved with the utilization of high signal MRI as well as new surface coils.

MRI OF THE NORMAL SPINE

In general, when spin-echo technique is used, the sequence of signal intensities in descending order is as follows: fat, nucleus pulposus (especially with T2-weighted spin-echo images generated with a long excitation time [TE]), the marrow cavity and cancellous bone, spinal cord, muscle, cerebrospinal fluid (with T1-weighted images with short TR and TE), annulus fibrosus, ligaments, and compact cortical bone.[18] Normal spinal anatomy is presented in Figures 9–1 through 9–18.

A minimal soft-tissue thickening has been described in the C1–C2 region of the cervical spine on sagittal images and is presumed to represent a combination of the synovial joint and the transverse ligament. The anterior and posterior longitudinal ligaments generally are not apparent on T1-weighted images (using spin-echo technique), because they are of low signal intensity and are not readily separable from adjacent vertebral cortical bone. On T1-weighted images using spin-echo technique, the lumbar intervertebral

Text continued on page 488

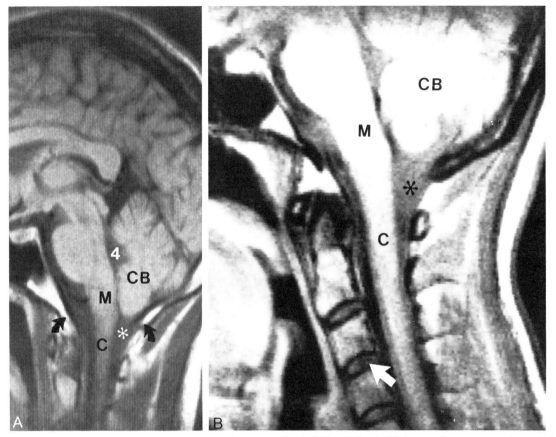

Figure 9–1. *A*, Normal brain and craniocervical juncture. Sagittal T1-weighted MR image demonstrates the spinal cord (**C**) and midbrain (**M**) and their relationship to the foramen magnum (arrows). *Key*: **CB** = cerebellum; **4** = fourth ventricle; **asterisk** = subarachnoid space. *B*, Normal craniocervical juncture. Sagittal T2-weighted MR image demonstrates spinal cord (**C**), the medulla oblongata (**M**), the cerebellum (**CB**), and the surrounding cerebrospinal fluid (asterisk). Additionally, the upper cervical vertebral bodies as well as their intervening discs (arrow) are readily apparent. Notice the diminished signal of cortical bone.

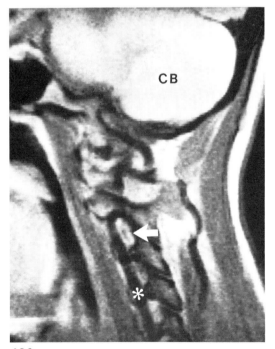

Figure 9–2. Normal cervico-occipital junction. Parasagittal MR image demonstrates the cerebellum (**CB**) as well as the oval-shaped neural foramen (arrow) of the upper cervical spine. The vertebral artery is also well delineated as a region of low signal intensity (asterisk).

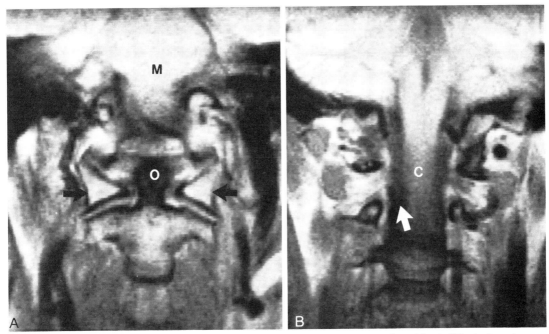

Figure 9–3. *A,* Normal craniocervical juncture. Coronal MR image demonstrates the midbrain (**M**), the lateral masses of C1 (black arrows), the C2 vertebra, and the odontoid process (**O**). *B,* Normal craniocervical juncture. Coronal image (slightly posterior to the level of Figure 9–3A) demonstrates the upper cervical spinal cord (**C**) and the cerebrospinal fluid, which is seen bilaterally adjacent to the spinal cord (arrow).

Figure 9–4. Normal cervico-occipital region. Axial MR image demonstrates the high signal intensity of the odontoid process (**O**) and spinal cord (**C**). *Key:* **L** = lateral masses of C1; **asterisk** = subarachnoid space.

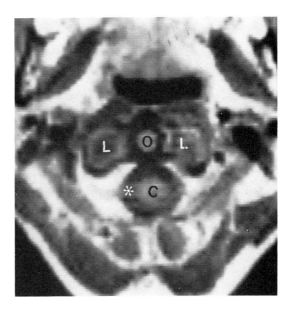

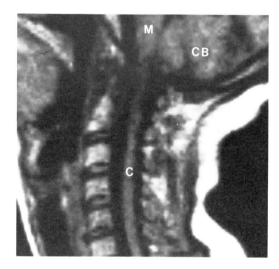

Figure 9–5. Normal cervical spine. T1-weighted sagittal MR image demonstrates the cerebellum (**CB**), midbrain (**M**), and cervical spinal cord (**C**). The cervical vertebrae and intervening discs are well delineated.

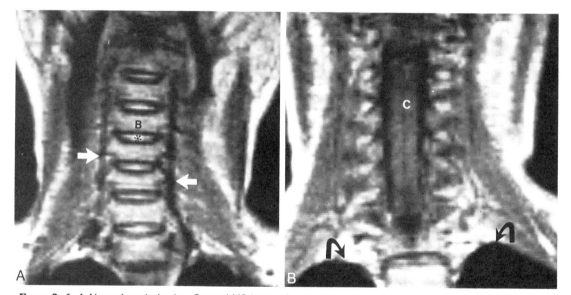

Figure 9–6. *A,* Normal cervical spine. Coronal MR image demonstrates the vertebral arteries (arrows), vertebral body (**B**), and intervertebral disc (asterisk). *B,* Normal cervical spine. Coronal MR image demonstrates lateral articulating pillars of the cervical vertebrae as well as the spinal cord (**C**). The pulmonary apices are also visible (curved arrows).

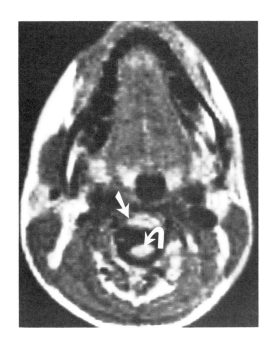

Figure 9–7. Normal upper cervical spine. Transaxial MR image demonstrates the high signal intensity of the fat-rich marrow of C2 (straight arrow) as well as the high signal intensity of the spinal cord (curved arrow).

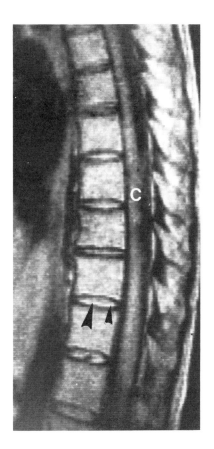

Figure 9–8. Normal thoracic spine. Sagittal MR image demonstrates the high signal intensity of the subcutaneous adipose tissue of the fat-rich bone marrow and permits direct visualization of the spinal cord (C). The moderately high signal intensity of the nucleus pulposus (large arrowhead) can be easily distinguished from the low signal intensity of the surrounding annulus fibrosus (small arrowhead). The cortical bone surrounding the bone marrow is also of very low signal intensity.

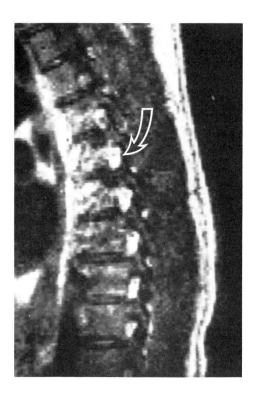

Figure 9–9. Normal thoracic spine. Parasagittal T1-weighted MR image demonstrates the neural foramen filled with high signal intensity fat (arrow). Within the neural foramen is the lower signal intensity region of the exiting nerve root.

Figure 9–10. Normal thoracic spine. Coronal MR image demonstrates the intermediate to high signal intensity of the marrow space within the thoracic vertebral bodies. Note the relatively high signal intensity of nucleus pulposus surrounded by the lower signal intensity of the annulus fibrosus. The normal kyphosis of the thoracic spine explains the demonstration of a portion of the upper thoracic spinal cord (arrow) in the same coronal plane as the middle and lower thoracic vertebral bodies.

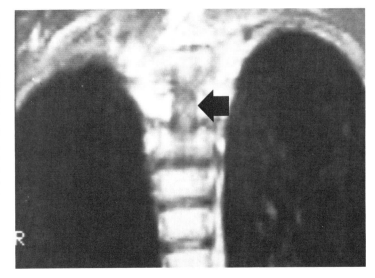

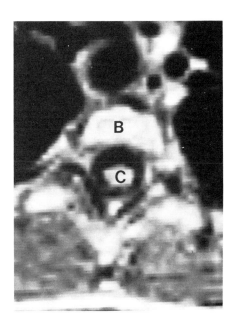

Figure 9–11. Normal thoracic spine. Axial MR image demonstrates the vertebral body (**B**), the relatively high signal intensity of the spinal cord (**C**), and the great vessels anteriorly.

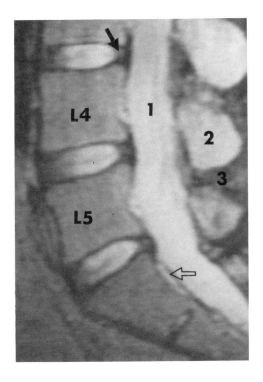

Figure 9–12. Normal lumbar spine. Sagittal scan. Spin-echo. TR 2000/TE 60. *Key*: **1** = thecal sac; **2** = spinous process; **3** = interspinous ligaments; **closed arrow** = annulus fibrosus; **open arrow** = epidural fat. Notice the increased signal intensity of the nucleus pulposus and CSF, the darker annulus fibrosus and nerve roots within the thecal sac, and the normal darker slit within the disc.

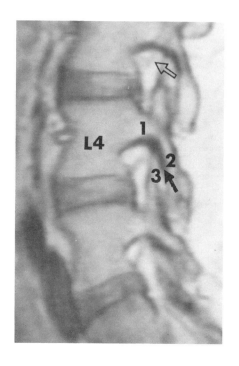

Figure 9–13. Normal lumbar spine. Parasagittal scan through the neural foramina. TR 2000/TE 20. Notice that the fat tissue is brighter and the intervertebral discs are normally darker with a shorter TE than with the longer TE observed in Figure 19–12. *Key:* **1** = pedicle; **2** = inferior articular process; **3** = superior articular process; **open arrow** = nerve root within the neural foramen (notice the surrounding brighter fat tissue); **black arrow** = facet joint.

Figure 9–14. *A,* Normal lumbar spine. Sagittal T1-weighted MR image demonstrates the relatively high signal intensity of the vertebral bodies, the intermediate to high signal intensity of the nucleus pulposus, and the low signal intensity of the annulus fibrosus. The thecal sac is not well demonstrated. There is a focal intraosseous herniation of the disc tissue (Schmorl's node) (arrow). *B,* Normal lumbar spine. Sagittal T2-weighted MR image of the same patient reveals the greater signal intensity of the cerebrospinal fluid within the thecal sac, now allowing for demonstration of the interface between the posterior aspect of the annulus fibrosus and the anterior aspect of the thecal sac (arrow).

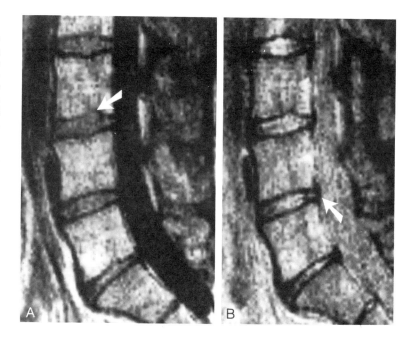

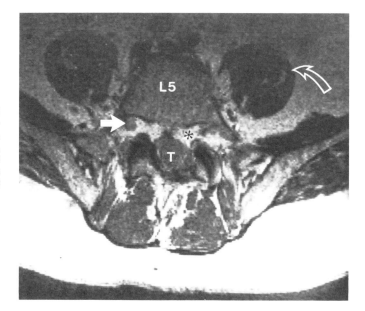

Figure 9–15. Normal L5 intervertebral level. T1-weighted axial MR image demonstrates the psoas muscle (open arrow), the L5 vertebral body, the thecal sac (**T**), and the anterior epidural fat (asterisk). The exiting right L5 nerve root (closed arrow) is particularly well demonstrated. The facet joints demonstrate dark signal.

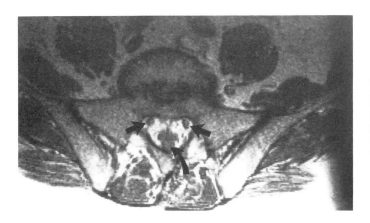

Figure 9–16. Normal lumbosacral junction. T1-weighted axial MR image demonstrates the intermediate signal intensity of both the thecal sac (curved arrow) and the S1 nerve roots (straight arrows) and the high signal intensity of the intervening epidural fat. The sacroiliac joints are noted as well.

Figure 9–17. Normal lumbar spine. Coronal MR image demonstrates the psoas muscle (arrows) and retroperitoneum as well as the vertebrae and intervertebral discs.

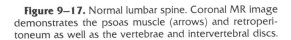
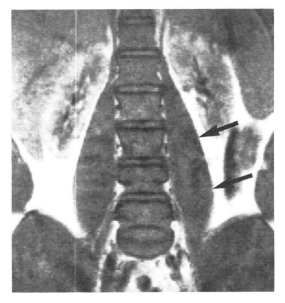

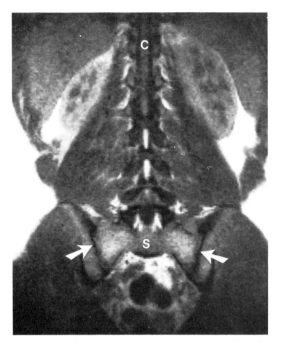

Figure 9–18. Normal lower abdomen and pelvis. Coronal MR image demonstrates the thoracic and upper lumbar spinal cord (**C**). Note the sacrum (**S**) and sacroiliac joints (arrows).

discs are of intermediate signal intensity. With T2 weighting, the nucleus pulposus demonstrates a bright linear, axially oriented signal or, in patients who have reached the age of 30 years, two adjacent axially oriented regions of high signal intensity surrounded by the low signal intensity of the annulus fibrosus.[1] Cervical discs usually appear brighter than lumbar discs with T1 weighting, and when the TE is lengthened, the central part of the cervical intervertebral disc demonstrates a subtle increase in signal intensity.[18] On T1-weighted images the spinal cord is clearly visualized and exhibits intermediate signal intensity that is surrounded by an area of low signal intensity obtained from the cerebrospinal fluid, dural membranes, and epidural structures. In the lumbar spine, the darker cerebrospinal fluid is surrounded by the high signal intensity of the epidural fat, which is usually abundant in this region. The nerve roots may sometimes be visualized separately from the surrounding cerebrospinal fluid. With T2-weighted images, the cerebrospinal fluid becomes brighter, giving a "myelographic" effect on sagittal scans of the lumbar spine. Nerve roots within the thecal sac may be

identified. Although the posterior elements are best visualized on the axial images, the intervertebral neural foramina are usually best demonstrated on the direct parasagittal images. The low to intermediate signal intensity of the exiting nerve root is surrounded by a small collar of CSF, which in turn is surrounded by a larger amount of high signal intensity from epidural fat.

MRI OF SPINAL DISORDERS

Pitfalls in Diagnosis

At present the major pitfalls in diagnosis are related to uncertainty about the optimal technique to display the suspected pathology. As a satisfactory regimen of parameters that will "cover the waterfront" of pathology emerges, the possibility of unwittingly masking an abnormality should become less of a legitimate concern.

Chronic Neck Pain Syndromes

The paucity of epidural fat in the cervical spine generally precludes an adequate search for intervertebral disc disease in this region by CT without the introduction of intrathecal contrast material. Magnetic resonance imaging provides the unique opportunity to examine this region in a noninvasive manner. Differentiation of the nucleus from the surrounding annulus is possible in the normal disc, and degeneration of a disc is readily demonstrated by reduction in the amplitude of the signal intensity from the nucleus pulposus. Intervertebral disc herniation and the osteophytic overgrowth of spondylosis deformans are readily demonstrable (Fig. 9–19). Oblique MR images may better delineate the cervical neural foramina.[16b] MRI is also particularly helpful in the cervicothoracic junction, where beam-hardening artifacts often degrade CT imaging.

Low Back Pain Syndrome and Lumbar Disc Disease

The last 5 years have revealed an efficacious application of computed tomography to the evaluation of the patient with low back pain. Many patients who previously had to undergo myelography have now been

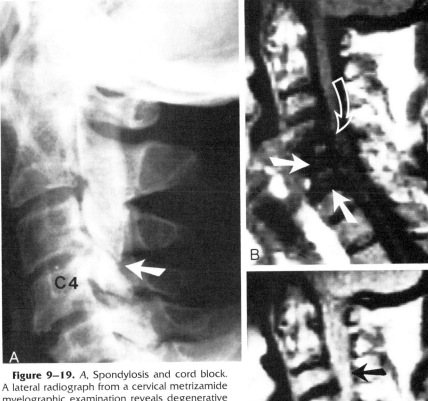

Figure 9–19. *A*, Spondylosis and cord block. A lateral radiograph from a cervical metrizamide myelographic examination reveals degenerative disc disease at the C4–C5 and C5–C6 and C6–C7 levels (not shown), with osteophytes emanating both anteriorly and posteriorly from the C3 through C7 vertebral bodies. A complete myelographic block (arrow) at the C3–C4 level is evident. *B*, A sagittal T1-weighted MR image of the same patient reveals a reduction in bone marrow signal (straight arrows) in the C4, C5, C6, and, to a lesser extent, C7 vertebral bodies, reflecting the encroachment of the hypertrophic bony sclerosis on the high signal intensity, fat-rich marrow. Additionally, irregularity of the anterior aspect of the spinal cord (curved arrow) in the lower cervical spine reflects osteophytic impingement. *C*, Same patient. Sagittal T2-weighted MR image. The cerebrospinal fluid (arrow) is now demonstrated, allowing for a more precise depiction of the posterior extent of the low signal intensity osteophytes (arrowheads).

evaluated by computed tomography, obviating the use of intrathecal contrast material. Some patients, primarily those with extensive postoperative changes, have been studied by CT following the introduction of water-soluble contrast agent into the subarachnoid space. The opportunity to evaluate such patients with magnetic resonance imaging, which does not require the use of ionizing radiation and intrathecal contrast material, is very attractive.

In the process of disc degeneration, the high-intensity MRI signal of the nucleus pulposus appears to diminish. This reduction suggests an intrinsic abnormality. When seen in a nonruptured disc, the finding is presumed to indicate deterioration of the disc. The loss of high signal intensity of the nucleus pulposus is thought to represent the desiccation of the nucleus that occurs with degeneration and also in general with the extrusion of nuclear material at the time of herniation[3] (Figs. 9–20 to 9–22). Chemonucleolysis rapidly leads to a similar appearance. How frequently such a disc will, with time, rupture is uncertain. Because digital

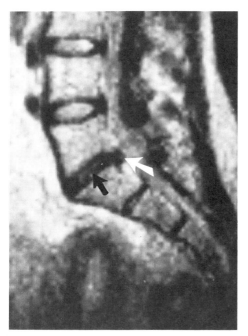

Figure 9–20. Degenerated disc. A parasagittal MR image of the lumbar spine reveals the high signal intensity of the nucleus pulposus of the normal L1 through L4 discs. The low signal intensity of the L5–S1 (black arrow) disc is an indication of the typical desiccation that occurs in the nucleus pulposus of a degenerated disc. The posterior extent of the low signal intensity annulus fibrosus suggests a broad-based disc protrusion (white arrow).

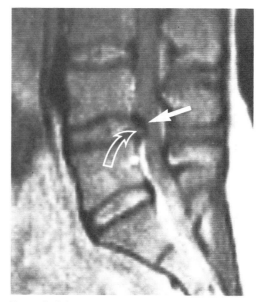

Figure 9–21. Herniated disc. A parasagittal MR image through the lower lumbar spine of an individual with low back pain reveals an abnormality at the L4–L5 level. Effacement of the anterior portion of the thecal sac (straight arrow) at this disc level and a posterior tongue-like protrusion of the nuclear material (curved arrow) are indicative of a herniated nucleus pulposus.

scout images similar to those routinely obtained at the beginning of a CT examination have not been uniformly available with MRI, the direct sagittal MRI image has been most useful in determining anatomic location in the spine. It is also on the sagittal image that the intensity of the nucleus pulposus at one level can be most readily compared with that at other levels. Furthermore, a narrow L5–S1 disc space may be optimally evaluated by direct MRI sagittal images Figs 9–23 and 9–24. The partial volumes of the adjacent vertebrae may render this area difficult to evaluate with axial images on both CT and MRI. Herniation of disc tissue can be identified in the sagittal and axial images (Figs. 9–20 through 9–24).

With spin-echo technique, the differentiation between the nucleus pulposus and the annulus fibrosus becomes more apparent as TR and TE values are increased. Occasionally, a "free fragment" in the epidural space may demonstrate high signal intensity on both T1- and T2-weighted images. Such high signal intensity abnormalities are more easily recognized on T1-weighted images

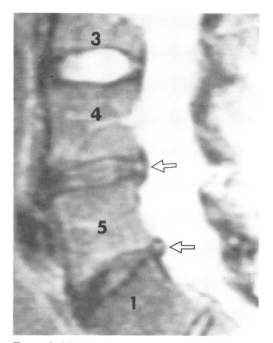

Figure 9–22. Disc degeneration. Sagittal scan of the lumbosacral spine. TR 2000/TE 60. A less than normal signal intensity is noted in the nucleus pulposus of both the L4–L5 and L5–S1 discs. Compare with the normal brighter disc of L3–L4. The decreased signal in the intervertebral discs indicates degeneration. There is herniation of the intervertebral discs (arrows). Notice that brighter nuclear tissue has herniated posteriorly.

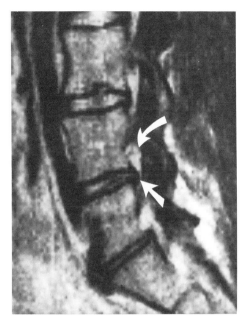

Figure 9–23. Lateral disc herniation. A parasagittal MR image through the neural foramen (curved arrow) demonstrates effacement of a portion of the anterior epidural fat (straight arrow) within the L4 neural foramen. This was due to a far lateral disc herniation.

Table 9–2. MRI CRITERIA FOR DIAGNOSIS OF DISC DISEASE

Disc space narrowing
Decrease in nucleus pulposus signal
Effacement of epidural fat
Posterior protrusion of nucleus
Defect in CSF contour
Distortion of thecal sac

At this time, surface coil MRI is comparable to CT in the identification of disc ruptures.[16a] However, many patients with low back syndromes have nondiscogenic bony stenoses that are either isolated or present in combination with discogenic abnormalities. CT is more efficacious in diagnosis of these bony abnormalities, and therefore it is likely, in the immediate future, to remain the modality of choice in the assessment of the patient with low back pain.

(whereas the similar high signal intensity of CSF on T2-weighted images can render the identification of the free fragment difficult). Criteria for the MRI diagnosis of disc disease are given in Table 9–2. Focal fat replacement of red marrow is related to age and the presence of spondylosis and spondylitis and is commonly noted.[9c]

Spinal Stenosis

In the depiction of bony overgrowth seen in the spinal stenoses (lateral recess and central canal stenoses) as well as of the arthritic changes seen in facet disease, MRI has been reported to be as accurate as myelography and CT in quantifying narrowing of the spinal canal (Fig. 9–25); however, CT has been found to be more accurate in separating bony from soft-tissue impingement because of the low signal intensity obtained from cortical bone with MRI.[17]

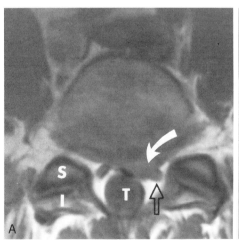
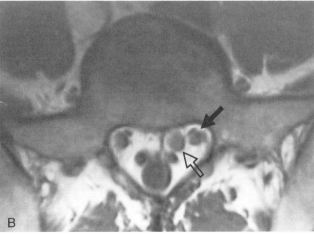

Figure 9–24. Disc herniation with sequestered fragment. Axial scans. TR 1500/TE 20. *A,* There is a herniated L5–S1 intervertebral disc (curved arrow), which has displaced the left nerve root (straight arrow) and distorted the thecal sac (**T**). Notice the sharp contrast between the nerve root and thecal sac with the surrounding brighter epidural fat. *Key:* **I** = inferior articular process; **S** = superior articular process. *B,* Same patient, wtih a more caudal axial scan through the lateral recess of S1. There is a sequestered disc fragment (open arrow) surrounded by fat, which demonstrates a brighter signal. The nerve roots within the lateral recess (closed arrow) are not compressed.

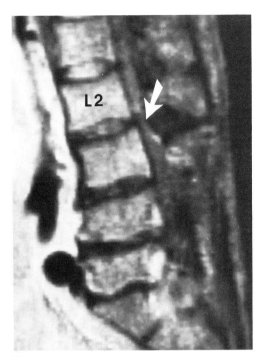

Figure 9–25. Spinal stenosis and degenerated discs. Parasagittal MR image of an elderly male with a previous lumbar fusion and recurrent back pain. Multiple degenerated discs in the lower lumbar spine are evident. Additionally, narrowing of the thecal sac in the anteroposterior diameter is evident at the L2–L3 level (arrow). This is due to formation of bony overgrowth from the posterior lumbar fusion, which has caused central canal stenosis.

Postoperative Spine

Recurrent Disc Rupture Versus Scarring

The difficulty distinguishing postoperative fibrosis from recurrent disc rupture on CT imaging has led investigators to try intravenous[4] and intrathecal contrast agents. On the basis of preliminary findings, it appears that postoperative fibrosis may be readily distinguished from disc and other adjacent epidural structures with MRI[5] (Figs. 9–26, 9–27). This differentiation is generally best seen with more T2-weighted techniques. Scar that has resulted from recent surgery within the previous 2 years demonstrates intermediate to high signal intensity on T2-weighted images. In contrast, signal intensity of a recurrent disc appears very low on similar images.

The Postchemonucleolysis Disc

Signal intensity has also been shown to be increased in the subchondral bone near the vertebral end-plates of some patients following chymopapain injection, suggesting inflammation.[5] Such injections are followed by rapid dehydration, collapse, fibrosis, and rigidity of the disc. The success of treatment may be causally related to destruction of the cartilaginous end-plates, with subsequent ingrowth of granulation tissue and rapid scarring of the disc space.[5] Rapid loss of the signal intensity of the nucleus pulposus following chemonucleolysis has been demonstrated.[7]

Surrounding Soft Tissues

Another preliminary observation is the differentiation on magnetic resonance imaging of atropic muscle or fatty infiltration of muscular tissue from normal muscle. Should this observation be confirmed in other patients, the determination by MRI of the extent of involvement of motor neuron disease may be possible.

Spinal Cord Tumors and Soft-Tissue Tumorlike Conditions

Soft-tissue tumors are well demonstrated by magnetic resonance imaging.[9a, 11, 13, 19] MRI can delineate the extent of tumor and the association with cyst formation or hemorrhage. The high signal intensity of lipomas makes them particularly easy to identify. The intermediate to high signal intensity of neurofibromas (above that of the CSF) has permitted their recognition within the thecal sac, the neural foramen, or the paraspinal tissues (Fig. 9–28). The lower signal intensity of CSF (with T1 weighting) allows distinction between the soft-tissue fibromas and both dural ectasia and meningoceles.[11]

The increase in the girth of the spinal cord associated with an intramedullary tumor has been described in cystic astrocytoma, ependymoma, intramedullary lipoma, and metastasis to the cord.[11, 13] The zone of transition between normal and neoplastic tissue has generally been demonstrable. Most promising is that the extent of involvement in the

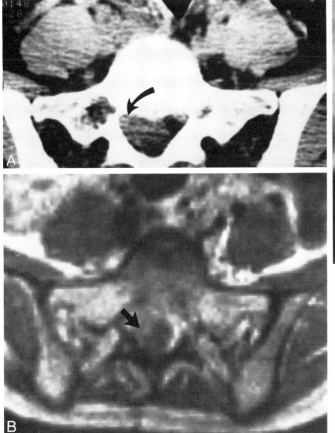

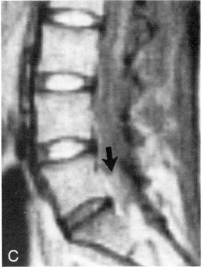

Figure 9–26. *A,* Axial CT images at the superior aspect of the S1 level reveal effacement of the right anterolateral epidural fat by a soft-tissue mass (curved arrow) of uncertain etiology. Postoperative fibrosis, recurrent disc rupture, and a conjoined nerve root were all clinical possibilities in this young woman with recurrent back pain following laminectomies in the lower spine. *B,* An axial MR image in this region reveals intermediate signal intensity of the thecal sac and an intermediate to high signal intensity in the right anterolateral region (arrow) corresponding to the abnormalities seen in 9–26A. *C,* Postoperative scar and degenerated disc, same patient. A parasagittal MR image to the right of the midline reveals degeneration of the L5–S1 nucleus pulposus as well as the intermediate to high signal intensity region (arrow) corresponding to that seen on the CT and the axial MR images. Subsequent surgery revealed that this region contained only postoperative scar.

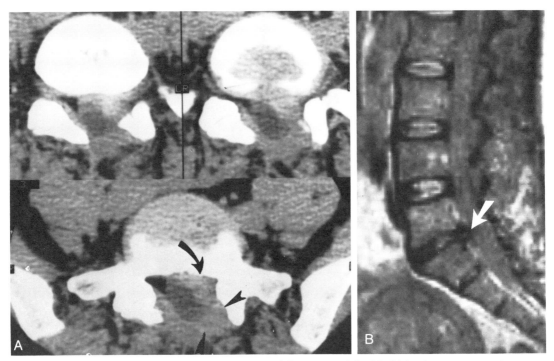

Figure 9–27. *A,* Recurrent herniated disc. Sequential axial CT images of the L5–S1 level in a patient with recurrent postoperative left-sided low back pain demonstrate the posterior laminectomy defect and accompanying scar (arrowheads). Distortion of the left anterolateral aspect of the thecal sac by a mass of intermediate radiographic density (curved arrow) raises the diagnostic possibilities of postoperative scar versus recurrent disc. *B,* Recurrent herniated disc. T2-weighted sagittal MR image of the same patient reveals subnormal signal intensity of the L5–S1 nucleus pulposus and posterior protrusion of both the annulus and the nucleus pulposus, which are deforming the anterior aspect of the thecal sac (arrow). A recurrent disc rupture was found at surgery.

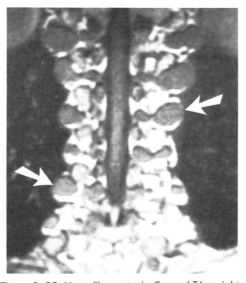

Figure 9–28. Neurofibromatosis. Coronal T1-weighted MR image of the thoracic spine of a patient with neurofibromatosis. Multiple bilateral soft-tissue masses extend laterally from the spinal canal. They pass through and expand the neural foramina. These dumbbell-shaped masses (arrows) are typical of neurofibromas.

spinal canal, spinal cord, and the brain stem (in the case of some astrocytomas) can be depicted without the use of an intrathecal contrast agent. Spinal cord tumors often enhance to a greater extent than surrounding CSF on long TR-weighted images.[9a]

Syringohydromyelia

Syringohydromyelia has been one of the abnormalities most easily depicted by magnetic resonance imaging of the cervical spinal cord.[8, 12, 14, 23a, 26] The syrinx cavity containing cerebrospinal fluid within the spinal cord has been easily demonstrable without the use of intrathecal contrast agent and without the delay following intrathecal introduction of contrast agent that is sometimes required with CT. A cystic cord lesion has low intensity with a T1-weighted imaging sequence (Fig. 9–29). With a T2-weighted imaging sequence, the intensity of a CSF–filled syrinx increases and may become isointense with the spinal cord,

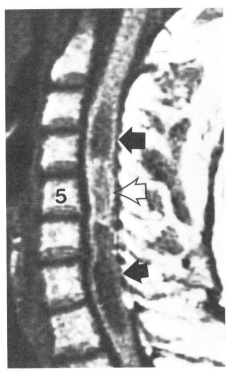

Figure 9–29. Cystic astrocytoma and syringohydro-myelia. Sagittal T1-weighted MR image of the cervical spine reveals an intramedullary high signal intensity lesion at the level of C5, representing an astrocytoma (open arrow). Associated cystic components are noted both above and below the lesion (black arrows).

thereby masking the presence of a syrinx cavity.[9a]

Demyelinating Disorders

MRI has become the modality of choice for imaging the spinal cord. Demyelinating disorders such as multiple sclerosis (Fig. 9–30) can easily be demonstrated on the first echo of the long TR sequences. Plaques of multiple sclerosis have been depicted in the brain and upper cervical spinal cord.[15] They appear as areas of high signal intensity. MR is more sensitive in detecting plaques than CT.[23] Demonstration of more distal sites of involvement await technologic advances that are likely to be forthcoming in the near future.

Chiari Malformation

Magnetic resonance imaging has success-fully delineated the extent of Chiari malfor-mation; it can be performed noninvasively on a routine, outpatient basis.[19] The caudal herniation of cerebellar tonsils, the low po-sition of the fourth ventricle, and the relation of the brainstem and cervical medullary junction to the upper cervical canal and foramen magnum are easily recognized[8, 18, 19, 25] (Fig. 9–31). Tonsillar herniation is best demonstrated on sagittal images; however, occasionally, asymmetric tonsil herniation may be identified only on coronal images.[25] Hydromyelia can also be demonstrated. The association of Chiari I malformation and hydromyelia is important in treatment plan-ning. Ventricular decompression of cysts that do not communicate with the ventricu-lar system in the presence of Chiari I mal-formation does not cause the clinical symp-toms to resolve.[14]

Osseous Lesions

Metastasis

Normal cancellous bone characteristically demonstrates high signal intensity. Blastic metastases, like cortical bone, demonstrate low signal intensity and thus can be readily

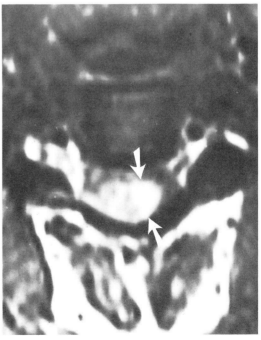

Figure 9–30. Multiple sclerosis. Axial T2-weighted MR image of the cervical spine demonstrates large, high signal intensity MS plaques (arrows).

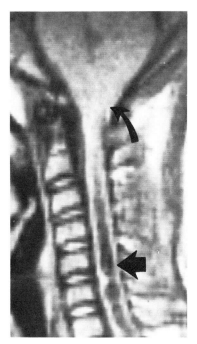

Figure 9–31. Chiari malformation and syringohydromyelia. Parasagittal midline cervical MR image reveals a Chiari malformation (curved arrow) and an associated cervical syrinx (straight arrow). (Courtesy of Dr. H. Newton and Dr. D. Haas, San Francisco, California.)

recognized amidst the high signal intensity medullary space[20] (Fig. 9–32). Lytic metastases are usually readily detected, as they demonstrate dark signals on T1-weighted images and bright signals on T2-weighted images. In some instances, lytic metastases demonstrate a relatively high signal intensity similar to the normal medullary space on T1-weighted images and therefore are more readily identified on T2-weighted images. Focal vertebral involvement as demonstrated by MRI is not specific for metastatic disease and may be caused by benign processes that replace marrow such as eosinophilic granuloma.[6] Most important, magnetic resonance imaging can delineate direct extension of tumor to the spinal canal[1a, 21] (Fig. 9–33). Widespread replacement of normal marrow has been demonstrated by MRI in patients with marrow iron deposition, thalassemia, and osteopetrosis[22a] and can be anticipated in any marrow replacement disorder[20] (Fig. 9–34).

In children with acute lymphocytic leukemia, MR evaluation of lumbar spine bone marrow has demonstrated longer T1 relaxation times in those with recently diagnosed tumor than in those with tumor in remis-

sion.[20a] This may be helpful in the staging of this disorder[1a] as well as in the assessment and treatment of chronic granulocytic leukemia and aplastic anemia.[15b]

Infection

Magnetic resonance imaging has been used to demonstrate both spinal osteomyelitis[16, 24] and disc space infection.[8a, 17] The MRI appearance of vertebral osteomyelitis has been described as characteristic. The affected vertebrae and discs are lower in signal intensity than normal on T1-weighted images and greater in signal intensity than normal on T2-weighted images (Fig. 9–35). The MRI appearances of disc infection, disc degeneration, and the disc following chemonucleolysis are described in Table 9–3. The absence of the intranuclear cleft described as normal in patients over 30 years, especially in the presence of increased signal intensity within the disc, is regarded as compatible with infection. MRI has been shown to be as accurate and sensitive as radionuclide scanning in the assessment of vertebral osteomyelitis.[16] Magnetic resonance imaging was also able to demonstrate involvement of the paravertebral soft tissues and bone when routine radiographs and CT were negative or equivocal. Disc space infection and paravertebral abscess formation are best demonstrated in the coronal plane.[8a]

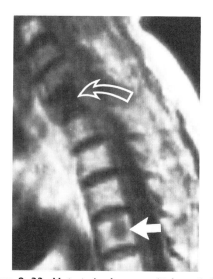

Figure 9–32. Metastasis. A parasagittal cervical and upper thoracic MR image demonstrates destruction of the C7 vertebral body (curved arrow) and a lesion in the fourth thoracic vertebral body (straight arrow) in a patient with metastatic prostate carcinoma.

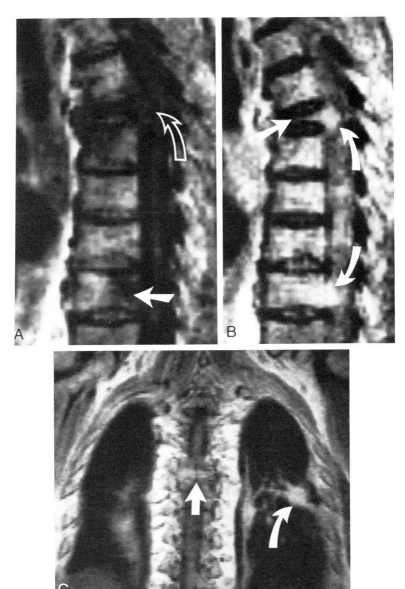

Figure 9–33. *A*, Metastasis. A T1-weighted sagittal MR image of the thoracic spine demonstrates a soft-tissue mass (curved arrow) in the spinal canal anterior to the spinal cord. The low signal intensity defects in the adjacent vertebral bodies (straight arrow) indicate replacement of the fat-rich, high signal intensity marrow by the tumor. *B*, A sagittal T2-weighted MR image of the same patient obtained at the same examination in a nearly identical location demonstrates the high signal intensity of the tumor (curved arrows), which has become enhanced beyond the intensity of the cerebrospinal fluid. The midthoracic vertebral collapse (straight arrow) and sparing of the adjacent disc spaces are apparent. *C*, A direct coronal MR image demonstrates the midthoracic spinal metastasis (straight arrow) and the left mid-lung field primary carcinoma (curved arrow).

However, small calcifications within an abscess cannot be identified with MRI.

Primary Bone Tumors and Tumorlike Conditions

MRI is particularly well suited to the demonstration of both the presence and the soft-tissue extent of benign and malignant bone tumors.[1a, 20] The soft-tissue contrast of magnetic resonance imaging permits a more definitive delineation of the boundaries of the tumor. This separation of soft-tissue structures, when coupled with direct multiplanar imaging, helps determine the aggressiveness of the tumor and facilitates the approach of the surgeon or radiotherapist (Figs. 9–36). Vertebral hemangiomas demonstrate a bright signal on both T1- and T2-weighted images (Fig. 9–37).

Congenital Abnormalities

The evaluation of patients with dysraphism can be aided by MRI. Tethered cord, diastematomyelia, lipomyelomeningocele, and Chiari malformation can be easily evaluated.[8, 10, 11, 21, 25] The position of the low-

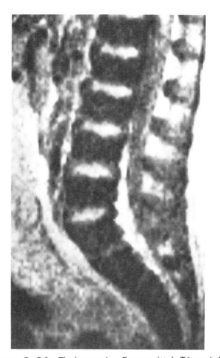

Figure 9–34. Thalassemia. Parasagittal T1-weighted MR image reveals low signal intensity of all vertebrae in this patient. Replacement of high signal intensity medullary fat by both hemosiderin and red marrow has occurred in this patient with thalassemia. (Courtesy of Dr. R. Brasch, San Francisco, California.)

lying spinal cord in patients with spinal dysraphism and tethered spinal cord and the extent of an accompanying lipoma are easily demonstrated with MRI[11] (Fig. 9–38). Lipomas give off a bright, high-intensity signal. In diastematomyelia, the divided spinal cord can be imaged in its entire craniocaudal extent as well as axially.[10] In addition, the bony septum, when containing enough fat marrow, may also be identified in part.[10] The spicule appears as an intermediate- to high-intensity signal. Associated abnormalities such as syringohydromyelia are also easily recognized. In one case of diastematomyelia, syringohydromyelia has been observed without Chiari malformation.[10] Nerve roots and the filum terminale are not consistently visualized; this is a current limitation of MRI in the evaluation of dysraphism.

In one individual with Sprengel's deformity, the presence of the anomalous omovertebral bone has been readily demonstrated (Fig. 9–39).

Trauma

There is a limited experience in magnetic resonance imaging of the acute trauma vic-

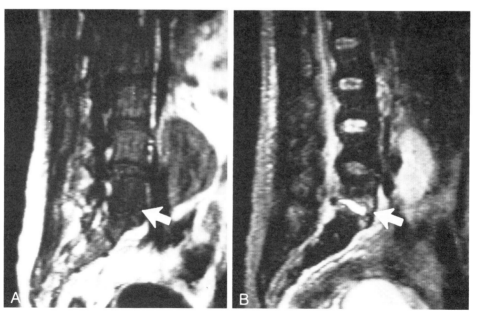

Figure 9–35. Osteomyelitis. *A,* Parasagittal T1-weighted MR image of the lumbar spine of a patient with L5–S1 disc infection and adjacent L5 and S1 osteomyelitis demonstrates lower than normal vertebral and disc signal intensity (arrow). *B,* On the T2-weighted MR image this intensity becomes greater than normal (arrow). (Courtesy of Dr. M. T. Modic, Cleveland, Ohio.)

Table 9–3. APPEARANCES OF DISC INFECTION, DISC DEGENERATION, AND CHEMONUCLEOLYSIS ON MAGNETIC RESONANCE IMAGING

Disorder	Short TR and TE	Long TR and TE
Infection	Decreased vertebral body and nucleus pulposus signals	Increased disc and vertebral end-plate signals
Degeneration	Decreased nucleus pulposus signal	Even more decreased nucleus pulposus signal
Chemonucleolysis	Decreased nucleus pulposus signal	Increased vertebral end-plate signal and persistently decreased nucleus pulposus signal

tim. MRI provides excellent soft-tissue discrimination, so that rapid assessment of the spinal cord for contusion, compression, or edema,[9b] as well as identification of hematoma, herniated disc, and spinal malalignment, may be accomplished. Such investigations have undoubtedly been hampered by the limited access to MRI scanners and the restrictions that proximity to the magnet place on basic life support apparatuses. Edema appears bright and the contusion site appears dark on T2-weighted images experimentally 3 to 5 hours after cord injury.[9b]

In patients who sustained prior cervical spinal cord injury and quadriplegia and who have developed new or progressive neurologic symptoms, MRI can accurately demonstrate abnormalities within the spinal cord.[21a] Myelomalacia can be differentiated from a post-traumatic spinal cord cyst. However, differentiation may at times be difficult when the two conditions coexist. Myelomalacia demonstrates low signal intensity on T-1 weighted images and signal intensity resembling that of normal spinal cord on moderate T2-weighted images.

Bone Mineralization

At this time, magnetic resonance imaging cannot be used for this assessment,[6] although progress is being made in this area.

Post-Radiation

Increased signal intensity of the vertebral body demonstrated on both T1- and T2-weighted images is another finding characteristically observed in a region that has previously been irradiated[22] (Fig. 9–40). This finding is believed to reflect replacement of red marrow with fat.[22]

Sacroiliac Joints

If sacroiliac joint disease is suggested by clinical symptomatology and nuclear medicine scanning yet is not confirmed by conventional radiography, it can be optimally, though somewhat expensively, depicted by computed tomography. To date, CT remains superior to MRI in the depiction of the cortical bony changes that occur in sacroiliitis.

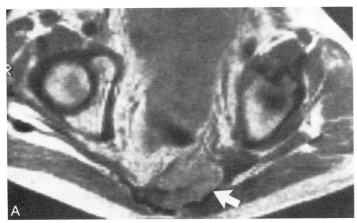
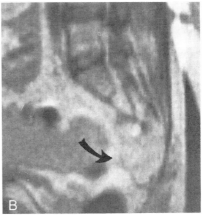

Figure 9–36. Chordoma. Axial (A) and direct (B) parasagittal MR images reveal the bony and soft-tissue extent of a sacral chordoma (arrows).

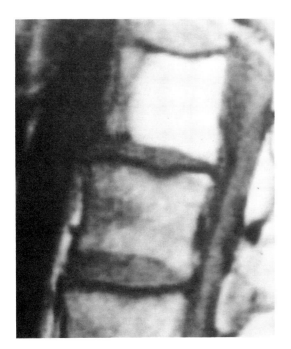

Figure 9–37. Hemangioma. Sagittal scan. Spin-echo technique. TR 2000/TE 20. The increased signal intensity in the entire vertebral body represents hemangioma. Persistent increased signal of the hemangioma was also noted with TR 2000/TE 70.

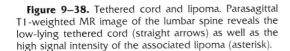

Figure 9–38. Tethered cord and lipoma. Parasagittal T1-weighted MR image of the lumbar spine reveals the low-lying tethered cord (straight arrows) as well as the high signal intensity of the associated lipoma (asterisk).

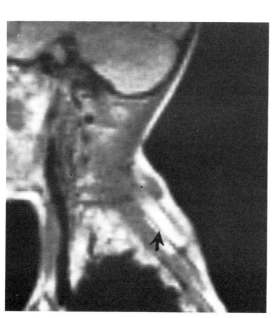

Figure 9–39. Parasagittal MR image of the cervicothoracic region in a patient with Klippel-Feil syndrome and Sprengel's deformity demonstrates posterocervical soft-tissue fullness and a high signal intensity posterocervical abnormality (arrow) believed to represent the fat-rich marrow in the associated omovertebral bone.

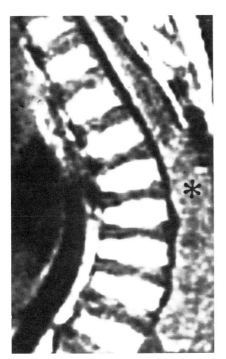

Figure 9–40. After radiation. Parasagittal T1-weighted MR image of the thoracic and lumbar spine reveals high signal intensity of the lower thoracic and upper lumbar vertebrae following radiation for an astrocytoma (asterisk).

COMPARISON WITH OTHER IMAGING MODALITIES

CT remains the imaging modality for the assessment of low back pain of arthritis and disorders involving predominantly the cortical bone. However, when a scout image, contiguous scanning (currently available on some scanners), and widespread accessibility to MRI scanners become available, MRI will assume a premier role in the diagnosis and extent of soft-tissue tumors, disorders of the cervical spinal region, spinal osteomyelitis, and perhaps intervertebral disc disease.[9] Its role in the assessment of spinal stenosis and facet joint disease, however, has yet to be established.

References

1. Aguila LA, Piraino DW, Modic MT, et al: The intranuclear cleft of the intravertebral disk: Magnetic resonance imaging. Radiology 155:155–158, 1985.
1a. Beltran J, Noto AM, Chakeres DW, et al: Tumors of the osseous spine: staging with MR imaging versus CT. Radiology 162:565–569, 1987.
2. Berquish TH: Magnetic resonance imaging: Preliminary experience in orthopedic radiology. Magn Reson Imaging 2:41–52, 1984.
3. Brandt-Zawadzki M, Mills CM, Davis PL: CNS application of NMR imaging. Appl Radiol 12:25–30, 1983.
4. Braun IF, Hoffman JC Jr, Davis PC, et al: Contrast enhancement in CT differentiation between recurrent disc herniation and post-operative scar: Perspective study. AJR 145:785–790, 1985.
5. Brown MD: The pathophysiology of disc disease. Orthop Clin North Am 2:359–370, 1971.
6. Cann CE, Genant HK: Precise measurement of vertebral mineral content using computed tomography. J Comput Assist Tomogr 4:493–500, 1980.
7. Chafetz NI, Genant HK, Moon KL, et al: Recognition of lumbar disk herniation with NMR. AJR 141:1153–1156, 1983.
8. DeLaPaz RL, Brady TJ, Buonanno FS, et al: Nuclear magnetic resonance (NMR) imaging of Arnold-Chiari type I malformation with hydromyelia. J Comput Assist Tomogr 7:126–129, 1983.
8a. deRoos A, van Persijn van Meerten EL, Bloem JL, et al: MRI of tuberculous spondylitis. AJR 146:79–82, 1986.
9. Edelman RR, Shoukimas GM, Stark DD, et al: High resolution surface-coil imaging of lumbar disk disease. AJR 144:1123–1129, 1985.
9a. Goy AMC, Pinto RS, Raghavendra BN, et al: Intramedullary spinal cord tumors: MR imaging, with emphasis on associated cysts. Radiology 161:381–386, 1986.
9b. Hackney DB, Asato R, Joseph PM, et al: Hemorrhage and edema in acute spinal cord compression: demonstration by MR imaging. Radiology 161:387–390, 1986.
9c. Hajek PC, Baker LL, Goobar JE, et al: Focal fat deposition in axial bone marrow: MR characteristics. Radiology 162:245–249, 1987.
10. Han JS, Benson JE, Kaufman B, et al: Demonstration of diastematomyelia and associated abnormalities with MR imaging. AJNR 6:215–219, 1985.
11. Han JS, Kaufman B, El Yousef SJ, et al: NMR imaging of the spine. AJR 141:1137–1145, 1983.
11a. James TL, Margulis AR (eds): Biomedical Magnetic Resonance. San Francisco: Radiology Research and Education Foundation, University of California Printing Department, 1984.
12. Kokmen E, Marsh WR, Baker HL Jr: Magnetic resonance imaging in syringomyelia. Neurosurgery 17:267–270, 1985.
13. Kucharczyk W, Brant-Zawadzki M, Sobel D, et al: Central nervous system tumors in children: Detection by magnetic resonance imaging. Radiology 155:131–136, 1985.
14. Lee BCP, Zimmerman RD, Manning JJ, et al: MR imaging of syringomyelia and hydromyelia. AJR 144:1149–1156, 1985.
15. Maravilla KR, Weinreb JC, Suss R, et al: Magnetic resonance demonstration of multiple sclerosis plaques in the cervical cord. AJR 144:381–385, 1985.
15a. Margulis AR, Higgins CB, Kaufman L, et al (eds): Clinical Magnetic Resonance Imaging. San Francisco: Radiology Research and Education Foundation, University of California Printing Department, 1983.
15b. McKinstry CS, Steiner RE, Young AT, et al: Bone marrow in leukemia and aplastic anemia: MR imaging before, during, and after treatment. Radiology 162:701–707, 1987.

16. Modic MT, Feiglin DH, Piraino DW, et al: Vertebral osteomyelitis—assessment using MR. Radiology 157:157–166, 1985.

16a. Modic MT, Masaryk T, Boumphrey F, et al: Lumbar herniated disk disease and canal stenosis: perspective evaluation by surface coil MR, CT, and myelography. AJR 147:757–765, 1986.

16b. Modic MT, Masaryk TJ, Ross JS, et al: Cervical radiculopathy: value of oblique MR imaging. Radiology 163:227–231, 1987.

17. Modic MT, Pavlicek W, Weinstein MA, et al: Magnetic resonance imaging of intervertebral disk disease. Radiology 152:103–111, 1984.

18. Modic MT, Weinstein MA, Pavlicek W, et al: Magnetic resonance imaging of the cervical spine: Technical and clinical observations. AJR 141:1129–1136, 1983.

19. Modic MT, Weinstein MA, Pavlicek W, et al: Nuclear magnetic resonance imaging of the spine. Radiology 148:757–762, 1983.

20. Moon KL, Genant HK, Helms CA, et al: Musculoskeletal applications of nuclear magnetic resonance. Radiology 147:161–171, 1983.

20a. Moore SG, Gooding CA, Brasch RC, et al: Bone marrow in children with acute lymphocytic leukemia: MR relaxation times. Radiology 160:237–240, 1986.

21. Norman D, Mills CM, Brant-Zawadzki M, et al: Magnetic resonance imaging of the spinal cord and canal: Potentials and limitations. AJR 141:1147–1152, 1983.

21a. Quencer RM, Sheldon JJ, Post MJD, et al: MRI of the chronically injured cervical spinal cord. AJR 147:125–132, 1986.

22. Ramsey RG, Zacharias CE: MR imaging of the spine after radiation therapy: Easily recognizable effects. AJR 144:1131–1135, 1985.

22a. Rao VM, Dalinka MK, Mitchell DG, et al: Osteopetrosis: MR characteristics at 1.5T. Radiology 161:217–220, 1986.

23. Sheldon JJ, Siddharthan R, Tobias J, et al: MR imaging of multiple sclerosis: Comparison with clinical and CT examinations in 74 patients. AJR 145:957–964, 1985.

23a. Sherman JL, Barkovich AJ, Citrin CM: The MR appearance of syringomyelia: new observations. AJR 148:381–391, 1987.

24. Smith FW, Runge V, Permezel M, et al: Nuclear magnetic resonance (NMR) imaging in the diagnosis of spinal osteomyelitis. Magn Reson Imaging 2:53–56, 1984.

25. Spinos E, Laster DW, Moody DM, et al: MR evaluation of Chiari I malformations at 0.15T. AJNR 6:203–208, 1985.

26. Yeates A, Brant-Zawadzki M, Norman D, et al: Nuclear magnetic resonance imaging of syringomyelia. AJNR 4:234–237, 1983.

10

Gerald Mandell, M.D.

Radionuclide Imaging

Bone scanning (scintigraphy) is a noninvasive imaging modality that utilizes radiopharmaceuticals to detect pathophysiologic abnormalities in the skeletal system by virtue of its extreme sensitivity to any disturbance in vascularity or osteogenesis.

INDICATIONS

Skeletal scintigraphy contributes to the detection of neoplastic, infectious, ischemic, traumatic, degenerative, and even metabolic disorders of the spine.

LIMITATIONS

The major limitation of radionuclide imaging is the lack of specificity, since a number of bone disorders may have similar scintigraphic appearances. Thus, specificity of the scintigraphic interpretation depends greatly upon the incorporation of pertinent historical information, plain radiographic observations, and in some instances adjunct scanning with other imaging agents. A lesion must be metabolically active to be detected. Highly osteolytic lesions with little or no osseous reparative response, such as myeloma, may not be visualized. Radionuclide scans cannot usually detect disease processes limited to disc or cartilage tissues.

RADIOPHARMACEUTICALS

General Principles

Bone-seeking radiotracers are usually analogues of calcium, hydroxyl groups, or phosphates. Technetium-99m phosphates are the most widely used. Strontium-85 and strontium-87m, analogues of calcium, are no longer used because of the large radiation burden of the former and the restricted availability of the latter. The short half-life (1.87 hours) and the positron emission of fluorine-18, the hydroxyl analogue, limit its clinical application. Other radiopharmaceuticals, such as gallium-67 citrate, technetium-99m sulfur colloid, and indium-111–tagged white blood cells, can be used to image the spine to further define certain more specific pathologic processes.

Technetium-99m Phosphate

The technetium-99m phosphate compounds have evolved into the most widely used radiopharmaceuticals for bone scanning because of their wide availability, ease of preparation, excellent skeleton-to-background ratios, and rapid plasma clearance. The monoenergetic gamma rays (140 kilo electron volts [keV]) of technetium permit rapid high-resolution imaging on the scintillation camera, which is also called an Anger camera or a gamma camera. The relatively short half-life (6 hours) and lack of beta rays limit the radiation dose and permit imaging in both adults and children. Of all the technetium phosphate complexes, technetium-99m methylene diphosphonate (Tc-99m MDP) probably produces the best image because it clears rapidly from the plasma and has the shortest imaging time. Diagnostic imaging can be performed approximately 2 to 4 hours after intravenous injection. Approximately 50% of the administered dose is excreted by the kidneys.

503

The initial accumulation of technetium-labeled phosphates is determined by blood supply. Increased blood flow causes increased delivery of the isotope, and interference with blood flow reduces skeletal activity. Capillary permeability, reactive bone formation, metabolic activity, and increased tracer extraction efficiency are other factors contributing to the accumulation of the radiotracer at a site of abnormal bone. The initial mechanism of binding is the chemisorption of bone-seeking tracers to immature collagen, whereas subsequent binding is to bone crystal or to organic matrix.

Gallium

Gallium-67 citrate (gallium) can be used as an adjunct to bone scintigraphy in the detection of ongoing infection.[36] Gallium is cyclotron produced, with principal energy peaks of 93, 184, and 296 keV and a physical half-life of 77.9 hours. The intravenous injection of gallium results in its initial binding to plasma transferrin, lactoferrin, and some haptoglobin, with the subsequent transfer of gallium complexes to the cell surfaces of bacteria and neutrophils. Gallium also has an affinity with the intracellular protein lactoferrin and the lysozomes of neutrophils.[36] Migration of labeled white cells may also contribute to the detection of inflammatory processes such as cellulitis, septic arthritis, and osteomyelitis. Unfortunately, gallium is nonspecific and also binds to the lysozomes of tumors such as hepatomas and lymphomas.

During the first 12 to 24 hours, gallium is excreted from the body primarily by the kidneys (20% to 30% of administered dose in the first 24 hours).[53] The intestinal mucosa then becomes the major route of excretion, with some contribution by the liver, biliary tract, and spleen. In addition, normal accumulation may be seen in lacrimal glands, breasts, external genitalia, and salivary glands.

Delayed imaging (24 to 48 hours after injection) is sometimes helpful in differentiating mobile bowel activity from the stationary activity of an infectious or neoplastic focus. However, inflammatory lesions may be detected with early scanning prior to bowel activity (6 to 8 hours after injection) if the target to nontarget ratios are high enough. Renal activity persisting 24 hours after injection may be indicative of renal disease such as pyelonephritis, interstitial nephritis, tubular necrosis, or abscess.

The disadvantages of gallium scintigraphy include the nonspecificity mentioned previously as well as gallium's mimicry of the technetium phosphate compounds' ability to distribute in areas of bone formation. This increases the difficulty in diagnosis of postoperative infection at osseous sites, since there is activity at those sites normally. The overlap of hepatic-splenic activity with the lower thoracic–upper lumbar spine reduces the accuracy of interpretation of gallium scintigraphic images in this area. Another disadvantage is the increased radiation burden of this radiotracer because of its long half-life and relatively high energy.

Technetium-99m Sulfur Colloid

Marrow scanning can be used to identify marrow replacement by tumor, fibrosis, or bone infarction.[25] The most common imaging agent is technetium-99m sulfur colloid, which localizes predominantly in the reticuloendothelial system of the bone marrow. Marrow scanning can also be performed readily, without fear of excessive radiation burden, since the radioactive properties of the imaging agent are similar to those of technetium phosphate compounds used in bone scanning. Marrow scanning in adults is more limited than in children because marrow distribution is restricted to the skull, ribs, sternum, vertebral bodies, pelvis, and proximal femora and humeri. In the adult spine, marrow scanning is currently reserved for localization of tumor biopsy site. The younger the child, the greater the application of marrow scanning, since distribution of red marrow is more extensive. Primary or hematogenously spread neoplasms that replace bone marrow in children include neuroblastoma,[40] leukemia, lymphoma,[70] and Ewing's sarcoma. Neuroblastoma occasionally infiltrates the marrow without destroying bone, and thus marrow scanning predates radiographic and histologic evidence of disease.[25] Marrow scanning can help differentiate symmetric metastatic disease from normal activity and also can locate a suitable site for biopsy.

In chronic hemolytic anemia such as sickle cell disease, the scintigraphic appearance of acute infarction is a focus of photopenia on both bone and marrow scans.[1, 19] In osteomyelitis the bone scan is usually quite active. The marrow was originally purported to be normal in acute osteomyelitis, differentiating it from acute infarction. However, recent advances in imaging with computed tomography and magnetic resonance imaging have refuted the former claim by demonstrating alterations in marrow with infection.[21] Gallium scintigraphy may help differentiate infarction from infection because the affinity of bone for gallium is decreased in acute infarction and increased in infection.[4] Marrow replenishment can occur after bone infarction, chemotherapy, or irradiation of less than 3000 rad. Sometimes the defects in the marrow scan produced by fibrosis persist permanently.

Bone marrow scintigraphy does have some disadvantages. Technetium sulfur colloid uptake by the liver and spleen prevents the lower thoracic and upper lumbar areas from being satisfactorily evaluated. Metastases are not able to be detected in regions physiologically devoid of red marrow. The production of defects by fibrosis and metastasis reduces the specificity of marrow scanning.

Indium

Autologous and heterologous white blood cell scans with indium-111 oxine offer encouragement for the usage of a more specific, earlier localizer of pyogenic sites.[64] The white blood cell scan can specifically detect infection in bone, soft tissues, or joints, without localizing in noninfected nonunions, degenerative arthritis, heterotopic ossification, metabolic bone disease, and inactive chronic osteomyelitis.[64, 65]

Predominantly polymorphonuclear leukocytes are separated from venous blood, labeled with indium-111 oxine, and reinjected into the patient's blood stream. The labeling efficiency is approximately 75% to 99%.[64] Indium-111 is an accelerator-produced isotope with a physical half-life of 67.5 hours. The patient can be scanned up to 72 hours after injection. The peaks of activity are 173 and 247 keV, which is satisfactory for imaging on the scintillation camera. All white blood cell scans are initiated before antibiotic therapy. The sensitivity and specificity of the leukocyte scan are high, and the overall accuracy is 93%. However, very few reports of the usage of the indium-tagged white cells in osteomyelitis of vertebrae have appeared in the literature, and it is premature to predict the value of this study in this locale. Early reports indicated that the leukocyte scan was positive only in acute osteomyelitis and was not superior to gallium in the detection of chronic osteomyelitis.[1a, 64] A recent report indicated that indium-111 white blood cell scintigraphy was superior to sequential technetium-gallium scanning in the diagnosis of low-grade musculoskeletal sepsis.[52a] The sensitivity, specificity, and accuracy of indium-111 white blood cells was reported to be 83%, 86%, and 83% compared with 48%, 86%, and 57%, respectively, of the technetium-gallium combination.

Unfortunately, in most cases the results of the study take at least 18 to 24 hours to determine. When a patient is neutropenic, labeled donor white blood cells can be substituted satisfactorily. Activity normally is physiologically greatest in the spleen and liver. Visualization of the thoracolumbar junction area may present a problem because of the overlap of activity in the liver and spleen. Occasional false positive reports have appeared because of accessory spleens. Accumulation of activity can also occur in bowel infarction and inflammatory bowel disease. False positive pulmonary infection can be produced by embolized clumps of white blood cells resulting from poor preparatory techniques.[12] The adoption of indium-111 white blood cells as a routine study for evaluating osteomyelitis will depend upon development of a labeling technique that is inexpensive, readily available, and easily performed.

Indium can be compared with other radionuclides. Bone scanning with technetium-99mm phosphate compounds is sensitive but not specific for infection. Sometimes infection can be present with normal or photopenic bone scintigrams because of compromise of vascular supply (usually purulent material under pressure). Gallium, because of its affinity with bone, has not been very successful in the detection of concurrent infection in the reparative osseous state.

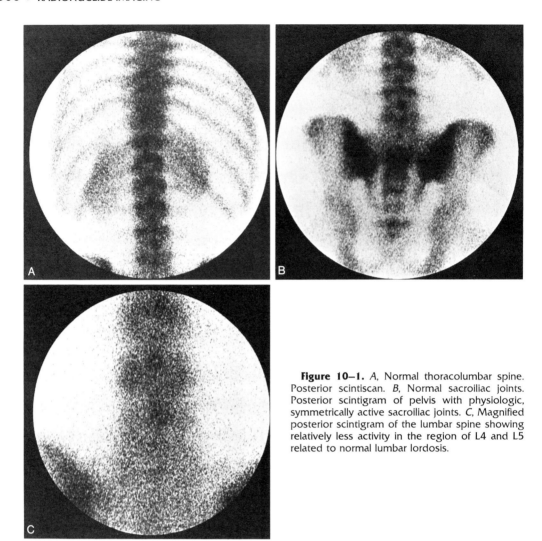

Figure 10–1. *A*, Normal thoracolumbar spine. Posterior scintiscan. *B*, Normal sacroiliac joints. Posterior scintigram of pelvis with physiologic, symmetrically active sacroiliac joints. *C*, Magnified posterior scintigram of the lumbar spine showing relatively less activity in the region of L4 and L5 related to normal lumbar lordosis.

TECHNIQUE

Technetium-99m Phosphate

The method of scanning varies according to the information desired. Adults receive 20 millicuries (mCi) of Tc-99m phosphate compound, such as Tc-99m MDP, intravenously in an extremity for routine bone scanning. In adults, the radiation dose to bone is approximately 0.7 rad (20 mCi). In children, the usual dose is 200 microcuries (μCi) per kg, and the radiation burden is from 0.3 to 0.5 rad (ages 1 to 15 years) with an administered dose of 200 μCi per kg.[72] Metaphyses with active bone formation receive approximately 6 times the radiation dose received by other portions of the immature skeleton. Fifty percent of the administered dose of

radioactivity is excreted by the kidneys. Two to five percent renal retention allows visualization of the kidneys on the bone scintigram. Hydration of patients is encouraged, and voiding prior to scanning is recommended to avoid obscuring the bony pelvis. Skeletal imaging 2 to 4 hours after injection of the radiopharmaceutical usually allows sufficient osseous uptake. Scanning is performed with a gamma camera that has a low-energy, all-purpose collimator, utilizing multiple spot or whole body format. Usually 500,000 counts are obtained per spot image.

The entire skeleton, except for hands and feet, is scanned for metastatic surveys. The spine is scanned posteriorly, and the pelvis is scanned both posteriorly and anteriorly (Fig. 10–1). Sometimes oblique and lateral views of the lumbar spine are taken to obtain

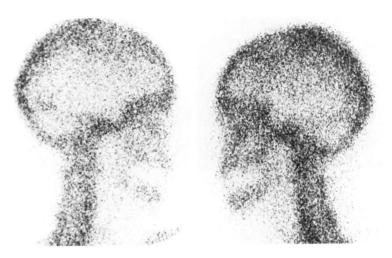

Figure 10–2. Normal scan. Left and right lateral oblique views of the cervical spine.

better visualization of the posterior elements. These additional views are of no value in the thoracic region, where rib activity is superimposed over thoracic vertebrae. The cervical spine is usually examined in the anterior and lateral oblique views as part of the skull examination on the metastatic survey (Fig. 10–2).

Selective pinhole imaging of areas of interest permits enhanced resolution and magnification. Pinhole imaging is quite applicable to focal lesions such as osteoid osteoma, spondylolysis, or pseudoarthrosis of a bone fusion.

Dynamic bone imaging may be added in evaluating a benign bone tumor or an infectious process of the spine.[51] The three-phase dynamic study consists of a radionuclide angiogram, an immediate extracellular space image (blood pool), and a delayed image.

Single photon emission computed tomography (SPECT) makes it possible to measure radioactive emission from different angles and, with the use of sophisticated software, SPECT makes possible the compilation of transaxial, coronal, and sagittal images of the spine.[41] With this method, a focus of increased activity can probably be localized to the pedicle, facet, lamina, transverse process, or spinous process. The time it takes for the examination is increased substantially with SPECT and, therefore, the relative benefit of the additional scintigraphic images remains to be seen. Certainly, because of the lack of anatomic specificity, it cannot sup-

plant the CT radiograph in transaxial imaging.

Gallium

Gallium-67 citrate is administered to adults in a dosage ranging from 3.5 to 5 mCi.[53] In children without malignancy, the standard intravenous dose is 30 to 50 μCi per kg. In children with known malignancy, the dose can be elevated to 50 to 100 μCi per kg. The imaging for the detection of inflammatory disease can commence as early as 6 to 8 hours after injection. Additional scintigrams should be performed at 24 and 48 hours after injection to allow for increased blood stream clearance when searching for tumor or when looking for infections in patients with an early negative or equivocal image. This improves target to nontarget ratios. Images typically consist of 250,000 to 500,000 counts and are collected on the scintillation camera with the medium-energy, parallel-hole collimator summating the major photopeaks (93, 184, and 300 keV).

Posterior images of the spine are most helpful. The pelvis is viewed anteriorly and posteriorly. The decision to use gallium should be carefully considered because of the significant radiation burden of this radionuclide. Adults receive 1.6, 1.9, and 1.5 rad to the liver, spleen, and skeleton, respectively. In children, radiation dose is 2.8 and 4.8 rad to the liver and spleen. It is strikingly higher in the metaphyses, where radiation doses from 2.1 to 21.6 rad have been estimated.[72]

Technetium-99m Sulfur Colloid

Marrow scanning with technetium-99m sulfur colloid is performed with an adult dose of 10 to 12 mCi. The children's dose (6.0 mCi per 1.7 m²) is twice the amount used in the liver-spleen scan.[74] The liver is the critical organ, receiving 0.2 to 0.4 rad per mCi. Imaging of the liver and spleen is performed with the low-energy, all-purpose, parallel-hole collimator on the scintillation camera 20 to 30 minutes after intravenous injection. The photopeak setting is at 140 keV. The time to collect a 200,000 to 300,000 count image of the anterior or posterior pelvis is used to obtain subsequent images of the spine, chest, or extremities. The liver and spleen should be lead-shielded to reduce their interference in imaging of the marrow. A complete study may take up to 2 hours owing to the extent of the marrow distribution in children.

Indium

With indium-111 white blood cell scanning, the medium-energy collimator is used, and the camera is set to summate the gamma emissions of 173 and 247 keV. In children, the recommended dose is 10 to 12 μCi per kg, with a maximum dose of 500 μCi.[27] Scanning can be performed as early as 6 hours and as late as 72 hours after injection.[64] The patient's venous blood is withdrawn in amounts of 40 to 80 ml (lower amounts in children), and the labeling process takes approximately 1.5 to 2 hours. The details of labeling are beyond the scope of this chapter and are described in the literature. Radiation exposure is high but acceptable in specific clinical situations. The spleen is the critical organ and receives approximately 18 rad per mCi in the adult. The radiation burden to the liver is 1 to 5 rad per mCi, and the whole-body dose is 0.5 rad per mCi.[27]

COMPLICATIONS

Radionuclide imaging is a safe procedure with a negligible risk of untoward reactions.

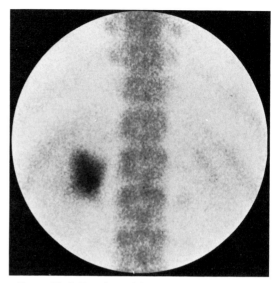

Figure 10–3. Two-hour delayed posterior image of the spine in a patient with low back pain. Increased activity in the left collecting system is seen, indicating a ureteropelvic obstruction. (Courtesy of Dr. S. Heyman, Philadelphia, Pennsylvania.)

The only contraindications to radionuclide scanning are pregnancy and breast feeding.

THE NORMAL BONE SCAN

In a normal patient, radionuclide uptake is evenly and symmetrically distributed throughout the skeleton (Figs. 10–1 and 10–2). In children, uptake is diffuse in the skeleton, with most of the activity in the metaphyseal growth regions, where bone production is the greatest. In the spine, the pedicles and posterior spinous processes are usually easily seen. The lordosis of the lumbar spine produces relatively less activity at the apex of the curvature on the posterior image because of the increased distance from the camera. There is usually symmetric increased activity in the sacroiliac joints.

The kidneys are readily visible on the posterior images of the lumbar spine. Urinary tract obstruction (Fig. 10–3) or renal tumor may be incidentally observed and could be the cause of the patient's back pain.

RADIONUCLIDE IMAGING IN SPINAL DISORDERS

Neck and Low Back Pain Syndromes

Degenerative changes in the bony spine are frequently detected by bone scan during

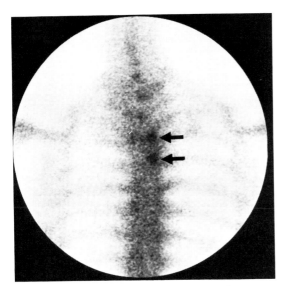

Figure 10–4. Posterior bone scan image of degenerative hypertrophic changes on the right side of T4–T5 and T5–T6 evidenced by eccentric foci of increased uptake (arrows).

the search for other disorders and could be mistaken for metastatic disease. The scintigraphic appearance of degenerative disease is mild to moderate increased uptake eccentrically placed and bridging two vertebrae (Fig. 10–4). The most frequent location of increased activity is in the cervical spine.[46] Plain radiographic correlation is necessary to differentiate increased uptake of degenerative disease from metastatic disease of the spine. Bone scanning plays no role in the detection of soft tissue abnormalities of the spine such as herniated disc.

Tumors and Tumorlike Conditions

Bone scanning is extremely sensitive in detecting the presence of malignant and benign tumors and tumorlike conditions. Any malignant or benign tumor is capable of producing an active bone scan.

Benign Lesions

Primary bone tumors and tumorlike conditions of the spine other than myeloma are infrequent and usually benign. Ten percent of osteoid osteomas occur in the spine, where 75% are located in the neural arch in the following order of frequency: laminae, facets, pedicles, and spinous processes.[39] Os-

teoid osteoma is one of the most scintigraphically active bone lesions because of its avid uptake of radiotracer (Fig. 10–5).[47] This allows detection of a very small nidus, which could go undetected by conventional radiography and conventional tomography.[49] The bone scan usually reveals a round, well-demarcated area of intense, increased activity (the nidus) and less intense surrounding activity (reactive sclerosis). This pattern is typical but not pathognomonic. Magnification views may also be included to identify the sometimes minute focus (Fig. 10–5). The hyperemia of the tumor is reflected by its increased uptake on the early angiographic and blood pool images. Once osteoid osteoma is located by spinal scintigram, computed tomography can be performed to evaluate its anatomic location and extent.[28] Bone scanning can also be utilized intraoperatively to locate the osteoid osteoma.

Scintigraphic differential diagnosis includes osteoblastoma,[39] aneurysmal bone cyst,[43] metastasis, and fracture, all of which may be very active and may not be differentiated from osteoid osteoma on the scintigram.

Osteoblastoma (Fig. 10–6) and aneurysmal bone cyst (Fig. 10–7) are two other disorders that involve the posterior elements of the spine[43] and may extend into the adjacent vertebral body. Osteoblastomas may calcify and are often destructive, and aneurysmal bone cysts are osteolytic and expansile. Plain radiographs and other imaging modalities may help differentiate and delineate these disorders.

Bone scanning is less sensitive than plain radiography in the detection of histiocytosis of the spine, with bone scan sensitivities varying from 35% to 94%.[61, 68, 71] "Cold" scintigraphic foci occur in 12% of patients and are usually located in the spine.[16] It may be difficult to detect these foci by radionuclide scanning because they are small, slow-growing lesions that have little effect on bone metabolism. Sometimes lesions can be relatively photopenic. Radiographic and scintigraphic skeletal surveys should probably be utilized concurrently in defining the distribution of histiocytosis (Fig. 10–8).[2]

Malignant Tumors

Metastasis. The most common use of bone scintigraphy is in the detection of metastatic disease. The bone scan is extremely sensitive

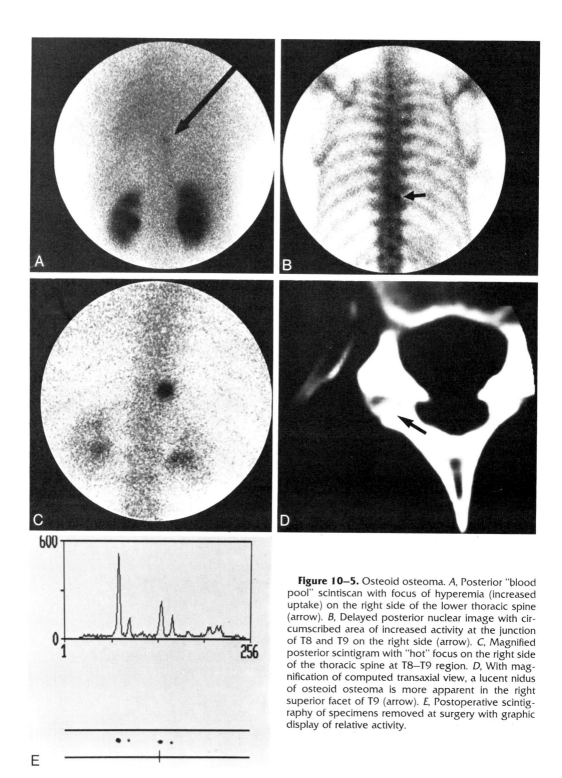

Figure 10–5. Osteoid osteoma. *A*, Posterior "blood pool" scintiscan with focus of hyperemia (increased uptake) on the right side of the lower thoracic spine (arrow). *B*, Delayed posterior nuclear image with circumscribed area of increased activity at the junction of T8 and T9 on the right side (arrow). *C*, Magnified posterior scintigram with "hot" focus on the right side of the thoracic spine at T8–T9 region. *D*, With magnification of computed transaxial view, a lucent nidus of osteoid osteoma is more apparent in the right superior facet of T9 (arrow). *E*, Postoperative scintigraphy of specimens removed at surgery with graphic display of relative activity.

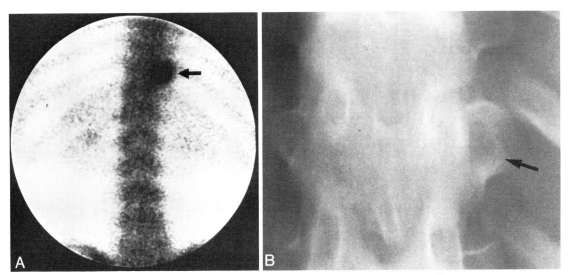

Figure 10–6. Osteoblastoma. *A*, Increased activity on the right side of T10 on posterior bone scan image (arrow). *B*, Linear tomographic view with lytic expansion of the left transverse process (arrow). Results of biopsy were consistent with osteoblastoma.

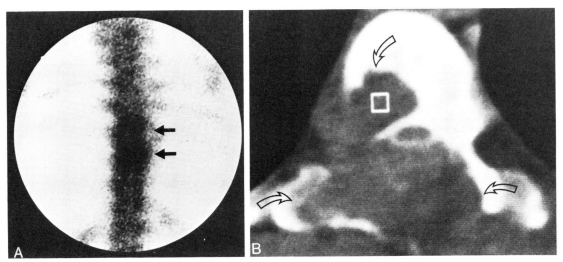

Figure 10–7. Aneurysmal bone cyst. *A*, Posterior scintigraphic image of the lumbar spine showing increased activity at T12 and L1 (arrows). *B*, Computed tomography (CT) demonstrating an expansile lytic process of an aneurysmal bone cyst in body and posterior elements of T12 (arrows).

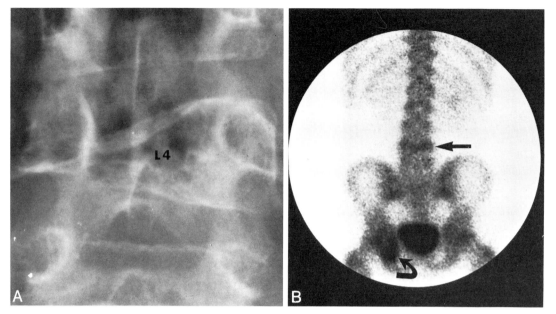

Figure 10–8. Histiocytosis. *A,* Posteroanterior radiograph of L4 with depression of the right side secondary to histiocytosis. *B,* Posterior scintigram with band of increased uptake at L4 (straight arrow). In addition, the left acetabulum is increased in activity secondary to another focus of histiocytosis (curved arrow). (Courtesy of Dr. S. Heyman, Philadelphia, Pennsylvania.)

in detecting osseous metastasis and has a false negative rate of only 2%. Conventional radiography, by comparison, has a false negative rate of 50% (Fig. 10–9).[56] Positive radionuclide scans can predate plain radiographic detection of metastasis by weeks or months, since approximately 30% to 50% of

calcium loss is necessary for plain radiographic appreciation of a metastatic lesion.[59]

The bone scan usually demonstrates multiple areas of increased radionuclide uptake, although single foci or increased uptake exists.[14] Eighty percent of all osseous metastases are located in the central skeleton,[44, 85]

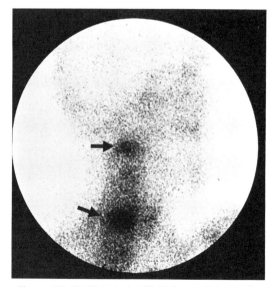

Figure 10–9. Metastasis. Multiple cervical vertebrae with increased uptake secondary to metastatic breast cancer (arrows).

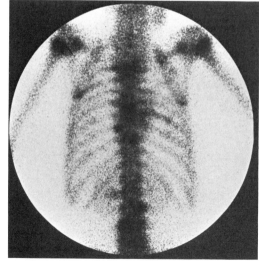

Figure 10–10. Metastasis. Diffuse metastatic involvement of vertebrae and ribs on posterior scintigraphic image in a patient with widely disseminated neuroblastoma.

with 40% of these in vertebrae, 29% in the ribs and sternum, and 11% in the pelvis. The remaining 20% are divided equally among the skull and extremities. Carcinomas of the breast, prostate, lung, kidney, and thyroid are the most frequent primary neoplasms that develop bone metastases in the adult. Carcinoma of the breast and prostate tends to metastasize predominantly to the axial skeleton.[78] Forty percent of patients with metastatic disease and positive bone scans have normal serum chemistries such as calcium, phosphate, and alkaline and acid phosphatase.[15] Thirty to sixty percent of patients with positive bone scans for metastasis are asymptomatic. Neuroblastoma is the most frequent tumor that metastasizes to bone in young children (Fig. 10–10).

Occasionally, in 15% of patients, metastatic disease can appear as a single focus, although a single site of increased activity on bone scan is most often related to benign disease, such as fracture, Paget's disease, infection, and other disorders.[14]

Detection of skeletal metastasis may obviate surgery, particularly in patients with carcinoma of the breast or lung. Patients who present with stage 1 and stage 2 breast carcinoma have positive scintigrams in less than 5% to 38% of cases.[56] Also, patients with stage 1 and stage 2 disease will ultimately develop bone metastases in 7% to 25% of cases. Five to thirty-five percent of patients with lung cancer will have osseous metastases detected at the time of initial diagnosis.[56]

Serial scans are excellent methods for following patients with breast carcinoma because 50% of patients will develop osseous metastases within the first year. Serial bone scanning is also a reliable way of following bone metastases in patients with advanced prostatic carcinoma.[62] In 6% of cases, there is a "flare" phenomenon in which the bone scan demonstrates increased radionuclide uptake in existing lesions in patients with concurrent clinical improvement.[63] This phenomenon is caused by increased blood flow at the site of tumor destruction associated with osteoblastic activity from reparative new bone formation.

Bone scintigraphy aids in localizing a lesion for biopsy, since the overlying skin can be marked during scanning. Bone scanning can also help define the portals for subsequent radiation therapy.

False negative bone scans in patients with bone metastases are due to slow growth of the lesion, minimal reactive bone formation, diffuse involvement throughout the skeleton, and obscuration of a pelvic focus by overlying radionuclide in the bladder.

Extreme care must be exercised on skeletal scintigraphy in the detection of metastases. Often slight blurring of the growth plate or a subtle change in intensity is indicative of metastatic disease.

Myeloma. Myeloma is the most frequent primary tumor of the spine in the adult and represents a disease with atypical findings on bone scintigraphy. There is a preponderance of osteoclastic activity coupled with relatively little osteoblastic response that results in a negative scan in about 40% of cases (compared with 25% for plain radiographs).[89] Many positive foci detected on the bone scan of patients with myeloma are related to superimposed pathologic fractures or impending fracture. Gallium scanning is less sensitive than radiography and bone scanning in patients with myeloma.[80]

Other Primary Malignant Tumors. Primary malignant tumors of the spine, other than myeloma, are rare. Radionuclide scanning can detect primary malignancies but cannot differentiate one from another. Radionuclide activity is markedly increased in the region of any primary malignant tumor. Ewing's sarcoma rarely occurs in the spine but, nevertheless, is the most frequent primary malignant tumor of the spine in children.[43] Ewing's sarcoma has increased uptake secondary to reactive bone formation. Osteosarcoma rarely involves the spine. Osteosarcoma may appear as a "hot" lesion owing to the excessive amount of tumor–new bone formation.

Superscan

Sometimes the distribution of disease is so widespread and uniform that the scan can be falsely interpreted as negative.[77] This so-called superscan results from relatively increased uptake of radiotracer by almost every bone in the body (Fig. 10–11).[59] This phenomenon can be detected in metastasis, renal osteodystrophy, myelofibrosis, and, less frequently, in Paget's disease and fibrous dysplasia.

The "superscan" phenomenon in patients

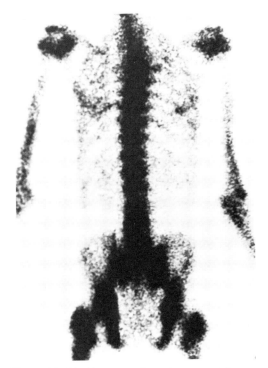

Figure 10–11. Metastasis. Posterior scan. Diffuse increased uptake of the axial skeleton as well as distal humeri and proximal femora in a patient with disseminated prostatic cancer. Note that visualization of the kidneys is faint with the "superscan."

with metastatic disease demonstrates uptake in the spine, pelvis, and proximal femora and humeri. Uptake in the kidneys and bladder is diminished or absent. This is due to

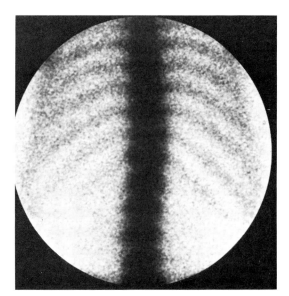

Figure 10–12. Superscan. Nonvisualization of the kidneys on a posterior scintigraphic image of the spine in osteomalacic patient with renal failure. The spine is diffusely increased in its activity.

a technical feature, most likely related to enhanced uptake by pathologic bone relative to normal uptake by normal kidneys and bladder. Prostatic carcinoma is the tumor that most frequently produces the superscan, but metastases from carcinoma of the breast, lymphoma, and leukemia may have a similar scintigraphic pattern. Patients with myelofibrosis, Paget's disease, and fibrous dysplasia who demonstrate a superscan also have diminished or absent renal activity on the bone scan. In renal osteodystrophy, the superscan phenomenon may be present, but renal and bladder activity are absent (Fig. 10–12).[76]

Recognition of the superscan by the lack of renal activity may be misleading. A false negative superscan may occur with diffuse bone metastasis and associated obstructed kidneys. A false positive superscan can develop in patients with renal failure. To avoid a misleading diagnosis of a superscan, a ratio of the radioactive uptake of T12 vertebral body to the uptake of adjacent soft tissues ("T12 index") has been generated from computerized skeletal images.[13] The highest ratios were recorded in the true superscan of disseminated bone metastasis from carcinoma of the prostate.

"Cold" Lesions

Bone lesions with decreased radionuclide uptake ("cold" or "photopenic" lesions) have been described with tumor, osteomyelitis, infarction, and irradiation. Metastatic disease is the most frequent cause of photon-deficient bone lesions, with 1% to 2% of osseous metastases in adults reported as "cold" on bone scintigraphy.[82] Carcinomas of the breast and lung are the most frequent primary tumors associated with photon-deficient metastatic foci (Fig. 10–13),[76] whereas neuroblastoma is the most frequent tumor to produce this phenomenon in children (Fig. 10–14).[82] Most photopenic lesions occur in the spine, where contrast with adjacent normal vertebrae enhances detection.

The photon-deficient areas most likely result from the combination of less bone mass due to bone destruction, lack of sufficient time for reactive response, and decreased blood supply secondary to infiltrating tumor, which compromises cortical nutrient vessels.[82] Replacement of marrow by tumor pro-

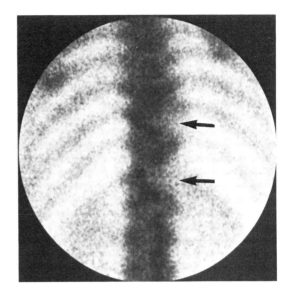

Figure 10–13. "Cold" lesions. Posterior scan of the spine demonstrating photopenic areas (arrows) on the right side of T10 and T12 in a patient with metastatic oat cell carcinoma of the lung. Renal activity is absent.

duces photopenia on marrow scans (Fig. 10–15). Other causes of decreased activity include avascular necrosis or infarction of bone, radiation therapy (Fig. 10–16), and artifacts. Infarction is frequent in the hemoglobinopathies—the decreased uptake is related to decreased perfusion and usually occurs in the acute phase of disease.[1] Acute infarction also devitalizes the bone marrow

(Fig. 10–17). Slight to moderate decrease in activity can be detected in portions of the skeleton included in radiation portals several months to years following radiation therapy.[88] Artifacts, such as belt buckles or metallic currency, may produce localized photopenia secondary to their blockage of detection of gamma rays by scintillation camera (Fig. 10–18).

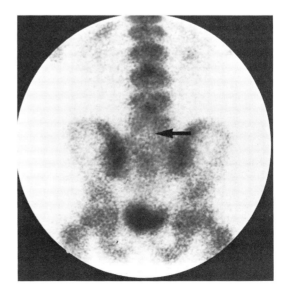

Figure 10–14. "Cold" metastatic lesion. Posterior scintigraphic image of the spine and pelvis. "Cold" lesion of metastatic neuroblastoma at the L5–S1 level (arrow).

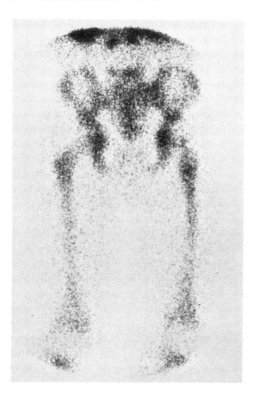

Figure 10–15. Photopenia of L4 and L5 on marrow scan representing replacement of marrow by metastatic Ewing's sarcoma in a 5 year old patient. (Courtesy of Dr. Aslam S. Siddiqui, Indianapolis, Indiana.)

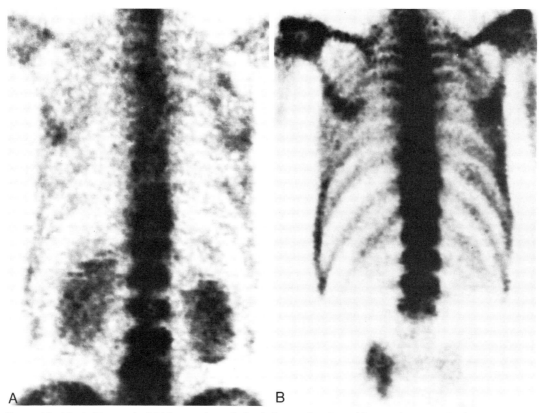

A   B

Figure 10–16. *A,* Metastasis. Initial posterior spinal scintigram showing widespread metastatic disease. *B,* "Cold" lesion. Photopenia of radiation portal to lower lumbar spine and right side of pelvis on posterior scintiscan of the spine.

Skull

Pelvis

Knees

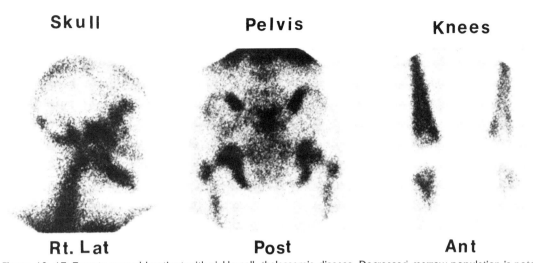

Rt. Lat

Post

Ant

Figure 10–17. Twenty year old patient with sickle cell–thalassemia disease. Decreased marrow population is noted in the lower spine, the distal left femur, and the right iliac bone. Bone marrow expansion is present in the base of the skull, the mandible, and the lower extremities. Bone marrow biopsy at this time revealed extensive necrosis. The patient was treated with intravenous fluids and recovered from the aplastic crisis. (Courtesy of Dr. Henry N. Wagner, Baltimore, Maryland.)

Paget's Disease

Paget's disease is usually detected incidentally in adults while the physician is searching for other disorders, or it is found in patients who have an elevated level of serum alkaline phosphatase. The scintigraphic appearance is dictated by the stage of disease.

Paget's disease is characterized histologically by an initial period of focal osteoclastic

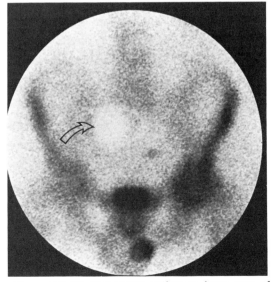

Figure 10–18. Photopenic artifact on bone scan of anterior pelvis caused by metal belt buckle (arrow).

activity resulting in bone resorption, followed by osteoblastic activity that results in new soft-bone production—bone produced in a disorganized manner.[26] Continued new-bone formation may lead to osseous enlargement and compression fractures in the spine.

Paget's disease is ideally suited for detection by bone scintigraphy, since both increased blood flow and increased osteogenesis occur in this disorder. The bone scan is more sensitive in detecting Paget's disease than plain radiography.[45] The early lytic phase is the most positive phase of the disease detected on bone scan. The mixed sclerotic and lytic radiographic lesion of healing pagetoid bone exhibits some increased activity but not to the extent of the purely lytic phase. In the totally sclerotic phase of Paget's disease, osteoblastic and osteoclastic activity may cease, and the bone scan may appear normal. Two thirds of all lesions are detected by both scintigraphy and plain radiography.[83]

The characteristic bone scan appearance of Paget's disease in the vertebrae consists of multiple or single areas of increased activity, which may be localized to the posterior spinous process or transverse process, appearing concurrently with an enlarged vertebral body (Fig. 10–19). This should help differentiate Paget's disease from metastasis. In addition, there are often large active areas in the calvarium and whole-bone involvement of the iliac and pubic

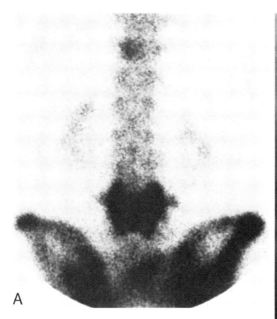

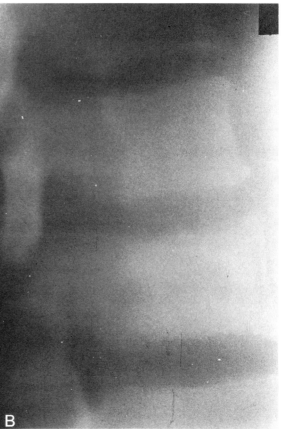

Figure 10–19. Paget's disease. *A,* Increased activity in the body, superior and inferior facets, and transverse processes of the L4 vertebra. The vertebra appears enlarged in the scintigram, and its appearance is compatible with the characteristics of Paget's disease. *B,* Lateral linear tomographic view of L4 showing thickened cortex and enlargement of the body—the appearance of Paget's disease.

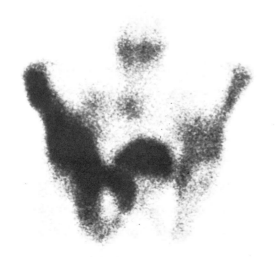

Figure 10–20. Paget's disease. On an anterior pelvic scintigraphic image, increased uptake is noted on the right iliac and pubic bones, which is indicative of Paget's disease. There is also increased activity in L5.

bones in Paget's disease (Fig. 10–20) These patterns are not usually found with metastatic disease. Plain radiographs should be correlated with the bone scan to confirm the diagnosis of Paget's disease.

Bone scintigraphy can be used to assess the response of pagetoid bone to calcitonin, diphosphonate, or mithramycin therapy.[79] With the assistance of computer technology, ratios of abnormal to normal bone can be generated for each area affected by Paget's disease. These results can be used to compare subsequent serial scans and objectively assess improvement. Bone scanning is useful in following patients who are in remission for recurrence, since an elevated serum alkaline phosphatase level may not be evident. Gallium-67 citrate is more accurate than technetium in assessing the response of Paget's disease to calcitonin.[81] Gallium scans improve concurrently with the reduction in the level of serum alkaline phosphatase.

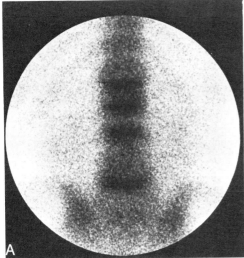

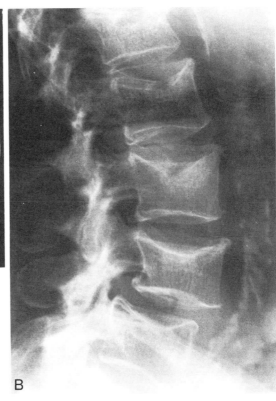

Figure 10–21. Osteoporosis. *A,* Multiple linear bands of increased activity on a posterior image representing compression fractures. *B,* Lateral radiographic view of the lumbar spine with superior end-plate indentations with adjoining sclerosis.

Sarcomatous degeneration in Paget's disease is rare and cannot usually be differentiated from the primary disease since both disease processes are active on bone scan. Recently, gallium-67 citrate scanning in conjunction with bone scanning was found to be helpful in the differentiation of the two processes.[90] Sarcomatous degeneration is suspected when the activity of gallium is greater than the bone scanning activity.

Metabolic Disease

Some of the metabolic diseases encountered include osteoporosis, primary hyperparathyroidism, renal osteodystrophy, and osteomalacia. In osteoporosis, bone scans are usually normal except when pathologic fractures occur, causing a linear band of increased activity in vertebrae (Fig. 10–21).

Diffuse symmetric increase of radionuclide uptake in the axial skeleton and long bones should suggest an underlying metabolic disorder, such as renal osteodystrophy, primary hyperparathyroidism, or osteomalacia.[10] There may be an additional increase in activity in the calvarium, mandible, sternum, patella, and wrist, producing the superscan appearance (Fig. 10–22).[24] The superscan of renal osteodystrophy (see Fig. 10–12) or osteomalacia can generally be differentiated from the superscan of diffuse metastasis or Paget's disease by the presence of activity in the bladder in the latter two disorders.[57] In osteomalacia, there are often associated pseudofractures of the ribs and scapulae, which present as additional focal areas of increased uptake (Fig. 10–22).

Many patients with metabolic bone disease can be differentiated from the normal population by increased skeletal to soft tissue ratios,[37] but there is a significant degree of overlap between normal patients and some patients with metabolic disease.[22] A value for whole body–bone radiotracer retention has been derived and is quite sensitive to the presence of metabolic disease.[23] More sensitive detecting methods using a whole-body monitor can differentiate patients experiencing conditions of increased bone turnover (renal osteodystrophy, osteomalacia, primary hyperparathyroidism) from the normal population.[23] Patients with osteoporosis could not be separated from the normal population by this method.

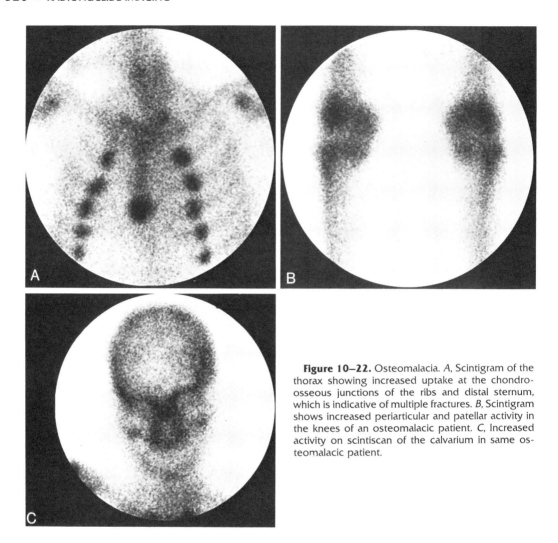

Figure 10–22. Osteomalacia. *A*, Scintigram of the thorax showing increased uptake at the chondro-osseous junctions of the ribs and distal sternum, which is indicative of multiple fractures. *B*, Scintigram shows increased periarticular and patellar activity in the knees of an osteomalacic patient. *C*, Increased activity on scintiscan of the calvarium in same osteomalacic patient.

Infection and Inflammation

Radionuclide scanning is ideal for the early detection of infection and inflammation in the spine, paraspinal regions, and sacroiliac joints. Initial scanning is usually performed with technetium-99m phosphate. If the scan is negative and suspicion of infection remains high, gallium is utilized. If the index of suspicion is very high at the onset, scanning may be initiated with gallium. At present, indium is reserved for problem cases.

Discitis versus Scheuermann's Disease

Discitis is inflammation of the intervertebral disc occurring in children and pre-sumed to be caused by blood-borne infection of low virulence. *Staphylococcus aureus* is the most frequent causative organism.[67, 84] Traumatic and viral etiologies have also been implied. The most frequent location is the lumbar spine, particularly L4–L5.

Early in the course of disease, plain radiographic examination may be normal. Disc narrowing may not occur until 2 to 4 weeks after initiation of symptoms (Fig. 10–23). Therefore, when there is clinical suspicion, bone scintigraphy plays an important role in early detection of this disorder.

The scintigraphic appearance is quite typical, with intense focal accumulation of activity in the disc space and in the two adjacent vertebral bodies. The scan may be positive as early as 9 days following onset of symptoms (Fig. 10–23).[6, 29] Gallium-67

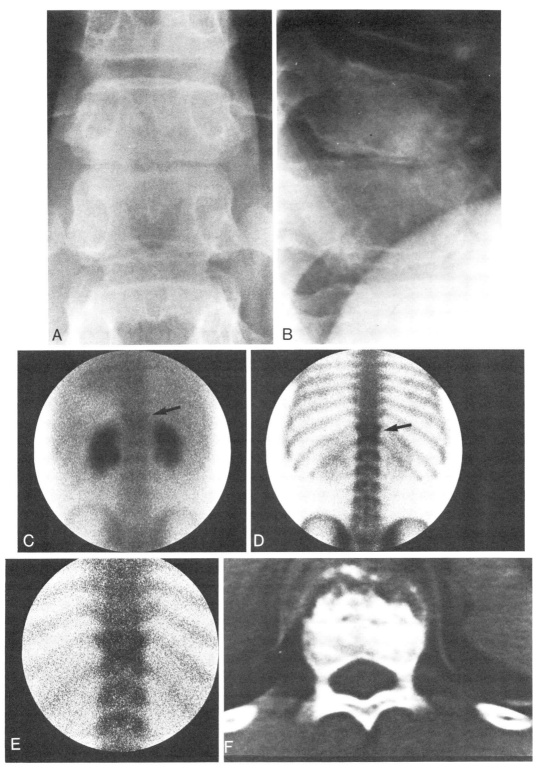

Figure 10–23. Discitis. *A, B,* Coned down anteroposterior and lateral plain radiographic views of T11–T12 demonstrating narrowed disc space and accompanying bilateral paravertebral soft tissue mass. *C, D,* Posterior scintigraphic "blood pool" (*C*) and delayed (*D*) images of the T11–T12 region displaying increased activity (arrows) of the two vertebral bodies and the intervening disc space characteristic of discitis. *E,* Magnified posterior scintigram of increased activity at T11, T12, and the intervening disc space. *F,* Computed transaxial tomographic image of a fragmented end-plate and associated soft tissue fullness of the vertebrae involved in discitis.

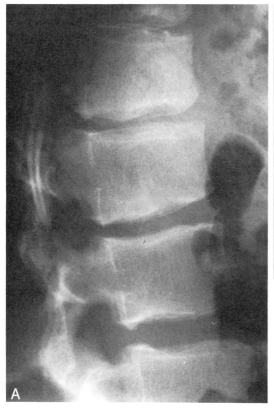
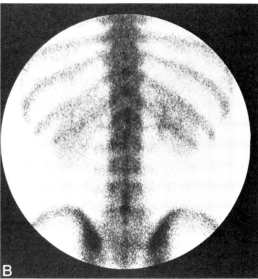

Figure 10–24. Scheuermann's disease. *A*, Lateral plain radiographic view of the lumbar spine with some irregularity of the end-plates, disc space narrowing, and anterior wedging of the upper two vertebral bodies. *B*, Normal posterior scintigraphic image.

citrate has also been used to demonstrate discitis. It has been extremely sensitive and specific, with an accuracy of 86%.[8] However, in most cases, bone scintigraphy is sufficiently diagnostic so that a gallium scan with its extra radiation burden is not necessary.

Scheuermann's disease (juvenile kyphosis) results from multiple, small focal herniations of disc tissue into adjacent vertebrae. In some instances, this disorder may present with plain radiographic changes similar to discitis, such as irregular endplates and disc space narrowing. However, the history of back pain is more prolonged and less well localized than with infection, and the bone scintigram, which should be reserved for problem cases, is uniformly negative (Fig. 10–24).[87]

Osteomyelitis

The bone scan is extremely sensitive in detecting early vertebral osteomyelitis, with positive findings predating radiographic alterations by several days to 1 week. The scanning pattern of osteomyelitis consists of localized increased radioactivity on both the immediate and delayed images and may be similar to that seen with neoplasm or fracture (Fig. 10–25). Clinical and plain radiographic correlations are necessary for proper interpretation of the bone scintigram. Computed tomography can help determine the extent of disease.

Acute osteomyelitis of the spine is rare in children[7] and more frequent in adults, even though osteomyelitis overall is more frequent in children.[57] In one series, 95% of children with subsequently confirmed early osteomyelitis had abnormal bone scans, whereas only 5% had abnormal plain radiographic findings.[20]

The sensitivity and specificity of bone scintigraphy in osteomyelitis are 95% and 92%, respectively, compared with plain radiography, which has 32% sensitivity and 89% specificity.[58] The specificity of scintigraphy increases with the addition of blood-pool imaging to the routine delayed images.[51]

In infants less than six weeks of age, bone

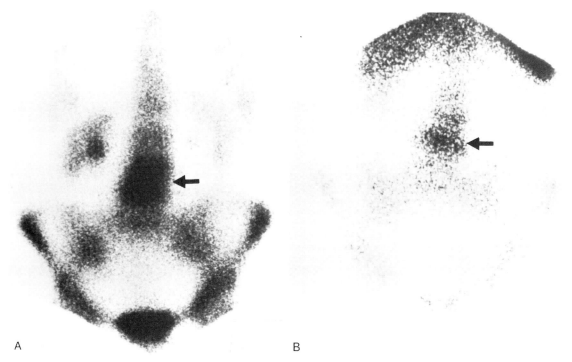

A   B

Figure 10–25. Osteomyelitis. *A*, Older patient with suspected osteomyelitis involving the lumbar spine. Anterior bone scintiscan displays increased uptake of L4 and L5 (arrow). *B*, Indium-111–tagged scan of white blood cells with accumulation of activity in same regions as bone scan is indicative of infection (arrow). (Courtesy of Dr. J. Ross McDougall, Stanford, California.)

scanning is not as sensitive, and only one third of the cases of osteomyelitis are positive on the phosphate scans.[5] Sometimes, in very early infection, relatively "cold" areas may appear and are related to vasospasm or the presence of purulent tissue under pressure.

Gallium-67 citrate should be administered in any patient with a negative bone scan who is highly suspected of having osteomyelitis. The images should be obtained within the first 24 hours, followed by delayed images up to 48 hours after injection. Gallium-67 citrate is often helpful in these situations because of its affinity with polymorphonuclear cells and bacteria.

Leukocytes labeled with indium-111 have been advocated recently in the detection of acute osteomyelitis (Fig. 10–25), but the reported cases have been mainly infected extremities. The usage of this radiotracer tagged to the white cell in the spine has not yet been reported sufficiently to estimate its sensitivity and specificity.

The normal uptake of isotope in the liver and spleen makes it difficult to detect infection in the lower dorsal and upper lumbar spine. To overcome this problem, a dual radionuclide subtraction technique combining indium-111–labeled leukocyte images and technetium-99m colloid liver-spleen scans is performed.[55] The infected area of the spine with its localized, actively tagged leukocytes is visualized once the activity of the technetium in the reticuloendothelial system is subtracted from the image. Indium-111 is very helpful in differentiating infection from metastases and traumatic lesions.

Sacroiliac Joints

Infection

The radionuclide scan is the imaging modality of choice for the early detection of infection of the sacroiliac joints. The bone scan demonstrates increase in isotope uptake most frequently in one joint (Fig. 10–26).[54] Plain radiographs are often negative in the early stages. Later, bone destruction about the sacroiliac joint could even be obscured on the plain radiograph by overlying bowel contents. Conventional tomography

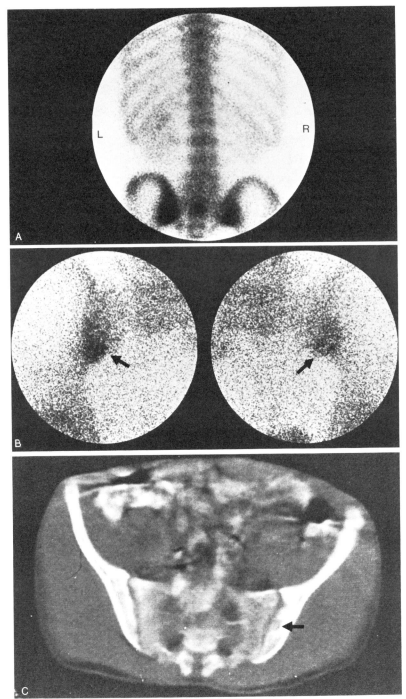

Figure 10–26. Osteomyelitis. *A,* Posterior scintiscan of the lumbosacral spine demonstrating increased uptake in the left sacroiliac joint in a patient with pain and fever. *B,* Gallium scintigraphy illustrates increased uptake in the left sacroiliac joint (arrows). Posterior scan (left); anterior scan (right). *C,* Computed transaxial image showing destruction of ilium caused by osteomyelitis along the left sacroiliac joint (arrow).

or computed tomography can demonstrate the degree of destruction if the plain radiographs are unrewarding.

Sacroiliitis

Asymmetry of isotope uptake in the sacroiliac joints may indicate an inflammatory disorder, and these changes are readily detected on the anterior and posterior pelvic scintiscans (Fig. 10–27). However, in some arthritides with bilateral, symmetric, increased uptake of activity (ankylosing spondylitis, Reiter's disease, and so forth), evaluation may be difficult.

Sometimes it may be difficult to differentiate normal sacroiliac joints from an infected or inflamed joint. This can be overcome by comparing the ratios of the peak count in the sacroiliac joint with the peak count in the sacrum. A modification of this quantitation method consists of evaluating the counts in the upper, middle, and lower portions of the sacroiliac joint and subtracting the soft tissue background activity (Fig. 10–28). This method is felt to be more sensitive in the detection of an abnormal sacroiliac joint. Some feel that at times it may be extremely difficult to separate controls from patients with sacroiliitis.[32] The procedure lacks sensitivity in detecting early stages of infection or inflammation in patients with minimal or absent plain radiographic changes.[18] Perhaps the sacrum is not the appropriate choice to serve as a neutral reference point for the sacroiliac joint to sacrum ratios since it too can be involved in the inflammatory process. The quantitation methods appear to need a more reliable reference point in order to establish a higher degree of sensitivity.

Trauma

Subtle or Radiographically Undetected Fractures

Bone scintigraphy is ideal for detecting fractures that may not be visible on plain radiographs because it is extremely sensitive to the hyperemia and osteoblastic activity occurring at a fracture site. Overlying bowel contents, which may obscure bone detail on the plain radiograph, do not interfere with bone scanning (Fig. 10–29). Compression fractures appear scintigraphically as linear bands of intense radioactivity (see Fig. 10–21). The etiology of the fracture (trauma, osteomalacia, or tumor) cannot be reliably determined from the scintigraphic pattern.

Ninety-five percent of fractures produce an abnormal scan 24 hours after the traumatic event. The optimum time for bone scintigraphy is 48 hours after the injury to assure more complete detection.[50] The scan could take up to 72 hours to become positive in osteopenic individuals over 65 years of age or in debilitated patients. The average

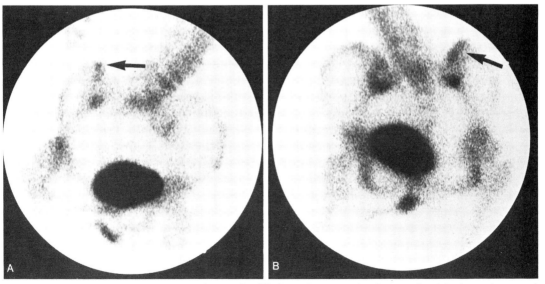

Figure 10–27. Sacroiliitis. Anterior (A) and posterior (B) views demonstrating increased uptake in posterosuperior portion of the right sacroiliac joint (arrow) in a patient with early Reiter's syndrome.

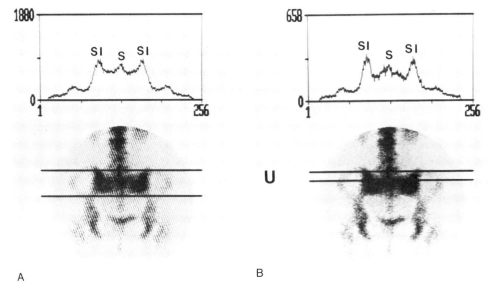

Figure 10–28. A, Wide-band profile slices of the full height of the sarcoiliac joints in a normal individual. Ratios are taken of peak sacroiliac joint (**SI**) uptake to the peak sacrum uptake (**S**). B, Triple-band profiles divide the sacroiliac joints into thirds. Illustration of the upper third (**U**).

time for a vertebral fracture to revert to a normal scan is 7 months. Ninety percent of all fractures return to a normal scan within 2 years.[50] Structural deformity, orthopedic fixation devices, and osteoporosis have a tendency to prolong the healing process.

Three characteristic stages of fracture healing have been described with bone scanning. The acute phase shows diffuse concentration of activity about the fracture site in the first 3 to 4 weeks after injury. The subacute phase consists of a linear collection of radiotracer at the fracture location in approximately 8 to 12 weeks of healing time. The third phase shows a gradual decrease of activity to normality.

Stress Fractures

Bone scanning plays an important role in the early detection of stress fractures. Stress fractures can be divided into fatigue and insufficiency fractures. Fatigue fractures occur when bones of normal elasticity undergo abnormal muscular stress (spondylolysis of the pars interarticularis).[86] Insufficiency fractures occur when normal physiologic stress is applied to bone with decreased elastic resistance (osteomalacia, osteoporosis, Paget's disease, fibrous dysplasia, and other disorders).[17]

There are various stages in the evolution of fatigue fractures involving the pars inter-

articularis that can be detected radiographically as well as scintigraphically and result from increasing levels of stress.[66] In an early stage, there is a poorly defined, slightly increased area of radioactivity that occurs during remodeling, when rapid osteoclastic resorption exceeds osteoblastic formation. At this stage, plain radiographs are normal, and cessation of physical activity reverses the process.[38] With continued stress, reactive bone formation reinforces the weakened osseous site. The bone scan exhibits a focal, well-circumscribed zone of increased activity. At this stage, the plain radiograph may be positive. Further continued stress results in bone exhaustion, inadequate reinforcement, and thus a cortical fracture. Therefore, the increased uptake of the radiotracer on the scintigram may predate the onset of fracture or lysis on the plain radiograph (Fig. 10–30).[30]

Thus, early detection by bone scan not only may prevent spondylolysis but helps determine the physiologic status of activity of a pars defect seen on the plain radiograph.

In some patients with a sclerotic pars interarticularis indicative of repeated stress, rest and nonparticipation in stressful activities allows the bone scan to revert to normal (average 7.3 months) and the patients to become asymptomatic (Fig. 10–31). Patients with a lytic defect in the pars interarticularis and associated increased uptake have also had bone scans revert to normal with ces-

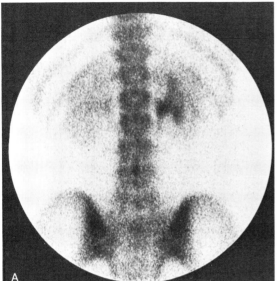
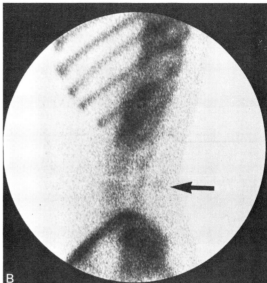
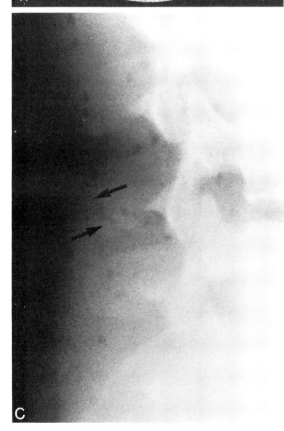

Figure 10–29. Patient with low back pain. *A,* Posterior scintigraphic image shows increased uptake in the posterior spinous process of L4. *B,* Lateral scintiscan with focal increased uptake in the spinous process of L4 (arrow). *C,* In orthoplast jacket, evidence of a linear fracture of the spinous process (arrows) on a plain radiographic image (lateral view).

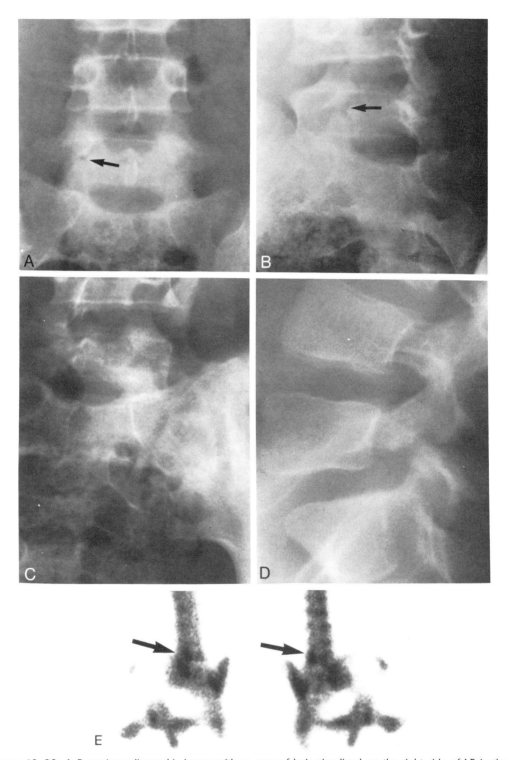

Figure 10–30. *A,* Posterior radiographic image with an area of lysis visualized on the right side of L5 in the pars interarticularis (arrow). *B,* Right posterior oblique radiograph. There is a defect in the pars interarticularis on the right (arrow). *C,* Left posterior oblique radiograph. There is no visible defect in the pars interarticularis on the left. *D,* Lateral radiographic view of the L5–S1 region demonstrating minimal slippage. A lucent defect in the pars interarticularis is noted. *E,* Posterior oblique scintigraphic images show increased uptake unilaterally on the left side (arrows), the opposite side of the radiographic defect.

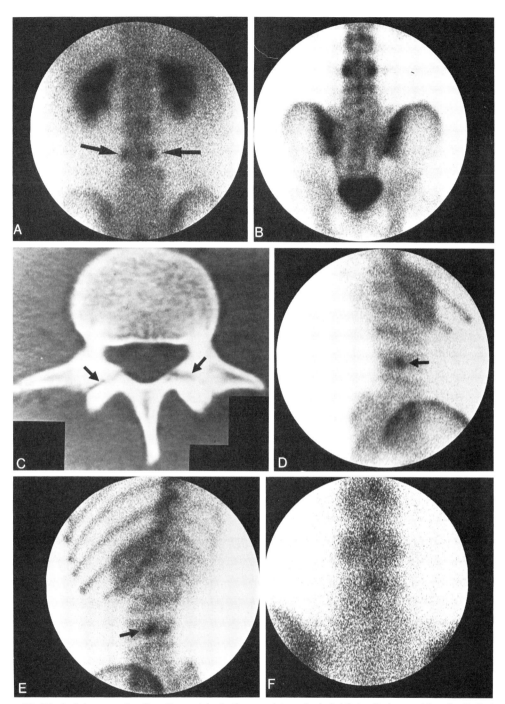

Figure 10–31. *A, B,* Increased radioactive uptake in the pars interarticularis bilaterally (arrows) in a football player on posterior scintigraphic "blood pool" (*A*) and delayed images (*B*) following acute trauma. *C,* Computed tomography demonstrating sharp linear defects representing bilateral fracture lines in the pars interarticularis (arrows). *D, E,* Left (*D*) and right (*E*) posterior oblique scintigraphic views with demonstration of increased activity bilaterally in the region of the pars interarticularis (arrows). *F,* After the patient rested for six months, the posterior image of the bone scan returned to normal.

sation of activities. Some feel that the scintigraphic findings in patients with spondylolysis do not correspond well to the radiographic findings.[30] This may be explained by stabilization of an old spondylolysis with normal bone metabolism (negative scan, positive radiograph) (Fig. 10–32) and an unapparent stress fracture (positive scan, negative radiograph).

Sometimes, the bone scan is positive on the side opposite the radiographic defect, implying stabilization of a spondylolysis in one pars and activity of a stress fracture in the contralateral pars (see Fig. 10–30).

Increased activity in the region of the pars interarticularis can be further localized with oblique views and SPECT (single photon emission computed tomography). The transaxial image of the spine on SPECT can more accurately localize a lesion in the anteroposterior plane (Fig. 10–33).

Most pars defects involve the fourth or fifth lumbar vertebrae and are rarely seen in patients under the age of five years. The incidence rises to 5% in children averaging 6.5 years.[86]

The most common demonstration of insufficiency fractures are compression fractures of the osteopenic spine (see Fig. 10–21). Bone scans are helpful in detecting stress fractures of the sacrum—an area difficult to evaluate on plain radiograph. A bow tie appearance has been described in stress fractures of the sacrum (Fig. 10–34).[48]

NONOSSEOUS RADIOPHARMACEUTICAL UPTAKE

During the examination of the axial portions of the skeletal scintigram for spinal aberrations, the bone-seeking agent may be visualized outside of the spinal column. The etiology of the extraosseous accumulation of activity may be physiologic, post-traumatic, postischemic, metabolic, neoplastic,[35] or artifactual.

Radiotracer is most frequently detected in normal kidneys and bladder following urinary excretion (approximately 50% of skeletal radiotracer is excreted in this manner). It is also deposited whenever there is excess tissue calcium, new collagen or osteoid formation, tissue necrosis, or altered vascular supply (ischemia).

It is interesting that 15% of urinary tract abnormalities are detected on bone scintigraphy and include bilaterally small kidneys with decreased uptake from end-stage renal disease and enlarged irregularly functioning kidneys from polycystic kidney disease or infiltration by tumor, such as lymphoma. Bilateral increased renal uptake occurs in nephrocalcinosis or in patients with metastatic calcifications from hypercalcemia and uremia,[3] acute bilateral urinary obstruction,[69] acute tubular necrosis, and interstitial inflammatory change produced by toxins[42] or radiation[88] (Fig. 10–35). Sickle cell disease in children may demonstrate renal find-

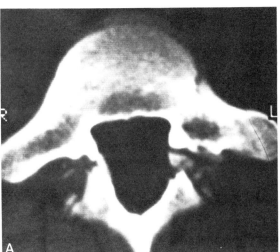
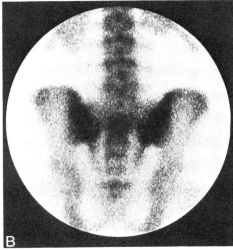

Figure 10–32. A, Computed tomography of L5 with areas of lysis and fragmentation of the pars interarticularis bilaterally. B, Normal bone scan of L5 implying stabilization of previous spondylolyses.

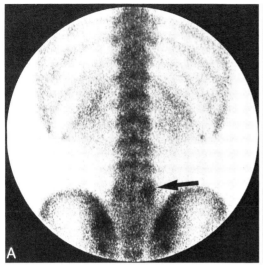

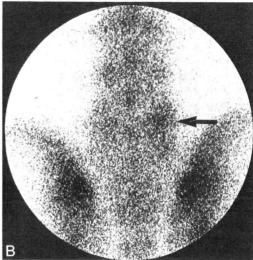

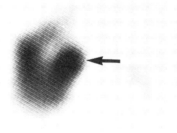

Figure 10–33. *A*, Subtle increase in activity on the right side of L5 (arrow) on a posterior scintigram. *B*, Magnified posterior image again showing increased activity on the right side (arrow). *C*, Single photon emission computed tomographic transaxial (SPECT) imaging shows increased activity adjacent to the region of the transverse process (arrow) posterior to the vertebral body.

C

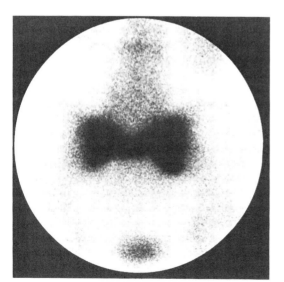

Figure 10–34. Posterior scintiscan of the sacrum with increased activity in the center mimicking a bow tie appearance. (Courtesy of Dr. J. Morales, Philadelphia, Pennsylvania.)

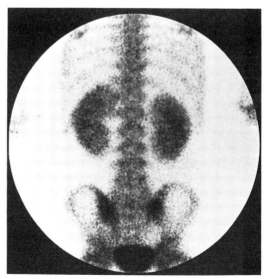

Figure 10–35. Bilaterally enlarged kidneys with increased uptake secondary to chemotherapy visualized on posterior scintigraphic image of the spine.

ings on the bone scan similar to acute tubular necrosis.[73] Iron overload from repeated transfusions, hemochromatosis, or iron supplement causes increased deposition of iron in soft tissues and delay of osseous uptake, leading to increased renal excretion.[9, 11, 60] Focal areas of increased uptake may be due to overlying rib or stasis in the upper pole collecting system. Focal decrease in uptake is usually caused by tumor, cyst, abscess, or metastatic disease. Congenital anomalies such as absent kidney, ectopic kidney, or horseshoe kidney (Fig. 10–36) are easily recognized. Patients undergoing chronic renal dialysis usually exhibit little renal function.[75]

Technetium-phosphate complexes may accumulate in tumors such as neurofibroma, hamartoma, lipoma, desmoid, mucinous carcinomas, carcinoma of the lung, and particularly neuroblastoma in children (Fig. 10–37). Metastatic pulmonary nodules from osteosarcoma concentrate radionuclide because of their osteoid formation.

Artifactual causes of extraskeletal radionuclide activity include urine contamination, equipment contamination, infiltrated injection site, and poorly prepared radiopharmaceutical.

INTRAOPERATIVE SCANNING

Radionuclide scanning may be used to detect lesions intraoperatively. The treat-

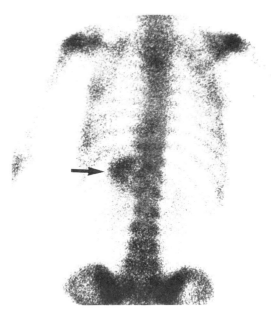

Figure 10–37. Extraosseous uptake in primary left suprarenal tumor, neuroblastoma (arrow), in a child surveyed for metastatic disease.

ment of osteoid osteoma usually consists of en bloc excision of the nidus and surrounding bone. Bone scintigraphy allows intraoperative control with accurate localization and, therefore, minimal bone resection, thus avoiding instability in the postoperative result.[31]

Several methods are utilized to achieve intraoperative control. The portable gamma camera can be moved to the operating suite after the patient has been injected with technetium-phosphate compound. The lesion is located during the operation. Following resection, the area can be scanned to assure complete removal of the lesion. The major disadvantages of this technique are the bulkiness of equipment in the operating room and the difficulty in positioning the detector over the operative field. An alternative is to place a small sterilized probe with a 1 inch diameter collimator directly through the incision and upon the bone. The probe is attached to a count rate meter. Prior to the operation, the count ratio of the abnormal to the normal bone is obtained. These statistics are then utilized on the operating table to help localize the lesion. Postoperative counting of the operative site will assure the removal of the entire lesion, and the postoperative counting of the specimens will assist the pathologist in locating the nidus (see Fig. 10–5).

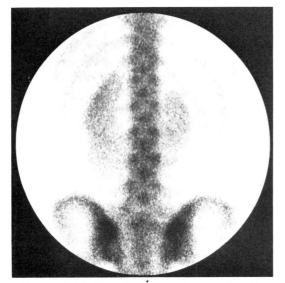

Figure 10–36. Horseshoe kidney discovered incidentally on a bone scan in a patient with back pain.

POSTOPERATIVE SCANNING

Pseudoarthrosis

Bone scintigraphy plays an important role in identifying the location of a postfusion pseudoarthrosis which is often difficult to detect on the plain radiograph (Fig. 10–38).[34] Pseudoarthroses represent nonunion of spinal fusion. This fusion procedure is performed in spondylolisthesis, in children with scoliosis and very progressive curvatures, and other disorders.

In general, mature bone graft is less active scintigraphically than the surrounding spine. However, in some patients with scoliosis, a small area of increased activity has been detected around Harrington hooks, but the hooks have been found to be firmly implanted (Fig. 10–39).[34] In patients with proven pseudoarthroses, approximately two thirds had increased activity on bone scan.[34]

The most accurate scans are obtained 1 year following surgery since there is a large amount of new bone still present six months after fusion, making interpretation diffi-

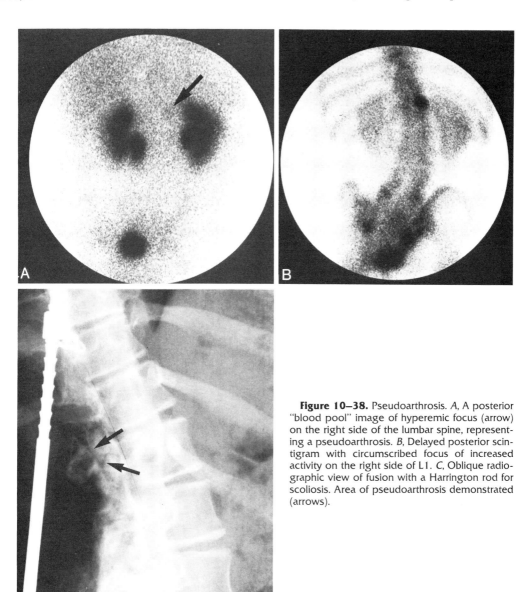

Figure 10–38. Pseudoarthrosis. *A*, A posterior "blood pool" image of hyperemic focus (arrow) on the right side of the lumbar spine, representing a pseudoarthrosis. *B*, Delayed posterior scintigram with circumscribed focus of increased activity on the right side of L1. *C*, Oblique radiographic view of fusion with a Harrington rod for scoliosis. Area of pseudoarthrosis demonstrated (arrows).

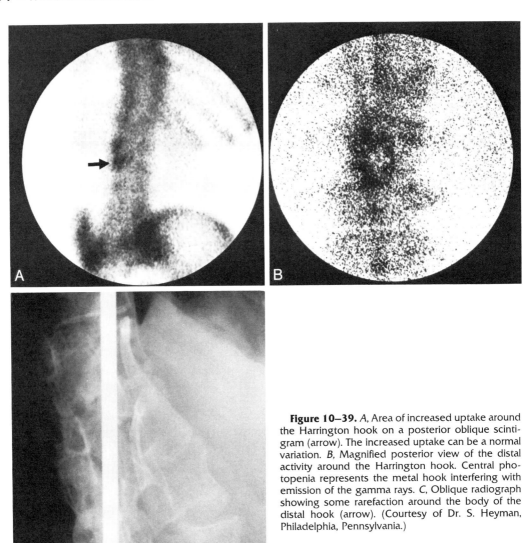

Figure 10–39. *A,* Area of increased uptake around the Harrington hook on a posterior oblique scintigram (arrow). The increased uptake can be a normal variation. *B,* Magnified posterior view of the distal activity around the Harrington hook. Central photopenia represents the metal hook interfering with emission of the gamma rays. *C,* Oblique radiograph showing some rarefaction around the body of the distal hook (arrow). (Courtesy of Dr. S. Heyman, Philadelphia, Pennsylvania.)

cult.[52] Movement of the site of pseudoarthrosis evokes a reactive bone response. Without the diffuse activity of reparative new bone, the local osteoblastic response of pseudoarthrosis with its increased activity becomes apparent. In many patients with pseudoarthrosis, the bone scan may become normal after a few years.[33] In patients with scoliosis and surgical fusion, there is slightly more activity on the convex side than on the concave side of the curvature, although there is no difference in the degree of healing or fusion.

DUAL PHOTON ABSORPTIOMETRY

Dual photon absorptiometry is a method by which the bone mineral content in the axial skeleton (particularly the lumbar spine) can be measured. It is based on measurements of the radiation transmission of two separate photoelectric peaks (gamma rays) through two different tissues, namely soft tissue and bone.[30a, 78a] Gadolinium-153 is utilized as the external energy source and has photoelectric peaks at about 44 keV and 100 keV. The patient lies in a supine position on the table, and the shielded radionuclide source is contained beneath the table. The 44 keV and 100 keV photons emitted by the radionuclide source are attenuated as they pass through the patient's body. A collimated, shielded scintillation detector (NaI crystal) is coupled to a single photomultiplier tube. A whole-body rectilinear scan of the lumbar spine is then performed.[78a] The advantages of dual photon absorptiometry are the direct measurement of axial bone mineral content, its high degree of accuracy and reproducibility,[30a] and the long half-life of gadolinium-153, which need be replaced only once a year.

The disadvantage of dual photon absorptiometry is that both cancellous and cortical bone are measured. Because cancellous bone is metabolically more active, measurement for mineral content in the spine should ideally be that of cancellous bone. Also, osteophytes of the vertebral body and articular processes, subchondral sclerosis, extraosseous calcification, and overlying barium in the gastrointestinal tract may cause inaccurate vertebral mineral measurements.[30a]

References

1. Alavi A, Bond, JP, Kuhl DE, et al: Scan detection of bone marrow infarcts in sickle cell disorders. J Nucl Med 15:1003–1007, 1974.
1a. Al-Sheikh W, Sfakianakis GN, Mnaymneh W, et al: Subacute and chronic bone infections: diagnosis using In-111, Ga-67 and Tc-99m MDP bone scintigraphy and radiography. Radiology 155:501–506, 1985.
2. Antonmattei S, Tetalman, R, Lloyd TV: The multiscan appearance of eosinophilic granuloma. Clin Nucl Med 4:53–55, 1979.
3. Arbona GL, Antonmattei S, Tetalman MR, et al: Tc-99m-diphosphonate distribution in a patient with hypercalcemia and metastatic calcifications. Clin Nucl Med 5:422, 1980.
4. Armas RR, Goldsmith SJ: Gallium scintigraphy in bone infarction: correlation with bone imaging. Clin Nucl Med 9:1–3, 1984.
5. Ash JM, Gilday DL: The futility of bone scanning in neonatal osteomyelitis. J Nucl Med 21:417–420, 1980.
6. Atkinson RN, Paterson DC, Morris LL, et al: Bone scintigraphy in discitis and related disorders in children. Aust NZ J Surg 48:374–377, 1978.
7. Bolivar R, Kohl S, Pickering LK: Vertebral osteomyelitis in children: Report of four cases. Pediatrics 62:549–553, 1978.
8. Bruschwein DA, Brown ML, McLeod RA: Gallium scintigraphy in the evaluation of disk-space infections: concise communication. J Nucl Med 21:925–927, 1980.
9. Byun HH, Rodman SG, Chung KE: Soft-tissue concentration of 99mTc-phosphates associated with injections of iron dextran complex. J Nucl Med 17:374–375, 1976.
10. Cheng TH, Holman BL: Increased skeletal:renal uptake ratio. Radiology 136:455–459, 1980.
11. Choy D, Murray IC, Hoschi R: The effect of iron on the biodistribution of bone-scanning agents in humans. Radiology 140:197–202, 1981.
12. Coleman RE, Welch D: Possible pitfalls with clinical imaging of indium-111 leukocytes: concise communication. J Nucl Med 21:122–125, 1980.
13. Constable AR, Crange RW: Recognition of the superscan in prostatic bone scintigraphy. Brit J Radiol 54:122–125, 1981.
14. Corcoran RJ, Thrall JH, Kyle RW, et al: Solitary abnormalities in bone scans of patients with extraosseous malignancies. Radiology 121:663–667, 1976.
15. Cowan RJ, Young KA: Evaluation of serum alkaline phosphate determination in patients with positive bone scans. Cancer 32:887–889, 1973.
16. Crone-Munzebrock W, Brassow F: A comparison of radiographic and bone scan findings in histiocytosis X. Skel Radiol 9:170–173, 1983.
17. Daffner RH. Stress fractures. Current concepts. Skel Radiol 2:221–229, 1978.
18. Dequeker J, Goddeeris T, Walravens M, et al: Evaluation of sacro-iliitis: comparison of radiological and radionuclide techniques. Radiology 128:687–689, 1978.
19. Dibos PE, Judisch JM, Spaulding MB, et al: Scanning the reticuloendothelial system (RES) in hematologic diseases. Johns Hopkins Med J 130:68–82, 1972.
20. Duszynski DO, Kuhn JP, Afshani, E, et al: Early radionuclide diagnosis of acute osteomyelitis. Radiology 117:337–340, 1975.
21. Fletcher BD, Scoles PV, Nelson AD: Osteomyelitis in children. Detection by magnetic resonance: work in progress. Radiology 150:57–60, 1984.
22. Fogelman I, Bessent RG, Gordon D: A critical assessment of bone scan quantitation (bone-to-soft-tissue ratios) in the diagnosis of metabolic bone disease. Eur J Nucl Med 6:93–97, 1981.
23. Fogelman I, Bessent RG, Turner JG, et al: The use of whole-body retention of 99m-Tc-diphosphonate in the diagnosis of metabolic bone disease. J Nucl Med 19:270–275, 1978.
24. Fogelman I, Carr D: Comparison of bone scanning and radiology in the evaluation of patients with metabolic bone disease. Clin Radiol 31:321–326, 1980.
25. Fordham EW: Radionuclide imaging of bone marrow. Semin Hematol 18:222–239, 1981.
26. Frame B, Marel GM: Paget Disease: A review of current knowledge. Radiology 141:21–24, 1981.
27. Gainey MA, McDougall IR: Diagnosis of acute inflammatory conditions in children and adolescents using In-111 oxine white blood cells. Clin Nucl Med 9:71–74, 1984.
28. Gamba JL, Martinez S, Apple J, et al: Computed

tomography of axial skeletal osteoid osteomas. AJR 142:769–772, 1984.

29. Gates GF: Scintigraphy of discitis. Clin Nucl Med 2:20–25, 1977.

30. Gelfand MJ, Strife JL, Kereiakes JG: Radionuclide bone imaging in spondylolysis of the lumbar spine in children. Radiology 140:191–195, 1981.

30a. Genant HK, Cann CE: Spinal osteoporosis: advanced assessment using quantitative computed tomography. In Genant HK, et al (eds): Spine Update 1984. San Francisco: Radiology Research and Education Foundation, 1983.

31. Ghelman B, Thompson FM, Arnold WD: Intraoperative radioactive localization of an osteoid osteoma: case report. J Bone Joint Surg 63A:826–827, 1981.

32. Goldberg RP, Genant HK, Shimshak R, et al: Applications and limitations of quantitative sacroiliac scintigraphy. Radiology 128:683–686, 1978.

33. Hannon KM, Wetta WJ: Failure of technetium bone scanning to detect pseudoarthrosis in spinal fusion for scoliosis. Clin Orthop 123:42–44, 1977.

34. Harcke HT, Larkin M, Clancy M: Evaluation of spinal fusions by bone scintigraphy. J Nucl Med 21:9, 1980. (Abstract)

35. Heck LL: Extraosseous localization of phosphate bone agents. Semin Nucl Med 10:311–313, 1980.

36. Hoffer P: Gallium mechanisms. J Nucl Med 21:282–285, 1980.

37. Holmes RA: Quantification of skeletal Tc-99m labeled phosphates to detect metabolic bone disease. [Editorial]. J Nucl Med 19:330–331, 1978.

38. Jackson DW, Wiltse LL, Dingeman RD, et al: Stress reactions involving the pars interarticularis in young athletes. Am J Sports Med 9:304–312, 1981.

39. Jackson RP, Reckling FW, Mants FA: Osteoid osteoma and osteoblastoma: similar histologic lesions with different natural histories. Clin Orthop 128:303–313, 1977.

40. Judisch JM, McIntyre PA: Recognition of metastatic neuroblastoma by scanning reticuloendothelial system (RES). Johns Hopkins Med J 130:83–86, 1972.

41. Keyes JW Jr: Perspectives on tomography. J Nucl Med 23:633–640, 1982.

42. Koizumi K, Tonami N, Hisada K: Diffusely increased Tc-99m MDP uptake in both kidneys. Clin Nucl Med 6:362–365, 1981.

43. Kozlowski K, Beluffi G, Masel J, et al: Primary vertebral tumours in children. Report of 20 cases with brief literature review. Pediatr Radiol 14:129–139, 1984.

44. Krishnamurthy GT, Tubis M, Hiss J, et al: Distribution pattern of metastatic bone disease. A need for total body skeletal image. JAMA 237:2504–2506, 1977.

45. Lentle BC, Russell AS, Heslip PG, et al: The scintigraphic findings in Paget's disease of bone. Clin Radiol 27:129–135, 1976.

46. Lin DS, Alavi A: Bone scan evaluation of degenerative joint disease of the spine. Int J Nucl Med Biol 9:63–64, 1982.

47. Lisbona R, Rosenthall L: Role of radionuclide imaging in osteoid osteoma. AJR 132:77–80, 1979.

48. Lourie H: Spontaneous osteoporotic fracture of the sacrum: an unrecognized syndrome of the elderly. JAMA 248:715–717, 1982.

49. Lutrin CL, McDougall R, Goris ML: Intense concentration of technetium-99m-methylene pyrophosphate in the kidneys of children treated with chemotherapeutic drugs for malignant disease. Radiology 128:165–167, 1978.

50. Matin P: The appearance of bone scan following fractures including intermediate and long-term studies. J Nucl Med 20:1227–1231, 1979.

51. Maurer AH, Chen DC, Camargo EE, et al: Utility of three phase skeletal scintigraphy in suspected osteomyelitis: concise communication. J Nucl Med 22:941–949, 1981.

52. McMaster MJ, Merrick MV: The scintigraphic assessment of the scoliotic spine after fusion. J Bone Joint Surg 62B:65–72, 1980.

52a. Merkel KD, Brown ML, Dewanjee MK, et al: Comparison of indium-labeled-leukocyte imaging with sequential technetium-gallium scanning in the diagnosis of low-grade musculoskeletal sepsis: a prospective study. J Bone Joint Surg 76A:465–476, 1985.

53. Mettler FA Jr, Guiborteau MJ: Essentials of Nuclear Medicine. New York: Grune & Stratton, 1983, pp 264–268.

54. Miller JH, Gates GT: Scintigraphy of sacroiliac pyarthrosis in children. JAMA 238:2701–2704, 1977.

55. Mountford PJ, Coakley AJ, Hall FM, et al: Dual radionuclide subtraction imaging of vertebral disc infection using an 111 In-labeled leukocyte scan and a 99mTc-tin colloid scan. Eur J Nucl Med 8:557–558, 1983.

56. Muroff LR: Optimizing the performance and interpretation of bone scans. Clin Nucl Med 6:68–76, 1981.

57. Musher DM, Thorsteinsson SB, Minuth JN: Vertebral osteomyelitis: still a diagnostic pitfall. Arch Intern Med 136:105–110, 1976.

58. Nelson HT, Taylor A: Bone scanning in the diagnosis of acute osteomyelitis. Eur J Nucl Med 5:267–269, 1980.

59. Osmond JD, Pendergrass HP, Potsaid MS: Accuracy of Tc99m-diphosphonate bone scans and roentgenograms in the detection of prostate, breast, and lung carcinoma metastases. AJR 125:972–977, 1975.

60. Parker JA, Jones AG, Davis MA, et al: Reduced uptake of bone-seeking radiopharmaceuticals related to iron excess. Clin Nucl Med 1:267–268, 1976.

61. Parker BR, Pinckney L, Etcubanas E: Relative efficacy of radiographic and radionuclide bone surveys in detection of skeletal lesions of histiocytosis X. Radiology 134:377–380, 1980.

62. Pollen JJ, Gerber K, Ashburn WL, et al: Nuclear bone imaging in metastatic cancer of the prostate. Cancer 47:2585–2594, 1981.

63. Pollen JJ, Witztum KF, Ashburn WL: The flare phenomenon on radionuclide bone scan in metastatic prostate cancer. AJR 142:773–776, 1984.

64. Propst-Proctor SL, Dillingham MF, McDougall IR, et al: The white blood cell scan in orthopedics. Clin Orthop 168:157–165, 1982.

65. Raptopoulos V, Doherty PW, Goss TP, et al: Acute osteomyelitis: advantage of white cell scans in early detection. AJR 139:1077–1082, 1982.

66. Roub LW, Gumerman LW, Hanley EN Jr, et al: Bone stress: a radionuclide imaging perspective. Radiology 132:431–438, 1979.

67. Sartoris DJ, Moskowitz PS, Kaufman RA, et al: Childhood diskitis: computed tomographic findings. Radiology 149:701–707, 1983.

68. Schaub T, Eissner D, Hahn K, et al: Bone scanning in detection and follow-up of skeletal lesions in histiocytosis X. Ann Radiol 28:407–410, 1983.

69. Siddiqui AR: Gamut: Increased uptake of technetium-99m labeled bone imaging agents in the kidneys. Semin Nucl Med 12:101–102, 1982.

70. Siddiqui AR, Oseas RS, Wellman HN, et al: Evaluation of bone marrow scanning with technetium-99m sulfur colloid in pediatric oncology. J Nucl Med 20:379–386, 1979.

71. Siddiqui AR, Tashjian JH, Lozarus K, et al: Nuclear medicine studies in evaluation of skeletal lesions in children with histiocytosis X. Radiology 140:787–789, 1981.

72. Silberstein EB: Bone Scintigraphy. Mount Kisco, New York: Futura Publishing Co 1983, pp 77–93.

73. Sty JR, Babbitt DP, Sheth K: Abnormal Tc-99m-methylene disphosphonate accumulation in the kidneys of children with sickle cell disease. Clin Nucl Med 5:445–447, 1980.

74. Sty JR, Starshak RJ, Miller JH: Pediatric Nuclear Medicine. Norfolk, Connecticut: Prentice-Hall, 1982, p 122.

75. Sy WM, Mittal AK: Bone scan in chronic dialysis patients with evidence of secondary hyperparathyroidism and renal osteodystrophy. Brit J Radiol 48:878–884, 1975.

76. Sy WM, Westring DW, Weinberger G: "Cold" lesions in bone imaging. J Nucl Med 16:1013–1016, 1975.

77. Thrupkaew AK, Henkin RE, Quinn JL: False negative bone scans in disseminated metastatic disease. Radiology 113:383–386, 1974.

78. Vider M, Maruyama Y, Navarez R: Significance of the vertebral venous (Batson's) plexus in metastatic carcinoma. Cancer 40:67–71, 1977.

78a. Wahner HW, Dunn WL, Riggs BL: Noninvasive bone mineral measurements. Semin Nucl Med 13:282–289, 1983.

79. Waxman AD, Ducker S, McKee PT, et al: Evaluation of 99mTc diphosphonate kinetics and bone scans in patients with Paget's disease before and after calcitonin treatment. Radiology 125:761–764, 1977.

80. Waxman AD, Siemsen JK, Levine AM, et al: Radiographic and radionuclide imaging in multiple myeloma: the role of gallium scintigraphy: concise communication. J Nucl Med 22:232–236, 1981.

81. Waxman AD, Siemsen JK, Singer FR: Gallium scanning in Paget's disease of bone: a superior parameter in following the response to calcitonin therapy. J Nucl Med 18:621–622, 1977. (Abstract)

82. Weingrad T, Heyman S, Alavi A: Cold lesions on bone scan in pediatric neoplasms. Clin Nucl Med 9:125–130, 1984.

83. Wellman HN, Schauwecker D, Robb JA, et al: Skeletal scintimaging and radiography in the diagnosis and management of Paget's disease. Clin Orthop 127:55–62, 1977.

84. Wenger DR, Bobechko WP, Gilday DL: The spectrum of intervertebral disc-space infection in children. J Bone Joint Surg 60A:100–108, 1978.

85. Wilson MA, Calhoun FW: Distribution of skeletal metastases in breast and pulmonary carcinoma: concise communication. J Nucl Med 22:594–597, 1981.

86. Wiltse LL, Widell EH Jr, Jackson DW: Fatigue fracture. The basic lesion isthmic spondylolisthesis. J Bone Joint Surg 57A:17–22, 1975.

87. Winter WA, Veraart B, Verdergaal WP: Bone scintigraphy in patients with juvenile kyphosis. Diagn Imaging 50:186–190, 1981.

88. Wistow BW, McAfee JG, Sagerman RH, et al: Renal uptake of Tc-99m-methylene diphosphonate after radiation therapy. J Nucl Med 20:32–34, 1979.

89. Woolfenden JM, Pitt MJ, Durie BGM, et al: Comparison of bone scintigraphy and radiography in multiple myeloma. Radiology 134:723–728, 1980.

90. Yeh SD, Rosen G, Benua RS: Gallium scans in Paget's sarcoma. Clin Nucl Med 17:546–552, 1982.

11

Bernard Ghelman, M.D.

Discography

Discography is a well-established diagnostic procedure for examination of the lumbar and cervical discs.[3, 11, 17] It is usually performed only after the results of other diagnostic imaging procedures prove to be either negative or of equivocal interpretation. Discography in general is an integral part of chemonucleolysis.

Discography should be performed by physicians who have familiarity with invasive diagnostic procedures of the spine (myelography, spinal bone biopsies, disc aspirations) and expertise with fluoroscopic equipment.

The integrity of a disc, or the lack of it, can be reliably evaluated by means of discography. The results are consistent, and, in competent hands, discography can be performed without great discomfort to the patient.

INDICATIONS

The most common indication for lumbar discography is persistent low back pain or radicular pain or both, with negative or equivocal myelogram findings.[14]

Often other imaging procedures of the lumbar and cervical spines are performed (CT scan without contrast agent, bone scan, magnetic resonance imaging), but, in general, discography should not be performed without previous myelography.

Discography is also performed, though not routinely, preceding lower lumbar spinal fusions.[6] The purpose of the test is to evaluate the integrity of the disc immediately above the level of planned fusion.

Discography can also be performed as part of chemonucleolysis[1] and disc aspiration.

The indications for cervical discography, in general, are the same as for lumbar discography. The cervical discogram, however, will often give positive results in patients over 40 years of age.[8] The annulus fibrosus of the cervical disc is weaker than the annulus of the lumbar disc, and contrast agent injected into the cervical region tends to extravasate from the disc space. As the patient grows older, the fragility of the cervical annulus becomes accentuated. Cervical discograms tend to be less informative than lumbar discograms.

Discography should be carried out only if surgery is being seriously considered.

LUMBAR DISCOGRAPHY

Technique

Equipment

Lumbar discography is ideally performed under biplane fluoroscopic control. The x-ray equipment might consist of a fixed installation of perpendicular fluoroscopes (Fig. 11–1) or a combination of a fixed fluoroscope (usually for the vertical beam) with a portable C-arm fluoroscope (horizontal beam) (Fig. 11–2). If the C-arm fluoroscope is used alone, the need to reposition the fluoroscope frequently during the procedure increases the amount of time necessary for completion of the test.

The standard myelographic tray is used. In addition, 25 gauge, 6 inch needles are

538

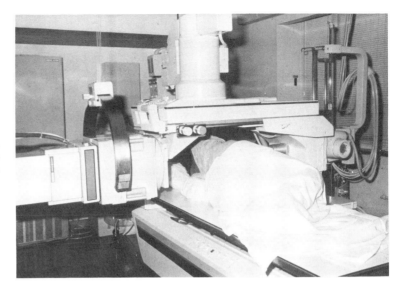

Figure 11–1. Fixed biplane fluoroscopic equipment. Patient in lateral decubitus position. If available, the "memory" (video recorder) is attached to the horizontal beam fluoroscope.

used for penetration into the disc (Fig. 11–3). Chemonucleolysis is performed using 20 gauge needles that are 7 or 8 inches long.

Approach for Injection

Lumbar discography can be performed from two approaches: transdural[12] and lateral.[4]

The transdural approach is used for diagnostic discography.

The lateral approach must be used if the discogram is part of chemonucleolysis or if there is a question of infection of the disc space.

Obtaining Patient Cooperation During Procedure

As with most invasive procedures in the radiology department, discography can be more easily performed if the radiologist manages to obtain the cooperation of the patient. This can be achieved, in most cases, by complete explanation about the test before it actually begins, including a step-by-step description of what is actually happening. To a large extent, the fear and anxiety that patients so often demonstrate are the result of ignorance of what is being done and poor rapport with the physician. The radiologist should be thorough in the ex-

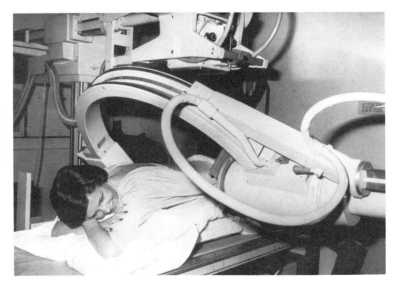

Figure 11–2. C-arm fluoroscope combined with overhead fluoroscope to achieve biplanar control. Lumbar lordosis is diminished by placing several pillows under patient's abdomen.

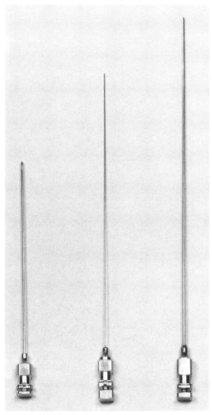

Figure 11–3. Standard, 20 gauge, 3.5 inch spinal needle, 25 gauge, 6 inch discography needle, and 18 gauge, 7 inch needle.

amination and also honest and straightforward with the patient. Most patients respond in a positive way to this reassuring and comforting attitude.

Position of Patient

The patient is placed in a prone position for the transdural approach (see Fig. 11–2). The degree of lumbar lordosis is decreased by placing pillows under the patient's abdomen.

The lateral approach can be performed with the patient in either the prone or the lateral decubitus position (see Fig. 11–1). The prone position is preferable if the procedure in question is mainly or only diagnostic in nature (diagnostic discography, disc aspiration, biopsy). If, however, the procedure in question is chemonucleolysis, the lateral decubitus position of the patient might facilitate the work of the anesthesiologist during the actual injection of enzyme

into the disc. Pillows should be placed under the recumbent flank of the patient when the lateral approach is used.

When the patient is in the prone position, he or she tends to remain immobile to a greater degree than in the lateral decubitus position. In this latter position, there is a tendency, especially if the placement of the needle is done with difficulty and pain, for the patient to move back and forth. The fluoroscopic recognition of the anatomic landmarks becomes difficult if the patient changes position. This author prefers the prone position.

Site of Injection

Under fluoroscopic control, indelible ink points that project over the discs to be injected are marked on the skin. For the transdural approach, these points, just as in myelography, are placed between the spinous processes of the corresponding vertebrae and as much as possible along the midline (Fig. 11–4). For the lateral approach, these points are marked 5 to 7 cm lateral to the midline, usually along the uppermost edge of the iliac crest (Fig. 11–5).

The lateral approach for the L2–L3, L3–L4, and L4–L5 discs is done with the needles being inserted in a plane essentially transverse to these disc spaces. This is not the case for the L5–S1 disc space, since the lumbosacral disc is positioned lower than the wing of the ilium. For the lumbosacral disc, the needle is inserted as close as possible to the uppermost edge of the iliac crest and aimed medially, anteriorly, and caudad.

Prior to actual needle insertion, the discographer makes sure that the disc spaces in question are well outlined in the lateral fluoroscope. If this is not the case, the patient should be repositioned until the lateral fluoroscopic beam is tangential to the vertebral end-plates and the disc spaces are well outlined. The clear display of the disc spaces is invaluable for proper orientation of the needle.

The use of a "memory" coupled with the fluoroscopic equipment not only makes the procedure easier but also greatly reduces the radiation exposure of both the patient and the personnel.

The lateral approach, if performed with the patient in a lateral decubitus position, is

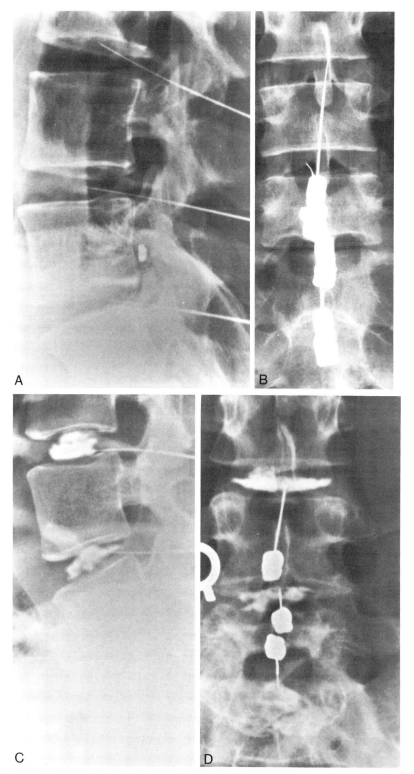

Figure 11–4. Transdural approach. Needles inserted into the L3–L4, L4–L5, and L5–S1 intervertebral discs. The 25 gauge needles have been inserted through the 20 gauge spinal needles. Two different cases are presented. Case 1: Prior to injection of contrast agent (A) lateral, (B) anteroposterior. Case 2: Following injection of contrast agent (C) lateral, (D) anteroposterior.

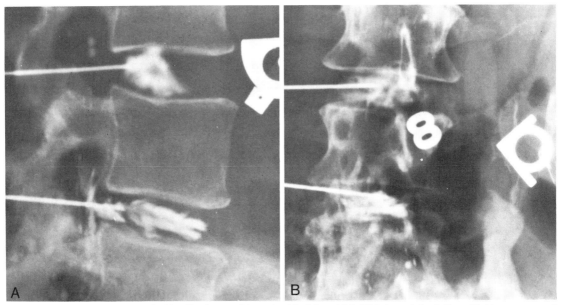

Figure 11–5. Lateral approach. Needles inserted into the L3–L4 and L4–L5 intervertebral discs. Eighteen gauge, 6 inch needles were used. These discograms were obtained prior to chemonucleolysis. A, Lateral, B, anteroposterior.

obviously done from the uppermost side of the patient.

Needle Placement

Transdural Approach. Most lumbar discograms are performed at L3–L4, L4–L5, and L5–S1 disc levels. These sites are marked between the corresponding spinous processes just as in myelography. Proper aseptic technique and local anesthesia are used. Twenty gauge spinal needles are advanced between the spinous processes, making sure with the anteroposterior fluoroscope that they remain in the midline as much as possible. Once the 20 gauge spinal needles fall in the space between the spinous processes, the lateral (horizontal) fluoroscope is used to make sure that these needles are properly aimed at the corresponding disc spaces. The deeper the 20 gauge needles are, the more difficult it becomes to change their position and orientation and, for this reason, it is better to aim these needles at the disc spaces before they penetrate the actual spinal canal.

The author prefers to give subcutaneous local anesthesia in the elected sites—the three lower lumbar disc levels, for instance—and then place the 20 gauge spinal needles at these levels. It is easier to proceed from top to bottom, working first at L3–L4, then at L4–L5 and L5–S1. Once the 20 gauge

spinal needles are in proper alignment with the disc spaces (which is checked with the lateral fluoroscope) and in the midline (checked with the vertical fluoroscope), the 25 gauge, 6 inch needles should be readied for use. In many cases, the 20 gauge needles penetrate the posterior aspect of the dura mater. The penetration of the dura by one or more of the 20 gauge needles, even though it should be avoided if possible, does not represent a major drawback in the procedure.

The stylets of the 20 gauge needles are removed, and the 25 gauge, 6 inch needles are inserted through them. These needles are advanced through the dura into the posterior aspect of the disc space. Once the disc material is penetrated, a "rubbery" resistance is encountered. The patient should be advised that the needles are being advanced into the disc, since pain is not unusual.[19]

The 25 gauge, 6 inch needles should be advanced as much as possible toward the center of the disc space. At times, the needles become impacted into the vertebral end-plate. The needle, in this case, should be withdrawn a few millimeters or the injection of contrast agent may be impossible because the bevel of the needle is blocked by cartilage.

The insertion of the needle at the L5–S1 level may be difficult with the transdural approach. The main reason for this difficulty is the angulation between the plane of the L5–S1 disc space and the plane between the corresponding spinous processes. Depending on the degree of lumbar lordosis and anterior wedging of these vertebral bodies, the angulation can be marked. In these instances, it is not unusual to have the 3.5 inch, 20 gauge spinal needle close to the posterior aspect of the L5–S1 disc space, but in a position that aims at the end-plates or corners of the adjacent vertebral bodies. In these cases, it may be helpful to curve the end of the 25 gauge, 6 inch needle gently before it is introduced into the 20 gauge, 3.5 inch needle. The purpose of this maneuver is to have the 6 inch needle reassume this curvature once it comes out of the 3.5 inch needle (Fig. 11–6). At this point, the 6 inch needle is inside the spinal canal and close to the posterior aspect of the disc space. If performed carefully, this maneuver allows the 6 inch needle to be introduced in many lumbosacral discs that otherwise could not be studied.

The curving or bending of the 6 inch needles should not be performed more than two or three times. Repeated bending maneuvers might result in a weak point in the stem of the needle, which might break either in the disc space or in the spinal canal.

Lateral Approach. Subcutaneous local anesthesia and proper aseptic technique are used in a fashion similar to that used for the midline approach. The 20 gauge spinal needles are advanced toward the lateral aspect of the disc spaces to be studied. The placement of the needle at L2–L3, L3–L4, and L4–L5 can, in most cases, be done without great difficulty. The 20 gauge spinal needles are inserted essentially at 45 degrees in relation to the surface of the skin and advanced along a transverse plane toward the corresponding disc. At times, the corresponding transverse process might obstruct the introduction of the needle. In these cases, it is advisable to remove the needle and reintroduce it in the skin a few millimeters above or below the original point. In general, small changes in the orientation of the needle are enough to make it avoid the adjacent transverse process (see Fig. 11–6).

The placement of the needle at the lum-

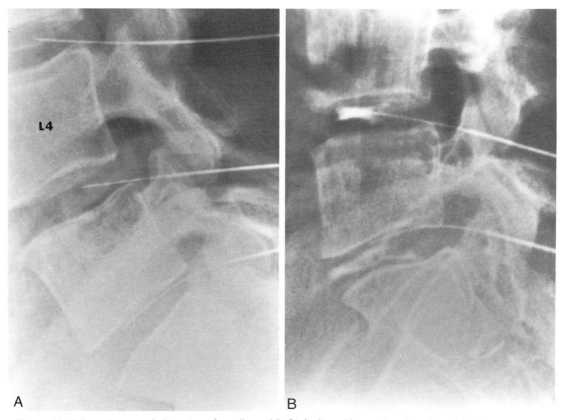

A   B

Figure 11–6. Lateral approach. Insertion of needles at L5–S1 facilitated by previous bending of the 25 gauge needle. Two different cases are shown (A, B). Notice lack of bending of the 25 gauge needles inserted at L3–L4 and L4–L5.

bosacral disc is done with greater difficulty because of the wing of the ilium. For the lumbosacral disc, the 20 gauge needle is introduced again at 45 degrees in relation to the skin but, in addition, it is aimed caudad from 30 to 45 degrees, depending on the degree of lumbar lordosis (Fig. 11–7). The use of biplane fluoroscopy should clearly determine the degree of angulation that is required for the needle to be introduced at L5–S1.

Once the 20 gauge spinal needles are close to the lateral aspect of the disc, the 26 gauge, 6 inch needles are threaded through to the spinal needles and advanced into the corresponding disc.

In the specific case of chemonucleolysis, the entire procedure can be performed by using 18 or 20 gauge, 7 or 8 inch needles, which are carried into the disc space.

The lateral approach for the placement of the needle should be performed with the patient under local anesthesia. General anesthesia should be avoided because of the danger of inadvertent damage to nerve roots. In general, percutaneous invasive tests of the spine should be performed with the patient awake and instructed to inform the physician of any pain or discomfort.

Injection of Contrast Agent

Once the needles have been placed inside the discs, positive water-soluble contrast agent is injected. A normal disc accepts only up to 1 or 1.5 cc of contrast agent (Fig. 11–8). The discographer will notice that to inject a normal disc there is need to exert moderate pressure on the plunger of the syringe. The injection of an abnormal (degenerated or ruptured or both) disc is done with greater ease, since less resistance is offered to the penetration of contrast agent (Fig. 11–9). The discographer should pay attention to the ease or difficulty found at the time of the injections, since this will help in the final interpretation of the findings.

The injection of the normal disc is painless. The injection of the abnormal disc is almost always accompanied by pain. The pain can vary from a mild, dull, low back ache to typical pain with radicular distribution.

The pain starts almost at the time of the injection and can last for several minutes. The pain caused by injection of an abnormal disc can be the result of distention of the disc, which then presses on the adjacent nerve root sleeves, or the result of leakage of contrast agent, which causes pain by coming in contact with the nerve root sleeves. Careful attention should be paid not only to the intensity but also to the distribution of pain. This information should be included in the final report of the procedure.

Removal of the Needles

After the injection of contrast agent, which might be painful or painless, posteroanterior

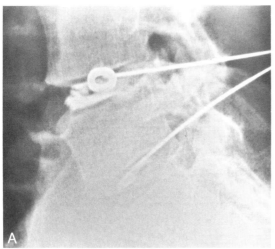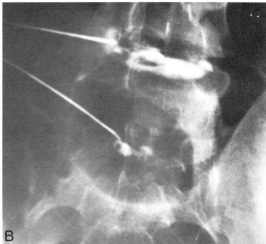

Figure 11–7. Lateral approach. Needles introduced at L4–L5 and L5–S1 through lateral approach. A, Lateral, B, anteroposterior.

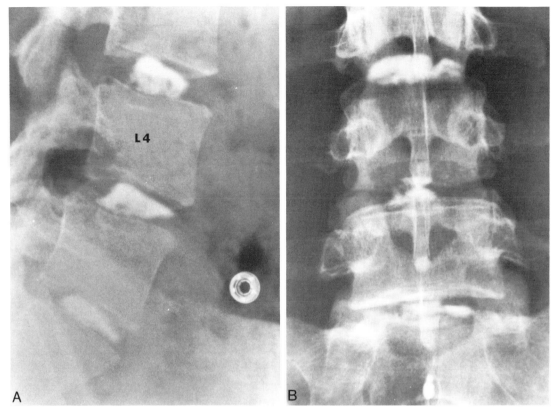

Figure 11–8. Normal lumbar discogram. Contrast agent injected at L3–L4, L4–L5, and L5–S1. The injected material collects in the central portion of the disc space. There was no pain at the time of injection. *A*, Lateral, *B*, anteroposterior.

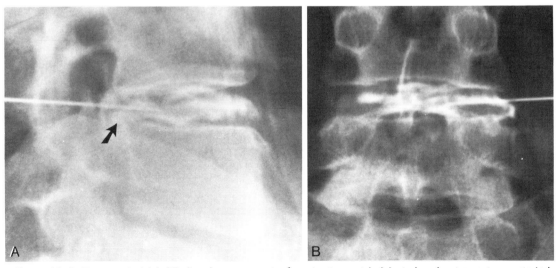

Figure 11–9. Degenerated L4–L5 disc. Large amount of contrast agent is injected and extravasates posteriorly (arrow). There was pain at the time of injection. *A*, Lateral, *B*, anteroposterior.

and lateral films of the spine should be obtained while the needles are in the discs. Once these two films are developed, the needles can be removed. The removal of the needles should be done with care. The 20 gauge spinal needles into which the 25 gauge needles have been inserted should be moved out as much as possible. The purposes of this maneuver are to free the tip of the 25 gauge needle and avoid the possible break of its stem by the sharp bevel of the 20 gauge needle. The removal of the needles might be accompanied by sharp pain.

Postdiscography Care

The instructions and orders to the patient are similar to those following Pantopaque (iophendylate) myelography. The patient should remain in bed for 24 hours, keep his or her head as flat as possible, and take pain medication only if required.

Complications

Discography is an invasive procedure in which different anatomic structures are penetrated. Therefore, the possibility of complications should always be taken into consideration, not only in the planning of the procedure but also during the actual performance of the test. We will discuss some of the common complications.

Infection

Poor sterile technique can lead to septic spondylitis and its usual complicated clinical course. The discographer should keep in mind the need to maintain the field sterile. Skill must be developed to maneuver all the needles as well as the fluoroscopic equipment without any contamination. Whenever there is a question about contamination, the physician in charge of the patient should be notified, and careful attention shoud be paid to the development of symptoms and signs of septic spondylitis (fever, white blood cell count shift, irregularity of vertebral endplates and narrowing of the disc space demonstrated by x-rays, localized increased uptake on radionuclide bone scan, and so forth).

Headaches

Since the dura is punctured several times during the discogram, especially if three levels are studied, the leakage of cerebrospinal fluid is expected to occur over a period of a few days. Headaches are not unusual, with the evolution and severity similar to those usually observed after spinal taps and myelography.

Radicular Pain

The lower lumbar nerve roots may be traumatized if the needle is not inserted along the midline in the case of the transdural approach, or if the needles are inserted too posteriorly in the case of the lateral approach. The patient invariably describes severe radicular pain at the time the needle is advanced. This can be followed by a dull ache, with the same radicular distribution, that can last for several days. This complication usually resolves without any significant residual effects.

Low Back Pain

Patients often describe a dull low back pain for several days following discography. This symptom is usually self-limited and disappears after 1 week to 10 days following the examination.

Needle Break

In one case in the author's experience, during the removal of the discogram needles, the distal end of the 26 gauge needle broke off, probably severed by the tip of the 20 gauge needle. Maximum care should be applied during the removal of the needles, and attention should be paid to the suggestions made earlier (see Removal of the Needles). Emergency surgery is necessary for removal of a broken needle fragment.

Anatomic Radiologic Correlation

The normal intervertebral disc is a structure formed by a thick annulus fibrosus, which surrounds a gelatinous nucleus pulposus.[11] As part of the normal aging process, the nucleus becomes dehydrated and loses its gelatinous character. In addition, the fibers of the annulus develop fissures and defects through which the nucleus might escape and herniate.

The normal annulus fibrosus offers a great deal of resistance to distention and, as a result, the normal disc accepts only 1.0 to 1.5 cc of contrast agent or saline solution during discography. The actual injection of the normal disc requires significant physical effort on the part of the discographer. In contrast, the degenerated disc can be injected without difficulty.[10] The fissures of the annulus allow injected contrast agent to escape from the intervertebral disc spaces and to reach the paraspinal spaces and the spinal canal. The injection of more than 2 cc of contrast agent into a disc is a sign that some degree of degenerative change is present in the annulus and nucleus.

Although the injection of a normal disc is painless, the introduction of contrast agent into the abnormal disc is often accompanied by severe pain.[2] The pain can be limited to the low back or have a radicular distribution or both. The symptoms that follow injection of the abnormal disc are probably due to distention of the disc and compression of the adjacent nerve roots and also to extravasation of contrast agent, which causes pain when in close contact with the nerve roots.

The escape of contrast agent occurs at the fissures of the annulus fibrosus. This is well demonstrated by CT examination of the injected disc.

The correlation between CT discography and the morphology of the disc can be made by the study of cadaver spines. The injection of the discs of cadaver spines with a mixture of radiographic contrast agent (sodium iodide) and chemical dye (aniline blue) allows a close comparison of discography, CT discography, and direct inspection of the disc material (Fig. 11–10).[10] There is a close correlation between the distribution of aniline blue and the distribution of contrast material. In addition, aniline blue is seen to leak at the points of the annulus where defects are present.

The CT scan of the injected disc provides an exact display of the fissures and defects in the annulus and the precise location of herniation of the nucleus pulposus. With the advent of microsurgery and chemonu-

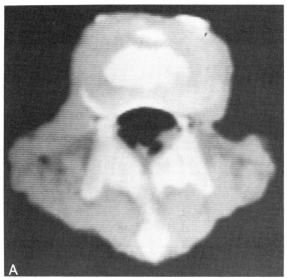

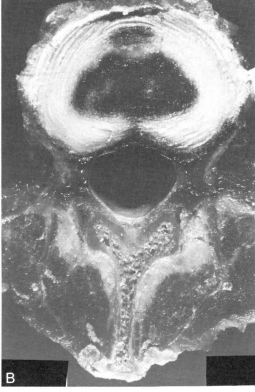

Figure 11–10. Discogram on a cadaver lumbar disc. The CT examination (A) shows central collection of contrast agent with swollen anterior collection. Similar distribution is seen on a photograph of specimen (B) in which aniline blue is seen as dark areas in the disc.

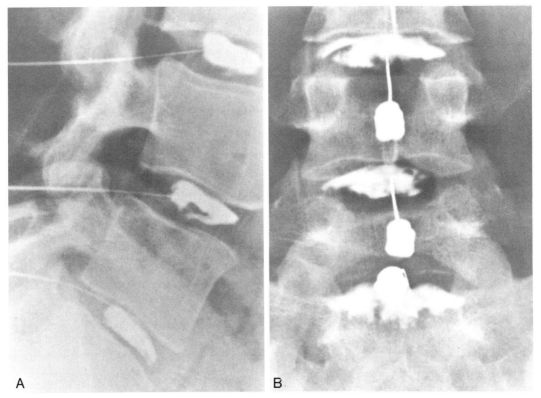

Figure 11–11. Normal discogram. Single central collection at L3–L4, L4–L5, and L5–S1. *A*, Lateral, *B*, anteroposterior.

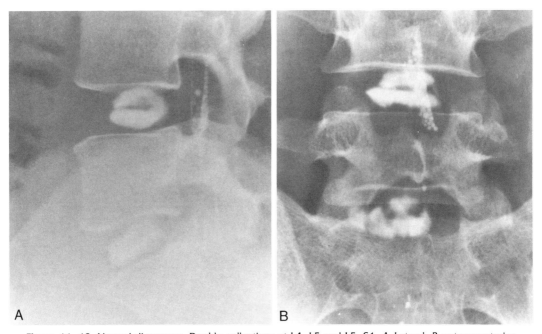

Figure 11–12. Normal discogram. Double collections at L4–L5 and L5–S1. *A*, Lateral, *B*, anteroposterior.

cleolysis, there is need for a more precise delineation of the anatomy of the degenerated and herniated disc.

THE NORMAL DISCOGRAM

Two basic appearances are seen after the injection of a normal disc:
1. Single contrast collection of contrast agent (Fig. 11–11).
2. Double contrast collections with an intervening lucent defect ("hamburger on a bun" appearance) (Fig. 11–12).

THE ABNORMAL DISCOGRAM

The abnormal discogram is seen as contrast agent extending to the periphery of the disc space. The extravasation can occur around the entire rim of the disc or it can be localized to a particular section of the annulus. The localized fissures of the annulus are better demonstrated by CT examination following discography (Figures 11–13 and 11–14).

PITFALLS IN DIAGNOSIS

Annulus Injection

At times, the needle is inserted in the annulus fibrosus (Fig. 11–15). If contrast agent is forced into this area, it will be seen to collect around the tip of the needle. These studies are inconclusive. While anteroposterior and lateral films are difficult to interpret at times, CT scans of the affected disc clearly demonstrate the annulus injection.

Vascular Escape of Contrast Agent

Sometimes, the contrast agent injected in the disc reaches subchondral vascular channels and rapidly disappears from the disc space.[16] The lack of opacification of the injected disc can be puzzling. The discographer should be aware of the possibility of injections into vascular spaces around the disc so as to avoid possible complications due to chemonucleolysis.

Schmorl's Node

These lucent defects in the vertebral endplates are the results of herniation of disc material into the vertebral bodies. This can be demonstrated with discography (Fig. 11–16). Limbus vertebra can be demonstrated in the same fashion.[5]

CHEMONUCLEOLYSIS

The role of discography in chemonucleolysis is controversial. In chemonucleolysis, a digestive enzyme (chymopapain, collagenase) is injected in the lumbar disc space for the purpose of interacting with proteoglycan or collagen or both. This procedure ultimately results in shrinkage of the disc material, especially if the fragments have herniated into the spinal canal.[13, 20, 21, 23]

The needle should be placed to the greatest extent possible in the center of the lumbar disc space; however, this is not always attainable—especially in the case of chemonucleolysis of the L5–S1 disc. As mentioned previously, the needles should always be inserted through a posterolateral approach.

The proper placement of the needle can be verified and documented with fluoroscopy and radiographs; only the injection of contrast agent, however, will allow the condition of the disc to become apparent. Questions such as, Is the disc normal or abnormal? Will the injected enzyme reach the herniated fragment or not? Will the enzyme reach the contents of the dural sac or not? can be answered only if the injection of contrast agent is performed prior to the injection of enzyme.

The combination of contrast agent and enzyme injections has been blamed as the cause of paraplegia observed in several patients following chemonucleolysis. One of the manufacturers of chymopapain[24] claimed that, once inside the lumbar dural sac, the mixture of enzyme and contrast agent can result in permanent damage to its neural contents.

It is the author's feeling that if the placement of the needle is done with care and skill, there is no reason to expect any injected substance, enzyme or contrast agent or both, to reach the lumen of the dural sac. Contrast agent and the digestive enzyme

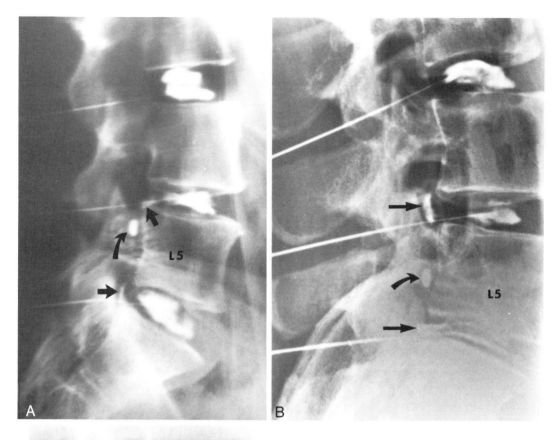

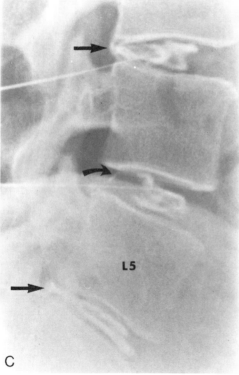

Figure 11–13. Abnormal discograms. *A,* Posterior extravasation at L4–L5 and L5–S1 (straight arrows). Normal discogram at L3–L4. Small amount of residual iophendylate (Pantopaque) is present behind the body of L5 (curved arrow). The extravasated contrast agent at L4–L5 is less dense than this residual oil drop. *B,* Posterior extravasation at L4–L5 and L5–S1 (straight arrows). Normal discogram at L3–L4. Minimal residual Pantopaque (curved arrow). *C,* Posterior extravasation at L5–S1 and minimal posterior extravasation at L3–L4 (straight arrows). Moderate degenerative changes at L4–L5 without extravasation (curved arrow).

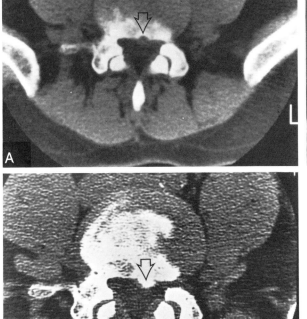

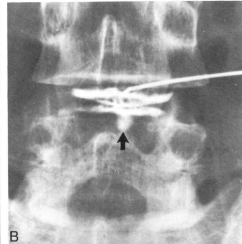

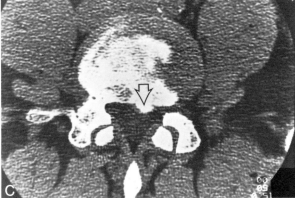

Figure 11–14. *A,* Plain CT examination at L4–L5. Small indentation in the posterior aspect of the L5 body close to the L4–L5 disc space (arrow). *B,* Anteroposterior projection of discogram at L4–L5. Small collection of contrast agent extending downward toward the body of L5 (arrow). *C,* CT discogram. Contrast agent opacifies the herniated fragment of the L4–L5 disc (arrow). The opacified fragment is located in the indentation of L5 seen on the plain CT.

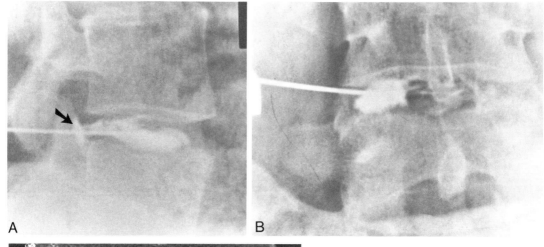

A

B

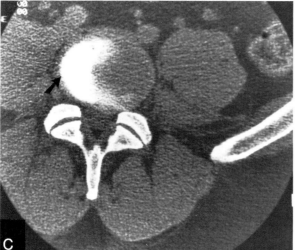

C

Figure 11–15. Annulogram. *A,* Lateral and *B,* anteroposterior projections of L4–L5 discogram. In the lateral projection, the L4–L5 disc appears to be extending posteriorly into the spinal canal (arrow). In the frontal projection, notice that the needle is placed close to the right edge of the disc space and that the contrast agent has unilateral distribution. *C,* CT discogram demonstrating opacification of the right side of the annulus fibrosus (arrow). There is no evidence of rupture of the annulus or herniation of nucleus pulposus.

Figure 11–16. Tomography following discography. Schmorl's node in the upper plate of L4 is partially opacified during discography (arrow).

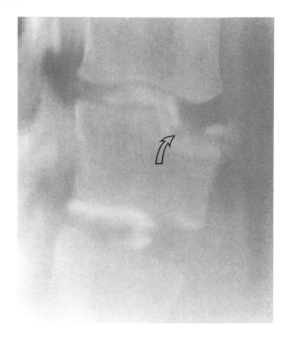

penetrate the dural sac only if an opening is present in the dura. These defects in the dura can be expected to exist if the patient has had recent spinal taps (diagnostic tap, myelography, transdural discography) and also if the placement of the needles during chemonucleolysis has been performed in a less attentive manner by a less experienced discographer.

The lack of familiarity with fluoroscopic imaging, the lack of experience with percutaneous procedures in the spine, the motion of the patient (especially if the procedure is performed with the patient in the lateral decubitus position), and the use of general anesthesia or heavy sedation during introduction of the needles can all result in penetration of the dural sac. The discographer will carry on the procedure, unaware that the dura has been punctured and that a route now exists for the materials injected in the disc to penetrate the dural sac. The discographer should note if there is return of cerebrospinal fluid through the needle, since this obviously indicates violation of the dura.

In my opinion, a discogram should be performed before chemonucleolysis. The discograms should be carefully analyzed before injection of enzyme, and the following questions should be answered at this point: Is contrast agent visualized? Is the disc normal or abnormal? Does contrast agent escape from the disc? Does the extravasated contrast agent collect in the herniated fragment or does it flow throughout the epidural space? Is there opacification of the dural sac?

Ideally chemonucleolysis should be performed in an abnormal disc only when contrast agent is seen to collect in the herniated fragment. In the case of a sequestered fragment, neither the contrast nor the digestive enzyme will reach it, and, therefore, the results are not gratifying.

The disc condition can also be assessed by the ease or difficulty with which it accepts saline solution. This is a reliable way to verify whether the disc is normal or abnormal; however, it fails to demonstrate the distribution of the injected materials. The rare cases in which there is penetration of vascular channels will not be verified if only saline is injected. It is conceivable, even though not proved, that some of the fatalities attributed to chymopapain injection were due to vascular escape of the injected enzyme.

In general, chemonucleolysis is used in younger individuals with clearly established herniation of the lumbar nucleus pulposus. With the proper patient selection and proper placement of needles, the procedure can be performed without discomfort, and the short- and long-term results can be gratifying.[1, 7, 15, 18, 22]

CERVICAL DISCOGRAPHY

Technique

In many respects, there is similarity between cervical and lumbar discography. The differences between these two studies are emphasized in the next paragraphs.

Equipment. Biplane fluoroscopic equipment should be used. The different possibilities have been discussed in the description of lumbar discography.

Position of Patient. The patient should be in the supine position, with the cervical spine in extension. This is easily achieved by placing a pillow behind the patient's shoulders.

Approach. The injection is done through an anterolateral approach. The needles are inserted in the skin anterior to the sternocleidomastoid muscle. The transdural approach obviously cannot be used for cervical discography.

Site of Injection. Under fluoroscopic control, indelible ink is used to mark points on the skin that project over the disc in question as seen in the lateral projection. The frontal projection is of little use in the determination of the point of needle insertion. The disc to be injected should be clearly outlined in the lateral fluoroscope, and end-plates should be seen tangentially by the x-ray beam.

Needle Placement. the discographer palpates the anterior edge of the sternocleidomastoid muscle. Pressure is applied, and the patient's skin is compressed until the cervical vertebra can barely be felt. Under local anesthesia, a 22 gauge spinal needle is inserted along a transverse plane and angled 45 to 30 degrees posteriorly in relation to the surface of the x-ray table. Once the needle is anchored in soft tissues, the position is checked with the fluoroscopes. Every effort should be made to avoid the front of the vertebral bodies and disc spaces.[9] If the

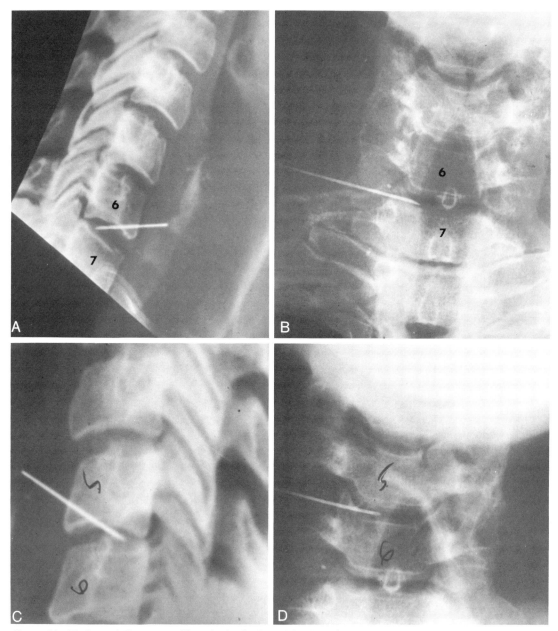

Figure 11–17. Cervical discograms. Films obtained prior to injection of contrast agent. *A, B,* Needle placed at C6–C7. *C, D,* Needle placed at C5–C6.

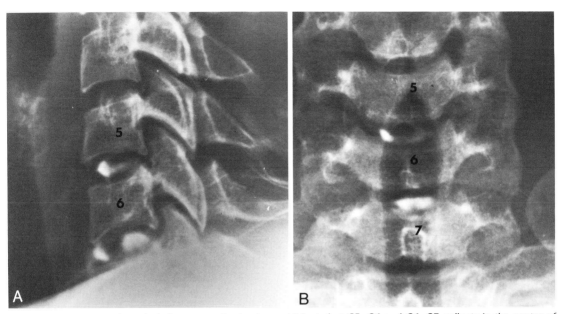

Figure 11–18. Normal cervical discogram. Contrast agent injected at C5–C6 and C6–C7 collects in the center of the disc space. *A,* Lateral, *B,* anteroposterior.

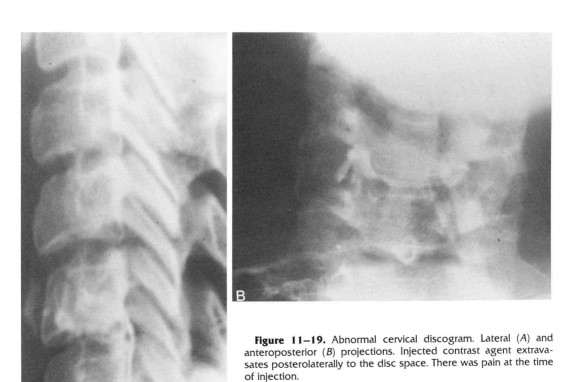

Figure 11–19. Abnormal cervical discogram. Lateral (*A*) and anteroposterior (*B*) projections. Injected contrast agent extravasates posterolaterally to the disc space. There was pain at the time of injection.

needle is oriented too much to the front of the spine, it might penetrate the esophagus and eventually cause infection in the spine, if the study is carried out with the same needle that penetrated the esophagus. Obviously, the area posterior to the body of the vertebra and disc space is also a dangerous one, since it corresponds to the spinal canal. The needle should always be aimed at the side of the vertebral body and disc space (Fig. 11–17), and for this reason the lateral fluoroscope is of paramount importance in this study.

Evaluation of Cervical Discogram

The cervical discogram is in essence evaluated in the same way as the lumbar discogram. Attention is paid to reproduction of pain, extravasation of contrast agent (Figs. 11–18 and 11–19), and extent of opacification of the disc space.[8] The value of cervical discography is limited by the fact that in patients over 40 years of age the cervical disc offers little resistance to the injection of contrast agent, and extravasation of contrast material can be easily achieved. Cervical discograms should be performed only after other studies such as CT examination,[16] cervical myelography, and CT myelography prove to be negative.

References

1. Brown MD: Chemonucleolysis with disease: Technique, results, case reports. Spine 1:115–120, 1976.
2. Brown MD: Technique of chemonucleolysis. In Brown MD (ed): Intradiscal Therapy. Chymopapain or Collagenase. Chicago: Year Book Medical Publishers, Inc, 1983, pp 84–91.
3. Collins HR: An evaluation of cervical and lumbar discography. Clin Orthop 134:133–138, 1975.
4. Edholm P, Fernstrom I, Lindblom K: Extradural lumbar disk puncture. Acta Radiol Diagn Scand 6:322–331, 1967.
5. Ghelman B, Freiberger RH: The limbus vertebra: An anterior disc herniation demonstrated by discography. AJR 127:854–855,1976.
6. Hartman JT, Kennrick LI, Lorman P: Discography

7. Javid M: Treatment of herniated lumbar disc syndrome with chymopapain. JAMA 243:2043–2048, 1980.
8. Kikuchi S, Macnab I, Moreau P: Localisation of the level of symptomatic cervical disc degeneration. J Bone Joint Surg 63-B:272–277, 1981.
9. Launa A, Lorenz R, Agnoli AL: Complications of cervical discography. J Neurosurg Sci 25:17–20, 1981.
10. Legre J, Serrano LR, Debaene A: Anatomo-radiological considerations about lumbar discography. An experimental study. Neuroradiology 17:77–82, 1979.
11. Lindblom K: Diagnostic puncture of intervertebral discs in sciatica. Acta Orthop Scand 17:231–239, 1948.
12. Lindblom K: Technique and results of diagnostic disc puncture and injection (discography) in the lumbar region. Acta Orthop Scand 20:315–323, 1950.
13. Mathews MB: The interaction of collagen and acid mucopolysaccharides: A model for connective tissue. Biochem J 96:710–716, 1965.
14. McCormick CC: Radiology in low back pain and sciatica. An analysis of the relative efficacy of spinal venography, discography and epidurography in patients with negative or equivocal myelogram. Clin Radiol 29:393–406, 1978.
15. McCullough, JA: Chemonucleolysis: Experience with 2,000 cases. Clin Orthop 146:128–135, 1980.
16. Merriam WF, Stockdale HR: Is cervical discography of any value? Eur J Radiol 3:138–141, 1983.
17. Patton JT: Discography in assessment of lumbar disc disease. Ann Rheum Dis 34:466–467, 1975.
18. Smith L, Brown JE: Treatment of lumbar intervertebral disc lesions by direct injection of chymopapain. J Bone Joint Surg 49-B:502–519, 1967.
19. Smyth MJ, Wright WW: Sciatica and the intervertebral disc. J Bone Joint Surg 40-A:1401–1409, 1958.
20. Sussman B, Bromley J, Gomez J: Injection of collagenase in the treatment of herniated lumbar disk. JAMA 245:730–732, 1981.
21. Thomas L: Reversible collapse of rabbits' ears after intravenous papain and prevention of recovery by cortisone. J Exp Med 104:245–252, 1956.
22. Wiltse LL, Widell EH, Hansen AY: Chymopapain chemonucleolysis in lumbar disc disease. JAMA 231:474–479, 1975.
23. Woessner JF Jr: Enzymatic mechanisms for the degradation of connective tissue matrix. In Owen P, Godfellow J, Bullough P (eds): Orthopedics and Traumatology. London: William Heinemann Medical Books, Ltd, 1980.
24. Correspondence regarding chemonucleolysis injection. Omnis Surgical Inc, July 19, 1984; p 2, paragraph 4.

12

Raziel Gershater, F.R.C.P. (C)
Eugene L. St. Louis, M.D.

Lumbar Epidural Venography

Epidural venography is an indirect technique for investigating intervertebral discs, vertebrae, the spinal cord, and other neural elements by visualizing the anterior epidural veins and their relationship to these structures. The anterior internal vertebral veins (aivv), which are important epidural veins in these studies, lie between the nerve roots and the intervertebral discs (Figs. 12–1, 12–2, 12–3) and may, therefore, be compressed by a herniating disc before there is impingement upon the dural sac.

INDICATIONS

The principal indication for lumbar epidural venography is to confirm the presence and location of a clinically suspected disc herniation. Lumbar epidural venography, high resolution computed tomography, outpatient myelography with nonionic water-soluble contrast agents,* and magnetic resonance imaging are all extremely accurate methods for diagnosing lumbar disc protrusions. However, utilization of lumbar epidural venography has dramatically declined with the increasing use of these other modalities. Although not widely used currently, lumbar epidural venography could still be a viable alternative and, in selected difficult cases, may be an ancillary examination.

TECHNIQUE

The epidural venous plexus can be opacified by catheterization and injection of con-

trast material into an ascending lumbar, presacral, pedicular (radicular, intervertebral), or internal iliac vein (Fig. 12–4).[4–8, 17, 36]

In those cases in which routine filming rather than digital subtraction is employed, the contrast material used is meglumine 76% mixed with lidocaine hydrochloride (injectable) in a ratio of 2 mg of lidocaine per 1 ml of contrast material.[8, 10, 41] The addition of lidocaine to the contrast material renders the injection relatively painless, but, to avoid toxic reactions, no more than 100 mg of lidocaine should be injected in a bolus, and no more than 200 mg should be used in an hour. When digital subtraction epidural venography is done, meglumine 15% is used, and an anesthetic agent is not required. If nonionic contrast material is used, an anesthetic agent is also not required.[1, 22]

A variety of catheterization techniques and routines have been reported,* and some authors use two catheters and inject two veins simultaneously.[23, 38, 39] We feel that this approach prolongs the examination unnecessarily and increases the possibility of a complication. Consequently, we use a single No. 5 Fr catheter (Fig. 12–5) and find that, with experience, selective cannulation of the left ascending lumbar vein or a presacral vein on either side can be accomplished quite simply.

The left femoral vein approach is used in all circumstances (regardless of the side of radicular symptoms) for the following reasons: (a) the left ascending lumbar vein is virtually always present and of good size

---

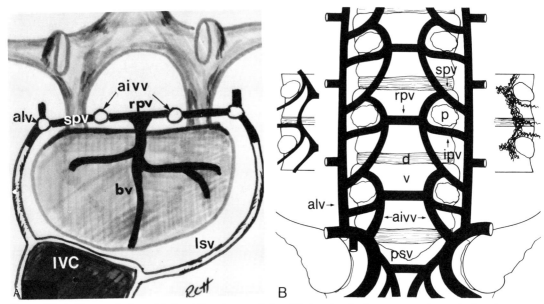

Figure 12–1. Diagram in the axial view (*A*) and coronal view (*B*) showing the intraosseous, intraspinal, and paraspinal venous complex. The intimate relationship of the anterior internal vertebral veins (**aivv**) to the posterior aspect of the vertebral bodies and intervertebral discs is demonstrated. The basivertebral vein drains from the vertebral body. *Key:* **aivv** = anterior internal vertebral veins; **alv** = ascending lumbar vein; **bv** = basivertebral vein; **d** = disc; **ipv** = infrapedicular vein; **ivc** = inferior vena cava; **lsv** = lumbar segmental vein; **p** = pedicle; **psv** = presacral vein; **rvp** = retrovertebral plexus of veins; **spv** = suprapedicular vein; **v** = vertebra. (From Gershater R, Holgate RC: Lumbar epidural venography in the diagnosis of disc herniations. AJR 126:992–1002, 1976. Copyright 1976 by the American Roentgen Ray Society.)

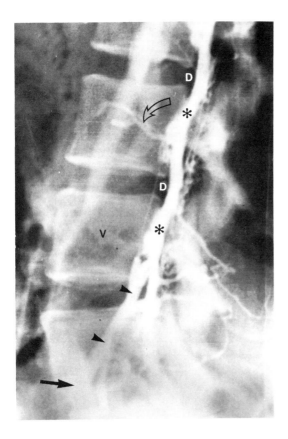

Figure 12–2. The lateral view of a lumbar epidural venogram shows the relationship of the aivv (asterisks) to the intervertebral discs (**D**) and vertebral bodies (**V**). Ascending lumbar veins (arrowheads) originate from the common iliac vein (straight arrow). The catheter is in the alv and, therefore, is pointing posteriorly. The basivertebral vein (curved arrow) drains into the rpv–aivv system. Note that there are no visualized posterior internal vertebral veins.

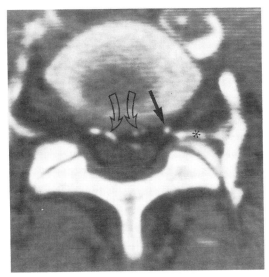

Figure 12–3. Normal L5–S1 computed tomographic epidural venogram in the cross axial projection. Contrast material was injected into the left ascending lumbar vein. Anterior internal vertebral veins are well demonstrated in the epidural fat adjacent to the disc (curved arrows). Note that at this level the aivv are fairly close to the midline and at some distance from the lateral aivv (straight arrow). Pedicular vein (asterisk) drains to the ascending lumbar vein.

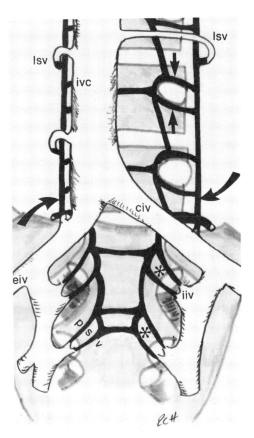

Figure 12–4. Diagram: Prevertebral abdominal veins (white) and paravertebral and epidural veins (black). *Key:* **civ** = common iliac vein; **eiv** = external iliac vein; **iiv** = internal iliac vein; **ivc** = inferior vena cava; **lsv** = lumbosacral vein; **psv** (asterisk) = presacral veins; curved arrows = ascending lumbar veins; straight arrows = pedicular veins. (From Gershater R, Holgate RC: Lumbar epidural venography in the diagnosis of disc herniations. AJR 126:992–1002, 1976. Copyright 1976 by the American Roentgen Ray Society.)

compared with the inconstant, often laterally directed, right ascending lumbar vein; (b) the left iliac vein is longer than the right, making catheterization of the contralateral internal iliac and presacral veins easier than catheterization with a right transfemoral approach (see Fig. 12–4).

Initially, while the natural catheter curvature is still well maintained, an ipsilateral

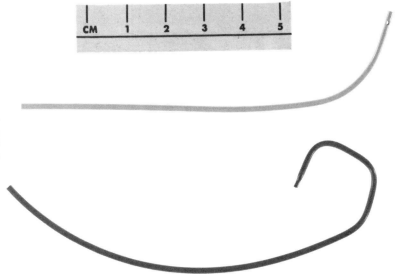

Figure 12–5. Catheters (Courtesy of Cook Inc., Bloomington, Indiana). These catheters can be used for catheterization of alv, iiv, psv, or pv (pedicular veins).

or contralateral presacral vein is catheterized, and filming is performed. Injection at these sites produces remarkably symmetric filling of the lumbar epidural plexus, particularly at L5–S1 and L4–L5 (Figs. 12–6 and 12–7).

In approximately half the cases, this single series of films will suffice. A second vessel is selectively studied in the remaining cases: (1) when there is inadequate filling on the symptomatic side; or (2) when in the presence of an occluded or displaced vein, it is essential to opacify venous channels proximal and distal to the occluded segment (Fig. 12–8). This second vessel may be either a presacral vein on the contralateral side or

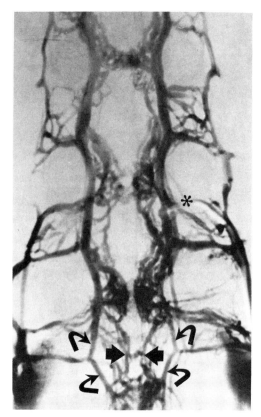

Figure 12–7. Normal epidural venogram (subtracted view). Catheter was inserted into the left L4 infrapedicular vein (asterisk) via the ascending lumbar vein. The medial aivv approach the midline at L5–S1 (straight arrows). The lateral aivv are undulant down to L5–S1, where they assume a more angular hexagonal configuration (curved arrows). (From Gershater R, St. Louis EL: Lumbar epidural venography—Review of 1,200 cases. Radiology 131: 409–421, 1979.)

the left ascending lumbar vein. If the latter is chosen, the catheter is usually advanced into a pedicular vein (see Fig. 12–6), and injection is performed at this site.[36]

Contrast material is injected at a rate of 5 to 8 ml per second, with a total volume of 40 to 50 ml. Five radiographs are taken over a 10 second period, with an initial plain film obtained for subtraction purposes. The radiographic tube is tilted 15 degrees craniad to demonstrate the two lowest intervertebral disc spaces to better advantage. Only anteroposterior filming is performed, as we have not found lateral or oblique projections helpful. Filling of the epidural veins is facilitated by application of a lower abdominal compression device (such as that used for intravenous urography) and performance of a Valsalva maneuver.

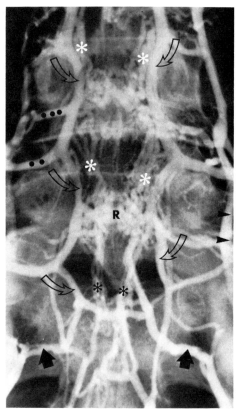

Figure 12–6. Normal epidural venogram. The retrovertebral plexus (**R**) is at the midvertebral level. The lateral aivv are single veins (curved arrows). The medial aivv appear as multiple irregular venous channels (white asterisks). At L5–S1, they leave the lateral aivv and come to lie closer to the midline (black asterisks). The catheter is in the ascending lumbar vein (arrowheads). The L4 infrapedicular vein is indicated by three black dots and the L5 suprapedicular vein by two black dots. The S1 presacral veins (solid arrows) drain to the internal iliac veins. (From Gershater R, St. Louis EL: Lumbar epidural venography—Review of 1,200 cases. Radiology 131: 409–421, 1979.)

Figure 12–8. Central L4–L5 disc herniation. *A*, Catheter inserted from the right side, with injection into the contralateral ascending lumbar vein (arrow). No epidural venous filling below L4. No conclusion can be drawn from this examination. *B*, A presacral vein injection shows a normal vein at the L5–S1 level and a complete block at L4–L5 (asterisk) from disc herniation.

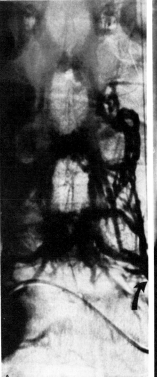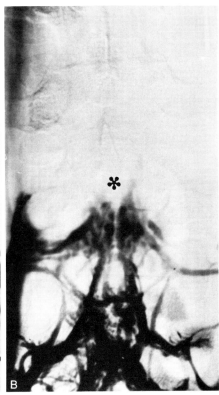

This combination promotes reversal of the normal venous flow such that contrast travels from the paravertebral veins to the epidural veins. When all lumbar veins on the symptomatic side have been shown, the examination is terminated. It is not necessary to do additional injections for the sole purpose of demonstrating the veins on the asymptomatic side.

The majority of the procedure are done in 30 minutes or less. Most are performed on outpatients[31] who are observed for 2 to 3 hours and then discharged. The examination is usually tolerated very well, and patients who have had both venography and myelography have invariably expressed a preference for the former.

COMPLICATIONS

The potential complications of this technique are identical to those encountered with any femoral vein catheterization and intravenous injection of iodinated contrast material.[8] Known allergy to contrast material is a contraindication to the procedure, as is the presence of deep vein thrombosis. Groin hematomas and thrombophlebitis are rare occurrences,[8] as are vein perforations and resultant extravasation, producing local pain for 5 to 10 minutes.[8, 21]

THE NORMAL VENOGRAM

Epidural venography is based on the fact that the anterior internal vertebral veins (aivv) have a constant relationship to the vertebral bodies and the intervertebral discs (see Figs. 12–1, 12–2, 12–3). The vertebral venous system consists of three communicating valveless networks: intraosseous vertebral veins, epidural venous plexus, and paravertebral veins.

Intraosseous Vertebral Veins. These veins drain each vertebral body and empty into a central venous sinus, the basivertebral vein, at the nutrient foramen of the posterior aspect of each vertebral body (see Fig. 12–1). The basivertebral vein connects at each vertebral level with a second network, the epidural plexus.

Epidural Venous Plexus. The basivertebral vein drains into the retrovertebral plexus, a serpiginous collection of venous channels that lies in the epidural space against the posterior aspect of the midvertebral body. Two vertical venous channels, the aivv, connect with each retrovertebral plexus and run the length of the spinal canal, hugging the posterior aspect of the vertebral bodies and intervertebral discs (see Figs. 12–1, 12–2, 12–3). Both the left and right aivv consist of medial and lateral components (see Figs. 12–6 and 12–7). The lateral components are usually single veins, whereas the medial ones vary considerably and are usually a group of rather irregular venous channels. The medial aivv are close to the lateral aivv at all levels in the lumbar spine except at L5–S1. At this level, the medial aivv leave the lateral aivv and come to lie close to the midline (see Figs. 12–6 and 12–7). The aivv lie medial to the pedicles and bulge laterally as they cross the intervertebral disc spaces. At every level, there are connections between the epidural venous plexus and the paravertebral veins. Usually, there are two connecting veins on each side at every intervertebral level, the supra- and infrapedicular (radicular) veins (see Figs. 12–6 and 12–7). Anatomy texts refer to a system of posterior internal vertebral veins.[2] We believe these veins either do not exist or are rudimentary. They are not opacified at epidural venography, which is, in fact, fortunate, as their existence and opacification would make assessment of the anterior veins difficult on frontal views.

Paravertebral Veins. The longitudinal paravertebral veins change their names as they run from clivus to coccyx. They are called vertebral veins in the neck, azygous and hemiazygous veins in the thorax, ascending lumbar veins in the abdomen, and internal iliac veins in the pelvis. In the pelvis, presacral veins that join the internal iliac veins to the epidural veins through the sacral foramina (see Fig. 12–4) are analogues of the infra- and suprapedicular veins in the lumbar region. The paravertebral veins connect with the caval system at many locations (see Fig. 12–4). The vertebral veins join the subclavian veins just medial to the internal jugular veins. The azygous and hemiazygous veins join the superior vena cava above the right atrium. The ascending lumbar veins join the common iliac veins as they cross the ala of the sacrum (see Fig. 12–4). The ascending lumbar veins sometimes connect directly with the inferior vena cava through

segmental veins, which course about the vertebral bodies (see Fig. 12–1).

Selective catheterization and epidural venography are possible because of these caval-paravertebral-epidural venous connections.

ANATOMIC VARIATIONS

As can be seen from the illustrations in this chapter, there is considerable variation in the configuration of the vertebral veins from patient to patient. In an individual, however, there is side-to-side and level-to-level symmetry from L1 to L5. At the L5–S1 level, the lateral aivv have a more hexagonal configuration, where they are undulant at higher levels. The medial aivv at L5–S1 are closer to the midline, whereas they lie adjacent to the lateral aivv above the L5–S1 level (see Fig. 12–6).

An important normal variant that can occur at the L5–S1 level is the absence of the inferior component of the lateral aivv. This can occur on either side or bilaterally and is really a transitional lumbar-to-sacral venous

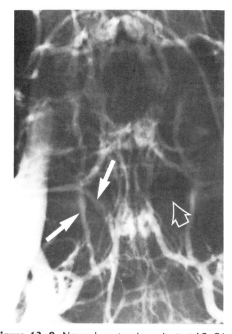

Figure 12–9. Normal anatomic variant at L5–S1. The usual hexagon of the lateral aivv is incomplete, with absence of the left inferolateral aivv (open arrow). This should not be interpreted as a venous occlusion due to disc protrusion. Another unusual feature of this patient's epidural plexus is that there is a double set of lateral aivv (white arrows).

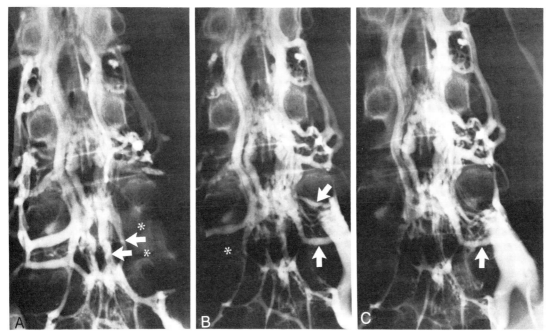

Figure 12–10. Normal venogram. Vagaries of pedicular vein filling are demonstrated. Nonfilling of a pedicular vein is of no clinical significance unless aivv are occluded as well. All injections were performed on the same patient during one examination. *A,* Left S3 presacral vein injection. Nonfilling of left S1 suprapedicular vein and left L5 infrapedicular vein (asterisks). The aivv are intact (arrows). *B,* Left ascending lumbar vein injection. Nonfilling of right S1 suprapedicular vein (asterisk). Left S1 suprapedicular and L5 infrapedicular veins are now opacified (arrows). *C,* Left S1 presacral vein injection (arrow). Nonfilling of all pedicular veins on the right. (From Gershater R, St. Louis EL: Lumbar epidural venography—Review of 1,200 cases. Radiology 131:409–421, 1979.)

pattern. Typically in this variant, the lateral aivv descend vertically, without completing the hexagonal shape (Fig. 12–9). This should not be interpreted as an occlusion of the infralateral aivv due to disc protrusion.

Nonfilling of a pedicular vein is of no clinical significance if the aivv are normal in appearance (Fig. 12–10). On occasion, the ascending lumbar veins are very small and difficult to catheterize; rarely, they do not arise directly from the common iliac vein and therefore cannot be cannulated.

THE VENOGRAM IN SPINAL DISORDERS

Disc Herniations

The venographic abnormalities that occur as a result of a disc herniation are caused by the disc compressing, displacing, and eventually occluding any or all of the adjacent anterior internal vertebral veins. Various combinations of venous displacement and

occlusion may be seen (see Fig. 12–8 and Figs. 12–11 through 12–17).*

Obstruction usually appears tapered owing to the compression of the lumen of the vein by the disc fragment. The lateral aivv are relatively mobile and are displaced laterally before being occluded. Sometimes they are displaced medially. The medial aivv are not mobile and are obstructed earlier than the lateral aivv. We should emphasize that we do not consider isolated pedicular vein occlusions to be of any significance. Disc herniations never occlude pedicular veins without occluding aivv as well (see Fig. 12–10). It should be remembered that asymptomatic disc protrusions can occlude veins, and careful clinical correlation is required.

Collateral flow may be observed about an obstructed segment of the aivv system (see Fig. 12–12).† These collateral veins can

*See references 4, 7, 8, 18, 38.
†See references 4, 7, 8, 18, 38.

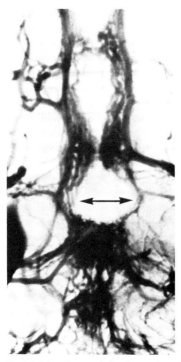

Figure 12–11. L4–L5 central disc herniation. Occlusion of the medial aivv. Slight lateral displacement of the lateral aivv, especially the left (arrows).

sometimes mimic the course of an epidural vein. If a vein is seen to cross a pedicle, it is clearly extravertebral.

On occasion, a small midline vein is opacified, lying posteriorly in the spinal canal (Figs. 12–18 and 12–19).[19] It has been postulated that this vein lies intradurally and is the continuation of the vena medulla spinalis.[19] We have observed it both in normal examinations and in patients with disc disease and, therefore, believe that, although it is a finding of interest, it should not be used as a diagnostic criterion for disc herniation.

Epidural venography has been shown to be more accurate than myelography in the diagnosis of far lateral disc herniation (see Fig. 12–16)[8, 17, 24, 25] and also in cases involving a large epidural space anteriorly at L5–S1, a short dural sac, or a very large dural sac (see Fig. 12–17).[8, 17, 18, 40]

Although epidural venography should be used only in primary investigation of patients suspected of having disc herniation, it is inevitable that other disorders will be encountered.[8, 20, 34, 45] Usually the pattern of venous occlusion raises suspicion that one is dealing with a disorder other than disc

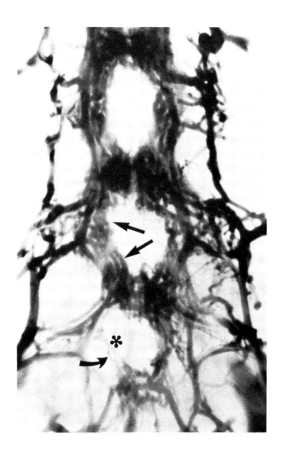

Figure 12–12. Right L5–S1 disc herniation. Occlusion of the right medial aivv (asterisk). Compare with normal medial aivv above (straight arrows). Small collateral veins (curved arrow).

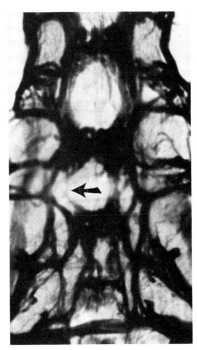

Figure 12–13. Right L5–S1 disc herniation. Compression of the right medial aivv (arrow). Note that there is a transitional pattern of the veins in the lower lumbar spine. The usual L5–S1 pattern is seen here at S1–S2.

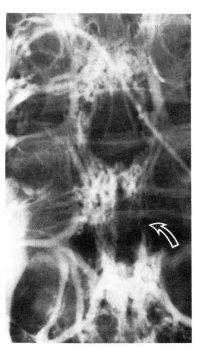

Figure 12–14. Left L5–S1 disc herniation. Occlusion of medial and lateral aivv (arrow).

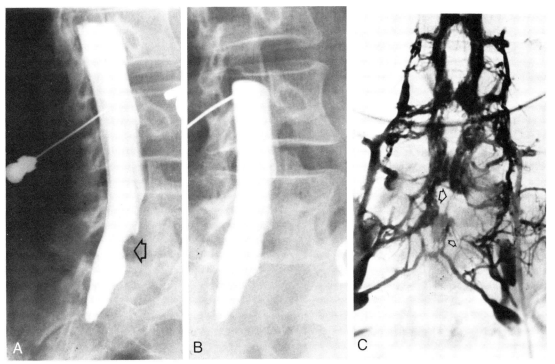

Figure 12–15. Sequestered disc fragment. *A*, Iophendylate (Pantopaque) myelogram showing left L5–S1 disc herniation (arrow). Chymopapain injection brought about immediate relief of symptoms. *B*, Same patient with a recurrence of symptoms two years later. Myelogram appears normal. *C*, A venogram obtained one day later (after 12–15*B*) shows occlusion of medial and lateral left L5–S1 aivv (large arrow) and attenuation of left S1 presacral vein (small arrow). At surgery, a sequestered disc fragment was found laterally on the left at L5–S1. (From Gershater R, and St. Louis EL: Lumbar epidural venography—Review of 1,200 cases. Radiology 131:409–421, 1979.)

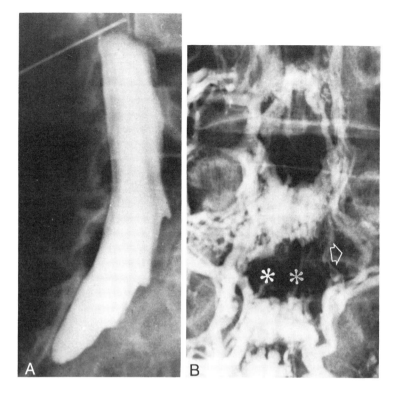

Figure 12–16. Central L5–S1 disc protrusion with herniation of a fragment into the foramen on the left. *A*, Normal myelogram. *B*, Occlusion of the medial aivv (asterisks). Deviation of the left lateral aivv into the left intervertebral foramen (arrow). (From Gershater R, St. Louis EL: Lumbar epidural venography—Review of 1,200 cases. Radiology 131:409–421, 1979.)

Figure 12–17. Disc protrusion. *A*, Normal myelogram. Unusually large epidural sac. *B*, Venogram. Occlusion of the medial aivv (arrowheads) and attenuation of left lateral aivv (arrow) at L5–S1 caused by a large disc protrusion.

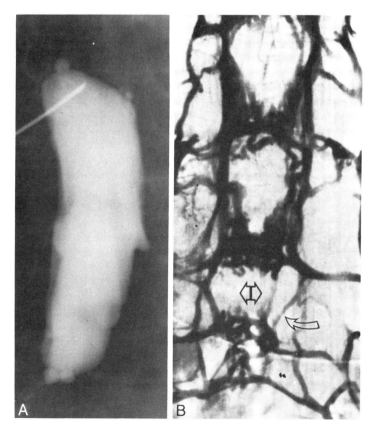

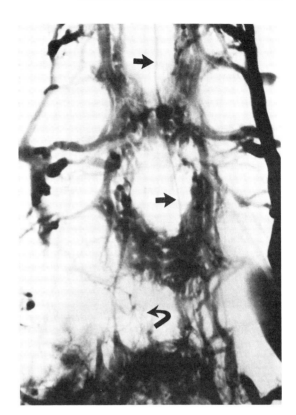

Figure 12–18. Disc herniation. Central vein (straight arrows). Right L5–S1 disc herniation with occlusion of medial and lateral aivv (curved arrow).

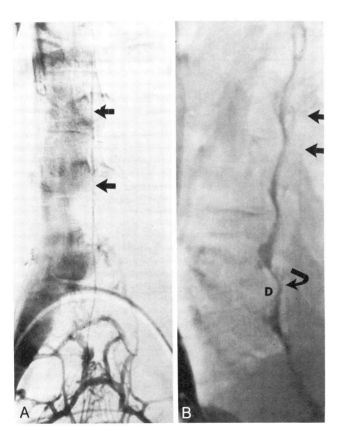

Figure 12–19. Large central L4–L5 disc herniation. *A,* Anteroposterior view. Initial presacral vein injection showed complete occlusion of the epidural plexus at L4–L5. The central vein is well demonstrated (arrows). *B,* A subsequent lateral view shows filling of the aivv with posterior displacement by a herniated disc (curved arrow, **D** = disc). The posterior location of the central vein is demonstrated (straight arrows).

herniation. Other possible disorders are outlined briefly here.

Discitis.[8] The findings can closely mimic those of disc herniation.

Lateral Nerve Root Entrapment.[8] This usually leads to occlusion of the pedicular veins only. Remember, disc herniation should never be diagnosed on the basis of pedicular vein occlusion only, that is, without aivv occlusion as well.

Spinal Stenosis. In lumbar spinal stenosis, the aivv tend to be thickened and are sheets of venous channels rather than discrete veins (Fig. 12–20) [8, 38] In concentric stenosis of the canal, these thickened aivv are closer together than normal (Fig. 12–21). This does not occur in anteroposterior stenosis with narrowing of the lateral recesses of the canal. In patients with spinal stenosis, a small, superimposed disc protrusion is frequently the precipitating cause of symptoms, and the aivv are thinned at the level of disc protrusion (see Fig. 12–20).

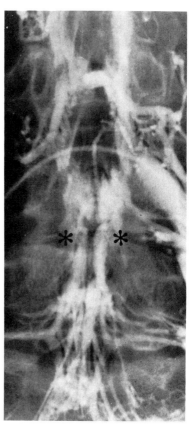

Figure 12–21. Spinal stenosis. This patient has localized, concentric spinal stenosis. The medial aivv at L4–L5 are thickened (asterisks), and the retrovertebral plexus is quite prominent. The aivv are closer to the midline than normal.

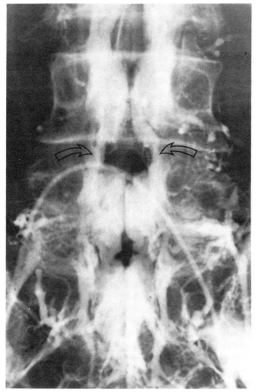

Figure 12–20. Spinal stenosis. In this patient with anteroposterior spinal stenosis, the aivv appear as sheets of veins rather than discrete channels. The aivv are thinned at L4–L5 owing to a small central disc protrusion (curved arrows).

Spondylolisthesis. The aivv can be stretched and even occluded on the posterosuperior edge of the lower vertebrae at a level of spondylolisthesis.[38]

Epidural Tumor, Primary or Secondary.[8, 220, 21, 38] Occasionally lumbar epidural venography may reveal an unexpected tumor when the clinical symptoms suggest a disc herniation. In these cases, the pattern of venous occlusion is usually different from that observed in cases of disc herniation. If a tumor is present, the pattern of aivv occlusion is abrupt compared with the tapered pattern seen in disc herniation. In cases of tumor, the occluded segment is usually much longer than in cases of disc herniation, and it is not localized to the disc space level (Figs. 12–22 and 12–23).

Epidural Venous Vascular Malformation. This disorder has been demonstrated by epidural venography.[34]

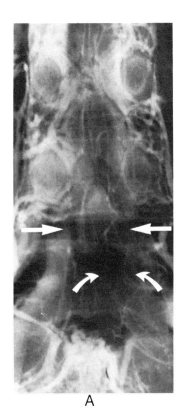

A

Figure 12–22. Sarcoma. This 35 year old woman had sciatica and was suspected clinically of having a disc herniation. *A,* Epidural venogram shows complete occlusion of the epidural venous plexus at the L4–L5 disc level (straight arrows) and over the entire region of the body of L5 (curved arrows). This is quite atypical for a disc protrusion and, therefore, a myelogram was performed. *B,* Myelogram shows large epidural mass (arrows). The histopathologic diagnosis was sarcoma.

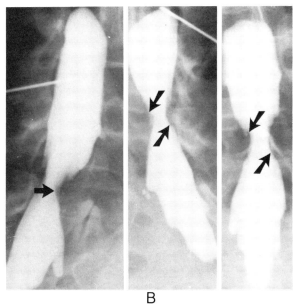

B

Sacral Neoplasms. Sacral neoplasms may mimic the clinical picture of the herniated intervertebral disc. A small number of patients referred for epidural venography will, in fact, have an unsuspected sacral neoplasm. Case reports describe extensive occlusion of epidural veins in the sacral region, with normal or relatively normal myelographic findings.[45]

Postoperative Patients. Following surgery, epidural veins are usually occluded at the level of procedure.

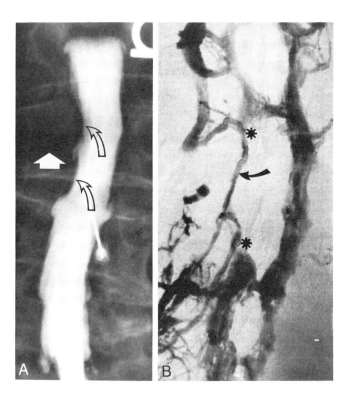

Figure 12–23. Epidural metastasis. *A,* Typical myelographic defect (curved arrows). Destruction of pedicle (straight arrow). *B,* Venogram shows occlusion of medial and lateral aivv by metastasis (between asterisks). The occlusion is too long to be caused by a disc herniation. The overlying vein (arrow) is not part of the aivv system. (From Gershater R, St. Louis EL: Lumbar epidural venography—Review of 1,200 cases. Radiology 131:409–421, 1979.)

DIGITAL SUBTRACTION EPIDURAL VENOGRAM (DSEV)

The use of digital subtraction instead of conventional film epidural venography is attractive for a number of reasons: DSEV allows for a more rapid examination because of the real-time production of the images; it is cheaper because of the use of less film and contrast material; and we have found radiation dose rates to be lower using digital techniques.[13] Another advantage of DSEV is the ability to manipulate the image by change of window level and width, pixel shift, edge enhancement, use of various filters, and so forth. For DSEV the technique of catheter placement is precisely the same as that used for the conventional study. The same volume of contrast material is injected. However, a much lower concentration is used, namely, 15% rather than 76%, and the injections are, therefore, painless. Our experience with a limited number of DSEV studies indicates that the results are very similar to those produced by the conventional technique (Fig. 12–24).

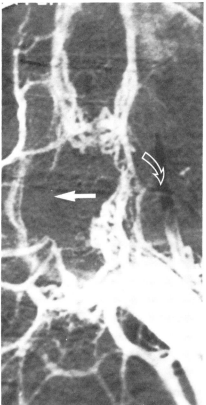

Figure 12–24. Digital subtraction venogram. Catheter is in the left L5 suprapedicular vein (curved arrow). Large right L4–L5 herniated disc fragment with occlusion of the medial and lateral aivv (straight arrow).

COMPUTED TOMOGRAPHIC EPIDURAL VENOGRAPHY

The method of injection used for the computed tomographic epidural venogram is precisely the same as that described for a conventional venogram. After selective placement of the catheter, the patient is moved to the CT scanning room, where thin axial sections are made through the intervertebral disc spaces that are suspected of being abnormal.[26] These scans are made during the injection of 40 cc of dilute 10% iodinated contrast material. A power injector is used, and the injection rate is 5 cc per second. The CT venographic images clearly show the location of the anterior internal vertebral veins in the anterior epidural fat adjacent to the vertebral bodies and intervertebral disc spaces (see Fig. 12–3).

An abnormal CT epidural venogram is shown in Figure 12–25, where a central and right L4–L5 disc hernation compresses and occludes the medial aivv and slightly attenuates the lateral vein.

There is clearly no place for routine CT epidural venography, as it is much too time consuming, but, in selected cases, this is a study that might be of some clinical use.[26]

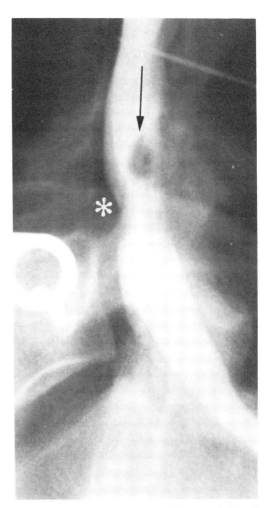

Figure 12–26. Ependymoma and herniated disc. Patient with symptoms of an L4–L5 disc herniation. Myelogram confirmed the diagnosis (asterisk) but, in addition, showed a small intrathecal tumor (arrow), which turned out to be an ependymoma. Epidural venogram demonstrated the disc herniation only. The tumor was not demonstrated through epidural venography because the location of the tumor was too posterior. Epidural venography visualizes veins in the anterior epidural space. (From Gershater R, St. Louis EL: Lumbar epidural venography—Review of 1,200 cases. Radiology 131:409–421, 1979.)

Large epidural veins can be mistaken for herniated disc fragments.

LIMITATIONS

The basic limitation of lumbar epidural venography is that the anterior epidural space (that is, the location of the aivv) is the only region within the spinal canal that can be adequately evaluated. For this reason, lesions in the anterior epidural space will alter the normal venous pattern, and in-

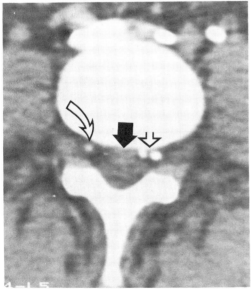

Figure 12–25. Disc herniation. L4–L5 computed tomographic epidural venogram. The contrast material was injected into a presacral vein. There is a central and right disc herniation (straight arrow). The medial and lateral aivv on the left at this level are close to each other and are normal (open arrow). The medial aivv on the right is occluded, and there is some attenuation of the lateral aivv (curved arrow).

trathecal neoplasms and extradural lesions located posteriorly may not be detected (Fig. 12–26).

The use of lumbar epidural venography should, therefore, be restricted to the evaluation of disc disease. If there is any clinical suspicion of additional or alternative pathology, another imaging method should be used.

Surgical procedures will often alter and usually occlude the aivv and render the procedure valueless at those levels previously operated upon. However, other levels may still be assessed by epidural venography. There are, of course, difficulties in evaluating postoperative sites with myelography and CT. Venography, although not technically difficult, does require expertise and experience in angiography. If venography is performed infrequently, high-quality examinations will not be produced.

References

1. Bacarini L, de Nicola T, Gasparini D, et al: Iopamidol (B 15000), a nonionic water-soluble contrast medium for neuroradiology. Part II: results of a double-blind study of the lumbar epidural venous plexuses. Neuroradiology 23:147–152, 1982.
2. Clemens HJ: Die Venensysteme der menschlichen wirbelsaule. Berlin: De Gruyter, 1961.
3. Drasin GF, Daffner RH, Sexton RF, et al: Epidural venography: diagnosis of herniated lumbar intervertebral disc and other diseases of the epidural space. AJR 126:1010–1016, 1976.
4. Gargano FP, Meyer JD, Sheldon JJ: Transfemoral ascending lumbar catheterization of the epidural veins in lumbar disk disease. Radiology 111:329–336, 1974.
5. Gargano FP: Extradural venography. In Shapiro R (ed): Myelography, 3rd ed. Chicago: Year Book Medical Publishers, Inc, 1975, pp 565–583.
6. Genant HK (ed): Spine Update 1984—Perspectives in Radiology, Orthopaedic Surgery and Neurosurgery. San Francisco: Radiological Research and Education Foundation, p 101.
7. Gershater R, Holgate RC: Lumbar epidural venography in the diagnosis of disc herniations. AJR 126:992–1002, 1976.
8. Gershater R, St. Louis EL: Lumbar epidural venography—Review of 1,200 cases. Radiology 131:409–421, 1979.
9. Giustra PE, Wickenden JW, Furman RS, et al: Epidural venography—Maine's first 75 examinations. J Maine Med Assoc 69:16–19 and 25, 1978.
10. Gordon IJ, Westcott JC: Intra-arterial Lidocaine. An effective analgesic for peripheral angiography. Radiology 124:43–45, 1977.
11. Haughton VM, Eldevik OP, Magnaes B, et al: A prospective comparison of computed tomography and myelography in the diagnosis of herniated lumbar disks. Radiology 142:103–110, 1982.
12. Hinshaw DB: Epidural venography for lumbar disk disease. West J Med 130:444–445, 1979.
13. Hynes DM, Gershater R, et al: Radiation dose implications of digital angiographic systems. AJR 143:307–312, 1984.
14. Iaccarino V, Spaziante R, de Divitiis E, et al: Dorsolumbosacral phlebography. Surg Neurol 15:198–203, 1981.
15. Kistler MW, Pribram HW: Epidural venography in the diagnosis of lumbar disc disease. Surg Neurol 5:287–291, 1976.
16. Le Page JR: Transfemoral ascending lumbar catheterization of the epidural veins. Exposition and technique. Radiology 111:337–339, 1974.
17. Macnab I, St. Louis EL, Grabias SL, et al: Selective ascending lumbosacral venography in the assessment of lumbar disc herniation. J Bone Joint Surg 58-A:1093–1098, 1976.
18. Meijenhorst GCH: Lumbar epidural double-catheter venography with metrizamide (Amipaque). Diagn Imaging 48:244–252, 1979.
19. Meijenhorst GCH: Epidural systematic double-catheter venography in the diagnosis of lumbar disc herniation; mysterious vein in the vertebral canal. Fortschr Rontgenstr 129:581–587, 1978.
20. Meijenhorst GCH, van Beeck JA, Hosea C: Infradiaphragmatic spinal tumours demonstrated by transfemoral epidural venography. Neuroradiology 19:95–100, 1980.
21. Meijenhorst GCH: Transfemoral Epidural Double-Catheter Venography in the Diagnosis of Lumbar Disc Herniation. The Netherlands: Drukkerij Nico B, De Bruijn BV, Deventer, 1980.
22. Meijenhorst GCH, de Bruin JNT: Hexabrix (Ioxaglate), a new low osmolality contrast agent for lumbar epidural double-catheter venography. Neuroradiology 20:29–32, 1980.
23. Meijenhorst GCH: Methods of transfemoral lumbar epidural venography in the diagnosis of lumbar disc herniation. Radiol Clin 46:439–457, 1977.
24. Meijenhorst GCH: Myelography and epidural double-catheter venography. BMJ 15:205–206, 1978.
25. Meijenhorst GCH: Systematic double-catheter epidural venography in the diagnosis of lumbar disc herniation. Neuroradiology 16:349–351, 1978.
26. Meijenhorst GCH: Computed tomography of the lumbar epidural veins. Radiology 145:687–691, 1982.
27. Miller MH, Handel SF, Coan JD: Transfemoral lumbar epidural venography. AJR 126:1003–1009, 1976.
28. Mosley GT: Technical considerations of epidural venography. Radiol Technol 52:371–374, 1981.
29. O'Dell CW, Coel MN, Ignelzi RJ: Ascending lumbar venography in lumbar disc disease. J Bone Joint Surg 59-A:159–163, 1977.
30. Raskin SP, Keating JW: Recognition of lumbar disk disease: Comparison of myelography and computed tomography. AJR 139:349–355,1982.
31. Rettig A, Jackson DW, Wiltse LL, et al: The epidural venogram as a diagnostic procedure in the young athlete with symptoms of lumbar disc disease. Am J Sports Med 5:158–164, 1977.
32. Roland J, Treil J, Larde D, et al: Lumbar phlebography in the diagnosis of disc herniations. J Neurosurg 49:544–550, 1978.
33. Roland J, Larde D, Schwartz JF, et al: Notes de Technique: Intérêt de la phlébographie dans le diagnostic des discopathies lombaires (Diagnosis of

lumbar disc herniation by transfemoral ascending lumbar venography). J Radiol 57:175–182, 1976.

34. Saibil EA, Rowed DW, Gertzbein SD: Case Report: Epidural vascular malformation demonstrated by epidural venography. AJR 132:987–988, 1979.

35. Smith P: Lumbar epidural venography. Can J Radiogr Radiother Nucl Med 7:129–132, 1976.

36. St. Louis EL, Grosman H, Gray RR, et al: Lumbar epidural venography in disk disease (L). AJR 140:406–407, 1983.

37. Tchang SPK, Howie JL, Kirkaldy WH. et al: Computed tomography versus myelography in diagnosis of lumbar disc herniation. J Can Assoc Radiol 33:15–20, 1982.

38. Theron J, Moret J: Spinal Phlebography. New York: Springer-Verlag, 1978.

39. Theron J, Houtteville JP, Ammerich H, et al: Lumbar phlebography by catheterization of the lateral sacral and ascending lumbar veins with abdominal compression. Neuroradiology 11:175–182, 1976.

40. Tournade A, Braun JP: Selective lumbar phlebography. Its diagnostic value when compared with radiculography. J Neuroradiol 7:199–207, 1980.

41. Widrich WC, Singer RJ, Robbins AH: The use of intra-arterial Lidocaine to control pain due to aortofemoral arteriography. Radiology 124:37–41, 1977.

42. Wilkie R, Beetham R: Trans-femoral lumbar epidural venography. Spine 5:424–431, 1980.

43. Wilmink JT, Penning L, Beks JWF: Techniques in transfemoral lumbar epidural phlebography. Neuroradiology 15:273–286, 1978.

44. Wittenberg J: Computed tomography of the body. New Engl J Med 309:1224–1229, 1983.

45. Zeit RM, Cope C: Diagnosis of sacral neoplasm by epidural venography. AJR 137:1045–1048, 1981.

13

Joachim F. Seeger, M.D.

Angiography

Initial and still classic anatomic research on the segmental blood supply of the spinal cord[1, 25] and more recent studies on the radiologic arterial anatomy of the spinal cord[3, 24, 28] stimulated the subsequent development of selective and superselective spinal cord angiography and therapeutic embolization procedures.[6, 10, 12]

INDICATIONS

Spinal angiography is used most frequently in the evaluation and possible embolization of arteriovenous malformations or fistulae of the spinal cord and its surrounding membranes. However, this technique is also useful in diagnosing and aiding in the surgical approach to hypervascular intraspinal tumors, particularly hemangioblastomas. Certain hypervascular osseous tumors, such as hemangiomas, giant cell tumors, and hypervascular metastases, may be diagnosed and even therapeutically embolized or perfused with chemotherapeutic agents by using selective spinal angiography. At times, the procedure is used to localize critical feeding arteries to the spinal cord prior to surgery of paraspinal vascular malformations and tumors, resection of aortic aneurysms, or correction of severe spinal scoliosis.

LIMITATIONS

Because selective spinal angiography may be associated with potentially devastating complications, the angiographer must have meticulous technique and a thorough knowl-

edge of the vascular anatomy of the normal spine and its variations. Spinal angiography should be performed only by expert angiographers. As will be described later in this chapter, the advent of digital subtraction angiography has increased the safety and decreased the morbidity of intra-arterial examinations and has allowed many screening examinations to be done intravenously and on an outpatient basis.

BLOOD SUPPLY OF THE SPINAL CORD AND VERTEBRAL COLUMN

A pair of segmental arteries to the vertebral column occurs at every vertebral level. In the neck, these arteries arise from the vertebral arteries and other branches of the subclavian artery; in the thoracic and lumbar regions, they arise from the aorta and are known as the intercostal and lumbar arteries; in the sacral region, they arise from the lateral sacral, middle sacral, and iliolumbar arteries. In addition to supplying the spinal cord via medullary feeders, the segmental arteries also provide nutrient branches to the vertebrae and to the paravertebral muscles (Fig. 13–1). Medullary arteries to the developing neural tube occur at every segmental level in the embryo, but many subsequently regress, so that at birth medullary branches arise from only some of the segmental arteries. These medullary feeders supply the three longitudinal arterial trunks of the spinal cord. The anterior median longitudinal arterial trunk lies along the anterior median sulcus of the spinal cord, superficial to its corresponding vein, extending from the medulla oblongata to the tip of the

574

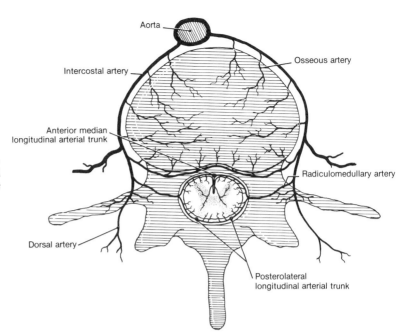

Figure 13–1. Schematic representation of a typical segmental pattern of blood supply to the thoracic spine and spinal cord.

conus medullaris. The other two paired trunks are situated posterolaterally and also run the entire length of the spinal cord. The posterolateral arterial trunks anastomose with each other at several levels. However, except for an anastomotic arcade in the conus medullaris region, only scanty, small communications exist between the anterior and the posterolateral arterial trunks.

The arterial pattern of the spinal cord varies greatly among individual patients. The anterior median longitudinal arterial trunk (referred to as the anterior spinal artery by most radiologists) is generally largest in the cervical and lower thoracic regions, corresponding to the cervical and lumbar enlargements, and is smallest between the T3 and T8 levels. Although medullary feeders may be found at any level, they occur with greatest frequency in the cervical and lower lumbar regions and are least numerous and most widely spaced at the level of the thoracic cord. The thoracic zone is thus most vulnerable to ischemia. An overall average of eight anterior medullary feeders has been observed in several anatomic studies, with a range of from 2 to 17.[15] Posterior medullary feeders are generally smaller and more numerous than anterior feeders, with an average of 12 and a range of from 6 to 25.[15] A typical pattern of blood supply to the spinal cord is demonstrated in Figure 13–2.

The anterior median longitudinal arterial trunk is extremely important to spinal cord function because it supplies the anterior two

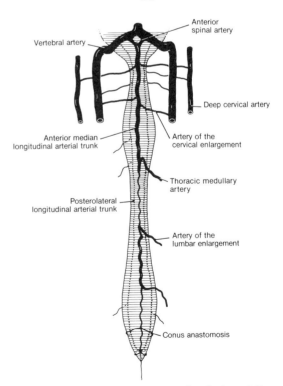

Figure 13–2. Schematic pattern of radiculomedullary feeding vessels to the anterior median and the posterolateral longitudinal arterial trunks of the spinal cord.

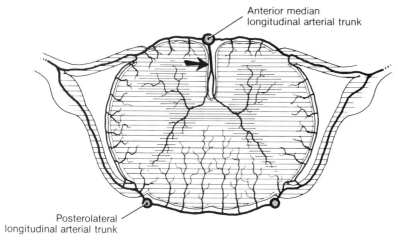

Figure 13–3. Sulcocommissural branches (arrow) arise from the anterior median longitudinal arterial trunk, pass through the anterior median sulcus, and supply the anterior two thirds of the spinal cord, including most of the gray matter.

ARTERIES

thirds to four fifths of the spinal cord (Fig. 13–3).[1, 4, 21] There is a virtual absence of capillary anastomoses within the substance of the spinal cord. The veins of the spinal cord are quite different from the arteries, with large anterior and posterior median veins draining into midline anterior and posterior longitudinal venous trunks, and radial veins draining into the pial plexus around the surface of the cord (Fig. 13–4). These veins then empty via medullary branches into Batson's plexus of veins, which includes the extradural vertebral venous plexus, intercostal, lumbar, and azy-gous communications, and the vertebral veins.[15] For a more detailed discussion of the blood supply and venous drainage of the spinal cord and vertebrae, the reader is referred to excellent textbooks on this subject.[4, 15]

TECHNIQUE

A thorough review of the technical aspects of spinal cord angiography is beyond the scope of this chapter, and the reader is referred to other sources.[7, 10, 17]

Spinal cord angiography should be per-

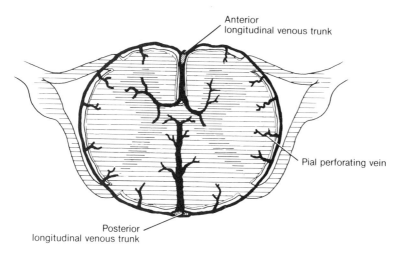

Figure 13–4. Prominent central veins drain the inner aspects of the gray columns into anterior and posterior longitudinal venous trunks. Smaller, radially oriented pial perforating veins drain the superficial spinal cord.

VEINS

formed only by individuals who are well trained in catheter techniques and who possess a thorough knowledge of blood supply of the spinal cord and its variations. The precise technique adopted depends on the preference of the individual angiographer. Whenever possible, spinal angiography is performed with selective catheterization of the segmental arteries, because of the greater sensitivity and accuracy of selective over nonselective techniques, such as midstream aortography. It is also felt that selective angiography is safer than nonselective techniques because the dose of contrast medium to the spinal cord can be better controlled. Furthermore, because the major anastomoses of the anterior and posterolateral longitudinal arterial trunks are vertical, with both ascending and descending currents, the period of contact between the contrast medium and the spinal cord is shorter with selective injections than with midstream aortography, in which all the radicular feeders are flooded at once.[7] In young infants, however, selective spinal angiography may be very difficult and sometimes impossible to perform. Fortunately, the feeding arteries to the spinal cord are relatively large in children, and vascular malformations, as well as other vascular lesions, can usually be localized quite accurately with aortography by using manual injections of contrast medium, after which limited selective catheterization may be performed.[35] In elderly patients, selective spinal angiography may also be difficult owing to extensive atheromatous plaques, stenoses, or occlusions of major vessels. Unfortunately, selective techniques are almost always mandatory when performing spinal angiography in the elderly.

Because spinal angiography usually produces only mild to moderate discomfort, we generally perform the procedure using local anesthesia and only mild sedation, so that the patient's neurologic status can be closely monitored throughout the examination. Although power injection may be used when performing vertebral or subclavian angiography to evaluate the segmental branches to the cervical spinal cord or vertebrae, contrast medium is always injected manually into the smaller arteries that may supply the spinal cord, such as the thyrocervical or costocervical trunks, the intercostal arteries, and the lumbar arteries. Three to five ml of

60% meglumine iothalamate per injection are generally adequate.

The conduct of each angiographic examination is influenced by the clinical presentation and the results of prior radiographic studies. When screening for a possible low thoracic spinal cord vascular malformation, for example, we generally "walk" the tip of the catheter up the lumbar and intercostal artery orifices on one side of the aorta and then down the other, using radiopaque markers on the patient's back to help localize the levels of injections. Anteroposterior filming is performed at a rate of 1 image per second for 6 to 7 seconds with each injection, using an injection delay so that the first film can be used as a subtraction mask. If an abnormality is demonstrated on review of these initial screening studies, the vessel or vessels of interest are recatheterized, and more detailed, biplanar imaging is performed, with the rate and duration of imaging determined by the type of lesion identified. If no abnormality is demonstrated, selective injections of the costocervical and thyrocervical trunks may be necessary so as not to overlook a radiculomedullary artery to the thoracic spinal cord arising from one of these vessels. Certain vascular lesions may require imaging for as long as 20 to 30 seconds in order to demonstrate slow-filling draining veins.

COMPLICATIONS

Spinal angiography carries a slightly higher risk of neurologic complications than does cerebral angiography.[7, 10, 17] Complications usually can be attributed either to the procedure of catheterization or to the effect of the contrast medium on the spinal cord. The risk of ischemic damage due to thrombosis, spasm, or simple mechanical occlusions of the injected artery by the catheter is generally minimal, provided the catheter is flushed frequently with heparinized saline and is left in the feeding artery only as long as necessary to perform the angiogram.

Selective spinal cord angiography often involves the injection of 20 to 30 vessels and should be done rapidly and with the least amount of contrast medium necessary to provide a high-quality study. A particular note of caution should be made regarding angiography in the midthoracic region, where the caliber of the anterior longitudinal trunk is very small. The superior thoracic medullary artery, which may arise from a common trunk with a bronchial artery from the third, fourth, or fifth intercostal artery, especially on the right, may be the only source of blood to the upper- and midthoracic spinal cord. Several spinal cord complications have been described in patients undergoing bronchial angiography, because of the inadvertent injection of a large quantity of contrast medium into this artery.[5, 26] Thus, when carrying out angiography of the midthoracic spinal cord or vertebrae, as little contrast medium as possible should be used.

The spinal cord can normally tolerate the relatively small concentrations of contrast medium required with selective techniques. In rare instances, transient paresthesias and spasm of the lower limbs may occur, particularly after injection into the artery of the lumbar enlargement (artery of Adamkiewicz).[10] Such complications can generally be controlled by the systemic administration of diazepam (Valium) directly through the catheter.[7, 10]

Methylglucamine iothalamate has been the contrast medium of choice for selective spinal cord angiography.[7] Some of the new water-soluble contrast agents such as iohexol and iopamidol may further diminish the occurrence of noxious effects of contrast medium. However, these new agents may prove to be prohibitively expensive for routine use.

RADIOGRAPHIC EQUIPMENT

Equipment for spinal angiography is determined to a considerable degree by the desires of the individual angiographer. Excellent spinal cord angiography usually requires high-quality image intensification fluoroscopy, biplanar filming capabilities, and film changers capable of 3 to 4 exposures per second. Magnification filming, using tubes with small focal spots (0.1 to 0.3 mm) may improve diagnostic accuracy. A comfortable floating table top that can also be moved in the vertical direction simplifies the procedure. Many institutions performing large numbers of spinal angiograms also utilize an electronic device for rapid film subtraction. Additional techniques which have been employed by certain investigators in-

clude angiotomography,[34] 4 × magnification,[37] and stereoscopic magnification.[40]

DIGITAL SUBTRACTION ANGIOGRAPHY

With the recent development of digital subtraction angiography (DSA) providing immediate logarithmic subtraction and the ability to enhance dilute intravascular contrast medium, spinal angiography can now be performed much more rapidly and with significantly lower doses of contrast medium than is the case with conventional techniques.[19, 20] This translates into less morbidity and greater safety for the patient. With DSA, it may also be possible to use nonselective techniques as a preliminary step, which may save precious time when screening a young child or an atherosclerotic adult for a suspected vascular lesion of the spinal column or spinal cord. The duration and dose of contrast medium of our last several spinal angiographies performed with arterial DSA were about one half of what would have been needed with conventional film-screen techniques.

A DSA system developed at our institution[33] has two separate C-arms, one of which is equipped with a 14-inch intensifier with up to 7.5 per second imaging capabilities using a 512 × 512 imaging matrix. With selective arteriography, this system has proved to be quite adequate for identifying the anterior median longitudinal arterial trunk and its various medullary feeders, defining arteriovenous malformations, and studying vascular spinal tumors (Fig. 13–5). However, clear definition of some of the smaller posterolateral spinal arteries may require supplementary investigation with higher-resolution conventional angiography. Some manufacturers are currently producing DSA systems with 1000 × 1000 matrices and up to 7 per second imaging capabilities. Such systems should obviate the need for conventional film-screen spinal angiography in essentially all cases.

As opposed to intra-arterial DSA, intravenous DSA is inadequate for evaluating the circulation of the spinal cord. However, when it is necessary to determine whether a bony spinal lesion is hypervascular (prior to surgery or biopsy), intravenous DSA has proved to be an excellent, safe, simple, and inexpensive screening study, which can be performed on an outpatient basis (Fig. 13–6).

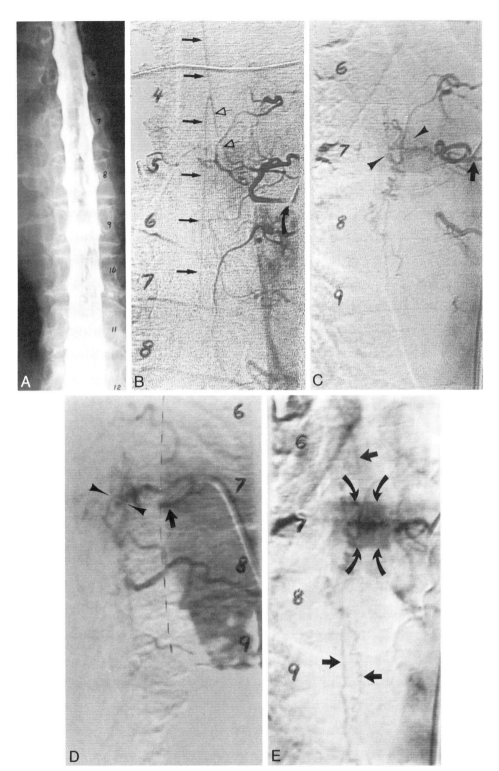

Figure 13–5. A 65 year old woman with progressive lower extremity weakness and a sensory level at T8. *A,* Complete myelogram suggests prominent vessels along the dorsal aspect of the thoracic spinal cord. *B,* Anteroposterior view of digital subtraction angiography (DSA) of the left T5 intercostal artery (curved arrow) shows a small medullary branch (open arrows) supplying a normal anterior median longitudinal artery (straight arrows) in the midthoracic region. Anteroposterior *(C)* and lateral *(D)* views of a left T7 intercostal injection (arrow at catheter tip) reveal a small arteriovenous malformation (AVM) (arrowheads) along the dorsal aspect of the spinal cord. Dashed line in *(D)* defines the anterior margin of the spinal canal. *E,* Later anteroposterior images of the left T7 injection show descending and ascending draining veins (straight arrows). Note the normal stain of the left T7 hemivertebra (curved arrows). Each injection required only 2 to 3 ml of 60% meglumine iothalamate, diluted with equal amounts of saline.

579

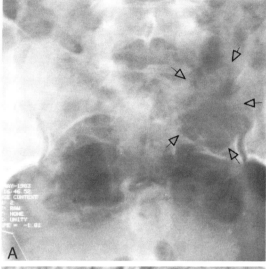

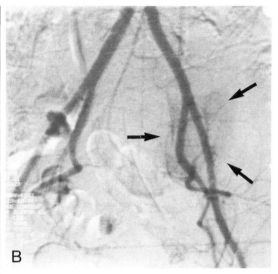

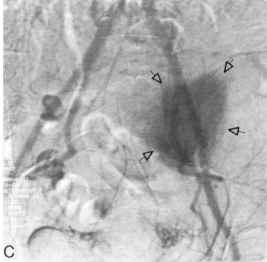

Figure 13–6. Giant cell tumor, sacrum. A 50 year old woman underwent intravenous DSA to evaluate a painful lytic lesion of the left sacrum. *A,* The scout image shows the bony defect (arrows). *B* and *C,* Images obtained 10 and 13 seconds after a superior caval injection of 40 ml of meglumine diatrizoate (Renografin-76) show the development of an intense tumor "blush" (arrows). A benign giant cell tumor was totally excised at subsequent surgery.

ANGIOGRAPHY IN SPINAL DISORDERS

Intraspinal Arteriovenous Malformations

Classification

Intraspinal vascular malformations occur in many shapes and sizes and can be found anywhere within the spinal canal.[2, 8, 9, 29] Their incidence varies between 3.4% and 11.5% of all spinal cord tumors.[38] The clinical presentations depend on many factors, including the location of the lesion; whether it is intramedullary, extramedullary, extradural, or mixed; its blood supply; and whether it is producing neurologic symptoms caused by vascular steal, venous en-gorgement, spinal cord compression, sub-arachnoid hemorrhage, or even thrombosis.

Although spinal vascular malformations are often studied first with myelography, angiography is necessary for precise diagnosis and classification. The basic vascular lesion, or nidus of the malformation or fistula, can generally be recognized at angiography.[16] Spinal vascular malformations are usually classified as intramedullary, extramedullary, or extradural. Recent investigations have shown that many of the lesions that previously were thought to represent arteriovenous malformations (AVMs) of the dorsal aspect of the spinal cord are in fact dilated medullary veins draining an AVM or fistula of the dorsal spinal dura.[27, 31, 32, 38]

Simple arteriovenous (AV) fistulae can also occur along the anterior aspect of the spinal cord.[8] These new discoveries have very significant ramifications regarding the appropriate treatment of these lesions.

Intramedullary Arteriovenous Malformations. Probably less than 20% of adult spinal cord vascular malformations are purely intramedullary, and another 20 to 25% are both intra- and extramedullary.[11] In children, on the other hand, over 80% of spinal AVMs are either purely intramedullary or mixed.[35] Most cervical AVMs are intramedullary. Fortunately, less than 20% of adult AVMs occur in the cervical region,[11] whereas 30% of childhood AVMs occur in this area.[34] Thoracic intramedullary AVMs carry the poorest prognosis, probably because there often is only one radicular artery available for collateral circulation in the upper thoracic region. The majority of intramedullary

or mixed AVMs occur in the thoracolumbar region in both children and adults. In children, there is a high association of cutaneous or osseous angiomatosis or both, including Osler-Weber-Rendu disease and the Klippel-Trenaunay-Weber syndrome.[9]

Intramedullary AVMs tend to have an early clinical presentation and a very rapid evolution. Eighty percent of patients present with sudden onset of acute myelopathy or subarachnoid hemorrhage or both.[30, 35] Because of their grave prognosis when left untreated, intramedullary AVMs must be treated as soon as the diagnosis is made, whatever the quality of remission.[30]

All of the intramedullary and nearly all of the mixed AVMs are fed at least in part by the anterior median longitudinal arterial trunk. Spinal cord AVMs have been classified according to their morphologic and hemodynamic features at angiography.[7] Type 1 is

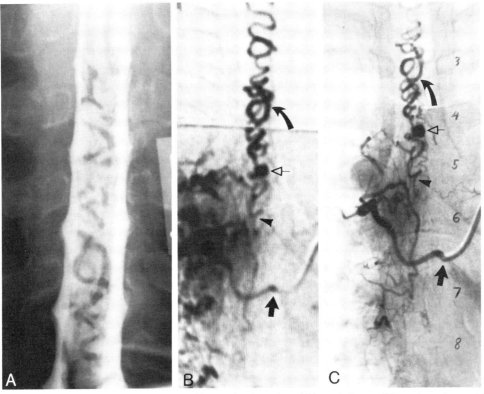

Figure 13–7. Arteriovenous fistula. A 40 year old man developed a midthoracic Brown-Séquard syndrome following heavy lifting. *A,* A thoracic myelogram shows serpentine filling defects consistent with an AVM. *B,* Using 2.5 ml meglumine iothalamate diluted with 2.5 ml saline, intra-arterial DSA of the right T6 intercostal artery (solid arrow) shows a simple arteriovenous fistula of the dorsal aspect of the spinal cord fed by a posterolateral longitudinal arterial trunk (arrowhead). A saccular aneurysm (open arrow) is seen at the site of the fistula. The vessels above the aneurysm are draining veins (curved arrow). *C,* A subtracted conventional angiogram shows the fistula and feeding arterial trunk to better advantage than the 256 × 256 matrix digital study of Figure 13–7B. (Courtesy of Dr. Jonathan Levy, Scottsdale, Arizona.)

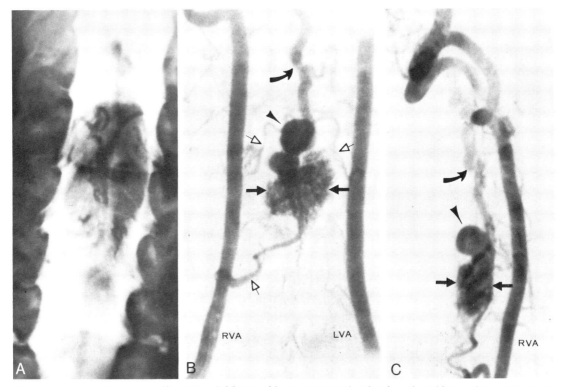

Figure 13–8. Arteriovenous malformation. A 30 year old man presented with subarachnoid hemorrhage and cervical myelopathy. *A,* A cervical myelogram shows an intramedullary mass with associated prominent vascular filling defects suggesting an AVM or vascular cord tumor. *B,* Superimposed anteroposterior views of a right (RVA) and left (LVA) vertebral angiogram show the glomus (nidus) of an intramedullary AVM (solid arrows) supplied by medullary branches (open arrows) arising from both vertebral arteries as well as an aneurysm on the venous side of the AVM (arrowhead). Note the large ascending draining vein (curved arrow). *C,* The lateral view of the right vertebral angiogram confirms the intramedullary location of the AVM (arrows) and aneurysm (arrowhead) and again shows the ascending draining vein (curved arrow).

a direct fistula between one or two longitudinal arteries and veins, and it generally shows a sluggish flow (Fig. 13–7). Type 2 is a localized plexus of vessels (glomus), which opacifies rapidly via a single or multiple arterial feeders, and from which one or several veins drain (Fig. 13–8). Type 3 (juvenile type) is seen more frequently in children. The hemodynamic features are reminiscent of cerebral AVMs, with multiple large arteries supplying a voluminous malformation, which drains rapidly into markedly dilated veins. Despite recent improvements in angiographic techniques, it is often very difficult to differentiate intramedullary from mixed or even purely extramedullary AVMs.

Extramedullary Arteriovenous Fistulae Fed by the Anterior Spinal Artery. These poorly understood lesions, which are often confused with intramedullary AVMs, were first described in 1977.[8] They are rare lesions and probably comprise only 6 to 7% of all AVMs supplied by the anterior median longitudinal arterial trunk. They tend to appear in persons 20 to 30 years of age, and they generally occur in the region of the conus medullaris.[34, 36]

These fistulae usually present clinically with slowly progressive myelopathy and radiculopathy, although there frequently is a history of antecedent subarachnoid hemorrhage, often with a long time interval between the hemorrhage and objective clinical findings.[34] They may be clinically indistinguishable from other medullary lesions, although the syndrome preferentially affects the territory of the anterior longitudinal trunk. Once impairment begins, there generally is an unremitting progression over a relatively short time to complete paraplegia. It is felt that the clinical symptoms are secondary to a steal phenomenon.[8]

Extramedullary AV fistulae differ from intramedullary AVMs in that they lie outside the spinal cord and constitute a direct shunt between the anterior median arterial and venous trunks. They have been divided into three types, based upon their angiographic features.[34] The first type is small and is supplied by a thin anterior arterial trunk. The second type is larger and is fed by an enlarged anterior arterial trunk. The third type is a giant fistula supplied by a very large anterior arterial trunk and often by accessory spinal feeders (Fig. 13–9).

Dural Arteriovenous Fistulae with Medullary Venous Drainage. Approximately 80% of all spinal angiomas in adults lie along the dorsal surface of the spinal cord, and over half of these are entirely extramedullary.[6, 32] The majority occur in the lower thoracic or thoracolumbar regions. It was discovered that many of these extramedullary angiomas (perhaps the vast majority) do not originate along the spinal cord but are in fact secondary to a small, localized, extradural arteriovenous fistula.[27] The component that for many years was mistakenly thought to represent the spinal cord AVM is nothing more than arterialized venous drainage of the fistula. These findings have subsequently been verified by others.[31, 32, 38]

Clinically, these lesions occur mostly in middle-aged or elderly men. They are insidious in onset, with relentless progression of spinal cord dysfunction manifested by motor weakness, sensory changes, sphincter disturbances, and, in half the cases, pain.[29] There are spontaneous fluctuations in severity, and the symptoms may be exacerbated by walking or other changes in posture, or by straining or coughing. Subarachnoid hemorrhage is very uncommon. Left untreated, nearly 20% of patients develop severe gait disability within 6 months of the onset of symptoms, and 50% are chairbound within 3 years.[29]

Provided supine as well as prone images are obtained, myelography is almost always positive in these patients, showing serpiginous filling defects along the dorsal aspect of the spinal cord but usually not revealing the nidus of the fistula. Selective spinal angiography is diagnostic. As opposed to a typical spinal cord angioma, which is supplied by one or more enlarged medullary branches to the anterior or posterolateral spinal arteries (see Fig. 13–8), the dural AV fistula is represented by a cluster of abnormal dural vessels projecting lateral to the spinal cord, often in the region of an intervertebral foramen and generally just below the pedicle (Fig. 13–10). The fistula is supplied by an artery (or arteries) that is almost always distinct from medullary vessels to the spinal cord. The fistula subsequently drains via a single dural vein into a tortuous and dilated "arterialized" venous plexus

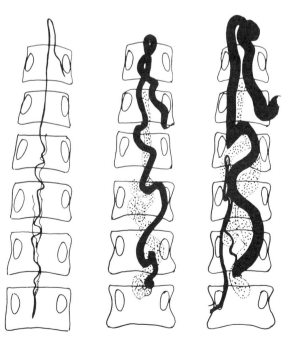

Figure 13–9. Three types of extramedullary arteriovenous fistulae involving the anterior median longitudinal arterial trunk. A small fistula (left) is an indication for surgical treatment. A larger fistula (center) can be treated with either surgery or embolization. A very large fistula (right) is treated best with detachable balloon embolization. (From Riché MC, Melki JP, Merland JJ: Embolization of spinal cord vascular malformations via the anterior spinal artery. AJNR 4:378–381, 1983. Copyright 1983 by the American Roentgen Ray Society.)

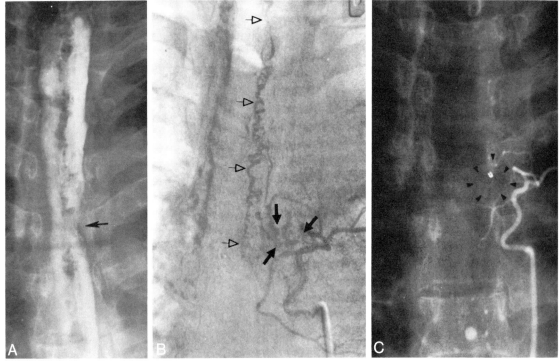

Figure 13–10. *A,* A myelogram shows a serpentine filling defect from T2 to T8. An extradural mass (arrow) is seen at T5–T6. *B,* A selective left fifth intercostal arteriogram shows an extradural cluster of vessels within the T5–T6 intervertebral foramen (solid arrows) and demonstrates early filling of spinal cord veins (open arrows), which, on later films, extend from T8 to T2. *C,* Postoperative arteriogram fails to opacify the previously demonstrated cluster of vessels (arrowheads) or the intradural veins. (From Oldfield EH, DiChiro G, Quindlen EA, et al: Successful treatment of a group of spinal cord arteriovenous malformations by interruption of dural fistulae. J Neurosurg 59:1019–1030, 1983.)

along the surface of the spinal cord (Fig. 13–11).

Increased blood flow and consequently higher intravascular pressure within the venous plexus presumably produce the chronic progressive myelopathy associated with these lesions.[27, 29] In support of this concept, two cases of an extradural AV fistula in the sacral sac have been described,[8, 29] presenting with signs of spinal cord damage presumably due to venous pressure elevation by a large draining vein passing up the film terminale and into the longitudinal venous plexus of the spinal cord. The reverse situation—lower cord symptoms produced by a dural AVM at the foramen magnum draining downward into the coronal venous plexus—has also been described.[38]

Because this condition is uncommon when compared with spinal cord tumors and is often insidious in onset, the diagnosis is frequently delayed, or the condition is misdiagnosed as multiple sclerosis, discogenic disease, or as secondary to cervical myelop-athy.[29] Myelography, which usually provides a clue to the correct diagnosis, may be deferred in the elderly or frail patient, or may be incomplete, especially if supine imaging is not obtained. The diagnosis of dural AV fistula should be suggested any time an elderly male develops a thoracolumbar cord syndrome involving all modalities and showing episodic exacerbation with a progressive downhill course occurring over a few months to a few years.

Treatment Modalities

Although the neurologic status of the patient is a significant factor in determining what, if any, treatment should be performed, the role of surgery vis-à-vis embolization is usually predicated on the angiographic findings. With intramedullary AVMs, it is important to define the number and location of the feeding vessels, the size and exact location of the nidus, the type (diffuse or com-

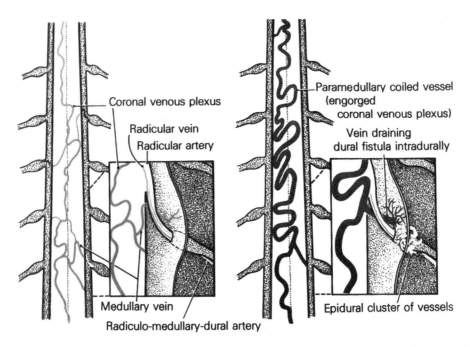

Figure 13–11. Schematic representation of normal vascular anatomy (left) and pathologic confirmation of the spinal cord venous plexus resulting from a dural AV fistula (right). (From Oldfield EH, DiChiro G, Quindlen EA, et al: Successful treatment of a group of spinal cord arteriovenous malformations by interruption of dural fistulae. J Neurosurg 59:1019–1030, 1983.)

pact), the length of the feeding sulcocommissural arteries arising from the anterior median longitudinal arterial trunk, the relationship between the AVM and the anterior trunk, and the degree and location of the venous drainage. If the lesion is focal and midline, is fed by long sulcocommissural arteries, is restricted to two vertebral segments, and has only minor posterior venous drainage, surgery is indicated.[34] If the AVM has a short afferent feeder, large sulcocommissural arteries, good collateral circulation to the anterior median longitudinal arterial trunk above and below the lesion, lacks

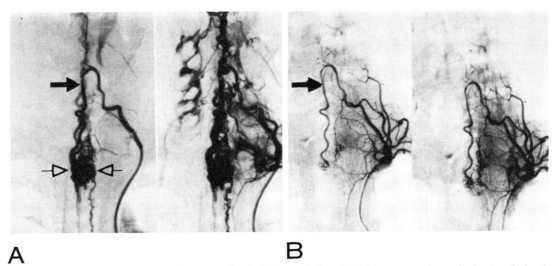

A   B

Figure 13–12. Arteriovenous malformation. Cervical intramedullary AVM (open arrows) supplied primarily by the anterior median longitudinal arterial trunk (solid arrow). Angiograms before (A) and six months after (B) embolization with particulate emboli. (From Riché MC, Melki JP, Merland JJ: Embolization of spinal cord vascular malformations via the anterior spinal artery. AJNR 4:378–381, 1983. Copyright 1983 by the American Roentgen Ray Society.)

extensive venous drainage, and does not meet the preceding criteria for surgery, embolization is indicated.[34] Often, only surgery can determine precisely whether an AVM is purely intramedullary, mixed or mostly extramedullary. Thus, exploratory surgery is often the first procedure performed after selective angiography.

The first case of embolization of a spinal cord AVM was described in 1968.[18] Since then, embolization techniques have become much more sophisticated. Depending on the type of lesion, particulate emboli, isobutyl-2-cyanoacrylate, silicone rubber, or detachable balloons can be employed.[13, 23, 34, 36] Because of numerous collateral anastomoses with radicular arteries, inoperable AVMs of the cervical spinal cord may be treated relatively safely with embolization via the anterior median trunk, provided this artery is large enough to allow the emboli to reach the angiomatous network (Fig. 13–12). Controlled embolization with particulate solids appears to be the method of choice at this time.[34] Because of the poor collateral circulation to the upper thoracic region, intramedullary AVMs in this area do not lend themselves well to embolization procedures.

With extramedullary AV fistulae fed by the anterior median trunk (see Fig. 13–9), the small fistulae can often be treated surgically, and embolization is contraindicated. The larger fistulae may be treated with macroemboli or with surgery. Surgical extirpation may be aided by temporary occlusion of the anterior median trunk with a balloon catheter. Surgery is contraindicated in the very large fistulae, some of which have been treated successfully with detachable balloon embolization.[36]

Some investigators have had considerable success treating dural AV fistulae with isobutyl-2-cyanoacrylate instead of surgery.[34] However, others favor surgical resection of the fistula and interruption of the draining vein.[32, 38] Although surgical disconnection of the dural AV fistula from its draining spinal cord veins seems relatively simple, there presumably are cases in which the fistula is located anterior to the exiting nerve root sleeves, and it would seem that such lesions could be treated more quickly and easily with liquid polymer embolization. Either form of treatment is certainly a marked improvement over the old methods of stripping the entire venous plexus from the dorsal

aspect of the spinal cord, often depriving it of its normal venous drainage, thinking that the arterialized veins represented the malformation.

SPINAL TUMORS

For many years, myelography has been the first diagnostic procedure of choice when a lesion involving the spinal cord is suspected. The role of spinal angiography as a supplement to myelography in defining the exact size, location, and intra- or extraspinal extent of many spinal tumors, such as neurinomas, certain cauda equina tumors, and various bony lesions, especially hemangiomas and vascular metastases, has recently been supplanted by CT scanning, with or without intrathecal contrast enhancement. There is little doubt that, in the near future, magnetic resonance imaging, with its greater contrast sensitivity, multiplanar imaging capabilities, and lack of bone artifacts, will supplant much of spinal CT and reduce the need for spinal angiography even further. However, selective spinal angiography still plays an important role in providing a more precise preoperative diagnosis of intramedullary and extramedullary masses associated with prominent vascular filling defects at myelography. This is particularly true with the rare intraspinal hemangioblastomas, which can be diagnosed with certainty only with angiography. The precise blood supply to vascular tumors of the spine and spinal cord and the relationship of such tumors to the anterior median longitudinal arterial trunk can be discerned by angiography. Such information may be very critical in order to avoid vascular damage to the spinal cord at the time of surgery.

Hemangioblastomas

Although myelography is abnormal in the vast majority of spinal hemangioblastomas, findings are almost always nonspecific, and rare false negative studies may also occur.[14] If a vascular lesion is suspected on the basis of the myelogram, or if the clinical setting suggests hemangioblastoma (either by family history or the presence of other lesions), spinal angiography is the next procedure of choice and is the only examination that can reliably diagnose spinal hemangioblastomas as well as provide information as to size, shape, multiplicity, feeding arteries, and draining veins.

Most spinal hemangioblastomas are intramedullary, usually in the posterior half of the cord. Less than 10% are intradural extramedullary, usually along the posterolateral aspect of the cord. About 20% lie alongside nerve roots, especially in the cauda equina region. Only rarely are they purely extradural.[14]

Spinal angiography for hemangioblastoma requires the same meticulous technique and completeness as that required for an AVM. If one lesion is found, the entire spinal cord should be studied, since lesions may be multiple in over 20% of cases.[30] If one or more spinal hemangioblastomas are found, the posterior fossa and kidneys should also be studied with CT scanning in order to rule out the fairly high probability (50%) of more diffuse disease.[30]

Spinal hemangioblastomas are angiographically identical to their cerebellar counterparts. Usually moderate or small in size, they present as hypervascular nodules that opacify early, show a persistent, extremely dense, and well-defined vascular stain, and often have very prominent but slow-to-fill draining veins. Some tumors may be very large, extending over several vertebral segments, but nodules as small as 3 mm can be found angiographically.[14] Hemangioblastomas may be fed by both anterior and posterolateral arterial trunks (Fig. 13–13). Although often enlarged, the feeding vessels are rarely as large as those that supply spinal vascular malformations.

Intraspinal Neuromas

For a relatively brief period, selective spinal angiography played an important role in the preoperative assessment of intraspinal neuromas. This was especially true in those tumors that were mostly extradural or had a dumbbell configuration at myelography, since such tumors tended to be more vascular than intradural neuromas, and their full extraspinal extent could often be defined

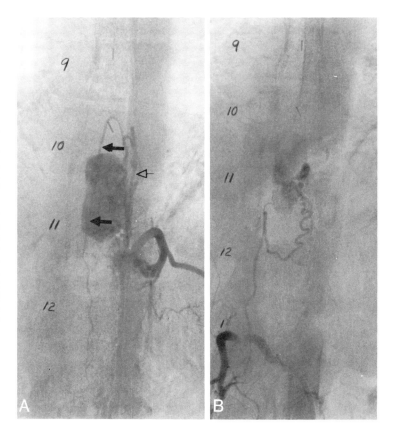

Figure 13–13. Hemangioblastoma. A 20 year old man presented with paraplegia. Myelography at another hospital showed a complete block at T11, and a "vascular spinal tumor" could not be surgically resected. *A,* An anteroposterior view of a subsequent selective left T11 intercostal arteriogram shows a typical hemangioblastoma supplied by a posterolateral (open arrow) and an anterior median (solid arrows) longitudinal arterial trunk. The latter was displaced to the right by the tumor. *B,* An anteroposterior view of a right L1 arteriogram reveals additional contribution to the caudal pole of the tumor. The tumor was subsequently successfully resected.

by a superficial tumor stain.[14] This particular
role of spinal angiography has now been
superseded by high-resolution CT scanning,
which will no doubt be replaced by nuclear
magnetic resonance imaging in the future.
However, spinal angiography may still be
useful in showing the relationship of the
tumor to the arteries supplying the spinal
cord, especially in the lower thoracic and
conus regions with regard to the artery of
Adamkiewicz. In rare instances, spinal angiography may be necessary to establish a
precise preoperative diagnosis of a conus or
cauda equina region tumor, since myelography in this area may be confusing not only
in differentiating a tumor from a vascular
malformation with an associated myelographic block but also in providing specificity as to the type of tumor. Even CT scanning
may not provide adequate information in
this regard. Spinal angiography can defini-
tively diagnose hemangioblastoma or AVM
and can frequently help differentiate an intradural neurofibroma (faint or absent tumor
stain and associated displacement of the
anterior median arterial trunk) from ependymoma (tumor stain, no displacement of
the anterior median trunk). Obviously, each
case requires individual evaluation, and the
need for angiography is often contingent
upon the information needed by the neurosurgeon.

Vertebral Hemangiomas

Most vertebral hemangiomas occur in the
mid to lower thoracic and thoracolumbar
regions. The diagnosis is usually made with
plain film studies, either as an incidental
finding or because the patient presents with
back pain or clinical symptoms of spinal
cord compression. Although spinal angiography has been employed to assess intra- or
paraspinal extension in the symptomatic patient, this function can now be performed
more safely and quickly with CT scanning.
However, angiography still may serve an
important function in confirming the diagnosis in a confusing case, and it may also be
used for therapeutic embolization prior to or
in place of surgical decompression.

The normal vertebral body is supplied
anteriorly by several small penetrating arteries arising from the proximal intercostal or
lumbar artery and posteriorly by lesser

branches from the arterial arcade along the
dorsal surface of the vertebral body that
connects the two radicular arteries (see Fig.
13–1). At spinal angiography, the normal
vertebra usually shows only a faint, homogeneous stain limited to the hemibody on
the side of injection (see Fig. 13–5E).

The clinical picture as well as the angiographic appearance of spinal hemangiomas
is probably determined mostly by the stage
of angiomatous development. Those patients
with long-standing signs of spinal cord
compression are usually the ones with an
advanced stage disease, and plain film studies show an expanded, striated vertebral
body or arch or both. Angiography typically
shows a dense stain that does not respect
the midline of the body, contrast pooling
that persists into the venous phase, only
slightly enlarged feeding arteries, and minimal or no arteriovenous shunting. Extravertebral extension of the stain is seen in most
cases, correlating with the CT findings. Less
advanced lesions, presenting clinically only
with pain to the patient, will show a typical
striated appearance of the vertebral body
without expansion on plain radiographs,
and they will generally show less staining,
smaller contrast pools, and no extravertebral
extension at angiography. Embolization of
some of these painful hemangiomas to relieve symptoms has been suggested.[30] In certain instances, angiography may show no
evidence of hemangioma despite typical
plain film findings.[14] These may represent
very early hemangiomas, thrombosed hemangiomas, or perhaps some other lesion.
Biopsy may be required for definitive diagnosis.

In rare instances, coexistent arteriovenous
malformations affecting the vertebra, the
paraspinous soft tissues, and the spinal cord
may be found (Cobb's syndrome).[14] However, the bony lesions are not typical hemangiomas in that they do not show characteristic plain film findings, and at angiography
they show features more in keeping with an
arteriovenous malformation, with dilated
feeding arteries and draining veins and arteriovenous shunting.

Other Bone Tumors

Other spinal tumors, such as plasmacytoma (Fig. 13–14), aneurysmal bone cysts,

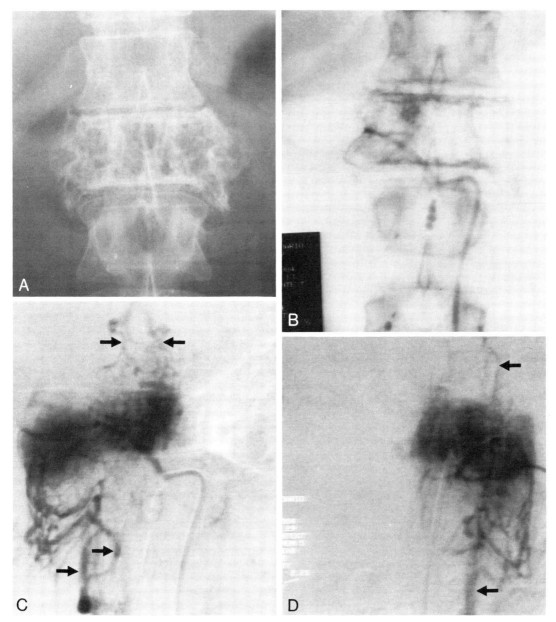

Figure 13–14. Plasmacytoma. A 30 year old man had a four year history of upper lumbar back pain and more recent lower extremity weakness. *A,* The L1 vertebra is diffusely expanded, with a coarse, honeycomb texture. Unsubtracted (*B*) and a later subtracted (*C*) DSA image of a right L1 injection and (*D*) a left L1 injection show intense staining of L1, with paraspinal extension and marked arteriovenous shunting into paraspinous and epidural veins (arrows). The degree of shunting and paraspinal extension is not typical of spinal hemangioma. Bilateral L1 particulate embolizations resulted in angiographic obliteration of the lesion. Subsequent biopsy showed plasmacytoma.

giant cell tumors, and certain metastases (hypernephroma, thyroid carcinoma), may be hypervascular and may require angiographic evaluation and embolization prior to planned resection or biopsy. The angiographic features of such tumors are varied and generally nonspecific. With the advent of digital subtraction angiography, the degree and pattern of vascularity of these tumors can be evaluated quickly, safely, and on an outpatient basis with intravenous contrast injection (see Fig. 13–5). Only rarely is selective angiography necessary for further evaluation.

Intra-arterial Chemotherapy

As is true in other organ systems of the body, angiography can also be employed for intra-arterial chemotherapy of certain nonresectable tumors involving the spine. It can be used in conjunction with or as an adjunct to radiation therapy. We have recently treated a large sacral ependymoma in this fashion, using intra-arterial DSA as a means of rapidly identifying the blood supply to the lesion for optimal catheter placement (Fig. 13–15).

TRAUMA

Spinal angiography has been employed only rarely in the evaluation of spinal fractures and dislocations with associated neurologic deficit, mainly to assess the status of the anterior median longitudinal arterial trunk. Angiographic demonstration of interruption of the anterior trunk opposite a fracture or dislocation carries a very poor prognosis for any return of spinal cord function, whereas interruption of an ascending radiculomedullary branch with preservation of

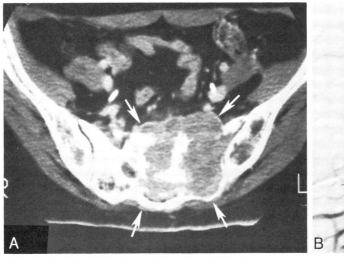
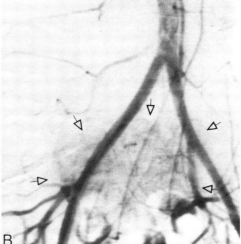
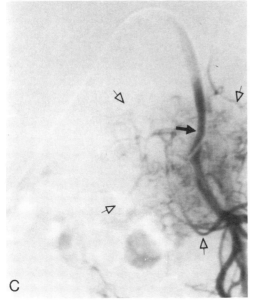

Figure 13–15. A 33 year old woman was referred for intra-arterial chemotherapy of an unresectable, previously irradiated ependymoma. A, A CT scan defines the large sacral tumor (arrows). B, Intra-arterial DSA of the lower abdominal aorta with 20 ml of 60% meglumine iothalamate shows a tumor "blush" (arrows). Subsequent selective injection of the right (not shown) and left (C) hypogastric artery (solid arrow) shows the neovascularity (open arrows) in greater detail. The patient underwent bilateral, hypogastric, intra-arterial infusion treatments.

continuity of the anterior trunk has a better prognosis.[39] From a practical management standpoint, however, angiography appears to play no significant role in the diagnosis and treatment of the patient with spinal cord injury.

SCOLIOSIS

If an anterior approach for the surgical reduction of a patient with a scoliotic spine is planned, selective spinal angiography can be very helpful in demonstrating the origins of the radiculomedullary arteries. This demonstration is helpful because the surgery will be very close to the segmental arteries. In a series of 33 consecutive patients studied angiographically prior to scoliosis surgery, 25% demonstrated only one feeder to the anterior median longitudinal arterial trunk between T4 and L2.[22] Should that vessel be traumatized during surgery, a significant neurologic deficit could be expected. Obviously, the risk of angiography must be weighed against the need for the surgeon to have this information preoperatively.

References

1. Adamkiewicz AA: Die Blutgefässe des menschlichen Rückenmarkes. I Teil. Die Gefässe der Rückenmarkssubstanz. Sitzungsb. d.k. Akad. d. Wissensch. Math.-naturw. Cl. 3 Abt., Vienna 84:469–502, 1882.
2. Aminoff MJ: Spinal Angiomas. Oxford: Blackwell Scientific Publications, 1976.
3. Corbin, JL: Anatomie et Pathologie Artérielles de la Moelle. Paris: Masson, 1961.
4. Crock HV, Yoshizawa H: The Blood Supply of the Vertebral Column and Spinal Cord in Man. New York: Springer-Verlag, 1977.
5. DiChiro G: Unintentional spinal cord arteriography: a warning. Radiology 112:231–233, 1974.
6. DiChiro G, Doppman J, Ommaya AK: Selective arteriography of arteriovenous aneurysms of the spinal cord. Radiology 88:1065–1077, 1967.
7. DiChiro G, Wener L: Angiography of the spinal cord. A review of contemporary techniques and applications. J Neurosurg 39:1–29, 1973.
8. Djindjian M, Djindjian R, Rey A, et al: Intradural extramedullary spinal arterio-venous malformation fed by the anterior spinal artery. Surg Neurol 8:85–94, 1977.
9. Djindjian R: Angiography in angiomas of the spinal cord. In Pia HW, Djindjian R (eds): Spinal Angiomas. Advances in Diagnosis and Therapy. Berlin: Springer-Verlag, 1978, pp. 98–136.
10. Djindjian R: Angiography of the Spinal Cord. Baltimore: University Park Press, 1970.
11. Djindjian R: Angiomas of the spinal cord. In Vinken PJ, Bruyn GW, (eds): Handbook of Clinical Neurology. Amsterdam: Elsevier, 1978, vol 32, chapter 16, pp. 465–510.
12. Djindjian R, Fauré C, Houdart R, et al: Exploration angiographique des malformations vasculaires de la moelle épinière. Acta Radiol [Diagn] 5:145–162, 1966.
13. Djindjian R, Merland JJ: Place de l'embolisation dans le traitement des malformations arterio-veineuses médullaires. À propos de 38 cas. Neuroradiology 16:428–429, 1978.
14. Djindjian R, Merland JJ, Djindjian M, et al: Angiography of Spinal Column and Spinal Cord Tumors. New York: Thieme-Stratton, 1981.
15. Dommisse GF: The Arteries and Veins of the Human Spinal Cord From Birth. Edinburgh: Churchill Livingstone, 1975.
16. Doppman JL: The nidus concept of spinal cord arteriovenous malformations. A surgical recommendation based upon angiographic observations. Br J Radiol 44:758–763, 1971.
17. Doppman JL, DiChiro G: Selective Arteriography of the Spinal Cord. St. Louis: Warren H. Green, 1969.
18. Doppman JL, DiChiro G, Ommaya A: Obliteration of spinal cord arteriovenous malformation by percutaneous embolization. Lancet 1:477, 1968.
19. Doppman JL, Krudy AG, Miller DL, et al: Intraarterial digital subtraction angiography of spinal arteriovenous malformations. AJNR 4:1081–1085, 1983.
20. Enzmann DR, Brody WR, Djang WT, et al: Intraarterial digital subtraction spinal angiography. AJNR 4:25–26, 1983.
21. Gillilan LA: The arterial blood supply of the human spinal cord. J Comp Neurol 110:75–103, 1958.
22. Hilal SK, Keim HA: Selective spinal angiography in adolescent scoliosis. Radiology 102:349–359, 1972.
23. Hilal SK, Sane P, Mitchelson WJ, et al: Embolization of vascular malformations of the spinal cord with low viscosity silicone rubber. Neuroradiology 16:430–433, 1978.
24. Houdart R, Djindjian R, Hurth M: Vascular malformations of the spinal cord: the anatomic and therapeutic significance of angiography. J Neurosurg 24:583–594, 1966.
25. Kadyi H: Über die Blutgefässe des menschlichen Rückenmarkes. Nach einer im XV. Bande der Denkschriften d. math.-naturw. Cl. d. Akad. d. Wissensch. in Krakau erschienenen Monographie, aus dem Polnischen übersetzt vom Verfasser. Lemberg: Gubrynowicz und Schmidt, 1889.
26. Kardjiev V, Symeonov A, Chankov T: Etiology, pathogenesis and prevention of spinal cord lesions in selective angiography of the bronchial and intercostal arteries. Radiology 112:81–83, 1974.
27. Kendall BE, Logue V: Spinal epidural angiomatous malformations draining into intrathecal veins. Neuroradiology 13:181–189, 1977.
28. Lazorthes, G: La vascularisation artérielle de la moelle. Recherches anatomiques et application à la pathologie médullaire et aortique. Neurochirurgie 4:3–19, 1958.
29. Logue V: Angiomas of the spinal cord: review of the pathogenesis, clinical features, and results of surgery. J Neurol Neurosurg Psychiat 42:1–11, 1979.

30. Merland JJ, Djindjian M, Chiras J, et al: Recent advances in spinal cord arteriography. In Post MJD, (ed): Radiographic Evaluation of the Spine. New York: Masson, 1980, pp. 623–645.

31. Merland JJ, Riché MC, Cheras J: Intraspinal extramedullary arteriovenous fistulae draining into the medullary veins. J Neuroradiol 7:271–320, 1980.

32. Oldfield EH, DiChiro G, Quindlen EA et al: Successful treatment of a group of spinal cord arteriovenous malformations by interruption of dural fistulae. J Neurosurg 59:1019–1030, 1983.

33. Ovitt TW, Christenson PC, Fisher HD III, et al: Intravenous angiography using digital video subtraction: x-ray imaging system. AJNR 1:387–390, 1980.

34. Riché MC, Melki JP, Merland JJ: Embolization of spinal cord vascular malformations via the anterior spinal artery. AJNR 4:378–381, 1983.

35. Riché MC, Modenesi-Freitas J, Djindjian M, et al: Arteriovenous malformations (AVM) of the spinal cord in children. A review of 38 cases. Neuroradiology 22:171–180, 1982.

36. Riché MC, Scialfa G, Gueguen B, et al: Giant extramedullary arteriovenous fistula supplied by the anterior spinal artery: treatment by detachable balloons. AJNR 4:391–394, 1983.

37. Shiozawa L., Tanaka Y, Makino N, et al: Spinal cord angiography using 4× magnification. Radiology 127:181, 1978.

38. Symon L, Kuyama H, Kendall B: Dural arteriovenous malformations of the spine. Clinical features and surgical results in 55 cases. J Neurosurg 60:238–247, 1984.

39. Theron J, Derlon JM, dePreux J: Angiography of the spinal cord after vertebral trauma. Neuroradiology 15:201–212, 1978.

40. Vogelsang H, Dietz K: Stereoscopic magnification in spinal angiography. AJNR 4:588–589, 1983.

14

David C. Kushner, M.D.
Robert H. Cleveland, M.D.

Digital Imaging in Scoliosis

Digital radiography is the most recent technologic advance for the diagnosis and follow-up examination in patients with scoliosis.[6, 7a] It is an imaging modality that is easy to perform and, compared with routine radiographs, employs relatively little radiation to acquire an image of the spine.[5, 11] A patient can undergo dozens of images before receiving the x-ray exposure required for a single routine radiograph of the spine.[1, 9, 12, 13]

INDICATIONS

Digital radiography is indicated as one of the imaging components necessary in the evaluation and follow-up of patients suspected of having scoliosis.[8]

TECHNICAL CONSIDERATIONS

The sophisticated technical information regarding the process of low-dose digital examination is beyond the scope of this chapter. Additional information may be sought by the interested reader.[1, 3, 11]

Basically, low-dose digital radiography of the spine is performed on a commercially available device that consists of four major components: an x-ray source, a detector, an image processor/computer, and an image display system.[10] The x-ray source and detector are positioned in an "upright gantry," so that the images of the patient can be acquired in the erect position.[7] As in standard radiography, the standing patient is positioned between the x-ray source and the detector. In contrast to standard radiography, the scanning system creates less distortion and magnification of the image when the patient is positioned as close as possible to the x-ray source rather than to the detector.[10] The x-ray source consists of a high-output x-ray tube matched with both rotating and fixed collimators. As the x-ray beam emerges from the x-ray tube, it is intercepted by a rapidly rotating lead collimator wheel, which allows only a tiny "point" of x-ray beam to enter the patient. The rotating wheel sweeps the scanning beam across the patient's width, producing a "line" of scan formation.[7a] As the x-ray tube is moved caudad, additional consecutive horizontal lines of scanned information are acquired. The time required for the scanning device to complete a spinal image of a patient is 20 msec per line, 10 sec total duration.[1, 3, 5]

The x-ray scanning beam emerges from the collimator housing, passes through the patient across an air-gap, and then is intercepted by a detector that moves simultaneously with the scanning beam so that each consecutive scan line of information is detected. The detector is a very efficient x-ray absorber, and, because of the tiny x-ray beam size and the air-gap, the detection system is virtually 100% efficient and free of image degradation by scatter.[2, 3] Following the scan, the accumulated analog data are converted to digital data and entered into computer memory for processing and display.[2] Careful calibration is used to ensure that the visual image is an accurate representation of the geometry of the patient's spine.[6]

The visual display of the digital image requires the use of an image processor and

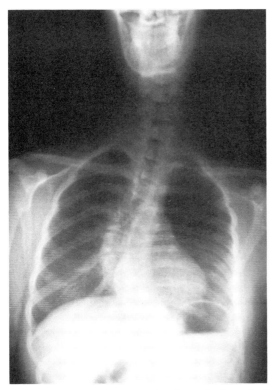

Figure 14–1. Low-dose digital radiograph of a patient who has scoliosis. Image displayed as it appears on the video display terminal (negative mode, only upper half displayed) in real time.

a high video display monitor. The image processor permits the viewing physician to select which data (window width and level) to display, so that the visual image of highest quality will be represented and the most useful information will be presented. The image can be recorded on film and stored on magnetic tape.[5, 10] The image appears on the video display monitor immediately after the scan is completed, and it can be manipulated immediately (Fig. 14–1). The image can be recorded on a multiformat camera as a single image of the entire spine (26 inches [66 cm] of patient spinal length presented on a single 8 × 10 inch sheet of film) (Fig. 14–2). Alternatively, the upper half of the spine (cephalad 13 inches [33 cm]) can be presented on one sheet of 8 × 10 inch film (Fig. 14–3A), and the lower half of the spine (caudad 13 inches [33 cm]) can be presented on a second sheet of 8 × 10 inch film (Fig. 14–3B). These sheets can be manually taped together so that the entire spine can be viewed in continuity.[6]

The images of each of the two halves of

the spine possess twice the spatial resolution of a single image of the entire spine. Therefore, the half-spine images can be utilized to search for intrinsic skeletal anomalies or other causes of scoliosis. The single image of the entire spine, although of lower spatial resolution, permits excellent analysis of the general shape of the curve and the relation-

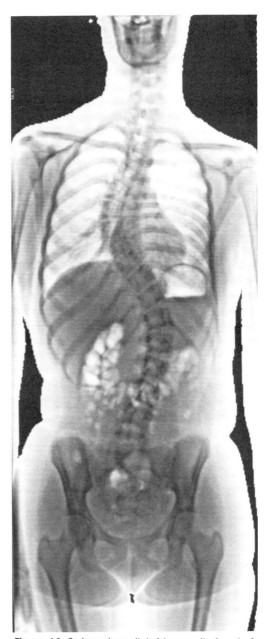

Figure 14–2. Low-dose digital image displayed after computer processed contrast enhancement and reduction of image size, permitting the entire spine (30 inch [76.2 cm] image length) to be displayed on a single terminal.

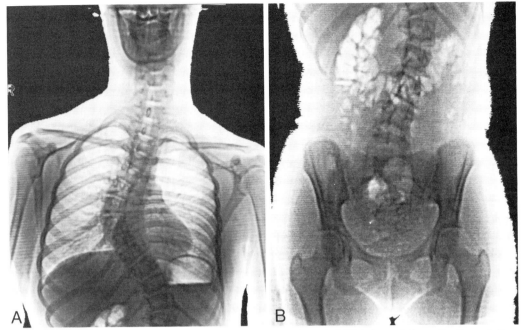

Figure 14–3. Low-dose digital images of the cephalad (*A*) and caudad (*B*) halves of the patient's scoliotic spine, displayed after computer processed contrast enhancement.

ship of the thoracic and lumbar components to each other.[3, 6]

ADVANTAGES

There are several advantages to using low-dose digital radiography in the evaluation of patients suspected of having scoliosis. The most significant advantage is the relatively low radiation dose.[1, 5, 6] A dose of only 2 mR (milliroentgen) of skin exposure is required for a digital scoliosis image as compared with 980 mR for a plain radiograph of the lumbosacral spine or 48 mR for the anteroposterior chest examination.[9, 12, 13]

Operation of the scanner requires basic skills in radiologic technology, with additional minimal training to manage the computer. An image of a patient can be made as long as he or she is able to remain stationary and erect for 10 seconds. Normal breathing motion will not interfere with the image.

Digital imaging permits the entire spine to be viewed following a single exposure just by altering window settings.[7a] No image, therefore, is judged uninterpretable because of over- or underpenetration. The physician can always compensate for varying levels of darkness or lightness of contrast seen on the initial image by changing the image as it appears on the video display terminal (Fig. 14–1.)[5, 6]

Another advantage of digital imaging is that the image appears instantaneously on the video display terminal at the end of the scan (Fig. 14–1). This image, which can be manipulated immediately, can be displayed at several sites simultaneously. Thus, physicians in remote viewing sites, such as the orthopedic clinic, can observe the image, while one physician at the central console alters the window settings.[5, 6] The high level of contrast resolution inherent in digital imaging permits selection of optimal window settings for the upper portion of the spine (where there is little soft tissue absorption) in the scoliosis examination, followed by selection of window settings appropriate for viewing the thoracolumbar junction and lumbosacral regions (where more absorption of x-ray beam has occurred owing to thicker soft tissue and bony structures).[3, 6, 10]

Another advantage of digital processing is the application of software programs that allow the radiologist to generate a *scoliosis angle* rapidly by applying cursors to the scoliotic regions of the spine, thus obviating the use of manual measurement (Fig. 14–4).[6] In addition, software programs can be

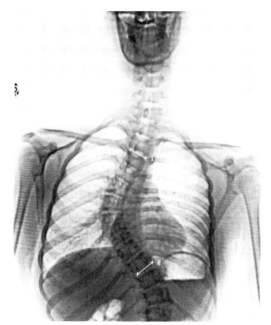

Figure 14–4. Low-dose digital image displayed with scoliosis angle software program demonstration. Image margin describes a scoliosis angle of 28.8 degrees.

selected that allow skeletal structures to display more contrast than they do in the initial visual image. This may help to partially compensate for the intrinsic low spatial resolution of digital radiography[3] (see Figs. 14–1 and 14–2).

LIMITATIONS

There are several limitations to digital radiography. The low radiation exposures, although adequate for anteroposterior views of the spine, are not sufficient for the evaluation of the lateral spine because of the increase in soft tissue absorption in the lumbar region (Fig. 14–5). In the clinical setting, the lateral images have not, as yet, been satisfactory enough to replace plain lateral radiographs. However, new detector systems may eliminate this problem in the near future.[6]

The spatial resolution of digital imaging systems is of far lower quality than the spatial resolution of plain radiographs.[7a] Thus, the digital image should not be a substitute for the plain radiograph, particularly in those individuals suspected of having a structural, inflammatory, or neoplastic etiology for the scoliosis. Small neoplasms and areas of destruction and malformation

may not be detected with the digital system but may be detected on a higher-resolution standard radiograph.[3]

Additionally, the time needed to acquire a scoliosis image is 10 seconds, during which the patient must remain still. A lateral body motion will cause a deformity in the scanning image, which may be misinterpreted as intrinsic scoliosis. The technician, observing the patient closely during the

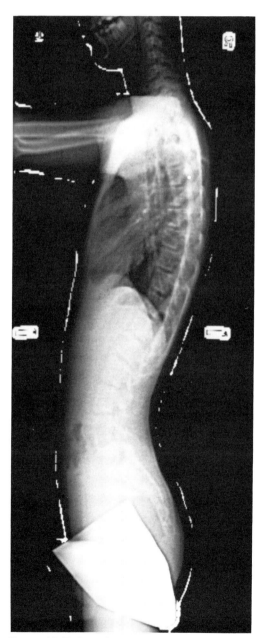

Figure 14–5. Low-dose digital image performed in lateral projection and displayed after computer processed image enhancement.

scan, can reject any image if patient movement has occurred.[6]

COMPLICATIONS

There are no known complications of digital radiography when used in the evaluation and follow-up of patients suspected of having scoliosis.

UTILIZATION

Scoliosis is a common curvature deformity of the spine, with the potential to progress to severe disfigurement, morbidity, and even mortality.[4] The current standard of pediatric practice is to attempt to detect scoliosis early in its course, in as large a childhood population as possible, with the goal of applying early therapy and, it is hoped, thereby preventing progression. Physical examination screening is usually accomplished by health professionals during the secondary school years. When scoliosis is detected, the child is usually referred for further evaluation.[8] Previously, this evaluation included routine radiographic film examination, sometimes with multiple radiographs. The availablility of low-dose digital radiography permits significant reduction in the radiation dose to the patient during both the initial evaluation and the follow-up phase of care. If scoliosis is confirmed by radiography, follow-up examinations during therapy are performed every 6 to 12 months until the age of skeletal maturity is reached. Occasionally, scoliosis continues to progress beyond skeletal maturity, in which case additional radiation exposure is necessary. In a case requiring multiple radiographic examinations over long periods of time, there is a dramatic reduction in radiation exposure from digital technology compared with that from standard radiography.

Low-dose digital radiography allows scoliosis to be evaluated with a relatively low radiation burden. In addition, the degree of curvature can be measured quickly and easily. Only anteroposterior views are used routinely. If lordosis or kyphosis are concomitant problems, the digital lateral image may be useful only for very thin or small patients. Older and larger patients (over 10 years old) demonstrate unacceptable lateral digital images because their relatively thicker soft tissues act as x-ray absorbers in this projection.

If the digital lateral examination is not adequate, routine radiographic film examination is performed. Also, if the etiology for the scoliosis of a child is suspected of being structural, neoplastic, or inflammatory, he or she is evaluated with higher-resolution standard radiographs in place of or in addition to the digital examination.

References

1. Annis M, Bjorkholm P, Frederick E, et al: Dose reduction using digital radiography. Presented at the Health Physics Society 14th Mid Year Topical Symposium. December 8–12, 1980.
2. Bjorkholm PJ, Annis M, Frederick EE: Digital radiography. Proceedings of application of optical instrumentation in medicine VIII. Proc SPIE 233:137–144, 1981.
3. Bjorkholm P, Annis M, Frederick E, et al: Digital radiography: spatial and contrast resolution. Proceedings of application of optical instrumentation in medicine IX. Proc SPIE 273:103–107, 1981.
4. Brooks HL, Azen SP, Gerberg E, et al: Scoliosis: a prospective epidemiological study. J Bone Joint Surg 57A:968–972, 1975.
5. Heller RM, Erickson JJ, Price RR: Pediatric nonangiographic applications of digital radiography. In Price RR, Rollo FD, Monahan WG, et al (eds): Digital Radiology: A Focus on Clinical Utility. New York: Grune & Stratton, 1982, pp 267–277.
6. Kushner DC, Cleveland RH, Herman TE, et al.: Scanning beam low dose digital radiography: initial clinical trials relevant to pediatric radiography. AJR 141:847, 1983.
7. Kushner D, Cleveland R, Herman TE, et al: Detection and evaluation of chest abnormalities with low-dose scanning beam digital radiography: comparison with standard radiographs. Radiology 149:64, 1983. Presented at the 69th Scientific Assembly and Annual Meeting of the RSNA. November, 1983.
7a. Kushner DC, Cleveland RH, Herman TE, et al: Radiation dose reduction in the evaluation of scoliosis: an application of digital radiography. Radiology 161:175–181, 1986.
8. Ozonoff MB: Pediatric Orthopedic Radiology. Philadelphia: WB Saunders Company, 1979, pp 30–69.
9. Radiation Protection in Pediatric Radiology. Recommendations of the National Council on Radiation Protection and Measurements. NCRP Report No. 68. Washington DC. February 15, 1981, p 56 (Appendix A).
10. Stein JA: X-ray imaging with a scanning beam. Radiology 117:713–716, 1975.
11. Tateno Y, Tanaka H: Low-dosage x-ray imaging system employing flying spot x-ray microbeam (dynamic scanner). Radiology 121:189–195, 1976.
12. Webster EW, Alpert NM, Brownell GL: Radiation doses in pediatric nuclear medicine and diagnostic x-ray procedures. In James AE, Wagner HM Jr, Cooke RE (eds): Pediatric Nuclear Medicine. Philadelphia: WB Saunders Company, 1974, p 34.
13. Whalen JP, Balter S: Radiation Risks in Medical Imaging. Chicago: Year Book Medical Publishers, Inc, 1984, pp 26 and 107 (Appendix B).

15

Matthew E. Pasto, M.D.
Barry B. Goldberg, M.D.

Sonography

Sonography, or ultrasonography, is a versatile and highly accurate imaging modality when used to study soft tissue and fluid areas.[3] Sonography has generally not been used in the evaluation of the adult spine, because the ultrasound beam, at standard frequencies and intensities, does not penetrate bone to any significant degree. However, ultrasonography is currently used in the examination of the fetal spine in search of neural tube defects, and it is also used in the neonatal spine to search for and document spinal dysraphism and associated soft tissue tumors.[*] Ultrasonography is also gaining popularity as an aid to the orthopedic and neurologic surgeon in evaluation of the brain and spinal cord in the operating room as well as in following these patients postoperatively.[†]

TECHNICAL CONSIDERATIONS

The ultrasonographic examination involves directing sound waves into tissues to produce an image of the organ or structure being studied. Ultrasonographic examinations are performed using static (or contact) or real-time equipment or both. In static scanning, the ultrasound beam is directed by the sonographer, and its position is recorded by an articulated arm attached to the transducer. Static scanners can give an overview of a large area and can demonstrate relationships between one organ or mass and another. Real-time scanning is useful in

small areas of interest and when observing internal motion is critical to the examination. Two different transducer formats are available for real-time scanning. One is sector real-time scanning, in which the sound beam is steered in an arc of 60 to 100 degrees. This produces a pie-shaped image and requires only a small area of contact with the patient. The second format, linear array scanning, produces a rectangular field of view. This type of transducer works best when a flat surface is available for transducer contact. Both formats allow for demonstration of motion and easy orientation of scan plane.

The sound wave frequency used in ultrasonographic examinations varies from 1,000,000 to 12,000,000 cycles per second, abbreviated 1.0 to 12.0 MHz (megaHertz). The lowest frequencies are capable of the greatest penetration; they can penetrate the skull and have been used in obtaining the reflections from the ventricles and midline structures of the brain (echoencephalography).[30, 31] The highest frequencies are used for delineating superficial structures such as the thyroid, eye, and carotid arteries. They also have better resolution than the lowest frequencies. Echoes are returned to the transducer whenever the sonic beam reaches an interface between tissues of varying acoustic impedance, which is related to the structure and elasticity of the tissues.

Solid tissues have homogeneous to slightly granular reflectivity (echogenicity) of varying intensity, depending on their internal structure. Fluid areas, however, have no internal structure, and therefore no echoes return to the transducer. In addition,

---

*See references 5, 9, 13, 16, 18, 20, 23, 25–27.
†See references 1, 2, 7, 10, 12, 17, 21, 22, 24.

598

the reflectivity distal to fluid areas is greater than that seen when the sound beam passes through solid areas. Brightness of the returning echoes is related to (1) the mismatch and acoustic impedance from one tissue to the next, (2) the angle of incidence of the sound beam—the more perpendicular the angle, the greater the reflection, and (3) the smoothness of the interface—the smoother the boundary, the more sound will be reflected back to the transducer.

Ultrasound is calculated to travel at a speed of 1540 m per sec in soft tissue and body fluids. The "time of flight" of the echo then corresponds to the depth of the structure visualized. The speed of sound in air and in bone is significantly different from that in soft tissues, resulting in a great acoustic mismatch. Therefore, nearly all of the sound beam is reflected when soft tissues interface with air or bone. Thus structures deep to bone or air cannot be visualized by using ultrasound. Cartilage and bone that have not yet ossified transmit a significant portion of the sound beam; therefore, the fetal brain as well as the neonatal and fetal spine can be examined easily by ultrasonography. The fluid surrounding the spinal cord serves as an aid in identifying the margins of the cord itself. The neural tissue is very homogeneous and reflects only a small amount of the ultrasound beam, giving its typical hypoechoic appearance.

SONOGRAPHY OF THE PRENATAL SPINE

Cursory imaging of the fetal spine is part of the routine obstetric ultrasonographic examination.[5, 16, 20, 29] However, if there is a familial history of neural tube defects, the fetus is at increased risk for spinal dysraphism. If maternal blood sampling reveals an elevated alpha-fetoprotein level (AFP), an ultrasonographic examination is done to date the pregnancy accurately and to search for severe fetal defects. In many cases, amniocentesis is performed at 15 to 16 weeks' gestational age. Elevated AFP levels in the amniotic fluid almost always indicate a severe fetal abnormality, but only 40% of these are neural tube defects.[14]

Other abnormalities causing an elevated AFP level are encephaloceles, omphaloceles, and gastroschisis. A false negative finding concerning AFP level occurs when a neural tube defect is completely covered by intact skin, since only "open" defects cause an elevation of the fetoprotein concentration. Another biochemical compound related to neural tube defects is acetylcholinesterase. Abnormally high acetylcholinesterase levels occur in 99.4% of the open neural tube defects but may occur also with severe nonneurologic fetal abnormalities, including exomphalos.[32] Because of the high false positive and false negative rates and the nonspecificity of these chemical markers, sonography is used to evaluate further the possibility of neural tube defects in utero.[29] Most meningoceles and meningomyeloceles larger than 1 to 2 cm in diameter are usually visualized, and some smaller than 1 cm may be detected. Amniograms (film contrast studies of the uterine contents) are very rarely done in the evaluation of neural tube defects because of the current accuracy of real-time ultrasonograms. The larger neural tube defects have been detected as early as 14 weeks with the aid of high-resolution ultrasonographic equipment.

Technique

Sonography of the uterus of the pregnant patient is generally performed with real-time equipment prior to the 20th week of gestation. After the 20th week of gestation, in addition to real-time equipment, static ultrasonographic imaging of the uterus can be used to visualize the entire uterine contents in order to estimate the uterine volume. Real-time scanning, because of its ability to orient scan planes rapidly and to follow fetal movements, is then used to evaluate fetal anatomy in detail. A transducer of the highest frequency possible is used. Thus in thin patients and in those in the early stages of pregnancy, 5 MHz transducers are most frequently used because of their higher resolution. In heavier patients and in those in the later stages of pregnancy, 3.0 to 3.5 MHz transducers are used. The fetal spine is visualized in transverse, coronal, and sagittal views if possible. The fetal back should also be evaluated for absence or distortion of the normal posterior soft tissues or the presence of a paraspinal mass.

Ultrasonographic Findings

In transverse view, the normal spine is visualized as three strongly reflecting ossifi-

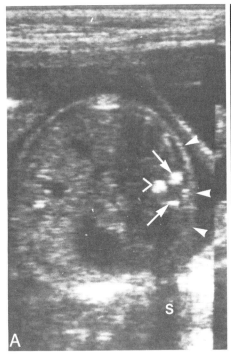

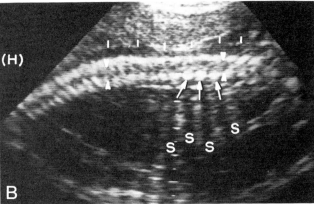

Figure 15-1. Normal fetal spine. *A*, A transverse view of the fetal abdomen demonstrates the fetal spine. The vertebral body ossification center (open arrowhead) is seen at the apex of a triangle formed by the two posterior ossification centers (arrows). The spine casts an acoustic shadow (**S**). The normal posterior soft tissues can also be delineated (solid arrowheads). *B*, Long axis sagittal view demonstrates two rows of brightly echogenic ossification centers, some of which are indicated by arrows. Acoustic shadows (**S**) are visualized distal to these centers. The spinal canal (arrowheads) is visualized between the echogenic rows. Note the normal fetal soft tissues posterior to the spine (lines). **H** = toward fetal head. (From Pasto ME, Kurtz AB: The prenatal examination of the fetal cranium, spine and central nervous system. Semin Ultrasound, CT, MR 5:170–193, 1984. Reprinted by permission.)

cation centers at each vertebral level: one for the vertebral body and one for each adjacent pars interarticularis (Fig. 15–1*A*). These three echogenic foci form a triangular appearance. Echoes forming parallel lines represent the spine in longitudinal view (Fig. 15–1*B*). Usually only two lines are visualized in any one image plane; the spinal canal is located between the two posterior (pars foci) echogenic lines. The canal should be parallel throughout the length of the spine, except for a slight widening of the canal in the cervical region. A mild kyphosis is often noted in the thoracic region. Often a longitudinal view of the spine in sagittal projection demonstrates a smooth line, which represents the posterior soft tissues. It must be emphasized that each vertebral level must be imaged carefully to rule out divergence of the two posterior ossification centers, a finding that would indicate spinal dysraphism.

A meningocele is visualized as a cystic mass projecting posteriorly from the spine, with divergence of the adjacent posterior ossification centers (Fig. 15–2). The meningoceles are rarely larger than 3 to 4 cm in diameter. Septations and echogenic material within the meningocele indicate the pres-

ence of neural tissue, making it possible to diagnose a meningomyelocele. Occasionally a meningocele will rupture, leaving only an area of soft tissue absence or irregularity associated with a widening of the canal. These areas will be more difficult to detect if each vertebral level is not imaged carefully for widening of the canal. Diastematomyelia has also been diagnosed in utero.[33]

Mass lesions may originate from the spine; several have been documented sonographically in utero. The most common is a teratoma, which is a benign lesion usually located in the sacrococcygeal area (Fig. 15–3).[28] Teratomas typically project caudally from the sacrum and contain both solid and cystic elements. Prenatal, ultrasound-guided needle aspiration of a teratoma has been performed as a debulking procedure in order to ease delivery of the fetus.[15]

Another abnormality of the spine that can be detected by ultrasound is deficient skeletal ossification, such as that which occurs in hypophosphatasia.[11, 20] This has been reported in severe forms of osteogenesis imperfecta and in some cases of achondrogenesis. Ultrasonically, the vertebral bodies lack their normal bright echogenicity and usually will not produce distal acoustic shadowing

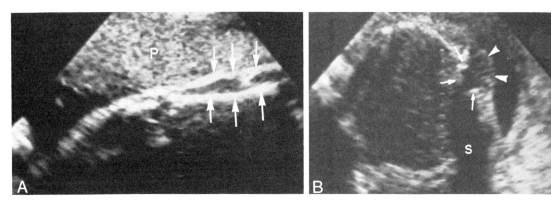

Figure 15–2. Lower thoracic meningomyelocele. *A*, Long axis view demonstrates widening of the spinal canal (arrows). The placenta (**P**) is seen adjacent to the back so that the posterior soft tissues are not well delineated. *B*, Transverse view demonstrates the thoracic meningomyelocele (arrowheads) extending posteriorly out of the widened spinal canal. The splayed vertebral ossification centers (arrows) still cast an acoustic shadow (**S**). (From Pasto ME, Kurtz AB: The prenatal examination of the fetal cranium, spine and central nervous system. Semin Ultrasound, CT, MR 5:170–193, 1984. Reprinted by permission.)

(Fig. 15–4). The echogenicity of the skull is also diminished. In these cases, the echoes arising from the falx cerebri will be as bright or brighter than the echoes arising from the bones.

SONOGRAPHY OF THE INFANT SPINE

Overt spinal abnormalities are easily recognized at birth; however, the internal structure of these anomalies is often not so easily demonstrated by any methodology. An ultrasound transducer can be applied directly to the surface of a meningocele or meningomyelocele to help delineate the internal contents.[19] The more insidious lesion may be an occult spinal dysraphism or spinal cord tethering, the signs of which can be voiding difficulties or lower limb neurologic problems as the child matures. Sonography enables us to see the neonatal spinal cord and to detect the presence of tethered cord syndrome as well as the often associated lipoma.* Ultrasonography has been used as a screening modality in patients with sacral cutaneous abnormalities such as hairy nevus, hypertrichosis, hemangiomas, and dermal sinus tracts, because of its ease of use, availability, and lack of ionizing radiation.

---

*See references 9, 13, 18, 19, 25, 27.

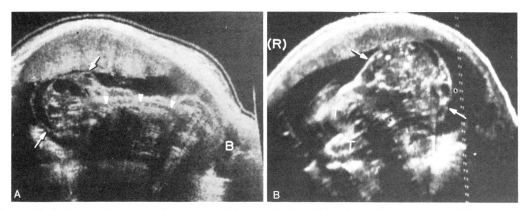

Figure 15–3. Large sacrococcygeal teratoma. *A*, Long axis view of the fetal spine (arrowheads) demonstrates a complex mass (arrows) extending caudally from the lower lumbar region. **B** = maternal bladder. *B*, Transverse view of the mass (arrows) again demonstrates its cystic and solid components. **T** = fetal thighs; **R** = toward maternal right. (From Pasto ME, Kurtz AB: The prenatal examination of the fetal cranium, spine and central nervous system. Semin Ultrasound, CT, MR 5:170–193, 1984. Reprinted by permission.)

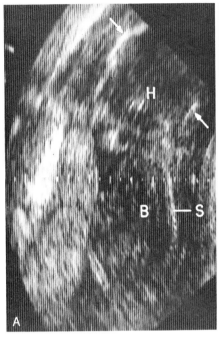
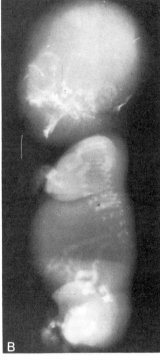

Figure 15–4. Achondrogenesis. *A*, This long axis view shows decreased bone brightness in the fetal spine **(S)** and calvarium (arrows). (Compare with 15–1 *B*.) **H** = fetal head; **B** = fetal body. *B*, Lateral radiograph of fetus following elective termination of pregnancy. Note the very poor ossification of the calvarium and spine. (From Kurtz AB, Wapner RJ: Ultrasonographic diagnosis of second-trimester skeletal dysplasias: A prospective analysis in the high-risk population. JUM 2:99–106, 1983.)

Technique

Scanning is easily accomplished over the area of interest using either real-time or static ultrasonographic equipment. A transducer of the highest frequency possible should be utilized. Transducers of from 7.5 to 10 MHz have been used successfully for very superficial lesions. Since the neonatal spine is still somewhat poorly ossified, the ultrasound beam will usually penetrate the lamina. Adjacent cutaneous and subcutaneous abnormalities have also been documented. One investigator has used an automated water path scanner.[13] This equipment was able to produce an image of a long section of the spine, making it easier to demonstrate its curvature and the overlying soft tissues. In infants, myelography is often risky, and computed tomography often requires sedation. Sonography that is performed at diagnostic energy levels has no proven deleterious effects in the human, and it can be done in the neonatal intensive care unit if necessary, which is a distinct advantage over other imaging methods.

Ultrasonographic Findings

Longitudinal images of the cord are often the best for delineating abnormalities. Any variations in the echogenicity or size of the cord usually can be seen as the successive laminae are traversed by the sound beam. The dural sac is well demonstrated as two brightly echogenic parallel lines. Fluid is noted around the spinal cord, which is itself hypoechogenic. Linear areas of echogenicity demarcate the ventral and dorsal aspects of the cord.

Meningoceles can be scanned to determine the presence or absence of neural elements within them. In one case, a large fluid-filled meningocele contained only a thin band of tissue, which represented the filum terminale. The lower cord/conus was deviated posteriorly (Fig. 15–5). In another patient exhibiting neurologic symptoms, a dimple was noted over the lower back, and the tethered cord syndrome was suspected. Longitudinal ultrasonograms demonstrated a focal echogenic enlargement of the lumbar cord, which represented a lipoma (Fig. 15–6). The ultrasonographic diagnosis of tethered cord syndrome was aided by utilizing real-time equipment to demonstrate that the conus medullaris was fixed dorsally within the distal thecal sac. The normal conus is located centrally and exhibits a mild undulating motion when observed on real-time examination.[9, 25] A soft tissue deformity over the lower back in another child was shown

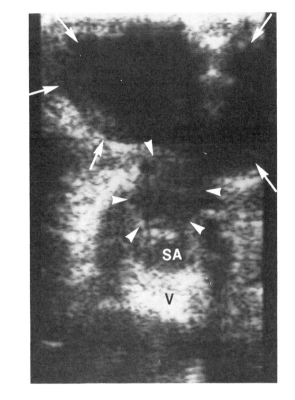

Figure 15–5. Large meningocele. This transverse magnified view demonstrates a large cystic mass (arrows) located posteriorly. The conus (arrowheads) is deviated posteriorly, enlarging the subarachnoid space (**SA**) between the thecal sac and the adjacent vertebral body margin (**V**).

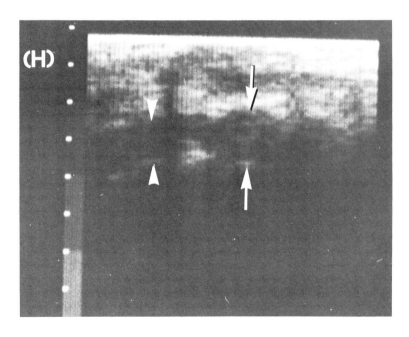

Figure 15–6. Spinal cord lipoma. This longitudinal view of the lumbar canal (arrowheads) demonstrates focal enlargement (arrows) in the region of the conus medullaris. Normal excursion of the distal thecal sac was not observed. **H** = toward patient's head.

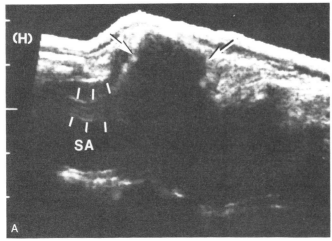

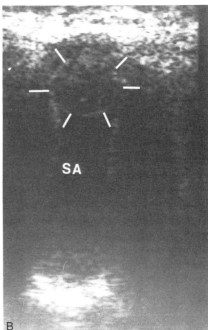

Figure 15–7. Dysraphism with large lipoma. *A*, A longitudinal posterior scan demonstrates a large lipoma (arrows) and posterior deviation of the cord (lines). **H** = towards patient's head; **SA** = subarachnoid space. *B*, A magnified transverse view of the cephalad margin of the mass demonstrates the posteriorly deviated cord (lines) enlarging the ventral subarachnoid space **(SA)**.

to represent a solid mass (lipoma) with posterior tethering of the conus (Fig. 15–7).

SONOGRAPHY OF THE ADULT SPINE

Technique and Limitations

Sonographic examination of the adult spine is fairly limited by the ossified neural arch. Posterior views of the spinal canal can be obtained by angling the transducer 15 degrees centrally from either side of the true median sagittal plane.[8] Visualization of the depth of the canal can be obtained between each successive lamina (Fig. 15–8A). Static contact scanning was the first method of investigation implemented, but real-time scanning also has been used to perform this procedure (Fig. 15–8B, C, D). Limitations include (1) calcification of the ligamentum flavum, which prevents the ultrasound beam from penetrating into the canal, and (2) any cause of narrowing of the intralaminar distance, that is, exaggerated lordosis, hypertrophic spurring, and degenerative disease.[6] Although knowledge of the anteroposterior dimensions of the canal is important in the work-up of spinal neuralgia, free extruded disc fragments and nerve root compression cannot be evaluated by sonographic techniques. An image of the spinal canal can

also be made from an anteroabdominal approach by directing the beam through a disc space that is intact (Fig. 15–9). Usually with this approach, only several disc levels in the lumbar region can be delineated in any one patient. Obesity, bowel gas, and spurs bridging the disc space all limit implementation of this technique; therefore, it is also not widely used.

INTRAOPERATIVE ULTRASONOGRAPHY

Sonography has recently become an important supportive procedure in the orthopedic or neurosurgical theater.* Ultrasonography is helpful in identifying abnormalities anterior to the spinal cord, thus minimizing complications of cord retraction.[21A] Sonography can be used during surgery to identify spinal cord enlargement and whether it is cystic or solid in nature. It can also differentiate mass from normal cord tissue. The dimensions of the abnormality can be documented easily in both longitudinal and transverse planes. Ultrasonographic examination can delineate the most direct surgical approach to the tumor, cyst, or collection, with the least trauma to normal

---

*See references 1A, 2, 7, 10, 17, 21–24, 26.

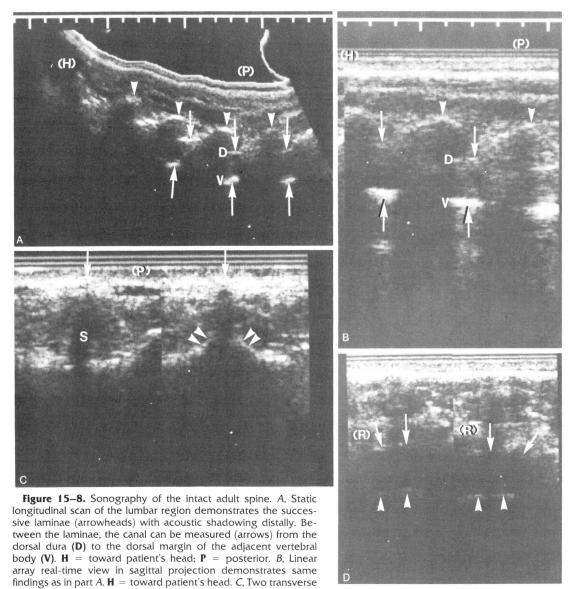

Figure 15–8. Sonography of the intact adult spine. *A*, Static longitudinal scan of the lumbar region demonstrates the successive laminae (arrowheads) with acoustic shadowing distally. Between the laminae, the canal can be measured (arrows) from the dorsal dura (**D**) to the dorsal margin of the adjacent vertebral body (**V**). **H** = toward patient's head; **P** = posterior. *B*, Linear array real-time view in sagittal projection demonstrates same findings as in part *A*. **H** = toward patient's head. *C*, Two transverse real-time views of the spinous process (arrows). The view at one level is shown on the left, and the spinous process and the laminae (arrowheads) in a slightly different projection are shown on the right. **P** = posterior; **S** = acoustic shadow. *D*, Two transverse real-time views angled cephalad in order to avoid the spinous process and the lamina. The dorsal dura (arrows) demarcates the posterior boundary of the spinal canal, and the dorsal aspect of the vertebral body (arrowheads) delineates the ventral extent of the canal. **R** = patient's right.

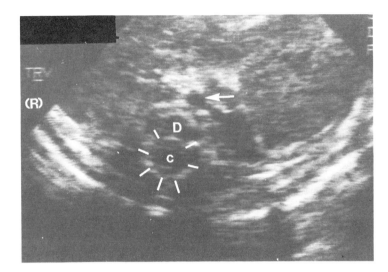

Figure 15–9. Anterior view of the lumbar canal. This transverse view demonstrates the aorta (arrow) and the area of the disc space (**D**). More posterior to this, the spinal canal can be outlined (lines). The spinal cord (**c**) is seen to be centrally placed in this child. **R** = patient's right.

neural tissue. Tumors adjacent to the dura can be visualized using ultrasound, and, in most cases, intradural extension of the tumor can be demonstrated accurately or excluded. Through sonography, the physician can confirm the removal of intradural extramedullary and extradural tumors and also can determine whether spinal cord or cauda equina decompression was adequate. Intraoperative ultrasonography can facilitate tumor biopsy, thus limiting the possibility of spinal cord damage and subsequent neurologic complications. In cases of vertebral body fractures, the dorsally protruding bone fragments (not easily visible from the posterior approach) can be identified readily, allowing for the least possible manipulation of the spinal cord during the surgical reduction. Follow-up imaging can be used to confirm that the cord lies free of impinging bony fragments. Intervertebral discs and herniation of disc tissue can be identified, and, following removal of the herniated tissue, nerve roots can be demonstrated to be free of compression.[21A]

Technique

Five and 7.5 MHz real-time sector scanners are the most commonly used in spinal cord surgery. When the cord is adequately exposed and only the canal and cord need be studied, a 10 MHz transducer can also be used. Transducer size is not critical when multiple laminectomies are performed. However, smaller probes are usually needed when single or keyhole laminectomies are performed. The gloved or sterilized transducer head can be applied directly on the dura once a laminectomy has been performed.[4] Most commonly, however, the open soft tissues of the back, when the patient is prone, form a trough, which can be filled with saline to act as an acoustic coupling agent for the ultrasound beam. This pool of fluid allows for scanning in many orientations, without fear of impinging upon the neural elements.

Ultrasonographic Findings

The normal cord is visualized as a well-defined band of hypoechoic tissue located within the dural sac, with subarachnoid spaces on either side (Fig. 15–10A).[21, 22] A bright line centrally placed in the cord represents the opposed walls of the central canal. In transverse views, the subarachnoid space is seen circumferentially, occasionally with dentate ligaments emanating laterally (Fig. 15–10B). On examination using a real-time scanner, arterial pulsations from the anterior spinal artery can be visualized. The dorsal aspect of the adjacent vertebral body is seen as a brightly echogenic line with distal acoustic shadowing. The conus medullaris and cauda equina may be identified.

Syringomyelia appears as a well-defined fluid space located centrally within the spinal cord (Fig. 15–11).* Its maximum transverse dimension and maximum length

---

See references 1A, 7, 10, 21A, 24, 26.

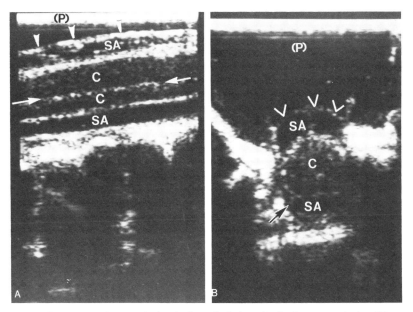

Figure 15–10. Normal intraoperative cervical spinal cord. *A,* Longitudinal scan posterior **(P)** approach, the dura (arrowheads) is the first line encountered. The spinal cord **(C)** is of uniform low-level echogenicity, with the central canal (arrows) visualized as a line of echoes within it. The subarachnoid spaces **(SA)** are noted on either side of the cord. *B,* This transverse view through the posterior **(P)** water-filled trough again demonstrates the subarachnoid spaces **(SA)** surrounding the cord **(C)**. The posterior dura (open arrowheads) and a dentate ligament (arrow) are noted.

can be determined easily. Sonographic examination of the cord following catheterization of a syrinx can confirm the proper positioning of the catheter within the cord (Fig. 15–12). Minimal dilatation of the central canal can be detected, since the axial resolution of the ultrasound beam is less than 1 mm. Atrophy of the cord is no hindrance, nor are subarachnoid adhesions. Computed tomography, even with delayed metrizamide studies, cannot detect all cystic areas, and 2 mm cysts may be below the resolution of magnetic resonance imaging.

Ultrasonography can identify the level of maximum widening of the spinal cord due to an intramedullary tumor and can differentiate mass from normal cord tissue. Intramedullary tumor is suspected if the low-level echoes of the spinal cord are increased, the central canal echo is not seen, or the highly reflective surfaces of the spinal cord are not visible.[23] It should be noted that a

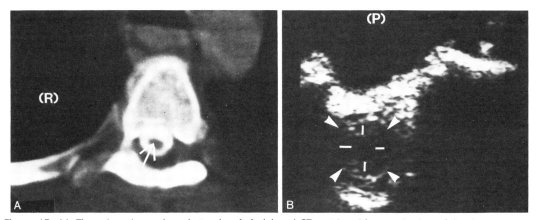

Figure 15–11. Thoracic syrinx and cord atrophy. *A,* A delayed CT metrizamide examination of the thoracic spine in the transaxial projection demonstrates an atrophic thoracic cord (arrow) surrounded by contrast material in the thecal sac. There is no filling of an intramedullary cyst. **R** = patient's right. *B,* Transverse intraoperative ultrasonography through the posterior **(P)** water trough. A syrinx is clearly identified (lines) within the spinal cord (arrowheads).

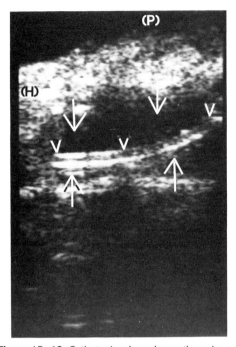

Figure 15–12. Catheter in a large lower thoracic syrinx. This longitudinal view through the posterior water trough (**P**) demonstrates the large syrinx (arrows). The drainage catheter (open arrowheads) enters posteriorly at the inferior margin of the scan plane, and the tip is seen well within the syrinx. **H** = toward patient's head.

traumatized spinal cord may produce similar findings.[24]

Displacement of the cord is commonly caused by extramedullary tumors. An intradural-extramedullary tumor such as neurofibroma or meningioma may be visualized as a solid echogenic mass displacing the spinal cord markedly to one side of the canal (Fig. 15–13). If the spinal cord demonstrates uniform homogeneous echogenicity, involvement by tumor is excluded. The intradural extent of tumor or lack of intradural extension can also be shown ultrasonically (Fig. 15–14).[10, 21, 26] Conventional myelography, and at times CT myelography, usually show only an obstruction and, therefore, fail to assess involvement of the individual tissue planes.

In vertebral body fractures, the ventral aspect of the cord is difficult to visualize via the posterior approach. However, sonography can easily demonstrate fracture fragments impinging upon the cord ventrally (Fig. 15–15), and thus it guides the neurosurgeon to them with the least disturbance of the cord. Ultrasonic imaging can also be used to confirm reduction of these fragments (Fig. 15–15D) and alignment of the vertebral

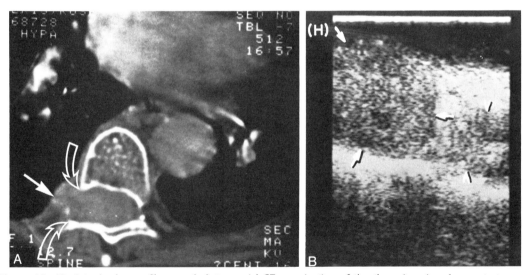

Figure 15–13. Extradural neurofibroma. *A*, A transaxial CT examination of the thoracic spine demonstrates a soft tissue mass filling the canal, expanding the right neural foramen (curved arrows), and extending into the extraspinal space (straight arrow). The mass cannot be distinguished from the spinal cord. *B*, A sagittal view of an intraoperative sonogram demonstrates the soft tissue mass (arrows) occupying the large portion of the canal and compressing the cord. Distally the spinal cord (arrowheads) is seen in its normal location. The echogenicity of the cord was uniform throughout, ruling out direct involvement by the tumor. At surgery, the tumor was easily stripped from the dura. **H** = toward patient's head. (From Pasto ME, Rifkin MD, Rubenstein JB, et al: Real-time ultrasonography of the spinal cord: intraoperative and postoperative imaging. Neuroradiology 26:183–187, 1984.)

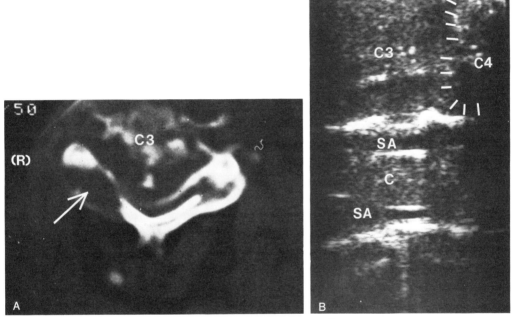

Figure 15–14. Extradural metastasis. *A,* A transaxial CT through the level of C3 demonstrates near complete destruction of the vertebral body. A metastatic lesion is also noted in the posterior elements (arrow) on the right **(R)**. There is compression of the spinal canal. *B,* An intraoperative sagittal view of the cord from the anterior oblique approach was performed after decompression of the canal. The sound is transmitted through the lytic vertebral body **(C3)** delineating the more posterior cord **(C)**. The subarachnoid spaces **(SA)** are clearly seen on both sides of the cord, indicating no intradural extent of tumor. The edge of fourth cervical vertebra **(C4)** is outlined (lines).

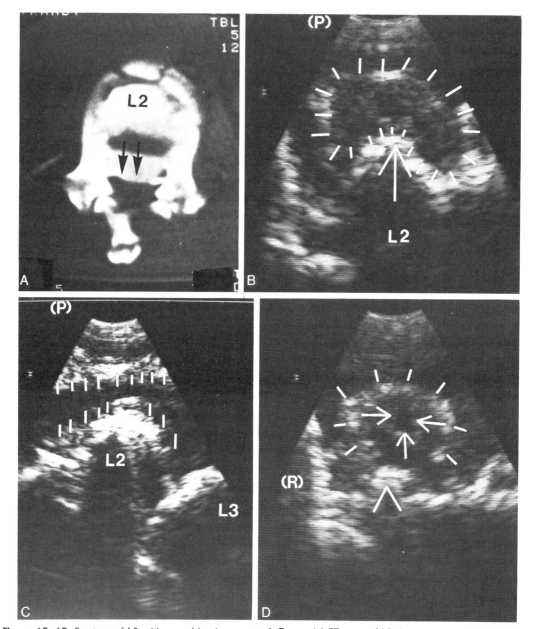

Figure 15–15. Fracture of L2 with neural impingement. *A,* Transaxial CT scan of L2 demonstrates the comminuted fracture as well as dorsal impingement into the spinal canal (arrows). *B,* A transverse intraoperative ultrasound examination demonstrates distortion of the thecal sac (lines) as it drapes over the dorsally protruding fracture fragment (arrow). **P** = posterior. *C,* A sagittal intraoperative ultrasound view demonstrates dorsal displacement and compression of the thecal sac (lines) by the fragments of L2. A normally positioned L3 is noted. *D,* Transverse ultrasound view following near complete reduction of the fracture. The thecal sac (lines) is no longer distorted. However, a small area of hemorrhage (arrows) is noted within. Ventral to the cord, a small fragment of bone (arrowhead) remains dorsally displaced. This fragment was removed on further surgical exploration. **R** = patient's right.

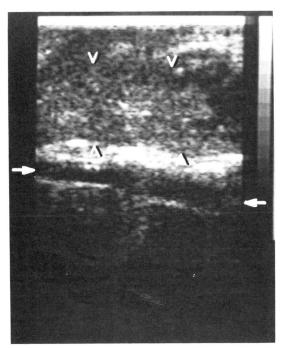

Figure 15–16. Edema or contusion of the spinal cord. A sagittal intraoperative view of the spinal cord (arrowheads) demonstrates an overall increase in its echogenicity, which is the result of contusion during trauma. Vertebral body realignment has been performed, as noted by the normal ventral subarachnoid space (arrows). (From Pasto ME, Rifkin MD, Rubenstein JB, et al: Real-time ultrasonography of the spinal cord: intraoperative and postoperative imaging. Neuroradiology 26:183–187, 1984.)

bodies during the placement of Harrington rods or other fixation devices. In areas of compression (with resultant edema) or contusion of the spinal cord or both, the echogenicity of the cord itself is moderately increased (Fig. 15–16). Further work will be necessary before nerve roots can be confidently delineated to rule out such abnormalities as avulsion.

Iatrogenically introduced substances may be detected by sonography during the surgical procedure and may obscure anatomic detail or cause a confusing ultrasonic image.[22] These include the Harrington rod, oil droplets from a previous myelogram, cottonoid pledgets, or gel foam powder.

Postoperative sequelae also can be visualized at subsequent operations. A large dural scar may be discovered at the site of previous surgical closure (Figs. 15–17 and 15–18).

POSTOPERATIVE ULTRASONOGRAPHY

As stated previously, the spinal cord can generally be well visualized by sonography once several laminae have been removed.[1, 21] A laminectomy of two or more segments provides an adequate window for viewing the underlying spinal cord. The cord itself can be measured to rule out enlargement or atrophy. Postoperative sequelae such as intramedullary cysts and postoperative pseudomeningoceles are ideally suited to ultrasonographic evaluation. Recurrent tumors in an area of prior resection can also often be delineated. Sonography may often provide additional information in areas of subarachnoid adhesions, which often result in inadequate myelographic studies and are less than optimally evaluated by CT. Limitations to the ultrasonic technique include gas in the subcutaneous tissues in the immediate postoperative state or as the result of a gas-forming infection. Also, desmoplastic tissue or calcification in the back following spinal surgery can cause significant attenuation of the sound beam, preventing adequate visualization.

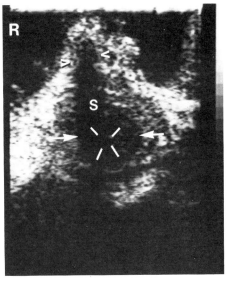

Figure 15–17. Dural scar. Patient with recurrent syringomyelia. A transverse intraoperative view demonstrates a soft tissue mass (arrowheads) that attenuates the sound beam. The mass is adherent to the posterior dural surface and represents a scar from previous surgery. The distal acoustic shadowing (**S**) prevents optimal visualization of the spinal cord (arrows), which contains a dilated central spinal canal (lines). **R** = patient's right.

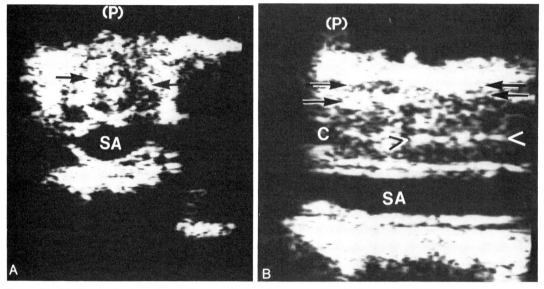

Figure 15–18. Dural adhesion of cord. Same patient as the one in 15–17, 1 year later. Patient developed recurrent symptoms. *A*, Transverse intraoperative view demonstrates an eccentric subarachnoid space **(SA)** that was much larger ventrally. The spinal cord (arrows) was fixed posteriorly **(P)** within the canal. There is no evidence of syringomyelia. *B*, The sagittal view through the posterior **(P)** water path demonstrates an area of dural adhesion (arrows). The cord **(C)** could not be separated from the dorsal dura. The central spinal canal (arrowheads) is not dilated. The ventral subarachnoid space **(SA)** is prominent. The adhesions were surgically lysed.

Technique

The patient is placed in the prone position, and the examination is performed through the soft tisues of the back, using gel or mineral oil as the acoustic coupling agent. Real-time scanning facilitates identification of the spinous processes, the area of the laminectomy, and the cord. A combination 3–5–7.5 MHz mechanical sector scanner placed directly on the back or positioned over a water bag or similar standoff has proved to be a useful approach in our facilities. However, other types of high-frequency transducers, both linear and sector, have been used successfully. Transverse, sagittal, and sagittal oblique views can be easily obtained. Static scanners can also be used. In cases of open skin wounds over the back, sterile sheaths can be used over the transducers.

Ultrasonographic Findings

The spinous processes are visualized as bright echoes with distal acoustic shadowing. They are located immediately beneath the skin surface in the midline. The laminae are visualized more deeply to either side (see Fig. 15–8C). The area of laminectomy is noted by loss of these echogenic areas and

visualization deeper into the body. In the region of the laminectomy, the spinal cord should be delineated as a hypoechoic structure with parallel echoes recorded from its dorsal and ventral walls (Fig. 15–19). Deeper than this would be the posterior aspect of the adjacent vertebral body. A varying amount of subarachnoid fluid usually can be detected around the spinal cord.

A common postsurgical phenomenon, the pseudomeningocele, can be seen as a fluid-filled space located dorsal to the normal dural interface (Fig. 15–20).[1, 12, 21] These actually serve as an aid to the penetration of the ultrasound beam, allowing better visualization of the more ventrally located cord. Adhesion of the cord to the dura can be noted by the lack of imaging of a fluid space around the circumference of the cord. Recurrent tumors appear as echogenic masses that displace (extra- or intradural) or enlarge (intramedullary) the cord itself. One relatively simple application of sonography is in diagnosing or excluding recurrent syringomyelia. When the intramedullary canal remains decompressed, it measures less than 2 mm in diameter and is visualized as a single echogenic line. A cystic space within the cord indicates either recurrent syringomyelia or the development of an intramedullary cyst. In the patient with

Figure 15–19. Postoperative examination of the spinal cord. A sagittal view of the cervical region demonstrates the moderately echogenic posterior soft tissues (P). The canal is defined by thick echogenic lines (arrowheads) representing the posterior dura and the posterior margins of the vertebral bodies. The spinal cord is noted by weakly echogenic parallel walls (lines). The central spinal canal (small arrows) is not significantly dilated.

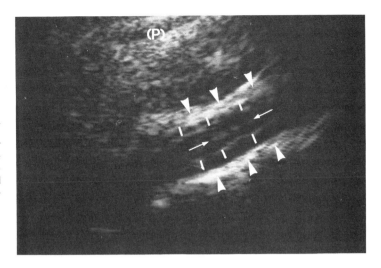

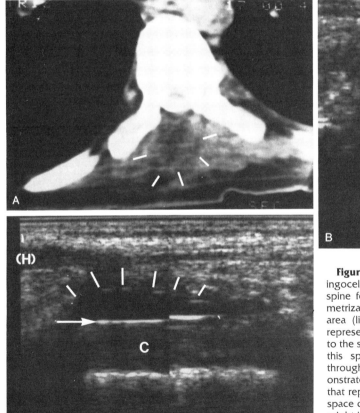

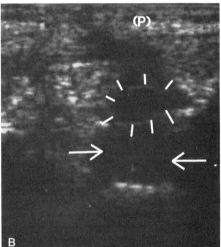

Figure 15–20. Postoperative pseudomeningocele. *A,* Transaxial CT scan of the thoracic spine following administration of intrathecal metrizamide demonstrates a poorly defined area (lines) of low attenuation values that represents a pseudomeningocele posterior to the spinal canal. Metrizamide did not enter this space. *B,* Transverse ultrasonography through the posterior soft tissues (P) demonstrates a well-defined fluid space (lines) that represents the pseudomeningocele. The space does not contain echoes or debris that might indicate an infection or a hematoma. It is located immediately posterior to the thoracic canal (arrows). *C,* Longitudinal scanning with linear array equipment demonstrates the sagittal extent of the pseudomeningocele (lines). (Two real-time images are pictured side by side to give this panoramic view.) The dorsal dura (bright horizontal line, arrow) clearly separates the pseudomeningocele from the spinal canal and cord (**C**). **H** = toward patient's head.

spinal fracture, ultrasonography has been used to check on the positioning of ventral bony fragments. This approach, however, is limited if metallic stabilization devices such as Harrington rods are present, since they may prevent the penetration of the ultrasound beam. CT examination can also be degraded by the presence of these metallic rods.

ACKNOWLEDGMENTS

The authors wish to thank Dr. Alfred B. Kurtz for manuscript review and for the use of Fig. 15-4. We would also like to acknowledge the departments of orthopedics and neurosurgery at Thomas Jefferson University Hospital for their cooperation in obtaining cases. Thanks also go to Donna Marandola for manuscript preparation.

References

1. Braun IF, Raghavendra BN, Kricheff II: Spinal cord imaging using real time high resolution ultrasound. Radiology 147:459–465, 1983.
1a. Chadduck WM, Flanigan S: Intraoperative ultrasound for spinal lesions. Neurosurg 16:477–482, 1985.
2. Dohrmann GJ, Rubin JM: Intraoperative ultrasound imaging of the spinal cord: syringomyelia, cysts, and tumors—a preliminary report. Surg Neurol 18:395–399, 1982.
3. Goldberg BB: Abdominal Gray Scale Ultrasonography. New York: John Wiley & Sons, Inc, 1977.
4. Gooding GAW: Use of an ultrasound transducer in a sterile field. Radiology 147:276, 1983.
5. Hobbins JC, Grannum PAT, Berkowitz RL, et al: Ultrasound in the diagnosis of congenital anomalies. Am J Obstet Gynecol 134:331–345, 1979.
6. Howie DW, Chatterton BE, Honi MR: Failure of ultrasound in the investigation of sciatica. J Bone Joint Surg 65B:144–147, 1983.
7. Hutchins WW, Vogelzang RL, Neiman HL, et al: Differentiation of tumor from syringohydromyelia: Intraoperative neurosonography of the spinal cord. Radiology 151:171–174, 1983.
8. Kadziolka R, Asztely M, Hanai K, et al: Ultrasonic Measurement of the Lumbar Spinal Canal. J Bone Joint Surg 63B:504–507, 1981.
9. Kangarloo H, Gold RH, Diament MJ, et al: High resolution spinal sonography in infants. AJR 142:1243–1247, 1984.
10. Knake JE, Gabrielsen TO, Chandler WF, et al: Real-time sonography during spinal surgery. Radiology 151:461–465, 1984.
11. Kurtz AB, Wapner RJ: Ultrasonographic diagnosis of second-trimester skeletal dysplasias: a prospective analysis in the high-risk population. JUM 2:99–106, 1983.
12. Laffey PA, Kricun ME: Sonographic recognition of postoperative meningocele. AJR 143:177–178, 1984.
13. Miller JH, Reid BS, Kemberling CR: Utilization of ultrasound in the evaluation of spinal dysraphism in children. Radiology 143:737–740, 1982.
14. Milunsky A: Prenatal detection of neural tube defects. JAMA 244:2731–2755, 1980.
15. Mintz MC, Mennuti M, Fishman M: Prenatal aspiration of sacrococcygeal teratoma. AJR 141:367–368, 1983.
16. Miskin MS, Baim RS, Allen LC, et al: Ultrasonic assessment of the fetal spine before 20 weeks' gestation. Radiology 132:131–135, 1979.
17. Montalvo BM, Quencer RM, Green BA, et al: Intraoperative sonography in spinal trauma. Radiology 153:125–134, 1984.
18. Naidich TP, Fernback SK, McLone DG, et al: Sonography of the caudal spine and back: congenital anomalies in children. AJR 142:1229–1242, 1984.
19. Naidich TP, McLone DG, Shkolnik A, et al: Sonographic evaluation of caudal spine anomalies in children. AJNR 4:661–664, 1983.
20. Pasto ME, Kurtz AB: The prenatal examination of the fetal cranium, spine and central nervous system. Semin Ultrasound, CT, MR 5:170–193, 1984.
21. Pasto ME, Rifkin MD, Rubenstein JB, et al: Real-time ultrasonography of the spinal cord: intraoperative and postoperative imaging. Neuroradiology 26:183–187, 1984.
21a. Rubin JM, Dohrmann GH: The spine and spinal cord during neurosurgical operations: real-time ultrasonography. Radiology 155:197–200, 1985.
22. Quencer RM, Montalvo BM: Normal intraoperative spinal sonography. AJR 143:1301–1305, 1984.
23. Quencer RM, Montalvo BM, Green BA, et al: Intraoperative spinal sonography of soft-tissue masses of the spinal cord and spinal canal. AJR 143:1307–1315, 1984.
24. Quencer RM, Mose BMM, Green BA, et al: Intraoperative spinal sonography: adjunct to metrizamide CT in the assessment and surgical decompression of posttraumatic spinal cord cysts. AJR 142:593–601, 1984.
25. Raghavendra BN, Epstein FJ, Pinto RS, et al: The tethered spinal cord: diagnosis by high-resolution real-time ultrasound. Radiology 149:123–128, 1983.
26. Rubin JM, Dohrmann GH: Work in progress: intraoperative ultrasonography of the spine. Radiology 146:173–175, 1983.
27. Scheible W, James HE, Leopold GR, et al: Occult spinal dysraphism in infants: screening with high-resolution real-time ultrasound. Radiology 146:743–746, 1983.
28. Seeds JW, Mittelstaedt CA, Cefalo RC, et al: Prenatal diagnosis of sacrococcygeal teratoma: an anechoic caudal mass. J Clin Ultrasound 10:193–195, 1982.
29. Slotnick N, Filly RA, Callen PW, et al: Sonography as a procedure complimentary to alpha fetoprotein testing for neural tube defects. J Ultrasound Med 1:319–322, 1982.
30. Tenner MS, Wodraska GM: Diagnostic Ultrasound in Neurology—Methods and Techniques. New York: John Wiley & Sons, Inc, 1975.
31. Uematsu S, Walker AE: A Manual of Echoencephalography. Baltimore: Williams & Wilkins Company, 1971.
32. Wald NJ, Cuckle HS: Amniotic fluid acetycholinesterase electrophoresis as a secondary test in the diagnosis of anencephaly and open spina bifida in early pregnancy. Lancet 15:321–324, 1981.
33. Williams RA, Barth RA: In utero sonographic recognition of diastematomyelia. AJR 144:87–88, 1985.

16

Judy M. Destouet, M.D.
William A. Murphy, M.D.

Arthrography and the Facet Syndrome

Recently there has been a resurgence of interest in facet arthropathy as an etiology of low back and leg pain. Attention was first focused on the facet joint as a source of sciatica in 1911;[8] 16 years later, the concept that anomalies of the facet joints were a major cause of sciatica was reinforced.[18] The term "facet syndrome" was coined in 1933 to describe those patients who had acute or chronic low back pain with or without sciatica.[6] However, one year later, the concept of vertebral disc herniation was introduced,[14] and it soon overshadowed facet arthropathy as the principal diagnosed cause of low back pain. Attention was refocused on the lumbar facet joint in 1971, when a 99.8% success rate in treating back and leg pain with percutaneous transection of the nerve supply to the facet joints was reported.[19] However, other investigators could not duplicate these results, and to avoid the morbidity associated with rhizotomy, radiofrequency coagulation of the nerves supplying the articular facets was introduced in 1976.[21] While attempting to delineate the pattern of pain radiation from facet syndrome, others injected saline and lidocaine into lumbar facet joints, thereby developing the technique of intra-articular facet block as a diagnostic and therapeutic method.[15]

The clinical importance of the facet syndrome has not been fully recognized. Many patients with low back pain without clinical or radiographic evidence of herniated disc disease are diagnostic and therapeutic problems. Indeed, some of these patients may have facet syndrome, but their condition is not diagnosed and may be inappropriately treated. The clinical and radiographic criteria for the diagnosis of facet syndrome, along with the technique of facet arthrography and block, are presented in this chapter.

SYMPTOMS AND SIGNS

The symptoms of facet arthropathy are nonspecific and, in some patients, mimic those of disc herniation. Many patients complain of a deep-seated dull ache instead of the sharp pain generally associated with a herniated disc.[11] In most patients, the onset of back pain is acute and related to specific circumstances at the time of injury, that is, a twisting motion with hyperextension or hyperflexion of the spine.[6] Duplication of these motions may reproduce the pain. Other patients relate a direct blow to the lower back during a fall. In a small number of patients, pain onset is insidious. Occasionally, patients describe a "catching" sensation in the back during the initial attempt to straighten up immediately following the injury.[11]

Clinically, the facet joint is implicated in those patients who experience focal low back pain or pain radiating into the buttocks and the posterolateral aspect of the thigh. The L1–2 and L4–5 facet joints were injected bilaterally in six healthy male volunteers, and it was found that in no instance did the referred pain extend beyond the knee.[13] In a similar clinical trial, the L3 through S1 facet joints were injected in 15 patients with chronic back pain, and it was found that in three patients pain radiation included the entire leg and foot.[15] As a general rule, patients with facet syndrome rarely have pain radiating to the foot.[21] Review of our clinical experience with pain distribution in 54 patients with facet syndrome showed that 21 patients had focal back pain and 29 complained of referred pain. Of these 29 patients, 11 had pain radiating to the buttocks, hip, or thigh, 5 had pain to the knee, and 13 had pain radiating to the calf. Only one patient had pain extending to the foot. In four patients the pain pattern was not precisely recorded.

On physical examination, patients may have focal tenderness over an affected facet joint or joints. The pain may increase with rotation, forward bending, or hyperextension of the spine. There may be a slightly diminished straight leg raising test, but this finding alone does not necessarily implicate nerve root compression from disc protrusion and should not be used as evidence against the presence of facet syndrome.[15] Specific dermatome sensory loss, motor weakness, or a positive crossed leg–straight leg raising test implicate disc herniation. When these findings are present, a herniated disc should be carefully excluded before other etiologies for low back pain are considered.

INDICATIONS

The prime indication for facet injection is focal low back pain with or without tenderness to palpation over a facet joint or joints. Patients who have low back pain and sciatica with a normal radiographic work-up are good candidates for facet arthrography and block. Additionally, facet injection may help those patients with persistent low back pain after laminectomy or a stable posterolateral spine fusion, provided there is no evidence of arachnoiditis or recurrent disc disease. Patients with back pain, facet joint osteoarthritis, and normal neurologic examinations are also good candidates for facet arthrography and treatment. Arthrography and block may be performed to evaluate for possible facet syndrome in selected patients who have computed tomographic evidence of a small central disc protrusion without associated nerve root impingement.

PATIENT EVALUATION

The radiologic work-up for those patients with clinically suspected facet syndrome begins with conventional radiographs of the lumbar spine. Those patients who have focal low back pain, no objective neurologic deficit, and normal lumbar spine radiographs need no further work-up prior to facet block. In those patients with sciatica or any clinical evidence of nerve root compression, myelography or computed tomography (CT) or both should be performed to exclude disc herniation or neural foraminal nerve impingement. Patients with radiographic evidence of degenerative disc disease or severe facet joint osteoarthritis should also undergo myelography or spinal CT prior to facet injection to exclude nerve root impingement from disc herniation or osteophyte formation.

ANATOMY

The functions of the facet joints are to permit movement between vertebrae and to guide and limit that excursion. In conjunction with the intervertebral discs, the facet

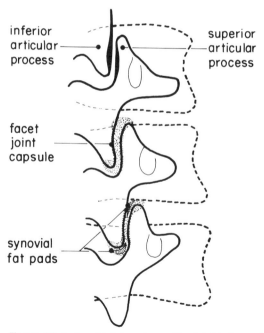

Figure 16–1. Facet joint anatomy. The joint is formed by the superior and inferior articular processes of adjacent vertebrae. Hyaline cartilage covers the articular surface of the joint processes. Each joint is encapsulated by a thin fibrous layer, which is redundant superiorly and inferiorly to form recesses. Contained within the recesses are meniscus-like protrusions or synovial villi.

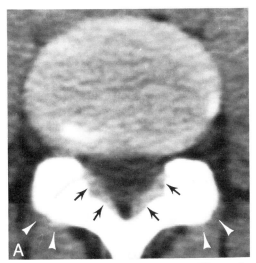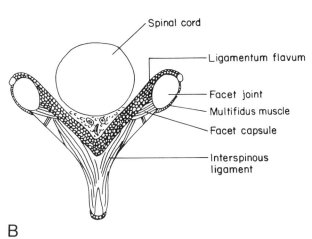

Figure 16–2. *A*, Facet joint anatomy. CT scan through the L4 disc shows the ligamentum flavum (arrows) forming the anteromedial margin of the facet joint capsule. The multifidus muscle forms the posterior margin of the facet joint capsule (arrowheads). *B*, A diagram of the posterior elements shows the ligamentous and muscular structures that maintain the integrity of the joint capsule and prevent entrapment of soft tissues. Note the proximity of the joint to the epidural space and spinal cord. Distention of the joint capsule or degenerative osteophyte formation of the articular processes could compress the spinal nerve.

joints offer load support to the spine. Each facet joint is formed by the inferior articular process of one vertebra and the superior articular process of the subjacent vertebra (Fig. 16–1). The joint processes are short and stout; the concave articular surface of the superior process appears to embrace the inferior process, which is slightly convex[20] (Figs. 16–2 and 16–3). This congruent configuration results in a locking mechanism that helps resist the shearing motion produced by forward bending and the compression loading produced by rotation.

The facet joint is a true synovial joint, encapsulated by a thin fibrous layer. Hyaline cartilage covers the articular surfaces of the joint processes, and a synovial membrane lines the joint capsule (see Fig. 16–1). The size and shape of the joint capsule permit rotation and forward bending of the spine. The capsule has a medial extent and forms both superior and inferior recesses (see Fig. 16–1). The anteromedial portion of the fibrous capsule is formed almost totally by the ligmentum flavum (see Fig. 16–2), which exerts a constant pull on the anterior capsule, probably preventing entrapment of capsular fibers between the articular processes.[15] At the lateral extent of the ligamentum flavum, just as it borders the intervertebral foramen, there is a strong fibrous band called the superior articular ligament.[9] Just medial

to this fibrous band there is a recess in the ligamentum flavum through which the synovium of the facet joint may bulge and encroach upon the mixed spinal nerve as it passes through the intervertebral foramen.[15] Adipose tissue contained within the superior recess is continuous with that around the spinal nerve in the intervertebral foramen. The multifidus muscle completely cov-

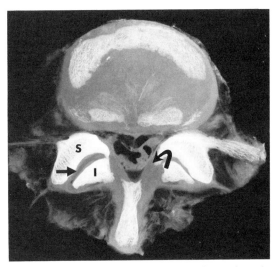

Figure 16–3. Radiograph of an anatomic specimen in the transaxial plane. *Key:* **I** = inferior articulating facet; **S** = superior articulating facet; **straight arrow** = facet joint; **curved arrow** = ligamentum flavum.

ers the posterior aspect of the facet joint and provides structural support (see Fig. 16–2).

The lining of the facet joint capsule is unique in that it forms meniscuslike inclusions called synovial villi, or fat pads, which are contained within the superior and inferior recesses[7] (see Fig. 16–1). Two types of intra-articular synovial protrusions have been observed in the lumbosacral facet joints in cadavers: a fat-filled vascular synovial pad and a dense, fibrous protrusion project from the recesses into the space between the articular processes. It has been postulated that with age the fat-filled vascular protrusion becomes fibrotic in response to the long-continued pressure upon it from the opposed articular surfaces.[7] Although the exact function of these synovial villi is unclear, one investigator maintains that these protrusions simply fill the space between peripheral, noncongruent parts of the articular surfaces and that the villi move in and out of the joint freely in response to joint movements and forces.[22] Others feel that the menisci function to displace the capsule, thereby preventing entrapment between the apposed articular surfaces.[16]

The capsule of the facet joint is richly innervated by the dorsal ramus of the lumbar spinal nerve (Fig. 16–4), but no nerve fibers have been found to penetrate the joint capsule.[17] Triple-level innervation of each joint has been described in anatomic studies.[16] A very small, deep branch of the dorsal ramus loops under the transverse process and supplies the joint capsule of the adjacent superior articular facet. A second larger descending branch passes medially and downward to innervate the superior and medial aspects of the joint capsule below. In addition, an ascending branch arises from the dorsal ramus of the spinal nerve just anterior to the intertransverse fascia and ascends through the soft tissues to innervate the posterior aspect of the facet joint above. This ascending nerve is somewhat larger than the deep branch but is smaller than the descending nerve. Therefore, a single lumbar spinal nerve supplies three facet joints, and each facet joint has trisegmental innervation.

ETIOLOGY OF FACET SYNDROME

Although the etiology of the facet syndrome remains unclear, the unique anatomy

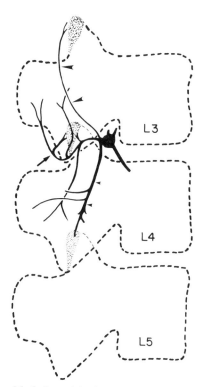

Figure 16–4. Facet joint innervation. The dorsal ramus of a lumbar spinal nerve divides into several branches. A deep branch loops under the transverse process to innervate the facet joint at the same level (arrow) as the spinal nerve. A descending branch innervates the subjacent joint capsule (small arrowheads). An ascending branch arises from the dorsal ramus and courses through the soft tissues to reach the joint above (large arrowheads).

of this joint provides many possibilities. For example, with rotation and hyperextension of the spine, multifidus muscle weakness could predispose the posterior joint capsule to painful entrapment between the articulating processes.[16] Laxity of the ligamentum flavum, either developmental or postoperative, could result in the pinching of the anterior aspect of the facet capsule between the articular processes.[16] Facet pain may be due to entrapment of the synovial villi between the articular processes.[7, 11] This entrapment could cause the "catching" sensation[11] and the "vertebral block" syndrome.[10] As in other joints, a nonspecific synovitis could result in pain. Osteoarthritis of the articular processes may contribute to development of pain not only from cartilage loss and osteophyte formation but also from the ligament laxity that frequently accompanies degenerative joint disease.

TECHNIQUE

The long-axis planes of facet joints vary from near sagittal in the upper lumbar spine to near coronal at the lumbosacral junction. This intrinsic curve and oblique orientation of the apophyseal joints must be considered when arthrography is attempted. It is important to remember that with a standard 45 degree oblique radiograph of the lumbar spine, the anterior portion of the joint space is in profile[1] (Fig. 16–5). However, only the posterolateral portion of the joint is accessible to percutaneous puncture from a posterior approach. In most cases, the posterior joint space is profiled by slowly rotating the patient from a prone position into a shallow oblique position, with the affected side up (see Fig. 16–5A). However, in steeply curved joints the posterior joint space lies in or near a sagittal plane and can be entered with the patient in the prone position (see Fig. 16–5B).

With fluoroscopic guidance, a metal pointer is moved on the skin so that it lies directly over the facet joint, and the skin is marked. Following this, the skin is aseptically prepared and draped. The skin and subcutaneous tissue are infiltrated with 1%

lidocaine. Under fluoroscopy, a 22 gauge, 3.5 inch spinal needle is directed vertically into the facet joint. In obese patients or when postoperative scars are present, a 20 gauge, 3.5 or 4.0 inch spinal needle provides better control in guiding the needle into the joint. If the needle tip has been placed correctly, it will move with the facet joint when the patient is rotated into a steep oblique position (Fig. 16–6). Approximately 0.5 ml of a water-soluble contrast agent, iothalamate meglumine (Conray-60), is injected to confirm intra-articular needle position. Following this, 1.0 ml of 0.25% bupivacaine hydrochloride (Marcaine) and 40 mg of methyl prednisolone acetate (Depo-Medrol) or 20.0 mg of triamcinolone hexacetonide (Aristospan) suspension are injected for treatment.

COMPLICATIONS

To date, no important complications of lumbar facet injection have been reported. In our experience, approximately 4% of patients have had exacerbation of their back pain for approximately 24 hours after the procedure. Presumably, this increased pain is due to an acute inflammatory reaction

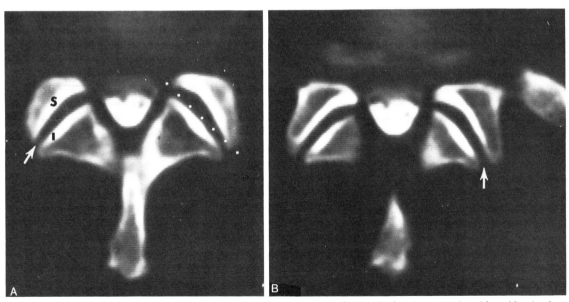

Figure 16–5. *A,* Facet joint anatomy. The congruent configuration of the articular processes is evident (that is, the concave superior process of L5 [**S**] appears to embrace the slightly convex inferior process of L4 [**I**]) in this bone-windowed CT image. The anterior facet joint space is usually in profile with a routine 45 degree oblique projection (dotted line). Since the posterior joint space can be entered only from a posterior approach (arrow), the patient should be put in an oblique position under fluoroscopy just enough to profile this joint space. *B,* With steeply curved joints, the posterior joint space (arrow) can be punctured if the patient is in the prone position.

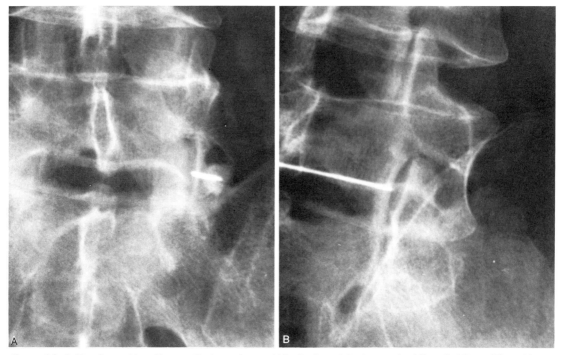

Figure 16–6. Needle position. The needle tip projects within the facet joint in anterior (*A*) and oblique (*B*) positions.

related to the injection of corticosteroid. Transient numbness of a lower extremity occurred in one patient and may have been secondary to the effect of the local anesthetic agent on the dorsal ramus of the spinal nerve. In postoperative patients with extensive laminectomy defects, care must be taken to avoid the subarachnoid space, since paresthesia may develop.

ARTHROGRAPHIC APPEARANCE

The normal joint capsule is smooth and oval in the frontal position and sigmoid-shaped in the oblique projection (Fig. 16–7). In most patients, the inferior articular recess is substantially larger than the superior recess.[4] With injection of contrast material or medication, either recess may rupture, resulting in medication diffusing around branches of the spinal nerve or into an intervertebral foramen where a nerve passes. In some patients, the joint capsule has marginal irregularities and nodular filling defects in the recesses, probably secondary to synovial proliferation or synechiae

(Fig. 16–8). Intra-articular filling defects, which probably represent enlarged synovial fat pads, are sometimes observed (Fig. 16–9).

Pars interarticularis defects have been demonstrated arthrographically by injection of one facet joint, followed immediately by opacification of a tract or lobulated connection through the pars defect and concurrent opacification of the adjacent facet joint[5] (Fig. 16–10). In our series, three cases of clinically unsuspected and radiographically undetected pars interarticularis defects were found by facet arthrography (Fig. 16–11). A patient with bilateral L5 pars interarticularis defects had an associated disruption of the ligamentum flavum demonstrated by facet arthrography (Fig. 16–12).

Opacification of lymphatic drainage occurs occasionally as a result of overdistention of the joint capsule or from synovial inflammation (Fig. 16–13). In severe osteoarthritis, the joint capsule may be constricted, resembling adhesive capsulitis (Fig. 16–14) seen in other joints. Patients who have had a laminectomy or a spinal fusion or both frequently have distorted and irregular joint capsules (Fig. 16–15).

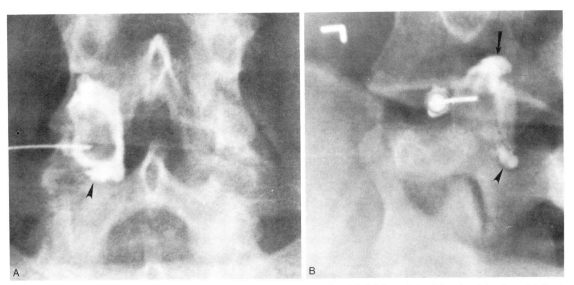

Figure 16–7. *A*, Normal facet arthrogram. Posteroanterior view of an L4–L5 facet joint following injection of 1.0 ml of iothalamate meglumine (Conray-60) shows an oval-shaped joint capsule. The slightly irregular appearance (arrowhead) probably represents rupture of the inferior recess. *B*, Oblique view of the same facet joint shows a normal joint capsule that has a smooth, sigmoid configuration. The superior (arrow) and inferior (arrowhead) recesses are evident.

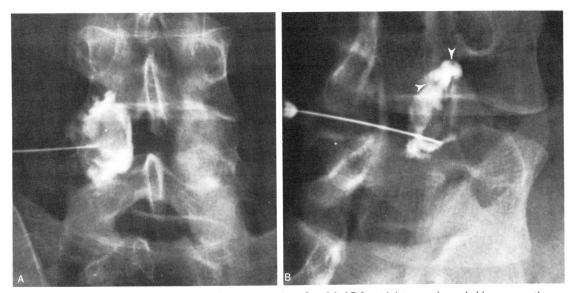

Figure 16–8. *A*, Probable synovitis. Irregular joint margins of an L4–L5 facet joint capsule probably representing a synovitis. *B*, Note the small peripheral nodular filling defects (arrowheads).

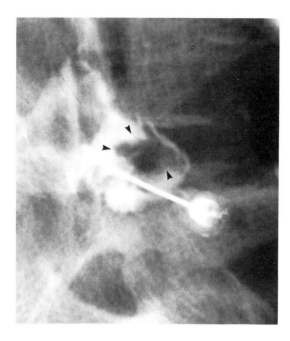

Figure 16–9. Probable synovitis. Irregular filling defect that may represent an enlarged, synovial fat pad (arrowheads) is located in the inferior recess of the left L4–L5 joint capsule. Entrapment of the fat pad between the articular processes can cause low back pain.

Figure 16–10. Spondylolysis. After injection of the L4–L5 facet joint (small arrowheads), a large lobulated pars defect tract (arrows) is noted with concurrent opacification of the L5–S1 facet joint (large arrowheads).

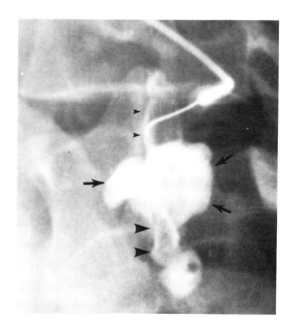

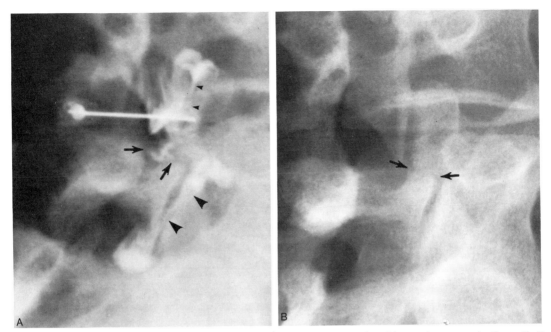

Figure 16–11. *A*, Spondylolysis. L4–L5 facet joint arthrogram (small arrowheads) reveals communication with the L5–S1 facet joint (large arrowheads) via an unsuspected pars defect (arrows). *B*, Analysis of the oblique view of the lumbar spine confirms a subtle L5 spondylolysis (arrows).

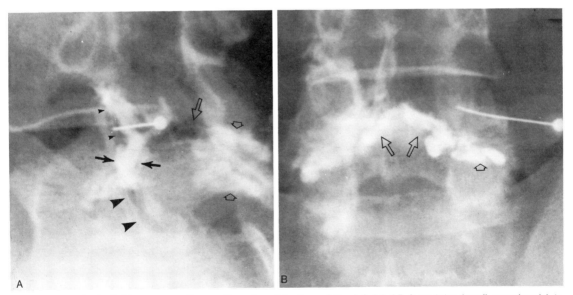

Figure 16–12. *A, B,* Ligamentum flavum disruption. Injection of the left L4–L5 facet joint (small arrowheads) is followed by opacification of a pars defect (solid arrows) and immediate filling of the L5–S1 facet joint (large arrowheads). Contrast also crosses the midline through the disrupted ligamentum flavum (open arrow) to fill the contralateral L5–S1 facet joint (open arrowheads).

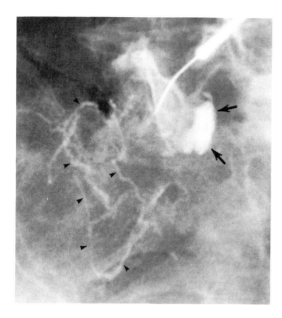

Figure 16–13. Lymphatic filling. After the injection of 1.5 ml of Conray-60 into the L5–S1 facet joint, several curvilinear lymphatic channels (arrowheads) are opacified. Rupture of the inferior recess (arrows) is present.

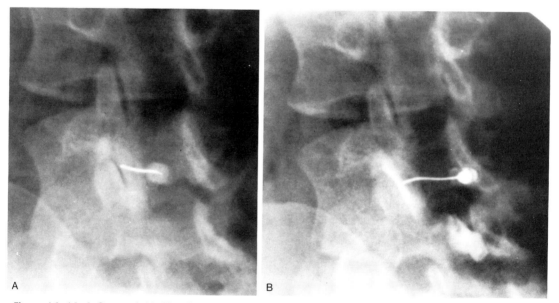

A   B

Figure 16–14. *A,* Osteoarthritis. Needle projects into the L4–L5 facet joint, which is markedly narrowed and sclerotic from osteoarthritis. *B,* Injection of 0.5 ml of Conray-60 fills a small attenuated joint capsule, suggesting adhesive capsulitis.

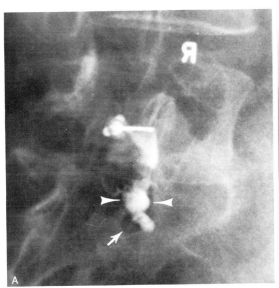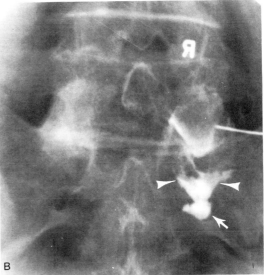

Figure 16–15. *A, B,* Postlaminectomy arthrogram. Following injection of 2 ml of Conray-60 into an L5–S1 facet joint, an irregular capsule is noted. There is inferior extension of the joint capsule (arrowheads) into the S1 neural foramen (arrow).

TREATMENT OF FACET SYNDROME

Conservative treatment including bed rest, traction, physical therapy, and nonsteroidal, anti-inflammatory agents should be exhausted before any invasive procedure is performed. In the early 1900s, facetectomy or posterolateral fusion of the lumbar spine or both was the recommended therapy for facet syndrome if conservative methods failed.[6] Percutaneous rhizolysis of the nerve supply to the facet joint[19] is seldom used today. Instead, radiofrequency coagulation and phenol chemolysis of the nerves supplying the facet joint are current treatment methods.[15, 20, 21] The diagnostic role and therapeutic benefit of the intra-articular injection of corticosteroid have been detailed in the literature.[1–3, 11, 12]

Prior to facet arthrography, each patient is fully evaluated regarding onset of symptoms, pain pattern, and the clinical or radiographic work-up that has been performed. The level or levels of injection should encompass the patient's back pain; therefore, detailed information regarding pain distribution is helpful in determining exactly where to inject. Also, review of lumbar spine roentgenograms and radionuclide and CT scans may aid in the decision of which level or levels to inject. Concerning our patients, choice of injection level was based primarily on clinical evidence, especially focal tenderness over a joint or joints. With focal tenderness at one level, three joints were routinely injected, the site of tenderness as well as the joints immediately above and below that site. In those patients who had no focal tenderness and unilateral back pain, the ipsilateral L3 through S1 facet joints were injected. In those patients with bilateral low back pain, the L3 through S1 facet joints were injected bilaterally. If there was no focal tenderness but osteoarthritis was present at a particular site on roentgenograms or CT scan, that level and the joints above and below were injected. In those patients who had no specific clinical findings and no radiographic evidence of osteoarthritis, the L3 through S1 facet joints were injected bilaterally. In patients who had undergone spinal fusion, the level above the fusion mass was injected.

RESULTS

We reviewed our clinical experience with 100 consecutive patients who underwent intra-articular facet block for acute or chronic low back pain (Table 16–1). Eighty-one patients had had no previous surgery, and 19 patients had previously undergone laminectomy, diskectomy, chemonucleolysis, or posterolateral fusion. There were 46

Table 16–1. LUMBAR FACET ARTHROGRAPHY RESULTS

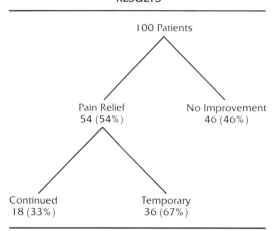

women and 54 men, and their ages ranged from 20 to 83 years. Of the 100 patients injected, 54 experienced pain relief immediately; the remaining 46 patients did not benefit from the injection. Thirty-two of the 54 responding patients experienced relief of their symptoms for 6 months or less (Table 16–2). Seven patients had pain relief for approximately 1 year. Two patients who had been asymptomatic for 18 months were lost to follow-up. Eighteen patients have had continued relief; six of them have been free of pain for over 2 years.

In our series, 33% of 54 patients with facet syndrome remain free of pain 6 to 30 months after injection. Although this success rate is less than the 46% success rate previously reported,[2] it compares favorably with the 20% long-term pain relief reported by others.[12, 15] Thus, lumbar facet arthrography is both a diagnostic and therapeutic procedure. In those patients with facet syndrome, prolonged pain relief may result from the intra-articular injection of corticosteroid. Al-

though the cause of the facet syndrome is unknown, pain relief following corticosteroid injection suggests an inflammatory etiology. During facet arthrography, rupture of the articular capsule results in diffusion of medication around the branches of the spinal nerve, allowing the anesthetic and corticosteroid to affect the synovial membrane, the adjacent nerves, and other periarticular structures. Fluoroscopically controlled intra-articular facet arthrography and block are reliable techniques for diagnosing and treating low back pain caused by lumbar facet syndrome.

References

1. Carrera GF: Lumbar facet joint injection in low back pain and sciatica: description of technique. Radiology 137:661–664, 1980.
2. Carrera GF: Lumbar facet joint injection in low back pain and sciatica: preliminary results. Radiology 137:665–667, 1980.
3. Destouet JM, Gilula LA, Murphy WA, et al: Lumbar facet joint injection: indication, technique, clinical correlation, and preliminary results. Radiology 145:321–325, 1982.
4. Dory MA: Arthrography of the lumbar facet joints. Radiology 140:23–27, 1981.
5. Ghelman B, Doherty JH: Demonstration of spondylolysis by arthrography of the apophyseal joint. AJR 130:986–987, 1978.
6. Ghormley RK: Low back pain with special reference to the articular facets, with presentation of an operative procedure. JAMA 101:1773–1777, 1933.
7. Giles LGF, Taylor JR: Intra-articular synovial protrusions in the lower lumbar apophyseal joints. Bull Hosp Joint Dis Orthop Inst XLII:248–255, 1982.
8. Goldthwait JE: The lumbosacral articulation: an explanation of many cases of "lumbago," "sciatica" and paraplegia. Boston Med Surg J 164:365–372, 1911.
9. Hadley LA: Anatomico-roentgenographic studies of the posterior spinal articulations. AJR 86:270–276, 1961.
10. Kos J, Wolf J: Les menisques intervertébraux et leur role possible dans les blocages vertébraux. Ann Med Physique 15:203–218, 1972.
11. Kraft GL, Levinthal DH: Facet synovial impingement. A new concept in the etiology of lumbar vertebral derangement. Surg Gynecol Obstet 93:439–443, 1951.
12. Maldague B, Mathurin P, Malghem J: Facet joint arthrography in lumbar spondylolysis. Radiology 140:29–36, 1981.
13. McCall IW, Park WM, O'Brien JP: Induced pain referral from posterior lumbar elements in normal subjects. Spine 4:441–446, 1979.
14. Mixter WJ, Barr JS: Rupture of the intervertebral disc with involvement of the spinal canal. New Engl J Med 211:210–215, 1934.

Table 16–2. DURATION OF IMPROVEMENT FOR 54 PATIENTS

Number of Months	Number of Patients	Percentage of Patients
6	32	59
6–12	7	13
12–18*	4	8
18–24	5	9
24–30	6	11

*Two patients were lost to follow-up.

15. Mooney V, Robertson J: The facet syndrome. Clin Orthop 115:149–156, 1976.
16. Paris SV: Anatomy as related to function and pain. Orthop Clin North Am 14:475–489, 1983.
17. Pedersen HE, Blunck CFJ, Gardner E: The anatomy of lumbosacral posterior rami and meningeal branches of spinal nerves (sinu-vertebral nerves): with an experimental study of their functions. J Bone Joint Surg 38A:377–391, 1956.
18. Putti V: New conceptions in the pathogenesis of sciatic pain. Lancet 2:53–60, 1927.
19. Rees WES: Multiple bilateral subcutaneous rhizol-
ysis of segmental nerves in the treatment of the intervertebral disc syndrome. Ann Gen Pract 16: 126–127, 1971.
20. Selby DK, Paris SV: Anatomy of facet joints and its clinical correlation with low back pain. Contemp Orthop 3:1097–1103, 1981.
21. Shealy CN: Facet denervation in the management of back and sciatic pain. Clin Orthop 115:157–164, 1976.
22. Tondury G: Anatomie fonctionnelle des petites articulations du rachis. Ann Med Physique 15:173–191, 1972.

17

Rubem Pochaczevsky, M.D.

Thermography

Thermography is a unique, noninvasive diagnostic imaging procedure that detects thermal changes produced by physiologic responses to sensory nerve abnormalities—particularly from nerve root compression syndromes and nerve irritating disorders. The thermal changes form characteristic and diagnostic thermographic patterns that are associated with irritation of fibers of specific spinal nerve roots, thus enabling localization of the disorder. In addition, thermography can detect focal thermal changes due to inflammatory and other hyperemic conditions.

INDICATIONS

Thermography is indicated as a useful screening procedure whenever a patient is suspected of having nerve root compression syndromes or nerve irritating disorders. It is helpful in the evaluation of patients with clinical complaints of pain in the neck, back, or extremities, whose routine spine radiographs are negative or nonspecific. Thermography may be the first and only imaging modality that can document the subjective complaint of pain or offer a clue as to its origin by establishing the existence of abnormal skin temperature in a dermatome of a relevant extremity (Fig. 17–1). It may prove to be a valuable and objective means of distinguishing true somatic from psychosomatic complaints. A positive thermogram should eliminate consideration of malingering. In the face of a negative thermogram, the index of suspicion for malingering is increased significantly, and it is increased

even more so in the face of other negative diagnostic procedures. Thermography can also detect the presence of inflammatory musculotendinous as well as focal hyperemic disorders.

Thermography may play an important role in the selection of those patients with suspected nerve root compression syndromes who require myelography. In this author's experience, a negative thermogram in patients with low back pain syndromes is almost invariably associated with a negative myelogram and a more benign clinical course. Thermography is also helpful in the evaluation of patients with negative or questionable myelograms and may complement myelography and CT by helping determine whether a myelographic or CT finding of herniated disc, for example, is clinically or physiologically significant.

The most important role of thermography in spinal disorders is to detect nerve root compression or nerve irritating disorders from any cause, but thermography is capable of detecting heat-producing musculotendinous disorders as well as osteomyelitis, metastatic disease, and fractures of the spine.

Thermography may be useful in pre-employment examinations in helping to identify and document occult or latent nerve root syndromes. Applicants may then be steered away from potentially hazardous occupations or from strenuous athletic activities. It establishes a baseline pattern for future reference or comparison and may help separate recent occupational injuries from previously existing disorders.

In the postoperative patient, thermography may help document pain and establish

628

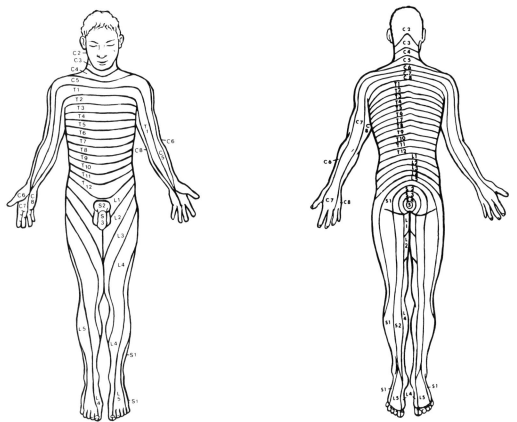

Figure 17–1. Schematic drawings indicate the location of the body dermatomes. (Modified from Keegan JJ, Garrett FD: The segmental distribution of the cutaneous nerves in the limbs of man. Anat Rec, 102:409–437, 1948.)

a probable level of spinal nerve involvement, but it cannot determine the etiology of the nerve root compression syndrome or nerve irritating disorder.

LIMITATIONS

Thermography reflects the physiologic responses to sensory nerve root abnormalities. Its chief limitation is that it does not diagnose the structural abnormalities responsible for nerve fiber irritation. For example, a herniated disc or lateral recess stenosis, both of which cause nerve root entrapment, may produce identical thermographic findings. In the postoperative patient, thermography can diagnose spinal nerve entrapment by either recurrent disc or postoperative scarring, but it cannot differentiate between these disorders. On the other hand, structural abnormalities detected by either myelography or CT may be shown by thermography not to be responsible for the patient's clinical symptoms.

COMPLICATIONS

There are no complications associated with thermography.

TECHNICAL CONSIDERATIONS

The liquid crystals used in thermography (LCT) are cholesterol derivatives that selectively reflect polarized light in a spectrum of narrow wavelengths. They have strong molecular rotatory power and specific color-temperature responses that are utilized in color thermography.[2, 5]

The adaptation of liquid crystals to thermography in previous years was hampered by the necessity of skin preparation with black, water-based paint in the form of a spray prior to the actual application of liquid crystals to the skin.[2, 22, 23] Rigid plastic plates subsequently replaced skin preparation and spraying, but the unyielding plates precluded uniform contact between the liquid crystals and the skin, particularly when ap-

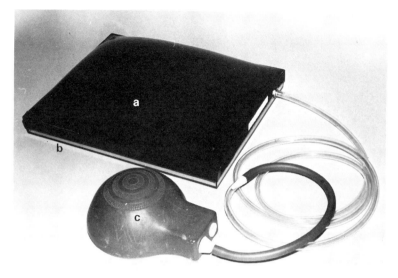

Figure 17–2. Apparatus consists of liquid crystals in elastameric sheets (*a*) mounted on "air pillow" boxes (*b*) inflated by a small pump (*c*). The inflated "air pillow" contours to any body surface. (From Pochaczevsky R, Wexler CE, Myers PH, et al: Liquid crystal thermography of the spine and extremities. Its value in the diagnosis of spinal root syndromes. J Neurosurg, 56: 386–395, 1982.)

plied to the spine or extremities. The resultant thermograms were, therefore, inadequate.

A new contact thermographic technique using liquid crystals embedded in elastomeric Flexi-Therm* was first adapted clinically for breast thermography by the au-

thor.[23, 24] The method was further refined for use with the extremities and torso by mounting the elastic sheets, which had been impregnated with liquid crystals, on inflatable frames or boxes. The resultant liquid crystal "air pillows" could then be closely contoured to any shape or body surface (Figs. 17–2 and 17–3). Six or more "air pillow" boxes are used and are progressively numbered from 24 to 35 to correspond to the median Celsius temperature ranges of their

*Flexi-Therm, Inc., 117 Magnolia Avenue, Westbury, NY 11590.

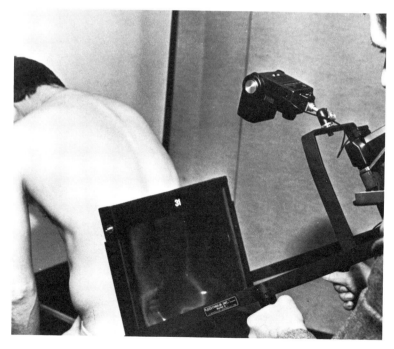

Figure 17–3. Recording system. (Courtesy of Flexi-Therm, Inc., Westbury, New York.)

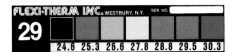

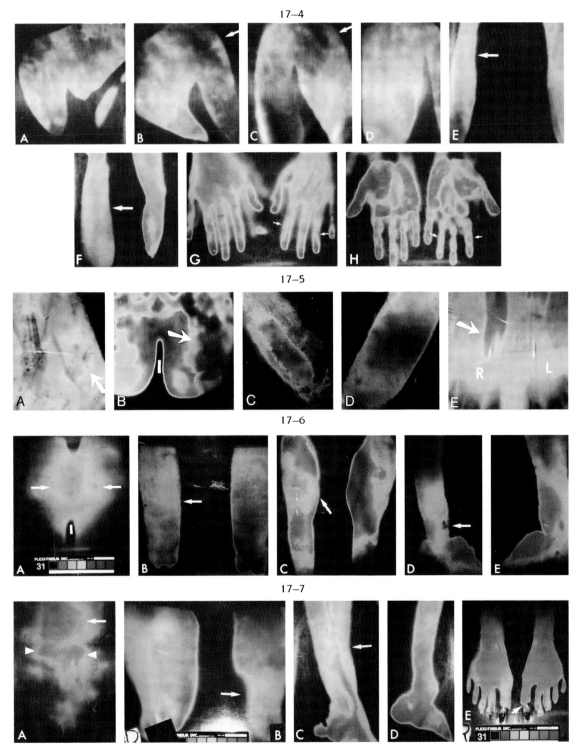

17–4

17–5

17–6

17–7

17–8

incorporated liquid crystal Flexi-Therm sheets. Liquid crystals have accurate and reliable color responses to specific temperature changes. The lowest temperature in the liquid crystal thermal gradient is displayed as dark brown. As temperature rises, the color changes from dark brown to tan, reddish brown, yellow, green, light blue, and then dark blue. The highest temperature (hyperthermia) is indicated by a dark blue color and the lowest temperature (hypothermia) by a dark brown color (Fig. 17–4).

THE THERMOGRAPHIC EXAMINATION

Patients are prepared by disrobing and waiting in an air-conditioned, draft-free room for 15 minutes. The "air pillow" selected is the one with the widest display for the patient's skin temperature. A 30°C box is initially used. If brown colors seem to predominate, skin temperature is too cold for that particular box, since brown represents the lowest temperature on the liquid crystal color scale (see Fig. 17–4). A 28°C box is then substituted. If blue colors predominate with the 30°C box, the skin temperature is too warm, since blue indicates the highest temperature on the liquid crystal color scale. A 32°C box is then used. The appropriate box is then firmly pressed against the patient's skin (see Fig. 17–3). A colored image promptly appears on the liquid crystal sheet. The box is then lifted slightly from the skin surface to eliminate distortion and glare, and the image is immediately photographed by an instant camera with color film, electronic flash system, and cross-polarized filter. A fixed distance frame attached to the camera provides support for the "air pillow" and facilitates photography (see Fig. 17–3).

Routine thermographic images of the cervical spine and upper extremities include separate images of the anterior and posterior shoulders, including the proximal arms; ulnar, radial, dorsal, and volar aspects of the forearms; and dorsal and palmar aspects of the hands and fingers.

Routine thermographic images of the lumbosacral region and lower extremities include separate images of the lumbar spine and buttocks; anterior, lateral, and posterior aspects of both thighs; anterior, lateral, medial, and posterior aspects of both lower legs, including the ankles; and dorsal aspects of the feet, including the toes.

Abnormal thermographic images are successively repeated at least three times in order to confirm their consistency. Particular attention is also given to body dermatomes (see Fig. 17–1).[14] It is this author's opinion that thermographic accuracy in diagnosing spinal nerve root compression syndromes is greatly improved when a simultaneous study of extremity dermatomes is included as part of the routine LCT evaluation of the spine.

COMPARISON OF THERMOGRAPHIC TECHNIQUES

Advantages of LCT over electronic infrared telethermography include its simple mechanics and ease of operation, its contrast and sensitivity, and its low cost. Liquid crystals also have the added advantage of displaying the actual skin temperature to 0.3°C resolution. Temperature differentials, even in patients with particularly cold extremities, may be imaged by using specially calibrated detectors. Infrared thermography of the hands and feet of such patients is usually of limited value. The chief advantages of telethermography are that skin contact is not required and larger body surfaces can be encompassed on each view.

Figure 17–4. Liquid crystal "Flexi-Therm" color calibration chart (thermal detector No. 29). See color plate and text for description. (Courtesy of Flexi-Therm, Inc., Westbury, New York.)

ANATOMIC AND PATHOPHYSIOLOGIC CONSIDERATIONS

The sympathetic system, which regulates the microcirculation of the dermis, and the sudomotor system play important roles in maintaining skin temperature.[29a, 30]

When a spinal root compression or irritation syndrome is present, the ensuing pain initiates complex sympathetic reactions. As a result, the thermal symmetry, which normally exists between both sides of the body and the paired extremities, is disrupted.

Although there are no white preganglionic sympathetic rami communicating directly with the spinal cord below L2, 8% or more of the fibers of an average skeletal nerve are sympathetic fibers.[11] Therefore, the sympathetic fiber disturbances that occur in spinal root compression or irritation and the resultant thermographic abnormalities must be attributed to a reflex action. This may occur at any point distal to the junction between the postganglionic gray sympathetic fibers and the spinal nerves. A possible explanation for this reflex action must take into account that abnormal stimuli carried by peripheral afferent nerves or dorsal spine root in cases of spinal root compressions are propagated to dorsal root ganglia. It has been shown that impulses arriving at or arising in spinal root ganglia can be propagated both orthodromically into the root and antidromically into the peripheral nerve.[31] Antidromic stimulation of nociceptive fibers causes dilatation of small skin vessels, perhaps owing to local release of vasoactive chemical mediators into the subcutaneous territory of the nerve fiber dermatome. The latter is a well-established phenomenon called the cutaneous axon reflex.[17a] Subsequently, however, a somatosympathetic[27] reflex vasoconstriction may occur. As a result, zones of hypothermia may be visualized in the corresponding extremity dermatomes of a particular spinal root or peripheral nerve.

The sciatic nerve itself also carries a large number of postganglionic sympathetic fibers to the lower extremity. It has been found that a significant correlation exists between decreased temperature of the affected distal limb and the probability of spinal nerve root compression in 174 patients with sciatica.[15a] Follow-up of operated patients also showed a significant correlation between normaliza-tion of the affected limb temperature and the relief of subjective and clinical findings. They suggested that mechanical pressure on the root, as in a herniated disc, could result in a derangement of the antegrade axoplasmic transport of neuropeptides to the chemical mediators of the subcutaneous perivascular sympathetic fibers emanating from the sciatic nerve. A disturbance of skin temperature in patients with sciatica could thereby be created. The relationship between extremity skin temperature, sympathetic activity, and the presence of pain has also been demonstrated.[1] Significant increases in the extremity skin temperatures occurred in 15 patients who had relief of limb pain following therapeutic transcutaneous electrical stimulation. There was no significant change in the extremity skin temperatures of 18 patients who had no pain relief.

A possible alternate, but more complex, pathway could be that of abnormal sensory stimuli, which also reach the spinal cord and then travel via the ascending spinothalamic tracts, reticular formation, hypothalamus, limbic system, periaqueductal gray matter, and descending reticulospinal tract to reach the sympathetic system at several levels via the lateral horn.[16a, 29a] This would account for the fact that thermographic abnormalities corresponding to a known level of dermatomal pattern may mimic root involvement at one level or even two levels above or below the actual site of root compression. Another possible cause of dermatome overlap is that postganglionic sympathetic fibers may vary their site of entry into skeletal nerve trunks.

Another pathway of sympathetic action is the sinuvertebral nerve—a recurrent branch of each spinal nerve. It originates just distal to the dorsal nerve root ganglion, where it frequently unites with a branch from the sympathetic chain, the ramus communicans. Thus, it has a dual spinal and autonomic composition.[27] The sinuvertebral nerve passes through the superior part of the intervertebral foramen between the dorsolateral surface of the vertebral body and its respective spinal roots. It also innervates the posterior longitudinal ligament, the dura, and the periosteum.[27]

Osteophytes and herniated or bulging discs may irritate fibers of the sinuvertebral nerve even prior to actual compression of spinal nerve roots.

Thus, reflex sympathetic vasoconstriction causes temperature changes, and the pattern and anatomic level of these changes can be detected by thermography. Disorders such as metastasis, infection, and spinal fractures are associated with focal hyperemia and, therefore, may be detected by thermography as focal areas of hyperthermia. If these disorders also irritate nerve roots, the reflex sympathetic vasoconstrictive changes mentioned previously will be detected as well.

THE NORMAL THERMOGRAM

Normally, there is a symmetric temperature distribution at all paraspinal levels as well as upper and lower extremities.* There is a distinct continuous vertical midline zone of heat emanating from the spinous processes of the cervical spine down to the upper lumbar spine, at which point the pattern may be interrupted. There is a zone of hypothermia that may normally exist between the lower lumbar spine and the intergluteal fold.[7, 26] The intergluteal folds are reflected as hypothermic areas, since they do not come in contact with the liquid crystal sheets. The sacroiliac joints usually show symmetric, localized, increased heat emission.[7, 26]

In a thermographic survey of the cervical spine and upper extremities of 100 actively employed manual factory workers, 94 showed either exact thermal symmetry or a minor thermal difference of less than 1°C between comparable sides of the body.[9] The remaining six cases were considered as showing false positive findings, although the presence of subclinical abnormalities or old trauma could not be excluded. Their statistics showed that an asymmetry of 0.6°C over 25% of an examined area is presumptive evidence of an abnormality. An asymmetry of more than 1°C is definitely abnormal.

In normal individuals, it has been shown that skin temperatures of opposite sides of the body vary by approximately 0.24°C ± 0.073°C.[29b]

THERMOGRAPHY IN SPINAL DISORDERS

Any clinical disorder that causes nerve root compression or nerve fiber irritation,

*See references 4, 9, 16, 18–21, 25, 26.

such as herniated disc, spinal stenosis (canal, lateral recess, neural foramen), facet syndrome, and spondylolisthesis, produces similar abnormal thermographic patterns at the same nerve root level (Table 17–1).* Other nerve root or nerve irritating disorders, such as tumor, inflammation, hemorrhage, cysts, or scarring, may produce thermographic patterns similar to those of herniated disc. These patterns differ from focal inflammatory and hyperemic conditions, such as spinal metastasis, infection, fractures, and musculoligamentous injuries, which will be discussed subsequently.

Thermographic Patterns of Nerve Root Compression

Nerve root compression, sinuvertebral nerve irritation without root compression, or irritation of branches of the posterior spinal nerves that innervate the facet joints will produce a characteristic thermographic pattern that is dependent on the anatomic level involved (Figs. 17–5 through 17–8).

In the cervicothoracic spine (see Fig. 17–5), there is decreased heat emission in the ipsilateral paraspinal myotomes, whereas in the lumbar spine, there is increased heat emission in ipsilateral paraspinal myotomes (see Figs. 17–6 and 17–7).† The hyperther-

*See references 3, 6–9, 11, 15, 18–21, 26, 30, 32.
†See references 3, 7, 18–21, 25, 26, 32.

Table 17–1. ROOT COMPRESSION SYNDROMES (SURGICAL FINDINGS IN 48 PATIENTS*)

Level of Root Compression	Cause	Cases
L5	Herniated discs, facet entrapment, osteophyte impingement, and/or spinal stenosis	32
S1	Herniated discs, facet entrapment, osteophyte impingement, and/or spinal stenosis.	15
S1	Neurofibroma	1
C6–T3	Neurofibroma	1
S1	Extradural metastasis	2
L3	Ependymoma	1
C3–C7	Syringomyelia	1
L4	Spinal stenosis and facet entrapment	4

*Some findings were at two or more levels.
(Modified from Pochaczevsky R.: Back pain assessment by contact thermography of extremity dermatomes. Orthop Rev *12*:45–58, 1983.)

Text continued on page 638

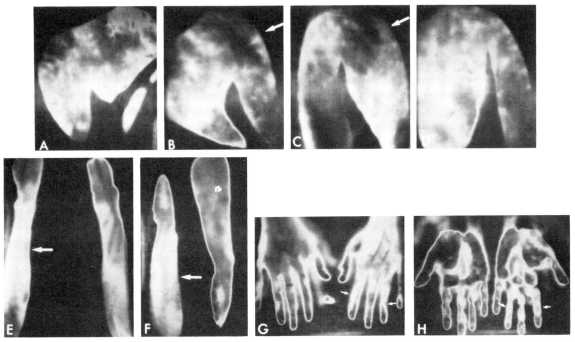

Figure 17–5. Cervical spine trauma with reflex sympathetic dystrophy involving left C5–C8 spinal roots and dermatomes. Patient is a 22 year old male with painful left shoulder and numb left hand. An auto accident 3 years prior resulted in a C7 spinous process fracture. See color plate. *A, B,* Liquid crystal thermogram (LCT) of anterior shoulders. The left shoulder (*B*) shows decreased heat emission (darker brown, arrow) compared with the right shoulder (*A*). *C, D,* Posterior shoulders. The left (*C*) shows decreased heat emission (darker brown, arrow) compared with the right (*D*). *E,* Anterior forearms. The left (arrow) shows decreased heat emission (less green). *F,* Radial forearms. The left (arrow) shows decreased heat emission (less green) compared with the right. *G,* Dorsal and (*H*) palmar view of hands. The left hand and second, third, and fourth fingers (arrows) show decreased heat emission (less green) compared with the right.

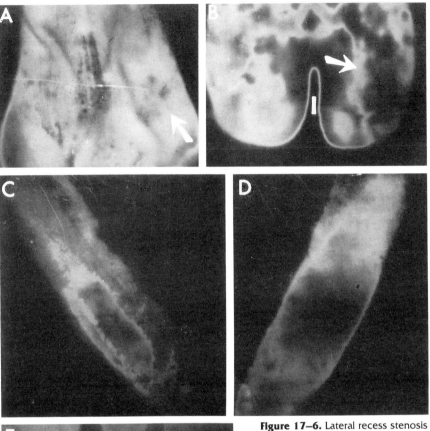

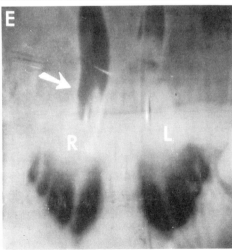

Figure 17–6. Lateral recess stenosis causing right L5 root compression syndrome. A 20 year old female with low back pain radiating to the right leg. See color plate. *A,* LCT of lower back shows a right paralumbar zone of increased temperature (arrow, green). *B,* Gluteal regions. Note right midgluteal zone of decreased heat emission (arrow, dark brown). The "I" represents intergluteal folds. *C, D,* Lateral thighs. The lateral right thigh *(C)* is colder (less green) than the left *(D). E,* Both feet. Note increased heat emission (arrow, green) from dorsum of the right foot **(R)** as compared with the left **(L)**. Myelogram and CT scan were normal. An electromyogram revealed dysfunction of the right L5 root. At surgery, a lateral recess spinal stenosis compressed the right L5 root. Thermographic findings closely followed the right L5 root dermatome. (From Pochaczevsky R: Liquid crystal thermography in the diagnosis of pain. Its value in spinal root compression syndromes. Mod Med Can 38:185–194, 1983.)

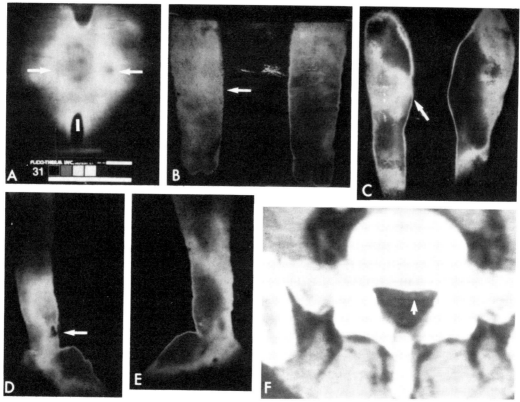

Figure 17–7. Herniating disc producing bilateral S1 root compression syndrome. A 55 year old male with back pain radiating to both gluteal regions and thighs for 2 months. See color plate. LCT shows: (*A*) Increased heat emission (green) radiating to right and left of midline (arrows) ("I" represents intergluteal folds). (*B*) Posterior thighs show decreased heat emission (less green) on left (arrow). (*C*) Posterior legs show decreased heat emission (less green and blue) on left (arrow). (*D*) Lateral right leg (arrow) is colder (less green) than (*E*) lateral left leg. (*F*) CT shows bulging central disc (arrow) and prominent ligamentum flavum at the L5–S1 level and narrowing of the spinal canal. *Comment:* Findings on left *A*, *B*, and *C*, as well as on right *A* and *D*, are compatible with a bilateral S1 root compression syndrome and were confirmed by CT.

Figure 17–8. Metastasis to L4 vertebra with left L4 root compression syndrome. See color plate. LCT shows: (A) Central heat increase (green) in lower lumbar (arrow) and upper sacral levels (arrowheads), representing focal hyperthermia from metastasis and not necessarily part of the nerve root compression pattern. B, Anterior thighs: lower left thigh (arrow) is colder (less green) than the right. C, Medial left leg (arrow) is colder than (D) medial right leg. E, Dorsum feet: first left toe (less green) and second left toe (arrow) are warmer (greener) than the right. F, CT: A destructive metastatic lesion involves the left L4 body with an associated soft tissue mass (arrow).

Comment: LCT findings at the L4 level in the back, anterior left thigh, medial left leg, and left first and second toes correspond to a left L4 root dermatome distribution. CT confirmed L4 root compression. Other thermographic findings not illustrated showed hypothermia of the posterior right thigh and posterior and lateral left leg compatible with bilateral S1 root compression syndrome. This was also correlated with the lumbosacral view (A).

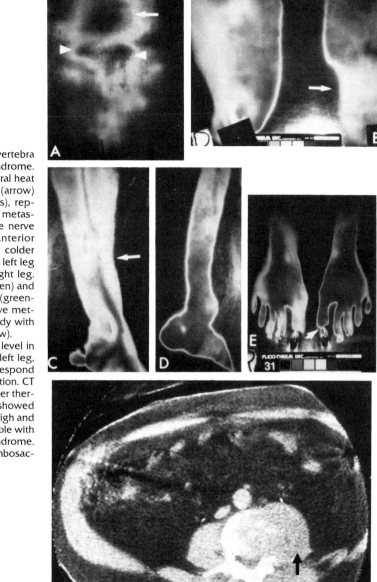

mia in the lumbar spinal myotomes may be due to metabolic change, muscle spasm, or reflex vasodilatation of the skin[18-21, 25] and appears as hyperthermic streaks radiating from the spine along myotome distributions. The midline heat pattern may remain unchanged except for small coin-shaped or fusiform foci of hyperthermia.

However, in the upper and lower extremities, the thermographic changes of nerve root compression are similar: decreased heat emission in the dermatomes of the involved extremity and increased or decreased heat emission in the hands or feet (see Figs. 17–5, 17–6, 17–8).*

An asymmetric increase or decrease in temperature in the extremity dermatomes is considered abnormal if the temperature dif-

*See references 3, 6, 9, 11, 14, 17, 18–21, 25, 30, 32..

ferential is 1°C and involves at least 25% of two dermatome regions studied. If only one dermatome is affected, the existence of an abnormality is thought to be questionable.

Thermography can, in most cases, pinpoint the exact level of spinal root irritation.[3, 4, 18-21, 25] Occasionally, as noted above, thermographic changes are found at one or two levels above or below the site of the lesion.

Distinctive heat patterns associated with nerve root compression or nerve fiber irritation have been established and follow known dermatome distribution (Figs. 17–1 and 17–9).[2a, 3, 3a, 18-21, 25, 32] The thermographic findings of the most frequently involved spinal nerve roots are described here.

C6 Nerve Root. Hypothermia of the ipsilateral posterior cervical muscles, posterior shoulder, and radial side of the forearm.

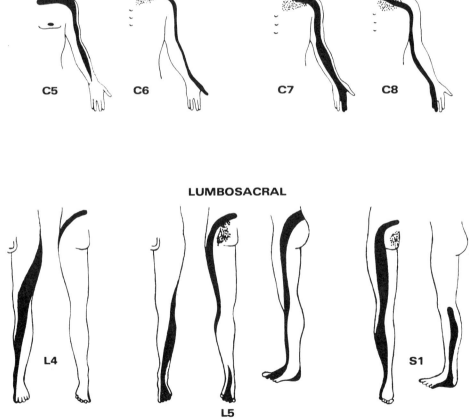

Figure 17–9. Dermatome chart shows the single nerve distribution of the most frequent cervical and lumbosacral nerve root syndromes. (From Pochaczevsky R: Liquid crystal thermography in the diagnosis of pain. Its value in spinal root compression syndromes. Mod Med Can 38:185–194, 1983. Modified from Keegan JJ, Garrett FD: The segmental distribution of the cutaneous nerves in the limbs of man. Anat Rec 102:409–437, 1948.)

Hyperthermia or hypothermia of the thumb (see Figs. 17–5 and 17–9).

C7 Nerve Root. Hypothermia of the ipsilateral posterior cervical spine muscles, posterior shoulder, and dorsal aspect of the forearm. Hyperthermia or hypothermia of the ipsilateral second and third fingers in most cases (see Figs. 17–5 and 17–9).

L4 Nerve Root. Hyperthermia of the lateral aspect of the lumbar spine. Hypothermia of the ipsilateral lower anterior thigh and medial aspects of the leg and ankle. Hyperthermia or hypothermia of the medial aspect of the foot, including the first toe (see Figs. 17–8 and 17–9).

L5 Nerve Root. Hyperthermia of the ipsilateral lumbar spine, usually radiating laterally. Hypothermia of the ipsilateral midgluteal region, lateral thigh, and anterior leg. Hyperthermia or hypothermia of the dorsum of the foot and first, second, third, and fourth toes (see Figs. 17–6 and 17–9).

S1 Nerve Root. Hyperthermia of the affected side of the lumbosacral region. Hypothermia (in most cases) of the ipsilateral posterior thigh and posterior and lateral aspects of the leg. Hyperthermia or hypothermia along the lateral aspects of the foot and fifth toe. Hypothermia of the ipsilateral buttock, with inferomedial extension (see Figs. 17–7 and 17–9).

Thermographic Patterns of Focal Inflammation and Hyperthermia

Inflammatory, infectious, and other hyperemic disorders involving the vertebrae, paravertebral areas, or musculoligamentous structures[12] may result in local hyperthermic zones anywhere along the spine or torso.

Metastasis, osteomyelitis, inflammation, and fractures are focal disorders that cause increased midline heat patterns in the cervical and thoracic spine that are superimposed on the normal spinal midline heat pattern (Fig. 17–10).[1a, 12] This pattern is usually not seen in root compression syndromes except in the lumbar spine. However, when metastasis, infection, and fracture fragments extend to and irritate nerve fibers, thermographic heat patterns typically associated with nerve root compression will develop in addition to the midline focal hyperthermic zone (see Fig. 17–8). Clinical correlation usually helps to identify the underlying etiology.

Thermographic Patterns of Musculotendinous Inflammatory Disorders

Musculotendinous inflammatory disorders in the torso and extremities cause localized thermographic changes. Back muscle spasm and musculoligamentous injuries may produce thermographic patterns indistinguishable from those produced by spinal nerve root compression syndromes or other nerve fiber irritation syndromes. Again, clinical correlation and clinical course are important considerations in determining the final diagnosis. Clinical findings in back muscle strain should reveal localized pain, tenderness, and musculoligamentous spasm.[12, 13]

Clinically tender anatomic sites ("trigger" points) usually produce focal hyperthermic zones in the acute phase of disease and hypothermic zones during the chronic phase of the disease.[10] "Trigger" points do not follow a dermatome distribution.

THE POSTOPERATIVE PATIENT

Thermography may be useful in the postoperative patient by documenting pain and helping to establish the probable level of spinal nerve involvement. In patients who have positive myelographic or CT findings or both, thermography may be particularly helpful in determining whether those radiographic findings are the cause of the patient's pain. Thermography cannot differentiate among recurrent disc, postoperative scarring, or spinal stenosis as the cause of the nerve root compression syndrome. Diagnosing postoperative scarring without nerve root impingement requires further clinical investigation.

DIFFERENTIAL DIAGNOSIS

The thermographic differential diagnosis of spinal root irritation syndromes includes deep venous thrombosis,[4, 24] ischemic arterial disease, local trauma, reflex sympathetic dystrophy,[20a, 20b, 29a] and arthropathies of extremity joints.[24, 29] These disorders usually cause a local hyperthermic pattern. They can be differentiated from spinal root irritation syndromes in most cases by their distinct clinical pictures and by the focal thermographic patterns.

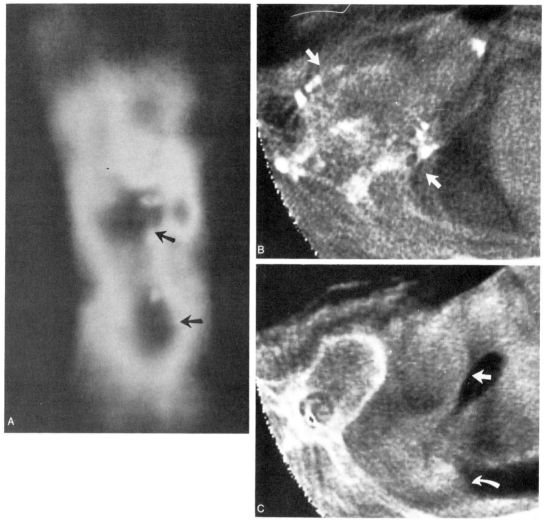

Figure 17–10. Osteomyelitis of a lower thoracic vertebra with right paravertebral abscess. A 75 year old female with recently drained lower thoracic epidural abscess. LCT shows: (*A*) Increased lower thoracic spine heat emission (arrows). (*B*) CT at T11 level shows extensively destroyed vertebral body (arrows). (*C*) CT at T10 level shows a left paravertebral mass (straight arrow), pleural effusion (curved arrow), and contrast material in spinal canal from previous myelogram. Paravertebral aspiration yielded purulent material. *Comment:* Localized lower thoracic hyperthermia correlated precisely with the presence of osteomyelitis.

In normal extremities, there is a proximal to distal decreasing longitudinal thermal gradient in both upper and lower extremities. In an acute ischemic disorder, there may be a decrease in heat emission of the affected limb. However, if the arterial occlusion is not complete, or if collateral circulation develops, or both, skin temperature may, in fact, increase, thus masking signs of ischemia. Focal hyperthermia and hypothermia may be abnormal for a particular area, since there should be a decreasing thermal gradient in all extremities. Therefore, in addition to asymmetry, hypothermia or hyper-

thermia for a particular segment of a symptomatic limb may raise the index of suspicion of whether ischemia exists.

On thermograms, varicose veins can be distinguished by their serpentine course.[24]

In the upper extremities, differential diagnosis also includes the ulnar nerve entrapment syndrome[15] and the carpal tunnel syndrome with median nerve irritation. With median nerve involvement, there may be temperature changes in the thumb, second and third fingers, and the radial side of the fourth finger (author's unpublished data). The ulnar nerve entrapment syndrome is usually associated with a cold dorsal forearm and temperature changes in the fourth and fifth fingers. In leprosy, hypothermic areas noted on thermograms are the sites of most marked sensory loss.[28]

COMPARISON WITH OTHER IMAGING MODALITIES

Thermography is a harmless, noninvasive imaging modality that is free of complications. There is a high correlation with myelography, electromyography, and clinical and surgical findings.[3, 18–21, 25, 32] LCT has an accuracy rate of 92% (Table 17–2).[18–21, 25] The author's subsequent experience confirmed these results and also showed high correlation with computed tomography (see Figs. 17–7, 17–8, 17–10). A high correlation of thermography with clinical symptoms in patients with back pain, as well as with electromyography, myelography, and computed tomography has been reported.[11b] In a study of 80 patients with back pain, good correlation was found with computed tomography as well as with thermographic changes along spinal root extremity dermatomes.[5a] It was felt that thermography was a sensitive method, but one of relative specificity, since in a small number of cases with positive thermograms, the tomogram was negative. Conversely, because those patients were symptomatic, thermography could be regarded as being more sensitive than computed tomography, since thermograms more closely reflected clinical findings. LCT is an excellent screening procedure in suspected nerve root compression disorders, not only in correlating the existence of pain but in localizing the level as well. It may help determine whether a myelographic or CT observation is clinically significant.

Table 17–2. LIQUID CRYSTAL THERMOGRAPHY AND MYELOGRAPHY COMPARISON (RESULTS IN 48 OPERATED PATIENTS)

Findings	LCT	Myelography
True positive	43	40
True negative	1	1
False positive	3	0
False negative	1	7
Total	48	48
Accuracy	92%	85%

(From Pochaczevsky R: Back pain assessment by contact thermography of extremity dermatomes. Orthop Rev *12*:45–58, 1983.)

References

1. Abram SE: Increased sympathetic tone associated with transcutaneous electrical stimulation. Anesthesiology 45:575–577, 1976.
1a. Agarwal A, Lloyd KN, Dovey P: Thermography of the spine and sacroiliac joint in spondylitis. Rheumatol Phys Med 10:349–355, 1970.
2. Archer F: Utilization des cristaux liquides en thermographie medicale. These Medicine (Strasbourg) No. 53, 1969.
2a. Brelsford K, Uematsu S: Thermographic presentation of cutaneous sensory and vasomotor activity in the injured peripheral nerve. J Neurosurg 62:711–715, 1985.
3. Ching C, Wexler CE: Peripheral thermographic manifestations of lumbar disc protrusions. Appl Radiol 100:53–59, 1978.
3a. Comstock W, Marchettini P, Ochoa J: Thermographic mapping of skin of the human hand during intrafascicular nerve microstimulation. Paper presented at Peripheral Nerve Study Group Meeting. Muerren, Switzerland. Sept. 9–12, 1985.
4. Cooke ED, Pilcher MF: Deep vein thrombosis: preclinical diagnosis by thermography. Br J Surg 61:971–978, 1974.
5. Crissy JJ, Gordy E., Fergason JL, et al: A new technique for the demonstration of skin temperature patterns. J Invest Dermatol 43:89–91, 1970.
5a. Delcour C, Sztencel J, Vander Elst A, et al: Tele-thermography selection of patients for computed tomography exploration of herniated lumbar disks. J Radiol 65:443–447, 1984.
6. Duensing F, Becker P, Rittmeyer K: Thermographic findings in lumbar disc protrusions. Arch Psychiatr Nervenkr 217:53–70, 1973.
7. Edeiken J, Wallace JD, Curley RF, et al: Thermography and herniated lumbar disks. AJR 102:790–796, 1968.
8. Epstein JA, Epstein BS, Rosenthal AD, et al: Sciatica caused by nerve root entrapment in the lateral recess: the superior facet syndrome. J Neurosurg 36:584–589, 1972.
9. Feldman F, Nickoloff EL: Normal thermographic standards in the cervical spine and upper extremities. Skeletal Radiol 12:235–249, 1984.
10. Fischer AA: Thermography and pain. Paper presented at the Annual Meeting of the American Academy of Physical Medicine & Rehabilitation, San Diego, California, 1981.
11. Freyschmidt J, Rittmeyer K, Kaiser G: Vergleichende thermographische und myelographische Untersuchungen beim lumbosakralen Diskusprolaps. In: Gemeinsamer Kongress der deutschen und österreichischen Roentgengesellschaft 1973. Stuttgart: Roefo Suppl Georg Thieme Verlag, 1974, pp 366–367.
11a. Guyton AC: Textbook of Medical Physiology, 7th ed. Philadelphia: WB Saunders Company, 1986, p 687.
11b. Hubbard JE, Hoyt C: Pain evaluation by electronic infrared thermography: correlations with symptoms, EMG, myelogram and CT scan. Thermology 1:26–35, 1985.
12. Karpman H, Knebel A, Semel CJ, et al: Clinical studies—application of thermography in evaluating musculo-ligamentous injuries of the spine—a preliminary report. Arch Environ Health 2:412–417, 1970.

13. Karpman HL, Kalb IM, Sheppard JJ: The use of thermography in a health care system for stroke. Geriatrics 27:96–105, 1972.
14. Keegan JJ, Garrett FD: The segmental distribution of the cutaneous nerves in the limbs of man. Anat Rec 102:409–437, 1948.
15. Koob S: Thermography in hand surgery. Hand 4:64–67, 1972.
15a. Lindholm RV, Myllyla MT, Savaranta J: The cold foot symptom in sciatica. A clinical and thermographic study. Am Chir Gynecol 70:176–181, 1981.
16. Lovisatti L, Mora L, Pistolesi GF: Thermographic patterns of lower limb disease. Bibl Radiol 6:107–114, 1975.
16a. Melzack R, Wall PD: Pain mechanisms. A new theory. Science 150:971–979, 1965.
17. Meyer DA, Meyers PH: Would you like to know what pain looks like? Louisiana Bar Journal 28:77–81, 1980.
17a. Milnor WR: Autonomic and peripheral control mechanisms. In Mountcastle VB (ed): Medical Physiology, 13th ed. St. Louis: CV Mosby Company, 1974, pp 944–957.
18. Pochaczevsky R: Back pain assessment by contact thermography of extremity dermatomes. Orthop Rev 12:45–58, 1983.
19. Pochaczevsky R: Liquid crystal thermography in the diagnosis of pain. Its value in spinal root compression syndromes. Mod Can Med 38:185–194, 1983.
20. Pochaczevsky R: The value of liquid crystal thermography in the diagnosis of spinal root compression syndromes. Orthop Clin N Am 144:271–288, 1983.
20a. Pochaczevsky R: Thermography in skeletal and soft tissue trauma. In Taveras JM, Ferucci F, Norman A (eds): Radiology: Diagnostic Imaging and Intervention. Philadelphia: JB Lippincott Company, 1987.
20b. Pochaczevsky R: Thermography in posttraumatic pain. Am J Sports Med 15:243–250, 1987.
21. Pochaczevsky R, Feldman F: Contact thermography in the diagnosis of spinal root compression syndromes. AJNR 3:243–250, 1983.
22. Pochaczevsky R, Meyers PH: The value of vacuum contoured, liquid crystal dynamic breast thermoangiography as an aid to mammography in the detection of breast cancer. Clin Radiol 30:405–411, 1979.
23. Pochaczevsky R, Meyers PH: The value of vacuum contoured, liquid crystal dynamic thermoangiography. Acta Thermographica 4:8–16, 1979.
24. Pochaczevsky R, Pillari G, Feldman F: Diagnosis of deep vein thrombosis by liquid crystal contact thermography. AJR 138:717–723, 1982.
25. Pochaczevsky R, Wexler CE, Meyers PH, et al: Liquid crystal thermography of the spine and extremities. Its value in the diagnosis of spinal root syndromes. J Neurosurg 56:386–395, 1982.
26. Raskin MM: Peripheral vascular disease. In Raskin MM, Viamonte M, (eds): Clinical Thermography. Chicago: American College of Radiology, 1977, pp 51–55.
27. Rothman, R, Simeone F (eds): The Spine, 2nd ed. Philadelphia: WB Saunders Company, p 35.
27a. Sato A, Schmidt RF: Somatosympathetic reflexes: Afferent fibers, central pathways, discharge characteristics. Physiol Rev 53:916–947, 1985.
28. Sobin TD: Temperature-linked sensory loss: a unique pattern in leprosy. Arch Neurol 20:257–262, 1969.
29. Tiselius P: Studies on joint temperature, joint stiffness and muscle weakness in rheumatoid arthritis. Acta Rheumatologica Scand Supp 14:12–44, 1969.
29a. Uematsu S: Telethermography in the differential diagnosis of reflex sympathetic dystrophy and chronic pain syndrome. In Rizzi R, Visentin M (eds): Pain Therapy. New York: Elsevier Medical Press 1983, pp 63–72.
29b. Uematsu S: Thermographic imaging of cutaneous sensory segment in patients with peripheral nerve injury. Skin-temperature stability between sides of the body. J Neurosurg 62:716–720, 1985.
30. Uematsu S, Long D: Thermography in chronic pain. In Uematsu S (ed): Medical Thermography, Theory and Clinical Applications. Los Angeles: Brentwood Publishing Corp, 1976, pp 52–67.
31. Wall PD, Devor M: Sensory afferent impulses originate from dorsal root ganglia as well as from the periphery in normal and nerve injured rats. Pain 17:321–339, 1983.
32. Wexler CE: An overview of liquid crystal and electronic lumbar, thoracic and cervical thermography. Tarzana, CA: Thermographic Services, Inc, 1981, pp 34–35.

18

William A. Murphy, M.D.
Judy M. Destouet, M.D.

Percutaneous Biopsy of the Spine

Percutaneous biopsy of the vertebral column is a diagnostic method available for obtaining a tissue specimen prior to making management or treatment decisions. Since there are several possible therapeutic choices for each inflammatory or neoplastic disease affecting the spine, a precise bacteriologic or histopathologic diagnosis is necessary. In many cases, the appropriate regimen of medical, surgical, and radiation therapy cannot be formulated until such a diagnosis is made. Since Martin and Ellis[12] reported their successful series of percutaneous needle biopsies in 1930, the technique has gained progressively greater acceptance. This continued success of the percutaneous method is attributable to its simplicity, safety, and low morbidity rate as well as refinements or developments in needle design, procedural technique, radiologic technology, and specimen evaluation.

Advantages of the percutaneous needle biopsy are fairly obvious when compared with the two alternatives: (1) no tissue confirmation of diagnosis, and (2) open surgical biopsy. In modern medical practice, it is usually unacceptable to make treatment decisions without a tissue diagnosis. The various medical, surgical, and radiation therapies are specific for certain diseases. Each therapy has its own risks, which are acceptable if the correct disease is treated but unacceptable if applied to normal tissue or an incorrect disease. Percutaneous needle biopsy can provide specimens for tissue diagnosis.

Open surgical biopsy usually requires a general or regional anesthetic, a substantial incision, tissue dissection for visualization, and a large specimen. Notwithstanding all of this, open biopsy may lack precision, especially for small lesions of vertebrae. Percutaneous needle biopsy, performed with radiologic control, has none of these disadvantages. First, it is highly accurate if sufficient tissue is obtained. Second, it can be performed with only a local anesthetic and has little associated morbidity. The incision is only large enough to admit the needle, and the only tissue disturbed is that along the needle tract. Because it is radiologically guided, precision should be very high, even for small or barely discernible lesions. Finally, because general anesthesia and operating room time are not required, the cost of a percutaneous biopsy should be substantially lower than that of open biopsy.

Finally, it must be realized that percutaneous biopsies require a team approach. The result is only as good as the cooperation among the referring clinician, the radiologist, and the pathologist. Each must be cognizant of the others' needs in order to provide the best service possible for the patient.[15, 16]

INDICATIONS AND CONTRAINDICATIONS

A percutaneous vertebral biopsy is indicated when there is evidence that infection

643

or neoplasm may be present in the spinal column and a specific diagnosis is required prior to choosing and beginning appropriate therapy. Any time a tissue diagnosis is desired, a percutaneous procedure should be considered as an alternative to an open surgical procedure. The indications are broad and include all benign and malignant neoplasms as well as all infections. Vertebrae of any stage of collapse or destruction, with or without a soft tissue mass, may be sampled. Patients in almost any condition are candidates for percutaneous biopsy—even those too seriously ill for an open biopsy procedure.

There is only one absolute contraindication for a percutaneous biopsy: When the potential information gained from the biopsy makes no contribution to management or therapy. Under these conditions there is no reason to subject a patient to the procedure. Otherwise, all potential contraindications are relative, as long as the need for a diagnosis outweighs the risks of the procedure. A biopsy can be performed even on patients with lesions adjacent to important neural or vascular structures or those with potentially hypervascular tumors or systemic coagulation defects, if appropriate precautions and techniques are observed.

These liberal indications and restricted contraindications may seem aggressive to some, but they are reasonable if used sensibly. Each case must be evaluated individually and the risks and benefits assessed. The risks of percutaneous biopsy must be weighed against the risks of alternative diagnostic methods and against the risks incurred if no specific diagnosis is made. In each case, the alternative providing maximum benefit to the patient must be chosen.

PROCEDURE

Guidelines. Several basic principles serve as important general guidelines. If these principles are followed, spinal biopsies can be completed rapidly, easily, and safely. Each principle will be discussed more fully in subsequent sections, but all are presented here now for clarity and continuity. First, the patient should have had an imaging work-up that adequately shows that the spine is the most appropriate biopsy site. Second, the patient should be psychologi-

cally prepared for the biopsy and physically comfortable during the procedure. Third, a needle or needles appropriate for the anticipated specimen or specimens should be selected. Fourth, the needle should be positioned perpendicular to the bone that will be examined and away from vital structures. Fifth, the entire procedure should be carefully monitored, using imaging techniques that assure precision of the biopsy and safety for the patient. Sixth, the needle tip position at the time of the biopsy should be documented with images appropriate for a permanent medical record. Finally, the specimen must be obtained in adequate quantity and quality, prepared appropriately for the test to be performed, and handled efficiently.

Patient Work-up. It is necessary to know enough about the patient to anticipate the most likely pathologic abnormality in the vertebra undergoing biopsy. Often, the conventional spine films provide enough information to permit general categorization of the abnormality—such as neoplasm or infection. At other times, only a compression deformity is present, without evidence of a focal destructive lesion (Fig. 18–1). In these

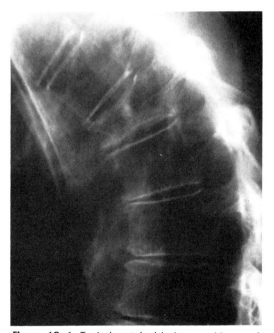

Figure 18–1. Typical vertebral lesion requiring work-up. A new compression deformity of the T5 vertebral body developed in this 75 year old woman with known lung cancer and osteopenia. Confirmation of the presence or absence of metastasis is important for a correct treatment decision. An adequate work-up is required prior to undertaking the thoracic vertebral biopsy.

cases, it is useful to know whether there is evidence of a malignancy elsewhere in the body.

When the conventional films show an abnormal vertebra but do not disclose a likely etiology, other imaging methods may be used to resolve the problem. The two most useful studies are radionuclide bone scans and computed tomography. The bone scan is used to survey the skeleton for other sites of involvement that may help categorize the vertebra under consideration for biopsy. The bone scan may also disclose another skeletal site that might be easier to sample. Conversely, in patients undergoing evaluation for a known malignancy, the bone scan may be the first test to indicate the possibility of osseous metastases. In some cases, conven-

tional films fail to show a corresponding abnormality or do not define the extent of the lesion fully (Fig. 18–2). Computed tomography is used to evaluate the vertebra under consideration and may show characteristics such as a soft tissue mass or focal bone destruction that help in either the categorization of the lesion or, by showing the extent of the lesion, in the determination of the best approach and location for the biopsy (see Fig. 18–2).

In summary, the patient's problem should be understood well enough that it is certain that there is not a more accessible biopsy site, that no less invasive manner of obtaining the necessary diagnostic information exists, and that the best technical approach to the biopsy is discovered.

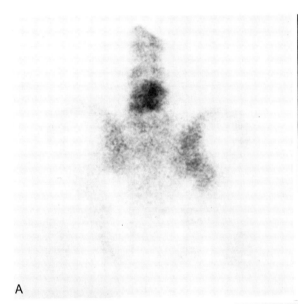
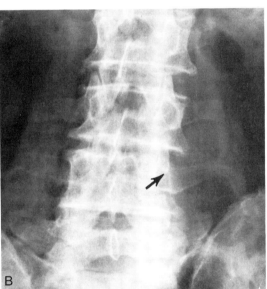
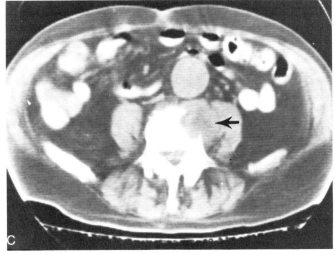

Figure 18–2. Typical sequence of imaging studies preceding a percutaneous biopsy. The patient is an 86 year old man with known epidermoid carcinoma of the lung. *A,* The bone scan shows a focal abnormal radionuclide accumulation in the L4 region. *B,* The subsequent lumbar spine films show subtle cortical destruction (arrow). *C,* The CT scan clearly documents the location and extent of the metastasis; this information was valuable when the percutaneous biopsy was planned. Metastatic epidermoid carcinoma was confirmed.

Choice of Biopsy Site. It is best to perform a biopsy of the spine on the lowest vertebra possible. This is because the lumbar vertebrae are larger and farther away from vital structures than are the thoracic vertebrae. It is better to perform a biopsy from the right than from the left side in order to avoid the aorta, but this is only a rule of thumb. It is more important to do the biopsy on the side of a vertebral body that has the most involvement. Finally, if a paravertebral soft tissue mass is present, it is better to approach the vertebra on the side of the mass (Fig. 18–3). Thus a soft tissue biopsy of the mass might be obtained in addition to a bone biopsy. It is also possible to take advantage of the soft tissue mass by passing the needle through it to avoid putting the needle through a more critical region, such as the pleura or lung.

Patient Preparation. Prior to the procedure, a physician, preferably the person who will do the biopsy, should counsel the patient. The patient should be reassured concerning the need for the biopsy, and the general aspects of the procedure should be explained. The risks and benefits should be discussed. A frank but sensitive discussion will prepare the patient psychologically so that he or she will be more cooperative during the biopsy.

During the procedure, the patient should be positioned in as comfortable a position as possible. For vertebral biopsies, this is usually the prone position. A pillow can be provided for the head, and another pillow or sponge can be placed between the ankle and the table to elevate the toes from the tabletop, thereby eliminating forced plantar flexion and direct pressure on the toes. The patient should be kept warm.

Spinal biopsies should be considered a minor surgical procedure, and appropriate aseptic precautions should be taken. Minimally, this includes a thorough scrub of the patient's skin as well as sterile drapes, gowns, and gloves.

Needle Choice. A limited number of needles will suffice for vertebral biopsies. These include an aspiration needle, a soft tissue needle (Tru-Cut), a short trephine needle (Ackermann), and a long trephine needle (Craig) (Fig. 18–4). From these, one or more can be chosen according to the biopsy site or the specimen anticipated (Table 18–1). In general, it is best to combine aspiration and cutting biopsies for most lesions. The aspiration needle can be used both for deep infiltration of a local anesthetic agent and for aspiration of a specimen. We prefer to use an Ackermann needle for the

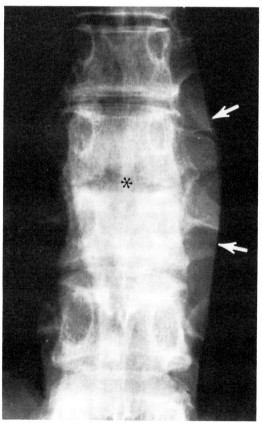

Figure 18–3. Paravertebral soft tissue mass. A percutaneous biopsy needle should be inserted through the paravertebral soft tissue mass (arrows) and into the destroyed disc space (asterisk) in order to obtain samples of both the mass and the disc space. The pleura and lung can be avoided. Diagnosis: *Staphylococcus aureus* disc space infection.

Table 18–1. NEEDLE SELECTION ACCORDING TO SITE OR SUSPECTED LESION

Site or Lesion	Aspiration	Tru-Cut	Trephine Ackermann	Craig
Thoracic spine	*	—	**	*
Lumbar spine	*	—	—	**
Sacrum	*	—	—	**
SI joint	**	—	—	**
Disc space infection	**	—	—	*
Osteomyelitis	**	—	—	**
Blastic metastases	—	—	—	**
Lytic metastases	*	*	—	**
Soft tissue mass	*	**	—	—
Paget's disease	—	—	—	**

**Primary needle
*Secondary needle

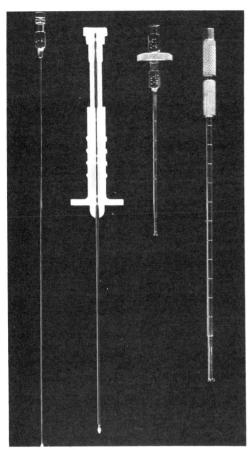

Figure 18–4. Basic needles for spinal biopsies. Four needles should suffice for all vertebral biopsies. From left to right, they are aspiration/anesthesia needle, Tru-Cut soft tissue needle, Ackermann trephine needle, and Craig trephine needle. Needles are pictured here in their assembled states.

bone biopsy in the thoracic spine, but we prefer the Craig in the lumbar spine. For disc space infection and vertebral osteomyelitis, both aspiration and trephine needles are necessary. For blastic metastases the trephine needles are most useful, whereas for lytic metastases the aspiration, Tru-Cut, and trephine needles may be of equal utility. In this instance, the Tru-Cut is used to obtain a soft tissue core from the lytic focus within the vertebra. Biopsies of soft tissue masses are best performed with a Tru-Cut needle. It is best to use trephine needles if Paget's disease is suspected.

Anesthesia. General anesthesia is almost never required, except in young children and extremely apprehensive adults. All others can be managed with standard sedation. In fact, it is an advantage to have the patient alert enough to follow commands

and to inform the operator of pain that might indicate irritation of a nerve. The needle can then be redirected, avoiding nerve damage. It is also useful to have the patient able to assume a certain position or sustain respiration for a few seconds.

An adequate local anesthetic is all that is necessary to keep the patient relatively free of pain during the biopsy. The skin should be well infiltrated. Deep to the skin, there are few nerve endings except at fascial planes. It is necessary to inject local anesthetic agents only when specific painful areas are approached, rather than along the entire needle tract. Beyond the skin, the only other truly painful region is the surface (periosteum) of the vertebra, and this must be adequately anesthetized. Once this is accomplished, the patient should be free of sharp pain and should experience pressure only when a needle is advanced.

Needle Placement. For spinal biopsies in general, it is important to enter the disc space or vertebral body from a dorsolateral approach. This approach results in a needle position that is nearly perpendicular to the rounded contour of the cylindric spinal column. It also assures that the needle is at a safe distance from the spinal canal and the more ventral great vessels. Finally, this approach makes the greatest vertebral diameter available for a trephine core.

For thoracic spine biopsies, it must be remembered that the regional anatomy is very restrictive (Fig. 18–5). First, there is little paraspinal soft tissue; the pleura and lung are juxtaposed to the spinal column. For this reason, it is necessary to place the needle close enough to the midline to avoid the pleural space and a resultant pneumothorax but far enough laterally to enter the dorsolateral aspect of the body or disc space. Unfortunately, when the needle is correctly placed 3 to 4 cm from the midline, ribs, transverse processes, and costotransverse joints are normally encountered. These present an obstruction that can be avoided by angling the needle cranially or caudally following insertion through an intercostal space (Fig. 18–6). This requires a little planning to choose the correct interspace. One interspace too high or too low may render a correct angle impossible. Although it is more difficult to obtain optimal needle placement for thoracic spine biopsies than those of the lumbar spine, with a little planning, thoracic

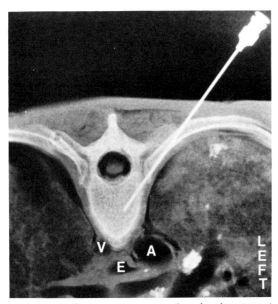

Figure 18–5. Cadaver cross-section showing correct needle placement for thoracic spine biopsy. The needle is inserted close to the midline and between adjacent costotransverse joints. This technique permits sampling of thoracic vertebrae and disc spaces while avoiding the pleura, lung, and major vessels. *Key:* **A** = aorta; **E** = esophagus; **V** = azygous vein. (Courtesy of James W. Debnam, St. Louis, Missouri and Tom W. Staple, Long Beach, California.)

spine biopsies can be completed easily and efficiently.

Lumbar anatomy is not as restrictive; thus, whenever possible, spinal biopsies should be in the lumbar region (Fig. 18–7). Vital structures are further away, and the vertebrae are larger. Needle placement should begin about 8 cm from the midline but may be even further lateral in larger patients. No osseous obstructions are encountered unless a biopsy of the lumbosacral junction is to be performed or a transitional lumbosacral vertebra with large transverse processes is in the way. There are no reported cases of renal trauma from this approach.

For the sacroiliac joints, it is useful to have the patient in the prone position and rolled toward the side from which the specimen will be taken. A pillow or bolster under the contralateral hip will provide stability. A needle can then be inserted parallel to the main anteroposterior axis of the joint. Generally, it is easier to enter the inferior aspect of the joint rather than a more cranial part.[10] The sacrum is usually approached with the patient in the prone position and the needle perpendicular to the tissue to be sampled (Fig. 18–8).

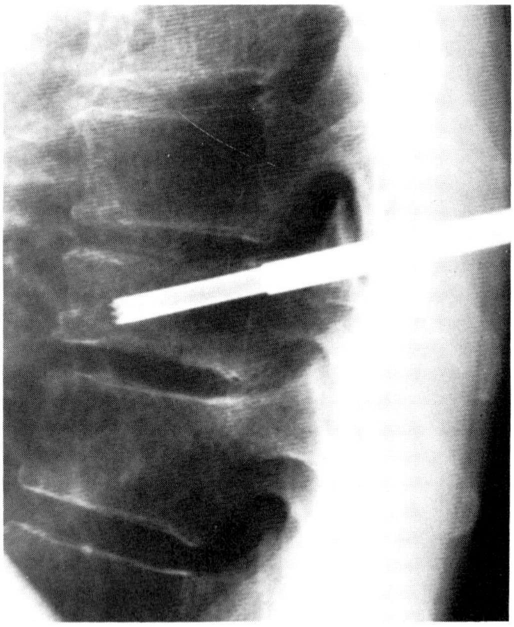

Figure 18–6. Craig needle biopsy of T9. Following insertion through the T8–T9 intercostal space, the needle is directed caudally so that a core can be obtained from the center of the collapsed vertebra.

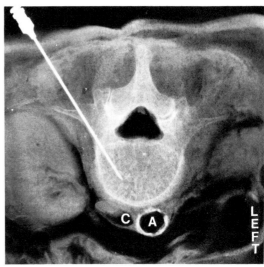

Figure 18–7. Cadaver cross-section showing correct needle placement for lumbar spine biopsy. The needle is inserted 8 cm or more from the midline, and just above or below the transverse process. The aorta (**A**) and vena cava (**C**) are juxtaposed to the ventral aspect of the vertebra, but they are not at risk if the needle does not pass anterior to the vertebra. Similarly, the spinal canal is avoided by ensuring that the needle enters the vertebra from its posterolateral aspect. (Courtesy of James W. Debnam, St. Louis, Missouri and Tom W. Staple, Long Beach, California.)

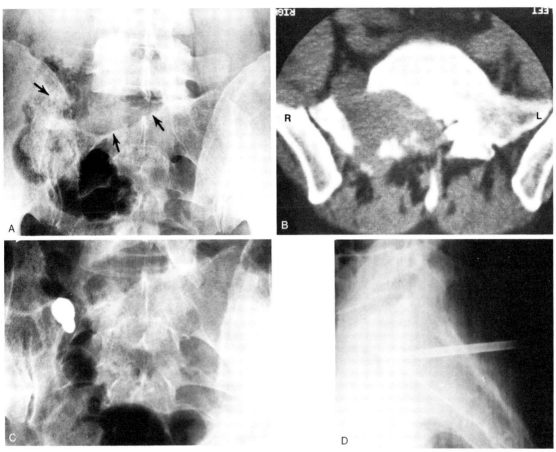

Figure 18–8. Craig needle biopsy of sacrum. *A*, Conventional radiograph shows focal destruction of the right side of S1 (arrows). *B*, CT confirms the destructive lesion and shows its extent. *C, D*, With the patient prone, the Craig needle is inserted perpendicular to the destructive lesion. Part *C* is reversed here to correlate with parts *A* and *B*. Diagnosis: plasmacytoma.

Technique. Following skin preparation and anesthesia, a small incision (generally 5 to 8 mm in length) is created. All subsequent needles will be inserted through this incision. The needle used for deep anesthesia may serve two additional purposes: first, as an aspiration instrument and, second, as a guide for placement of subsequent cutting needles. In the thoracic spine, a standard 3.5 inch, 18 to 20 gauge spinal needle (used for deep anesthesia) is long enough to reach a disc space or the center of a vertebral body. For the lumbar spine, a 7 to 9 inch, 18 to 20 gauge obstetric anesthesia needle is necessary. Either needle may be suitable for sacroiliac joint aspirations.

Once an aspiration needle is in place, there are several methods available for obtaining a specimen. If the lesion is fluid-filled (blood or pus), simple aspiration will provide a sample. If not, a core can sometimes be obtained by applying negative pressure with a syringe partially filled with non-bacteriostatic, sterile saline. If this is unsuccessful, 1 to 3 ml of the saline can be instilled and reaspiration attempted. Sometimes, a rapid back and forth motion on the syringe plunger will loosen tissue that can then be recovered. Movement of the needle tip can shear off small pieces of tissue for aspiration. In general, these techniques are best suited to infections and lytic metastases. They are recommended only as adjunctive techniques to core biopsy of solid tumors.

The Ackermann[1] trephine biopsy needle is our first choice for thoracic spine core biopsies. It consists of a sharp trocar, a cannula, a cutter, and a blunt stylet (Fig. 18–9). For insertion, the trocar is fitted snugly within the cannula. The two are then pushed through the skin incision immediately adjacent to the anesthesia-aspiration needle. Using the anesthesia needle as a guide, the combined trocar-cannula is then advanced

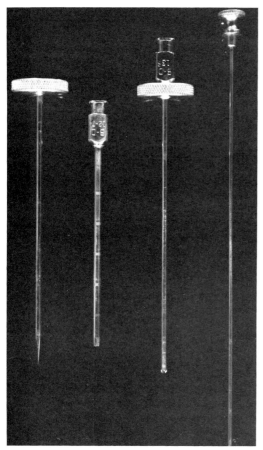

Figure 18–9. Ackermann trephine biopsy needle. From left to righ., the components are the trocar, cannula, cutter, and stylet.

until the sharp trocar tip is embedded in the region to be sampled. The cannula is advanced over the trocar until its blunt end rests on the surface of the lesion. Both the anesthesia needle and the trocar are removed, leaving only the cannula in place. At this point, everything is ready for a core biopsy. The cutter is inserted through the cannula and advanced to the surface of the lesion. Using clockwise turns and constant pressure, the cutter is twisted into the tissue to be sampled (Fig. 18–10). When the cutter has advanced beyond the cannula by the desired distance, it is time to remove the core. First, the entire needle should be wiggled back and forth by small increments to separate the core within the needle from its deep tissue attachments. If this is not done, when the cutter is retracted, the core will most likely remain behind. Second, a syringe should be attached to the cutter, and a small amount of negative pressure should be ap-

plied as the needle is slowly withdrawn from the cannula, which remains in place so that another biopsy can be performed. The specimen can then be gently pushed out of the cutter with the blunt stylet. It should be transferred immediately to an appropriate specimen container. If these simple methods are followed, cores 1.5 mm in diameter and 10 to 25 mm in length should be obtained routinely.

The Craig[4] trephine biopsy needle is favored for the lumbar spine and as the backup instrument should an aspiration or Ackermann needle fail to retrieve a specimen in the thoracic spine. The Craig needle is similar to the Ackermann but has several more components and is operated slightly differently. The Craig consists of a semiblunt trocar, a cannula, a cutter, a blunt-ended stylet, a double-pronged, sharp-toothed

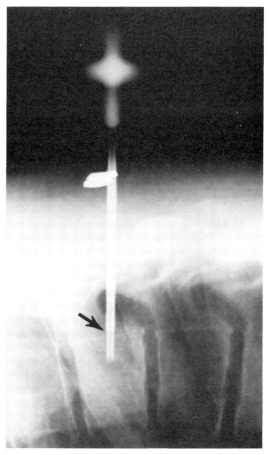

Figure 18–10. Ackermann needle biopsy of T6 vertebra. The edge of the cannula rests against the posterolateral aspect of the vertebral body (arrow), and the cutter extends into the sclerotic body. Diagnosis: Hodgkin's disease.

worm, and a wrench (Fig. 18–11). Using the anesthesia needle as a guide, the trocar is placed through the previously anesthetized tract until its tip rests in precise position against the area to be sampled (Fig. 18–12).

The cannula is passed over the trocar and advanced through the tissue, with alternating clockwise and counterclockwise rotation. Rotation makes insertion of the cannula easier, and the alternating direction keeps

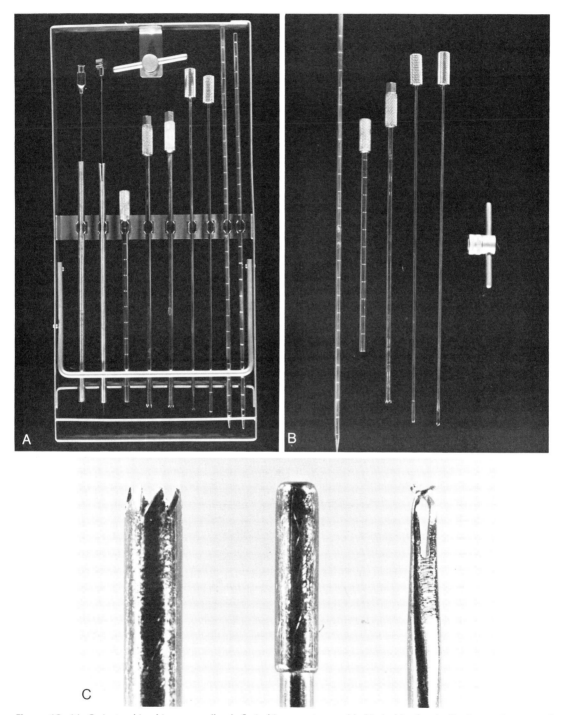

Figure 18–11. Craig trephine biopsy needle. *A,* Craig biopsy set assembled in holder for sterilization and storage. *B,* From left to right, the components are the trocar, cannula, cutter, stylet, worm, and wrench. *C,* Close-up view of the tips of the cutter (left), blunt stylet (center), and sharp-toothed worm (right).

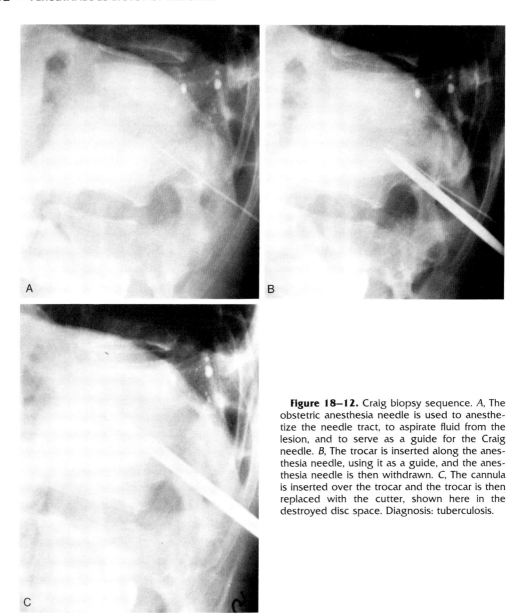

Figure 18–12. Craig biopsy sequence. *A*, The obstetric anesthesia needle is used to anesthetize the needle tract, to aspirate fluid from the lesion, and to serve as a guide for the Craig needle. *B*, The trocar is inserted along the anesthesia needle, using it as a guide, and the anesthesia needle is then withdrawn. *C*, The cannula is inserted over the trocar and the trocar is then replaced with the cutter, shown here in the destroyed disc space. Diagnosis: tuberculosis.

tissue from binding the cannula. Once the cannula is on the surface of the lesion, the trocar is removed. The cutter is passed through the cannula, and a core is trephined (Fig. 18–13). The cutter-cannula combination is wiggled to shear the core free, and the cutter is retracted, leaving the cannula in place. A syringe attached to the cutter can be used to create a gentle suction as the cutter is removed. Alternatively, the worm may be inserted while the cutter is in the lesion. The worm is carefully rotated until the teeth engage the specimen. Once the worm has snagged the core, it is used to maintain the core in the cutter as all three

are slowly withdrawn from the cannula. Once outside the patient, the worm is disengaged from the specimen and withdrawn from the needle. The blunt stylet is used to push the specimen from the cutter. Finally, the core is transferred to a waiting specimen container. For cortical or sclerotic bone, a wrench is provided to improve mechanical advantage while advancing the cutter. If these methods are followed, cores 3.5 mm in diameter and 10 to 20 mm in length are retrieved (Fig. 18–14).

The Craig set worm has one other use. If the cannula is in place but no core can be obtained with the cutter, the worm may be

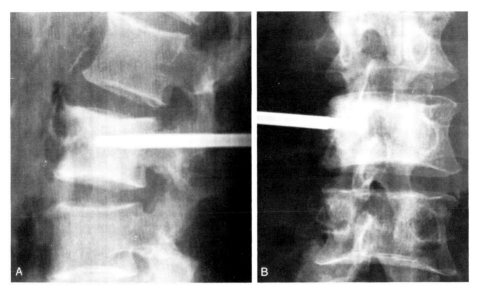

Figure 18–13. Craig needle biopsy of L3 vertebra. *A*, Lateral view shows cannula and cutter in place. *B*, Frontal view confirms that cutter is within sclerotic vertebral body. Diagnosis: metastatic epidermoid cancer.

used instead.[8] These are always cases of soft tissue mass or lytic bone lesion. The worm is passed through the cannula and into the abnormal tissue. The tool is gently rotated to engage soft tissue and is then retracted through the cannula, pulling soft tissue fragments with it (Fig. 18–15). Care must be exercised with this maneuver to avoid bending or breaking the teeth. In a small percentage of cases, this simple technique provides the only diagnostic specimen.

It should be emphasized that, with either the Ackermann or the Craig needle, the angle of the cannula can be changed in order to obtain a specimen from an adjacent site through the same anesthetized tract. Because there is a fulcrum, or pivot point, at or just deep to the skin, moving the needle hub will cause a correspondingly opposite motion of

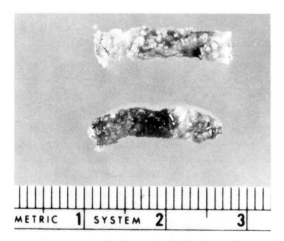

Figure 18–14. Typical bone cores obtained with a Craig needle biopsy.

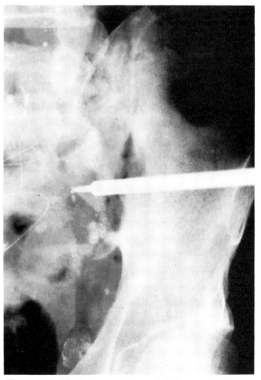

Figure 18–15. Accessory use of Craig worm. Worm is extended through cannula into lytic lesion of sacrum and sacroiliac joint. Diagnosis: *Escherichia coli* infection.

the tip. This can be used to advantage in order to obtain multiple samples from slightly different sites in the region of interest (Fig. 18–16).

The Tru-Cut disposable needle is favored for biopsy of soft tissue (paraspinal) masses and for the center of lytic lesions. It is a very simple tool, consisting of a cannula and stylet (Fig. 18–17). The cannula and stylet are inserted beside the anesthesia needle, and the anesthesia needle is then removed. Once on the surface of the site to be sampled, the stylet, with its specimen slot, is advanced beyond the cannula. Alternatively, the engaged needle can be advanced into the center of the lesion and the cannula pulled back, thereby exposing the slotted stylet.

Local tissue pressure causes tissue to fill the slot in the stylet. The cannula is then advanced over the stylet, cutting a piece of tissue, which is trapped in the stylet slot now enclosed within the cannula. The stylet can then be withdrawn from the cannula, and the specimen retrieved from the slot. The procedure can be repeated as many times as necessary to ensure adequacy of the sample (Fig. 18–18).

Radiologic Monitoring. Spinal biopsies require a three-dimensional appreciation of needle position to ensure precision and safety of the biopsy. There are several ways to accomplish this: (1) overhead fluoroscopy with cross-table radiography, (2) biplane fluoroscopy, or (3) computed tomography.

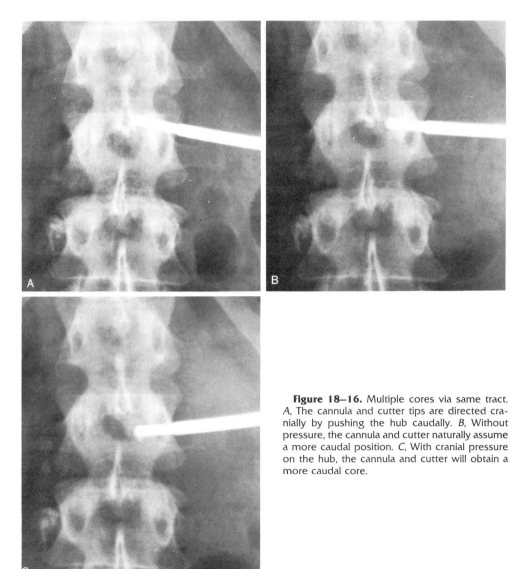

Figure 18–16. Multiple cores via same tract. A, The cannula and cutter tips are directed cranially by pushing the hub caudally. B, Without pressure, the cannula and cutter naturally assume a more caudal position. C, With cranial pressure on the hub, the cannula and cutter will obtain a more caudal core.

We find biplane fluoroscopy to be the most advantageous method of monitoring our biopsies. If a biplane angiographic or myelographic suite is available, it is the optimal location for performing the biopsy, because the television chain and monitor are likely to be the best in the department. Also, the arrangement of this equipment tends to be convenient. A good alternative, and one we often employ, is an overhead angiographic fluoroscope, with portable C-arm fluoroscopy for the cross-table image (Fig. 18–19). Although this arrangement is also convenient, it requires more time to set up. Biplane fluoroscopy provides instantaneous confirmation of needle position in two planes 90 degrees to one another. This assures accurate knowledge of needle position at all times. Such immediate visual feedback allows rapid adjustment of needle position.

Computed tomography[2] can also be used to provide a cross-sectional image that accurately displays the needle position (Fig. 18–20). With modern fast scanners, the image feedback is almost as fast as fluoroscopy. However, there are disadvantages to CT monitoring of spine biopsies. First, it is less convenient to perform the procedure in a CT gantry than it is in the open space available on an angiographic table. Second, CT scanners tend to be in high demand, and some spinal biopsies may require an hour or more to complete. Therefore, it is more efficient to use equipment other than CT scanners.

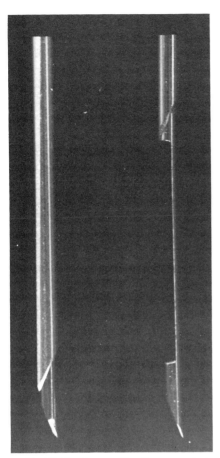

Figure 18–17. Tru-Cut needle. Close-up photograph of needle tip in two positions. On the left, the slotted stylet is enclosed in the cannula. On the right, the cannula has been withdrawn, exposing the slot in the stylet.

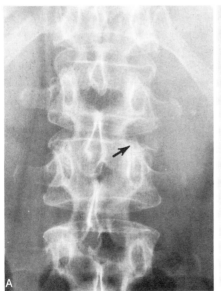
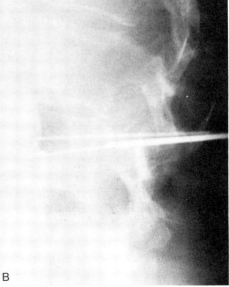

Figure 18–18. Tru-Cut needle biopsy of lumbar paraspinal mass. *A,* Frontal radiograph shows a left paraspinal mass and focal destruction of L2 vertebra (arrow). *B,* Lateral radiograph shows anesthesia needle and unsheathed Tru-Cut needle in the paraspinal mass. Diagnosis: metastatic cancer of cervix.

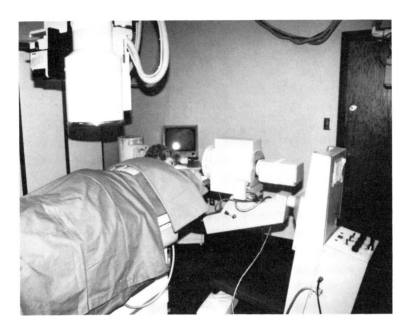

Figure 18–19. Biplane fluoroscopy for monitoring biopsies. Overhead angiographic fluoroscope combined with portable C-arm fluoroscope provides simple, efficient biplanar imaging for precise needle positioning.

For these reasons and because we have considerable experience with fluoroscopically guided biopsies, we rarely monitor them with CT scanners.

Computed tomography has other important uses in the work-up of patients who may undergo spinal biopsy.[9] CT may help confirm the presence of a lesion suspected but not proved by radionuclide scans or conventional films. It may provide information that helps determine needle choice or placement or that is sufficient to alter management without a biopsy. In these ways, CT makes important contributions to spinal biopsies.

Regardless of the imaging technique used for monitoring the procedure, it is necessary to obtain an image of the final needle position. Again, this may be by CT or some conventional film method. Whatever the method, the final film provides permanent documentation of the sample site. This information can become important during histologic evaluation or future care of the patient.

Specimen Handling. Since the pathologist

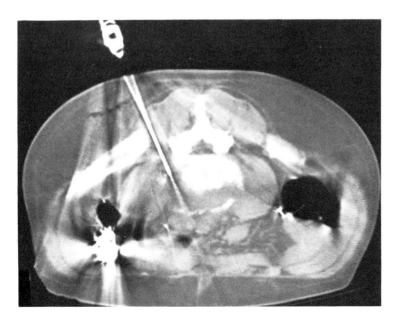

Figure 18–20. Computed tomography for monitoring biopsies. CT confirms aspiration needle position in destroyed vertebral body endplate. Diagnosis: anterior Schmorl's node.

must analyze the specimen obtained, he or she deserves the best specimen possible and one that is appropriate for the tests that must be performed. If there are any questions as to the type or quantity of specimen, the appropriate tubes or solutions, or the personal preferences of the pathologist, these should be answered before rather than after the procedure. Correct and timely handling of the specimen is particularly important.

Fluid aspirates for possible infections should be transferred immediately to appropriate culture tubes and delivered rapidly to the microbiology laboratory for incubation or plating or both. Rapid, efficient handling is of utmost importance if anaerobic organisms are to be recovered. When an infection is suspected and no fluid can be aspirated, several milliliters of nonbacteriostatic, sterile saline may be instilled and reaspirated. If this fails, tissue fragments are suitable for making a culture. Any combination of these techniques may be utilized to assure an adequate specimen. The clinical microbiologist should be consulted if special problems are anticipated.

Tissue aspirates are very important and can improve the accuracy of percutaneous biopsies.[11] These aspirates may be processed in several ways. They may be smeared for cytologic examination or collected and embedded in paraffin for routine histologic sections. Specific handling depends on the likely disease process and on the personal preference of the pathologist.

Trephine tissue cores are subject to creation of artifacts as a result of crushing during the biopsy or during specimen transfer. Crushing is minimized by use of larger inner-diameter needles and by care in handling once the core is removed from the patient (Fig. 18–21). When pushing the trephine core out of the needle, excessive pressure should be avoided. It is best not to pick up the core with one's fingers. Rather, the specimen should be extruded from the cutting needle directly into a sterile specimen container or into a loose, sterile, half-opened 4 × 4 in (10 × 10 cm) gauze pad and then teased into the formalin-containing specimen jar. The pathologist must also treat the specimen gently. Touch preparations can be prepared prior to placing a specimen in formalin, but this increases the likelihood of crush artifacts.

Diagnostic accuracy depends on the adequacy of the specimen. It is rarely necessary to terminate a procedure prior to obtaining sufficient fluid, cells, or cores. A combination of techniques and retrieval of several specimens at each biopsy will optimize the accuracy of percutaneous biopsy (Fig. 18–22).

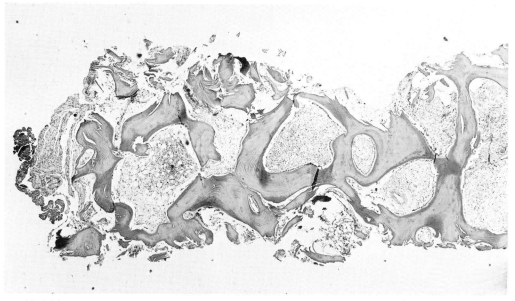

Figure 18–21. Typical histologic section of bone biopsy core. This low power photomicrograph shows a portion of a core with many trabeculae and marrow spaces. There is very little crush artifact. Original magnification 33 ×. Diagnosis: acute and chronic inflammation. (Courtesy of Michael Kyriakos, St. Louis, Missouri.)

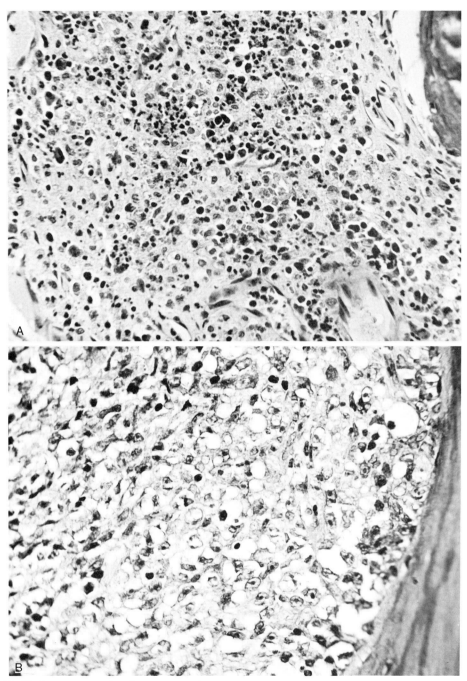

Figure 18–22. Representative histologic sections from percutaneous spinal biopsies. *A,* Osteomyelitis; *B,* Lymphoma; *C,* Metastatic carcinoma of the breast; *D,* Metastatic epidermoid carcinoma. These examples show that diagnostic specimens can be routinely obtained by the percutaneous method.

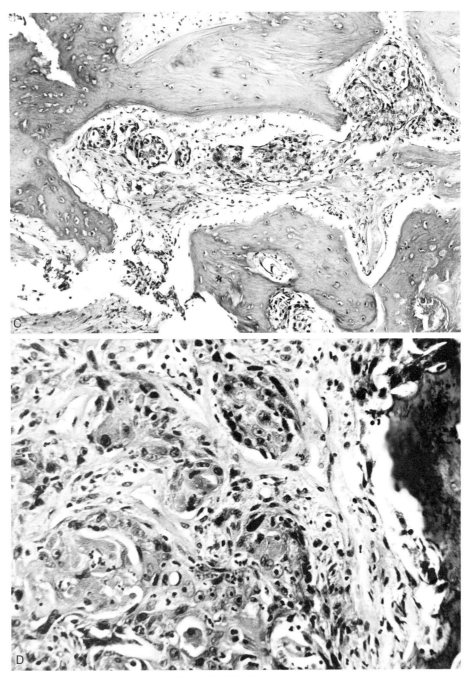

Figure 18–22 *Continued*

COMPLICATIONS

Complications of percutaneous spinal biopsies are few, if the biopsies are performed with standard technical care. The most common complication of spinal biopsy is pneumothorax. This results from inadvertent needle entry into the pleural space or through the lung tissue. If the pneumothorax is small, it can be managed conservatively. Otherwise, a chest tube is necessary.

The serious complications are those involving nerve injury and include transient or permanent paraplegia or quadriplegia.[13, 14, 17, 19] Footdrop has resulted from spinal nerve injury.[14] There have been two deaths recorded following spinal biopsy.[17, 18]

Overall, for approximately 10,000 percutaneous aspirations and trephine biopsies of the spine and appendicular skeleton, the raw estimate for all complications is 0.2%. Serious neurologic injury has occurred in 0.08% and death in 0.02%.

RESULTS

The results of percutaneous biopsy of the spine have been very good.[3, 5–7, 14, 20] Both aspiration and trephine techniques have high rates of accuracy. Biopsies yielding true negative results have not been as well documented as those producing true positive findings, but it seems that a biopsy with a negative result has a high predictive value for a negative diagnosis. It is important to emphasize two points here. First, accuracy is absolutely dependent on technical precision and specimen adequacy. The accuracy of percutaneous biopsy is only as good as the technical performance of the procedure. Second, good clinical judgment must be exercised. If the test result does not match the clinical impression, further procedures must be undertaken to resolve the conflict. For example, if a patient has a destructive lesion of a vertebral body and the pathologist finds only necrosis, another biopsy is indicated. This may be a repeat percutaneous biopsy or an open biopsy, although the percutaneous biopsy is still preferred for the same reasons it was chosen initially.

CLINICAL EXAMPLES

Our experience indicates that requests for percutaneous needle biopsy of the spine

originate from one of five general clinical circumstances: (1) to confirm a metastasis when the patient has a known primary tumor, (2) to confirm a metastasis when the patient has no known primary tumor, (3) to evaluate a compressed vertebra in an osteopenic patient with no known primary tumor, (4) to confirm an infection, or (5) to confirm a miscellaneous group of diseases such as Paget's disease or sarcoidosis. Although high accuracy of percutaneous biopsy techniques has been shown for primary tumors of the appendicular skeleton, not many percutaneous procedures have been performed for primary tumors of the spine. The major reasons are that primary osseous tumors of the spine are rare and are generally sampled by open biopsy.

The most common clinical situation involving percutaneous needle biopsy of the spine is in confirming or excluding a metastasis in patients who have a known primary tumor (Fig. 18–23). This information contributes to major management and treatment decisions, such as a choice between radical surgery or a combination of radiation and chemotherapy. In these circumstances, the

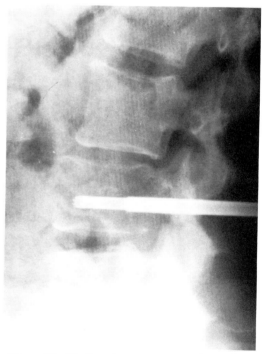

Figure 18–23. Breast cancer metastasis confirmed. Percutaneous spinal biopsy confirmed metastatic disease in this 43 year old woman and contributed to a correct treatment decision.

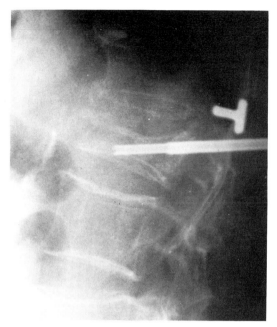

Figure 18–24. Exclusion of metastasis. In this 68 year old man with colon cancer, osteopenia, and a recent compression fracture of L1, the percutaneous biopsy excluded metastatic disease and contributed to a correct management decision.

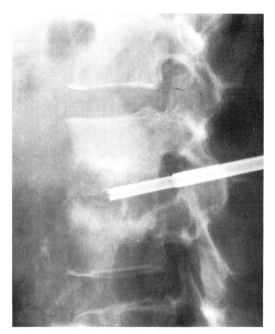

Figure 18–25. Confirmation of infection. Percutaneous aspiration and core biopsy were combined to confirm the disc space infection in this 64 year old woman.

negative predictive value is very important. The operator must have confidence in the performance of the prebiopsy work-up and

the choice of biopsy site. Likewise, the biopsy must be performed with precision, and the specimen must be representative of the

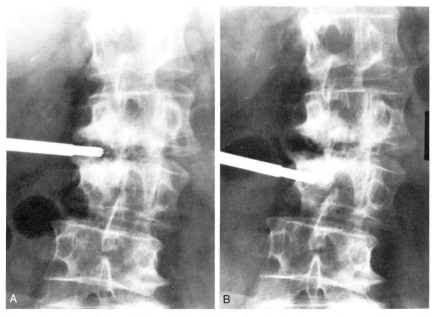

Figure 18–26. Confirmation of degenerative disc disease and discogenic sclerosis. Core biopsy of both the disc space (A) and the sclerotic vertebral body (B) confirmed the degenerative process in this 62 year old woman with rapidly progressive disc destruction associated with severe pain.

abnormal vertebra. If these criteria are met, the accuracy of a negative finding is dependable.

The clinical situation of a new vertebral abnormality in a patient who might have a malignancy is almost as common as the one involving a search for a metastasis in a patient who has a known neoplasm. The same concerns for precision and accuracy apply. Here, the biopsy result may mean the difference between a complete cancer work-up and no further work-up. The result must be reliable. A subgroup of these patients includes those who have an osteopenic spinal column with a new wedge deformity. Here, the specimen must be sufficient for differentiation of osteopenic bone from tumor (Fig. 18–24).

Finally, percutaneous techniques are important for documenting infections (Fig. 18–25) and miscellaneous diseases (Fig. 18–26). The organism or specific diagnosis is often suspected. Under these circumstances, the specimen and its handling should be tailored to optimize recovery of an organism or documentation of the suspected histologic pattern.

SUMMARY

Percutaneous aspiration-trephine biopsy of the spine has many advantages and few disadvantages. It can be done rapidly, accurately, economically, and nearly painlessly. The safety and low morbidity of such closed biopsies compare very favorably with open surgical techniques. The procedure can be optimized by careful attention to choice of lesion for biopsy, selection of biopsy technique, precision of needle placement, and assurance of specimen adequacy. The decision to perform a biopsy should be considered a team effort involving the referring clinician, the pathologist, and the radiologist. A percutaneous spinal biopsy procedure is indicated any time a specific diagnosis is needed prior to a management decision.

References

1. Ackermann W: Vertebral trephine biopsy. Ann Surg 143:373–385, 1956.
2. Adapon BD, Legada BD Jr, Lim EVA, et al: CT–guided closed biopsy of the spine. J Comput Assist Tomogr 5:73–78, 1981.
3. Ayala AG, Zornosa J: Primary bone tumors: percutaneous needle biopsy: radiologic-pathologic study of 222 biopsies. Radiology 149:675–679, 1983.
4. Craig FS: Vertebral-body biopsy. J Bone Joint Surg 38A:93–102, 1956.
5. Debnam JW, Staple TW: Trephine bone biopsy by radiologists. Radiology 116:607–609, 1975.
6. deSantos LA, Lukeman JM, Wallace S, et al: Percutaneous needle biopsy of bone in the cancer patient. AJR 130:641–649, 1978.
7. El-Khoury GY, Terepka RH, Mickelson MR, et al: Fine-needle aspiration biopsy of bone. J Bone Joint Surg 65A:522–525, 1983.
8. Gilula LA, Destouet JM, Murphy WA: Valuable use for the "worm" of the Craig skeletal biopsy set. Radiology 142:778, 1982.
9. Hardy DC, Murphy WA, Gilula LA: Computed tomography in planning percutaneous bone biopsy. Radiology 134:447–450, 1980.
10. Hendrix RW, Lin PJP, Kane WJ: Simplified aspiration or injection technique for the sacro-iliac joint. J Bone Joint Surg 64A:1249–1252, 1982.
11. Hewes RC, Vigorita VJ, Freiberger RH: Percutaneous bone biopsy: the importance of aspirated osseous blood. Radiology 148:69–72, 1983.
12. Martin HE, Ellis EB: Biopsy by needle puncture and aspiration. Ann Surg 92:169–181, 1930.
13. McLaughlin RE, Miller WR, Miller CW: Quadriparesis after needle aspiration of the cervical spine. J Bone Joint Surg 58A:1167–1168, 1976.
14. Moore TM, Meyers MH, Patzakis MJ, et al: Closed biopsy of musculoskeletal lesions. J Bone Joint Surg 61A:375–380, 1979.
15. Murphy WA, Destouet JM, Gilula LA: Percutaneous skeletal biopsy 1981: a procedure for radiologists—results, review, and recommendations. Radiology 139:545–549, 1981.
16. Murphy WA: Radiologically guided percutaneous musculoskeletal biopsy. Orthop Clin North Am 14:233–241, 1983.
17. Nagel DA, Albright JA, Keggi KJ, et al: Closer look at spinal lesions: open biopsy of vertebral lesions. JAMA 191:975–978, 1965.
18. Ramgopal V, Geller M: Iatrogenic klebsiella meningitis following closed needle biopsy of the lumbar spine: report of a case and review of literature. Wis Med J 76:41–42, 1977.
19. Stahl DC, Jacobs B: Diagnosis of obscure lesions of the skeleton: evaluation of biopsy methods. JAMA 201:83–85, 1967.
20. Tehranzadeh J, Freiberger RH, Ghelman B: Closed skeletal needle biopsy: review of 120 cases. AJR 140:113–115, 1983.

19

Morrie E. Kricun, M.D.
Norman E. Leeds, M.D.

Algorithms

The technologic advances in medical imaging over the past few years have enabled the physician to evaluate patients more accurately, more thoroughly, and with less morbidity. With these advances has come a change in the way certain clinical conditions are evaluated. Some modalities that were once the first line of attack have now been dropped from the initial work-up for certain clinical conditions, and newer technologies have found an ever-increasing role. For instance, imaging of the spinal canal has been significantly improved with the introduction of high signal magnetic resonance imaging (1.5 Tesla) and new surface coils. With so many modalities available, there is often confusion as to which imaging study should be performed for a particular clinical condition.

The purpose of this chapter is to guide the reader toward an appropriate diagnostic work-up when faced with a particular clinical problem that may require imaging. Having a working protocol aids in the work-up, eliminates unnecessary diagnostic studies, minimizes unnecessary radiation to the patient, and contributes to lowering the cost of medical care.

The guidelines presented here are recommended ideas and, thus, are amenable to change. Such changes may occur during the work-up of the patient as new information is acquired or as the clinical condition alters, and also in the future as current technologies improve and new techniques develop. The patient's age and clinical condition may also affect the imaging approach.

The work-up of each patient should be individualized and should vary according to the training and experience of the imaging physician as well as the equipment available to the imager. What works best for some may not work best for others. If a particular modality is unavailable, another can be substituted easily.

The goal of imaging is to locate the lesion anatomically, determine its extent and relationship to surrounding structures or its association with other disorders, and establish a diagnosis or differential diagnosis when possible. Some imaging modalities are principally locators (for instance, radionuclide scan for bone lesions, myelography and magnetic resonance imaging for intraspinal lesions); some determine the extent of the lesion (for instance, magnetic resonance imaging and myelogram for intraspinal lesions, computed tomography for paraspinal and intraspinal extent); some establish the diagnosis in some instances (plain radiograph, magnetic resonance imaging, computed tomography); still others are therapeutic (angiography, arthrography). Imaging modalities may have several functions. Computed tomography and magnetic resonance imaging should not be utilized principally as locators of metastasis to bone.

The clinical situations presented in this chapter are some of the more common situations encountered by the imaging physician. The imaging modalities cited in the algorithms are the ones currently in frequent use. The physician in charge of the patient should make every attempt to locate the lesion clinically and establish a working diagnosis. Communication between the attending physician and imaging physician is essential for a more precise work-up and

663

accurate diagnosis with a minimum expense to the patient. The reader is referred elsewhere in this text for more specific information and detail regarding the disorders and imaging modalities discussed in this chapter as well as those not discussed here.

The format of each section of this chapter is as follows: A brief discussion of the goals of imaging in the given clinical situation is followed by a description of an algorithmic approach to the use of various imaging modalities. Again, it should be stressed that these are guidelines and not rules. The numbers listed in the algorithms indicate priority or preference between two or more choices (again, the reader's preference may differ according to physician experience, equipment available, etc). When the imaging modalities are rated about the same, no designations are used. The modality with number 1 is preferred to that with number 2. If there is a slight preferential difference, then 1A and 1B are used. The absence of a number indicates a clear-cut pathway. When the diagnostic work-up is completed for that clinical problem, then an "X" indicates stop (the work-up is complete). We are not saying that care of the patient is completed when we place an X at the end of the algorithm branch. We are saying to stop at that point— that no other imaging studies are necessary to solve the problem. Obviously, patients must be followed (for instance, for fractured spine or infection) and the clinical situation may change, requiring new diagnostic pathways (for instance, development of a post-traumatic hematoma with sudden cord block in a patient who has sustained a fracture).

We recognize that not all possible variations can be discussed in a given clinical setting; when these variations are encountered in practice, the algorithmic pathways can be modified and new ones added.

KEY TO ABBREVIATIONS

The abbreviations used in this chapter are as follows:

CT = conventional computed tomography
CTIV = conventional computed tomography with intravenous contrast agent
CTM = computed tomographic myelography with intrathecal water-soluble contrast agent
M = conventional myelography with water-soluble contrast agent
MRI = magnetic resonance imaging
PR = plain (conventional) radiograph
RI = radionuclide imaging (isotope)
T = conventional tomography
U = ultrasonography
X = stop

RULE OUT BONE METASTASIS
(Figure 19–1)

The Asymptomatic Patient

The goal of imaging is to locate any osseous metastatic disease. This may be performed preoperatively (carcinoma of the lung, breast) or as a follow-up for metastatic disease. The radionuclide bone scan is the superior locator modality to accomplish this goal, for it is extremely sensitive to the presence of metastatic disease. It should be recalled that the radionuclide bone scan yields false-negative results in only 3% of cases of metastasis but in up to 50% of patients with myeloma. Once the lesion(s) is detected by the scan, a plain radiograph may demonstrate the metastasis. If the conventional radiograph is negative in the presence of a positive bone scan, and metastasis is suspected or the patient is at high risk for metastasis, CT with its superior resolution may detect bone destruction, and magnetic resonance imaging can demonstrate marrow invasion by metastatic disease. One should remember that although the radionuclide scan is very sensitive, it is nonspecific, reflecting hyperemia or active bone turnover.

The Symptomatic Patient

The goal is to detect the presence and extent of metastatic disease and, if there are neurologic signs, to establish the presence and extent of a block of the spinal cord or cauda equina. Radionuclide bone scan is the locator of choice for metastasis to bone. If the patient's symptoms do not include neurologic signs, the work-up is similar to that for the asymptomatic patient. If there are symptoms and signs of spinal cord block, however, myelography with a water-soluble contrast agent is utilized to locate the level of block and examine the entire canal for

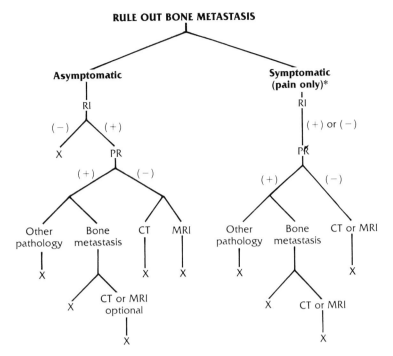

RULE OUT BONE METASTASIS

Figure 19–1. Algorithm for ruling out bone metastasis. * = If signs of cord or cauda equina block are present, see Figure 19–4. For explanation of other symbols and abbreviations, see text.

other sites of intraspinal metastasis. CT myelography with a water-soluble contrast agent can better delineate the morphology of the intraspinal block, the extent of bone destruction, and paravertebral extension. It may be utilized without a complete conventional myelographic examination if the level of block is known beforehand. Magnetic resonance imaging can also be utilized as a primary imaging modality to establish the level of block and presence of tumor in the spine.

RULE OUT SPINAL INFECTION
(Figure 19–2)

The goal of imaging is to establish the presence and location of infection and to determine any intraspinal or paravertebral extension. The radionuclide bone scan is the superior study to determine the presence and locate the site of infection. The plain radiograph can usually establish the diagnosis and the degree of disc narrowing. CT is indicated to delineate the presence and extent of bone destruction as well as the presence of paravertebral or intraspinal extension. Magnetic resonance imaging can demonstrate vertebral and disc involvement as well as intraspinal or paravertebral extension. If the patient has signs of intraspinal

block, then either myelography with a water-soluble contrast agent followed by CT myelography or magnetic resonance imaging can locate the level of block. CT myelography can delineate the bony changes more satisfactorily than magnetic resonance imaging.

SPINAL TRAUMA (Figure 19–3)

The work-up for patients who sustain trauma to the spine varies, depending on the

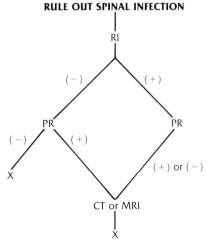

RULE OUT SPINAL INFECTION

Figure 19–2. Algorithm for ruling out spinal infection. For explanation of abbreviations, see text.

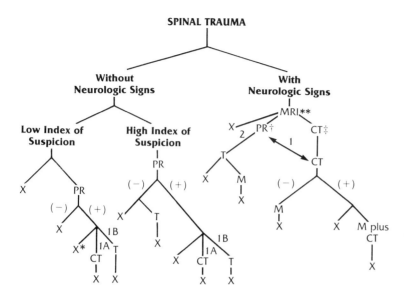

Figure 19–3. Algorithm for use in spinal trauma.
1 = Preferable to 2. **1A** = Slightly preferable to 1B.
* = May be all that is required in some clinical settings.
** = If MRI is not available or if life support mechanisms and the patient's clinical condition preclude evaluation with MRI, begin with PR† or CT‡. † = Depends on clinical presentation and availability of CT scanner. ‡ = Lateral spine on CT localizer. For explanation of abbreviations, see text.

type of injury and the presence and severity of clinical signs and symptoms. Three categories may be established.

In the first category, patients have no neurologic symptoms or signs and there is a low index of clinical suspicion for fracture. In this situation, either no imaging is performed or the plain film is the initial examination. If the radiograph is negative, the patient may be followed clinically. If the conventional radiograph is positive for fracture, then CT or conventional tomography is performed to better define the extent of fracture and its possible association with other lesions.

In the second category, patients have no neurologic symptoms, yet there is a high index of clinical suspicion for fracture. A cross-table lateral plain film and additional views may be obtained, followed by CT if the level of injury is detected or by conventional tomography if the level of injury is unknown. An anterior wedge fracture may need no additional studies other than the plain film. In the presence of a normal plain film, radionuclide scan may demonstrate the presence of a fracture, but the scan is more effective if performed at least 24 to 48 hours after trauma (and at least 3 days in patients whose bones appear osteopenic).

In the third category, the patient has neurologic signs and symptoms and, obviously, an extremely high index of clinical suspicion for fracture. If the level of injury can be determined clinically, the first study of choice could be magnetic resonance imaging, which can detect spinal cord compres-

sion, spinal cord edema, malalignment, and disc herniation. This modality may thus aid the surgeon in making the clinical decision of surgical versus nonsurgical management. If necessary, conventional radiographs may then be obtained. If magnetic resonance imaging is unavailable, or if life support mechanisms and the patient's clinical condition preclude evaluation with MRI, then the initial imaging procedure could be evaluation of the lateral spine on the CT localizer, followed by plain CT, which can diagnose the presence and extent of fracture. If the intraspinal pathology is clearly delineated, the examination may be terminated or myelography plus CT myelography can be performed to better define its extent and morphology. If CT and magnetic resonance imaging are unavailable, then myelography can locate the level of pathology, and the plain radiograph and conventional tomography can delineate the extent of fracture.

SUSPECT INTRASPINAL LESION
(Figure 19–4)

The goal is to locate the lesion, determine its extent and relationship to surrounding structures, and if possible diagnose the type of tissue (syrinx versus tumor, lipoma). The pathway of work-up depends on whether the lesion can be localized clinically. One must remember that myelopathies can have similar clinical presentations, so that the work-ups for these two situations may be similar initially.

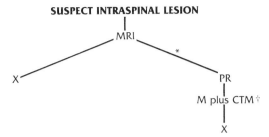

SUSPECT INTRASPINAL LESION

Figure 19—4. Algorithm for suspicion of an intraspinal lesion. * = If MRI is unavailable. † = Angiography if vascular tumor or AVM is suspected. For explanation of abbreviations, see text.

If the lesion cannot be localized clinically, then magnetic resonance imaging is the preferred method of investigation; however, if magnetic resonance imaging is unavailable, then a plain radiograph is obtained in an attempt to locate the lesion by the alterations on the bony spinal canal. Myelography with a water-soluble contrast agent follows, to locate the lesion and its extent within the spinal canal and to determine whether there is any partial block. Magnetic resonance imaging should be the superior technique, since it offers the ability to visualize within the spinal canal. If myelography is used to locate the lesion, CT myelography is then performed to better delineate the morphology and extent of the lesion. If magnetic resonance imaging and CT myelography are unavailable, conventional myelography becomes the primary locator and diagnostic study.

If the lesion can be located clinically, then magnetic resonance imaging is the preferred imaging modality. However, if it is unavailable, then conventional radiography followed by myelography plus CT myelography can be performed to evaluate the extent of the lesion. Again, if magnetic resonance imaging and CT are unavailable, conventional myelography becomes the primary locator if the plain film is unrewarding. It should be emphasized that an intraspinal lesion may be many levels above the clinical site of presentation.

One has several options when utilizing CT in the presence of intraspinal lesions. CT myelography is preferred to CT for the additional information it establishes. It is a localizer and can also determine the morphology of the lesion. Delayed CT myelography can diagnose almost all cases of syringomyelia (only 5% are detected by immediate CT myelography). If a syrinx is discovered, a search for associated disorders such as Chiari malformation (best accomplished with CT myelography or magnetic resonance imaging) and the possible association of syrinx with tumor or arachnoiditis should be accomplished. If tumor is suspected (because of slower partial filling of the cyst, irregular walls of the syrinx cavity, or only a partial cavity), an intravenous contrast agent can enhance a tumor, hematoma, arteriovenous malformation, and other vascular lesions.

DYSRAPHISM (Figure 19–5)

The imaging of a patient with occult or overt dysraphism depends on the clinical condition of the patient and the disorder. The decision to image patients with overt dysraphism is variable. Most meningoceles are easily diagnosed at birth, and since surgery is relatively uncomplicated and patients do not usually have a tethered cord or Chiari malformation, imaging other than conventional radiography is often not obtained. If the diagnosis of meningocele is uncertain, then sonography, magnetic resonance imaging, or myelography plus CT myelography can be performed. Myelomeningocele is readily diagnosed at birth; however, patients with such lesions are often not imaged preoperatively, because surgery is performed as soon as possible and because it is known that patients with myelomeningocele almost invariably have a tethered cord and Chiari malformation.

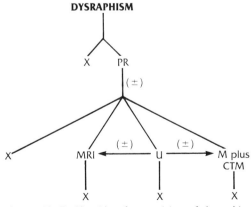

DYSRAPHISM

Figure 19–5. Algorithm for suspicion of dysraphism. The choice of MRI, U, or M plus CTM may vary with the suspected diagnosis and clinical condition of the patient (see text). For explanation of abbreviations, see text.

On the other hand, patients with occult spinal dysraphism should be imaged as soon as possible so that appropriate surgery may be performed to correct the underlying defect.

The goal of imaging is to establish the level and extent of the underlying dysraphic lesion(s) and evaluate the presence and extent of abnormalities of bone (spina bifida, spinal cord tethering or splitting), as well as the presence of thecal sac defects, syringo-hydromyelia, Chiari malformation, intra-spinal masses, and other abnormalities.

The plain radiograph is usually the initial imaging modality. It can sometimes locate lesions such as diastematomyelia and some intraspinal lesions and can demonstrate the presence and extent of spina bifida. Magnetic resonance imaging is a superior imaging modality, for it can delineate fat (lipoma), cord (tethering), and fluid (syringohydromyelia, meningocele) abnormalities as well as the Chiari malformation.

Ultrasonography can be helpful when meningocele, lipomyelomeningocele, or myelomeningocele is present, because the dorsal bony defect acts as a window to allow location of cord position (tethering, placode, and, occasionally, nerve roots). This modal-

ity also can delineate the size and shape of the protruding sac and its relationship to the spinal column and skin surface.

Myelography with a water-soluble contrast agent is an excellent localizing modality for intraspinal pathology. Following myelography, CT myelography can then better define the morphology of the intraspinal lesions, Chiari malformation, and bony defects. If syringohydromyelia is suspected on CT myelography, delayed scanning is in order. The brain may be scanned for hydrocephalus with either CT or magnetic resonance imaging.

NECK PAIN (Figure 19–6)

With Radiculopathy

The goal is to locate the level and cause of radiculopathy and, if possible, determine whether other additional causes of the radiculopathy are present. The plain radiograph may be a guide, as it may demonstrate the site of pathology. However, one must remember that the radiographic signs of aging seen on the plain radiograph may not represent the cause of the patient's symp-

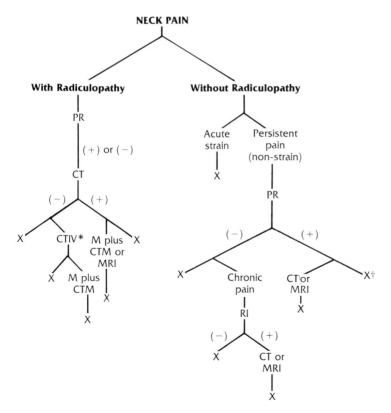

Figure 19–6. Algorithm for use in patient with neck pain. * = At level of radiculopathy. † = Spondylosis, etc. For explanation of abbreviations, see text.

toms. If the plain radiograph is unrevealing in the presence of radiculopathy, the investigation should be continued. CT has the advantage of evaluating both the intraspinal contents and the surrounding spine and its ligaments. Abnormalities in any of these may contribute to the patient's symptoms. If a disc is suspected but not delineated, particularly in the lower cervical region, intravenous administration of a contrast agent and CT at the affected levels may demonstrate a disc. Magnetic resonance imaging and conventional myelography or CT myelography can adequately define the intraspinal pathology. CT myelography alone may be used in the older patient, in whom mobility is somewhat restricted, since images obtained during routine myelography may be inadequate because of poor patient cooperation resulting from the continued manipulations required.

Without Radiculopathy

The goal is to establish the etiology of the pain. Since radiculopathy is absent, it is more difficult to narrow the differential diagnosis. Muscle and ligament pain are often responsible for the patient's symptomatol-

ogy, and radiographic findings may be unrewarding. Patients with typical acute neck strain do not necessarily require a radiographic examination. The plain radiograph is the initial imaging study for patients with pain not due to mild strain. Radionuclide imaging can be reserved for patients with chronic bone pain and negative plain radiograph. CT provides increased anatomic detail about affected vertebrae and enables assessment of the spinal canal, disc space, and posterior elements. If metastasis, fracture, or another lesion is suspected, however, one should proceed with the imaging investigation as for those situations.

LOW BACK PAIN (Figure 19–7)

With Radiculopathy

In evaluating patients with low back pain, it is extremely important to establish whether a true radiculopathy is present. If it is, then the goal of imaging is to determine the etiology of the radiculopathy, its location, and its association of other spinal abnormalities that may contribute to the symptomatology, since more than one cause of

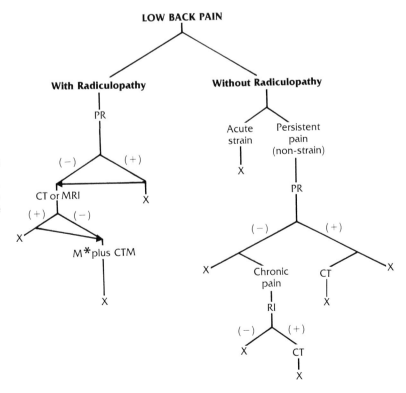

Figure 19–7. Algorithm for use in patient with low back pain. * = Utilized for unexplained, complex, or multiple findings. For explanation of abbreviations, see text.

the radiculopathy may be present simultaneously.

One should recall that the etiology of the radiculopathy can occur anywhere along the course of the nerve root. Thus, it is important to evaluate the relationship of the nerve root to the intervertebral disc, lateral recess, neural foramen, and spinal canal. It should also be remembered that a lesion in the region of the conus medullaris could produce a radiculopathy at a lower level.

The plain radiograph is performed as a screening technique. In some instances, the etiology of radiculopathy can be strongly suspected, and the physician may choose to conclude the work-up. In many instances, however, further clarification may be required. CT without a contrast agent is the next imaging modality utilized, because it delineates the bony structures and the spinal contents to advantage. The only limiting factor is its failure to distinguish structures within the thecal sac.

Conventional myelography with a water-soluble contrast agent and CT myelography, either alone or combined, as well as magnetic resonance imaging are excellent modalities for the evaluation of intraspinal structures. The limitation of conventional myelography is difficulty in detecting far lateral disc herniation and disc protrusion at the L5–S1 level. Nerve compressions at the lateral recess and neural foraminal levels are difficult to appreciate as well. These deficiencies in conventional myelography can be overcome with CT and magnetic resonance imaging. On the other hand, conventional myelography and magnetic resonance imaging allow for evaluation of a larger segment of the thecal sac than CT, so a tumor of the conus medullaris can be detected.

Without Radiculopathy

The goal in this clinical setting is to establish the location and etiology of low back pain. This goal is often difficult to achieve clinically, since the cause of low back pain in many patients is chronic musculotendinous strain and the exact location of the etiology of the pain is not as clear-cut as when a radiculopathy is elicited. In addition, the conventional radiograph is unrewarding in patients who present with musculotendinous strain. One should also remember that the plain radiographic features of aging (spondylosis, disc degeneration, etc.) may not be the cause of the patient's pain. Therefore, the plain radiograph is frequently unrewarding, although it often demonstrates bony abnormalities. Also, there are nonspinal causes of low back pain, such as ureteral colic.

The plain radiograph should be obtained initially to rule out a number of disorders. In patients with prolonged bone pain in whom the plain radiograph is normal, radionuclide imaging may detect the site of abnormality. If the scan is positive and the plain radiograph is normal in appearance, then further evaluation with CT can better delineate bony morphology. If an intraspinal cause of pain is suspected, one should proceed as for an intraspinal lesion.

Index

Note: Page numbers in *italics* refer to illustrations; page numbers followed by t refer to tables.

671

Paraplegia, fracture dislocation and, 252
  osteomyelitis and, 144
  tuberculosis and, 147
Parathyroid hormone, 180
Paresthesias, in lumbar disc herniation, 393t
Pars interarticularis, 21
  facet arthrography and, 620, 622, 623
  fracture of, 322, 526, 528–531, 530
  spondylolisthesis of, 123–125, 124
  spondylolysis of, 122–123, 123
    CT of, 407–408, 407
Pediatrics. See Children.
Pedicle(s), 20
  aplasia of, 95–96, 95, 360, 388
    congenital vs. pathologic, 96
    neural foramen and, 101
  distance between, 97, 98–100, 99–100, 110
  hypoplasia of, 95, 95, 95t
  in rotation measurement, 217–218, 218
  large, 96
  metastases to, 126–127, 126, 127
  myeloma and, 129
  narrow, 96, 96
  osteomyelitis of, 144
  radiation effects on, 209
  radiography of, 94–97, 94–99, 99–100
  sclerotic, 96–97, 97, 207, 207
    vs. nidus, 414, 414
  short, 97, 97
  tuberous sclerosis and, 207, 207
Percutaneous biopsy, anesthesia for, 647
  complications of, 660
  contraindications to, 644
  CT with, 645, 645, 655–656, 656
  indications for, 643–644, 660, 662
  needles for, 646–647, 646t, 647, 649–654, 650–655
    placement of, 647–648, 648, 649
  of disc disease, 661
  of infection, 646, 652, 653, 657, 658, 661
  of metastases, 644, 645, 653, 655, 659, 660
  patient preparation for, 646
  radiologic monitoring of, 654–656, 656
  site for, 646, 646
  specimen handling in, 656–657, 657–659
  technique of, 649–654, 650–655
  vs. surgical biopsy, 643
  work-up for, 644–654, 644, 645
Perineurial cyst, 385
Peripheral nerve, 39
Pia-arachnoid, 9–10
  lipoma and, 15
Pia mater, 36–37, 36
"Picture frame" appearance, in Paget's disease, 205, 206
Pillar fracture, 231, 441–442, 442
Pillar view, 64, 65
Plasmacytoma, 129–130, 471, 649
  angiography of, 589
Platybasia, 156
Platyspondyly, in Morquio's syndrome, 169
  in spondyloepiphyseal dysplasia, 174, 174
Pluridirectional tomography, equipment for, 291
  false shadows in, 290, 291
  indications for, 289
    in trauma, 317, 319, 321
  limitations of, 289–290

Pluridirectional tomography (Continued)
  normal anatomy in, 293–294, 293–303, 298, 303
    cervical, 299
    cervicothoracic, 300
    craniovertebral junction, 293–298
    lumbar, 302
    sacral, 303
    thoracic, 301
  of arthritides, 310, 311, 312, 312
  of congenital abnormalities, 303–304, 303–309, 308–309
  of degenerative disorders, 309–310, 309, 310
  of infection, 313, 314, 315
  of trauma, 313, 315–317, 316–323, 319, 321
  of tumors, 312–313, 313, 314
  postoperative, 321, 323, 324, 324
  technique for, 291, 291–292, 293
POEMS syndrome, 130, 412
Poliomyelitis, scoliosis and, 214
"Polka dot" appearance, 415, 415
Posterior cervical line, 75, 75
Posterior longitudinal ligament, ossification of. See Ossification of posterior longitudinal ligament (OPLL).
  osteophytes and, 117
  rupture of, 363
Posterior vertebral line, 72, 72
Postoperative evaluation, CT, 445, 447–452, 448, 450, 452
  3D, 473, 473
  MRI, 492, 493, 494
  myelographic, 344–348, 346–349
  pluridirectional tomographic, 321, 323, 324, 324
  radiographic, 219–224, 221–224
  thermographic, 628–629, 639
  ultrasonographic, 611–612, 612–613, 614
Pregnancy, ultrasonography in, 599
Prenatal diagnosis, 599–601, 600–602
Prevertebral fat stripe, 71, 71
Primitive streak, 2–4, 3
Prochordal plate, 2
Pseudoarthrosis, 533–534, 533, 534
Pseudodisplacement of odontoid process, 74, 74
Pseudoherniation of disc, 383–384, 383
  spondylolisthesis with, 408, 408
Pseudohypoparathyroidism, radiography of, 183–184
Pseudomeningocele, 348, 349, 449–450, 450, 613
Pseudospread of atlas, 73–74, 73
Pseudosubluxation of axis, 74–75, 74
Psoas margin, trauma and, 227
Psoriatic arthritis, radiography of, 191–192, 192
  vs. DISH, 121
Pycnodysostosis, 172, 172
Pyogenic osteomyelitis, 143–144, 143, 144
  vs. tuberculosis, 148t

Quantitative computed tomography, bone loss evaluation by, 453–455, 453–455

Spondylosis deformans, 44–45, 47, 48,
116–117, *117*
MRI of, 488, *489*
stenosis and, 113
three-dimensional CT of, 473
vs. intervertebral osteochondrosis, 48
Sprains, hyperextension, 242, *242*
hyperflexion, 243–244, *244*
Squared vertebra, in ankylosing spondylitis,
188, *188*
in psoriatic arthritis, 192
Stability, trauma and, 233–234, *234, 235*
Staphylococcus aureus. 143, 646
Stenosis, spinal, 111, 113–114
acquired, 113–114, 400t
classification of, 398t
congenital, 113, 399t
CT of, 398–404, *399–403,* 499
3D, *472, 473, 474, 475*
degenerative, 400–401, *400,* 400t, *402*
ligamentous hypertrophy and, 400–401,
401
MRI of, 491, *492*
myelography of, 341–344, *341–344,* 401
vs. metastases, *372*
pluridirectional tomography of,
309–310, *309*
preoperative evaluation of, 449
vs. herniated disc, *341*
"Step ladder" appearance, in rheumatoid arthritis, 195, *196*
Steroid therapy, vertebral sclerosis and, 91
Stress fracture, radionuclide imaging of, 526,
528–531, 530
Strut graft, 220, *224*
Stylohyoid ligament, calcification of, 108,
108, 169
Subarachnoid space, 37
embryogenesis of, 9–10, *9, 10*
lesions of, 365, *365*
vs. herniated disc, 371
Subdural space, 37
Subluxation, apophyseal, 406, 442, *444*
atlantoaxial, 72–73, 236, 425
differential diagnosis of, 425
in osteomyelitis, 144
in psoriatic arthritis, 192
in rheumatoid arthritis, 193, *193, 311,
312*
CT of, 425, *425*
in trisomy 21, 175
surgery for, 220–221
pathologic vs. physiological, 74–75, *75*
spondylolisthesis and, 123
Sulcus limitans, 7
Superscan, 513–514, *514*
Supraspinous ligament, 36
Surgery, arachnoiditis after, 336, 346, *346,
347,* 449
disc, 224, 447–450
evaluation after, CT, 445, 447–452, *448,
450, 452*
3D, 473, *473*
MRI, 492, *493, 494*
myelographic, 344–348, *346–349*
pluridirectional tomographic, 321, *323,
324,* 324
radiographic, 219–224, *221–224*

Surgery (*Continued*)
evaluation after, thermographic, 639
ultrasonographic, 611–612, *612–613,
614*
of arteriovenous malformation, 585–586
pseudomeningocele after, 348, *349,*
449–450, *450,* 613
radionuclide imaging during, 532
scarring after, *348,* 447–449, *448,* 492, *493,
611*
symptoms after, 344–345, 449–450, *450*
ultrasonography during, 604, 606–608,
607–612, 611
Swimmer's view, 64, 66, *66*
myelographic, 334, *335*
Synchondrosis, vs. fracture, *306*
Syndesmophyte, 121
in ankylosing spondylitis, 188–189, *188,
189*
in colitic arthritis, 198, *198*
in psoriatic arthritis, 192, *192*
vs. osteophyte, 48
Synovial osteochondromatosis, 428
Synovitis, *621, 622*
Syphilis, arthropathy in, 199–200, *200*
Syringohydromyelia, 152–153, 435–438,
436, 437
cord size in, 436–437
intraoperative ultrasonography in,
607–608, *607, 608*
MRI of, 494–495, *495, 496*
myelography of, 353, *353*
myelomeningocele with, 430
tumors and, 437
Syrinx, 437–438
CT of, 418
MRI of, *495, 496*
posttraumatic, 447
tumors and, 437–438
ultrasonography of, 606–607, *607, 608*
Systemic lupus erythematosus, sacroiliitis
in, 200

Tarlov cyst, 385
"Teardrop" fracture, 228, 246–247, *247,* 442
Technetium-99m phosphate, 503–504
technique with, 506–507
Technetium-99m sulfur colloid, 504–505
technique with, 508
Tectorial membrane, 33
Teratoma, ultrasonography of, 600, *601*
Tethered cord, 432–433, *433*
causes of, 433
embryogenesis of, 15–16
lipoma with, 366–367, *367,* 431, 433, 500,
603
MRI of, *500*
myelography of, 365–367, *365, 367*
ultrasonography of, 602, *603,* 604, *604*
Thalassemia, 205
marrow hyperplasia in, 202–203, *203*
MRI of, 496, *497*
sickle cell disease with, 204
vertebrae in, 89, *90,* 203
Thanatophoric dwarfism, 174, *175*